PHYSICAL THERAPY MANAGEMENT OF PATIENTS WITH **SPINAL PAIN**

AN EVIDENCE-BASED APPROACH

PHYSICAL THERAPY MANAGEMENT OF PATIENTS WITH **SPINAL PAIN**

AN EVIDENCE-BASED APPROACH

Deborah M. Stetts, PT, DPT
Orthopaedic Clinical Specialist
Fellow, American Academy of Orthopedic and Manual Physical Therapists
Associate Professor
Department of Physical Therapy Education
Elon University
Elon, North Carolina

J. Gray Carpenter, PT, DPT, COMT
Orthopaedic Clinical Specialist
Fellow, American Academy of Orthopedic and Manual Physical Therapists
Adjunct Assistant Professor
Department of Physical Therapy Education
Elon University
Elon, North Carolina

Routledge
Taylor & Francis Group
NEW YORK AND LONDON

First published 2014 by SLACK Incorporated

Published 2024 by Routledge
605 Third Avenue, New York, NY 10158

and by Routledge
4 Park Square, Milton Park, Abingdon, Oxon OX14 4RN

Routledge is an imprint of the Taylor & Francis Group, an informa business

Deborah M. Stetts, J. Gray Carpenter, and Mary C. Hannah have no financial or proprietary interest in the materials presented herein.

Library of Congress Cataloging-in-Publication Data

Stetts, Deborah M., - author.
Physical therapy management of patients with spinal pain : an evidence-based approach / Deborah M. Stetts, J. Gray Carpenter.
p. ; cm.
Includes bibliographical references and index.
ISBN 9781556429323
I. Carpenter, J. Gray, 1968- author. II. Title.
[DNLM: 1. Back Pain--therapy. 2. Spine--physiopathology. 3. Evidence-Based Practice. 4. Physical Therapy Modalities. WE 725]
RD771.B217
617.5'6406--dc23

2013017308

ISBN: 9781556429323 (hbk)
ISBN: 9781003525738 (ebk)

DOI: 10.4324/9781003525738

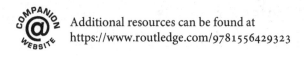

Additional resources can be found at
https://www.routledge.com/9781556429323

Dedication

To my parents, Michael and Sophia, who have provided unconditional support and encouragement throughout my professional life. Thank you for instilling a strong work ethic and the merits of education, self-discipline, and patience.

—Deborah M. Stetts, PT, DPT

To my wonderful wife, Darice, whose patience, caring, and guidance made this possible.

To my parents, who gave me examples and foundations on how to live.

—J. Gray Carpenter, PT, DPT, COMT

Contents

Acknowledgments

The authors wish to express their gratitude and recognize the contributions of those individuals whose kindness and dedication made this work possible:

- To our instructors and colleagues who have shown us the way forward.
- To the clinicians, researchers, and clinician-researchers who spend long hours producing the evidence that supports the efficacy of our profession.
- To the Elon University Department of Physical Therapy Education and Alamance Regional Medical Center for the opportunity to teach and serve.
- To Elon University for financial support from a faculty research and development grant.
- To Ben Fisher for his countless hours behind the camera.
- To George Wentz, Sara Fleming, and Dr. Jane Freund for their modeling expertise and perseverance with early morning weekend photo shoots.
- To Darice Carpenter for her photo and copy editing savvy and countless other actions.
- To Dr. Mary Kay Hannah for content review, expert editing, and writing the foreword.
- To the students we have the privilege to teach, who, as they translate evidence to practice, will challenge mediocrity and pave the way forward.
- To the professionals at SLACK Incorporated for giving us the opportunity to write this book.

About the Authors

Deborah M. Stetts, PT, DPT is an associate professor in the Department of Physical Therapy at Elon University, NC, where she teaches professional students in the area of musculoskeletal management. Current research interests involve the use of real-time ultrasound imaging to examine abdominal muscle performance in select patient populations. Dr. Stetts is board certified in orthopedic physical therapy and a Fellow of the American Academy of Orthopedic and Manual Physical Therapists. She has over 23 years of service as a physical therapist in the United States Army working in a variety of clinical, academic, and administrative positions. Dr. Stetts completed her DPT from Arizona School of Health Sciences, A.T. Still University, Mesa, AZ, in 2003; a master of physical therapy from the U.S. Army–Baylor University Graduate Program in Waco, TX in 1981; and a bachelor of science in health and physical education from Pennsylvania State University, State College, PA in 1976. She completed a residency in advanced orthopedic manual therapy at the Kaiser Physical Therapy Program, Hayward, CA, in 1990. Her professional experience and training have been primarily in orthopedic and manual physical therapy.

J. Gray Carpenter, PT, DPT, COMT graduated with a bachelor's degree in physical therapy from East Carolina University, Greenville, NC in 1992 and completed his doctor of physical therapy from the University of North Carolina at Chapel Hill in 2006. Dr. Carpenter also completed the Certificate in Orthopedic Manual Therapy from Manual Concepts, Curtin University, Perth, Western Australia, in 2002. He became a board-certified specialist in orthopedics through the American Physical Therapy Association in 2008 and became a Fellow of the American Academy of Orthopedic and Manual Physical Therapists in 2009. During his career, Dr. Carpenter has primarily worked in outpatient orthopedic settings but has experience in several settings such as acute care, home health, inpatient rehab, and wound care. He currently works as a staff physical therapist at Alamance Regional Medical Center in Burlington, NC as well as serving as associate faculty at Elon University in the musculoskeletal module. Dr. Carpenter has been very active in the North Carolina Physical Therapy Association (NCPTA) and has held several positions with the NCPTA.

Preface

The purposes of *Physical Therapy Management of Spinal Pain: An Evidence-Based Approach* are (1) to provide a supplement for neuromusculoskeletal management courses in academic settings and (2) to provide a reference text for recent graduates and clinicians to aid in translating evidence into practice. The book systematically and eclectically approaches the evaluation and management of spinal pain using a clinical reasoning framework that allows for continual integration of emerging evidence and biopsychosocial concepts based on patient response, current best practice, and a clinician's knowledge. The goal is to reach an informed decision that balances the best available evidence with what is safe and, most important, for the patient to reach an optimal outcome.

Chapter 1 discusses the process of making evidence-based physical therapy a reality. Commitment to integrating patient-oriented research into clinical practice involves seeking answers to clinical questions through emerging research, accepting and adopting new clinical practice guidelines, applying research as appropriate by communicating well with patients and colleagues, and assessing performance using standardized outcomes.[1]

Chapter 2 presents a detailed overview of the subjective examination and patient history. The systematic format is adaptable to different body regions and is designed to meet specific goals that aid in differentiating between musculoskeletal and nonmusculoskeletal disorders, planning an appropriate examination, and implementing effective interventions.

Chapter 3 outlines a physical examination process and basic components that are also adaptable to different body regions. The objectives of the physical examination are highlighted to provide an overall strategy for testing procedures and interpretation of a patient's response.

Chapters 4, 5, and 6 present evidenced-based physical therapy practices related to low back pain, thoracic spinal pain, and neck pain, respectively. Each chapter pursues an in-depth focus of the history and physical examination for each region. Key history and exam findings are used to place the patient into either a diagnostic classification and/or an impairment-based category. To inform clinical decision making, each diagnostic classification integrates current best evidence, clinical reasoning, and clinical practice guidelines related to specific low back pain, thoracic spinal pain, and cervical pain subgroups and the importance of characteristics that are likely to respond to initial physical therapy management strategies. Supported by current best evidence, initial management strategies are presented for each diagnostic subgroup as a guide to an informed decision for initial treatment agreed upon by the clinician and patient. Continual assessment and reassessment of the patient's response to treatment guide treatment progression targeting the patient's functional recovery.

Each examination and intervention section has accompanying video demonstrations to assist in learning the procedures. A password-protected Web site is provided at www.routledge.com/9781556429323/books/spinalvideos.

The Appendices provide case studies for each region to illustrate the clinical reasoning framework. Each case study allows for practice taking a history and planning a physical examination. The data from the history and physical examination are then synthesized using current best evidence to determine appropriate diagnostic classification, prognosis, and initial management strategies. The case study process provides an opportunity to practice using clinical reasoning and an evidence-based framework.

Reference

1. Herbert R, Sherrington C, Masher C, Moseley A. Evidence-based practice: imperfect but necessary. *Physiother Theor Pract.* 2001;17:201-211.

Foreword

As a clinical physical therapist trained in evidence-based medicine, I know as every year passes that I am getting further away from the current best evidence despite trying to stay informed. With my busy life of part-time private practice, part-time teaching in a doctoral physical therapy program, and full-time family, I try to stay up to date with recent evidence. I read two professional journals that arrive monthly, attend continuing education, and receive the American Physical Therapy Association's *Hooked on Evidence*. Even with that, I am reluctant to make major changes to my practice based on a single article or study. What I need is a collection, a compilation that will guide me toward evidence-based changes to my practice. One area that deserves this treatment is the spine because it is the bread and butter of physical therapy.

Fortunately for our profession, Dr. Deborah Stetts and Dr. J. Gray Carpenter provide exactly this kind of volume in *Physical Therapy Management of Spinal Pain: An Evidence-Based Approach*. With great thoroughness, the authors describe the best practice for evaluating and treating the lumbar spine, the thoracic spine, and the cervical spine, providing a detailed review of evidence-based evaluation and treatment complete with considerations for different diagnoses and different patient personalities. Their work provides a thorough literature review of all aspects and regions of the spine that serves as an encyclopedic text for physical therapy students and also a superb resource for practicing physical therapists at all experience levels. It provides what no physical therapy clinician realistically can do on his or her own—a comprehensive literature review of current best evidence for evaluating and treating pain and dysfunction related to the spine arranged into a clinically useful structure and context. Though designed for students and new clinicians, I predict this work will be an essential resource for experienced clinicians as well.

This book stands out among textbooks because it provides comprehensive coverage of all spine-related regional pathologies, dysfunctions, and complaints from evaluation to treatment. It will be an essential go-to resource because of its structure that follows a smart outline starting with Chapter 1 on the importance of evidence-based medicine and how best to learn and practice using evidence-based medicine. Chapter 2 follows with instruction on performing a subjective exam using best practice according to the available literature. Chapter 3 logically covers the objective portion of the exam with an extensive look at how tests and measures are evaluated, highlighting which tests and measures are the most valid, reliable, and able to help increase or decrease the probability of a patient's likely diagnosis. On top of learning which tests and measures are currently best practice, the authors provide detailed step-by-step descriptions with how-to pictures and figures to present a method by which therapists can perform these tests.

The rest of the book covers each region from evaluation through treatment. Chapter 4 covers the lumbar spine, Chapter 5 the thoracic, and Chapter 6 the cervical. Within each chapter, Dr. Stetts and Dr. Carpenter carefully distinguish between chronic and acute pain literature and between medical disease pathologies and neuromusculoskeletal dysfunctions and how they relate and contribute to each other. Furthermore, each region chapter includes all issues related to the spine such as sacroiliac joint dysfunction, shoulder pain, headaches, and temporomandibular complaints. The full coverage in each chapter comes directly from a comprehensive collection, selection, and analysis of an extensive amount of research literature right up to and including studies published in 2012. Best of all, the authors contextualize the otherwise overwhelming amount of evidence in a way that makes it useful for clinical practice.

Dr. Stetts and Dr. Carpenter have tackled the problem of a massive literature review, integrating current concepts with specific detail in a well-organized structure that goes beyond a mere collection or sampling of the variety of ideas and techniques. There are other books available that discuss all regions of the body or specialty books on different schools of treatment of the spine, but none brings everything together in the context of a treatment-based classification. I only wish I had learned how to evaluate and treat the spine with this book when I was a student, but I am glad to have it now as an experienced therapist. It will be open on my desk daily.

Mary C. (Mary Kay) Hannah, PT, DPT
Board Certified in Sports Physical Therapy
Associate Faculty, Elon University
Elon, North Carolina
Mary Kay Hannah Physical Therapy, LLC
Cary, North Carolina

Chapter 1

Evidence-Based Practice in Physical Therapy

Evidence-based medicine is most commonly described as the integration of the best research evidence with clinical expertise and patient values in order to achieve the highest level of excellence in clinical practice.[1] The American Physical Therapy Association's (APTA) *Statement for Physical Therapy Vision 2020* states that physical therapists, as autonomous practitioners, will render evidence-based services throughout the continuum of care to guide clinical decision making and provide best practice for the patient/client.[2] Responsibility for clinical decision making requires more use of research to look for the most current and effective interventions and less reliance on anecdotal evidence, the basis of traditional physical therapy practice. Continued dependence on personal preference, trial and error, and authority provides opportunities to select less effective or inappropriate treatments. Increased emphasis on the critical appraisal of research as part of the decision-making process supports the effectiveness and safety of physical therapy practice and is likely to produce the best outcomes through a patient-centered approach.[3,4] With ease of online access to relevant journals, a structured approach to reviewing the literature provides a sound path to becoming an evidence-based physical therapist.

The Practice of Evidence-Based Physical Therapy

The process of evidence-based physical therapy (EBPT) begins with each patient encounter and results in a practice that is guided by scientific research. EBPT follows a well-known, 5-step process.[1,4-6] For an in-depth discussion, clinicians are referred to excellent resources.[1,7] The 5 steps are reviewed as follows.

Step 1: Ask a Focused Clinical Question About a Patient Problem

A well-built clinical question increases the likelihood of finding the best available evidence.[8] The clinical focus of the questions may be in the form of "background" or "foreground" questions. Background questions seek general information about the problem and ask who, what, where, when, and why. For example, what causes ankylosing spondylitis? Foreground questions seek specific information about optimal treatment for the problem. Table 1-1 shows examples of foreground questions. For example, in a 27-year-old male with a 5-year history of ankylosing spondylitis, is a supervised exercise program more effective than a home exercise program for increasing lumbar spinal mobility? Foreground questions include 4 factors related to the problem, often referred to as PICO:

- **P**: Patient and characteristics (age, gender) or problem (diagnosis, acuity)
  - 27-year-old male with a 5-year history of ankylosing spondylitis
- **I**: Intervention or test
  - Supervised exercise program more effective than

Stetts DM, Carpenter JG. *Physical Therapy Management of Patients With Spinal Pain: An Evidence-Based Approach (pp 1-29).*

TABLE 1-1. FOREGROUND CLINICAL QUESTIONS RELATED TO PHYSICAL THERAPY DIAGNOSIS, PROGNOSIS, INTERVENTION, AND OUTCOMES

	FOREGROUND CLINICAL QUESTIONS
DIAGNOSIS	In a 27-year-old male with acute onset of low back pain and sciatica, is a lumbar lateral shift more accurate than a positive straight leg raise in detecting a lumbar disc herniation?
PROGNOSIS	In a 32-year-old female who is 6 months postpartum, is abdominal muscle strength or endurance a better predictor of chronic pelvic girdle pain?
INTERVENTION	In a 45-year-old male with chronic neck pain, is thoracic manipulation more effective than thoracic mobilization in decreasing pain and increasing range of motion?
OUTCOME	In a 25-year-old female with acute low back pain, is the Roland-Morris Disability Questionnaire better than the Modified Oswestry Disability Questionnaire for detecting change in disability over a 4-week period?

- **C**: Comparison intervention or test (as needed)
    - Home exercise program
- **O**: Outcome (therapist or patient)
    - Increasing lumbar spinal mobility

Therapists can ask questions related to diagnosis, prognosis, intervention, prevention, or outcomes. Questions about diagnosis investigate the reliability and accuracy of specific tests to determine whether the test has the ability to discriminate between patients with and without a specific disorder.[9] Diagnostic accuracy studies help to determine the best tests and interpret their meaning on specific patients.[10] Questions about intervention identify patient-centered clinical research to provide current information about the best possible treatment options for a specific patient to maximize patient outcomes. Questions about outcomes ask for information about the end result of an intervention or appropriate methods for measuring the end results. Outcomes inform the clinician and patient about what to expect at the close of an episode of care.

Step 2: Find the Best Available Evidence to Answer the Question

This step involves the ability to accurately and efficiently search and access the health care literature. The most practical way to find relevant evidence is to use electronic databases. Several electronic databases are available to assist in this process. The most frequently used are PubMed,[11] the Cumulative Index of Nursing and Allied Health Literature (CINAHL),[12] the Cochrane Library,[13] Physiotherapy Evidence Database (PEDro),[14] and the APTA's *Hooked on Evidence*.[15]

PubMed,[11] the National Library of Medicine journal literature search system, is a free service that provides access to the MEDLINE database for biomedical literature. Access to full text articles may be free or pay-per-article.[11] This database is complex due to its size and search strategies. However, PubMed[11] offers tutorials to learn and improve the essential skill of online database searching at http://www.nlm.nih.gov/bsd/disted/pubmedtutorial/020_010.html.

Within PubMed,[11] Clinical Queries[16] uses predetermined evidence-based practice search strategies to find the best evidence to answer questions related to etiology, diagnosis, therapy, and prognosis. Additional features also seek clinical prediction guides and systematic reviews.[17] Clinical Queries[16] is an efficient method for the initial search for the highest quality of evidence available.[17] The CINAHL database,[12] a comprehensive index of nursing and allied health journal, is a valuable source of many physical therapy journals not indexed through MEDLINE.[18]

The Cochrane Library[13] is a collection of evidence-based medicine databases that provide high-quality, independent evidence summaries. Within the Cochrane Library, the Cochrane Reviews[19] database offers free access to abstracts and summaries of all systematic reviews and meta-analyses about health care interventions for prevention, treatment, and rehabilitation. Using predefined criteria, the reviews are based on randomized controlled trials (RCTs) and published every 3 months.[19]

PEDro[14] is a free, Web-based database of RCTs, systematic reviews, and evidence-based clinical practice guidelines (CPGs) focused on physical therapy research. The RCTs are rated for methodological quality on a scale of 0 to 10.[20,21] The PEDro total score has good reliability (intraclass correlation coefficient [ICC] = 0.58 to

0.91).[22,23] Macedo et al[24] provided preliminary evidence of PEDro[14] total score and convergent and construct validity. The PEDro[14] scale is a guide to the quality of each trial and is only one database that stores research on the effectiveness of physical therapy interventions.[20] Other databases, such as the Cochrane Library[13] and the APTA's *Hooked on Evidence*,[15] present a different set of reports or scoring criteria.

Hooked on Evidence[15] is a database of article extractions related to physical therapy interventions. Though the database provides fast, easy access to current research, it does not provide a comprehensive search of any topic. The service is provided by contributions from APTA members and is available free to APTA members.[15]

SUMSearch[25] is a public site that performs live searches of other Web sites such as PubMed.[11] This free service selects the best resources for the question, formats the question for each resource, and routinely makes additional searches based on results. Additional resources are available at the Health Sciences Online Library Web site of McMaster University.[26]

Even though many online services are available, no one database provides all of the resources for a comprehensive search. The search may identify an abundance of literature or only a few articles when evidence is lacking. To find the best answer to the question, it is important to systematically target all relevant high-quality articles rather than limit the search to articles that only support predetermined ideas. Whether evidence is abundant, limited, or uncertain, use of the current best evidence in combination with clinical expertise and patient preference is desired. A skillful search often provides the best information about how useful a diagnostic test is or what interventions are effective and ineffective for a specific patient.[4]

Step 3: Critically Appraise the Available Literature

As defined by Sackett et al,[1] this step requires the clinician to independently review the best evidence for its validity, applicability, and impact. This process requires an analysis of the quality of the study design (internal validity), an ability to generalize the results to the clinical situation (external validity), and consideration of the diagnostic accuracy of a test or the size of the treatment effect (impact) prior to making changes in clinical practice.[1,17,20]

Critical appraisal of research is a skill that helps the clinician identify effective diagnostic tests and interventions and requires practice and an understanding of research design and statistical analyses. One way for clinicians to develop this skill is to use forms that provide a structured process to evaluate articles.[27] The Oxford Centre for Evidence-Based Medicine[28] (OCEBM) offers online forms to guide the critical appraisal process for an RCT, diagnostic accuracy study, or systematic review. These forms provide a systematic approach to evaluate whether a given study can report true, statistically significant, and clinically important conclusions.[27] Clinicians are referred to a 2-part clinical commentary series for a detailed review of this process with emphasis on studies of interventions in orthopedic and sports physical therapy.[17,29]

Another concept that assists the clinician with the critical appraisal process is the hierarchy of evidence, a classification system based on scientific rigor and quality. Though many classifications exist, one system, recognized in the United States by the Agency for Healthcare Research and Quality (AHRQ), is available for free on the OCEBM Web site.[28,30] Evidence ranges from expert opinion to systematic reviews. OCEBM levels of evidence[28] are shown in Table 1-2 along with grades of recommendations on the strength of the supporting evidence. Grades of recommendation are associated with levels of evidence but report only on the validity of a study, not on its relevance to clinical care. Revised OCEBM levels of evidence have been introduced as a shortcut to finding the likely best evidence and are available at the OCEBM Web site.[31]

Within the hierarchy of evidence, the RCT is the most common study design for determining treatment effectiveness. Despite its potential to produce high-quality evidence, the RCT can be conducted soundly or poorly. Because not all RCTs meet all of the critical appraisal criteria, it is essential for clinicians to render an independent decision regarding the relevance of the study findings. As the number of RCTs increases, systematic reviews, CPGs, and meta-analyses are emerging as valuable sources of the best available evidence related to specific clinical questions.

A systematic review is a structured, exhaustive search for and critical appraisal of all relevant studies that address a specific clinical question.[17,27,32] A systematic review with homogeneity of results from multiple RCTs is consistent with a higher level of evidence (Level 1A) than a single RCT with narrow confidence intervals (CIs; Level 1B; see Table 1-2). A systematic review that uses statistical methods to combine and summarize results across studies is a meta-analysis.[27,32] A meta-analysis result is a synthesis of the overall body of best evidence to provide an overall estimate of the question of interest, diagnostic accuracy, or treatment effectiveness. Through pooling of data and statistical analysis from multiple trials, the meta-analysis can provide estimates and enhanced precision in deciding if a diagnostic test or a treatment is clinically meaningful.

CPGs often incorporate the results of systematic reviews to develop summary recommendations about the relative effectiveness of patient management strategies. One critical difference between systematic reviews, CPGs, and meta-analyses is that CPGs make a recommendation based on expert opinion related to general societal, cultural, and patient interests in addition to the best

TABLE 1-2. OXFORD CENTRE FOR EVIDENCE-BASED MEDICINE—LEVELS OF EVIDENCE

LEVEL 1A	*THERAPY/PREVENTION, ETIOLOGY/HARM*	Systematic review (SR) (with homogeneity*) of RCTs
	PROGNOSIS	SR (with homogeneity*) of inception cohort studies; CDR" validated in different populations
	DIAGNOSIS	SR (with homogeneity*) of Level 1 diagnostic studies; CDR" with Level 1B studies from different clinical centers
	DIFFERENTIAL DIAGNOSIS/SYMPTOM PREVALENCE STUDY	SR (with homogeneity*) of prospective cohort studies
	ECONOMIC AND DECISION ANALYSES	SR (with homogeneity*) of Level 1 economic studies
LEVEL 1B	*THERAPY/PREVENTION, ETIOLOGY/HARM*	Individual RCT (with narrow CI"¡)
	PROGNOSIS	Individual inception cohort study with >80% follow-up; CDR" validated in a single population
	DIAGNOSIS	Validating** cohort study with good""" reference standards; or CDR" tested within one clinical center
	DIFFERENTIAL DIAGNOSIS/SYMPTOM PREVALENCE STUDY	Prospective cohort study with good follow-up****
	ECONOMIC AND DECISION ANALYSES	Analysis based on clinically sensible costs or alternatives and systematic review(s) of the evidence, but includes multi-way sensitivity analyses
LEVEL 1C	*THERAPY/PREVENTION, ETIOLOGY/HARM*	All or none§
	PROGNOSIS	All or none case series
	DIAGNOSIS	Absolute SpPins and SnNouts""
	DIFFERENTIAL DIAGNOSIS/SYMPTOM PREVALENCE STUDY	All or none case series
	ECONOMIC AND DECISION ANALYSES	Absolute better-value or worse-value analyses""""
LEVEL 2A	*THERAPY/PREVENTION, ETIOLOGY/HARM*	SR (with homogeneity*) of cohort studies
	PROGNOSIS	SR (with homogeneity*) of either retrospective cohort studies or untreated control groups in RCTs
	DIAGNOSIS	SR (with homogeneity*) of Level >2 diagnostic studies
	DIFFERENTIAL DIAGNOSIS/SYMPTOM PREVALENCE STUDY	SR (with homogeneity*) of Level 2B and better studies
	ECONOMIC AND DECISION ANALYSES	SR (with homogeneity*) of Level >2 economic studies
LEVEL 2B	*THERAPY/PREVENTION, ETIOLOGY/HARM*	Individual cohort study (including low-quality RCT; eg, <80% follow-up)
	PROGNOSIS	Retrospective cohort study or follow-up of untreated control patients in an RCT; derivation of CDR" or validated on split-sample§§§ only
	DIAGNOSIS	Exploratory** cohort study with good""" reference standards; CDR" after derivation, or validated only on split-sample§§§ or databases
	DIFFERENTIAL DIAGNOSIS/SYMPTOM PREVALENCE STUDY	Retrospective cohort study, or poor follow-up
	ECONOMIC AND DECISION ANALYSES	Analysis based on clinically sensible costs or alternatives and limited review(s) of the evidence or single studies, but includes multi-way sensitivity analyses
LEVEL 2C	*THERAPY/PREVENTION, ETIOLOGY/HARM*	Outcomes research; ecological studies
	PROGNOSIS	Outcomes research
	DIAGNOSIS	
	DIFFERENTIAL DIAGNOSIS/SYMPTOM PREVALENCE STUDY	Ecological studies
	ECONOMIC AND DECISION ANALYSES	Audit or outcomes research

See Key on page 6

(continued)

TABLE 1-2 (CONTINUED). OXFORD CENTRE FOR EVIDENCE-BASED MEDICINE—LEVELS OF EVIDENCE

LEVEL 3A	THERAPY/PREVENTION, ETIOLOGY/HARM	SR (with homogeneity*) of case-control studies
	PROGNOSIS	
	DIAGNOSIS	SR (with homogeneity*) of Level 3B and better studies
	DIFFERENTIAL DIAGNOSIS/SYMPTOM PREVALENCE STUDY	SR (with homogeneity*) of Level 3B and better studies
	ECONOMIC AND DECISION ANALYSES	SR (with homogeneity*) of Level 3B and better studies
LEVEL 3B	THERAPY/PREVENTION, ETIOLOGY/HARM	Individual case-control study
	PROGNOSIS	
	DIAGNOSIS	Nonconsecutive study, or without consistently applied reference standards
	DIFFERENTIAL DIAGNOSIS/SYMPTOM PREVALENCE STUDY	Nonconsecutive cohort study, or very limited population
	ECONOMIC AND DECISION ANALYSES	Analysis based on limited alternatives or costs and poor quality estimates of data, but includes sensitivity analyses incorporating clinically sensible variations.
LEVEL 4	THERAPY/PREVENTION, ETIOLOGY/HARM	Case series (and poor quality cohort and case-control studies§§)
	PROGNOSIS	Case series (and poor quality prognostic cohort studies***)
	DIAGNOSIS	Case-control study, poor or non-independent reference standard
	DIFFERENTIAL DIAGNOSIS/SYMPTOM PREVALENCE STUDY	Case series or superseded reference standards
	ECONOMIC AND DECISION ANALYSES	Analysis with no sensitivity analysis
LEVEL 5	THERAPY/PREVENTION, ETIOLOGY/HARM	Expert opinion without explicit critical appraisal, or based on physiology, bench research, or "first principles"
	PROGNOSIS	Expert opinion without explicit critical appraisal, or based on physiology, bench research, or "first principles"
	DIAGNOSIS	Expert opinion without explicit critical appraisal, or based on physiology, bench research, or "first principles"
	DIFFERENTIAL DIAGNOSIS/SYMPTOM PREVALENCE STUDY	Expert opinion without explicit critical appraisal, or based on physiology, bench research, or "first principles"
	ECONOMIC AND DECISION ANALYSES	Expert opinion without explicit critical appraisal, or based on economic theory or "first principles"

Notes: Users can add a minus-sign "–" to denote the level that fails to provide a conclusive answer because:

- EITHER a single result with a wide CI
- OR an SR with troublesome heterogeneity

Such evidence is inconclusive and therefore can only generate Grade D recommendations

GRADES OF RECOMMENDATION	
A	Consistent Level 1 studies
B	Consistent Level 2 or 3 studies or extrapolations from Level 1 studies
C	Level 4 studies or extrapolations from Level 2 or 3 studies
D	Level 5 evidence or troublingly inconsistent or inconclusive studies of any level

"Extrapolations" are where data are used in a situation that has potentially clinically important differences than the original study situation.

See Key on page 6 *(continued)*

TABLE 1-2 (CONTINUED). OXFORD CENTRE FOR EVIDENCE-BASED MEDICINE—LEVELS OF EVIDENCE

KEY	
*	By homogeneity, we mean a systematic review that is free of worrisome variations (heterogeneity) in the directions and degrees of results between individual studies. Not all systematic reviews with statistically significant heterogeneity need to be worrisome, and not all worrisome heterogeneity need to be statistically significant. As noted previously, studies displaying worrisome heterogeneity should be tagged with a "–" at the end of their designated level.
"	Clinical decision rule. These are algorithms or scoring systems that lead to a prognostic estimation or a diagnostic category.
"i	See note for advice on how to understand, rate, and use trials or other studies with wide confidence intervals.
§	Met when all patients died before the prescription became available, but now some survive on it; or when some patients died before the prescription became available, but now none die on it.
§§	By poor quality cohort study, we mean one that failed to clearly define comparison groups and/or failed to measure exposures and outcomes in the same (preferably blinded) objective way in both exposed and nonexposed individuals and/or failed to identify or appropriately control known confounders and/or failed to carry out a sufficiently long and complete follow-up of patients. By poor quality case-control study, we mean one that failed to clearly define comparison groups and/or failed to measure exposures and outcomes in the same (preferably blinded) objective way in both cases and controls and/or failed to identify or appropriately control known confounders.
§§§	Split-sample validation is achieved by collecting all of the information in a single tranche, then artificially dividing this into "derivation" and "validation" samples.
""	An "Absolute SpPin" is a diagnostic finding whose specificity is so high that a positive result rules in the diagnosis. An "Absolute SnNout" is a diagnostic finding whose sensitivity is so high that a negative result rules out the diagnosis.
"i"i	Good, better, bad, and worse refer to the comparisons between treatments in terms of their clinical risks and benefits.
"""	Good reference standards are independent of the test and applied blindly or objectively to all patients. Poor reference standards are haphazardly applied but still independent of the test. Use of a nonindependent reference standard (where the "test" is included in the "reference," or where the "testing" affects the "reference") implies a Level 4 study.
""""	Better-value treatments are clearly as good and cheaper, or better at the same or reduced cost. Worse-value treatments are as good and more expensive, or worse and cost as much or are more expensive.
**	Validating studies test the quality of a specific diagnostic test, based on prior evidence. An exploratory study collects information and trawls the data (eg, using a regression analysis) to find which factors are "significant."
***	By poor quality prognostic cohort study, we mean one in which sampling was biased in favor of patients who already had the target outcome; the measurement of outcomes was accomplished in <80% of study patients; outcomes were determined in an unblinded, nonobjective way; or there was no correction for confounding factors.
****	Good follow-up in a differential diagnosis study is >80%, with adequate time for alternative diagnoses to emerge (eg, 1 to 6 months acute, 1 to 5 years chronic).

Reprinted with permission from Centre for Evidence-Based Medicine. Levels of Evidence (March 2009). *University of Oxford.* http://www.cebm.net/?o=1025. Updated April 3, 2013. Accessed June 27, 2011.

available evidence.[27,33] These methods can greatly enhance a clinician's ability to interpret and apply the evidence to ultimately improve outcomes. The National Guideline Clearinghouse, a project of AHRQ, is a free, comprehensive, online database of evidence-based CPGs.[34] As an example, clinicians should review a physical therapy CPG on neck pain published by Childs et al.[35] Because the quality and completeness of systematic reviews, meta-analyses, CPGs, and RCTs are variable, the clinician is reminded to critically appraise this evidence and determine its applicability to individual patients.

The critical appraisal process results in the selection of the best available evidence. The clinician must now integrate the research data with clinical expertise and patient preferences to determine whether the evidence is relevant and applicable to an individual patient.

Step 4: Integrate the Critical Appraisal Into Clinical Practice

Applying research evidence to an individual patient is one of the most thought-provoking phases of EBPT, often requiring information and judgments that go far beyond the results of the study. Though specific procedures address steps 1 through 3, applying the evidence to individual patients requires sound clinical reasoning and expertise.[36] If a patient is reasonably similar to those in the study, a clinician should be able to integrate the evidence with considerable confidence.[29] When social, demographic, or pathological variables are so different from those in the study, the results are likely discarded in favor of an alternative.[1] Clinical reasoning and expertise are essential whether the valid evidence does or does not apply to a patient or where evidence is limited or inconclusive. The value of clinical expertise is indicated by Sackett et al[37(p72)]: "External clinical evidence can inform, but can never replace, individual clinical expertise, and it is this expertise that decides whether the external evidence applies to the individual patient at all and, if so, how it should be integrated into a clinical decision."

Each patient has a unique personality, cultural characteristics, and personal concerns. Each clinician has a distinct collection of knowledge, experiences, and values. In addition, the availability, accessibility, and cost of a rapidly changing health care system can influence the integration of best evidence. Good communication skills are essential to determine and understand patient preferences and concerns. Patient preferences and considerations such as a willingness to accept or comply with treatment, potential risks, and financial costs are highly variable and must be carefully factored into the decision.[29] The fourth step ends with implementation of the evidence into practice.

Step 5: Evaluate the Effectiveness of Performing Steps 1 Through 4

The final step is a reflection and self-evaluation of the EBPT process and development of a plan for improvement.[1,38] As discussed in detail by Sackett et al,[1] clinicians should reflect on their ability to perform each of the first 4 steps and their overall success in the execution of EBPT. Additionally, Noteboom et al[29] suggested that clinicians should formally assess patient outcomes to determine whether true, clinically important changes in daily activity limitations occur during and at the end of an episode of care. The use of reliable and valid outcome measures in addition to self-assessment of the effectiveness of the EBPT process will result in the best quality care and improved clinical practice.[29]

Critical Appraisal of Literature Related to Diagnostic Tests

Diagnosis

The process of diagnosis involves gathering data through taking a history and the performance of various tests and measures. All elements of the history and tests and measures are considered diagnostic tests. Based on the examination, working hypotheses are ruled in or ruled out and a diagnosis is established, which, in turn, directs the intervention. The accuracy of the diagnosis then relates to the purpose and the validity of the applied tests. Before selecting and applying a test or sequence of tests, an evaluation of the test's properties is required. This section discusses how to (a) determine the validity of a diagnostic study; (b) use the results to select the best tests; and (c) apply the results to individual patients.

In order to evaluate a potentially relevant article about a diagnostic test, 3 questions are typically asked about the evidence[1,39]:

1. Are the results valid? Is the evidence about the accuracy of a diagnostic test valid?
2. What are the results? Does the evidence accurately distinguish between patients who do and do not have a specific disorder?
3. Will the results help me in caring for my patients?

Are the Results Valid? Is the Evidence About the Accuracy of a Diagnostic Test Valid?

The validity of the evidence about the accuracy of a diagnostic test is affected by the reference standard, the diagnostic test, and the population studied. The accuracy of a diagnostic test is best established by comparing it to the reference or "gold" standard.[1,39] In a diagnostic study, a valid reference standard confirms or proves that the condition is present or absent. The results of the reference standard (ie, arthroscopy, magnetic resonance imaging) and the diagnostic test should be assessed independently of one another to avoid conscious or unconscious bias of the assessor related to interpretation.[1,39]

The study should apply the diagnostic test to patients with a range (mild to severe) of presentations of the condition of interest or other commonly competing diagnoses. If the study includes patients who clearly do or do not have the condition, the diagnostic accuracy of the test becomes inflated and the results are not informative.[1,10] To avoid spectrum bias and ensure a range of clinical presentations, a valid diagnostic study uses a prospective cohort design with a consecutive group of subjects from a clinical setting.[40] If the diagnostic study describes a spectrum of patients, a blind comparison of the test, and reference standard, the results most likely represent an unbiased estimate of the accuracy of the test.

If possible, the reference standard and the diagnostic test must be applied to every patient in the study to avoid verification or workup bias. For example, in cases where the reference standard is expensive or unnecessarily invasive (ie, arthroscopy), only those who are positive on the test will get arthroscopy; however, it is not likely to be performed on patients with negative test results. To overcome this bias, researchers include follow-up evidence to show that the patient does not have the condition.[1] Workup bias leads to an overestimation of the accuracy (increased sensitivity and decreased specificity) of the diagnostic test.[41]

Consideration of the validity of a diagnostic test also requires a detailed description of how to use it. The description should include the intended use or purpose, performance of the test, and the scoring criteria.[39,40] The purpose may be for differential diagnosis or selection of an intervention. In order to generalize the results to a clinical situation, the test should be performed in the clinic in the same manner as it was performed in the study.[39,40] For example, ligamentous stability tests performed under anesthesia may not have the same clinical utility when performed without anesthesia. Scoring criteria include the definitions of positive and negative results. To be reassured about accuracy, a final concern is to determine whether the results were replicated in a second independent set of patients. When the study is deemed a valid estimate of the test properties, the results are analyzed for clinical usefulness or accuracy.

Valid studies of diagnostic tests should include a blind comparison of the test, a valid reference standard, and application to a spectrum of patients, as well as a detailed description of the test. If these criteria are not met, the study may not provide an unbiased estimate of the accuracy of the test. If the study is unbiased, proceed to the next step.

What Are the Results? Does the Evidence Accurately Distinguish Between Patients Who Do and Do not Have a Specific Disorder?

The diagnostic process begins with consideration of the patient's presenting symptoms and signs. Each element of the history and tests and measures as a diagnostic test either increases or decreases the probability of a target condition.[42] Clinically, however, test properties of all information are not available. Prior to performing a diagnostic test or sequence of tests, all known information including prevalence statistics of the condition of interest, if available, is combined with clinical expertise to estimate a pretest probability of the target condition. The clinical utility of a diagnostic test rests in its ability to differentiate among patients with and without the target disorder.[42] That is, the diagnostic test must assist the clinician in moving closer to or farther away from a given diagnosis.[10] Clinically, the accuracy of a test rests in the ability of the test to change what we thought before the test (pretest probability) to what we think after the test (posttest probability). Diagnostic tests that have the potential to make big changes from pretest to posttest probability are important and likely useful in practice.[1,43]

Accuracy of a test is assessed by the measure of agreement between the diagnostic test and the reference standard.[39,40] Results obtained from the reference standard are compared with the test in question to determine the diagnostic accuracy or the percentage of people correctly diagnosed through the use of a 2 × 2 contingency table (Table 1-3). Positive and negative predictive values (PPVs and NPVs, respectively), sensitivity, specificity, and likelihood ratios (LRs)[1,10,40] are statistical measures used to interpret the results of diagnostic tests. Common descriptions of these measures are listed in Table 1-4.

Predictive Values, Sensitivity, Specificity, and Likelihood Ratios

A PPV is the chance that a patient who has a positive test result actually has the condition. An NPV is the chance that a patient who has a negative test result does not have the condition. In other words, given that a test result is positive or negative, the PPV or NPV is the probability that the test is correct.[10,40] Predictive values are affected by the prevalence of the condition. Unless the proportion of patients in the clinical setting is the same as that used in the study, these values should be interpreted with caution.[40] Sensitivity and specificity are not influenced by prevalence and may be more valuable in the decision-making process.[10]

Sensitivity describes the test's ability to classify those patients who actually have the condition (true positive rate).[1,40] A test with high sensitivity has relatively few false negatives.[40,43] The acronym SnNout is a reminder that a

TABLE 1-3. 2 × 2 CONTINGENCY TABLE

	REFERENCE STANDARD POSITIVE/PRESENT	REFERENCE STANDARD NEGATIVE/ABSENT
DIAGNOSTIC OR CLINICAL TEST POSITIVE/PRESENT	(a) True positive	(b) False positive
DIAGNOSTIC OR CLINICAL TEST NEGATIVE/ABSENT	(c) False negative	(d) True negative

TABLE 1-4. COMMONLY USED STATISTICAL COMPUTATIONS

STATISTICAL MEASURES	COMPUTATION	DESCRIPTION
PPV	a/(a+b)	Probability that the patient has the condition given a + test finding
NPV	d/(c+d)	Probability that the patient does not have the condition given a – test finding
Sensitivity	a/(a+c)	Proportion of people with the condition who have a + test (true + rate)
Specificity	d/(b+d)	Proportion of people without the condition who have a – test (true – rate)
Positive LR	Sensitivity/(1–Specificity)	The ↑ in odds favoring the condition given a + test result; helpful for ruling in the condition
Negative LR	(1–Sensitivity)/Specificity	The ↓ in odds favoring the condition given a – test result; helpful for ruling out the condition
Pretest probability	(a+c)/(a+b+c+d)	Probability of a target condition before the result of the diagnostic test is known
Pretest odds	Pretest probability/1–Pretest probability	The odds that the patient has a target condition before the test is performed
Posttest odds	Pretest odds × LR	The odds that the patient has a target condition after the test is performed
Posttest probability	Posttest odds/Posttest odds+1	Probability of a target condition after the result of the diagnostic test is known

test with a high sensitivity and a negative result is good for ruling out the condition but does not address the value of a positive test.[1,40] Specificity describes the test's ability to classify those patients who actually do not have the condition (true negative rate).[1,4] A test with high specificity has few false-positive rates.[40,43] The acronym SpPin is a reminder that a test with high specificity and a positive result is good for ruling in the condition.[1,40] Sensitivity and specificity do not provide information about the change in pretest probability if the test results are positive or negative.[40] Determining the LR using sensitivity and specificity (see Table 1-4) provides an accurate measure to indicate how much a given test will increase or decrease the pretest probability of the target disorder.[42]

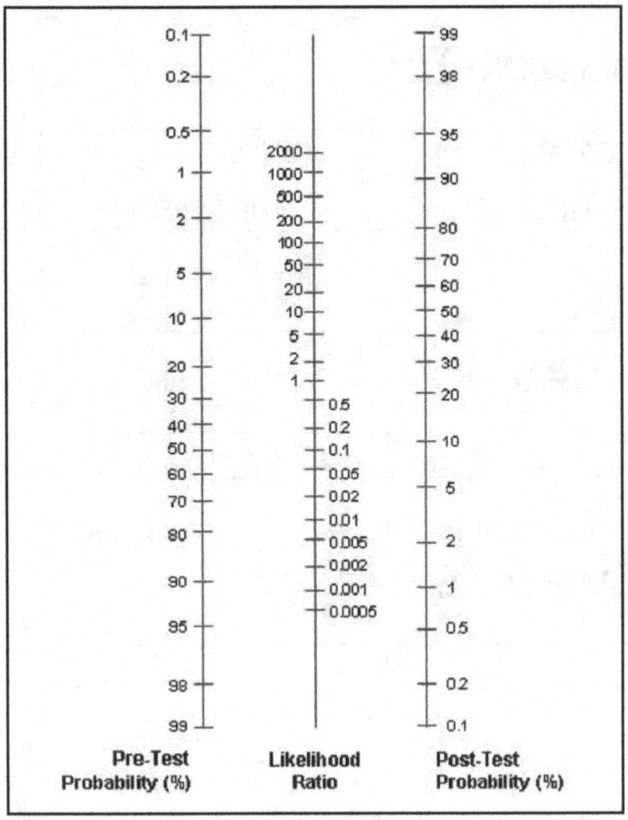

Figure 1-1. Fagan's nomogram for interpreting diagnostic test results. To obtain the posttest probability, draw a line from the pretest probability through the LR to the posttest probability line to observe the percentage. (Reprinted with permission from Fagan TJ. Nomogram for Bayes's theorem. *N Engl J Med.* 1975:293:257. Copyright © 1975, Massachusetts Medical Society. All rights reserved.)

LRs describe both directions of test performance or quantify how much a given test raises or lowers the pretest probability. A positive LR shifts the probability in favor of the presence of the condition when the test is positive, helpful for ruling in the condition. The higher the value, the better the ability of the test to determine the posttest odds that the condition is actually present if the result is positive. A negative LR shifts the probability in favor of the absence of the condition when the test is negative, helpful for ruling out the condition. The lower the value, the better the ability of the test to determine the posttest odds that the condition is actually absent if the result is negative. Because the magnitude of the shift in probability signifies the clinical usefulness of a test, an LR of greater than 1 increases the odds of the condition, whereas an LR of less than 1 lessens the odds of the condition.[40] An LR of 1 indicates that the test result has no effect on the pretest probability. Jaeschke et al[42] provided a guide to assist in interpretation of LR values for shifts from pretest to posttest probability.

- LRs > 10 or < 0.1 generate a large and often conclusive change.
- LRs of 5 to 10 and 0.1 to 0.2 generate a moderate shift.
- LRs of 2 to 5 and 0.5 to 0.2 generate a small but sometimes important change.
- LRs of 1 to 2 and 0.5 to 1 generate a small but rarely important change.

After the LRs are calculated, a nomogram[44] (Figure 1-1) is often used in the clinic to go from pretest to posttest probability, but a more precise calculation of the shift in probability is accessible.[45] Generally, diagnostic tests that have the most potential to make change from pretest to posttest probability are important and should be selected.[1,43] The findings of individual test results alone do not establish a probability that a patient has a specific condition. Figure 1-2 is a diagram of the process by which the pretest probability is constantly revised with each element of data from the history and tests and measures until it reaches a treatment threshold, the level at which examination stops and treatment begins.[46] The clinician decides when the posttest probability is high enough to establish a diagnosis or low enough to refute a diagnosis and consider alternative testing.[42,43]

To assist in interpretation of the findings of the study, the sensitivity, specificity, and LRs, usually reported as single values, represent an estimate of the true value of a sample population and should be reported with a CI.[1] The CI, the likely range of the true value and a measure of the precision of this value, is commonly supplied for diagnostic studies.[42] A 95% CI is a range of values within which there is a 95% probability that the true value is located. A 95% CI that does not capture a zero difference represents a difference that is statistically significant when comparing continuous data. A narrow CI is preferred for validity purposes. The CI width is related to the sample size and the variability in the test under investigation.[40] A larger sample size results in a narrower CI and a more precise study finding.[47] If the CI is wide, indicating that the estimate of the positive LR is not very precise, the usefulness of the measure may be questionable.[40]

In clinical practice, single tests are rarely used to establish a diagnosis. Clusters of symptoms and signs and clinical prediction rules (CPRs) are increasingly being presented as diagnostic tools in orthopedic physical therapy literature.[42,48-52] Beattie and Nelson[53] described CPRs as the combining of relevant clinical findings (history, physical examination, patient beliefs) to calculate a probability of the presence or absence of a condition or for patient classification for treatment. Development and testing of CPRs involves a 3-step process: (1) derivation or identification of predictive variables; (2) validation (evaluating the rule in a similar clinical setting and population and multiple clinical setting); and (3) impact analysis or the change in clinical behavior, outcomes, and economic benefits. Full validation is recommended before use in clinical practice.[54]

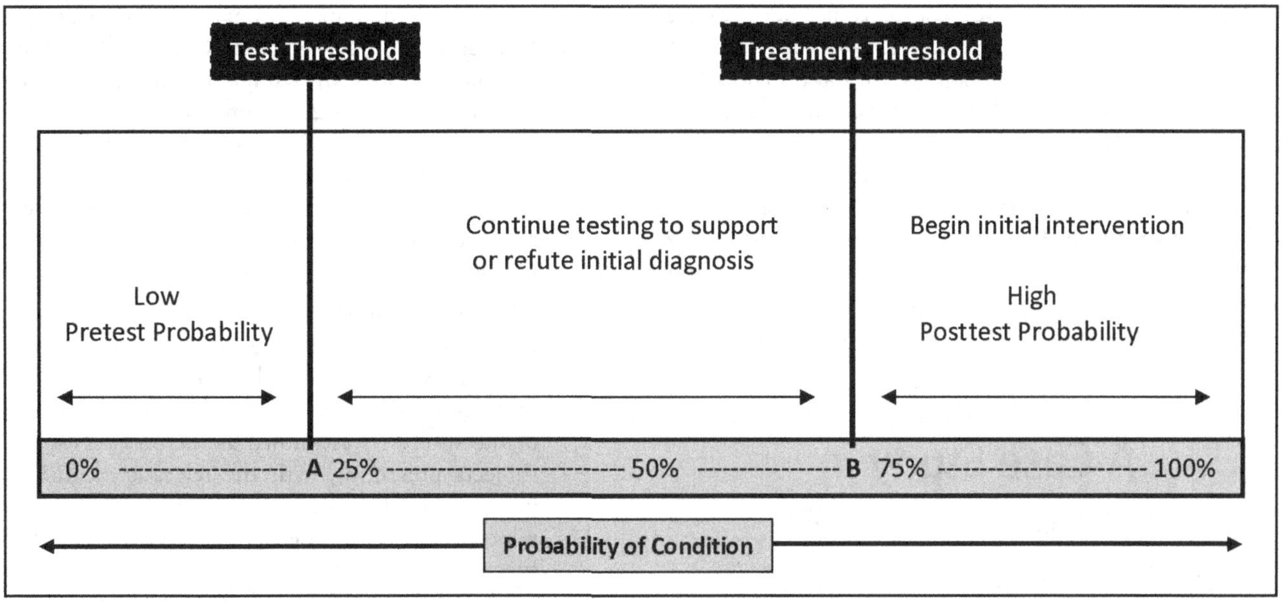

Figure 1-2. Probability of condition, test, and treatment thresholds.

CPRs are designed with the same statistical measures, sensitivity, specificity, and LRs used to interpret the results of diagnostic tests. The quality, strengths, and weaknesses of CPRs must be considered by the clinician when determining appropriateness for a specific patient.[55] CPRs can be used as an adjunct to the diagnostic process but do not necessarily advocate a decision.[56]

When evaluating diagnostic studies reporting measures of PPVs, NPVs, sensitivity, specificity, and LRs, use of the CI helps to interpret the results of diagnostic tests so that clinicians will know the precision of the estimate. A diagnostic test calculator is available at http://araw.mede.uic.edu/cgi-bin/testcalc.pl.[57] This calculator determines sensitivity, specificity, LRs, and the posttest probability of disease given the pretest probability and test characteristics. Given sample sizes, CIs are also computed.

Will the Results Help Me in Caring for My Patients?

Given that the results are valid, relevant to the patient, and have sufficient clinical accuracy, the final step is applying the test to the patient. If your patient meets the study inclusion criteria and the practice setting is similar to the study, the results are applied with confidence. If not, clinical judgment is needed. The test must be performed in a competent, reproducible manner. In order to minimize error, clinicians should perform and interpret the test exactly as the study described.

Prior to applying the test, the clinician decides on a sensible estimate of the patient's pretest probability using clinical experience, prevalence statistics, the study's prevalence, and regional studies or pretest probabilities.[1] If the result of the diagnostic test does not alter the pretest probability to meet the test threshold (see Figure 1-2), the probability below which no further testing is needed, the clinician should refute a diagnosis.[42] If the test result alters the pretest probability to the treatment threshold (see Figure 1-2), the clinician confirms a diagnosis and begins treatment.[42] When the probability lies between the test and treatment thresholds, further tests are required.[42] No absolute values exist for test or treatment thresholds. Test and treatment thresholds are different for different conditions and patient presentations and are an issue of clinical judgment.

The pretest probability is a key to the diagnostic process because it establishes the level of uncertainty prior to performing a test.[42] With a high pretest probability (75%) that a condition is present, one negative test result is unlikely to adequately reduce the probability to rule out the condition. Additional testing is needed.[58] Similarly, with a low pretest probability (20%), one positive test result is unlikely to increase the probability past the threshold to rule in the condition. Based on the test result, LRs quantify the direction and amount of change in the pretest probability to assist the clinician in moving across the test or treatment thresholds.[10,40] A sufficiently high posttest probability has a direct implication for moving beyond the treatment threshold and initiating treatment.[1,42]

The final consideration for the usefulness of a diagnostic test is its ability to add information beyond that which is available and whether this information leads to a change in management that benefits the patient.[1,10] Performing tests on patients who are either highly likely or unlikely to have the condition usually results in a small gain in information. Applying a test to a patient who has a low or high pretest probability of truly having the condition results in a moderate to high risk of a false-positive or false-negative finding, respectively.[10]

The systematic approach to appraising the evidence related to diagnosis is an important step in the practicing EBPT because a diagnosis leads to an appropriate intervention. A systematic worksheet for assessing diagnostic accuracy studies is available in Table 1-5.[28] Clinicians obtain diagnostic tests to lower the probability of the target condition below the testing threshold (ie, stop testing for it and eliminate it from further consideration) or to increase this probability above the treatment threshold (ie, stop testing for it and initiate appropriate therapy). The LR best captures the direction and magnitude of this change from pretest to posttest probability.[59]

A Case Study in Diagnosis Using the Critical Appraisal Criteria

The following is an example of a diagnostic study worksheet:

1. **Focused clinical question**: In a 45-year-old female who presents with unilateral neck pain and headache without side shift, is the cervical flexion-rotation test (CFRT) an accurate test in the differential diagnosis of cervicogenic headache?
2. **Selected search article**: Ogince M, Hall T, Robinson K, Blackmore AM. The diagnostic validity of the cervical flexion-rotation test in C1/2-related cervicogenic headache. *Man Ther.* 2007;12:256-262. The purpose of the study was to determine the sensitivity and specificity of the CFRT. A single-blind comparative group design was used to determine differences between asymptomatic subjects (n = 23; 8 males, 15 females), migraine with aura subjects (n = 12; 9 males, 3 females), and those with C1/2-related cervicogenic headache (n = 23; 3 males, 20 females). Subjects ranged in age from 18 to 66 years. A power of 80% with alpha at .05 required at least 10 subjects in each group. Subjects, 325 symptomatic and 23 asymptomatic, were recruited by advertisement. Eighty-two percent were rejected due to overlapping cervicogenic and migraine symptoms. A convenience sample of 23 cervicogenic headache, 23 asymptomatic, and 12 migraine subjects with aura were recruited into the study.
3. Are the results of this diagnostic study valid?
    a. Was there an independent blind comparison with an appropriate reference gold standard of diagnosis? Two examiners blinded to group allocation independently performed the CFRT on all subjects. The test was considered positive or not based on the therapist's interpretation of a 10-degree minimum reduction in range of motion and a firm end feel. The reference gold standard was manual diagnosis by a single independent assessor to identify C1/2 dysfunction. The method of assessment is a valid means of identifying the symptomatic cervical level. No other reference standards are available. Radiography is not effective and nerve block procedures are not practical in the upper cervical region.

    b. Was the diagnostic test evaluated in an appropriate spectrum of patients? Is it similar to those in whom it would be used in practice? Spectrum bias is evident because the diagnosis of the subjects was known at the onset. Not all subjects presenting with the relevant condition were included in order of entry, nor was the selection random. The authors argued that the spectrum bias and case control design are not limitations. Considering the subjective criteria of the International Headache Society, the subjects must either have a cervicogenic headache or not. Yet, a more likely clinical situation is a population whose symptoms overlap those of cervicogenic and migraine headache. The diagnostic accuracy of the CFRT is unknown in this population. The reported sensitivity and specificity may be falsely inflated.

    c. Was the reference standard applied to every subject regardless of the diagnostic test result? Only the cervicogenic group was manually examined for C1/2 dysfunction. The subjects in this study were divided into groups based on the International Headache Society criteria. The results of the test did not influence the decision to perform the reference standard.

    d. Were the methods for performing the test described in sufficient detail to permit replication? Yes. The purpose, performance of the test, and scoring criteria were described.
4. What are the results? Does the evidence accurately distinguish between patients who do and do not have a specific disorder?
    a. Interpret the results using a 2 × 2 contingency table. Data from therapist #2 were used for the calculation. CIs were not described in the article but were calculated using the CI calculator and the diagnostic test calculator.[57]

Cervicogenic Headache

	Positive/present	**Negative/absent**
CFRT Positive/present	True positive (a) = 21	(b) = 4 False positive
CFRT Negative/absent	False negative (c) = 2	(d) = 31 True negative

Table 1-5. Diagnostic Accuracy Study Appraisal Worksheet

Are the Results of the Study Valid?

R: Was the diagnostic test evaluated in a representative spectrum of patients (like those in whom it would be used in practice)?	
What Is Best?	*Where Do I Find the Information?*
It is ideal if the diagnostic test is applied to the full spectrum of patients—those with mild, severe, early, and late cases of the target disorder. It is also best if the patients are randomly selected or consecutive admissions so that selection bias is minimized.	The Methods section should tell you how patients were enrolled and whether they were randomly selected or consecutive admissions. It should also tell you where patients came from and whether they are likely to be representative of the patients in whom the test is to be used.
This paper: Yes ☐ No ☐ Unclear ☐ Comment:	

A: Was the reference standard ascertained regardless of the index test result?	
What Is Best?	*Where Do I Find the Information?*
Ideally, both the index test and the reference standard should be carried out on all patients in the study. In some situations where the reference standard is invasive or expensive, there may be reservations about subjecting patients with a negative index test result (and thus a low probability of disease) to the reference standard. An alternative reference standard is to follow-up with patients for an appropriate period of time (dependent on disease in question) to see if they are truly negative.	The Methods section should indicate whether the reference standard was applied to all patients or if an alternative reference standard (eg, follow-up) was applied to those who tested negative on the index test.
This paper: Yes ☐ No ☐ Unclear ☐ Comment:	

B: Was there an independent, blind comparison between the index test and an appropriate reference ("gold") standard of diagnosis?	
What Is Best?	*Where Do I Find the Information?*
There are 2 issues here. First the reference standard should be appropriate—as close to the "truth" as possible. Sometimes there may not be a single reference test that is suitable and a combination of tests may be used to indicate the presence of disease. Second, the reference standard and the index test being assessed should be applied to each patient independently and blindly. Those who interpreted the results of one test should not be aware of the results of the other test.	The Methods section should have a description of the reference standard used, and if you are unsure of whether this is an appropriate reference standard, you may need to do some background searching in the area. The Methods section should also describe who conducted the 2 tests and whether each was conducted independently and blinded to the results of the other.
This paper: Yes ☐ No ☐ Unclear ☐ Comment:	

(continued)

TABLE 1-5 (CONTINUED). DIAGNOSTIC ACCURACY STUDY APPRAISAL WORKSHEET

What Were the Results?

ARE TEST CHARACTERISTICS PRESENTED?

There are 2 types of results commonly reported in diagnostic test studies. One concerns the accuracy of the test and is reflected in the sensitivity and specificity. The other concerns how the test performs in the population being tested and is reflected in predictive values (also called posttest probabilities). To explore the meaning of these terms, consider a study in which 1000 elderly people with suspected dementia undergo an index test and a reference standard. The prevalence of dementia in this group is 25%. Two hundred forty people tested positive on both the index test and the reference standard, and 600 people tested negative on both tests. The first step is to draw a 2 × 2 table as shown below. We are told that the prevalence of dementia is 25%; therefore, we can fill in the last row of totals—25% of 1000 people is 250—so 250 people will have dementia and 750 will be free of dementia. We also know the number of people testing positive and negative on both tests, so we can fill in 2 more cells of the table.

Reference Standard

		+	−	
Index Test	+	240		
	−		600	
		250	750	1000

By subtraction we can easily complete the table:

Reference Standard

		+	−	
Index Test	+	240	150	390
	−	10	600	610
		250	750	1000

WHAT IS THE MEASURE?	*WHAT DOES IT MEAN?*
Sensitivity (Sn) = the proportion of people with the condition who have a positive test result.	The sensitivity tells us how well the test identifies people with the condition. A highly sensitive test will not miss many people.
In our example, the Sn = 240/250 = 0.96	10 people (4%) with dementia were falsely identified as not having it. This means the test is fairly good at identifying people with the condition.
Specificity (Sp) = the proportion of people without the condition who have a negative test result.	The specificity tells us how well the test identifies people without the condition. A highly specific test will not falsely identify many people as having the condition.
In our example, the Sp = 600/750 = 0.80	150 people (20%) without dementia were falsely identified as having it. This means the test is only moderately good at identifying people without the condition.
PPV = the proportion of people with a positive test who have the condition.	This measure tells us how well the test performs in this population. It is dependent on the accuracy of the test (primarily specificity) and the prevalence of the condition.
In our example, the PPV = 240/390 = 0.62	Of the 390 people who had a positive test result, 62% will actually have dementia.

(continued)

TABLE 1-5 (CONTINUED). DIAGNOSTIC ACCURACY STUDY APPRAISAL WORKSHEET

WHAT IS THE MEASURE?	*WHAT DOES IT MEAN?*
NPV = the proportion of people with a negative test who do not have the condition. In our example, the NPV = 600/610 = 0.98	This measure tells us how well the test performs in this population. It is dependent on the accuracy of the test and the prevalence of the condition. Of the 610 people with a negative test, 98% will not have dementia.

Application

WERE THE METHODS FOR PERFORMING THE TEST DESCRIBED IN SUFFICIENT DETAIL TO PERMIT REPLICATION?	
WHAT IS BEST?	*WHERE DO I FIND THE INFORMATION?*
The article should have sufficient description of the test to allow its replication and also interpretation of the results.	The Methods section should describe the test in detail.
This paper: Yes ☐ No ☐ Unclear ☐ Comment:	

Reprinted with permission from Centre for Evidence-Based Medicine. Levels of Evidence (March 2009). *University of Oxford.* http://www.cebm.net/index.aspx?o=1157. Updated April 3, 2013. Accessed June 27, 2011.

b. Calculations:

Sn = a/(a + c) = 0.91 (0.73, 0.97)

Sp = d/(b + d) = 0.89 (0.74, 0.95)

+LR = Sens/(1 – Spec) = 7.99 (3.1, 20.2)

–LR = (1 – Sens)/Spec = 0.1 (0.03, 0.37)

Pretest probability (prevalence) = (a + c)/(a + b + c + d) = 0.397 = 40%

If + test, posttest probability (odds) = 87% (6.6) [70%, 90%]

If – test, posttest probability (odds) = 6% (0.1) [2%, 20%]

PPV = a/(a + b) = 84.0

NPV = d/(c + d) = 93.9

Pretest odds = Pretest probability/(1 – Pretest probability)

Posttest odds = Pretest odds × LR

Posttest probability = Posttest odds/(Posttest odds + 1)

Note: Fagan's nomogram[44] (Figure 1-3) for interpreting diagnostic test results. The left-hand column is the pretest probability. The middle column is the LR. The right-hand column is the posttest probability. To obtain the posttest probability, draw a line from the pretest probability through the LR to the posttest probability line to observe the percentage.

5. Will the results help me in caring for my patients?
   a. Will the reproducibility of the test results and its interpretation be satisfactory in my setting? Yes. The test is easily reproducible but may require practice to determine end feel if this is not a routine part of the therapist's practice.
   b. Are the results applicable to my patient? Yes. With a pretest probability of 40% and a positive CFRT, the posttest probability is 87% (CI: 70%, 95%) surpassing the treatment threshold and establishing preliminary diagnosis. If the test is negative, the posttest probability is 6% (CI: 2%, 20%), effectively lowering the probability below the test threshold, and the diagnosis is ruled out or more testing is necessary. The test should assist in the differential diagnosis of C1/2-related cervicogenic headache.
   c. Will the results change my management? A positive CFRT might lead to further manual examination of the cervical spine for additional signs of cervicogenic headache and search for the most effective intervention for patients with cervicogenic headache.
   d. Will the patient be better off as a result of the test? Yes. The test is safe and may provide information to assist with a definitive diagnosis, which in turn guides the intervention.

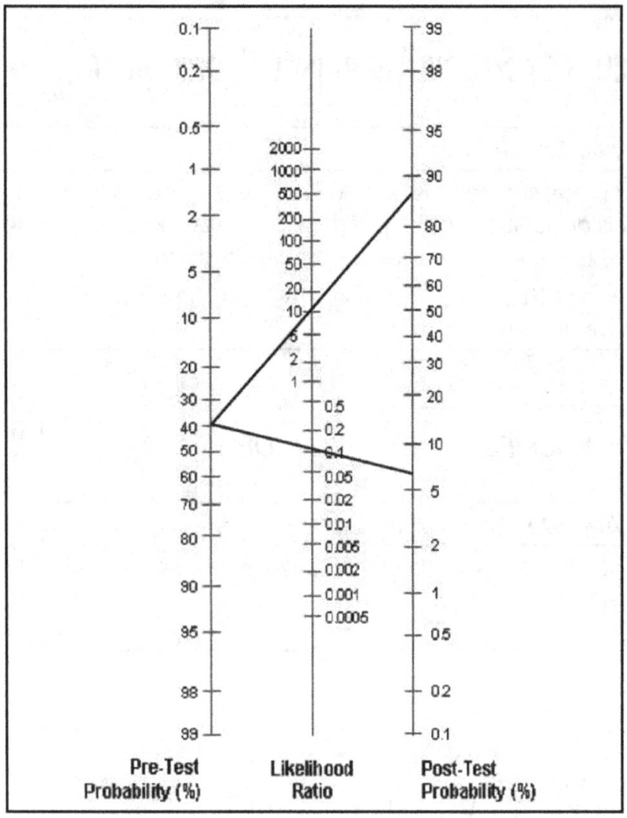

Figure 1-3. Fagan's nomogram for interpreting diagnostic test results. To obtain the posttest probability, draw a line from the pretest probability through the LR to the posttest probability line to observe the percentage. (Reprinted with permission from Fagan TJ. Nomogram for Bayes's theorem. *N Engl J Med.* 1975:293:257. Copyright © 1975, Massachusetts Medical Society. All rights reserved.)

Critical Appraisal of Literature Related to Intervention or Prevention

Intervention

When the treatment threshold is reached and the examination stops, the clinician must determine the best intervention to optimize patient outcomes. Within the hierarchy of evidence, a systematic review, when available, provides a higher level of evidence than the results of one RCT. Guides for appraising systematic reviews are available online.[28] In the absence of an RCT related to the intervention in question, the clinician must rely on weaker evidence from nonrandomized studies. The RCT, however, is the most common study design for determining treatment effectiveness because of its potential to control bias if appropriately designed and implemented. This section discusses the critical appraisal of a single RCT. When evaluating or critically analyzing a potentially relevant article on physical therapy intervention, the same 3 questions are typically asked about the evidence[1,60]:

1. Are the results valid?
2. What are the results? What is the size of the treatment effect? How precise is the estimate of the treatment effect?
3. Will the results help me in caring for my patients?

Are the Results Valid?

The first question is whether the allocation of patients to treatment was randomized. Randomization ensures that prognostic factors such as comorbidities and disease severity are evenly dispersed between treatment and control groups. However, randomization does not always occur, especially in studies with small samples.[1,60] Therefore, investigators should report the similarity of each group at baseline. If baseline differences exist between groups, statistical techniques such as the analysis of covariance may provide an adjusted comparison of the study results.[17,60] Prognostic factors that are unevenly dispersed between groups could enhance (ie, lead to false-positive results), cancel, or counteract (ie, lead to false-negative results) the effects of the intervention in question.[1] For similar reasons, randomization should be concealed from clinicians who enter patients into the trial.

After randomization is verified, validity is next questioned by looking to see whether all patients who entered into the trial were accounted for at the end of the trial and analyzed in the groups to which they were randomized.[1,60] Ideally, all patients who enter a trial should be accounted for at its end.[60] Patients lost to follow-up question the validity of the study because their outcomes (good or bad) would have affected the results of the study.[1] Patients lost to follow-up should be accounted for by assuming the worst-case scenario. All patients lost from the group that did well assume a poor outcome. All patients lost from the group that did poorly assume a good outcome. Accounting for patients lost to follow-up in this manner should allow researchers to support their original conclusions. If the conclusions change, the strength of the evidence is weakened.[1,60] Analyzing all patients in the groups to which they were assigned, an intention-to-treat analysis, preserves the unbiased comparison provided by randomization.[1,60] The outcome that results is then credited to the assigned treatment.[60] Clinicians should also determine whether the length of follow-up was sufficiently long to find a clinically important effect.[1]

Blinding of patients, clinicians, data collectors, and analysts is necessary in order to minimize subject and rater bias.[61] In situations where patients and clinicians cannot be kept blinded, as is often the case in physical therapy research, investigators should clearly explain all procedures related to blinding, especially those related to measuring outcomes. The clinician can then decide whether blinding was a serious threat to validity or not.[17]

The final consideration related to validity is to determine whether all patients were treated equally, apart from the experimental treatment itself.[1,60] Between-group differences in the overall experience may result in unintended beneficial cointerventions (ie, medications, etc).[60] Investigators minimize potential differences in care by structuring the study protocol with identical experiences (frequency, duration, treating clinicians). Acceptable cointerventions, if present, are described in the Methods section of the article.[17,60]

Valid clinical trials should randomly assign subjects to experimental and control groups, blind data collectors, and others if possible; account for all dropouts; and treat subjects equally except for the treatment itself. If these criteria are not present, validity could be compromised. The trial may not constitute strong evidence of treatment effectiveness or ineffectiveness.

What Are the Results? What Is the Size of the Treatment Effect? How Precise Is the Estimate of the Treatment Effect?

If the results are considered valid, the next step involves statistical analyses and a useful expression of the quantitative results to determine whether the potential benefits or harms are important.[1,29] Noteboom et al[29] provided a detailed review of basic statistical procedures commonly used in physical therapy research. Using selected hypothetical examples, this section will highlight some important concepts related to size and precision of the estimate of the treatment effect.

Statistical Significance and Power

Physical therapy research on intervention often makes use of the hypothesis testing approach for making decisions about statistical significance.[29,62] Hypothesis testing attempts to determine whether differences between or among sample means are due to chance or reflect a true difference in the target population.[29] In this form of hypothesis testing, the null hypothesis states that there is no difference between the sample means. For example, when comparing 2 types of exercises for increasing trunk strength in postmenopausal women with chronic low back pain, the null hypothesis states that a difference in strength gains will not exist between the 2 groups following treatment. The null hypothesis is assumed to be true until statistical tests prove otherwise. Based on the results of the statistical test, the null hypothesis is rejected or not rejected.[62] If the null hypothesis is rejected, observed differences between the groups are not likely due to chance. The difference is said to be statistically significant. However, a statistically significant result is not always a large effect or of clinical importance. Given a large enough sample, even small and unimportant differences can be found to be statistically significant.

Noteboom et al[29] stated that a statistical test provides an estimate of probability along a continuum. Therefore, researchers must declare a threshold for statistical significance. A traditional alpha (α) level is indicated with a P value $<.05$ or 5%, which means that there is a 5% probability that the study's results are due to chance.[63] Any result that achieves this threshold is statistically significant with confidence that a type I error (rejecting the null hypothesis when it is true) has not been committed. Therefore, the difference observed between the groups is a true difference but does not tell us about the size and precision of the difference.

In the hypothetical example, the critical question is whether one type of exercise is more effective than the other. Both groups increased trunk strength from pretreatment to posttreatment ($P=.04$), demonstrating that within-group improvements were significant; the null hypothesis is rejected with only a small risk (4%) of committing a type I error, rejecting a true null hypothesis. However, differences between the 2 groups were not significantly different ($P=.68$). The null hypothesis is not rejected; one type of exercise is not more effective than the other. The observed between-group difference in trunk strength improvement was due to chance, not due to a true difference in the effectiveness of the exercise program in postmenopausal women. However, even though the results are not significant, the probability still exists that a difference in the effectiveness of the exercise programs really does exist. Simply put, a nonsignificant outcome could mean that the available evidence is not strong enough to reject the null hypothesis and that a type II error (rejecting the null hypothesis when it is actually false) was committed.[63] The probability that a statistical test will reject a false null hypothesis or the probability of attaining statistical significance is determined by the power of the test.

The power of a statistical test is the probability that a test will reject a false null hypothesis or the probability of detecting an effect given that the effect actually exists. Power analysis can be done a priori (before) or post hoc (after) data collection.[63] The more powerful a test, the less chance there is to make a type II error (rejecting the null hypothesis when it is actually false). A power of 80% is the standard that represents a reasonable protection against a type II error when a study results in a nonsignificant finding.[64] Statistical power is the ability of a study to show a relationship or causal effect between 2 variables given that the relationship exists. If the power is low, the results are uncertain. Greater power means a higher likelihood of getting a statistically significant result.

Portney and Watkins[63] provided 4 factors that affect the statistical power of a test: the significance criterion, variance in the data, sample size, and effect size, a measure of the difference between groups.

1. *The significance criterion*: Lowering the significance level (α) decreases the probability of making a type I error and increases the probability of making a type II error (more difficult to demonstrate a significant difference); power is reduced. A study with low power is less likely to find a significant difference if one exists.
2. *Variance in the data*: A large variance within groups decreases the probability of detecting a change; power is reduced.
3. *Sample size*: A larger sample increases the probability of detecting a change; power is increased. A study with high power is likely to find a significant difference even if the size of the effect is of little value.
4. *Effect size*: The greater the effect size, the greater the power. Trying to detect a larger difference increases the likelihood that you will actually detect it.

Evidence of a statistically significant treatment effect is not enough information to make a decision about treatment. Statistical significance does not necessarily mean clinically important; the size of the effect determines the importance or usefulness. The treatment effect or measured outcomes must be meaningful and large enough to make the therapy advisable, and the beneficial effects should outweigh any small or uncommon harmful effects.

Effect Size and Confidence Intervals

Hypothesis testing and the P value provide a yes or no answer (whether the observed difference is real) to the question of statistical significance but do not provide the clinician with information about the size of the true treatment effect or how good an estimate it is of the true population difference. In addition to focusing on whether an intervention had an effect, how much of an effect the intervention had is equally important. The size of the intervention's effect is estimated by the average difference between comparison groups, also called the *raw effect size.*[65] The raw between-group effect size is calculated by subtracting one group mean from the other, retaining the units of the outcome scale.[65] Hypothetically, if neck pain, as measured on a 10-cm Visual Analogue Scale (VAS), was reduced by a mean of 4.5 cm in the treatment group and 1.5 cm in the control group, and the difference between groups is statistically significant ($P<.05$), the estimate of the mean effect of treatment or raw effect size is a 3-cm reduction in VAS (4.5 cm − 1.5 cm = 3 cm). This estimate is one way to determine whether the size of the reported treatment effect is large enough to be clinically meaningful. Clinicians must consider the CI about the treatment effect size to assess the precision or imprecision of the estimate.

CIs offer a means to determine how meaningful the results of a study are because they establish the precision of the effect size. The CI provides a range about the observed treatment effect size and is commonly reported as a 95% CI, a range of upper and lower limits of values within which there is a 95% probability that the true treatment effect is located.[43,62] The upper and lower limits tell us how big or small the true effect might be. A narrow CI width reflects greater precision around the point estimate of the treatment effect and greater certainty that the true effect and point estimate are similar, allowing greater confidence in deciding whether to administer the treatment.[29,59] If the CI is overly wide, estimates of the effect size are imprecise. The clinician may choose to administer the treatment selectively or not at all.[59] To determine the meaningfulness of the study results, the clinician examines the limits of the CI for the smallest plausible effect of the intervention and decides whether this effect is large enough to warrant change in practice.

Consider a hypothetical single-session RCT: the experimental treatment (thoracic mobilization, $n=22$) showed significantly better improvements ($P=.02$) in shoulder external rotation passive range of motion (PROM) in patients with primary shoulder impingement compared to a comparison treatment (trigger point release, $n=24$). Pretest to posttest measurements in the experimental group were 20 ± 11.2 degrees compared to 4.8 ± 7.4 degrees in the comparison group. The estimated difference between the mean group improvements (raw effect size) was 15.2 degrees favoring the treatment group. A 95% CI estimates the true population difference for mean improvement to be no less than 9.6 and no more than 20.8 degrees in favor of the treatment group. The 95% CI does not capture a zero difference representing a difference that is statistically significant when comparing continuous data and consistent with the reported value, $P=.02$. Because the smallest likely effect of a single-session intervention is 9.6 degrees, most clinicians would consider this increase in PROM a clinically meaningful change.

Another approach to assessing the size of an intervention's effect is to consider the relative size of the effects based on standardized estimates of effect size: (1) standardized mean difference measures, (2) correlation measures, and (3) odds ratios.[66,67] Using the standardized mean difference statistic, raw effect sizes are changed into unitless (numeric score) indices such as d for t-test and f for the analysis of variance method. The calculated effect size is a measure of the strength of the treatment effect[65] and may be positive or negative. For outcome measures such as the Roland-Morris Disability Scale where a lower value reflects a better outcome, the resultant calculated effect size is negative if the intervention group improves more than the control group.[67] If a higher value reflects a better outcome, the calculated effect size is positive.

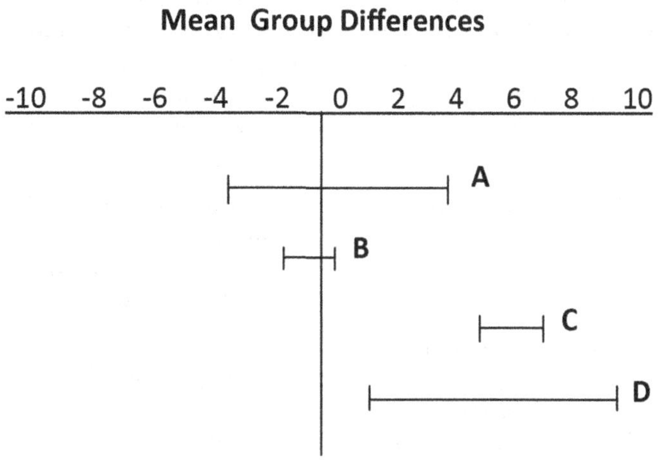

A: no significant difference (line crosses 0); small sample, wide width (less precise); upper limit is very positive, perhaps there is value to this intervention
B: no significant difference (line crosses 0); large sample size, narrow width (more precise)
C: statistically significant (line does not cross 0); large sample size, narrow width (more precise)
D: statistically significant (line does not cross 0); small sample, wide width (less precise); difficult decision because the true value may be close to 0 or very large

Figure 1-4. Interpretation of confidence intervals.

Cohen[65] described guidelines for interpretation of effect size outcomes as follows: (a) <0.20 trivial; (b) >0.20 to <0.50 small; (c) >0.50 to <0.80 medium; and (d) >0.80 large. These values relate to percentages of the control group that fall below the mean values of those in the experimental group.[67] Effect sizes of 0.9, 0.6, and 0.2 imply that 82%, 73%, and 58% of the control group, respectively, scored lower than the experimental group. The main limitation of standardized effect sizes is that they are less easily understood compared to raw effect sizes.[66]

CIs answer these 3 questions:

1. Is the difference between groups significant (ie, does not capture 0 for continuous data or 1 for dichotomous data)?
2. What is the precision of the study finding—how wide is it?
3. What is the clinical significance of the study findings—where is the upper and lower limit?

Figure 1-4 is a diagram to aid in the interpretation of CIs. The ability to analyze the CI is an important aspect of critical appraisal. In addition to assisting clinicians in understanding whether a study finding is statistically significant or not, the effect size and CI help to interpret the clinical usefulness of the findings. The CI allows greater confidence in deciding whether to administer the treatment.

Minimal Detectable Change and Minimal Clinically Important Difference

The minimal detectable change (MDC) and minimal clinically important difference (MCID) values can be used by clinicians to assist in determining whether a patient has experienced a real and meaningful change. The MDC is the smallest real difference that represents the smallest change in score that likely reflects true change rather than measurement change alone. Noteboom et al[29] proposed that the MDC only reflects a minimum score change but not necessarily the change that the patient would consider clinically meaningful. Jaeschke et al[68] reported the MCID of a therapy as the smallest treatment effect that would result in a change in patient management, given its side effects, costs, and inconveniences. Because many factors influence a patient's perception of change, the magnitude of the MCID may vary depending on circumstances.

The MCID estimate for different scales can be used to make decisions about clinical importance for individual and group differences.[68] If the MCID is less than the lower limit of the 95% CI, the results are statistically significant and very likely to be clinically meaningful.[69] If the MCID value is greater than the upper limit of the 95% CI, the results of the study are very unlikely to be clinically important.[69] If the MCID is within the 95% CI, the clinical importance is uncertain.[69] Using the concept of raw effect size, if the observed raw effect size is equal to or greater than the MCID, the treatment effect is clinically meaningful.[29] If not, the treatment effect is regarded as trivial even if statistical significance is achieved.[29]

Using Confidence Intervals to Interpret a Positive Trial (Continuous Outcomes)

A positive trial means that the results are statistically significant (chance is an unlikely explanation), and the experimental treatment is deemed more effective than the comparison. As previously stated, this information is not enough to determine clinical meaningfulness. A decision requires a comparison of the raw effect size and its CI to the MCID to assess whether the result is strong, weak, definitive, or not.[70] According to Guyatt et al,[71] a positive definitive trial results when the 95% CI excludes the MCID. The following scenario provides 2 examples related to interpretation of a positive trial.

In this hypothetical result, low back pain, as measured on the 11-point Numeric Pain Rating Scale (NPRS), was reduced by a mean of (6.1 ± 1.2) in the treatment group (n = 78; lumbar mobilization and exercise) and 2.5 ± 1.8 in the comparison group (n = 75; soft tissue mobilization and exercise). The difference between groups was statistically significant (P = .012). The estimate of the mean effect of treatment or raw effect size is a 3.6 reduction in NPRS (6.1 – 2.5 = 3.6). A 95% CI estimates the true population difference for mean improvement to be no less than 3.11 and no more than 4.09 cm in favor of the treatment group. The 95% CI does not capture a zero difference representing a difference that is statistically significant when comparing continuous data and consistent with the reported value, P = .012. MCID for the NPRS is a 2-point change.[72]

To assess whether the result is strong, weak, definitive, or not, comparison of the raw effect size and its CI to the MCID revealed the following:

- The raw effect size (3.6) is greater than the MCID (2). Though the results are clinically meaningful, the true size of the treatment effect may be greater than or less than the point estimate from the sample data.
- The next consideration is whether the MCID is within the CI. An MCID of 2 is not within the 95% CI (3.11 to 4.09). The results are definitive and provide strong evidence for benefit of treatment.

In the same study above, if the sample size was reduced to experimental group (n = 6) and comparison group (n = 6), the raw effect was still 3.6, but the 95% CI estimated the true population difference for mean improvement in pain to be no less than 1.63 and no more than 5.57. The 95% CI does not capture a zero difference representing difference that is statistically significant. To assess whether the result is strong, weak, definitive, or not, comparison of the raw effect size and its CI to the MCID revealed the following:

- The raw effect size (3.6) is greater than the MCID (2). The results are clinically meaningful.
- Because the MCID of 2 is within the 95% CI, the clinical importance is less uncertain. Within the 95% CI, some treatment effects (reduction in pain scores) are below 2.0, which is smaller than the MCID and therefore not clinically meaningful.
- The results are still statistically significant, favoring the experimental group, but not definitive. The raw effect size (3.6) remains clinically meaningful. The lack of precision due to the small sample size suggests that additional trials with larger samples are needed.

Using Confidence Intervals to Interpret a Negative Trial (Continuous Outcomes)

A negative trial means that the results are not statistically significant, suggesting the experimental treatment is no more effective than the comparison. Guyatt et al[71] noted that to determine whether a negative trial is definitive, the clinician must consider whether the upper limit of the CI falls below the smallest difference that the patient might consider important (ie, the 95% CI excludes the MCID). If yes, the sample size is adequate to conclude that the trial is definitively negative with 95% confidence that the treatment has no clinically meaningful benefit. If, however, the upper limit, the largest plausible effect, exceeds the smallest difference important to the patient, then the trial is not definitive (ie, the MCID is within the 95% CI).[71] A conclusion that the treatment is ineffective is not accepted. The trial has not ruled out the possibility that in a larger sample the intervention may be beneficial. Once again, a decision requires a comparison of the raw effect size and its CI to the MCID to assess whether the result is strong, weak, definitive, or not.[71]

In this hypothetical trial no significant difference (P = .29) was found for the modified Oswestry Disability Questionnaire (ODQ) outcome measure between 2 groups of patients 6 weeks post-lumbar microdiscectomy. A treatment group (n = 60) received supervised exercise 45 minutes 3 times per week; a comparison treatment group (n = 62) received advice to remain active and walk for 45 minutes 3 times per week. The MCID for the modified ODQ is 6 points.[73] At 6-week follow-up, the average ODQ for the supervised exercise group (22.1 ± 5.3) was not significantly different from the advice and walk group (21.2 ± 5.2). The difference between the means was 0.9 (95% CI: –2.78 to 0.98).

- The 95% CI (–2.78 to 0.98) captures a zero difference, indicating nonsignificant results.
- The 95% CI excludes the ODQ MCID of 6. The trial is definitively negative. The experimental treatment is no more effective than the comparison.

Considering a variation in the last hypothetical study in which the sample size is reduced to n = 5 in the experimental group and n = 5 in the comparison group, the difference between the means is 0.9 (95% CI: -8.56 to 6.76).

- The 95% CI (–8.56 to 6.76) captures a zero difference, indicating nonsignificant results.
- The MCID (6) is within the 95% CI. The upper limit (6.76), the largest plausible effect, exceeds the smallest difference important to the patient (MCID = 6) and the trial is not definitive. A conclusion that the experimental treatment is no more effective that the comparison is not accepted. The trial has not ruled out the possibility that in a larger sample the experimental intervention may be beneficial. A larger study is needed.

Results for Dichotomous Outcomes

Dichotomous outcomes are discrete events that either happen or do not (ie, undergo surgery or not, recurrent dislocation or not).[74] These outcomes are quantified in terms of the proportion of subjects who experience the event of interest within a specified time period, also known as the risk of the event for those patients.[74] In a hypothetical trial on the effects of 6 weeks of postsurgical rehabilitation, if 42 out of 175 subjects in the control group experienced a second surgery after lumbar discectomy, the risk of a second surgery is 23% (42/175). In clinical trials with dichotomous outcomes, the interest is whether the treatment reduces the risk of the event of interest (ie, Do the risks differ between treatment and control groups?).[74] The size of the risk reduction provides a measure of treatment effectiveness. Three commonly used measures of effect size for dichotomous outcomes are absolute risk reduction (ARR), relative risk reduction (RRR), and the number needed to treat (NNT) to prevent one bad outcome.

ARR states the difference in risk between treatment and control groups. In the hypothetical example of lumbar discectomy, 10/175 (6%) in the treatment group (postsurgical rehabilitation) versus 42/175 (23%) in the control group (no rehabilitation) experienced a second surgery. The ARR is 0.23 – 0.06 = 0.17 or 17%, which means that the rehabilitation group was at a 17% lower risk than the no rehabilitation group of having a second surgery. Large ARRs show that the treatment is very effective and negative ARRs indicate that risk is greater in the treatment group than in the control group and is therefore a harmful treatment.[74]

RRR expresses the risk reduction as a proportion of risk of untreated patients. The RRR equals the ARR divided by the risk in the control group.[74] Thus, the RRR produced by the rehabilitation is 0.17/0.23 = 0.72 (72%). The rehabilitation reduced the risk of a second surgery by 72% of the risk of the untreated patients. In other words, the risk of a second surgery in the no rehabilitation group (23%) can be reduced by 17% in absolute terms and by 75% in relative terms by providing rehabilitation to the patients in the no rehabilitation group.

The NNT is the inverse of the ARR.[74] In the hypothetical example above, the NNT or number of patients who would need to be treated on average to prevent one additional surgery is 1/0.17 or approximately 6 patients. A small NNT (such as 6) is better than a large NNT (such as 75) because it means that only a small number of people need to be treated before the treatment makes a difference to one of them.[74] The NNT is useful as a measure of the smallest clinically meaningful effect. In the example above, an NNT of 6 is meaningful because preventing a second surgery by the use of rehabilitation is a simple, low-risk, cost-effective treatment. Conversely, an NNT of 75 would be too costly to ineffectively treat 75 people for 6 weeks just to prevent one additional surgery. NNT is a concise, clinically useful presentation of the effect of an intervention. CIs for the AAR and NNT can be used in the same manner as described above for continuous outcomes.

EBPT practice requires each clinician to develop the skills to critically appraise clinical research. These skills allow the clinician to make self-directed professional decisions about the validity, strength, and relevance to individual patients. Clinical trials provide only an estimate of the most probable effects of treatment. When applying the findings to a specific patient, clinical expertise and patient preferences determine whether the results apply and how more or less likely the patient is to respond.[4]

Will the Results Help Me in Caring for My Patients?

Sackett et al[1] proceeded by asking 4 questions when determining whether valid, important results are applicable to the management of a specific patient.

Is the Patient so Different From Those in the Study That Its Results Cannot Apply?

If a patient is reasonably similar to those in the study, a clinician should be able to integrate the evidence with considerable confidence.[29] Clinicians should compare the patient characteristics to the inclusion and exclusion criteria to determine how likely the patient is to respond to the treatment. When these demographic, social, or pathological variables are so different from those in the study, the results may be discarded in favor of an alternative.[1] Clinical reasoning and expertise are essential to establish whether the valid evidence applies to a patient or does not apply to a patient or to make a decision in situations where evidence is limited or inconclusive.

Is the Intervention Feasible in This Practice Setting?

A determination must be made as to whether the intervention is cost-effective, whether or not the patient or health care system can afford it, and whether special services or equipment are needed.[1,29] Costs most obviously include monetary costs to the patient, health provider, or state, as well as the inconvenience, discomfort, and side effects of the intervention. If a treatment is to be clinically worthwhile, its positive effects must exceed its costs so that it does more good than harm. Thus, the evaluation of whether a treatment provides a clinically important effect usually requires a comparison of objective information about the benefits of treatment or alternatives provided by clinical trials against subjective thoughts of the costs and risks of treatment generated by therapists and patients.[1]

What Are the Patient's Potential Benefits and Harms From the Intervention?

When the study is applicable to the patient and the intervention is feasible, the clinician estimates what would happen to the patient if not treated.[1] As previously discussed, the NNT estimates the number of patients on average who must receive an intervention within a certain time frame to prevent one poor outcome or get one desired outcome.[75] Childs et al[76] provided an example of this estimate from the physical therapy research. The authors investigated whether patients who do not receive manipulation for their low back pain are at an increased risk for worsening disability compared to patients receiving an exercise intervention alone. The results were that patients who completed the exercise only intervention were 8 times (95% CI: 1.1, 63.5) more likely to experience a worsening in disability than patients who received manipulation.[76] The NNT with manipulation to prevent one additional patient from a worsening in disability was 9.9 (95% CI: 4.9, 65.3).

What Are the Patient's Values and Expectations for Both the Outcomes We Are Trying to Prevent and the Intervention That Is Offered?

A goal of every clinical encounter is to provide the best quality care and maximize positive patient outcomes. Therefore, outcomes measured in the clinical trial should be compatible with the patient's goals. The patient should be informed of the likelihood that the treatment will help versus harm and should be given time to value potential positive outcomes as well as the severity of potential negative outcomes. In this manner, the patient may establish a preference for either accepting or passing on the treatment. If the patient accepts, the selected intervention begins and the effects are measured. As an example, a critical appraisal sheet for randomized clinical trials related to intervention is shown in Table 1-6.[28]

A Case Study in Intervention Using the Critical Appraisal Criteria

The following is an example of an RCT intervention study worksheet:

1. **Focused clinical question**: In a 65-year-old female with a diagnosis of lumbar spinal stenosis, is manual therapy and exercise more effective than exercise alone in improving function and decreasing pain?
2. **Selected search article**: Whitman JM, Flynn TW, Childs JD, et al. A comparison between two physical therapy treatment programs for patients with lumbar spinal stenosis. *Spine.* 2006;31(22):2541-2549. Fifty-eight patients were randomized to one of two 6-week physical therapy programs: manual physical therapy exercise (MPTE), body weight-supported treadmill walking, and exercise (MPTE × walking group [WG]) or flexion exercises (FE), a treadmill walking program, and subtherapeutic ultrasound (FE × WG). Primary outcome was the Global Rating of Change (GRC) Scale. Secondary outcomes were Oswestry, a numerical pain scale, a measure of satisfaction, and a treadmill test. Testing occurred at baseline, 6 weeks, and 1 year.
3. Are the results valid?
   a. Was the assignment of patients to treatments randomized? Yes. Computer-generated randomization was prepared in blocks of 20 patients.
   b. Were the groups similar at the start of the trial? Yes. No significant baseline differences were identified for demographics, baseline physical impairment, or outcomes.
   c. Aside from the allocated treatment, were the groups treated equally? Yes. Subjects were allowed to continue previously prescribed medications but advised not to change the dosage of these medications in the 6 weeks before the baseline testing through the end of treatment period. Cointerventions were recorded at follow-ups.
   d. Were all patients who entered the trial accounted for and were they analyzed in the groups to which they were randomized? Yes. All subjects who met the inclusion/exclusion criteria were included in all analyses, regardless of their dropout status or completion of treadmill testing per intention-to-treat analysis by carrying the last available value forward. Losses to follow-up were accounted for at <20%.

Table 1-6. A Critical Appraisal Sheet for Randomized Clinical Trials Related to Intervention

Are the Results of the Trial Valid (Internal Validity)? What Question Did the Study Ask?

1A. R: Was the assignment of patients to treatments randomized?	
What Is Best?	*Where Do I Find the Information?*
Centralized computer randomization is ideal and often used in multicenter trials. Smaller trials may use an independent person (eg, the hospital pharmacy) to "police" the randomization.	The Methods section should tell you how patients were allocated to groups and whether randomization was concealed.
This paper: Yes ☐ No ☐ Unclear ☐ Comment:	

1B. R: Were the groups similar at the start of the trial?	
What Is Best?	*Where Do I Find the Information?*
If the randomization process worked (that is, achieved comparable groups) the groups should be similar. The more similar the groups, the better it is. There should be some indication of whether differences between groups are statistically significant (ie, P values).	The Results section should have a table of "baseline characteristics" comparing the randomized groups on a number of variables that could affect the outcome (ie, age, risk factors, etc). If not, there may be a description of group similarity in the first paragraphs of the Results section.
This paper: Yes ☐ No ☐ Unclear ☐ Comment:	

2A. A: Aside from the allocated treatment, were groups treated equally?	
What Is Best?	*Where Do I Find the Information?*
Apart from the intervention, the patients in the different groups should be treated the same (eg, additional treatments or tests).	Look in the Methods section for the follow-up schedule, permitted additional treatments, etc, and in the Results section for actual use.
This paper: Yes ☐ No ☐ Unclear ☐ Comment:	

2B. A: Were all patients who entered the trial accounted for? Were they analyzed in the groups to which they were randomized?	
What Is Best?	*Where Do I Find the Information?*
Losses to follow-up should be minimal—preferably less than 20%. However, if few patients have the outcome of interest, then even small losses to follow-up can bias the results. Patients should also be analyzed in the groups to which they were randomized—intention-to-treat analysis.	The Results section should say how many patients were randomized (eg, baseline characteristics table) and how many patients were actually included in the analysis. You will need to read the Results section to clarify the number and reason for losses to follow-up.
This paper: Yes ☐ No ☐ Unclear ☐ Comment:	

(continued)

TABLE 1-6 (CONTINUED). A CRITICAL APPRAISAL SHEET FOR RANDOMIZED CLINICAL TRIALS RELATED TO INTERVENTION

3. M: WERE MEASURES OBJECTIVE OR WERE THE PATIENTS AND CLINICIANS KEPT "BLIND" TO WHICH TREATMENT WAS BEING RECEIVED?	
WHAT IS BEST?	*WHERE DO I FIND THE INFORMATION?*
It is ideal if the study is double-blinded—that is, both patients and investigators are unaware of treatment allocation. If the outcome is objective (eg, death), then blinding is less critical. If the outcome is subjective (eg, symptoms or function), then blinding of the outcome assessor is critical.	First, look in the Methods section to see if there is some mention of masking treatments (eg, placebos with the same appearance or sham therapy). Second, the Methods section should describe how the outcome was assessed and whether the assessor(s) were aware of the patients' treatment.
This paper: Yes ☐ No ☐ Unclear ☐ Comment:	

What Were the Results?

1. HOW LARGE WAS THE TREATMENT EFFECT?	
Most often, results are presented as dichotomous outcomes (yes or no outcomes that do or do not happen) and can include such outcomes as cancer recurrence, myocardial infarction, and death. Consider a study in which 15% (0.15) of the control group died and 10% (0.10) of the treatment group died after 2 years of treatment. The results can be expressed in many ways, as shown below.	
WHAT IS THE MEASURE?	*WHAT DOES IT MEAN?*
Relative risk (RR) = Risk of the outcome in the treatment group/Risk of the outcome in the control group. In our example, the RR = 0.10/0.15 = 0.67	The RR tells us how many times more likely it is that an event will occur in the treatment group relative to the control group. An RR of 1 means that there is no difference between the 2 groups; thus, the treatment had no effect. An RR < 1 means that the treatment decreases the risk of the outcome. An RR > 1 means that the treatment increased the risk of the outcome. Since the RR < 1, the treatment decreases the risk of death.
ARR = Risk of the outcome in the control group − Risk of the outcome in the treatment group. This is also known as the *absolute risk difference.* In our example, the ARR = 0.15 − 0.10 = 0.05 or 5%	The ARR tells us the absolute difference in the rates of events between the 2 groups and gives an indication of the baseline risk and treatment effect. An ARR of 0 means that there is no difference between the 2 groups; thus, the treatment had no effect. The absolute benefit of treatment is a 5% reduction in the death rate.
RRR = AAR/Risk of the outcome in the control group. An alternative way to calculate the RRR is to subtract the RR from 1 (eg, RRR = 1 − RR) In our example, the RRR = 0.05/0.15 = 0.33 or 33% Or RRR = 1 − 0.67 = 0.33 or 33%	The RRR is the complement of the RR and is probably the most commonly reported measure of treatment effects. It tells us the reduction in the rate of the outcome in the treatment group relative to that in the control group. The treatment reduced the risk of death by 33% relative to that occurring in the control group.

(continued)

TABLE 1-6 (CONTINUED). A CRITICAL APPRAISAL SHEET FOR RANDOMIZED CLINICAL TRIALS RELATED TO INTERVENTION

WHAT IS THE MEASURE?	*WHAT DOES IT MEAN?*
NNT = Inverse of the ARR and is calculated as 1/ARR.	The NNT represents the number of patients we need to treat with the experimental therapy in order to prevent 1 bad outcome, and it incorporates the duration of treatment. Clinical significance can be determined to some extent by looking at the NNTs and by weighing the NNTs against any harms or adverse effects (numbers needed to harm) of therapy.
In our example, the NNT = 1/ 0.05 = 20	We would need to treat 20 people for 2 years in order to prevent 1 death.

2. HOW PRECISE WAS THE ESTIMATE OF THE TREATMENT EFFECT?

The true risk of the outcome in the population is not known; the best we can do is estimate the true risk based on the sample of patients in the trial. This estimate is called the *point estimate*. We can gauge how close this estimate is to the true value by looking at the CIs for each estimate. If the CI is fairly narrow, then we can be confident that our point estimate is a precise reflection of the population value. The CI also provides us with information about the statistical significance of the result. If the value corresponding to no effect falls outside of the 95% CI, then the result is statistically significant at the 0.05 level. If the CI includes the value corresponding to no effect, then the results are not statistically significant.

Will the Results Help Me in Caring for My Patient (External Validity/Applicability)?

The questions that you should ask before you decide to apply the results of the study to your patient are as follows:

- Is my patient so different from those in the study that the results cannot apply?
- Is the treatment feasible in my setting?
- Will the potential benefits of treatment outweigh the potential harms of treatment for my patient?

Reprinted with permission from Centre for Evidence-Based Medicine. Levels of Evidence (March 2009). *University of Oxford*. http://www.cebm.net/index.aspx?o=1157. Updated April 3, 2013. Accessed June 27, 2011.

e. Were measures objective? Were the patients and clinicians "blind" to which treatment was being received? Subjects and therapists were not blinded. Research assistants collected the outcomes measures and were blinded to group allocation.

4. What are the results?

a. What is the size of the treatment effect? How precise is the estimate of the treatment effect? Both nonsurgical physical therapy programs resulted in clinically important improvements at 6 weeks and 1 year. A dichotomized score of a difference of 30% or more in perceived recovery was considered to be clinically important. However, at 6 weeks, there was a significant association between MPTE × WG and perceived recovery (P = .0015); 79% MPTE × WG versus 41% FE × WG met perceived recovery threshold; 62% versus 41% at 1 year; and 38% versus 21% at long-term follow-up. Although the 1-year and long-term follow-ups were not significant, the NNT for benefit for perceived recovery was 2.6 (CI: 1.8 to 7.8) at 6 weeks, 4.8 (CI: –2.3 to 21.3) at 1 year, and 4.4 (CI: –2.1 to 22.7) at long-term follow-up. All of the secondary outcomes favored the MPTE × WG at 6 weeks and 1 year except improvement in NPRS for lower extremity symptoms, but the differences were not significant.

b. The NNT for benefit with the MPTE × WG was 2.6 at 6 weeks, meaning that about 3 patients need to be treated with the MPTE × WG program before the treatment makes a difference to one of them or to prevent 1 patient from not achieving perceived recovery on the GRC Scale. The authors did not report the ARR (38%) and RRR (65%) for the GRC outcome, but they can be calculated from the reported data.

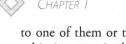

c. Seventeen of 29 (59%) patients in the FE × WG group failed to improve compared to 6 of 29 (21%) in the MPTE × WG group. Although the likelihood of not improving in the FE × WG group is high (59%), the risk of failure can be reduced by 38% (95% CI: 15% to 61%) in absolute terms (ARR) and by 65% (95% CI: 25% to 100%) in relative terms (RRR). Risk reduction is considered a positive outcome. In this scenario, the risk of failure in the comparison group (58%) can be reduced by 38% in absolute terms and by 65% in relative terms by providing manual therapy and exercise to patients in the FE × WG.

5. Will the results help me in caring for my patients?
   a. Is my patient so different to those in the study that the results cannot apply? No. The patient is similar based on inclusion/exclusion criteria.
   b. Is the treatment feasible in my setting? Yes. Both nonsurgical treatment programs are feasible in this setting except for the body weight-supported treadmill.
   c. Will the potential benefits of treatment outweigh the potential harms of treatment for my patient? Yes. Manual therapy and exercise for 12 sessions over 6 weeks may be a lower risk option for a patient with lumbar spinal stenosis when compared to the morbidity and mortality rates associated with surgical intervention for this population.

Critical Appraisal of Literature Related to Outcomes and Prognosis

RCTs are considered the best study design for providing evidence related to effectiveness of intervention. However, outcomes are also measured in real-world settings rather than experimental settings through cohort studies.[77] Cohort studies evaluate large groups of diverse individuals over a long period of time to gather information on outcomes. Like RCTs, they compare outcomes in groups that did and did not receive an intervention. Unlike RCTs, the assignment of subjects to groups is not by chance, leaving cohort studies vulnerable to selection bias, which is a threat to internal validity. In cohort studies, patients either choose a treatment or are preferentially assigned to receive a treatment. Baseline differences between groups may confound the assessment as to whether the treatment effect can be attributed to the intervention or other factors.[77]

During the critical appraisal of a cohort study, all potential confounding variables should be identified and their distribution between groups compared. Standardized differences or effect sizes can be used to show the relative magnitude of each confounder and the potential for bias.[78] Two statistical strategies—regression and stratification—are commonly used to assess and reduce confounding variables. Regression estimates how the confounding variables are related to the outcome, providing an adjusted estimate of the intervention effect.[79] Stratification divides the sample into similar subgroups and measures the effects of the intervention within each subgroup.[79] A series of articles provides a detailed review of the critical appraisal of cohort studies.[77-79]

Translating Research Into Practice

The process of making EBPT a reality in practice encounters many obstacles: (a) poor access; (b) not enough time; (c) not enough research; (d) not enough good research; and (e) lack of skills for critical appraisal.[4,80] However, all of these issues can be overcome with commitment to integrate patient-oriented research into daily practice. Four simple steps will help to close the gap between what is known and what is actually practiced: (a) seek to answer clinical questions through emerging research; (b) accept and adopt new CPGs; (c) apply research as appropriate by communicating well with patients and colleagues; and (d) assess performance using standardized outcomes.[4] Herbert et al[4(p211)] concluded that "evidence-based practice is imperfect, but necessary...in the sense that it is likely to produce the best outcomes with available resources."

Summary

EBPT follows a 5-step process: (1) ask a clinical question; (2) find the best research to answer the question; (3) critically appraise the evidence; (4) implement into clinical practice; and (5) assess your performance.[1] EBPT practice requires each clinician to develop the skills to critically appraise clinical research. These skills allow the clinician to make self-directed professional decisions about validity, strength, and relevance to individual patients. Clinical trials provide only an estimate of the most probable effects of treatment. When applying the findings to a specific patient, clinical expertise and patient preferences determine whether the results apply and how more or less likely the patient is to respond.[74]

The systematic approach to appraising the evidence related to diagnosis is an important step in practicing EBPT because a definitive diagnosis leads to an appropriate intervention. Valid studies of diagnostic tests should include a blind comparison of the test, a valid reference standard, and application to a spectrum of patients, as well as a detailed description of the test. If these criteria are met, the study may provide an unbiased estimate of the accuracy of the test. Given that the results are valid, relevant to the patient, and have sufficient significant clinical accuracy, the final step is applying the test to the patient. If a patient meets the inclusion criteria and the practice setting is similar to the study, a clinician may apply the results with confidence. If not, clinical judgment is needed. The test must be performed in a competent, reproducible manner. In order to minimize error, clinicians should perform and interpret the test exactly as the study describes. Clinicians use diagnostic tests to lower the probability of the target condition below the testing threshold (ie, stop testing for it and eliminate it from further consideration) or to increase this probability above the treatment threshold (ie, stop testing for it and initiate appropriate therapy).

When the treatment threshold is reached and the examination stops, the clinician must determine the best intervention to optimize patient outcomes. Valid clinical trials of intervention should randomly assign subjects to experimental and control groups, blind data collectors, and others if possible; account for all dropouts; and treat subjects equally except for the treatment itself. Evidence of a statistically significant treatment effect is not enough information to make a decision about treatment. Statistical significance does not necessarily mean clinically important; the size of the effect determines the importance or usefulness. The treatment effect or measured outcomes must be meaningful and large enough to make the therapy advisable, and the beneficial effects should outweigh any harmful effects.

EBPT provides a systematic framework, consisting of the current best scientific evidence, clinical experience, and patient preferences. From this platform, clinicians, instructors, and researchers seek to reach informed decisions that balance the best available research with what is most important to the patient.

References

1. Sackett DL, Straus SE, Richardson WS, Rosenberg W, Haynes RB. *Evidence-Based Medicine: How to Practice and Teach EBM.* 2nd ed. London, England: Harcourt Publishers Ltd; 2000.
2. America Physical Therapy Association. Vision 2020. http://www.apta.org/Vision2020. Updated September 18, 2012. Accessed April 20, 2009.
3. Schreiber J, Stern P. A review of the literature on evidence-based practice in physical therapy. *Internet J Allied Health Sci Pract.* 2005;3(4):1-10.
4. Herbert R, Sherrington C, Masher C, Moseley A. Evidence-based practice: imperfect but necessary. *Physiother Theor Pract.* 2001;17:201-211.
5. Cormack JC. Evidence-based practice...what is it and how do I do it? *J Orthop Sports Phys Ther.* 2002;2:484-487.
6. Johnson C. Evidence-based practice in 5 simple steps. *J Manipulative Physiol Ther.* 2008;31:169-170.
7. Guyatt G, Rennie D, eds. *User's Guide to the Medical Literature: Essentials of Evidence-Based Practice.* Chicago, IL: American Medical Association; 2002.
8. Richardson WS, Wilson MC, Nishikawa J, Hayward RS. The well-built clinical questions: a key to evidence-based decisions. *ACP J Club.* 1995;123:A12-A13.
9. Schwartz JS. Evaluating diagnostic tests: what is done—what needs to be done. *J Gen Intern Med.* 1986;1:266-267.
10. Stratford PW. Applying the results from diagnostic accuracy studies to enhance clinical decision-making. *Physiother Theor Pract.* 2001;17:153-160.
11. National Center for Biotechnology Information. PubMed. http://www.ncbi.nlm.nih.gov/pubmed. Accessed February 3, 2009.
12. EBSCO Publishing. Cumulative Index of Nursing and Allied Health Literature. http://www.ebscohost.com/cinahl. Accessed February 3, 2009.
13. The Cochrane Collaboration. http://www.cochrane.org. Accessed February 3, 2009.
14. Centre for Evidence-Based Physiotherapy. PEDro. http://www.pedro.org.au. Updated May 6, 2013. Accessed February 3, 2009.
15. American Physical Therapy Association. Hooked on Evidence. http://www.hookedonevidence.com. Accessed February 3, 2009.
16. US National Library of Medicine. PubMed Clinical Queries. http://www.ncbi.nlm.nih.gov/pubmed/clinical. Accessed May 26, 2013.
17. Cleland JA, Noteboom JT, Whitman MJ, Allison SC. A primer on selected aspects of evidence-based practice relating to questions of treatment, part 1: asking questions, finding evidence, and determining validity. *J Orthop Sports Phys Ther.* 2008;38:476-484.
18. Walker-Dilks C. Searching the physiotherapy evidence-based literature. *Physiother Theor Pract.* 2001;17:137-142.
19. The Cochrane Collaboration. Cochrane Reviews. http://www.cochrane.org/cochrane-reviews. Accessed May 26, 2013.
20. Maher CG, Sherrington C, Elkins M, Herbert RD, Moseley AM. Challenges for evidence-based physical therapy: accessing and interpreting high-quality evidence on therapy. *Phys Ther.* 2004;84:644-654.
21. Maher CG, Moseley AM, Sherringnon C, Elkins MR, Herbert RD. A description of the trials, reviews and practice guidelines indexed in the PEDro database. *Phys Ther.* 2008;88:1068-1077.
22. Maher C, Sherrington C, Herbert R, Moseley A, Elkins M. Reliability of the PEDro scale for rating quality of randomized controlled trials. *Phys Ther.* 2003;83:713-721.
23. Foley NC, Bhogal SK, Teasell RW, Bureal Y, Speechley MR. Estimates of quality and reliability with the physiotherapy evidence-based database scale to assess the methodology of randomized controlled trials of pharmacological and non-pharmacological interventions. *Phys Ther.* 2006;86:817-824.
24. Macedo LG, Elkins MR, Maher CG, Mosely AM, Herbert RD, Sherrington C. There was evidence of convergent and construct validity of Physiotherapy Evidence Database quality scale for physiotherapy trials. *J Clin Epidemiol.* 2010;63:920-925.
25. The University of Kansas Medical Center. SUMSearch2. http://www.sumsearch.org. Accessed May 26, 2013.
26. McMaster University. Health Sciences Library. http://hsl.mcmaster.ca. Accessed April 20, 2009.

27. MacDermid JC. An introduction to evidence-based practice for hand therapists. *J Hand Ther.* 2004;17:105-117.
28. Centre for Evidence-Based Medicine. *University of Oxford.* http://www.cebm.net/index.aspx?o=1000. Accessed June 27, 2011.
29. Noteboom JT, Allison SC, Cleland JA, Whitman JM. A primer on selected aspects of evidence-based practice relating to questions of treatment, part 2: interpreting results, application to clinical practice, and self-evaluation. *J Orthop Sports Phys Ther.* 2008;38:485-501.
30. Robey RR. Levels of evidence. *The ASHA Leader.* http://www.asha.org/Publications/leader/2004/040413/f040413a2.htm. Published April 13, 2004. Accessed February 14, 2009.
31. Centre for Evidence-Based Medicine. OCEBM Levels of Evidence System. *University of Oxford.* http://www.cebm.net/index.aspx?o=5653. Updated April 30, 2013. Accessed June 29, 2011.
32. Cook DJ, Mulrow CD, Haynes RB. Systematic reviews: synthesis of best evidence for clinical decisions. *Ann Intern Med.* 1997;126:376-380.
33. Scalzitti DA. Evidence-based guidelines: application to clinical practice. *Phys Ther.* 2001;81:1622-1628.
34. Agency for Healthcare Research and Quality. National Guideline Clearinghouse. http://www.guideline.gov. Accessed February 14, 2009.
35. Childs JD, Cleland JA, Elliott JM, et al. Practice guidelines. Neck pain. *J Orthop Sports Phys Ther.* 2008;38(9):A1-A34.
36. Jones M, Grimmer K, Edwards I, Higg J, Trede F. Challenges in applying best evidence to physiotherapy practice: part 2—health and clinical reasoning models to facilitate evidence-based practice. *Internet J Allied Health Sci Pract.* 2006;4(4):1-9.
37. Sackett DL, Rosenberg MC, Gray JAM, Hans RB, Richardson WJ. EBM: what it is and what it isn't. *BMJ.* 1996;312:71-72.
38. Childs JD, Flynn TW, Fritz JM. A perspective for considering the risks and benefits of spinal manipulation in patient with low back pain. *Phys Ther.* 2006;11:316-320.
39. Jaeschke R, Guyatt G, Sackett DL. Users' guides to the medical literature. III. How to use an article about a diagnostic test. A. Are the results of the study valid? *JAMA.* 1994;271:389-391.
40. Fritz JM, Wainner RS. Examining diagnostic tests: an evidence-based perspective. *Phys Ther.* 2001;81:1546-1564.
41. Reid MC, Lachs MS, Feinstein AR. Use of methodological standards in diagnostic test research: getting better but still not good. *JAMA.* 1995;274:645-651.
42. Jaeschke R, Gordon H, Guyatt G, Sackett DL. Users' guides to the medical literature. III. How to use an article about a diagnostic test. B. What are the results and will they help me in caring for my patients? *JAMA.* 1994;271:703-707.
43. Cleland JA. *Orthopaedic Clinical Examination: An Evidence-Based Approach for Physical Therapists.* Carlstadt, NJ: Icon Learning Systems; 2005.
44. Fagan TJ. Nomogram for Bayes's theorem. *N Engl J Med.* 1975:293:257.
45. Bernstein J. Decision analysis. *J Bone Joint Surg Am.* 1997;79:1404-1414.
46. Bernstein J. Test indication curves. *Med Decis Making.* 1997;17:103-106.
47. Guyatt GH, Sackett DL, Cook DJ. Users' guides to the medical literature. II. How to use an article about therapy or prevention. B. What were the results and will they help me in caring for my patients? *JAMA.* 1994;271:59-63.
48. Wainner RS, Fritz JM, Irrgang JJ, et al. Reliability and diagnostic accuracy of the clinical examination and patient self-report measures for cervical radiculopathy. *Spine.* 2003;28:52-62.
49. Flynn T, Fritz J, Whitman J, et al. A clinical prediction rule for classifying patients with low back pain who demonstrate short-term improvement with spinal manipulation. *Spine.* 2002;27:2835-2843.
50. Fritz JM, Childs JD, Flynn TW. Pragmatic application of a clinical prediction rule in primary care to identify patients with low back pain with a good prognosis following a brief spinal manipulation intervention. *BMC Fam Pract.* 2005;6:29.
51. Tseng YL, Wang WTJ, Chen WY, Hou TJ, Chen TC, Lieu FK. Predictors for the immediate responders to cervical manipulation in patients with neck pain. *Man Ther.* 2006;11:306-315.
52. Cleland JA, Childs JD, Fritz JM, Whitman JM, Eberhart SL. Development of a clinical prediction rule for guiding treatment of a subgroup of patients with neck pain: use of thoracic spine manipulation, exercise, and patient education. *Phys Ther.* 2007;87:9-23.
53. Beattie P, Nelson R. Clinical prediction rules: what are they and what do they tell us? *Aust J Physiother.* 2006;52:157-163.
54. McGinn TG, Guyatt GH, Wyer PC, et al, for the Evidence-Based Medicine Working Group. Users' guides to the medical literature, XXII: how to use articles about clinical decision rules. *JAMA.* 2000;284:79-84.
55. Beneciuk JM, Bishop MD, George S. Clinical prediction rules for physical therapy interventions: a systematic review. *Phys Ther.* 2009;89:114-124.
56. Reilly BM, Evans AT. Translating clinical research into clinical practice: impact of using prediction rules to make decisions. *Ann Int Med.* 2006;144:201-210.
57. Schwartz A. Diagnostic test calculator. http://araw.mede.uic.edu/cgi-bin/testcalc.pl. Accessed March 30, 2009.
58. Ross JM, Sox HC. If at first you don't succeed: clinical problem-solving. *N Engl J Med.* 1995;333:1557-1560.
59. Montori VM, Kleinhart, J, Newman TB, et al, for the Evidence-Based Medicine Teaching Tips Working Group. Tips for learners of evidence-based medicine: 2. Measure of precision (confidence intervals). *CMAJ.* 2004;171:611-615.
60. Guyatt GH, Sackett DL, Cook DJ. Users' guides to the medical literature. II. How to use an article about therapy or prevention. A. Are the results of the study valid? *JAMA.* 1993;270:2598-2601.
61. Schultz KF, Chalmers I, Altman DG. The landscape and lexicon of blinding in randomized trials. *Ann Intern Med.* 2002;136:254-259.
62. Sim J, Reid N. Statistical Inference by confidence intervals: issues of interpretation and utilization. *Phys Ther.* 1999;79(2):186-195.
63. Portney LG, Watkins MP. *Foundations of Clinical Research: Applications to Practice.* Upper Saddle River, NJ: Prentice Hall Health; 2000.
64. Chan YH. Randomised controlled trials (RCTs)—sample size: the magic number? *Singapore Med J.* 2003;44(4):172-174.
65. Cohen L. *Statistical Power Analysis for the Behavioral Sciences.* 2nd ed. Hillsdale, NJ: Lawrence Erlbaum Associates; 1988.
66. Valentine JC, Cooper H. *Effect Size Substantive Interpretation Guidelines: Issues in the Interpretation of Effect Sizes.* Washington, DC: What Works Clearinghouse; 2003.
67. Cook C. Clinimetrics corner: use of effect sizes in describing data. *J Man Manip Ther.* 2008;16(3):129-135.
68. Jaeschke R, Singer J, Guyatt GH. Measurement of health status: ascertaining the minimal clinically important difference? *Control Clin Trials.* 1989;10:407-415.
69. Chan KBY, Man-Son-Hing M, Molnar F, Laupacis A. How well is the clinical importance of study results reported? An assessment of randomized controlled trials. *CMAJ.* 2001;165:1197-1202.

70. Guyatt G, Jaeschke R, Heddle N, Cook D, Shannon H, Walter S. Basic statistics for clinicians; interpreting study results: confidence intervals. *Can Med Assoc J.* 1995;152(2):169-173.
71. Guyatt G, Walter S, Cook D, Jaeschke R. Therapy and understanding the results: confidence intervals. In: Guyatt G, Rennie D, eds. *User's Guide to the Medical Literature: Essentials of Evidence-Based Practice.* Chicago, IL: American Medical Association; 2002:104-107.
72. Childs JD, Piva SR, Fritz JM. Responsiveness of the numerical pain rating scale in patients with low back pain. *Spine.* 2005;30:1331-1334.
73. Fritz JM, Irrgang JJ. A comparison of a modified Oswestry Low Back Pain Questionnaire and the Quebec Back Pain Disability Scale. *Phys Ther.* 2001;81:776-788.
74. Herbert RD. How to estimate treatment effects from reports of clinical trials. II: dichotomous outcomes. *Aust J Physiother.* 2000;46:309-313.
75. Dalton GW, Keating JL. Number needed to treat: a statistics relevant to physical therapists. *Phys Ther.* 2000;80:1214-1219.
76. Childs JD, Fritz JM, Flynn TW, et al. A clinical prediction rule to identify patients with low back pain most likely to benefit from spinal manipulation: a validation study. *Ann Intern Med.* 2004;141:920-928.
77. Rochon PA, Gurwitz JH, Sykora K, et al. Reader's guide to critical appraisal of cohort studies: 1. Role and design. *BMJ.* 2005;330:895-897.
78. Mamdani M, Sykora K, Li P, et al. Reader's guide to critical appraisal of cohort studies: 2. Assessing potential for confounding. *BMJ.* 2005;330:960-962.
79. Normand ST, Sykora K, Li P, Mamdani M, Rochon PA, Anderson GM. Readers guide to critical appraisal of cohort studies: 3. Analytical strategies to reduce confounding. *BMJ.* 2005;330:1021-1023.
80. Cook C. Trample the weak, hurdle the dead: the tribulations of integrating research into clinical practice. *J Man Manip Ther.* 2008;16(4):194-196.

Chapter 2

Subjective Examination
A Patient's History

The American Physical Therapy Association's *Guide to Physical Therapy Practice*[1] outlines 5 elements of patient management that guide the decision-making process to maximize patient health and quality of life. The 5 elements are listed in Table 2-1 and schematically drawn in Figure 2-1. The clinician obtains both subjective and objective data from the patient, evaluates the data, and makes judgments leading to a physical therapy diagnosis or classification. The diagnosis guides the choice of physical therapy intervention and helps formulate a prognosis. In contrast to a medical diagnosis based on anatomical and clinical pathology, a physical therapy diagnosis is based on key subjective and objective findings such as impairments and activity limitations.

Most diagnoses or diagnostic hypotheses emerge during the patient history, but others emerge during the physical examination.[2] Clinicians agree that 80% of the information needed to explain the cause of a patient's problem is extracted during the interview.[3] In primary care, Crombie[4] recognized that a brief history and physical examination established 88% of diagnoses. In a general medicine clinic, Sandler[5] reported that by the end of the history and physical examination, 56% and 73% of patients, respectively, received a correct diagnosis. A thorough history and skilled interpretation of examination findings should provide sufficient data to make a decision on the appropriateness of physical therapy intervention and/or referral to another medical provider. A logical and methodical approach demands attention to detail in all aspects of the examination and calls for a personal commitment to understanding and respecting the suffering of the patient.

The purpose of this chapter is to discuss the general components of the patient history. A systematic format, targeted to the individual patient, helps the clinician organize thoughts about the patient and assists in obtaining a complete and accurate database. Formal interview questions and the use of standardized questionnaires ensure that the clinician overlooks no content areas. The order and flow of questions varies from clinician to clinician, but a relevant, accurate exchange of information must take place between the patient and clinician. Components of the patient history specifically related to regional spinal pain are covered in later chapters.

Communication During the Patient Interview

Obtaining a detailed description of the patient's problem during the interview process depends on highly efficient and effective communication skills. Novice physical therapists tend to be more technical and procedurally oriented when communicating with patients. Clinical experts use a patient-centered approach; they listen intently, ensure understanding, and build on and respond to what the patient says.[6,7] Experience alone does not routinely result in superior performance; good communication and listening skills can be taught and learned.[8,9] Audiovisual recording of the examination process is highly recommended for self-assessment of communication skills. Interviewing is a highly refined skill that requires patience, focus, and the ability to be self-critical during the learning process.

Stetts DM, Carpenter JG. *Physical Therapy Management of Patients With Spinal Pain: An Evidence-Based Approach (pp 31-61).*

Table 2-1. Elements of the Patient Management Process

Examination: Process of obtaining the history, conducting a systems review, and performing tests and measurements to obtain data	
Evaluation: Process of making clinical judgments based on the data gathered from the history and tests and measures	
Diagnosis: Involves assigning a diagnostic classification, category, or syndrome based on clusters of signs and symptoms, which guides the treatment of the patient	
Prognosis: Process of making clinical judgments to determine the optimal level of attainable improvement and the time required to reach that level	
Intervention: Purposeful and skilled physical therapy intervention between the clinician and patient to produce changes in the condition consistent with the diagnosis and prognosis	

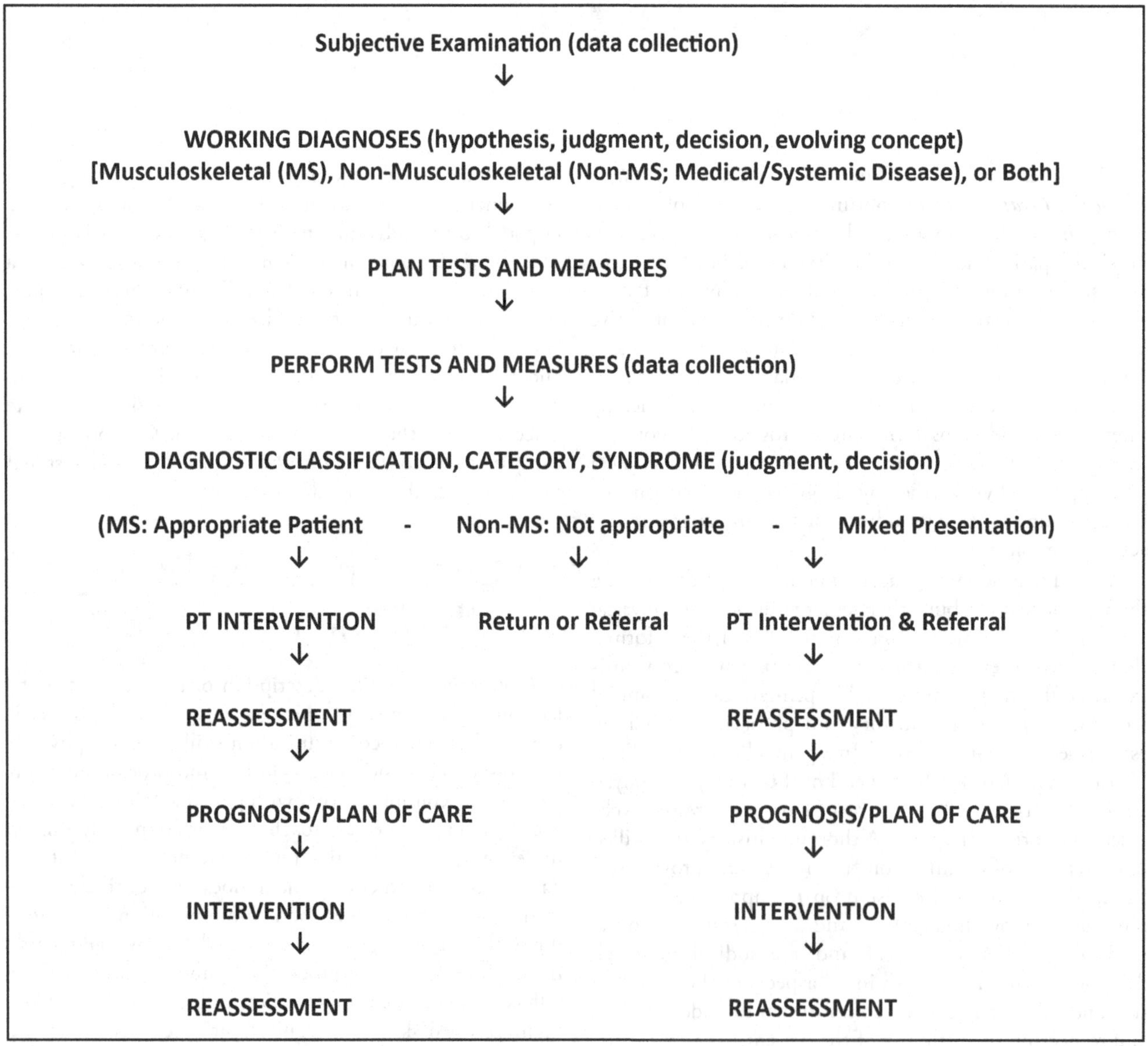

Figure 2-1. Neuromusculoskeletal examination and management process.

TABLE 2-2. OPEN-ENDED VERSUS CLOSED-ENDED QUESTIONS

OPEN-ENDED QUESTIONS	CLOSED-ENDED QUESTIONS
What makes your neck pain worse?	Does sitting make your neck pain worse?
How do you sleep at night?	Does your neck hurt at night?
What makes your neck pain better?	Does heat help your neck pain?
How would you describe the pain in your neck?	Is the pain a dull ache or sharp?
How did the exercise make you feel?	Did the exercise make your neck pain better?

The following simple interview techniques should be practiced:

- Speak slowly and deliberately.
- Keep questions short.
- Ask only one question at a time.
- Take notes while maintaining good eye contact.
- Give the patient time to answer.
- Provide nonverbal encouragement.
- Try not to interrupt.

Methods and styles of questioning vary from patient to patient because of common pitfalls associated with the transfer of information. Clinician interruptions, use of medical jargon, leading questions, illiteracy, cultural diversity, hearing impairments, and angry or depressed patients pose challenges to communication. When problems in communication occur, the clinician should ask questions in another way to help clarify or make it easier for the patient to find an answer. For example, the clinician might say, "I'm sorry I did not ask that question very well; what I meant to say was..." Basic interview strategies include open-ended (ie, allow more than a one-word response) and closed-ended (ie, allow yes or no responses) questions (Table 2-2). The interview typically begins with an open-ended question such as, "Please tell me what your problem is" versus "Do you have low back pain?" Opening in this manner allows the patient to present information that is most important and helps to establish effective patient-clinician rapport. The clinician then uses the open-ended patient response to present specific follow-up or closed-ended questions to clarify and obtain more precise and detailed information. If the clinician is unclear about a patient response, the clinician should restate the patient response or ask for an example to clarify. An open-ended approach initially avoids limiting yes or no answers, leading questions, or the possibility of omitting vital information.

Patient-centered interview skills result in improved patient outcomes,[10] improved efficiency,[11,12] increased patient and provider satisfaction,[13-17] and decreased malpractice claims.[18] During patient-centered communication, the clinician maintains control of the interview to ensure accurate and relevant information is obtained while carefully attending to personal and emotional concerns. Students and clinicians should continue to improve their communication skills and review detailed concepts of communication and the patient-centered interview process described in other references.[3,19-21]

Goals of the Subjective Examination

Obtaining accurate, relevant data from the patient history aids in differentiating between musculoskeletal (MS) and nonmusculoskeletal (non-MS) disorders, planning appropriate diagnostic tests, and implementing an effective intervention. Each question is regarded as a diagnostic test with a specific purpose that allows for early diagnostic hypothesis formation and differential diagnosis. The goals of the subjective examination as follows:

- Obtain patient demographics and answer the questions, "Who is the patient" and "What is the impact of the problem on the patient's life?"
- Make a preliminary decision as to whether the patient is appropriate for physical therapy intervention.
- Obtain a detailed description of all of the patient's symptoms and determine whether a link exists between the presenting symptoms.
- Determine the aggravating factors, easing factors, and the 24-hour behavior of each symptom.
- Determine contraindications or precautions to the examination and treatment process.
- Obtain a sequential history (present and past) of the patient's problem.
- Determine realistic patient expectations.
- Determine any barriers or facilitators of recovery.

- Develop a diagnostic hypothesis, classification, or pretest probability of the disorder.
- Evaluate the data from the patient history.
- Establish a baseline level of symptoms, activity limitations, and participation restrictions from which progress is measured.
- Establish a basis for planning the physical examination and selecting appropriate diagnostic tests (ie, determine what should be examined and in what detail).

Content Areas of the Patient History

Content areas for obtaining the patient history depend on the nature of the presenting disorder (eg, acute versus chronic, postsurgical versus nonsurgical, etc). Table 2-3 lists sample content for the patient history in an outpatient setting. Table 2-4 outlines sample content for the examination process in an inpatient setting. The general components of the patient history are discussed as follows for the outpatient setting as listed in Table 2-3. The organization of the patient history is varied across therapists and clinical settings, but a systematic approach is recommended.

Pre-Examination Questionnaires

Obtaining health history information during the initial visit in a timely manner is not an easy task. Patients often have extensive health histories with comorbidities, multiple surgical procedures, and substantial medication usage.[22,23] Accurate health history information is essential to establishing a diagnosis, identifying a patient problem that requires referral to another health care provider, and developing a safe and effective physical therapy intervention.[1,22] The self-administered health history questionnaire and standardized outcome measures provide evidence-based supplements to the patient interview.

Self-Administered Personal and Family Medical History Screening Questionnaire

The self-administered health history questionnaire is aligned with (1) more active and earlier patient participation in the interview; (2) more complete and thorough documentation in patient records; and (3) provider efficiency in data collection.[24-27] The patient usually completes the form prior to seeing the clinician. The clinician then reviews the form with the patient and clarifies all "yes" responses when ready to begin the review of systems inquiry. Boissonnault and Badke[28] concluded that a self-administered questionnaire can provide accurate information on illness, surgery, and medication use in an outpatient orthopedic setting. The mean percentage of agreement between the questionnaire data and the combined data from the patient interview and medical record across all items was 95.6% (range 57% to 100%) with a mean kappa of 0.69 (range 0.154 to 1.0). Open-ended and medication-related items on the questionnaire showed poor to fair agreement. Low false positive (1.84%) and low false negative (2.55%) findings suggest that patient self-report is an accurate tool to supplement the patient interview but should not be used as the only means to collect information.[28] Table 2-5 is an example of a medical screening questionnaire.[29]

Standardized Self-Report Outcome Measures

Standardized instruments measure various factors related to current level of function, activities, participation, and quality of life or health status. Reliable and valid outcome measures use closed-ended questions or specific procedures to provide a quantitative assessment of a patient's perceived activity limitations and participation in life restrictions.[30] The Oswestry Low Back Pain Disability Questionnaire and the Roland-Morris Disability Questionnaire are self-report measures used for patients with low back pain (LBP) to document baseline and functional status, which is then reassessed over time to determine whether clinically meaningful change has occurred. In addition to providing objective data related to meaningful change, outcome measures are used to identify patients at risk for poor outcomes,[31] assess clinician and clinic performance,[32] and ascertain the most effective interventions.[33,34]

Specific self-report outcome measures should possess the properties of reliability, validity, and responsiveness. Reliability describes the consistency with which a self-report instrument measures the variable of interest such as pain, health status, range of motion, function, or work status.[35] Reliability values close to 1 exhibit higher levels of consistency with values over 0.70 reported as acceptable.[36] If a reliable measure is used, any change that occurs over time is attributable to a real change in patient status. In clinical practice, the extent of reliability required for use of the outcome measure is often determined by the clinician.[37] Test-retest reliability describes the ability with which a self-report instrument measures similar scores over 2 separate test events given that the patient remains stable.[35]

Validity describes the extent to which the self-report instrument accurately quantifies what it intended to measure.[35] In addition to validity, functional self-report

TABLE 2-3. SAMPLE OUTLINE FOR THE SUBJECTIVE EXAMINATION IN AN OUTPATIENT SETTING

PRE-EXAMINATION QUESTIONNAIRES

Medical History Questionnaire; Self-Report Outcomes Measures

DEMOGRAPHIC PATIENT PROFILE (PP)

Age/gender/race, primary language, barriers to communication/learning

Occupation/work environment (What is your job? What is a typical day of activity at your job?)

Functional status/lifestyle (Regular exercise, hobbies, recreational activities?)

Psychosocial status (Family/social/behavioral/financial/cultural influences offering support or stress; health insurance, which influences treatment options; worker's compensation or litigation status)

Referring provider/diagnosis

CHIEF COMPLAINT

In your own words, please tell me what your main problem is

DESCRIPTION OF SYMPTOMS, ASSESSMENT OF PAIN AND OTHER SYMPTOMS, COMPLETE THE BODY CHART

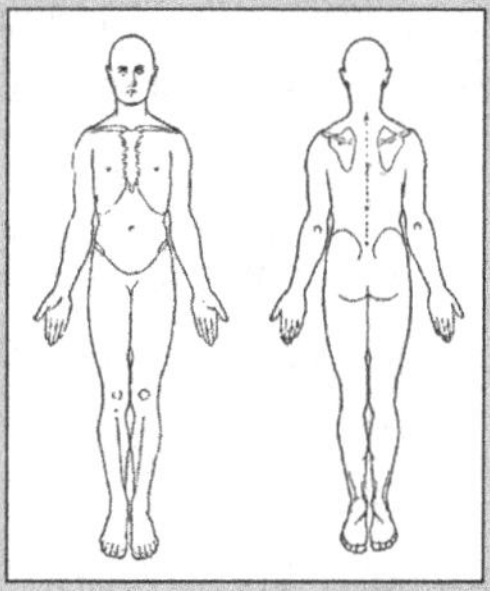

Location of symptoms (Show me exactly where you feel it)

Quality/type (What does it feel like?); Depth (superficial/deep)

Constant/intermittent/constant and variable

Multiple areas: establish relationship of symptoms

Other symptoms: numbness/tingling

Intensity (Numeric Pain Rating Scale or Visual Analogue Scale)

HISTORY (CURRENT EPISODE)

Mode and date of onset (traumatic versus nontraumatic) (How did this begin?)

Progression of symptoms (How have the symptoms changed since onset—location, severity?)

Treatments and effects (Have you had any treatment? What? And did it help?)

Compared to when this started, is it getting better, worse, or staying the same?

HISTORY (PREVIOUS EPISODE[S] OF SIMILAR PROBLEM)

Have you had this problem before? When/mechanism of Injury?

Previous treatment? Effects? Level of recovery?

SYMPTOM BEHAVIOR

Aggravating Factors: at least one aggravating factor for each symptom
What makes it worse? (Activity and amount, symptoms produced, time to settle)

Easing Factors
What makes it better? (Motion, position, medications, ice)

24-Hour Behavior
How does it feel at night? Do symptoms change during the day? What is it like when you first wake?

REVIEW OF MEDICAL SCREENING QUESTIONNAIRE

GENERAL HEALTH, SYSTEMS REVIEW, PAST MEDICAL/SURGICAL HISTORY, MEDICATION, IMAGING

PATIENT EXPECTATIONS AND GOAL

INTERVIEW SUMMARY

PLANNING THE EXAMINATION

Table 2-4. Sample Content for the Subjective Examination in an Inpatient Setting

CHART REVIEW

- Age, sex, date of admission (DOA)/date of surgery (DOS), medical diagnosis, physician, lab studies/special tests (RF, ESR, x-rays), secondary complications (cardiac, respiratory, etc), physician orders, meds, past medical history (diabetes, PVD), precautions (fluid restrictions, bed rest, weightbearing status, etc)

HISTORY

- Some information may be obtained from chart (may need to confirm with patient and family)
- Mental status, +/– marital status
- Home environment, family support systems, architectural barriers (stairs)
- Occupation, recreation, ADL (to assess work, play environments)
- Status prior to admission (ambulation, use of assistive devices, bed mobility, etc)
- Chief complaint
- Present history
- Brief aggravating/easing factors
- Activity level while in hospital (rolling in bed, sitting, etc)
- Patient goals/understanding of problem, precautions, discharge plan, etc

PHYSICAL EXAMINATION

- Communication: comprehension, speech
- Orientation (person, place, time), cooperative
- Observation: bed positioning, IVs, catheters, splints, etc
- Resting pain/symptoms
- CV endurance: heart rate, respiration/coughing, BP, O_2
- Functional/specific AROM, PROM
- Strength (gross/functional MMT)
- Palpation: erythema, swelling, warmth, pain, skin integrity, etc
- Sensation
- Functional assessment:
    - Mobility and assistance: self-care, rolling, supine to sit, sitting balance (dynamic and static), sit to stand, standing balance (dynamic and static), transfers, etc
    - Posture
    - Balance
    - Gait: assistive device, assistance, distance, surface level/stairs, deviations
    - Psychological status: depression/coping, attitude to rehab
    - Architectural barriers: work/home, assess need for change
    - Other: coordination, muscle tone, special tests, etc

DIAGNOSIS/ASSESSMENT/PLAN OF CARE

- Diagnosis
- Prognosis (risk factors, long-term goals/short-term goals)
- Impairments, functional limitation, disability as appropriate
- Plan of care—intervention
- Reassessment

RF indicates rheumatoid factor; ESR, erythrocyte sedimentation rate; ADL, activities of daily living; IV, intravenous; CV, cardiovascular; BP, blood pressure; AROM, active range of motion; PROM, passive range of motion; MMT, manual muscle test.

TABLE 2-5. MEDICAL SCREENING QUESTIONNAIRE

Instructions. Please answer the following questions.

NAME: ______________________________

OCCUPATION: ______________________________

LEISURE ACTIVITIES: ______________________________

Please check (✓) the medical providers who are currently providing you care:

_ Medical Doctor	_ Chiropractor	_ Osteopath
_ Dentist	_ Occupational Therapist	_ Pain Specialist
_ Orthopedic Surgeon	_ Psychiatrist/Psychologist	_ Physical Therapist
_ Other ______________		

If you have seen any of the above providers within the last 4 months, please describe the reason (surgery, medical illness, medication, tests):

____

____

Have you ever been diagnosed with any of the following disorders or problems?

YES NO Cancer. If yes, what kind: ______________

YES NO Heart problems	YES NO Stroke
YES NO High blood pressure	YES NO Asthma
YES NO Circulation problems	YES NO Anemia
YES NO Emphysema/bronchitis	YES NO Diabetes
YES NO Hepatitis	YES NO Epilepsy
YES NO Thyroid problems	YES NO Depression
YES NO Kidney disease	YES NO Headaches
YES NO Rheumatoid arthritis	YES NO Tuberculosis
YES NO Multiple sclerosis	YES NO Bowel/bladder
YES NO Osteoarthritis	YES NO Stomach
YES NO Chemical dependency (eg, alcohol)	

Has anyone in your immediate family (brother, sister, parent) ever been treated for any of the following?

YES NO Cancer	YES NO Arthritis
YES NO Diabetes	YES NO Stroke
YES NO Heart disease	YES NO Headaches
YES NO High blood pressure	YES NO Epilepsy
YES NO Kidney disease	YES NO Mental Illness
YES NO Tuberculosis	YES NO Chemical dependency (alcohol)

During the past month have you been:

1. Feeling down, depressed, or hopeless? YES NO
2. Bothered by having little interest or pleasure in doing things? YES NO
3. If yes, is this something you would like help with? NO YES YES, BUT NOT TODAY

Do you ever feel unsafe at home or has anyone hit you or tried to injure you in any way? YES NO

FOR WOMEN: Are you currently pregnant or do you think you might be pregnant? YES NO

(continued)

Table 2-5 (continued). Medical Screening Questionnaire

DATE REASON FOR SURGERY OR HOSPITALIZATION

_______ ____

_______ ____

_______ ____

DATE SIGNIFICANT INJURY (fracture, dislocation)

_______ ____

_______ ____

Which of the following OVER-THE-COUNTER medications do you take?

YES NO Aspirin	YES NO Decongestants
YES NO Tylenol	YES NO Antihistamines
YES NO Advil/Motrin	YES NO Vitamins/minerals
YES NO Laxatives	YES NO Antacid
YES NO Other ________________	

List Medications (pills, injections, patches)

________________________ ________________________

________________________ ________________________

________________________ ________________________

How many caffeinated coffee/beverages per day? _None _1-4 _5-8 _>8

Packs of cigarettes per day? _None _<½ _1 _2 _>2

Days per week you drink alcohol? __________

How many drinks at an average sitting? ______

Have you recently noticed any of the following?

YES NO Fever, chills, sweats	YES NO Fatigue
YES NO Dizziness/lightheaded	YES NO Weight loss/gain
YES NO Nausea/vomiting	YES NO Numbness or tingling
YES NO Other ________________	

Adapted with permission from *Primary Care for the Physical Therapist: Examination and Triage*, Boissonnault WG, Patient health history including identification of health risk factors, pp 61-65, Copyright Elsevier 2005.

measures must possess responsiveness, the ability to accurately detect whether a true or clinically meaningful change has occurred.[36,38] A clinically meaningful level of change is called the *minimal clinically important difference* (MCID). The MCID is the smallest meaningful change score that the patient perceives as beneficial. Another way of determining when meaningful change in an outcome measure has occurred is the minimal detectable change (MDC), the amount of change necessary to exceed measurement error.[38] For example, if the MDC for a specific self-report measure is 6, any change score below a 6 is attributed to measurement error and not a true change in patient status. Specific self-report outcome measures for each spinal region are discussed in later chapters.

Patient Demographic Profile

To place a patient's problem into a proper context, the initial inquiry should develop the patient's profile.

The patient profile includes information about patient demographics such as age, gender, race, occupation, lifestyle hobbies, exercise, recreation, marital status, primary language, referral source, barriers to communication, and learning preferences.

Age, Gender, Race, and Ethnicity (How Old Are You?)

Certain diseases have a higher incidence within specific age ranges, gender, and race categories. The most common primary risk factor for disease, illness, and comorbidities is age.[3] Women aged 60 and older have the highest risk for breast cancer; 99% of breast cancer occurs in women. Men aged 60 and older have the highest risk for developing prostate cancer. Prostate cancer accounts for one-third of all male cancers.[39] Lung cancer is currently the most common cause of cancer death in women. Approximately 1 in 3 women in the United States will develop cancer; the leading sites are breast, lung, colon, and rectum. The leading sites for men are prostate, lung, colon, and rectum.[40] Leukemia, almost 30% of all childhood cancers, is the most common cancer among children aged 0 to 14 years.[41] Health status related to race and ethnic background may also show a higher incidence of specific medical diseases. African Americans have a higher incidence of sickle cell disease, and basal cell carcinoma and melanoma are more common among Caucasians. Age-related pathology such as osteoporosis and degenerative joint disease may coexist with other disorders. Though some disease and associated risk factors are provided throughout this reference, students and clinicians should seek additional resources for more detailed information on pathology and medical disease.[40]

Occupation and Work Environment (What Is Your Job? What Does a Typical Day of Work Involve? Are You Currently Working?)

Patient data on employment should include activities, tasks, and work demands from current and previous occupations and factors related to the work environment, such as length of time at the present job, travel, perceived stressors, occupational hazards, hours, and type of work performed. Repetitive activities or prolonged postures may contribute to the etiology of the problem or affect the prognosis and potential for rehabilitation. In most instances, intervention and patient education related to work become integral components of the plan of care. The worker who sits 80% of the day in a poorly designed chair or repeatedly lifts for several hours per day may have an increased risk for LBP. Exposure to environmental toxins or high levels of mental and emotional stress might explain nonspecific neuromusculoskeletal symptoms such as fatigue, joint pain, headache, or myalgia.[40] The impact of the patient's symptoms on work, play, and social activities may give insight into motivation and fear-avoidance behavior. The cautious patient may fear movement and reinjury. The overactive patient may continue activities that aggravate the problem. Both behaviors may result in a slower recovery and require different management strategies.

Functional Status/Lifestyle (Do You Have a Regular Exercise Program, Recreational Activities, or Hobbies?)

An assessment of the patient's current activity or fitness level may provide information related to the etiology of the problem, relate to the amount of disability the patient experiences, or indicate a level of motivation or compliance with a prescribed intervention. For example, both the marathon runner and sedentary patient experiencing an acute episode of LBP may encounter difficulty with compliance. A patient with LBP caring for a disabled spouse with 2 small children and an elderly parent may have a different prognosis than someone who does not have those responsibilities. Current functional levels include self-care, home management, exercise, and sports activities. Documentation should include specific activities, frequency, duration, or percentage of performance currently and prior to problem.[40,42] Region-specific outcome measures are valuable as self-report measures for documenting functional status.

Psychosocial Status

Living environment, health habits, social activities, cultural beliefs, and caregiver support systems can be sources of both support and stress. Psychosocial factors related to depression, anger, stress, alcohol or drug abuse, tobacco use, or simply the need for assistance in the home often interfere with or influence the outcome. Workers' compensation, financial concerns, or health insurance issues may limit the options for intervention. Early identification of these issues is important and calls for early intervention by the physical therapist and/or referral to appropriate health care professionals to optimize the plan of care.[3,19]

Chief Complaint (In Your Own Words, Please Tell Me What Your Main Problem Is)

When the chief complaint is recorded on the body chart (Figure 2-2), the clinician asks specifically for symptoms in other areas of the body. Documenting the body chart with

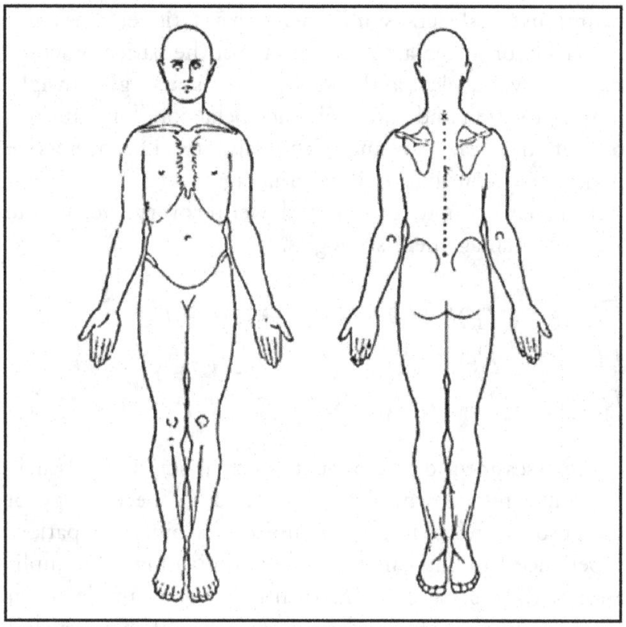

Figure 2-2. Body chart or diagram.

a check mark where the patient does not have symptoms is equally as important as noting where the patient does have symptoms.[43] For example, a patient with left-sided LBP may neglect to volunteer mild left-sided abdominal pain unless specifically asked because he or she thinks this is unrelated to the LBP. Through further questioning, the clinician attempts to establish a relationship between the LBP and abdominal pain to help differentiate if 1 or 2 problems are present.

The body chart is useful for visualizing symptom patterns and developing a working hypothesis regarding the nature of the disorder or identification of symptom-generating structures. The nature of the disorder can be a local or referred symptom, usually pain, associated with an MS disorder or systemic disease mimicking an MS disorder. Pain from visceral structures is typically located in the anterior chest wall or abdominal regions, but viscera located in the retroperitoneal region of the trunk may present as back pain rather than abdominal pain. Common visceral referral pain patterns are depicted in Figure 2-3.[3] Table 2-6[44-46] lists the segmental innervations of the viscera.[44-46] Visceral pain is referred to areas supplied by the associated spinal nerves.[44-46] The completed body chart (see Figure 2-2) and knowledge of pain patterns serve as a guide for further review of systems questioning and clarification as the examination process continues.

Completing the Body Chart or Symptom Diagram

To obtain an accurate and comprehensive picture of presenting symptoms, the clinician identifies the exact location of symptoms by stating, "Show me exactly where your pain or problem is"; further clarifies, "Does it travel anywhere?"; and clearly asks, "Are there any other areas that do not feel normal?" The clinician then pursues additional descriptors such as quality, depth (ie, superficial or deep), consistency (ie, constant or intermittent), and the relationship and intensity for the identified symptoms. Areas of abnormal sensations are also recorded:

- Anesthesia (loss of sensation)
- Hypesthesia (reduced touch sensation)
- Hyperesthesia (heightened perception to touch)
- Allodynia (pain provoked by stimuli that are normally not painful)
- Analgesia (absence of appreciation of pain)
- Paresthesia (sensations of tingling, pins and needles)

The sensory changes may be produced anywhere within a region innervated by a peripheral, cranial nerve, or nerve root. In the presence of sensory and/or motor deficits, a good understanding of dermatomes and cutaneous nerve distributions aids in the differential diagnosis of a nerve root lesion versus peripheral nerve lesion.[47] In addition, the location of pain or abnormal sensations may suggest spinal cord involvement, peripheral vascular disease (PVD), diabetes, or other pathology. Figures 2-4[48] and 2-5 depict dermatomal and peripheral nerve cutaneous distributions.

Description and Assessment of Pain and Other Symptoms

Pain

Pain, a frequent and routine symptom, is described as "an unpleasant sensory and emotional experience associated with actual or potential tissue damage, or described in terms of such damage."[49] Pain, an adaptive sensation or an alarm signal, provides an early warning sign that aids in repair after tissue damage, but pain can also be maladaptive (exaggerated or spontaneous), reflecting an abnormal function in the nervous system.[50] The patient's report of pain varies with levels of stress; social or cultural influences; and how he or she thinks, feels, and communicates. The subjective nature and complex pathophysiology of a patient's report of pain make assessment and differential diagnosis difficult.

Neuromatrix Theory of Pain

Traditionally, pain is thought of as a symptom due to pathology with the amount of pain being directly related to the amount of pathology. When the pathology resolves, the pain goes away. In some patients, however, pain is present even if the pathology resolves or no pathology can be found.

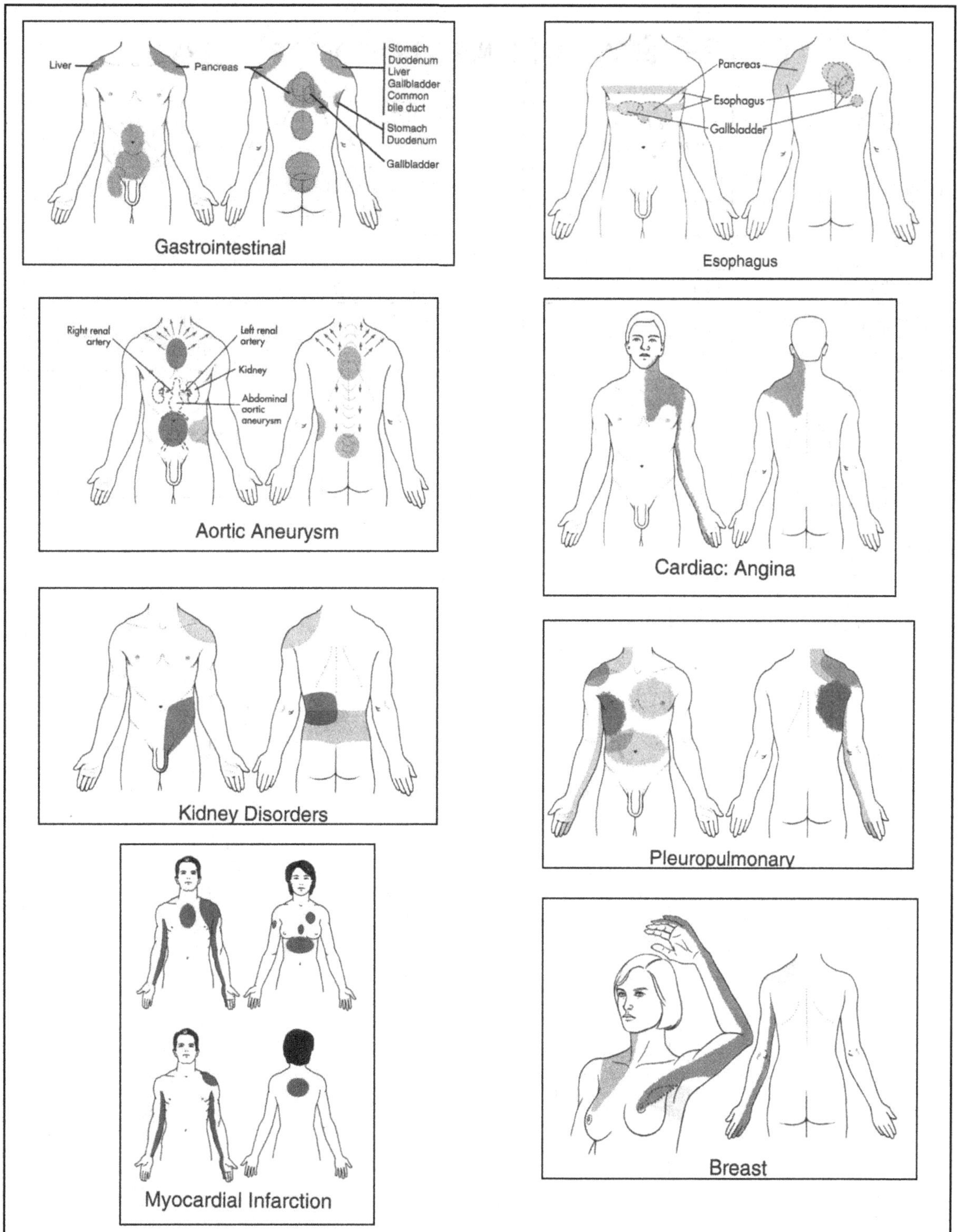

Figure 2-3. Common visceral referral pain patterns. (Reprinted with permission from *Differential Diagnosis for Physical Therapists: Screening for Referral, 4th edition*, Goodman CC, Snyder TE, Copyright Elsevier 2007.)

TABLE 2-6. SEGMENTAL INNERVATIONS OF THE VISCERA

VISCERA	*SEGMENTAL INNERVATION*
Heart	T1-5
Lungs	T5-6
Diaphragm	C3-5
Esophagus	T4-6
Stomach	T6-10
Pancreas	T10
Liver/gallbladder	T7-9

VISCERA	*SEGMENTAL INNERVATION*
Small intestine	T7-10
Large intestine	T11-L1
Kidney	T10-L1
Bladder/prostate	T11-12, S2-4
Uterus	T1-L1, S2-4
Ovaries/testes	T10-11

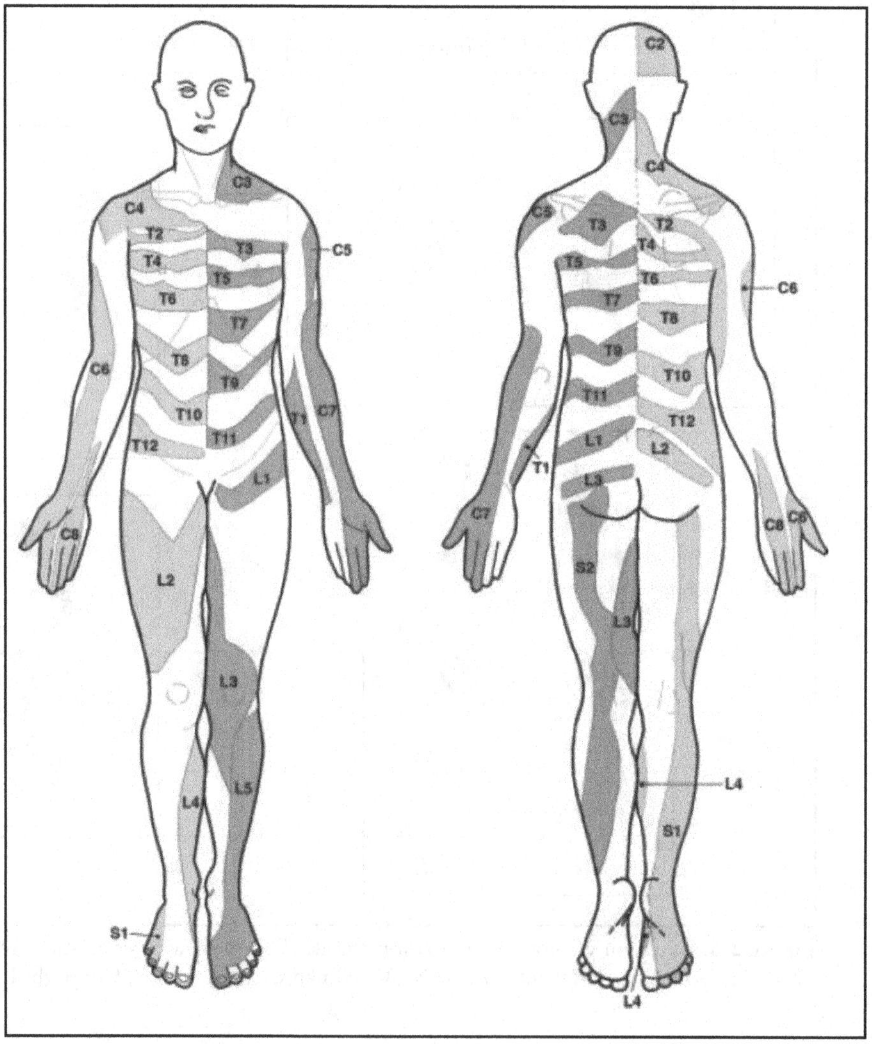

Figure 2-4. Dermatomes. (Reprinted with permission from Lee MWL, McPhee RW, Stringer MD. An evidence-based approach to human dermatomes. *Clin Anat.* 2008;21:363-373. Copyright John Wiley & Sons, Inc. 2008.)

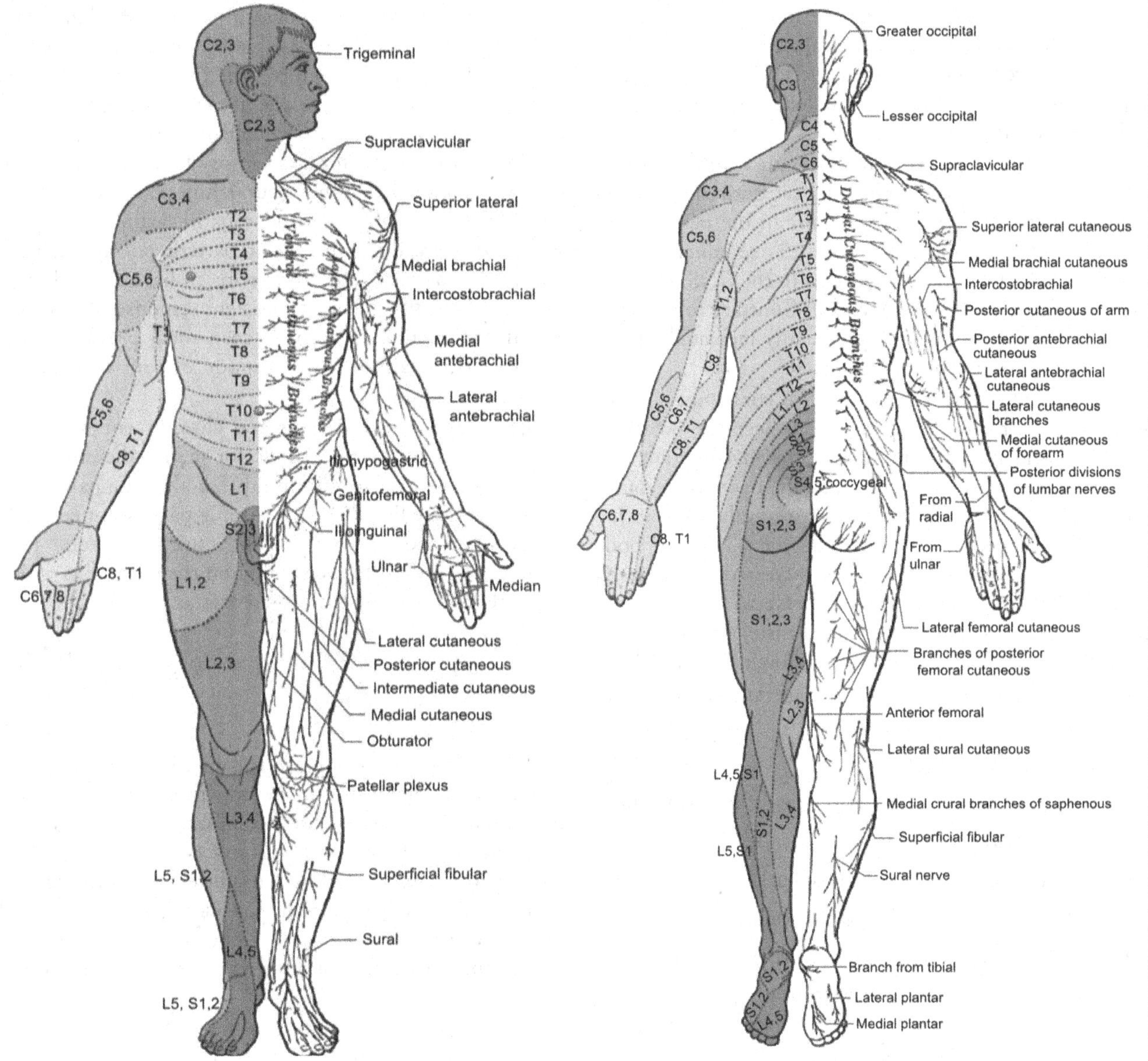

Figure 2-5. Dermatomal and peripheral nerve cutaneous distributions, anterior and posterior. (Reprinted with permission from the author: Mikael Häggström. Available at Wikipedia Commons, freely licensed media file repository. http://commons.wikimedia.org/wiki/File:Dermatomes_and_cutaneous_nerves_-_anterior.png and http://commons.wikimedia.org/wiki/File:Dermatomes_and_cutaneous_nerves_-_posterior.png. Accessed July 6, 2011.)

Pain is a multidimensional experience modulated by many influences. These influences are variable and depend on the meaning of pain to the individual.

Pain is generally thought of as a signal of injury or potential injury. When tissue is perceived to be under threat, central nervous system (CNS) outputs occur. However, it is the individual's perception of the degree of threat that determines the outputs, not the state of tissues or the actual threat to tissues.[51] The neuromatrix theory of pain proposes that pain is produced by output of a widely distributed neural network in the brain rather than purely by sensory input evoked by trauma, inflammation, or other pathology.[52] The neuromatrix is a combination of cortical mechanisms that produce pain when activated, but it requires no actual sensory input (ie, noxious stimulus) to produce pain experiences. Pain is produced by the brain when it perceives that body tissue is in danger and that action is required. Pain is a multifaceted, subjective, emotional experience produced by a characteristic neurosignature of a widely distributed brain neural network called the *body-self neuromatrix*.[52,53] This matrix integrates cognitive inputs (evaluative: past experience, context, beliefs), sensory inputs (discriminative: cutaneous, visual), and motivational inputs (affective: emotions, stress, immune system) and proposes that output patterns engage perceptual (cognition and emotions), behavioral (action patterns, coping strategies, social interaction), and homeostatic (cortisol and stress regulation) systems in response to injury and chronic stress.[54] Psychological stress and cognitive and sensory events modulate each person's neurosignature, resulting in an altered neuromatrix output often associated with chronic pain.

Multiple mechanisms or influences are involved in driving the pain experience and broadly categorized as peripherally mediated (ie, processing occurs in the periphery or related to somatic, visceral, or neural tissue injury) or centrally mediated (ie, processing occurs in the CNS related to cognitive and emotional influences). Contrary to common beliefs, all acute pain is not peripherally mediated and all chronic pain is not centrally mediated.

Two interdependent mechanisms contribute to the development of chronic pain: (1) nociceptive, which is peripheral and includes immune-related dysfunction that stimulates nociceptive structures, and (2) non-nociceptive, which is central and includes cognitive-evaluative mechanisms. These mechanisms persuade the CNS that body tissue is in danger, which causes increased neuromatrix activity and results in a lowered threshold for activation and sensitization occurs. Chronic, persistent pain provides the patient and clinicians with the following challenges[55]:

- Increased sensitivity to noxious and non-noxious stimuli
- Altered motor output
- An unclear relationship between pain and tissue input
- Unpredictable flare-ups
- Poor tolerance of normal therapeutic approaches
- Problems with physical and functional improvement
- Difficulty transferring gains to other activities.

The dominant processes vary from individual to individual, but they must be recognized when examining and treating a patient with MS pain.

Acute Versus Chronic Pain

As described by Waddell,[56] a careful assessment of pain has 4 categories: anatomic distribution, quality, time course, and severity or intensity. Although individuals vary, the anatomic distribution and quality of pain or other symptoms often display a recognizable pattern that may suggest either an MS or non-MS nature. Acute pain, whether somatic or visceral, is often referred to as *nociceptive pain*, or the normal response to noxious stimuli (mechanical or chemical) that are damaging or potentially damaging to normal tissue.[50] Nociceptive pain is associated with injury, inflammation, and repair and is identified by a predictable response to stretch, compression, and movement during examination.

As discussed earlier, chronic pain is more complex and not as well understood. Chronic pain, whether somatic or visceral, persists past the point of healing and appears to be associated with abnormal processing or sensitization within the peripheral and CNS, also called *neuropathic pain*.[3,50] Peripheral neuropathic pain results from injury to neural tissue such as spinal or peripheral nerves. Symptoms such as burning and paresthesia are consistent with corresponding innervation of motor and sensory fields and identified on examination by testing neural function and mechanics.[57] Symptoms of central neuropathic pain are atypical with a widespread nonanatomical pattern, poorly localized, and often unstable. The pain seems to have a mind of its own and is identified by inconsistent responses to physical examination, such as normal mechanical pressure being interpreted as pain or the perception of pain without any appropriate stimulus.

These definitions of acute and chronic pain are based on the mechanisms responsible for pain rather than just the symptoms, but keep in mind that all acute pain is not peripherally mediated and all chronic pain is not centrally mediated. Standard definitions of acute and chronic pain do not exist and differ depending on the context in which they are used and the cited references.

Mechanical, Chemical, Neuropathic Pain

Three types of stimuli are capable of producing pain: mechanical, chemical, or neuropathic.[3,58] Mechanical pain occurs as a result of sufficient compressive or tensile force on normal tissue such as end range muscle stretch and usually presents as an intermittent (ie, on/off) pattern. A mechanical pattern has clear aggravating and easing factors, a predictable response to examination, and is appropriate for physical therapy examination and intervention.[3,58]

Chemical pain is a result of chemical irritants in the tissue due to inflammation or infection. A chemical pattern is usually constant (ie, unremitting for 24 hours per day) and may have a mechanical component that varies with aggravating and easing factors, but pain is still present at rest. Further examination of the source of the chemical irritants guides the initial course of treatment. Pain that is constant and does not have a mechanical component—which means that it does not vary with aggravating and easing factors—suggests an acute disease state or serious pathology.[3,47,58]

In general, pain that persists beyond the time of normal healing is probably neuropathic in nature with components of peripheral and central sensitization. However, not all chronic pain is neuropathic. Patients often present with acute episodes of a chronic condition but are pain-free or able to manage their symptoms in between episodes. Specific sources of neuropathic pain such as a radiculopathy present with distinct clinical signs and symptoms due to a focal neurological insult. Neuropathic pain due to central or peripheral sensitization presents with a widespread distribution of symptoms; hyperalgesia; allodynia; inconsistent aggravating and easing factors; signs and symptoms of autonomic nervous system disruption such as poor appetite, depression, and anxiety; and an unpredictable or absent response to examination and physical therapy intervention.[47,59]

Quality and Depth of Symptoms

In obtaining a description of symptoms the clinician also asks, "Is the pain superficial or deep?" and "How would you describe it?" Somatic pain is felt in either the body surface or MS tissues and is mechanical in nature, aggravated by activity, and relieved by rest. Superficial pain is sharp, well localized, and involves superficial structures, skin, fascia, and tendon sheaths. However, superficial or cutaneous pain can also be referred from viscera or deep somatic structures. Deep somatic pain is dull or aching; poorly localized; involves bone, muscles, tendon, nerve, and blood vessels; and can be referred from some other sites. Deep somatic pain can be mechanical in nature or due to a pathological process such as metastasis in somatic structures. Visceral pain is pain felt in the internal organs and the heart muscle, has the ability to refer to distant sites, and is generally described as diffuse or poorly localized.[3] Visceral pain is usually not reproduced with movement and does not have a consistent mechanical pattern of aggravating and easing factors.[3,58] Visceral structures can refer pain to somatic tissue such as in a heart attack, which may refer pain to the jaw. Some somatic structures can refer pain to visceral locations (eg, a low back disorder may refer pain to the abdomen).

Magee[60] offered the following common descriptors of pain and possible related structures:

- Bone pain tends to be deep, boring, and localized
- Vascular pain tends to be diffuse, aching, poorly localized, throbbing, pounding, or pulsing and may be referred to other areas of the body
- Muscle pain is hard to localize, dull, cramping, aching, and may refer to other areas
- Ligament and joint capsule are dull and aching

The quality of the pain may suggest that certain anatomical structures or systems are at fault; however, like the depth of symptoms, the quality is often variable.

Local, Referred, and Radicular Pain

Assuming that the source of a local area of pain for symptoms is deep or under the area of symptoms may be misleading. For example, pain in the elbow may be produced by local structures or may be due to a problem in the cervical spine. In this situation, pain in the elbow is referred pain. Referred pain is either somatic or visceral pain felt in an area away from the site where it originates; is supplied by the same or adjacent neural segments; and can originate from any cutaneous, somatic, or visceral source. Referred pain is usually well localized but can spread or radiate from its point of origin and has tenderness and muscle hypertonus over the referred pain area.[3] Referred pain appears to be consistent within an individual but variable among individuals.

Radicular pain results directly from irritation of a spinal nerve or its roots and usually is experienced as a sharp, lancinating pain that is somewhat localized to the dermatome, an area of skin innervated by a single spinal nerve. In contrast, somatic referred pain is static, dull, aching, and hard to localize. Compression of normal nerve roots results in paresthesia or numbness but not pain. Current theory suggests that radicular pain is due to ischemic and inflammatory processes involved in nerve root compression, not compression alone.[61] Intermittent irritation or compression of a spinal nerve or nerve root causes local edema. Continued irritation and edema result in ischemia to the nerve and a sensory, motor, or combined conduction loss, producing paresthesia or anesthesia (dermatomal), muscle weakness (myotomal), and diminished muscle stretch reflexes commonly called *deep tendon reflexes*. A conduction deficit associated with the spinal nerve or its roots is called a *radiculopathy*.[61]

Relationship

If more than one symptom is present, the clinician should ask the patient whether the symptoms are related in any way or, for example, "If your low back pain gets worse, is there any change in your calf pain?" This dialogue helps to determine whether more than one problem exists. If the patient's chief complaint is LBP and posterior calf pain, posterior calf pain that occurs only when the LBP gets worse suggests a primary low back problem rather than 2 separate problems. Conversely, if the presence or intensity of LBP does not affect the onset of calf pain, then the 2 symptoms are less likely to be related. Clarifying questions to obtain details of pain behavior assist the clinician in refining the diagnostic hypothesis. Clinically, the location of symptoms helps to determine the extent and nature of the disorder but may mislead the clinician regarding the anatomic source. The initial diagnostic hypothesis related to the presenting pain pattern is continually refined as data is gained from the history, physical examination, and re-examination.

Duration of Symptoms or Time Course

The terms *acute*, *subacute*, and *chronic* do not have standard definitions. Traditionally, the definitions from onset of symptoms are as follows[62]:

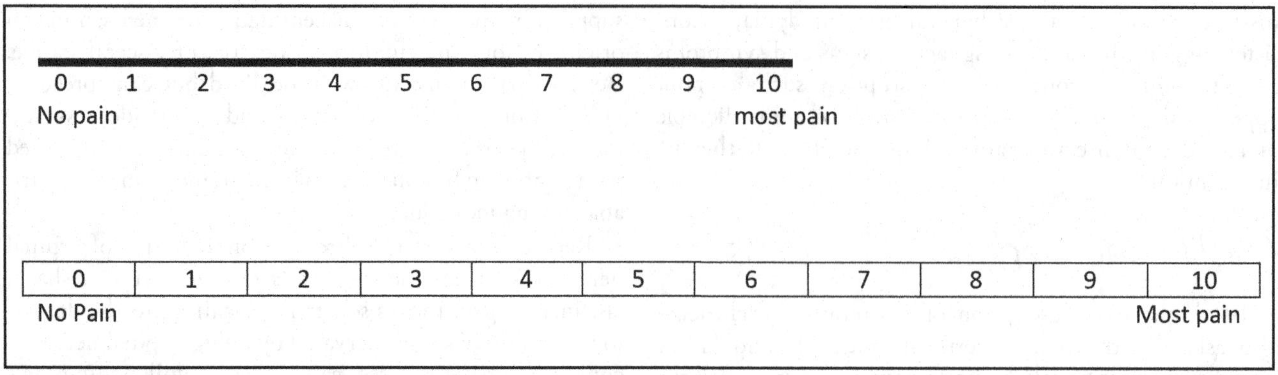

Figure 2-6. Numeric Pain Rating Scale.

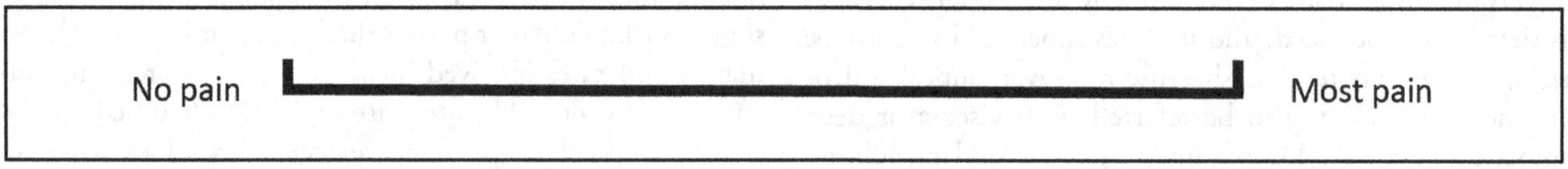

Figure 2-7. Visual Analogue Scale (usually 100 mm in length).

- Acute: less than 6 weeks
- Subacute: 6 to 12 weeks
- Chronic: more than 3 months of continuous pain

Other definitions for LBP are as follows[63]:

- Acute: present for less than 3 months
- Subacute: present for 5 to 7 weeks but not longer than 12 weeks
- Chronic: present for at least 3 months

Magee[60] listed acute pain as 7 to 10 days; subacute as 10 days to 7 weeks; and chronic as longer than 7 weeks. Not all patients fall neatly into these categories. Some patients have recurrent episodes over time and may fit the definition of acute on chronic if the recurrent episodes are pain-free. Differentiating among acute, subacute, and chronic LBP is important because the physiological basis, natural history, and response to therapy are different for each category. An acute condition often indicates the need for a brief and less vigorous initial examination. In general, interventions for acute LBP may not be appropriate for chronic LBP, and interventions for chronic LBP may not be indicated for acute LBP.

Severity or Intensity

Often difficult, measuring the intensity of pain or other symptoms is necessary to evaluate the effects of treatment and its underlying cause. Pain is assessed at rest and during movement using one-dimensional tools such as a numeric rating scale (NRS) or Visual Analogue Scale (VAS). Assessment of acute, chronic, or persistent pain additionally requires a multidimensional instrument such as the Roland-Morris Disability Questionnaire[64] to assess the physical, emotional, and social impact on quality of life.[65]

The Numeric Pain Rating Scale (NPRS; Figure 2-6) is usually an 11-point intensity, numeric scale (0 to 10), with 0 being no pain and 10 being the most pain imaginable. A 21-point scale (0 to 20) or 101-point scale (0 to 100) may also be used. The patient is asked to select a number verbally or graphically on a horizontal or vertical line that represents the subjective feeling of pain within a specific time frame, such as now or at present, at worst, at least, or an average over the last 24 hours. Reliability of the NPRS has been shown in patients ($n = 124$) with pain in the neck, back, upper extremity, and lower extremity.[66] Intraclass correlation coefficients varied from 0.64 to 0.86. The standard errors of measurement varied from 1.04 to 1.30 NPRS points.[66] For patients with MS problems, an estimate of the MDC at the 90% confidence interval is about 3 NPRS points.[66] In a review of multiple studies across 5 disease conditions of chronic pain of 12 weeks or less, Farrar et al[67] estimated a clinically important difference on the NPRS with scores of at least a 4 out of 10 by relating it to patient global impression of change (PGIC). The changes in pain intensity from baseline to the endpoint were compared to the PGIC for each subject. On average, a 2-point reduction in score or 30%, which means a PGIC of "much improved," represents a clinically meaningful improvement. A 50% improvement corresponded to a PGIC of "very much improved." The PGIC is tied to the concept of overall improvement, unlike the NPRS. The best indicator of improvement, raw change score or percentage change, remains controversial.[65]

The VAS (Figure 2-7) is a numerically continuous scale that requires the patient to mark perceived level of pain on a 100-mm line with anchors of no pain to the worst pain imaginable. The score is determined by measuring the distance in millimeters from the "no pain" anchor to the mark that the patient identified as his or her level of pain. Test-retest reliability of the VAS is between 0.95 and 0.97. In a sample of adults presenting to an urban emergency department, the minimum clinically significant difference for the VAS pain score is 12 mm ± 3 mm at a 95% confidence interval.[68]

Both the NPRS and VAS are clinically useful, easy to administer and score, and reliable, valid measures of pain intensity. For clinical practice, the NPRS is more practical than the VAS, generally easier to understand, quicker to administer, and does not require clear vision or pencil and paper.[65] Jensen and Karoly[69] stated that the sensitivity or ability to detect a treatment effect of the NPRS may be less relative to the VAS. The authors suggested that different pain scales may be more or less sensitive in different conditions, and that one measure will not consistently demonstrate higher statistical power than the other. When correlated with the VAS, the NPRS has 0.79 to 0.95 convergent validity,[70] meaning that the 2 measures assess the same event and provide similar results but are not interchangeable. Pain intensity is influenced by its context, expected duration, attitudes, and beliefs and is associated with, but not caused by, psychological factors such as fear, anxiety, and depression. Due to these many factors, patients interpret measurement scales differently and baseline scores vary broadly. Accurate and meaningful measurement of the multidimensional properties of pain remains a challenge to the clinician and may vary with clinical setting, duration of symptoms, MS region, and baseline scores.

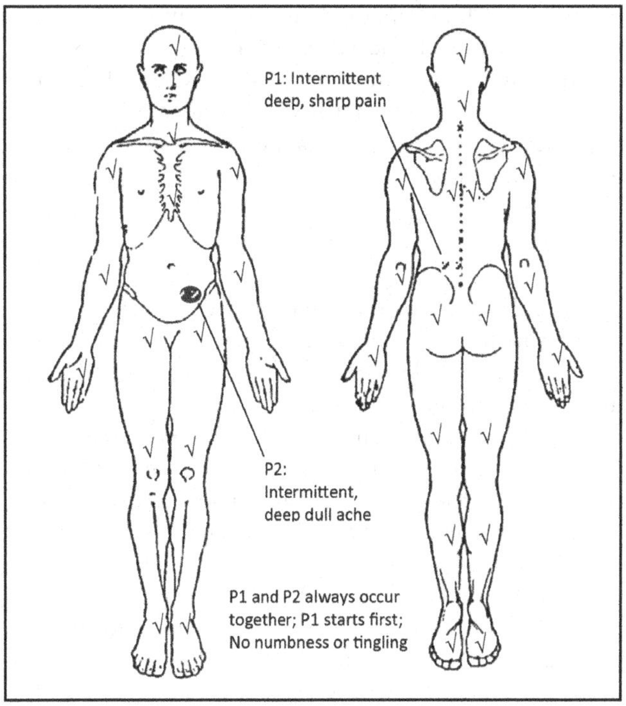

Figure 2-8. Example of a completed body chart or diagram.

Using the Completed Body Chart and Symptom Diagram

Pain patterns may be classified as MS or non-MS, or have components of both disorders. Knowledge of potential visceral pain patterns guides the review of systems toward detailed screening of specific organ systems. A recognizable MS pattern may suggest body structures or functions that must be examined independently or questioned in detail as to onset and behavior of aggravating or easing factors. For example, a patient may complain of a deep ache and a sharp, piercing pain in the shoulder. Patient responses to specific aggravating factors guide the clinician in selecting appropriate diagnostic test procedures. Shoulder movement that results in both the deep ache and sharp pain suggests that both symptoms are related to a shoulder problem. If the deep ache is produced by neck movement and the sharp pain by shoulder movement, the patient may have more than one problem. Additionally, the clinician should consider examination of the cervical and thoracic spine as either a referral source or a biomechanical contributor to the patient's problem. Figure 2-8 depicts a completed body chart.

The patient's description and pattern of pain or other symptoms form the initial impression or working diagnosis, which in turn focuses the rest of the history and identifies areas for further questioning and clarification. The working diagnosis is continuously refined and confirmed by a detailed history, physical examination, and the patient's response to intervention.

History (Present or Current Episode)

When the latest bout of symptoms is not the patient's first episode, the quickest way to obtain relevant data is to start with the present episode. Details of the current episode should establish the circumstances or manner in which the current symptoms began, the progression of those symptoms, and the stage and stability of the problem. The clinician should elicit details about the mode of onset or mechanism of injury (traumatic versus nontraumatic), date of onset, progression of each symptom, all treatments to date and their effects, and the overall progression of the problem. A thorough history helps to determine the nature (ie, MS or non-MS), stage (ie, acute, subacute, chronic), and stability (ie, getting better, worse, or staying the same) of the problem. In considering the nature of the patient's problem, the clinician looks for clusters of symptoms to establish the working diagnosis. The first determination is whether the patient is appropriate for physical therapy management. If not appropriate, the patient is referred to a medical specialist. If the working diagnosis is an MS disorder, the clinician identifies the body structures, functions, or regions and other contributing factors that must be examined as well as any precautions or contraindications to the examination.

Mode and Date of Onset

Careful inquiry by the clinician often reveals the cause of the patient's problem. Asking "How or when did the problem begin?" allows the clinician to explore the exact mechanism of injury or nature of the onset. If the onset is sudden or related to a specific event, the clinician should determine the activity, position, and direction and magnitude of forces related to the injury. Injury related to a fall, lifting, or a motor vehicle accident may provide information related to potential or extent of injured structures, severity of onset, and intervention. With an acute condition or recent onset, a full examination may not be possible due to severity or irritability. The clinician performs a limited examination with test procedures that provide the most information and minimize stress to the patient.

If the onset is gradual or insidious, which means that it occurred for no apparent reason or started without a specific incident, the clinician must ask for predisposing factors such as unusual activity, repetitive activities, changes in work, training, recent illness, or stress. Gradual may mean over one day or over weeks to months. A truly insidious onset merits concern about the underlying cause of the condition and raises the suspicion of a non-MS problem.

Progression of Symptoms

Using the completed body chart, the clinician asks for the progression of each symptom since onset. Changes in area and severity of symptoms provide clues about the relationship and stability of the problem. For example, if a patient reported the onset of right-sided LBP 3 days ago and now has lateral calf pain radiating to the right foot, the clinician may infer the condition is worsening. A condition may worsen if the pain or symptom distribution becomes more widespread and distal (ie, peripheralizes). Likewise, the patient whose lower extremity symptoms have resolved over the past week and now reports only right-sided LBP describes a condition that is likely improving with time. A condition may improve if the symptom distribution becomes more localized and moves proximally (ie, centralizes).

Treatment and Effects

To determine the effects of current or previous treatment, the clinician asks, "Have you had any treatment? Did it help?" If yes, "In what way?" Specific details of the exact treatment and patient response help with treatment planning. If the symptoms are better or worse, the clinician should ask, "In what way?" to determine both a symptom and functional response to the intervention. Symptoms unchanged, worsened, or improved and then worsened again despite physical therapy intervention are considered a red flag.

Stability (Getting Better, Worse, Staying the Same?)

Determining the stability of the problem is established by asking, "Compared to when this first started, is it getting better, worse, or staying the same?" If better or worse, the clinician should then ask, "In what way?" Changes in the intensity, severity, duration, and location of symptoms reveal the stability of the problem and assists with prognosis and the rate and level of recovery. Generally, symptoms that are worsening with the passage of time take longer to respond to intervention than symptoms that are beginning to resolve.

History (Previous Episode[s] of Similar Problem)

Knowledge of the current history helps the clinician to quickly identify relevant information from previous episodes. The history of previous episodes begins with the question, "Have you had this problem before?" If the patient is not sure, "Is it similar to what you are feeling now?" With a long history of recurrence, determine the initial manner of onset, severity, previous treatment and effects, frequency of recurrences, time to recover, level of recovery, and status between episodes.

The initial onset and mechanism of injury should be described in detail. Frequency and duration of episodes and level of recovery from the last episode or between episodes may affect the potential for recovery. Is there a pattern to the manner of onset? For example, if each episode of LBP is associated with prolonged sitting, an important aspect of intervention and recurrence involves addressing the activity of sitting. Previous treatment and effects and level of recovery put the present injury in perspective, help to establish reasonable goals for treatment and likelihood of recurrence, and provide data on the stability of the problem over time.[20] If the symptoms are easier to provoke or last longer with each episode and full recovery does not occur between episodes, then the clinician infers the problem is getting worse over time and potential for recovery may be limited. The chronicity of a problem has implications related to mechanism of pain, management, and prognosis.

Symptom Behavior

Aggravating factors, easing factors, and 24-hour behavior for each of the patient's symptoms provide insight into the impact on the patient's activities. Symptoms associated with an MS problem typically vary as mechanical loads on the body increase or decrease with time of day and onset or cessation of specific activities or postures.[43] Symptoms that show no response or inconsistent responses to mechanical loads are not likely MS in nature. In this instance, the clinician should suspect a non-MS disorder or one with a central sensitization component.[57] For example, constant LBP unchanged by activity, posture, or rest may be inflammatory or systemic in nature. However, the presence of symptoms that are altered by activity does not rule out a disease process. For example, pain in both lower extremities provoked by walking and relieved by rest may be due to PVD. Nonmechanical events such as night pain; changes with eating; or cyclical pain that gets worse, then better, and then worse again could indicate a non-MS source for the pain.

Pursuit of aggravating factors, easing factors, and 24-hour behavior may also bring out a pattern of activity avoidance. Unwarranted activity avoidance or fear of pain and movement may lead to withdrawal from work, recreational, and social activities and may affect rehabilitation. In-depth questioning regarding which postures or movements result in a change in the location, intensity, or quality of a patient's symptoms helps to determine the mechanical nature of the problem, provides an indication of activity limitations, and defines the problem's severity or impact on function and irritability (which means the ease with which symptoms are provoked and then subside). The severity of symptoms relates to the intensity and the degree to which the symptoms restrict movement or function. Knowing the severity and irritability of symptoms helps to identify patients who will not tolerate a full physical examination and provides a baseline of activity limitations.

Aggravating Factors (What Makes It Worse?)

The patient identifies the exact movement or posture and amount of time, distance, or repetitions it takes to produce or increase each symptom and how long it takes for the provoked symptom to ease. These details suggest how easy or difficult it may be to reproduce the patient's symptoms during the physical examination, provide an activity baseline against which to measure progress, and assist in setting functional goals for the patient. The aggravating movements and activity limitations should be meaningful to the patient, highlighted, and then reassessed during follow-up examination sessions to evaluate intervention effectiveness. The clinician also analyzes the aggravating movement or posture to hypothesize what body structures or functions are causing the symptoms, which provides guidance for the selection of specific tests and measures. To address specific needs of each patient, it is sometimes necessary to ask, "What would you like to do that you are not able to do because of this problem?"

After identifying a specific movement, the clinician pursues additional details to clarify severity and irritability. For example, the clinician asks, "When you walk for 5 blocks and get LBP, are you able to continue walking as long as you need to or do you have to stop?" If the patient is able to continue walking, the symptoms may not be severe. If the patient has to stop walking, the symptoms are likely severe. When movement provokes symptoms quickly and the symptoms persist for more than 2 to 3 minutes, the symptoms are likely irritable.[57] If the symptoms come on slowly and go away as soon as the movement stops, the symptoms are not irritable. To determine irritability, the clinician asks, "When you walk for 5 blocks and get LBP, does it go away immediately when you stop or does it take some time to go away?" If the LBP goes away immediately, the symptoms are not irritable and a full examination is possible. If the LBP lingers for several minutes, then the symptoms are likely irritable and the clinician considers a limited examination. A full examination is likely to make the patient worse. A limited examination avoids an unnecessary increase of the patient's symptoms.

In patients presenting with multiple areas of symptoms recorded on the body chart, the clinician must determine whether the symptoms are related to one another. If a patient reports LBP, anterior hip pain, and posterior thigh pain, the clinician must establish links between the symptoms areas. If the LBP and posterior thigh pain are produced with walking, the clinician must also ask, "Does the hip pain come on at the same time?" If the answer is yes, then the symptoms may come from the same body structures and functions. A reasonable hypothesis would be the lumbar spine. If the answer is no, then a reasonable hypothesis would be that the patient may have 2 separate problem areas. Aggravating factors for groin pain must be identified. Common aggravating factors for each region of the spine are discussed in later chapters.

Easing Factors (What Makes It Better?)

Movements, positions, medications, or other treatments that decrease or alleviate symptoms are easing factors. Similar to aggravating factors, details of positions, movements, or medications and the time it takes to ease symptoms are recorded. Symptoms that ease quickly are more likely to respond more quickly than symptoms that last longer. Easing factors should be sought for all symptoms as well as the effects of easing one symptom on other symptoms.

Most MS problems improve with a change in position and with rest. A systemic disease process is temporarily, minimally, or not affected by position or rest.[3] If the patient's symptoms do not improve with position, rest, or movement, the clinician suspects a non-MS problem, an acute, inflammatory condition, or a problem with a central sensitization component. Easing factors often guide the initial intervention or the overall management of the patient's problem. For example, a patient who reports walking as an easing factor for LBP may require a specific dosage of walking as a therapeutic exercise intervention. The patient with a chronic problem and a central sensitization component may require a multidisciplinary approach with a focus on resolving activity limitations rather than resolution of pain.

24-Hour Behavior

Clinicians must inquire about the behavior of symptoms over a 24-hour period with specific emphasis on a patient's ability to sleep through the night. The quality of sleep is important for restoring body function. With a disruptive sleep pattern, the body and mind are not capable of optimal function. In addition to pain, medication side effects, increased urination, and night sweats are a few factors related to sleep deprivation that can interfere with the rehabilitation process.[40]

Night (How Is the Pain at Night?)

Pain at night is often deemed a symptom of cancer, but further clarification is needed when a patient answers "yes" to the question, "Does it wake you at night?" The clinician might then ask, "What is it that wakes you?" Pain at night is typical of mechanical problems when the patient reports an inability to lie on the involved side or reports waking with symptoms that are simply relieved by a change of position and an easy return to sleep. If the pain is the most intense at night and the patient is unsure of what wakes him or her, reports he or she must get up and walk around, and has difficulty returning to sleep, the clinician should consider the possibility of an active inflammatory component or more serious pathology.[19] If night pain is a primary mechanical complaint, the clinician should determine the frequency, provocative position, and symptoms produced. This information is helpful to reassess at subsequent visits as one way to determine treatment effectiveness.

Morning (What Is It Like When You First Get up?)

Most MS problems are better in the morning when eased by rest. Some degenerative joint disorders are better or less painful in the morning, but patients often report pain and/or stiffness that are eased with movement within 30 to 60 minutes. Systemic inflammatory disorders such as ankylosing spondylitis are usually better with rest, but stiffness lasts longer than 60 minutes.[3] Symptoms that are worse in the morning may be due to poor sleeping posture. Symptoms that are unchanged in the morning may be nonmechanical or minor mechanical problems.

Evening (Do the Symptoms Change as the Day Progresses?)

Clinicians should ask patients how symptoms change throughout the day or vary with workdays versus activities over non-workdays. Changes throughout the day may highlight contributing factors that should be addressed. Symptoms that are improved in the morning and remain better with movement throughout the day are likely mechanical in nature. Symptoms that are improved in the morning but worsen with the activities of the day are mechanical. Symptoms that do not vary with daily activities are minor mechanical problems or suggestive of a more serious pathology.

Review of Medical Screening Questionnaire

Review of the medical screening questionnaire (see Table 2-5) is a limited discussion of general health; a systems review intake; and an evaluation of past medical, surgical, medication, and diagnostic test histories. Synthesis of this information helps the clinician formulate a diagnosis, prognosis, and plan of care, and select direct interventions. This review screens for systemic disease that may mimic MS conditions and requires referral to another medical provider or may identify precautions or contraindications related to physical therapy intervention.

The clinician must be alert for the presence of red or yellow flags during the history and physical examination. Red flags are symptoms and/or signs suggestive of serious pathology that require referral or consultation with a medical specialist. Yellow flags are factors noted, monitored by the clinician, that may or may not require immediate referral. Yellow flags are psychological risk factors such as fears and unhelpful beliefs.[71] Blue flags, or workplace environmental risk factors, have also been identified.[71] Yellow and blue flags (Table 2-7) may assist in identifying patients who are at risk of poor prognosis.[71] If identified, modifiable risk factors become potential targets for early cognitive-behavioral and workplace interventions and improved outcomes.[71]

The clinician should be aware of common characteristics of systemic disease (Table 2-8).[3] The following discussion is a brief systems review that may reveal red or yellow flags that indicate the presence of a systemic disease

TABLE 2-7. SUMMARY OF DIFFERENT TYPES OF FLAGS

FLAG	*NATURE*	*EXAMPLES*
Red	Signs of serious pathology	• Cauda equina syndrome, fracture, tumor
Orange	Psychiatric symptoms	• Clinical depression, personality disorder
Yellow	Beliefs, appraisals, and judgments	• Unhelpful beliefs about pain: indication of injury as uncontrollable or likely to worsen • Expectations of poor treatment outcome, delayed return to work
	Emotional responses	• Distress not meeting criteria for diagnosis of mental disorder • Worry, fears, anxiety
	Pain behavior (including pain coping strategies)	• Avoidance of activities due to expectations of pain and possible reinjury • Over-reliance on passive treatments (hot packs, cold packs, analgesics)
Blue	Perceptions about the relationship between work and health	• Belief that work is too onerous and likely to cause further injury • Belief that workplace supervisor and workmates are unsupportive
Black	System or contextual obstacles	• Legislation restricting options for return to work • Conflict with insurance staff over injury claim • Overly solicitous family and health care providers • Heavy work, with little opportunity to modify duties

Reprinted from Nicholas MK, Linton SJ, Watson PJ, Main CJ, "Decade of the Flags" Working Group. Early identification and management of psychological risk factors ("yellow flags") in patients with low back pain: a reappraisal. *Phys Ther.* 2011;91:737-753, with permission of the American Physical Therapy Association. Copyright © 2011 American Physical Therapy Association.

process or factors that may influence the examination or management of patients referred to physical therapy. An excellent reference by Goodman and Snyder[3] is available to assist in screening for systemic illness that can mimic neuromusculoskeletal conditions.

General Health

Patients are often asked, "In general, how would you rate your health?" The response choices are usually excellent, very good, good, fair, or poor. Self-assessment of general health is a complex process related to the patient's experience with and knowledge of disease causes and consequences. Health status rated as poor is predictive of future mortality,[72] functional limitations,[73] and the development of chronic conditions.[74] The patient's response to the general health question is a potential warning signal, but as with all risk factors or red flags should be considered in the context of the whole person and the clinical presentation. Exploring general health status gives insight into the patient's clinical presentation and the prognosis for rehabilitation.

Constitutional Symptoms

Fever, chills, night sweats, nausea, vomiting, diarrhea, pallor, dizziness, syncope, fatigue, and weight loss are the central signs and symptoms often present with systemic illness. These signs and symptoms can occur any time during an episode of care and are commonly associated with many diseases such as the common flu, occult infection, or cancer. Other constitutional symptoms and a persistent low-grade (< 95°F) or high-grade (99.5°F to 102°F or higher) temperature may indicate a serious illness or more urgent

Table 2-8. Common Signs and Symptoms Suggestive of Systemic Illness, Red or Yellow Flags

CONSTITUTIONAL	Fevers, chills, night or day sweats, nausea, vomiting, diarrhea, pallor, dizziness, syncope, fatigue, unexplained weight loss or gain; altered respiration, pulse, blood pressure, temperature; history of cancer
INTEGUMENT	Alterations of skins, nails, hair (eg, wounds, abrasion, bruises, edema, rashes, moles)
CARDIOVASCULAR AND PULMONARY	Chest pain, palpitations, diaphoresis, difficulty breathing; nausea, vomiting, persistent cough; calf pain (deep vein thrombosis); dizziness, headache; overweight or obese, abnormal vital signs; peripheral edema anemia, PVD (claudication)
GASTROINTESTINAL	Abdominal pain, swallowing difficulties, indigestion, heartburn, food intolerance; nausea/vomiting, bowel dysfunction (diarrhea, bloody, color or shape changes in stool)
GENITOURINARY	Pain with urination; blood in urine, increased or decreased frequency, urgency, force of urination; incontinence; impotence, pain with intercourse; reproductive status; pregnancy
NEUROLOGICAL	Numbness, paresthesia, weakness, radicular pain; altered vision, hearing, balance, cognitive status; dizziness, vertigo, tremors, headaches; history of falls
ENDOCRINE	History of diabetes or metabolic bone disorders: osteoporosis, osteomalacia; temperature intolerance
IMMUNOLOGICAL	History of inflammatory rheumatic disorders: rheumatic arthritis, psoriatic arthritis; human immunodeficiency virus, ankylosing spondylitis, multiple sclerosis; lymph node changes
PSYCHOLOGICAL	Depression, anxiety, history of posttraumatic stress disorder, sleep/personality/eating disorders; fear-avoidance beliefs or behavior
MUSCULOSKELETAL	Potential for bone infection, septic arthritis, cellulitis, fracture; history of cancer

Data adapted from Goodman CC, Snyder TE. *Differential Diagnosis for Physical Therapists: Screening for Referral.* Philadelphia, PA: Saunders; 2007.

nature and referral, respectively.[3,75] A sense of feeling "chilled" is often reported along with fever. Unexplained nausea or vomiting may be related to pregnancy, cancer, medications, gastrointestinal disease, and severe vestibular disorders and migraine headaches.[75]

Fever and night sweats are associated with systemic diseases and should be discussed with the primary care physician. Night sweats result from a gradual increase in body temperature followed by a rapid drop in temperature due to changes in immunologic, neurologic, or endocrine function. Night sweats are also associated with menopause, poor room ventilation, and other medications.

Changes in appetite and unexplained weight loss may be due to a variety of conditions such as gastrointestinal disorders, diabetes mellitus, malignancy, hyperthyroidism, and depression.[76] A 10% loss of weight during a 4-week period unrelated to intentional diet is suggestive of a neoplasm. A 5% to 10% unexplained weight loss or gain over a 6- to 12-month period is a warning sign of underlying disease.[77] Congestive heart failure, hypothyroidism, cancer, and renal or liver disease may result in significant unexplained weight gain.[3]

Fatigue or loss of energy is a common complaint that may result from depression, infection such as hepatitis, anemia, cancer, nutritional deficits, medications, or rheumatoid arthritis.[76] Fatigue becomes a red flag when the tiredness interferes with the patient's ability to carry out typical daily activities at home, work, social settings, school, or during rehabilitation and when the fatigue has lasted for 2 to 4 weeks or longer.[78]

Nausea and vomiting are usually associated with gastrointestinal disorders. Low-grade nausea may be linked with medication side effects or metastatic disease. The clinician must pursue an explanation of these symptoms and whether the symptoms seem to be getting worse, and consider referral for further investigation.

Dizziness, lightheadedness, and syncope may be related to adverse effects of medication, blood pressure problems, hypoglycemia, vestibular problems, or cervicogenic in origin. If dizziness is a symptom, the clinician must determine a baseline of its description and how and when it occurs. Lightheadedness or feeling faint is often associated with cardiac and vascular insufficiency that is worse with standing and better with lying down. Vestibular disease often presents with sensations of the head spinning or the room spinning around the patient.

Integumentary System

Observation of the skin is continuous throughout the interview and physical examination. The clinician examines for surgical wounds, abrasions, bruises, edema, rashes, or other suspicious alterations in skin, hair, and nail color or condition.

Cardiovascular and Pulmonary Systems

Body mass index (BMI), blood pressure, pulse, and respiratory rates are basic measures of general health that should be established at the initial visit. Baseline information obtained may result in a referral to a medical specialist or used to develop the plan of care. Overweight (BMI of 25.0 to 29.9 kg/m^2) or obese (BMI > 30 kg/m^2) adults are at risk of morbidity from hypertension, type 2 diabetes; stroke; gall bladder disease; osteoarthritis; sleep apnea and respiratory problems; and endometrial, breast, prostate, and colon cancer.[79]

Normal blood pressure ranges, resting pulse rates, and respiratory rates vary with age, but many factors can affect these values. Hypertension is defined as a resting systolic blood pressure of more than 140 mm Hg or a resting diastolic blood pressure of more than 90 mm Hg.[80] Hypotension is a systolic blood pressure of below 90 mm Hg or a diastolic pressure below 60 mm Hg.[3] Guidelines for initiating or terminating activity based on blood pressure, pulse rate, and respiratory rates vary according to practice setting and patient history. Students and clinicians are referred to additional references for an in-depth review of vital signs, exercise testing, and appropriate responses to exercise.[3,81]

Difficulty with breathing may indicate cardiovascular or pulmonary disease, asthma, anxiety, or anemia. If the patient reports a history of asthma or allergies, he or she should list the specific allergy, symptoms, and medications. Anemia is a result of diminished oxygen carrying capacity of blood due to a deficiency in erythrocytes and can lead to various symptoms in individuals. Due to a diminished exercise capacity in individuals with anemia, exercise prescription should proceed with caution in consultation with the physician.[82]

PVD is the presence of atherosclerosis below the bifurcation of the abdominal aorta with clinical features of intermittent claudication, decreased pedal pulses, and coolness in a distal extremity.[83] The likelihood of a patient having PVD, as defined by an ankle-brachial index of < 0.9, was increased by male gender (odds ratio [OR] 1.6), age > 60 (OR 4.1), ischemic heart disease (OR 3.5) or cerebrovascular disease (OR 3.6), smoking (OR 1.6), diabetes mellitus (OR 2.5), hyperlipidemia (OR 1.6), or intermittent claudication (OR 5.6).[84]

A presentation of calf pain, tenderness, warmth, or lower extremity edema requires the differential diagnosis of an MS problem from a deep vein thrombosis (DVT). DVT risk factors include pregnancy, oral contraceptive, surgery, malignancy, trauma, and prolonged immobilization of the extremities such as with a cast, immobilizer, or long plane or car ride. A validated clinical prediction rule (CPR)[85] aids in the clinical assessment of DVT. Using the Wells criteria,[85] clinical assessment involves 10 weighted items with the weight shown in brackets:

1. Active cancer (ongoing treatment or within previous 6 months or palliative) [1]
2. Paralysis, paresis, or recent plaster immobilization of the lower extremities [1]
3. Bedridden for 3 days or more or major surgery within the previous 12 weeks requiring general or regional anesthesia [1]
4. Localized tenderness along the distribution of the venous system [1]
5. Entire leg swelling [1]
6. Unilateral calf swelling at least 3 cm larger than the uninvolved leg (measured 10 cm below the tibial tuberosity) [1]
7. Unilateral pitting edema, symptomatic leg only [1]
8. Dilated superficial veins (non-varicose) [1]
9. Previously documented DVT [1]
10. An alternative diagnosis at least as likely as DVT [–2]

A total score of 3 or more points suggests a high risk (73% probability of DVT), 1 to 2 points suggests moderate risk (28% probability), and a 0 or less suggests a low risk (6% probability). In secondary care using the Wells criteria,[85] less than 5% of outpatients classified as low probability have DVT. A systematic review[85] concluded that in patients with low probability on the CPR and a negative D-dimer test, a diagnosis of DVT (< 1% probability) can be excluded without ultrasound. In patients with low probability, a positive D-dimer test and a normal ultrasound also excludes a DVT diagnosis (< 1% probability). An abnormal ultrasound is considered predictive of DVT. Patients with high clinical probability require diagnostic imaging.[85] In a primary care setting, Tagelagi and Elley[86] reported that the Wells CPR used alone has only moderate sensitivity

(82%; 95% CI: 67.3 to 91.0), poor specificity (22.5%; 95% CI: 18.1 to 27.7), and poor likelihood ratios (+LR 1.06; CI: 0.90 to 1.24; –LR 0.80; CI: 0.39 to 1.16), limiting their use in the diagnosis of DVT in primary care. Poor study design may have contributed to these findings. Additional studies are needed in the primary care setting.[85] The Wells criteria[85] to classify patients at risk for lower extremity DVT may aid in deciding whether a patient should be referred for further diagnostic testing.

Musculoskeletal System

MS disorders that require referral to a medical specialist include but are not limited to cancers, infections, fractures, and inflammatory arthritides. Analysis of the mechanism of injury should indicate if sufficient force occurred to cause a fracture. In the presence of decreased bone density, a minor force such as sneezing or opening a window is enough to cause a fracture. A variety of systemic diseases and medications are associated with diminished bone density. Clinicians should adjust examination and intervention procedures in the presence of compromised bone density. In instances of suspected fracture, appropriate referral for imaging is indicated prior to the physical therapy examination and/or intervention. Osteomyelitis or bone infection may spread from a wound, systemic infection, or injection site. The presence of local and systemic symptoms should raise the clinician's suspicion of a bone infection or septic arthritis. Constitutional symptoms or inability to bear weight, constant pain, and marked tenderness at the joint or site of infection are additional factors that suggest serious pathology of the MS system.

Risk of Falls

The screening process may reveal 4 patterns:

1. No falling pattern
2. Just starting to fall
3. Falls often or more than once every 6 months
4. Fear of falling

When the patient describes a potential balance impairment, a detailed neuromuscular and balance examination is indicated. Vital signs and medication should also be screened.

Gastrointestinal System

Reports of swallowing difficulties, indigestion, food intolerance, or bowel dysfunction are typically linked to the gastrointestinal system. Melena, the passage of black, tarry stools (sticky and shiny), suggests gastrointestinal bleeding. The passage of bright, blood-red stools suggests a problem in the left side of the colon or the anorectal area. A change in shape or caliber (pencil-like, flat, or ribbon-like) suggests carcinoma of the anus or distal colon. The color and shape of stool, constipation, and diarrhea require follow-up questioning about onset, progression, and additional symptoms and may warrant referral.

Even though most abdominal pain has a visceral origin, the MS system must be ruled out as a cause. Sparkes et al[87] have identified predictors of abdominal pain that are likely MS in origin. A "yes" response to 2 questions, "Does a cough, sneeze, or deep breath aggravate your symptoms?" and "Does bending, sitting, lifting, twisting, or turning over in bed aggravate your symptoms?" yields a sensitivity of 0.76, specificity of 0.84, positive LR of 4.2, and negative LR of 0.39. An added "no" response to all of the following questions: "Has there been a change in bowel habits since onset of symptoms?" "Does eating foods aggravate your symptoms?" and "Has your weight changed since onset of symptoms?" yields a sensitivity of 0.96, specificity of 0.96, positive LR of 16.8, and negative LR of 0.34. Asking these questions aids in differentiation and early recognition of patients with abdominal pain that is likely of MS origin.

Genitourinary System

Problems with the genitourinary system relate to both reproduction and urination. Blood in the urine is a common finding of many diseases of the genitourinary tract. Any change from usual patterns such as increased or decreased frequency, urgency, increased amount or reduced force, incontinence, and/or pain with urination requires additional questioning and physician consultation. If the patient is pregnant, a general discussion of progression, potential complications, or concerns should occur.

Neurological System

Reports of numbness, paresthesia, or weakness indicate the need for a detailed neurological screening examination for either a lower motor neuron or upper motor neuron disorder. The primary red flags for neurologic impairment in patients with spinal pain are progressive sensory or strength deficits, reports of "saddle" anesthesia, urinary retention, increased urinary frequency, overflow incontinence, bilateral extremity deficits, or combined upper and lower extremity deficits. Weakness is investigated to determine whether it is the result of spinal nerve root compression; peripheral nerve lesion; disuse; inhibition due to pain or swelling; injury to the contractile or inert tissues; or a more serious pathology such as a CNS disorder, fracture, or tendon avulsion. Weakness that prevents the performance of normal daily activities with no other neurological symptoms is likely to be a yellow flag. Observable weakness such as a drop foot may be a red flag, especially in the presence of other neurological symptoms including sensory changes, balance difficulties, or visual impairments.

Altered cognitive status may be the presenting problem associated with many underlying physical or neurological disorders in the elderly and should be differentiated from delirium and depression.[88] Memory loss, memory decline, or dementia is frequently screened using the Mini-Mental State Exam (MMSE).[89] The summed score of 2 questions from the MMSE—the time orientation and serial sevens test—is a simple predictor for cognitive impairment. The clinician first asks the patient the month, day of the month, day of the week, year, and season. The patient receives one point for each correct answer. Next, the patient is asked to count backwards from 100 by sevens with a maximum of 5 answers and one point for each correct answer. The maximum score for both tests is 10 points. Onishia et al[90] reported a cutoff score of 7 for the 2 tests as a good predictor of cognitive impairment, yielding a sensitivity of 0.98 and specificity 0.69 in older adults.

Endocrine System

Two common conditions related to the endocrine system are diabetes mellitus and metabolic bone disorders such as osteoporosis, osteomalacia, and Paget's disease. Because osteoporosis has no observable signs or symptoms, early identification of risk factors for men and women are important. Physical examination and selected interventions require careful planning in these individuals.

Immunologic Disease

Inflammatory rheumatic disorders related to immune system dysfunction such as rheumatoid arthritis, polymyalgia rheumatica, and psoriatic arthritis are systemic diseases, not simply local muscle and joint disorders like osteoarthritis. The symptoms of joint pain, stiffness, and swelling can mimic MS dysfunction similar to osteoarthritis. Unlike osteoarthritis, patients with rheumatoid arthritis often present with generalized weakness, constitutional systems, and morning stiffness lasting longer than 1 hour and usually affecting multiple joints symmetrically. Other disorders related to immune system dysfunction include human immunodeficiency virus, ankylosing spondylitis, multiple sclerosis, and Guillain-Barré syndrome.

Psychological System

Anxiety and depression are commonly noted in patients with MS pain. Acute pain is associated with anxiety whereas depression is more frequent in chronic pain. Depression, an indicator of poor prognosis for LBP, often prolongs the recovery process.[91] Therefore, early identification and intervention are important to prevent poor outcomes. Two questions for depression are effective in screening for depressive symptoms: "During the past month, have you often been bothered by feeling down, depressed, or hopeless?" and "During the past month, have you often been bothered by little interest or pleasure in doing things?"[91] Depression is unlikely if both questions are answered "no" (Sn 0.96, Sp 0.78; +LR 4.4, –LR 0.05). Patients who respond positively to the questions should be monitored closely. If satisfactory progress is not made, the clinician should consider referral for additional testing. To improve the accuracy of the 2 screening questions, Arroll et al[92] added an additional question that is asked only if the patient responded "yes" to either of the first 2 questions: "Is this something with which you would like help?" The possible responses were "No"; "Yes, but not today"; and "Yes." Any patient who answers "yes" to one or both of the screening questions or answers "yes" to the help questions is at high risk for major depression (Sn 0.96, Sp 0.89, +LR 9.1, –LR 0.05). The clinician should consider consultation with or referral to an appropriate specialist.

Individuals with a learning disability, personality disorder, posttraumatic stress disorder, sleep disorder, depression, or anxiety are at risk for substance abuse. Common substances that alter mood or behavior include alcohol, tobacco, coffee, caffeinated beverages, depressants, stimulants, opiates, and hallucinogens. The physiologic effects and unintended consequences of abuse depend on the substance itself and involve many of the body systems.

Risk factors for eating disorders include the White, female gender, perfectionist, or high-achieving personality traits; strong athletic participation; distorted body image; and a history of sexual abuse. Men with a distorted body image and eating disorders are often preoccupied with increasing body weight and size. Abuse of performance-enhancing drugs or anabolic steroids should be considered in this population.

Medications

A detailed discussion of side effects of medication is beyond the scope of this chapter. Goodman and Snyder[3] provided a list of medications and their common side effects: antibiotics (skin reactions, noninflammatory joint pain), diuretics (muscle weakness and cramping), nonsteroidal anti-inflammatory drugs (back and/or shoulder pain due to retroperitoneal bleeding, gastrointestinal symptoms), corticosteroids (avascular necrosis femoral head, osteoporosis, immunosuppression, steroid-induced myopathy), thorazine/tranquilizers (gait disturbances), antipsychotics or antidepressants (movement disorders), contraceptives (elevated blood pressure), opioids (nausea, constipation, dry mouth, dizziness), anticoagulants (bleed or bruise easily), and statins (muscle aches and pains, weakness, myositis).

Family, Past Medical, or Surgical History

Certain diseases such as rheumatoid arthritis, diabetes, cardiovascular disorders, or kidney disease have familial tendencies.[76] Recent illness, surgery, or diagnostic testing should be thoroughly documented. Results from diagnostic tests such as radiography, magnetic resonance imaging, computed tomography, and electromyographic or laboratory testing provide objective data related to the presence of pathology and potential precautions or contraindications to the physical therapy examination or intervention. Past medical history and previous surgery or surgery related to the patient's primary complaint require additional details including the date of surgery or illness, procedure, and physician follow-up.

A reported history of cancer and advancing age are considered red flags and require due diligence on the part of the health care provider to continuously monitor for recurrence or metastasis. Bone, liver, lung, brain, and lymph nodes are the most common sites of metastasis. The primary sites for most metastatic bone disease are lung, prostate, thyroid, breast, and lymphatic tissue. Cancer in its early stages often presents without signs and symptoms. Therefore, a careful history and review for risk factors are important for early detection. The following signs and symptoms of certain cancers are useful for screening purposes[93]:

- Changes in bowel and bladder habits
- Nagging cough or hoarseness
- Unusual bleeding or discharge
- Thickening or lump in breast or elsewhere
- Indigestion or difficulty in swallowing
- Obvious change in wart or mole
- A sore that does not heal in 6 weeks
- White patches inside the mouth or white spots on the tongue

Review of the medical screening questionnaire covers symptoms associated with multiple disease states and adverse drug reactions. The checklist helps to identify red or yellow flags and body systems that require more detailed questioning and examination. The main goals for review are early identification of a systemic disease process or factors that may influence the examination, referral or management of patients referred to physical therapy.

Patient Expectations and Goals

The clinician should discuss and document the patient's expectations of recovery after physical therapy intervention. Myers et al[94] concluded that higher expectations for recovery are associated with greater functional improvement in patients with acute LBP. Simple questions may assist in gaining the patient's positive or negative perspective about recovery. Bialosky et al[95] suggested asking, as an example, "At the end of 4 weeks, what do you think the pain associated with your low back will be?" or "What do you believe your ability to return to work will be?" The response is then attached to an NRS: 0, which is no better/no worse, or 10, completely better or completely worse. A link exists between predicted expectations and outcomes related to MS pain regardless of how expectations are measured.[95] In a systematic review of literature on expectations of recovery, positive patient expectations were associated with better health outcomes.[96]

Interview Summary

At the end of the formal interview, the clinician should ask, "Are there any other problems or concerns that you would like to tell me about or that we have not discussed?" In patients with chronic pain, further insight into the emotional state of the patient may be gained from a question such as, "How do you feel about your recovery at this point in time?" The clinician should then present a brief summary of the key findings from the interview and discuss the plan for the physical examination.

Planning the Physical Examination

After completing the subjective examination, the clinician interprets the details of the patient's story to increase the likelihood of an efficient and appropriate examination. The subjective examination reveals a core set of data commonly asked of all patients, but the details are specific to each patient. These details contribute to the working diagnostic hypotheses and direct the search for further information. The database from the subjective examination guides the focus and comprehensiveness of the physical examination, but the clinician continuously adjusts according to patient responses to further testing and intervention. To plan the extent and vigor of the physical examination, the clinician considers the severity, irritability, nature, stage, and stability of the patient's symptoms or problem.[20,42]

The physical examination is not simply the blanket application of routine tests, but instead intended for the collection of additional data to test the working diagnostic hypotheses.[97] The reliability and diagnostic accuracy of tests and measures must be considered before they are selected. As discussed in Chapter 1, the diagnostic usefulness of selected tests and measures is based on the test's diagnostic properties. The LR is the most useful property

Table 2-9. Clinical Reasoning Guide to Planning the Physical Examination

ANALYZE THE DATA FROM THE HISTORY TO PLAN THE PHYSICAL EXAMINATION.

1. Are the symptoms mild (0 to 3), moderate (4 to 6), or severe (7 to 10)? Provide an example for each symptom. Self-report outcome scores.
2. Is the presentation irritable or not irritable? Provide an example for each symptom.
3. What is the nature of the condition? Provide rationale.
   a. Musculoskeletal, nonmusculoskeletal, or components of both.
   b. What is your initial working diagnostic hypothesis or classification?
      - Primary hypothesis (body structures, functions, regions to examine in detail)
      - Secondary hypothesis (body structure, functions, regions to screen on sessions 1, 2, or 3)
      - Precautions or contraindications to your examination
4. What is the stage of the disorder? (Acute, subacute, chronic; acute on chronic)
5. What is the stability of the disorder? (Getting better, worse, or staying the same)
6. What tests and measures (region/structures) should be completed at the first session?
   - Functional activities (from history)
   - Specific active movements (region[s]: detailed exam or screen for session 1)
   - Neurological examination (lower or upper motor neuron)
   - Special tests
   - Limited or full examination (Severity, Irritability, Nature, Stage, Stability (SINSS), precautions/contraindications, easy/hard to produce symptoms
7. What is the physical therapy diagnosis/classification/prognosis at the end of the subjective/physical examination?
8. What is your intervention/reassessment for session 1?
9. What evidence (research, expertise, patient preferences) supports your decision?
10. Are there potential risk factors/concerns contributing to condition? Psychosocial issues, patient education, environmental, ergonomic, comorbidities, patient expectations, etc)

to assist in altering the probability that a patient has a specific condition.[98] Appropriate selection of examination procedures should result in the data to support or negate working hypotheses by altering the pretest probability beyond the treatment threshold or the point where the examination stops and treatment begins.

The clinician plans what needs to be examined and in what detail with consideration of the following content:

- Body structures or regions
- Functional activities or specific movements
- Specific tests
- Neurological examination
- Precautions or contraindications
- Performing a limited or full examination

Table 2-9 is a sample clinical reasoning guide used for planning the examination. The clinician also considers risk factors associated with the development of the patient's problem or other factors contributing to the condition such as posture, ergonomics, conditioning, depression, job requirements, body awareness and sensorimotor integrity, trauma, previous episodes, and other medical problems. Both inexperienced and experienced clinicians should find this form helpful to evaluate the detailed information gained from the history and to guide the physical examination. Additional planning forms with detailed questions to assist in planning the examination are available.[20,47,97]

Performing a Limited Examination

A decision to perform a limited or full examination is based on the severity, irritability, nature, stage, and stability of the presenting symptoms or disorder. Any factors that indicate a need for caution generally require a gentle, limited examination that can be performed safely without aggravating the symptoms. Factors that indicate caution include the following[97,99]:

- Symptoms at rest that increase quickly with movement and take a long time to settle
- Symptoms that are worsening
- History or recent traumatic onset or surgical history
- Subjective indications of loss of structural integrity (rheumatoid arthritis) or neurological or vascular compromise
- Symptoms that do not behave in a predictable pattern
- General health considerations such as osteoporosis or use of anticoagulant medications

The number of tests performed is limited to only a few, the most important, and taken only to the point of onset or increase in symptoms. Monitoring the return of symptoms to baseline between test procedures is critical to preventing a worsening due to the examination. Any movement or position that eases or relieves symptoms may be useful as treatment. Initial treatment is then directed at symptom reduction. Further examination takes place at subsequent visits. Appendix A provides a case history illustration to consider performing a limited examination.

Performing a Full Examination

If the subjective examination does not reveal factors that require caution, the clinician is able to perform a full examination to establish a diagnostic classification that guides the initial intervention and management. Because it is unlikely that the examination will exacerbate the patient's symptoms or problem, the clinician proceeds to the fullest extent needed, limited only by the time available at the initial visit. The extent and vigor needed is a complex decision determined by the findings of the subjective examination, clinical expertise, the most important test procedures, and the goals of the physical examination. In reality, the examination process results in a range of test procedures, some performed maximally, others limited or deferred to the next visit. The clinician prioritizes the region(s), functional activities, and movements to be examined, and the sequence of the test procedures. Appendix B provides a case history illustration to consider performing a full examination.

Summary

The subjective examination seeks to identify key information from patients and the context and details specific to the patient's presenting problems. This early information provides the basis to form initial diagnostic hypotheses or classifications that then guide the focus and comprehensiveness of the physical examination. Obtaining accurate, relevant data from the patient history aids in differentiating between MS and non-MS disorders, planning the physical examination, and implementing an effective intervention. Table 2-10 summarizes the elements of the history that assist in differentiating an MS from a non-MS disorder.

References

1. American Physical Therapy Association. Guide to Physical Therapy Practice, 2nd edition. *Phys Ther.* 2001;81:9-746.
2. Sackett DL, Rennie D. The science of the art of the clinical examination. *JAMA.* 1992;267:2650-2652.
3. Goodman CC, Snyder TE. *Differential Diagnosis for Physical Therapists: Screening for Referral.* Philadelphia, PA: Saunders; 2007.
4. Crombie DL. Diagnostic process. *J Coll Gen Pract.* 1963;6:579-589.
5. Sandler G. The importance of the history in the medical clinic and the cost of unnecessary tests. *Am Heart J.* 1980;100:928-931.
6. Jensen GM, Shepard KF, Hack LM. The novice versus the experienced clinician: insights into the work of the physical therapist. *Phys Ther.* 1990;70:314-323.
7. Jensen GM, Gwyer J, Shepard KF, Hack LM. Expert practice in physical therapy. *Phys Ther.* 2000;80:28-43.
8. Duffy DF. Dialogue: a core clinical skill. *Ann Intern Med.* 1998;128:139-141.
9. Simpson M, Buckman R, Stewart M, et al. Doctor-patient communication: the Toronto consensus statement. *BMJ.* 1991;303:1385-1387.
10. Roter DL, Hall JA, Katz NR. Patient-physician communication: a descriptive summary of the literature. *Patient Educ Couns.* 1988;12:99-119.
11. Evans BJ, Stanley RO, Mestrovic R, et al. Effects of communication skills training on student's diagnostic efficiency. *Med Educ.* 1991;25:517-526.
12. Stewart M, Brown JB, Donner A, et al. The impact of patient-centered care on outcomes. *J Fam Pract.* 2000;49:796-804.
13. Bates AS, Harris LE, Tierney WM, et al. Dimensions and correlates of physician work satisfaction in a Midwestern city. *Med Care.* 1998;36:610-617.
14. Levinson W, Stiles WB, Inui TS, et al. Physician frustrations in communicating with patients. *Med Care.* 1993;31:285-295.
15. Smith RC, Lyles JS, Mettler J, et al. The effectiveness of intensive training for residents in interviewing: a randomized, controlled clinical trial. *Ann Intern Med.* 1998;128:118-126.
16. Smith RC, Lyles JS, Mettler J, et al. A strategy for improving patient satisfaction by the intensive training of residents in psychosocial medicine: a controlled, randomized study. *Acad Med.* 1995;70:729-732.
17. Smith RC, Osborh G, Hoppe RB, et al. Efficacy of a one-month training block in psychosocial medicine for residents: controlled study. *J Gen Intern Med.* 1991;6:535-553.
18. Levinson W, Roter DL, Mullooly JP, et al. Physician-patient communication: the relationship with malpractice claims among primary care physicians and surgeons. *JAMA.* 1997;227:553-559.
19. Boissonnault WG, ed. *Primary Care for the Physical Therapist. Examination and Triage.* Philadelphia, PA: Saunders; 2005.
20. Maitland GD. *Vertebral Manipulation.* 6th ed. Woburn, MA: Butterworth-Heinemann; 2002.
21. Lyles JS, Dwamena FC, Lein C, Smith RC. Evidence-based patient centered interviewing. *J Clin Outcomes Manag.* 2001;8(7):28-34.

TABLE 2-10. SUBJECTIVE DATA THAT MAY AID IN DIFFERENTIATING A MUSCULOSKELETAL FROM A NONMUSCULOSKELETAL DISORDER

SUBJECTIVE DATA	MUSCULOSKELETAL	NONMUSCULOSKELETAL
Description of symptoms	Local symptoms, aching, cramping, stiffness with rest; constant and variable or intermittent (no pain at rest); deep or superficial; possible referral to distant sites	Stabbing, cutting, boring, throbbing, bone pain; constant nonvarying but may come in waves; tends to be deep; possible referral to distant sites
History (current and previous episodes)	Sudden or gradual onset usually precipitated by a trauma (micro- or macro-); may be chronic (off/on over months or years) in nature	Recent, sudden onset for no apparent reason; cycle nature (gets worse, better, then worse again)
Aggravating factors	Predictable pattern of response (getter better or worse) to position, rest, and activity	Unpredictable pattern (minimal, temporary, or no response) of response to position, rest or activity; may be related to eating, breathing, bowel or bladder function
Easing factors	Symptoms eased or abolished with rest or position change	Symptoms unchanged by rest or position change; however, may be organ dependent (eg, kidney pain is often eased by leaning to the painful side)
24-hour behavior	Infrequently awakens at night usually due to position, able to return to sleep quickly; usually better with rest	Awakens patient at night consistently, difficulty returning to sleep; may need to get up and walk around; most intense pain at night
Other	No constitutional symptoms or warning signs of cancer	• Constitutional symptoms • Warning signs of cancer • Red or yellow flags identified on systems review • Poor progress or worsening with physical therapy despite good prognosis • Abnormal vital signs

22. Boissonnault WG, Koopmeiners MB. Medical history profile: orthopaedic physical therapy outpatients. *J Orthop Sports Phys Ther.* 1994;20:2-10.
23. Boissonnault WG. Prevalence of comorbid conditions, surgeries, and medication use in a physical therapy outpatient population: a multicentered study. *J Orthop Sports Phys Ther.* 1999;29:506-519; discussion 520-525.
24. Gilkison CR, Fenton MV, Lester JW. Getting the story straight: evaluating the test-retest reliability of a university health history questionnaire. *J Am Coll Health.* 1992;40:247-252.
25. Inui TS, Jared RA, Carter WB, et al. Effects of a self-administered health history on new-patient visits in a general medical clinic. *Med Care.* 1979;17:1221-1228.
26. Katz JN, Chang LC, Sangha O, et al. Can comorbidity be measured by questionnaire rather than medical record review? *Med Care.* 1996;34:73-84.
27. Pecoraro RE, Inui TS, Chen MS, et al. Validity and reliability of a self-administered health history questionnaire. *Public Health Rep.* 1979;94:231-238.
28. Boissonnault WG, Badke MB. Collecting health history information: the accuracy of a patient self-administered questionnaire in an orthopedic outpatient setting. *Phys Ther.* 2005;85:531-543.
29. Boissonnault WG. Patient health history including identification of health risk factors. In: Boissonnault WG, ed. *Primary Care for the Physical Therapist. Examination and Triage.* Philadelphia, PA: Saunders; 2005:61-65.
30. Jette DU, Halbert J, Iverson C, Miceli E, Shah P. Use of standardized outcome measures in physical therapist practice: perceptions and applications. *Phys Ther.* 2009;89(2):125-135.
31. George SZ, Fritz JM, Childs JD. Investigation of elevated fear-avoidance beliefs for patients with low back pain: a secondary analysis involving patients enrolled in physical therapy clinical trials. *J Orthop Sports Phys Ther.* 2008;38(2):50-58.
32. Lansky D, Butler JBV, Waller FT. Using health status measures in the hospital setting: from acute care to outcomes management. *Med Care.* 1992;30:MS57-MS73.

33. Flynn T, Fritz J, Whitman J, et al. A clinical prediction rule for classifying patients with low back pain who demonstrate short-term improvement with spinal manipulation. *Spine.* 2002;27:2835-2843.
34. Childs JD, Fritz JM, Flynn TW, et al. A clinical prediction rule to identify patients with low back pain most likely to benefit from spinal manipulation: a validation study. *Ann Intern Med.* 2004;141:920-928.
35. Portney LG, Watkins MP. *Foundations of Clinical Research: Application to Practice.* 2nd ed. Upper Saddle River, NJ: Prentice Hall Health; 2000.
36. Binkley JM, Stratford PW, Lott SA, et al. The Lower Extremity Functional Scale (LEFS): scale development, measurement properties, and clinical application. North American Orthopaedic Rehabilitation Research Network. *Phys Ther.* 1999;79:371-383.
37. Wainner RS. Reliability of the clinical examination: how close is "close enough"? *J Orthop Sports Phys Ther.* 2003;33:488-491.
38. Resnik L, Dobrzykowski E. Guide to outcomes measurement for patients with low back pain syndromes. *J Orthop Sports Phys Ther.* 2003:33:307-316.
39. Jernal A, Tiwari RC, Murray T, et al. Cancer statistics. *CA Cancer J Clin.* 2004;54:8-29.
40. Goodman CC, Fuller KS. Pathology. *Implications for the Physical Therapist.* 3rd ed. St. Louis, MO: Saunders; 2009.
41. American Cancer Society. *Cancer Facts and Figures 2008.* Atlanta, GA: Author; 2008. http://www.cancer.org/acs/groups/content/@nho/documents/document/2008cafffinalsecuredpdf.pdf. Accessed May 20, 2013.
42. American Academy of Orthopaedic Manual Physical Therapists. *Orthopaedic Manual Physical Therapy: Description of Advanced Specialty Practice.* Tallahassee, FL: Author; 2008.
43. Godges JJ, Boissonnault WG. Symptom investigation. In: Boissonnault WG, ed. *Primary Care for the Physical Therapist. Examination and Triage.* Philadelphia, PA: Saunders; 2005:66-86.
44. Boissonnault WG, Bass C. Pathological origins of trunk and neck pain: part I—pelvic and abdominal visceral disorders. *J Orthop Sports Phys Ther.* 1990;12(5):192-207.
45. Boissonnault WG, Bass C. Pathological origins of trunk and neck pain: part II—disorders of the cardiovascular and pulmonary systems. *J Orthop Sports Phys Ther.* 1990:12(5):208-215.
46. Boissonnault WG, Bass C. Pathological origins of trunk and neck pain: part III—diseases of the musculoskeletal system. *J Orthop Sports Phys Ther.* 1990:12(5):216-221.
47. Petty NJ, Moore AP. *Neuromusculoskeletal Examination and Assessment. A Handbook for Therapists.* 2nd ed. New York, NY: Churchill Livingstone; 2002.
48. Lee MWL, McPhee RW, Stringer MD. An evidence-based approach to human dermatomes. *Clin Anat.* 2008;21:363-373.
49. International Association for the Study of Pain. IASP Taxonomy—Pain. http://www.iasp-pain.org/AM/Template.cfm?Section=Pain_Definitions&Template=/CM/HTMLDisplay.cfm&ContentID=1728#Pain. Accessed April 30, 2009.
50. Scholz J, Woolf CJ. Can we conquer pain? *Nat Neurosci.* 2002;5:1062-1067.
51. Moseley GL. Reconceptualising pain according to modern pain science. *Phys Ther Rev.* 2007;12:169-178.
52. Melzack R. Pain and the neuromatrix in the brain. *J Dent Educ.* 2001;65:1378-1382.
53. Melzack R. Evolution of the neuromatrix theory of pain. *Pain Pract.* 2005;5:85-94.
54. Melzack R, Casey KL. Sensory, motivational and central control determinants of pain: a new conceptual model. In: Kenshalo D, ed. *The Skin Senses.* Springfield, IL: Charles C. Thomas; 1968:423-443.
55. Moseley GL. A pain neuromatrix approach to patients with chronic pain. *Man Ther.* 2003;8(3):130-140.
56. Waddell G. *The Back Pain Revolution.* 2nd ed. New York, NY: Churchill Livingston; 2004.
57. Christensen N, Jones MA, Carr J. Clinical reasoning in orthopedic manual therapy. In: Grant R, ed. *Physical Therapy of the Cervical and Thoracic Spine.* 3rd ed. St Louis, MO: Churchill Livingstone; 2002:85-104.
58. Jefferson J. *Low Back Pain and the Evidence for Effectiveness of Physical Therapy Interventions. Independent Study Course 18.1.3. Lumbar Examination and Assessment.* Lacrosse, WI: Orthopedic Section, American Physical Therapy Association; 2008.
59. Strong J, Sturgess J, Unruh AM, Vincenzino B. Pain assessment and measurement. In: Strong J, Unruh AM, Wright A, Baxter GD, eds. *Pain: A Textbook for Therapists.* Edinburgh, UK: Churchill Livingstone; 2002:123-147.
60. Magee DF. *Orthopedic PhysicalAssessment.* 5th ed. Philadelphia, PA: Saunders; 2008.
61. Bogduk N, Twomey LT. *Clinical Anatomy of the Lumbar Spine.* 2nd ed. New York, NY: Churchill Livingstone; 1991.
62. Spitzer WO, Leblanc FE, Dupuis M, et al. Scientific approach to the assessment and a management of activity-related spinal disorders: a monograph for physicians: report of the Quebec Task Force on Spinal Disorders. *Spine.* 1987;12:7(suppl):s1-s59.
63. Bogduk N, McGuirk B. *Medical Management of Acute and Chronic Low Back Pain: An Evidence-Based Approach.* Amsterdam, The Netherlands: Elsevier Health Sciences; 2002.
64. Roland M, Fairbank J. The Roland-Morris Disability Questionnaire and the Oswestry Disability Questionnaire. *Spine.* 2000;25:3115-3124.
65. Breivik H Borchgrevink PC, Allen SM, et al. *Br J Anaesth.* 2008;101:17-24.
66. Stratford PW, Spadoni G. The reliability, consistency, and clinical application of a numeric pain rating scale. *Physiother Can.* 2001;53(2):88-91.
67. Farrar JT, Young JP, LaMoreaux L, Werth JL, Poole RM. Clinical importance of changes in chronic pain intensity measured on an 11-point numerical pain rating scale. *Pain.* 2001;94(2):149-158.
68. Kelly AM. The minimum clinically significant difference in visual analogue scale pain score does not differ with severity of pain. *Emerg Med J.* 2001;18:205-207.
69. Jensen MP, Karoly P. Self-report scales and procedures for assessing pain in adults. In: Turk DC, Melzack R, eds. *Handbook of Pain Assessment.* New York, NY: Guilford; 1992;135-151.
70. Good M, Stiller C, Zauszniewski JA, Anderson GC, Stanton-Hicks M, Grass JA. Sensation and distress of pain scales: reliability, validity, and sensitivity. *J Nurs Meas.* 2001;9:219-238.
71. Nicholas MK, Linton SJ, Watson PJ, Main CJ, "Decade of the Flags" Working Group. Early identification and management of psychological risk factors ("yellow flags") in patients with low back pain: a reappraisal. *Phys Ther.* 2011;91:737-753.
72. Idler EL, Benyamini Y. Self-rated health and mortality: a review of twenty-seven community studies. *J Health Soc Behav.* 1997;38:21-37.
73. Idler EL, Russell LB, Davis D. Survival, functional limitations, and self-rated health in the NHANES I Epidemiologic Follow-up Study 1992; First National Health and Nutrition Examination Survey. *Am J Epidemiol.* 2000;9:874-883.

74. Kopec JA, Schultz SE, Goel V, Williams JI. Can the Health Utilities Index measure change? *Med Care.* 2001;39:562-574.
75. Boissonnault WG. Review of systems. In: Boissonnault WG, ed. *Primary Care for the Physical Therapist. Examination and Triage.* Philadelphia, PA: Saunders; 2005:87-104.
76. Bates B. *A Guide to Physical Examination and History Taking.* 8th ed. Philadelphia, PA: Lippincott Williams & Wilkins; 2003.
77. Swartz MH. *Textbook of Physical Diagnosis.* 4th ed. Philadelphia, PA: WB Saunders; 2002.
78. Morrison RE, Keating HJ. Fatigue in primary care. *Prim Prev Care Obstet Gynecol.* 2001;28:225-240.
79. National Heart, Lung, and Blood Institute. Rationale. In: *Guidelines on Overweight and Obesity: Electronic Textbook.* http://www.nhlbi.nih.gov/guidelines/obesity/e_txtbk/ratnl/20.htm. Accessed June 22, 2009.
80. Boissonnault WG. Review of cardiovascular and pulmonary systems and vital signs. In: Boissonnault WG, ed. *Primary Care for the Physical Therapist. Examination and Triage.* Philadelphia, PA: Saunders; 2005:126-128.
81. American College of Sports Medicine. *ACSM's Guidelines for Exercise Testing and Prescription.* 8th ed. Philadelphia, PA: Lippincott Williams & Wilkins; 2009.
82. Callahan LA, Woods KF, Mensah GA, Ramsey LT, Barbeau P, Gutin B. Cardiopulmonary responses to exercise in women with sickle cell anemia. *Am J Respir Crit Care Med.* 2002;165:1309-1316.
83. Sontheimer DL. Peripheral vascular disease: diagnosis and treatment. *Am Fam Phys.* 2006;73:1971-1976.
84. Stoffers HE, Kester AD, Kaiser V, Rinkens P, Knottnerus JA. Diagnostic value of signs and symptoms associated with peripheral arterial occlusive disease seen in general practice: a multivariable approach. *Med Decis Making.* 1997;17:61-70.
85. Wells PS, Owen C, Doucette S, et al. Does this patient have deep venous thrombosis? *JAMA.* 2006;295(2):199-207.
86. Tagelagi M, Elley CR. Accuracy of the Wells Rule in diagnosing deep vein thrombosis in primary health care. *J N Z Med Assoc.* 2007;120.
87. Sparkes V, Prevost AT, Hunter JO. Derivation and identification of questions that act as predictors of abdominal pain of musculoskeletal origin. *Eur J Gastroenterol Hepatol.* 2003;15:1021-1027.
88. Wenker S, Euhardy M. The geriatric population. In: Boissonnault WG, ed. *Primary Care for the Physical Therapist: Examination and Triage.* 2nd ed. Philadelphia, PA: Saunders; 2011:367-368.
89. Folstein MF, Folstein SE, McHugh PR. "Mini-Mental State": a practical method for grading the cognitive state of patients for the clinician. *J Psychiatr Res.* 1975;12:196-198.
90. Onishia J, Suzukia Y, Umegakia H, Kawamurab T, Imaizumic M, Iguchia A. Which two questions of Mini-Mental State Examination (MMSE) should we start from? *Arch Gerontol Geriatr.* 2007;44:43-48.
91. Haggman S, Maher CG, Refshauge KM. Screening for symptoms of depression by physical therapists managing low back pain. *Phys Ther.* 2004;84:1157-1166.
92. Arroll B, Goodyear-Smith F, Kerse N, Fishman T, Gunn J. Effect of the addition of a "help" question to two screening questions on specificity for diagnosis of depression in general practice: diagnostic validity study. *BMJ.* 2005;331:884.
93. American Cancer Society. Signs and symptoms of cancer: what are signs and symptoms? http://www.cancer.org/Cancer/CancerBasics/signs-and-symptoms-of-cancer. Revised August 13, 2012. Accessed June 28, 2011.
94. Myers SS, Phillips RS, Davis RB, et al. Patient expectations as predictors of outcome in patients with acute low back pain. *J Gen Intern Med.* 2008;23(2):148-153.
95. Bialosky JE, Bishop MD, Cleland JA. Individual expectation: an overlooked, but pertinent, factor in the treatment of individuals experiencing musculoskeletal pain. *Phys Ther.* 2010;90:1345-1355.
96. Mondloch MV, Cole DC, Frank JW. Does how you do depend on how you think you'll do? A systematic review of the evidence for a relation between patients' recovery expectations and health outcomes. *Can Med Assoc J.* 2001;165(2):174-179.
97. Jones MA, Jones HM. Principles of the physical examination. In: Boyling JD, Jull GA, eds. *Grieve's Modern Manual Therapy: The Vertebral Column.* 2nd ed. London, England: Churchill Livingstone; 1994:483-501.
98. Cleland JA. *Orthoapedic Clinical Examination: An Evidence-Based Approach for Physical Therapists.* Carlstadt, NJ: Icon Learning System LLC; 2005.
99. Magarey M. Examination of the cervical and thoracic spine. In: Grant R, ed. *Physical Therapy of the Cervical and Thoracic Spine.* 3rd ed. St. Louis, MO: Churchill Livingstone; 2002:105-137.

Chapter 3

Components of the Basic Neuromusculoskeletal Examination
Tests and Measures

After completing the history, the clinician interprets the gathered information to increase the likelihood of performing an efficient and effective physical examination. The history reveals a core data set commonly asked of all patients, but the details are specific to each patient. These details contribute to the working diagnostic classification and direct the search for supporting or negating information during the physical examination. Data from the history guide the focus and comprehensiveness of the initial physical examination, but the clinician continuously modifies according to the patient's response to additional tests and intervention. As discussed in Chapter 2, planning the extent of the physical examination requires the clinician to judge the severity, irritability, nature, stage, and stability of the patient's symptoms or problem.[1]

The data obtained during the physical examination specifically tests the diagnostic hypotheses generated during the history until a treatment threshold or initial diagnosis is reached. The physical therapist's challenge is to select, perform, and interpret the necessary diagnostic tests along with key history data for each patient, and then integrate the findings into patient management. The process of selecting and interpreting diagnostic tests involves understanding why tests are performed. Diagnostic tests are performed to differentiate among competing diagnostic classifications, detect structural pathology, rule in or rule out contributing regions of interest, identify disorders not appropriate for physical therapy, and/or assist with selecting specific interventions.

Cook and Hegedus[2] identified clinical tests with the highest diagnostic utility for spinal conditions. These authors used a cutoff sensitivity of 0.90 or higher and negative likelihood ratio of <0.20 for screening or ruling out disorders for general musculoskeletal (MS) conditions. For ruling in a disorder or diagnosis, a positive likelihood ratio (LR) of at least 5.0 or higher is desirable.[3] Results from the Cook and Hegedus[2] review revealed only a few tests with adequate diagnostic utility.

- For the cervical spine, the upper limb tension sign (median nerve bias), a posterior-anterior passive accessory test, and Spurling's test are effective screening tests. Only the passive side glide test at C2-3 is considered a useful diagnostic test.
- No studies related to the thoracic spine met the inclusion criteria.
- For the lumbar spine, effective screening tests are the passive straight-leg raise (SLR) for nerve root compression and the extension-rotation test for zygapophyseal pain. Centralization was diagnostic for discogenic symptoms; posterior-anterior intervertebral movements and passive physiological intervertebral movements (PPIVM) for radiographic instability; and firm closed-fist percussion in standing and the supine sign (ie, the inability to lie supine due to severe pain) for osteoporotic compression fractures.

Students and clinicians are encouraged to review the section in Chapter 1 related to determining the accuracy and usefulness of diagnostic tests and interpreting the importance of negative and positive test results (positive and negative likelihood ratios) within the diagnostic process. The physical examination is a progressive process with

Stetts DM, Carpenter JG. *Physical Therapy Management of Patients With Spinal Pain: An Evidence-Based Approach (pp 63-111).*

Table 3-1. Physical Examination Objectives

- Reproduce the patient's complaint or symptoms
- Determine the impact of postures, movement, work, and recreational factors as causes or contributors to the patient's problem
- Establish the treatment threshold for a diagnosis or diagnostic classification
- Establish an accurate data baseline from which you can measure the outcome

tests applied based on clinical reasoning and diagnostic utility. Clinical decisions related to diagnosis or diagnostic classifications are usually based on the results of a cluster of signs and symptoms and not solely on the result of one test.[2]

Goals of the Physical Examination

The physical examination has several objectives (Table 3-1). The first goal is to reproduce the patient's complaint(s). The symptoms of most neuromusculoskeletal problems are related to changes in position, movement, or activity. These symptoms can usually be reproduced or changed with various tests and measures. Occasionally, nonmusculoskeletal (non-MS) or serious pathology may be produced with position or movement; however, additional testing combined with data from the history should clarify the likelihood of a non-MS problem. Failure to change a patient's symptoms during the examination may indicate a non-MS condition or one that requires added vigor such as combined or sustained movements or repeated movement such as walking or running. For example, a clinician may find it difficult to reproduce a patient's low back pain (LBP) if it only comes on after 2 miles of running. As discussed in Chapter 2 under Differential Diagnosis, establishing a diagnosis is an ongoing process that requires evaluation of the data from both the history and physical examination, as well as following the model of assessment, intervention, and reassessment.

The second goal is to determine the impact of posture, movement, work, and recreational factors as causes of, contributors to, or perpetuators of the patient's problem. Understanding the positive or negative effects of movement or activities on the patient's symptoms may assist in determining an appropriate intervention and the overall plan of care.

The third goal is to establish the treatment threshold for a diagnostic or impairment-based classification by identifying a cluster of signs and symptoms. The physical therapy classification or diagnosis is linked to the patient's subjective data and to impairments of the articular, muscular, neural, and/or sensorimotor (balance, joint position sense) control systems and their relevance to the patient's symptoms and activity limitations. Confirmation of a diagnosis is continued throughout the episode of care. Diagnostic classification and the use of classification-based treatment approaches (ie, identification of specific LBP subgroups and the evidence-based characteristics that are likely to be most responsive to management treatment strategies) are presented in detail in subsequent chapters on LBP, thoracic pain, and cervical pain.

The final goal is to establish an accurate baseline or outcome measures from which to evaluate and progress treatment. The outcome measures focus on identifying relevant impairments, activity limitations, or participation restrictions and facilitate an understanding of the relationship among symptoms, impairments, and function.

Conducting the Physical Examination

The clinician should provide a comfortable, caring, and respectful clinical atmosphere. Preparing the examination area with appropriate equipment and supplies prior to the patient's arrival provides an opportunity for efficient data collection. Explaining what is going to happen and why reduces anxiety, provides understanding of the process, and helps to gain consent to proceed. Continual communication throughout the hands-on portion of the examination builds patient rapport and helps in obtaining an accurate patient response to test procedures. For safety and effectiveness, the clinician should utilize efficient body mechanics and perform examination techniques in a standardized manner.

Based on the data from the history, the clinician initially selects specific tests and measures depending on the region(s) to be examined and/or screened. Many tests and measures have been described for patients with lumbopelvic, thoracic, or cervical pain. Clinicians have the potential to produce significant amounts of relevant and nonrelevant data and must keep in mind that not all tests are necessary for all patients. Tests are selected based on their diagnostic usefulness and as needed for problem solving. Appropriate selection of examination procedures should result in the key findings that support or negate the working diagnostic hypotheses.

This chapter presents an overall strategy for the examination of patients presenting with neuromusculoskeletal disorders who are appropriate for physical therapy management and general guidelines for interpreting a patient's response. Selected topics related to patients with spinal pain are also discussed. Tests and measures are typically performed according to patient position (standing, sitting, supine, prone, side-lying) but are not presented here in that sequence. The examination process for each spinal region is sequenced according to patient position in subsequent chapters. Where appropriate, the uninvolved side is examined first and compared to the involved side. The clinician documents the quality, quantity, and symptom response to all tests. Resting or baseline symptoms are obtained prior to and after all test procedures throughout the examination. Attention to these guidelines results in a clear understanding of the patient's response to each procedure and prevents a worsening of the patient's symptoms due to the examination. Anthropometric data (height, weight, body mass index) and vital signs (pulse, respiration, and blood pressure) should be obtained prior to the examination procedures listed below. Table 3-2 lists the basic components of the physical examination.

TABLE 3-2. BASIC COMPONENTS OF THE PHYSICAL EXAMINATION

- Observations
- Posture
- Gait
- Balance
- Functional tests
- Active range of motion
- Passive range of motion (physiological, accessory, segmental motion testing)
- Neurological screening examination
- Muscle length tests
- Muscle performance (motor control/strength/power/endurance)
- Screen region/joints above and below
- Special tests
- Palpation

Observation

Informal observation begins as soon as the clinician greets the patient. General appearance and well-being, facial expression, assistive devices, and willingness to move are noted. Movement patterns related to transitions from sitting to standing or the reverse as well as walking may generate early hypothesis formation. In addition to informal observation of movement, the clinician should be aware of the patient's attitudes and feelings (eg, fear, anger, depression, anxiety) that may influence posture, movement, development of rapport, and compliance throughout the rehabilitation process. The patient should be appropriately gowned for mandatory inspection of the region to be examined.

Posture

Static Standing Posture

Postural deviations may be nonprotective (structural or behavioral) and protective.[4] Long-standing scoliosis is a nonprotective, structural deformity if it is not correctable with movement and attempts to correct it do not alter symptoms. A nonprotective behavioral deformity may be due to emotional state, personality, or poor body awareness. This type of posture is correctable actively or passively by the clinician without a change in symptoms, although it may still be relevant to the problem. A sustained, repetitive slumped posture may contribute to or perpetuate cervical, thoracic, and/or low back problems. A protective posture is an attempt by the patient either consciously or unconsciously to lessen symptoms. For example, a left lateral shift (Figure 3-1) in a person with LBP may be a protective posture. Correction of the shift and the patient's response determine the relevance and may guide the initial intervention.

Standing postural analysis may expose patterns of tightness and weakness suggestive of muscle imbalance that require additional tests such as balance, gait, tests of muscle length, joint mobility or muscle performance (ie, endurance, strength, activation patterns), and specific movements. According to the theory of Janda et al,[5] muscle imbalance occurs between tonic muscles, which are prone to tightness or shortness, and phasic muscles, which are prone to weakness or inhibition (Table 3-3). Muscle imbalance may occur in any group of muscles or patterns, but it often occurs in the lumbopelvic hip region (eg, lower crossed syndrome) and neck-shoulder region (eg, upper crossed syndrome).

The lower crossed syndrome (Figure 3-2) presents as stiffness of the hip flexors or erector spinae (ES) and weakness of the gluteal and abdominal muscles. Typical postural deviations include anterior pelvic tilt, increased flexion of the hips, and increased lumbar lordosis.[5] The upper crossed syndrome (Figure 3-3) presents as stiffness in the upper trapezius (UT), levator scapulae, pectoralis major, and sternocleidomastoid and weakness of the deep neck flexors and lower trapezius and serratus anterior, stabilizers of the scapula.[5] Typical postural deviations include forward head, increased upper thoracic kyphosis, anterior translation of the cervical spine, and protracted, elevated scapulae, possibly affecting all movements of the cervical spine and upper extremity. Janda et al[5] suggested that this system is most reliable when the patient is pain free or almost pain free but not in the acute pain state. Clinically,

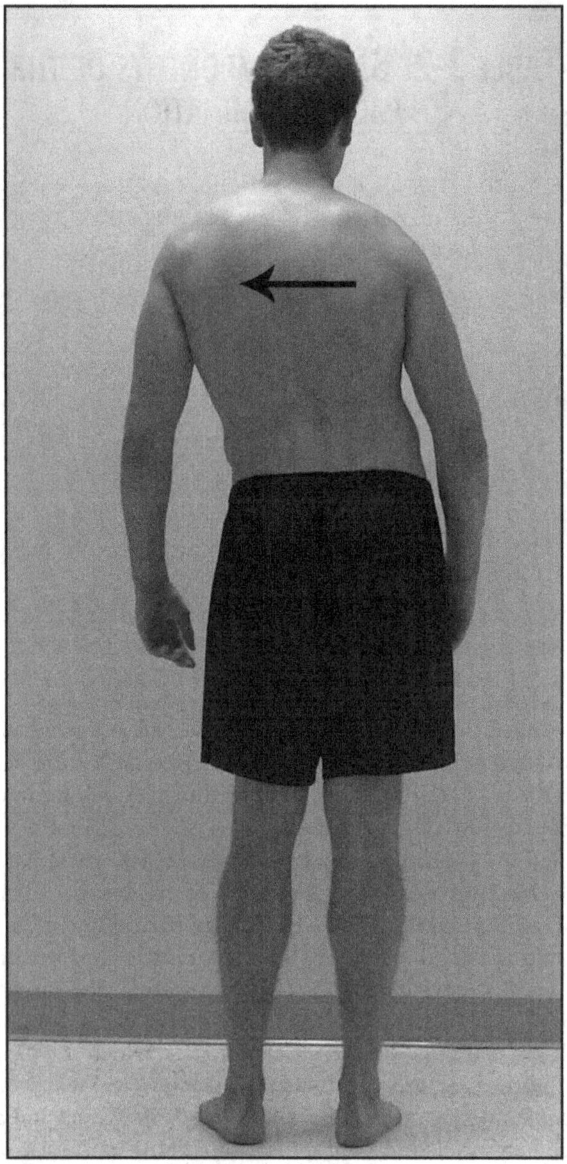

Figure 3-1. Left lateral shift.

TABLE 3-3. MUSCLE IMBALANCE

TONIC MUSCLES PRONE TO STIFFNESS OR SHORTNESS	PHASIC MUSCLES PRONE TO WEAKNESS OR INHIBITION
• Gastroc-soleus, tibialis posterior • Hip adductors • Hamstrings • Rectus femoris, iliopsoas, tensor fascia lata • Piriformis • Thoracolumbar extensors • Quadratus lumborum • UT, sternocleidomastoid • Levator scapulae, scalenes • Sternocleidomastoid • Pectoralis major, upper limb flexors	• Peroneus longus, brevis • Tibialis anterior • Vastus medialis, lateralis • Gluteus maximus, medius, minimus • Rectus abdominis • Serratus anterior • Rhomboids • Lower trapezius • Deep neck flexors • Upper limb extensors

muscle imbalance occurs in a variety of patterns and may be the cause or consequence of the patient's presenting complaint.

Kendall et al[6] described several common postures deviating from the ideal. The ideal represents "a minimal amount of stress and strain and that which is conducive to maximal efficiency in the use of the body."[7(p5)] The kyphosis-lordosis posture (Figure 3-4) is similar to the upper and lower crossed syndromes and is associated with weakness in the neck flexors, upper back ES, and external oblique (EO); stiffness in the neck extensors, hip flexors, and lumbar ES; and hamstrings may or may not be weak. The flat back posture (Figure 3-5) presents with a reduced or absent lumbar lordosis, posterior pelvic tilt, extension of the hip, slight plantarflexion of the ankle, a slightly extended cervical spine, flexion of the upper thoracic spine, and straight lower thoracic spine. Hip flexors are weak, hamstrings are stiff, and the lumbar paraspinals may be weak. A swayback posture (Figure 3-6) presents as a forward head, extended cervical spine, increased flexion and posterior displacement of the upper trunk, flexion of the upper spine, posterior pelvic tilt, hyperextension at the hips with anterior pelvis displacement, hyperextension at the knees, and neutral at the ankles.

Initially, standing posture is observed in a standardized, systematic manner including anterior, posterior, and right and left lateral views (Figure 3-7), beginning with a global screen with detailed focus on the regions of interest. The clinician looks for symmetry of body regions, trunk and extremity positions, bony and soft tissue contours (ie, scoliosis, cervical/lumbar lordosis, thoracic kyphosis, atrophy, edema), and skin, noting erythema, bruising, scars, etc. As suggested by aggravating and easing factors in the patient history, sustained or repetitive postures such as sitting, reaching, or squatting should be examined in a similar manner. A detailed description of the clinical examination of posture is described in other references.[8-10]

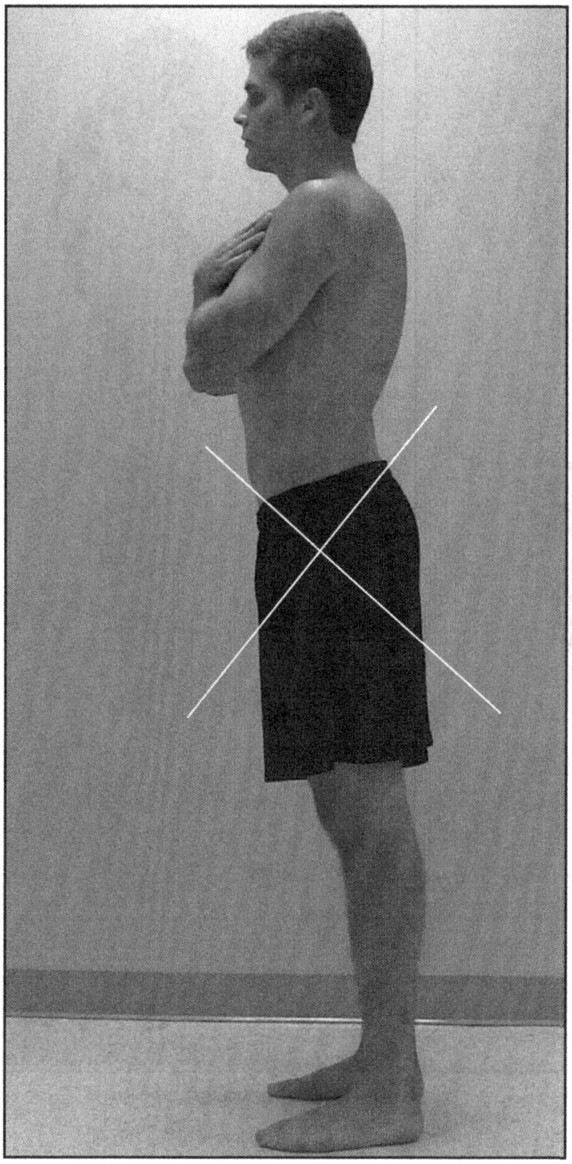

Figure 3-2. Lower crossed syndrome.

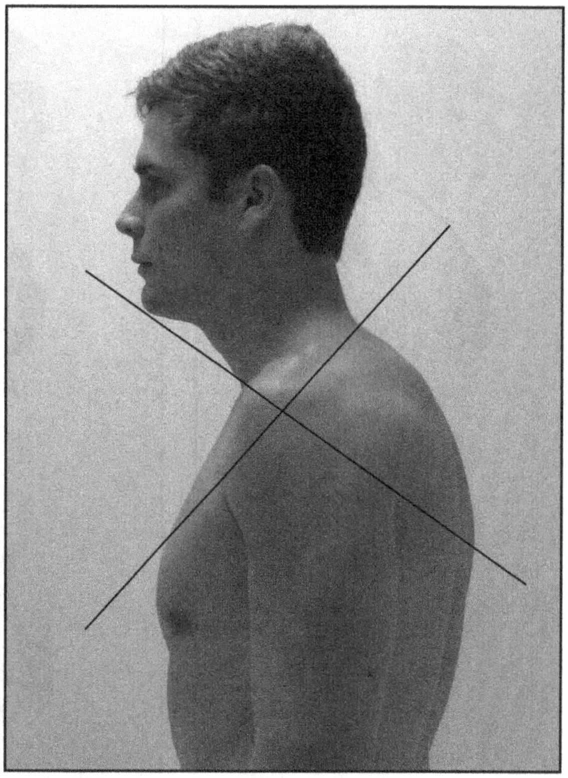

Figure 3-3. Upper crossed syndrome.

Static Sitting Posture

Evidence related to sitting as a risk factor for LBP is conflicting. Studies report no conclusive evidence[11] or report sitting as a major contributor.[12-14] Bakker et al[14] reported that strong evidence exists that prolonged standing, walking, and sitting at work are not associated with LBP. Limited evidence supports that sitting both exacerbates and perpetuates LBP.[15,16] In certain subgroups of nonspecific chronic LBP (CLBP) patients have difficulty assuming a neutral lumbar spine position in sitting. Patients with an extension pattern disorder actively hold themselves in hyperextension while patients with a flexion pattern disorder position themselves near the end of the available flexion range at the symptomatic region of the spine.[15,17,18] Despite conflicting evidence related to LBP, prolonged sitting posture is a risk factor for current and future LBP for some occupational subgroups. Bell et al[19] investigated sedentary workers who spent a mean proportion of 83% of time at work sitting and 17% of time sitting for more than 90 minutes without a break. The authors determined that current LBP (symptoms lasting >24 hours) is associated with a kyphotic posture (odds ratio [OR] 2.1, 1.1 to 4.1). For some individuals, sitting in a relatively static position and adopting a kyphotic posture significantly increases the risk of future LBP. The patient's history dictates whether assessment and ergonomic intervention are necessary.

Similarly, strong evidence is not available to support a relationship between posture and neck pain or neck pain and headache.[20-22] Research in adolescents failed to demonstrate a relationship between neck pain and posture.[23] During a 10-minute computer task, Falla et al[24] demonstrated that symptomatic persons with neck pain have an increased forward head posture compared to those without neck pain. Forward head postures were reported as more common in persons with neck pain than in those without neck pain.[25]

O'Sullivan et al[26] reported different trunk muscle activation patterns in 3 different upright sitting postures: lumbopelvic upright, thoracic upright, and slump sitting (Figure 3-8). In considering an optimal posture for sitting, lumbopelvic sitting (ie, anterior pelvic rotation, lumbar lordosis, and thoracic relaxation) is favored for the lumbar and thoracic regions because it does not involve end-range

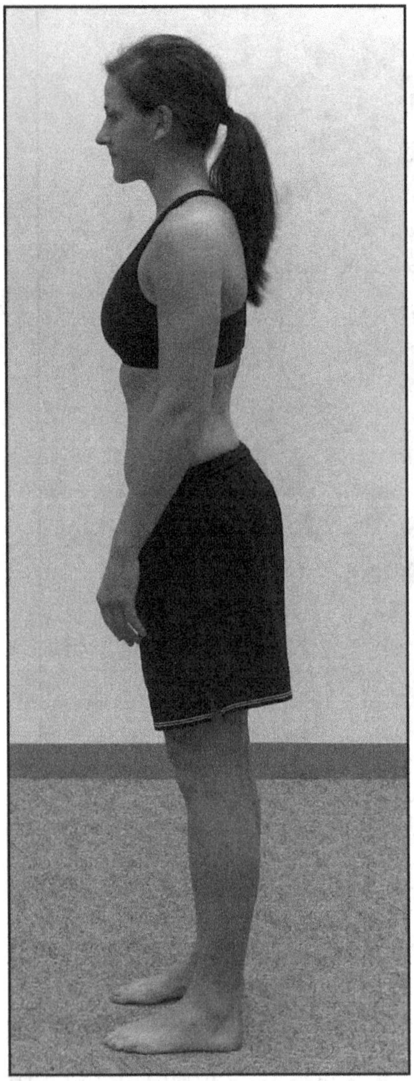

Figure 3-4. Kyphosis-lordosis posture.

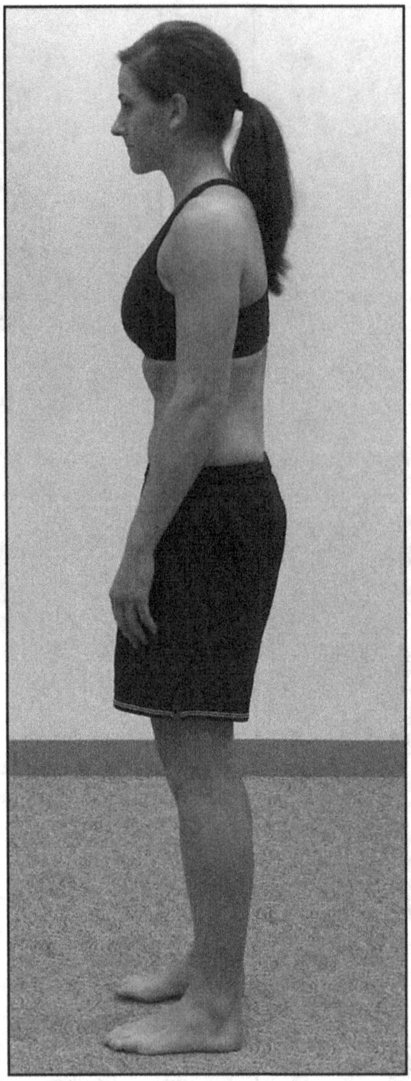

Figure 3-5. Flat back posture.

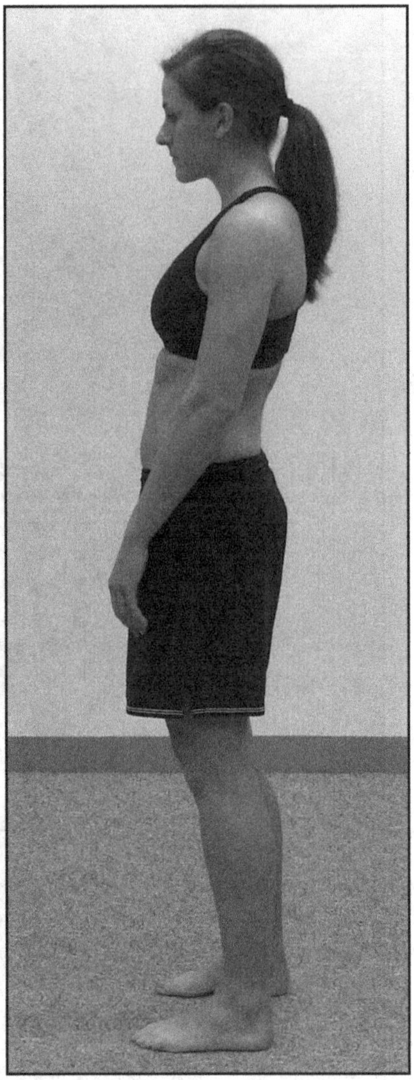

Figure 3-6. Swayback posture.

positions and results in preferential activation of local stabilizing muscles without high compressive loads of the thoracic extensor spinae (TES).[26] Thoracic upright sitting (ie, shoulder blades slightly retracted and thoracolumbar spine extended) results in high compressive axial loads from the TES and EO.[26]

Caneiro et al[27] reported altered muscle activity of the cervicothoracic region and altered head/neck kinematics during the 3 upright sitting postures reported previously, demonstrating a link between thoracolumbar posture, head/neck posture, and muscle activity. As expected, slump sitting resulted in greater head/neck flexion, anterior head translation, and increased cervical erector spinae (CES) activity compared to thoracic and lumbopelvic sitting. Thoracic upright sitting showed increased activity of the TES compared to lumbopelvic and slump postures. The favored posture for sitting is the lumbopelvic posture resulting in a relatively neutral head/neck alignment and diminished CES and TES compared to slump sitting.[27] These findings are consistent with research that demonstrated increased deep neck flexor and lumbar multifidus (LM) activity in a therapist-facilitated (ie, manually and verbally) lumbopelvic posture compared to the nonfacilitated thoracic upright sitting postures.[24,28] In other words, simply telling a patient to "sit up straight" does not facilitate an optimal position of the spine.

Jull et al[29] described the following process of assessing upright sitting posture in patients with neck pain. First, the patient's unsupported sitting posture is observed with the feet flat on the floor and hips in 80 degrees of flexion. The clinician manually assists anterior rotation of the pelvis, which results in neutral spinal posture as follows: (a) restoration of the normal low lumbar lordosis; (b) kyphosis in the thoracic spine adjusted with a slight sternal lift or depression; (c) scapulae sitting flush on the thoracic wall; and (d) head-on-neck posture adjusted with gentle occipital lift away from cervical extension. The clinician manually repositions the scapulae as needed. The patient is asked to

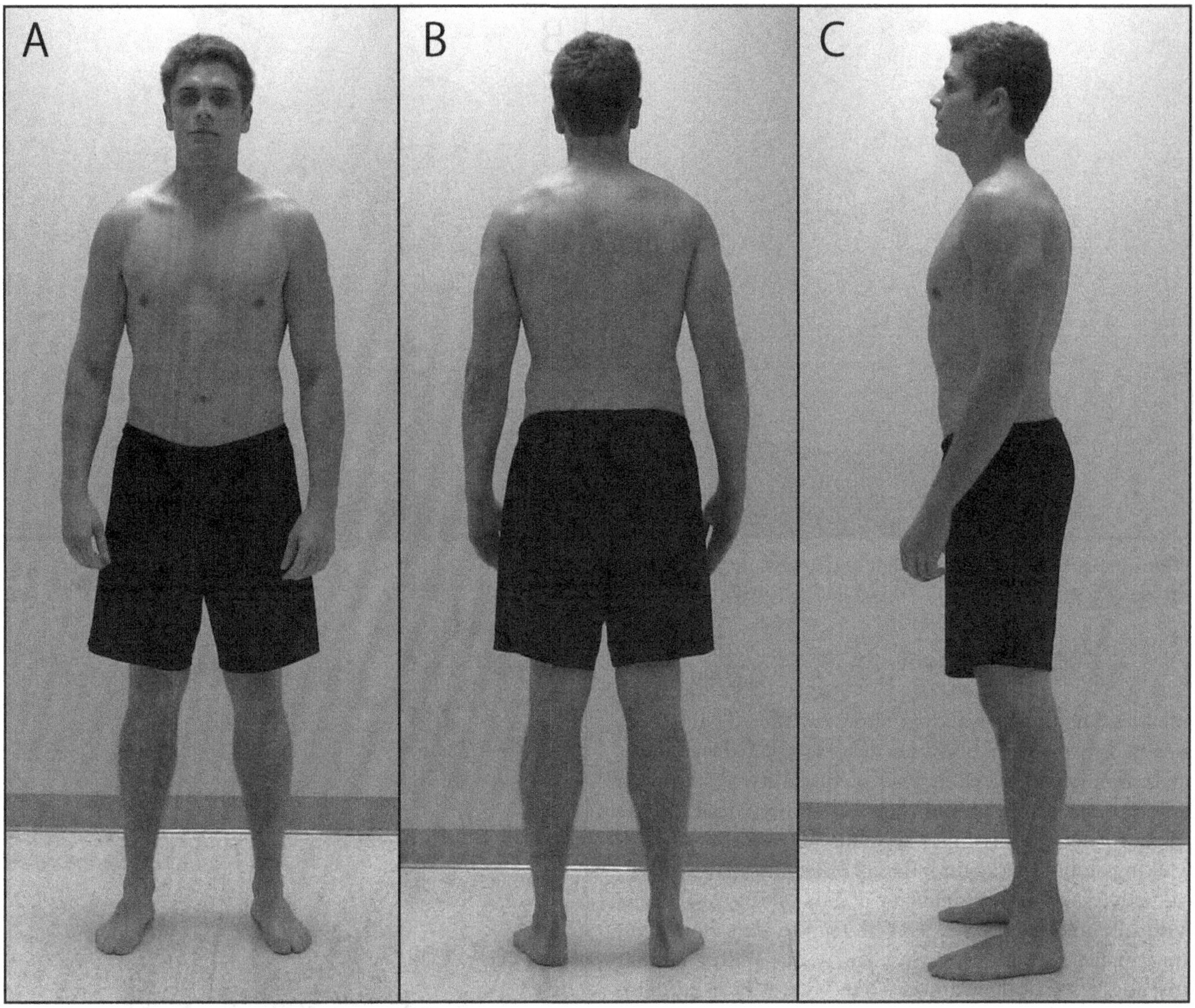

Figure 3-7. Standard standing posture views: (A) anterior; (B) posterior; and (C) left lateral.

actively maintain this position. The effect of postural correction on the patient's symptoms is assessed to determine relevance. Symptoms may increase, decrease, or remain the same or patients may have difficulty assuming the desired position, perhaps due to impaired spinal mobility.

Static postural alignment varies greatly among individuals. Widely accepted clinical viewpoints define good, bad, normal, or ideal postures, but little quantitative evidence is available to define these postures.[30] Qualitative descriptions tend to describe a spectrum of spinal curve combinations. Therefore, not all deviations from what is considered normal or ideal should be considered pathological, and some faulty postures should not always be corrected. For example, a patient with symptomatic lumbar spinal stenosis necessarily has a reduced lumbar lordosis. However, observed postural deformities should be corrected passively by the clinician or actively by the patient to note any change in the patient's symptoms and assist in establishing a provocative or easing link between the posture and the patient's problem. Provocative postures require further assessment of mobility, muscle activation patterns, and dynamic motor control. The patient must have sufficient range of motion (ROM) to correct deviations from normal. The posture should be comfortable and maintained with minimal activity of the superficial trunk muscles. The patient should be able to easily move in and out of functional postures as required by activities of daily living, work, or recreation.[31]

Gait Screen

Compared to age-matched controls without pain, most individuals with LBP walk slower, take shorter steps, and have asymmetrical step lengths.[32-37] In order to walk faster, persons with LBP increase cadence rather than stride length.[38-40] These differences may be attempts to limit motion about the spine and hips in order to modify

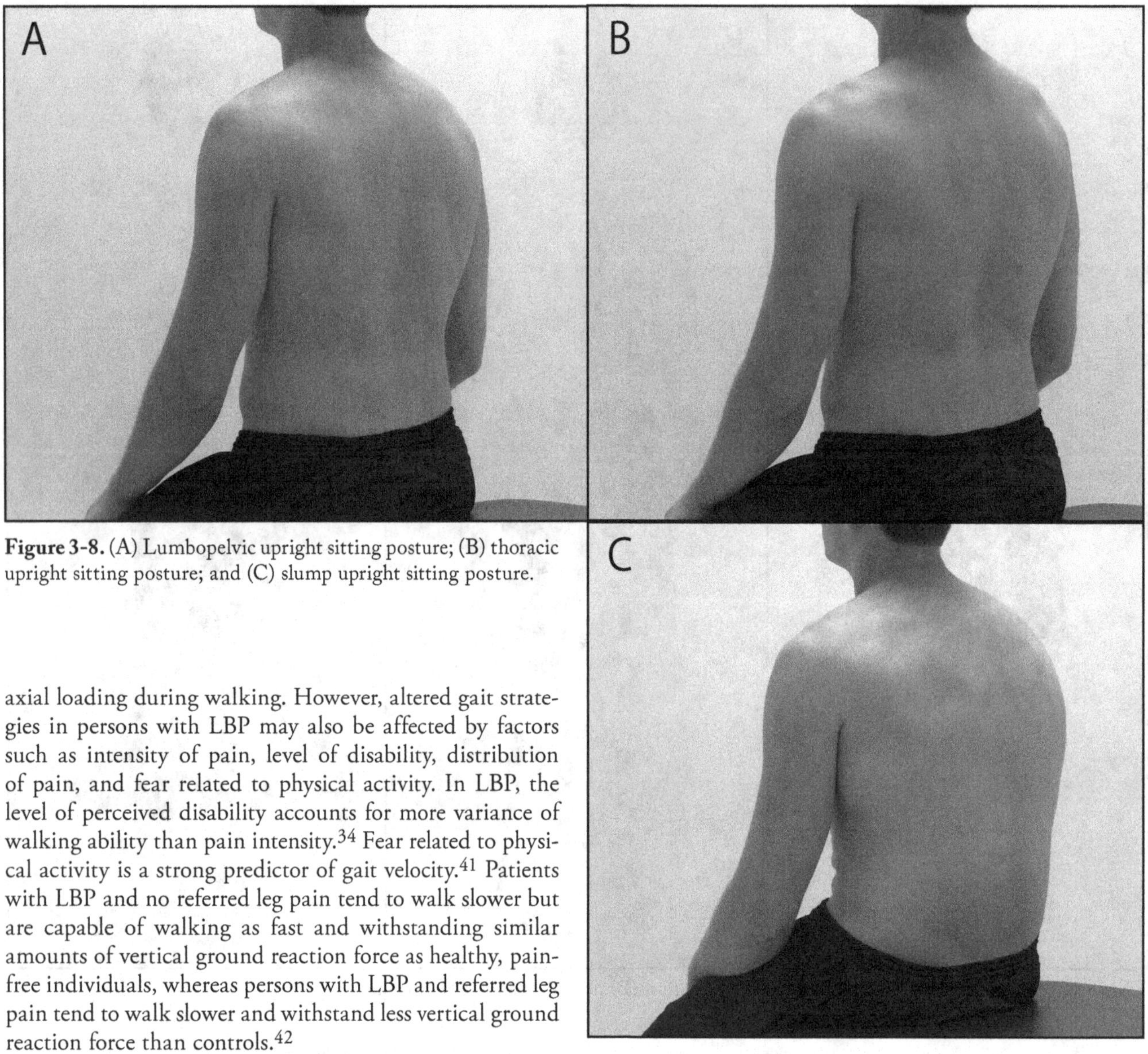

Figure 3-8. (A) Lumbopelvic upright sitting posture; (B) thoracic upright sitting posture; and (C) slump upright sitting posture.

axial loading during walking. However, altered gait strategies in persons with LBP may also be affected by factors such as intensity of pain, level of disability, distribution of pain, and fear related to physical activity. In LBP, the level of perceived disability accounts for more variance of walking ability than pain intensity.[34] Fear related to physical activity is a strong predictor of gait velocity.[41] Patients with LBP and no referred leg pain tend to walk slower but are capable of walking as fast and withstanding similar amounts of vertical ground reaction force as healthy, pain-free individuals, whereas persons with LBP and referred leg pain tend to walk slower and withstand less vertical ground reaction force than controls.[42]

Gait speed is a standard measure that has the potential to predict functional decline[43] and future health status.[44,45] Because self-selected walking speed is slower in patients with CLBP, walking speed should be assessed when appropriate to provide data relevant to the patient's future functional ability and safety. While variations exist related to age and gender (Table 3-4[46]), the normal range for walking speed is 1.2 to 1.4 m/s.[47]

The 10-meter walk test[48] is an easy, reliable test to measure walking speed. A straight, level 20-m path is used beginning with 5 m for acceleration, 10 m for timed walking at a comfortable pace, and ending with 5 m for deceleration. The average of 2 trials is scored. The amount of change needed for a small but meaningful improvement is 0.04 to 0.06 m/s and for a substantial change 0.08 to 0.14 m/s.[48] Gait speed of less than 1 m/s (ie, 6 seconds to complete a 6-m course) identifies well-functioning older persons at high risk of adverse health outcomes within 1 year.[49]

During walking, control of lumbopelvic motion and maintenance of stability is coordinated by all lumbopelvic muscles. In persons with LBP, investigators have described an integrated muscle system during walking.[50-52] The transversus abdominis (TrA) is tonically active throughout the gait cycle while the superficial abdominal muscles and all paraspinal muscles act phasically. Peak periods of activation of all muscles or coactivation occur with foot strike.[50] During walking in persons with recurrent LBP who are currently asymptomatic, Saunders et al[51] have provided preliminary evidence of loss of tonic activation of the TrA, periods of TrA silence during high lumbopelvic impact (ipsilateral foot strike), and increased duration of rectus abdominis activity (trunk rigidity). These data suggest that in some patients with a history of recurrent LBP, intersegmental control of the spine may be impaired providing rationale to assess specific muscle function.

TABLE 3-4. MEAN (X) AND STANDARD DEVIATION (S) OF COMFORTABLE GAIT SPEED PRESENTED BY SEX AND DECADE OF AGE

	COMFORTABLE GAIT SPEED (CM/S)				*MAXIMUM GAIT SPEED (CM/S)*			
	ACTUAL		*HEIGHT-NORMALIZED**		*ACTUAL*		*HEIGHT-NORMALIZED**	
SEX/DECADE	*X*	*S*	*X*	*S*	*X*	*S*	*X*	*S*
Men								
20s	139.3	15.3	0.788	0.093	253.3	29.1	1.431	0.162
30s	145.8	9.4	0.828	0.052	245.6	31.5	1.396	0.177
40s	146.2	16.4	0.829	0.090	246.2	36.3	1.395	0.197
50s	139.3	22.9	0.794	0.119	206.9	44.8	1.182	0.259
60s	135.9	20.5	0.777	0.116	193.3	36.4	1.104	0.198
70s	133.0	19.6	0.762	0.105	207.9	36.3	1.192	0.201
Women								
20s	140.7	17.5	0.856	0.098	246.7	25.3	1.502	0.142
30s	141.5	12.7	0.864	0.087	234.2	34.4	1.428	0.206
40s	139.1	15.8	0.856	0.098	212.3	27.5	1.304	0.160
50s	139.5	15.1	0.863	0.104	201.0	25.8	1.243	0.158
60s	129.6	21.3	0.808	0.131	177.4	25.4	1.107	0.157
70s	127.2	21.1	0.807	0.131	174.9	28.1	1.110	0.176

* actual speed (cm/s)/height (cm).

Data from Bohannon RW. Comfortable and maximum walking speed of adults aged 20-79 years: reference values and determinants. *Age Ageing.* 1997;26:15-19. Reprinted by permission of Oxford University Press.

Observation of the motion between the thoracic spine and ribs relative to the pelvis may reveal patterns of impaired postural control during walking.[53] If symptomatic, apparent excessive motion or movement with less control of the lumbar spine may suggest insufficient muscular stabilization and perhaps requires an intervention strategy to enhance stabilization, whereas a stiffened trunk posture or one with restricted movement with poor thoracic-pelvic dissociation suggests a coping strategy of enhanced muscular cocontraction in the presence of reduced or absent TrA activity and may require intervention to reduce the amount of muscular cocontraction.[53] In subjects with CLBP, van der Hulst and colleagues[54] demonstrated increased superficial muscle activity of the ES and rectus abdominis but not of the EO abdominals. These differences were present irrespective of gait velocity. Increased coactivation of the ES and rectus abdominis may serve to control spinal movement and support a hypothesis of muscle guarding or trunk rigidity.

Gait impairments are most commonly observed in persons with LBP with or without radiating pain into the lower extremity. However, activity limitations related to the upper body regions may also produce gait abnormalities due to upper quarter symptoms, posture, or movement impairments. Assessment of gait includes anterior, posterior, right lateral, and left lateral views with or without footwear. The clinician should perform a global screen of the gait cycle with focus around the point in the gait cycle that produces or alters the patient's symptoms as well as abnormal patterns and gait speed. A more detailed clinical examination of gait is available from these sources.[8,9]

Balance Screen

Patient complaints of dizziness, balance problems, unsteadiness with walking, and neck pain or LBP are indications for both static and dynamic balance screening.

The history, systems review, and patient's description and degree of the problem guide the required level and type of screening.

Postural control is a requirement for all activities of daily living. This very complex skill involves the ability to integrate various sensory inputs from somatosensory, vestibular, and visual systems, which all depend on the task, environment, and a person's ability to compensate for impairments.[55] On a stable surface in a well-lit environment, a healthy person uses somatosensory (70%), vision (10%), and vestibular (20%) information.[56] On an unstable surface, the use of visual and vestibular information is increased relative to somatosensory inputs.[56] Because multiple systems are involved, one balance test is not sufficient to understand why a person's balance is impaired.[55] Similarly, one treatment to improve balance is unlikely to be optimal for everyone. For example, if hip extensor weakness is the cause of a person who falls, sitting on a wobble board with eyes closed (EC) is likely to be an ineffective intervention. However, a person who has an impaired vestibular system may benefit from this added challenge.

Balance impairments have been demonstrated in individuals with LBP[57-61] and neck pain.[62,63] Byl and Sinnot[57] showed that LBP subjects had significantly increased postural sway, kept their center of force significantly more posterior, and were significantly less likely to be able to balance on one foot with EC. Mok et al[59] showed that when compared with age- and gender-matched controls, individuals with LBP had poorer standing balance with altered postural adjustment strategies (reduced hip strategy) and increased visual dependence. Mok et al[64] demonstrated that persons with LBP use a different lumbar spine movement strategy after sudden trunk loading (eg, catching a 1-kg weight dropped from a 30-cm height) when compared to healthy controls. Persons with CLBP require a longer recovery period with more postural adjustments to resume postural stability. This deficit in balance control relates to an unexpected external perturbation, which is consistent with previous studies. The authors suggest that poor use of lumbopelvic movement for postural control may be due to a maladaptive, cocontraction, or trunk stiffening strategy.[65-67]

Treleaven et al[62] showed that subjects with whiplash-associated disorders who do and do not complain of dizziness have standing balance deficits likely due to altered postural control mechanisms and not due to medications, anxiety, or compensation status. Compared to controls, patients with idiopathic and whiplash-induced neck pain demonstrate deficits in standing balance, with both groups being significantly less likely to complete the EC tandem test for 30 seconds.[63] These results also suggest a somatosensory impairment as the likely cause. These authors recommend a battery of balance tests including comfortable, narrow, and tandem stance with eyes open (EO) and EC for all neck pain patients.[63]

Using the one-leg stand test with EO and EC, Maribo et al[68] examined postural balance in 40 subjects ages 18 to 75 years (mean 51.5, standard deviation 12.35) with CLBP for more than 6 months. Patients were barefoot with eyes focused on a point 1.5 cm away, arms across their chest, and one foot lifted approximately 10 cm and placed behind the weightbearing leg. Timing was stopped at 60 seconds for EO or 30 seconds for EC or if it was impossible to maintain the position. During EO, a ceiling effect was seen as more than 48% of patients could stand for 60 seconds. For EC, intraobserver (standard error of the mean [SEM] 2.48 seconds; minimal detectable change [MDC] 6.88) and interobserver (SEM 1.42 seconds; MDC 3.95) reliability were acceptable (intraclass correlation coefficient [ICC] 0.86; ICC 0.91, respectively). Real change is indicated by 6.88 seconds, though the test might differ up to 2.48 seconds without any real difference in balance for EC. In this study, only 28% of patients less than 60 years of age could stand with EC for 10 seconds or more with a mean of 8.9 seconds.[68] Bohannon et al[69] reported normative data of a mean 21 ± 9.5 seconds for EC one-leg stand ages 50 to 59 years old. The variance between the 2 studies is likely due to different subjects, persons with CLBP compared to persons without orthopedic disorders. Comparing subjects with and without LBP, Sung et al[70] reported that core spine stability was significantly decreased when visual feedback was blocked for subjects with LBP during a one-leg stand test, suggesting that trunk muscle imbalance may contribute to unbalanced postural activity resulting in a decreased, uncoordinated bracing effect.

Springer et al[71] reported age- and gender-specific performance values (Table 3-5) in healthy individuals during the one-leg stand test. Subjects stood barefoot with arms crossed over chest on the limb of their choice with the other limb lifted so that it was near, but not touching, the ankle of the stance side. Each subject focused on a spot on a front wall at eye level throughout the EO test. The time the subject was able to stand on one limb was measured. Time ended when (1) the subject used his arms (ie, uncrossed arms), (2) the subject used the raised foot (ie, moved it toward or away from the standing limb or touched the floor), (3) the subject moved the weightbearing foot to maintain his balance (ie, rotated foot on the ground), (4) a maximum of 45 seconds had elapsed, or (5) the subject opened eyes on an EC test.[71] An EO, one-leg stand test of < 5 seconds is predictive of injurious falls[72] and < 10 seconds = 1.58 (95% confidence interval [CI]: 1.03, 2.41) relative risk of falls.[73]

Jull et al[74] recommended the following clinical examination of standing balance (Figure 3-9) in persons with neck pain. Balance is first tested in a comfortable and then narrow stance on a firm and then soft surface (eg, 10-cm dense foam) with EO and EC. These tests measure outcomes of time and abnormal responses such as large excessive sway, slow response to correct sway, and inability

TABLE 3-5. ONE-LEG STANCE TEST TIME BY AGE AND GENDER FOR EYES OPEN AND EYES CLOSED

AGE	*MEAN (SE) EYES OPEN (SECONDS)*		*MEAN (SE) EYES CLOSED (SECONDS)*	
	FEMALE	*MALE*	*FEMALE*	*MALE*
18 to 39	43.5 (3.8)	43.2 (6.0)	8.5 (9.1)	10.2 (9.6)
40 to 49	40.4 (10.1)	40.1 (11.5)	7.4 (6.7)	7.3 (7.4)
50 to 59	36.0 (12.8)	38.1 (12.4)	5.0 (5.6)	4.5 (3.8)
60 to 69	25.1 (16.5)	28.7 (16.7)	2.5 (1.5)	3.1 (2.7)
70 to 79	11.3 (11.1)	18.3 (15.3)	2.2 (2.1)	1.9 (0.9)
80 to 99	7.4 (10.7)	5.6 (8.4)	1.4 (0.6)	1.3 (0.6)

SE indicates standard error.

Data extracted from Springer BA, Marin R, Cyhan T, Roberts H, Gill NW. Normative values for the unipedal stance test with eyes open and closed. *J Geriatric Phys Ther.* 2007;30:8-15.

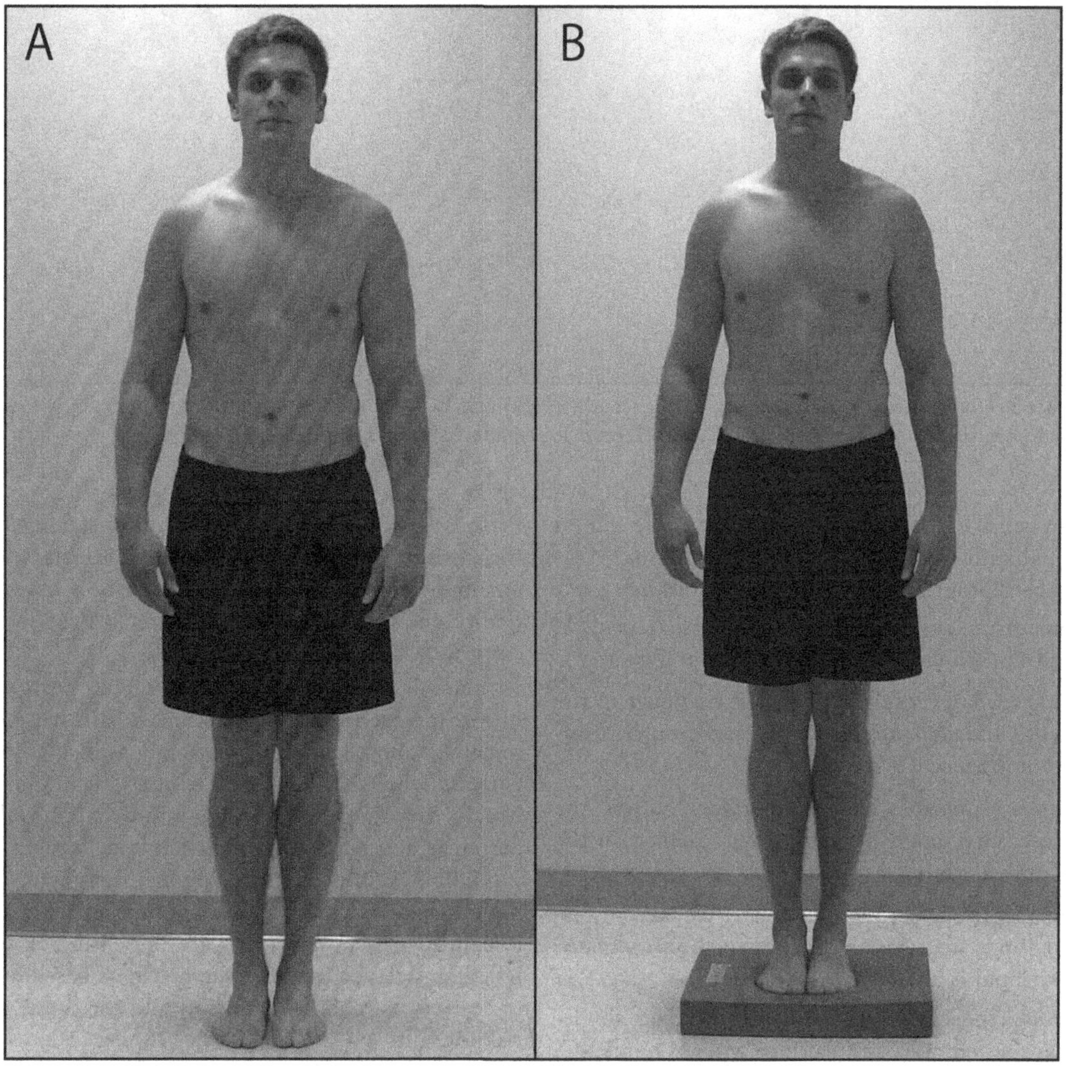

Figure 3-9. Selected standing balance tests—EO and EC on firm and soft surface (10-cm dense foam): (A) narrow stance on firm surface, EO; (B) narrow stance on a soft surface, EO. *(continued)*

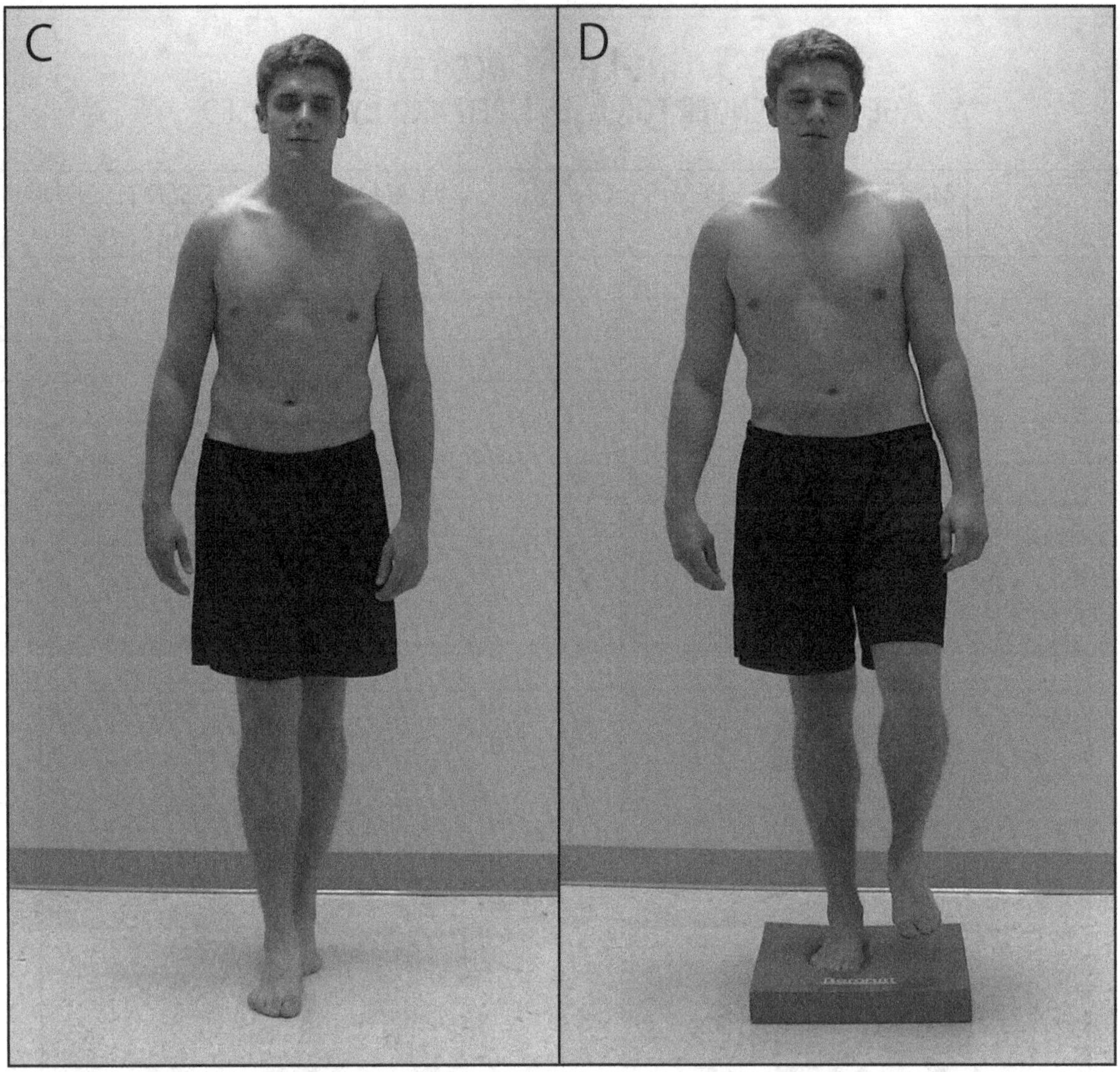

Figure 3-9 (continued). Selected standing balance tests—EO and EC on firm and soft surface (10-cm dense foam): (C) tandem stance on a firm surface, EC; and (D) one-leg standing test on soft surface, EC.

to maintain balance. Persons under 60 years of age should be able to maintain all of these conditions for up to 30 seconds. Balance is progressively challenged as follows:

- EO on a firm, level surface utilizes the visual, vestibular, and somatosensory systems for postural control.
- EC on a firm, level surface increases challenge to the vestibular and somatosensory systems through elimination of the visual system.
- EO on an unstable or foam surface changes the somatosensory input, placing greater reliance on the visual and vestibular systems.
- EC on a foam surface requires greater reliance on vestibular input since vision is eliminated and somatosensory input is altered.

To increase the challenge, tandem and then single-leg stance are tested on a firm surface with EO and EC. Persons under 45 years of age should be able to complete these tests.[62] As previously noted, patients with insidious or traumatic neck pain and dizziness have more difficulty completing tandem tasks on a firm surface than controls.[62,63]

Though the precise nature of altered postural mechanisms in persons with LBP and neck pain requires further research, simple clinical tests are available to identify patients who have problems with balance and who may benefit from intervention to improve postural control. Standing and single-limb balance tests with EO and EC should be examined at some point throughout the examination process but may not be appropriate if weightbearing is painful or the symptoms are presenting as severe and irritable. Balance tests may be useful as baseline measures to reassess as mobility improves and for those who are at risk for falls.

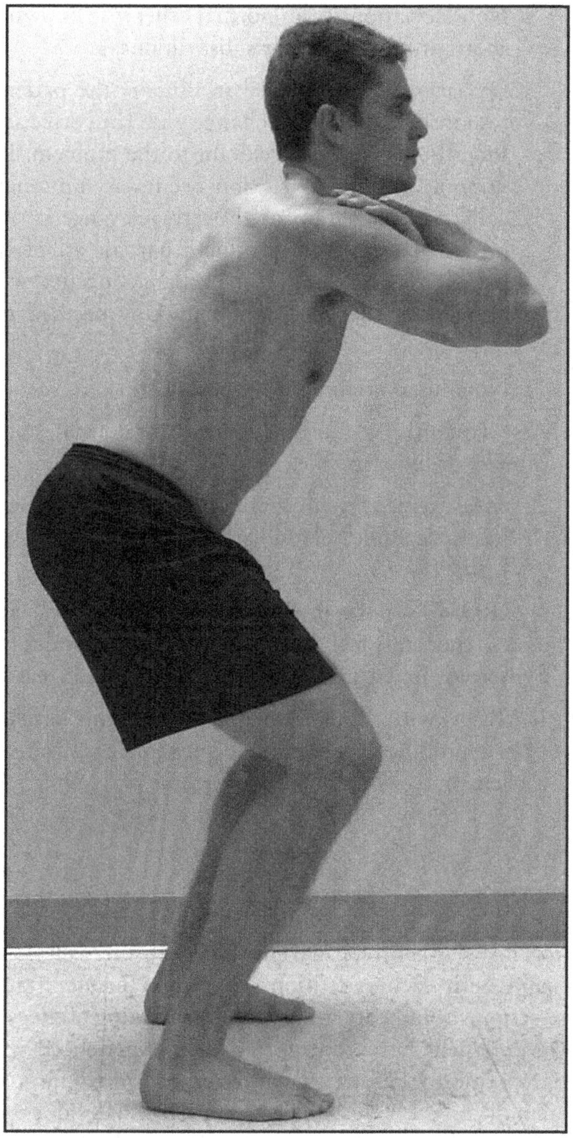

Figure 3-10. Functional movement test—squat, lateral view.

Movement Testing

Assessment typically includes detailed examination of functional, active, and passive movement tests. To minimize clinician error for within and between session reassessments, all tests must be performed in a standardized manner. Goals of functional or active movement testing are as follows:

- Reproduce all or part of the patient's symptoms
- Identify and document patterns of restricted or excessive movements
- Assess quality, quantity, and pain or symptom response for each direction of movement
- Gain baseline data from which to assess a treatment effect

Functional Movement or Performance Tests

Functional movements (Figure 3-10) ask the patient to perform a movement such as squat or sit-to-stand, an activity such as stair climbing, or a position such as sitting that reproduces or eases his or her symptoms. Often, this provocative or easing test can be analyzed biomechanically or altered actively or passively to assist in determining the source or cause of the change in symptoms. If functional movements are easing, the movement may assist in management. If provocative, the movement may be reassessed after intervention to determine a treatment effect. When appropriate, standardized physical performance tests related to the functional capacity of the patient are performed and used as outcome measures (eg, repeated sit-to-stand and the 6-minute walk test).[75]

Active Range of Motion or Active Movement Tests

Active range of motion (AROM) tests the integrity of articular, muscle, and neural systems as well as the patient's willingness to move. Active movements, typically standard cardinal plane movements, and then repeated, sustained, or combined movements as necessary are voluntarily performed by the patient. The clinician assesses resting symptoms prior to each test or procedure to accurately determine the effect of the movement on the patient's symptoms and analyzes each movement. Analysis of AROM results in a quantitative and a qualitative measure of movement control, patient symptomatic response, details related to function, willingness to move, and fear of movement. Generally, flexion, extension, lateral flexion, and rotation to both sides are tested in the spine. Patterns of motion restriction and pain response provide guidance for treatment and dosage. Active motion testing for the cervical, thoracic, and lumbar spine are covered in subsequent chapters.

Symptom Response to Movement Tests

Assessment procedures require the patient to report any change in symptoms as a result of movement or manual pressure.[76,77] The pain response is a useful finding in the initial diagnostic classification (pre- and postintervention within and between treatment sessions) as well as for long-term treatment evaluation.[77-80] Patient response on initial examination and after treatment is used to guide prognostic, diagnostic, and management decisions. For example, patient responses to repeated movement testing such as changes in pain location (eg, centralization or peripheralization) are used to guide diagnosis and prognosis in LBP and neck pain. Systematic review[81] supports the use of symptom response in the prognosis of spinal

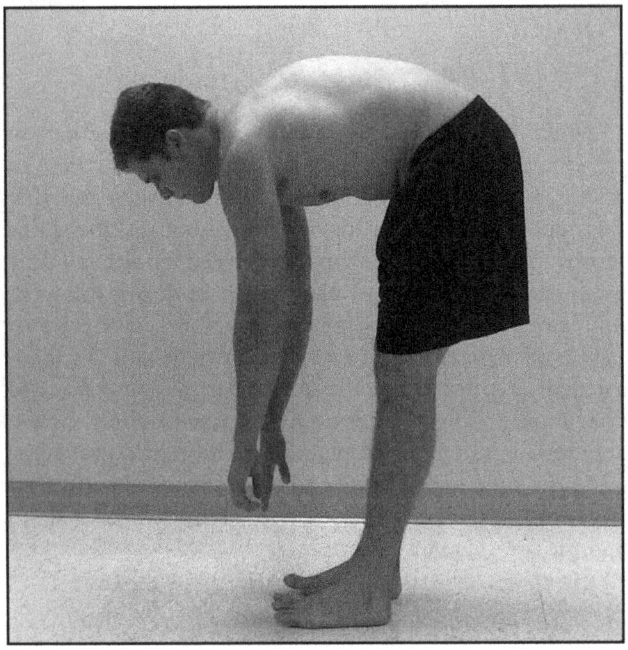

Figure 3-11. Active range of motion lumbar spine—flexion.

outcomes when changes in pain location and/or intensity occur with repeated spinal movement tests or as a response to treatment.

Active Range of Motion Testing Procedure

- Test uninvolved side first and compare to the involved side (Figure 3-11).
- Explain what you want the patient to do and ask for a response to the movement.
  - The patient should indicate where in the range symptoms are felt or increased if resting symptoms are present and which symptoms are affected by the movement.
- Establish symptoms at rest prior to movement.
- Assess pain or symptom response—seek to reproduce patient's symptoms.
  - Note pain rating using the Numeric Pain Rating Scale.
  - Note behavior of symptoms through movement: local or referred, type and location, and where in range the symptoms were produced (eg, pain at end-range, mid-range, painful arc).
  - Re-establish symptom baseline between tests to prevent a cumulative effect.
- Assess quality of movement by observing from front, back, or sides as needed.
  - Note smoothness, ease of movement, and control of movement.
  - Note deviations from normal otherwise known as aberrant movements or substitutions.
  - Deviations are corrected to observe the patient's response. If symptoms change with the correction, then the deviation is relevant to the problem. For example, if lumbar flexion occurs asymptomatically with deviation to the left, relevance is supported if correction produces part or all of the patient's symptoms. If no change occurs with correction, the deviation is initially deemed not relevant.
  - Note intervertebral movement.
- Assess quantity of movement grossly as normal, hypomobile, or hypermobile.
  - Measurement with gravity/bubble inclinometer has acceptable reliability for neck pain[82,83] and LBP.[84-87]
- If AROM is normal, apply overpressure (OP) and assess the end feel and the effect on symptoms. Symptoms may stay the same, increase, or decrease.
- If AROM with OP is normal and symptoms have not been reproduced, try repeated movements, sustained movements, or combined movements.

Repeated Movement Tests

According to the mechanical diagnosis and treatment approach,[88] "When repeated movements produce less and less pain with each repetition or produce greater range, these responses indicate an appropriate loading strategy… However, when more and more pain is experienced with each repetition, that particular exercise is inappropriate or premature."[88(p409)] A single repetition usually does not provide as clear an understanding of the mechanical effect of multiple repetitions.[88]

The repeated movement portion of the examination provides information on symptom response, initial data to support one or more diagnostic classifications, the need for additional testing, and/or guidance for intervention.[88] The patient's response to repeated movements may help to begin differentiating among 3 subgroups related to mechanical neck, thoracic, or lumbar spinal pain, which may assist in determining an initial treatment strategy: (a) derangement syndrome, also referred to as *direction-specific exercise classification*; (b) dysfunction syndrome suggesting limited mobility; or (c) postural syndrome. The most common subgroup is derangement or direction-specific exercise (cervical 82%, thoracic 87%, lumbar 80%), dysfunction (cervical 8%, thoracic 9%, lumbar 6%) and postural (cervical 3%, thoracic 0%, lumbar 1%).[89] Patients who initially do not fit 1 of the 3 subgroups require additional testing and subsequent classification outside of these 3 subgroups.[88,90]

1. *Derangement syndrome or direction-specific exercise classification*: The key finding for this subgroup is either centralization or peripheralization in response to mechanical loading strategies such as repeated movements. Symptoms that are decreased, abolished, or centralized in response to repeated movement in one direction reliably indicate a direction of movement that may be useful as an intervention strategy. Conversely, a response of increased or peripheralized pain suggests movements to avoid initially. As soon as centralization is identified and a directional preference (DP) is observed, no further examination may be needed. A DP is demonstrated by improvement in ROM and pain in one direction that is worse in the opposite direction but does not include centralization or peripheralization. In the absence of a response of centralization or peripheralization, additional testing is required, but DP may be considered for the initial treatment direction. Patients who demonstrate centralization have better outcomes than noncentralizers.[91-94] Of the individuals who do not centralize on the first day, 60% may become centralizers with further testing sessions.[95]
2. *Dysfunction or presentation of spinal pain and mobility deficits*: The key finding for this subgroup is reproduction of the patient's familiar pain at end-range possibly due to mechanical loading of adaptively shortened tissue (ie, loss of tissue mobility). On return to neutral, the pain is no longer present. The symptoms do not get progressively worse or peripheralize and ROM will not change rapidly, suggesting a preliminary hypothesis of spinal pain with mobility deficits that warrants further examination of segmental mobility and other test procedures. In general, the provocative limited, end-range movement or movements guide the initial treatment to reduce pain and improve mobility through application of manual techniques and exercise intervention. For example, if lumbar extension ROM was limited and painful consistently at end-range with painful, central, or unilateral segmental hypomobility, manual techniques and exercise are considered to decrease pain and restore motion in the restricted plane or planes.
3. *Postural syndrome*: In this less common subgroup, the response to repeated movements is not provocative. Theoretically, only sustained postures or positions reproduce the patient's symptoms as a result of mechanical deformation of normal soft tissues.[88,89] A postural component rarely presents in isolation but may be a factor in a variety of patients presenting with spinal pain.

Repeated Movement Testing Procedure[88]

- Establish baseline resting symptoms and explain what you want the patient to do.
- During the repeated movements, continually ask the patient about any change in symptom behavior (location or intensity during movement or at end-range).
    - The history may provide clues as to the movement that will worsen symptoms.
    - Sagittal plane movements are performed first (eg, extension or flexion).
    - Frontal plane or horizontal plane movements are tested as needed for lateral or rotational DP for the cervical, thoracic, or lumbar spine.
- After 10 to 15 movements or one set, the patient relaxes and reports current symptoms.
    - If the patient's response is worsening or peripheralization occurs, the movements are discontinued prior to completing all repetitions. A different loading strategy may be performed in an attempt to obtain centralization or a DP.
    - If the patient is centralizing or getting better, additional repetitions may be required or a different loading strategy performed (eg, moving from extension in standing to extension in lying).
- According to the following definitions, the patient's response is detailed and recorded as centralized, peripheralized, better, no better, worse, no worse, or no effect.[88]
    - **Centralized:** Pain in the extremity coming from the spine is abolished, progressively moves in a proximal direction, and remains abolished after testing. At the same time, proximal pain may develop or increase in the spine.
    - **Peripheralized:** The opposite of centralized. Pain coming from the spine is produced distally, spreads distally or increases distally, and remains in the extremity after testing.
    - **Better:** Symptoms decreased or abolished remain better after testing.
    - **No better:** Symptoms decreased or abolished return to baseline after testing.
    - **Worse:** Symptoms produced or increased with movement remain increased after testing.
    - **No worse:** Symptoms produced or increased with movement return to baseline after the test.
    - **No effect:** Symptoms do not change during or after testing.
- Specific repeated movement tests for the cervical, thoracic, and lumbar spine are detailed in subsequent chapters.

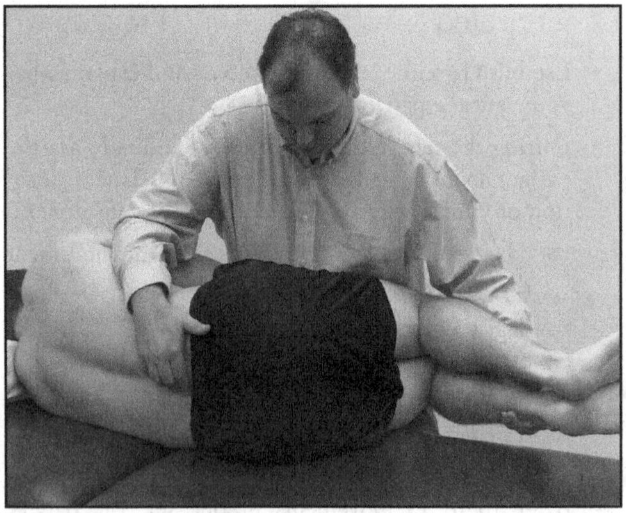
Figure 3-12. Lumbar flexion PPIVM.

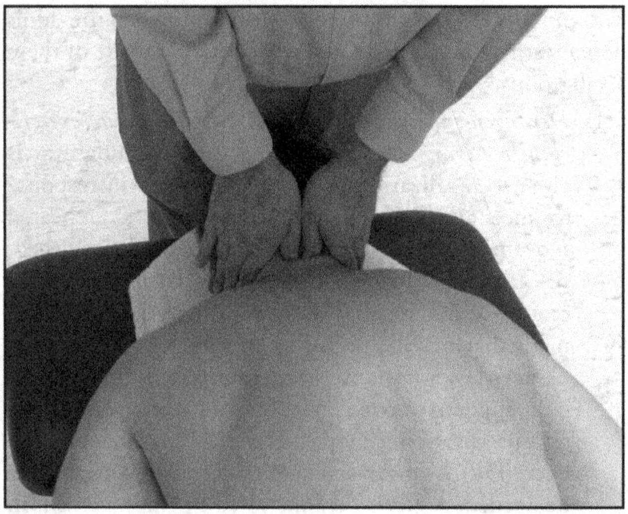
Figure 3-13. Cervical spine central posterior-to-anterior PAIVM.

Passive Range of Motion: Physiological and Accessory Movement Testing

In the peripheral joints, if AROM was painful and/or limited, the same motions that were tested actively are then tested passively by the clinician. Quality, quantity in degrees, and symptom response are recorded in addition to comparisons between AROM and passive range of motion (PROM). AROM and PROM that are limited and painful in the same direction suggest a joint mobility deficit. For example, hip flexion AROM and PROM that are limited and painful suggest a hip joint mobility deficit that requires additional testing of hip passive accessory motion and muscle length. AROM and PROM that are limited and painful in opposite directions suggest a contractile component of the patient's problem. For example, if the following findings are present, hip flexor muscle activation is suspected as a source of pain: active hip flexion is painful and limited (ie, hip flexor muscles contract), passive hip extension is limited and painful (ie, hip flexors are lengthened), and passive hip flexion is full range with no pain (ie, hip flexors do not contract). Testing of isometric hip flexion is used to confirm hip flexion activation as a source of pain. A final comparison of hip flexion AROM that is limited and not painful and hip flexion PROM that is full range and not painful indicates a finding of hip flexor muscle weakness but does not indicate the cause of the weakness.

Passive accessory movements (PAMs) are necessary for normal physiological movement at any joint. These movements occur both in the peripheral joints and in the spine at the joint surfaces. PAMs usually cannot be performed actively by the patient, but they can be performed by the clinician. The term *arthrokinematics* is used to describe motions of the bone at the joint surfaces such as gliding, sliding, translation, distraction, rolling, or spinning. The PAMs available at the peripheral joints vary but include distraction, anterior, posterior, superior, inferior, medial, or lateral glides of one bone on its adjacent partner. Passive accessory motions at the peripheral joints are performed by the clinician initially in the resting position of the joint and graded as hypomobile, normal, or hypermobile with or without a pain response in a specific direction. For example, hip PAM for anterior glide was hypomobile and produced anterior hip pain. PAMs are used to identify movement impairments and to guide clinical decision making for treatment.

PROM in the spine is produced by applying manual examination techniques, PPIVM, or passive accessory intervertebral movements (PAIVM) to the individual motion segments. PPIVM tests (Figure 3-12) involve physiological segmental motion palpation in the same planes as AROM such as flexion, extension, lateral flexion, and rotation. PAIVM tests (Figure 3-13) involve passive accessory segmental motion testing of gliding motions such as posterior to anterior gliding centrally over the spinous process.

Segmental motion tests are usually graded as normal, hypomobile, or hypermobile with or without a pain response and tested at each segment in a specific direction. As part of a thorough examination, passive segmental motion tests of the lumbar spine, thoracic spine, and cervical spine are used for classification purposes and to guide clinical decision making for treatment.[96] Using segmental motion palpation as a diagnostic test requires that the procedure is adequately reliable[97] and a valid indicator of dysfunction, and that a relationship between spinal pain and segmental dysfunction actually exists.

Reliability

Reliability studies of segmental motion tests are conflicting and controversial partly due to varied methodological design, varied techniques, and variable motion in asymptomatic subjects. In subjects with central LBP, Landel et al[98] reported that lumbar PAIVM intertester reliability for identifying the least mobile segment was good with agreement 82% (κ = 0.71, 0.48 to 0.94) but poor for identifying the most mobile segment (κ = 0.29, 0.13 to 0.71) despite good agreement. Validity of PAIVM tests was questioned as the assessment did not agree with sagittal plane motion measured on magnetic resonance imaging (MRI). Johansson[99] reported no acceptable interrater reliability for lumbar flexion and extension PPIVM when comparing 3 therapists with similar education but currently not working together and without coordination prior to the study. A systematic review[100] concluded that reliability of passive segmental mobility tests of the cervical and lumbar spine ranges from poor to substantial with overall reliability rated as poor to fair. A review[101] of reliability of cervical, thoracic, and lumbar segmental motion tests concludes the following:

- Intrarater agreement varies from less than chance to moderate or substantial.
- Interrater agreement rarely exceeds poor to fair.
- Rating scales of pain response or dichotomous scales of present or absent provide higher agreement.
- Firm conclusions regarding segmental motion tests required more research.

In a study of persons with neck pain, Cleland et al[102] reported the intertester reliability of segmental mobility tests (PAIVM for occiput on C1, C2-C7, and T1-T9) and pain provocation for the cervical (weighted κ =–0.26 to 0.74, –0.52 to 0.90, respectively) and thoracic spine (weighted κ = 0.13 to 0.82, –0.11 to –0.90, respectively). The overall findings for reliability of mobility assessment and pain provocation were highly variable and consistent with other studies.[103,104] Using a lateral glide segmental mobility test to detect only hypomobility, Piva et al[105] also reported variable reliability at different segments. Findings include substantial and moderate reliability for occipital-atlas mobility and symptom provocation of the lower cervical segments. Reliability for C2-C6 segmental motion tests revealed no agreement to fair for mobility (κ =–0.07 to 0.45) and slightly higher for pain provocation (κ = 0.29 to 0.76).[105] Jull et al[106] found excellent agreement (70%) between examiner pairs when using manual passive segmental examination to determine the presence of painful upper cervical joint dysfunction in 40 subjects with and without neck pain and headache.

Interrater reliability studies involving PAIVM or PPIVM of the thoracic spine are limited. Brismée et al[107] demonstrated fair to substantial interrater reliability for PPIVM at T5 to T7 with healthy subjects. Haas et al[108] examined T3-L1 rotation PPIVM to identify hypomobile segments resulting in fair reliability. Similar to the lumbar and cervical spine, uncertainty exists regarding the reliability of these manual assessments. No studies have examined validity in the thoracic spine.

Validity

Several studies[109-111] determined that PPIVM in sidelying for lumbar flexion (Sn 0.05, Sp 0.99; +LR 8.73, –LR 0.96) and extension (Sn 0.16, Sp 0.98; +LR 7.07, –LR 0.86) may have moderate validity for assessing intervertebral displacement. In a study of consecutive primary care patients with recurrent LBP, Abbott and Mercer[109] demonstrated an association between abnormal or hypomobile segmental sagittal rotation and LBP. Furthermore, lumbar segmental mobility disorders are present in greater numbers in persons with recurrent LBP compared to asymptomatic persons and may contain valid subgroups of nonspecific LBP. Lumbar segmental mobility disorders were defined as a segment(s) contributing significantly more or significantly less to total lumbar motion compared to other segments within the same individual.[111]

The patient's pain response to PAIVM is considered more important than both quantity and quality or stiffness of perceived motion and has shown generally good reliability for lumbar PAIVM.[96,112] Fritz et al[86] and Abbott et al[110] concluded that PAIVM may possess concurrent validity for detecting excessive sagittal translation or hypermobility predictive of radiographic instability. PAIVM has adequate specificity (0.81 to 0.89) and low sensitivity (0.29 to 0.46) for detecting excessive sagittal translation displacement. However, the magnitude of the association was small, suggesting weak diagnostic value if PAIVM are used as an isolated clinical finding.[96]

Segmental motion tests used in combination with other clinical findings demonstrate predictive validity and usefulness for determining treatment and outcome.[113-116] Lumbar hypomobility identified with PAIVM combined with key history and physical exam findings is useful in predicting which patients are most likely to improve with manipulation.[113,115] Lumbar hypermobility assessed with PAIVM, a factor in a multivariate clinical prediction rule, was predictive of a successful outcome with a stabilization program. Fritz et al[114] concluded that persons with LBP judged by PAIVM to have lumbar hypomobility experienced greater benefit from an intervention including manipulation, while those with hypermobility were more likely to benefit from a stabilization exercise program. Despite the low reliability associated with PAIVM tests, judgments of hypomobility or hypermobility provide useful and valid information for clinical decision making when combined with other examination findings.[114]

In the cervical spine, Jull et al[117] reported a correct diagnosis of symptomatic cervical zygapophyseal joint syndromes in 20 patients (Sn = 1.0, Sp = 1.0), demonstrating excellent validity for PAIVM and PPIVM. The reference standard for the symptomatic zygapophyseal joint was a radiological-controlled diagnostic nerve block. The examiner was blinded to patient condition and accurately identified the symptomatic joint in 15 patients and correctly identified 5 patients without joint dysfunction.

Manual examination of the spinal segments is a qualitative assessment of tissue compliance and pain response in an attempt to identify symptomatic and dysfunctional segments.[74] Most manual physical therapists accept the face validity of manual segmental motion testing when used in combination with the results of other examination procedures.[74] Despite some disagreement and a need for more research, a growing body of evidence supports the use of passive segmental motion tests in clinical decision making for diagnosis and intervention for spinal pain. Specific techniques for each region are described in detail in subsequent chapters.

Passive Range of Motion Testing Procedure

- Test uninvolved side first and compare to the involved side.
- Patient position is relaxed. Explain what you plan to do. Standardize commands and instructions.
- Establish resting symptoms prior to movement.
- Ask for response to movement.
- Always perform as an oscillation to assess quality of movement through range and at end-range to establish a pain-stiffness relationship.
- Assess quality, quantity, and pain or symptom response. Compare to adjacent levels or expectations of normal.
- Quality: assess amount of stiffness and displacement.
- Quantity: assess as normal, hypomobile, or hypermobile.
- Determine symptom response as type and location of symptoms.
- Assess relationship between pain and resistance.
- Symptom provocation may be more reliable than perception of movement.
- If the end of available range is reached, assess quality of resistance at end-range.
- Clinical uses: classification, treatment selection, and prognosis in combination with other historical and examination findings.

Neurological Examination

Persons with spinal pain and neurological impairment are more likely to have slower recovery rates, more recurrent episodes, and increased risk for surgery than individuals without neurological involvement. For those reasons, accurate and timely identification of neurological involvement are critical. History and physical examination findings related to cauda equina syndrome, lumbar spinal stenosis, cervical or thoracic myelopathy, and cervical or lumbar radiculopathy are covered in this chapter. Indications from the history for persons with LBP, thoracic pain, or neck pain that raise suspicion of neurological involvement include, but are not limited to, weakness, numbness, paresthesia (ie, sensations of tingling, prickling, pins and needles), loss of sensation or anesthesia, referred or radicular pain into the extremities, bowel and bladder dysfunction, and complaints of balance or gait disturbances such as ataxia or a wide-based gait.

A neurological examination is performed to identify the presence or absence of central nervous system (CNS) or peripheral nervous system (PNS) deficit. Current clinical practice guidelines[118] recommend that clinicians conduct a focused history and physical examination to classify patients with LBP into 1 of 3 broad categories: nonspecific LBP, LBP potentially associated with radiculopathy or spinal stenosis, or LBP potentially associated with another specific spinal cause. Similar guidelines exist for patients with cervical pain. If neurological signs are present, the clinician should inform the referring physician, refer appropriately, and/or assess neurological status at each visit before and after treatment in order to monitor improvement or deterioration. Progressive deterioration of neurological signs indicates serious pathology and requires immediate notification of the patient's physician. The most common neurological screening tests are manual muscle testing, deep tendon reflexes (DTRs) also known as *muscle stretch reflexes*, and sensory tests.

Sensibility Testing

For examining sensation, light touch (cotton wool) and/or pain (sharp/dull) stimulus are tested bilaterally in key segmental cutaneous areas usually representing a dermatomal (Table 3-6) distribution.[8] The clinician also examines specific areas of impaired sensation as described by the patient during the history. If a sensory deficit is present, the area should be mapped to determine if the loss corresponds to the distribution of a peripheral nerve or a spinal nerve root level. Dermatome and peripheral nerve cutaneous maps are shown in Chapter 2, Figures 2-4 and 2-5. Dermatomal maps in standard anatomy texts are variable in showing location, size, and overlap of dermatomes.[119]

Sensibility Testing Procedure: Upper Quarter (Figure 3-14) and Lower Quarter (Figure 3-15)

- Patient sitting with feet supported and area to be tested appropriately exposed.
- Explain the procedure and show patient what to expect. In an area of normal sensation, demonstrate light touch or break a sterile tongue depressor in half and test sharp/dull using the blunt or sharp edge of the blade or other instrument.

TABLE 3-6. KEY SEGMENTAL CUTANEOUS AREAS

UPPER QUARTER	LOWER QUARTER
• C2: Posterior occiput (scalp)	• L1: Groin
• C3: Anterior neck	• L2: Mid anterior thigh
• C4: Supraclavicular area	• L3: Medial aspect knee
• C5: Lateral arm over deltoid	• L4: Medial side of foot
• C6: Thumb/index finger pads	• L5: Dorsum of foot
• C7: Middle finger pad	• S1: Lateral border of foot and little toe
• C8: Ring finger, little finger pads	• S2: Posterior mid-leg
• T1: Medial arm, above elbow	

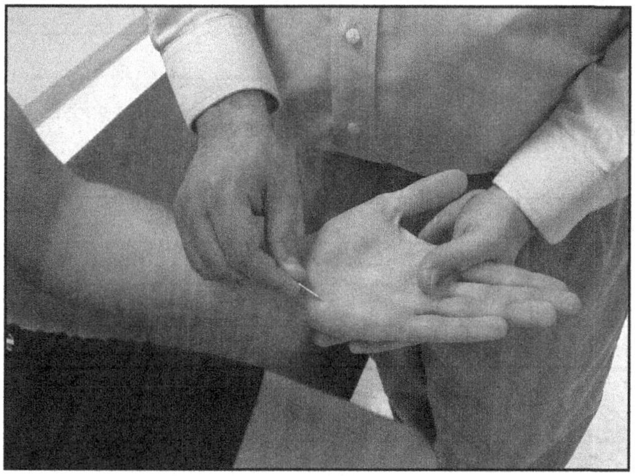

Figure 3-14. Upper quarter sensory testing. Sharp stimulus ulnar border of the left hand.

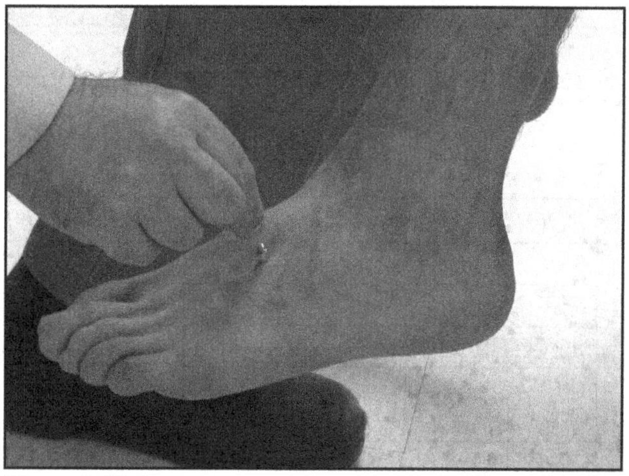

Figure 3-15. Lower quarter sensory testing. Dull stimulus dorsum of left the foot.

- Have the patient close his or her eyes and assess the response to each stimulus one segment at a time, alternating sides.
- Ask, "Does this feel the same as this?" or, "Does this feel sharp or dull?"
- Document, map, and record the location and response to stimulus.
  - o *Light touch*: Normal, reduced sensitivity to touch or hypoesthesia, absent, increased sensitivity to touch or hyperesthesia, or allodynia, which is a painful response to a normally innocuous stimulus.
  - o *Pain stimulus*: Normal, hyperalgesia or increased sensitivity to a painful stimulus; hypoalgesia or a decreased sensitivity to painful a stimulus; or anesthesia, which is a complete sensory loss suggesting a positive neurological finding.
  - o *Bilateral deficits*: May be suggestive of a CNS problem.

Manual Muscle Testing

Impairment in the ability of muscle to produce force suggests either a problem with nerve supply or muscle itself. If the nerve root is affected, then the group of muscles (myotome) supplied by that nerve root or segment are affected. If the peripheral nerve is affected, then only the muscles supplied by that nerve are affected. Tables 3-7 and 3-8 list myotomes and peripheral nerves for the lower and upper extremities, respectively.[8] Muscles of the extremities are innervated by more than one nerve root, but it is generally agreed that a primary or dominant segmental origin is present. Figure 3-16 shows the manual muscle test positions for the upper extremity. Figure 3-17 shows the manual muscle test positions for the lower extremity.

Muscle strength testing is performed to identify abnormalities using an isometric test of key muscles as representative of spinal nerve roots during a one-repetition manual muscle test. Specific muscular weakness, not associated with pain or disuse, is suggestive of a positive neurological finding. Weakness or substitution by other muscles requires

TABLE 3-7. KEY LOWER EXTREMITY MYOTOMES AND PERIPHERAL NERVES

ROOT: MOVEMENT	PERIPHERAL NERVE	MUSCLE
L2/L3: Hip flexion	Femoral nerve	Iliacus/psoas
L2/L3/L4: Knee extension	Femoral nerve	Quadriceps
L5/S1/S2: Knee flexion	Sciatic-tibial nerve	Hamstrings
L4/L5: Ankle dorsiflexion	Deep peroneal	Tibialis anterior
L4/L5: Great toe extension	Deep peroneal	Extensor hallucis longus
L5/S1: Toe extension	Deep peroneal	Extensor digitorum
L5/S1: Ankle eversion	Superficial peroneal	Peroneal longus/brevis
S1/S2: Plantarflexion	Tibial nerve	Gastrocnemius/soleus
L5/S1/S2: Hip extension	Inferior gluteal nerve	Gluteus maximus

TABLE 3-8. KEY UPPER EXTREMITY MYOTOMES AND PERIPHERAL NERVES

ROOT: MOVEMENT	PERIPHERAL NERVE	MUSCLE
C3/C4: Shoulder girdle elevation	CN XI	UT
C5/C6: Shoulder abduction	Axillary	Deltoid
C5/C6: Elbow flexion	Musculocutaneous	Biceps
C6/C7/C8: Wrist extension	Radial	Extensor carpi radialis longus and brevis/ extensor carpi ulnaris
C7/C8: Elbow extension	Radial	Triceps
C7/C8: Wrist flexion	Median/ulnar	Flexor carpi radialis/ulnaris
C7/C8/T1: Thumb interphalangeal extension	Radial	Extensor pollicis longus
C7/C8/T1: Finger flexion	Median/ulnar	Flexor digitorum superficialis/profundus
C8/T1: Finger abduction/adduction	Ulnar	Dorsal/palmar interossei

further testing of muscles that share the same innervation to differentiate spinal nerve root versus peripheral nerve compromise. For example, if a manual muscle test of the deltoid or abduction is weak and index of suspicion is high for a neurological impairment, additional testing is needed to differentiate a C5 radiculopathy from an axillary neuropathy. Standardized test positions and grading have been described in the clinical literature.[6]

Muscle Strength Testing Procedure

- Obtain baseline symptoms; explain and demonstrate a consistent test procedure.
- Assess the uninvolved side first for comparison to the involved side.
- Ask the patient to move through the test range against gravity and assess response.
- If no symptoms, repeat the motion through the range.
- Stabilize and prepare to apply resistance in a smooth and gradual manner.
- Say, "Hold, meet my resistance" or, "Hold, don't let me move you."
  - Use force appropriate to the patient and the specific muscle group.
  - Hold the contraction for at least 5 seconds.
  - Attempt to elicit a maximum contraction.
  - Observe for substitutions by other muscle groups.

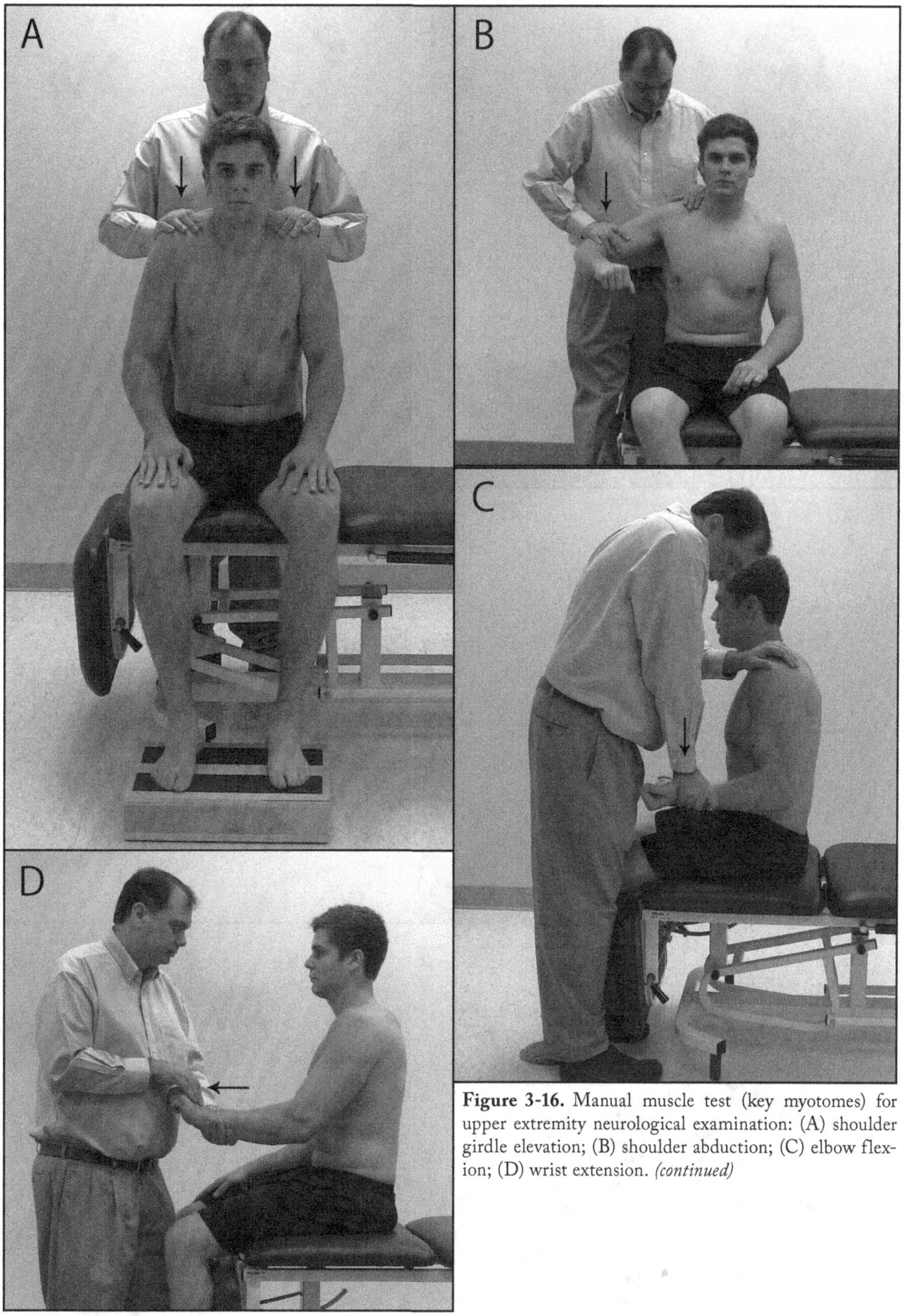

Figure 3-16. Manual muscle test (key myotomes) for upper extremity neurological examination: (A) shoulder girdle elevation; (B) shoulder abduction; (C) elbow flexion; (D) wrist extension. *(continued)*

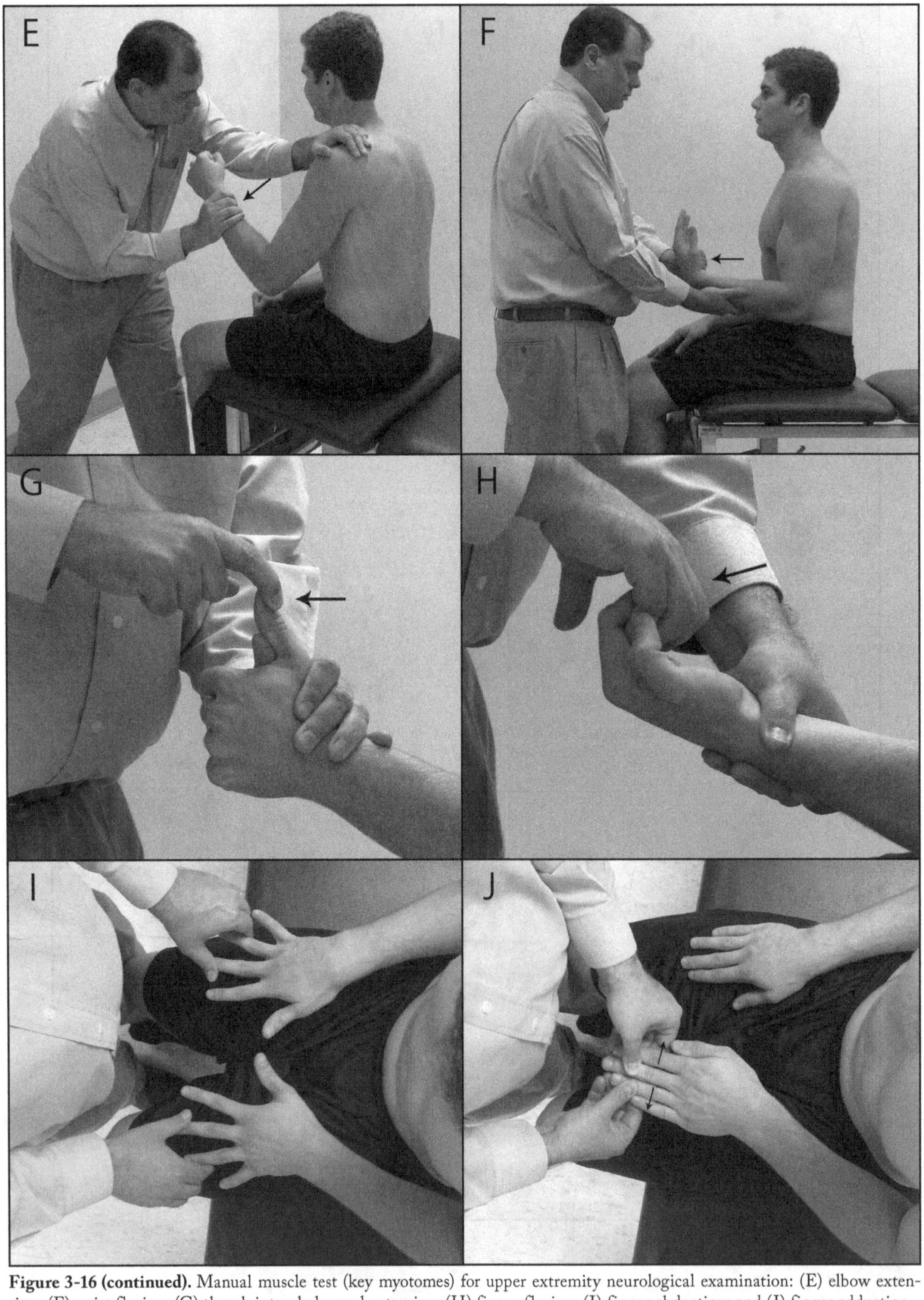

Figure 3-16 (continued). Manual muscle test (key myotomes) for upper extremity neurological examination: (E) elbow extension; (F) wrist flexion; (G) thumb interphalangeal extension; (H) finger flexion; (I) finger abduction; and (J) finger adduction.

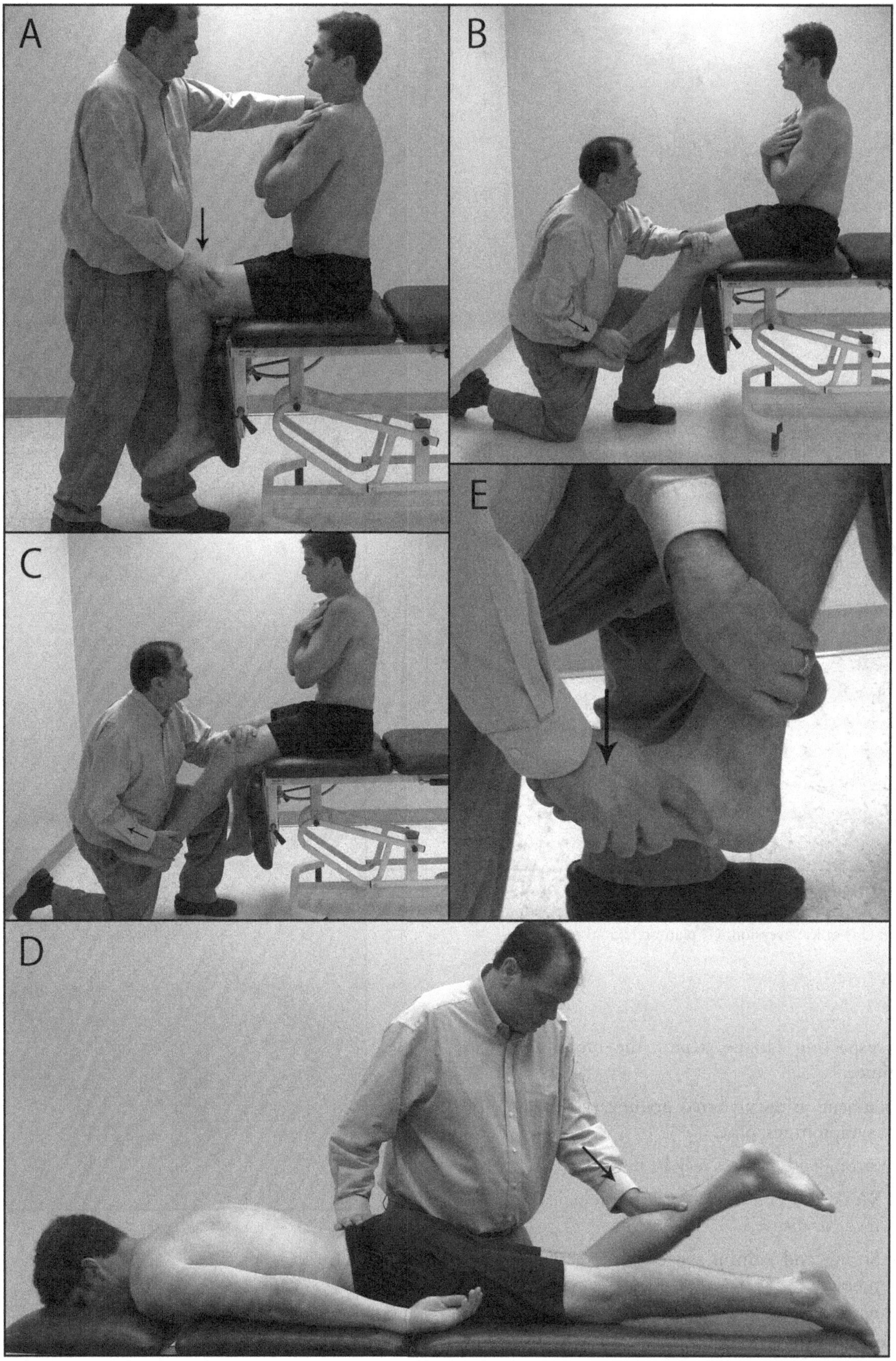

Figure 3-17. Manual muscle test (key myotomes) for lower extremity neurological examination: (A) hip flexion; (B) knee extension; (C) knee flexion (sitting); (D) knee flexion (prone); (E) ankle dorsiflexion. *(continued)*

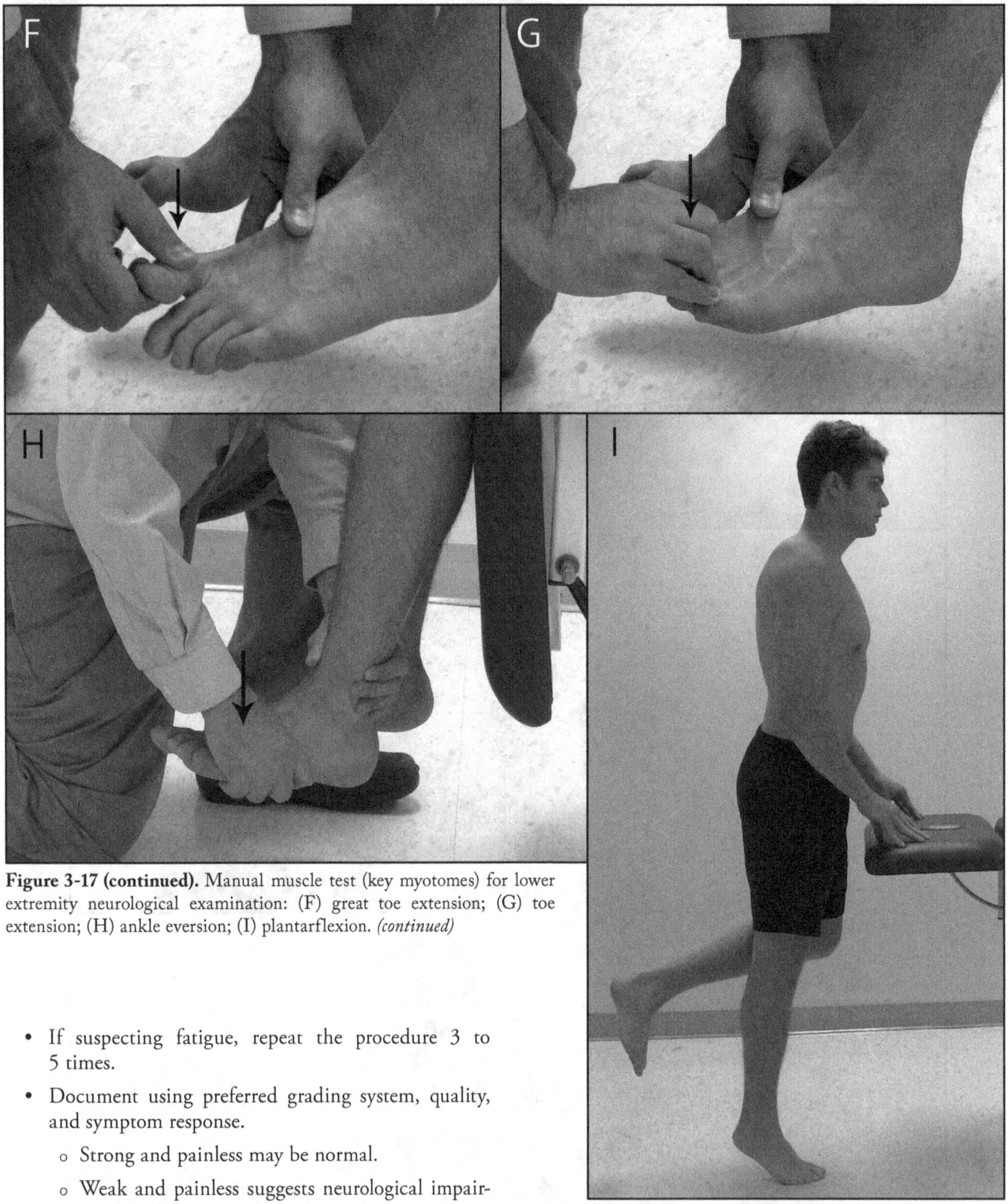

Figure 3-17 (continued). Manual muscle test (key myotomes) for lower extremity neurological examination: (F) great toe extension; (G) toe extension; (H) ankle eversion; (I) plantarflexion. *(continued)*

- If suspecting fatigue, repeat the procedure 3 to 5 times.
- Document using preferred grading system, quality, and symptom response.
  - o Strong and painless may be normal.
  - o Weak and painless suggests neurological impairment or disuse.
  - o Strong and painful suggests contractile or joint problem.
  - o Weak and painful suggests neurological, contractile and/or joint problem.
  - o Bilateral deficits at multiple levels may suggest a CNS problem.
- Grading system[6]:
  - o 5 = normal, able to hold position against strong pressure
  - o 4 = good, able to hold position against moderate pressure

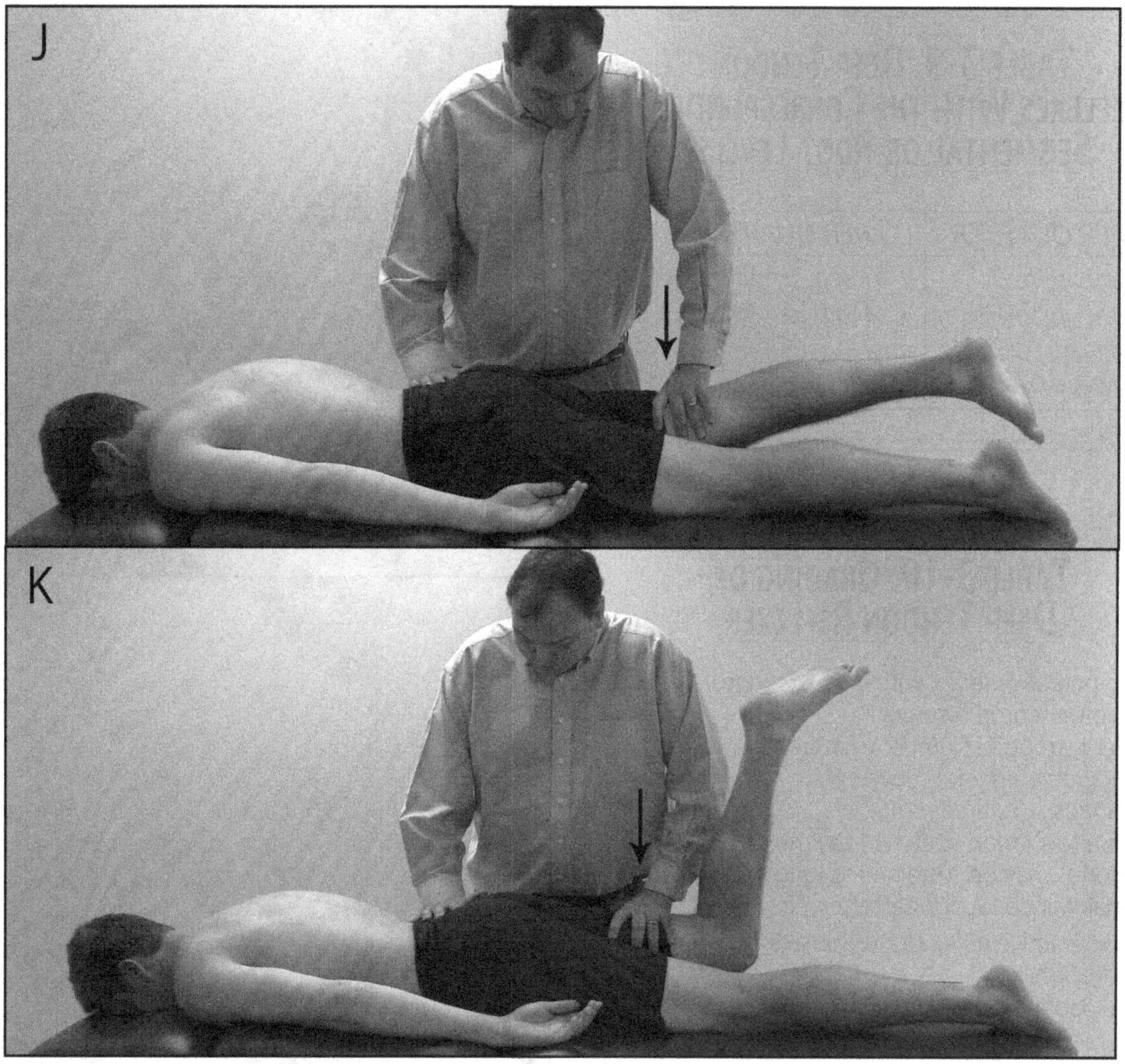

Figure 3-17 (continued). Manual muscle test (key myotomes) for lower extremity neurological examination: (J) hip extension (knee straight) and (K) hip extension (knee flexed).

- 3 = fair, able to hold position, but no pressure
- 2 = poor, moves through range gravity eliminated
- 1 = palpable contraction with no visible movement
- 0 = no evidence of muscle contraction

Deep Tendon Reflexes

DTRs, also known as muscle stretch reflexes, test the integrity of the spinal reflex arc and provide information on the integrity of the CNS and PNS via the spinal reflex arc. The most common reflexes are listed in Table 3-9, along with the corresponding segmental or root levels.[8,120] The DTR is elicited by tapping the muscle or tendon briskly, typically using a reflex hammer (Figure 3-18). The response is a contraction of the muscle. Each reflex is compared to the other side and graded appropriately (Table 3-10).[120]

Symmetry of responses between sides is important to correctly interpret the response. For example, bilaterally absent quadriceps tendon reflexes may be normal. In combination with the history, sensation, and muscle strength tests, an asymmetrical response between sides is suggestive of a problem. As a general rule, hypoactive or diminished reflexes or absent reflexes suggest lower motor neuron (LMN) pathology such as a peripheral nerve lesion or nerve root compression. LMN problems present with hyporeflexia or areflexia, weakness or atrophy, and diminished or absent sensation. Hyperactive or enhanced reflexes suggest upper motor neuron (UMN) pathology such as a symptomatic cervical myelopathy or traumatic brain injury. UMN problems present with hyperreflexia or clonus, spasticity, increased muscle tone, pathological reflexes such as Babinski's and Hoffmann's signs, and weakness in multiple muscle groups. If UMN pathology is suspected, additional tests (Babinski's, Hoffmann's, clonus, or cranial nerve (CN) screening) are performed as indicated.

Table 3-9. Deep Tendon Reflexes With the Corresponding Segmental or Root Levels

UPPER QUARTER	LOWER QUARTER
• Biceps: C5, C6 • Brachioradialis: C5, C6 • Triceps: C7	• Patellar tendon: L3, L4 • Medial hamstring: L5, S1 • Lateral hamstring: S1, S2 • Achilles tendon: S1, S2

Table 3-10. Grading of Deep Tendon Reflexes

4+ Hyperactive reflex with clonus, suggests upper motor neuron disorder.
Very strong brisk muscle contraction with exaggerated joint movement.
Clonus: involuntary muscular contractions due to sudden stretch of the muscle; the clonus may be sustained as long as stretch is maintained or stopped after a few beats.

3+ Hyperactive reflex but within a limit of normal variation.
Palpable contraction and exaggerated movement.

2+ Normal.
Palpable contraction with visible extremity movement.

1+ Hypoactive reflex, present but diminished.
Palpable muscle contraction with no extremity movement.

0 Absent, no visible or palpable muscle contraction with reinforcement.*

*The Jendrassik's maneuver is used to reinforce a DTR. For the upper extremity, ask the patient to clench his or her teeth. For the lower extremity, ask the patient to clasp his or her fingers and pull them apart

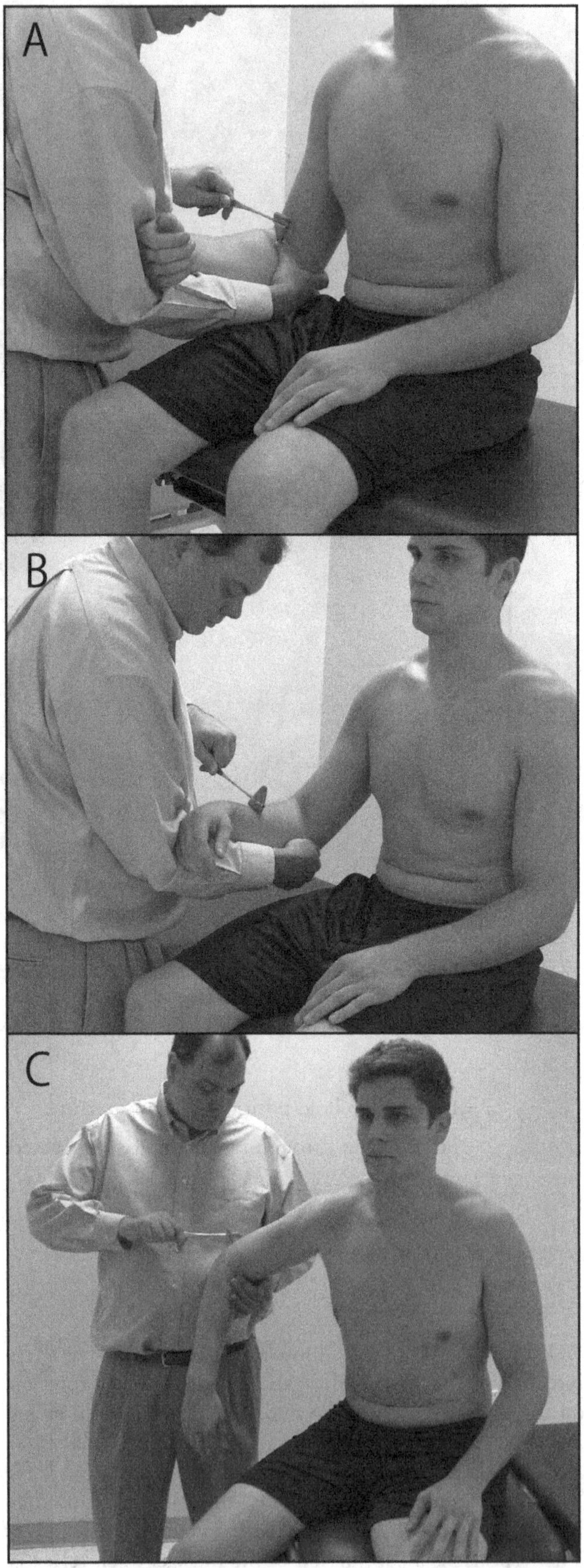

Figure 3-18. DTR testing for upper and lower extremities: (A) biceps: C5, C6; (B) brachioradialis: C5, C6; (C) triceps: C7. *(continued)*

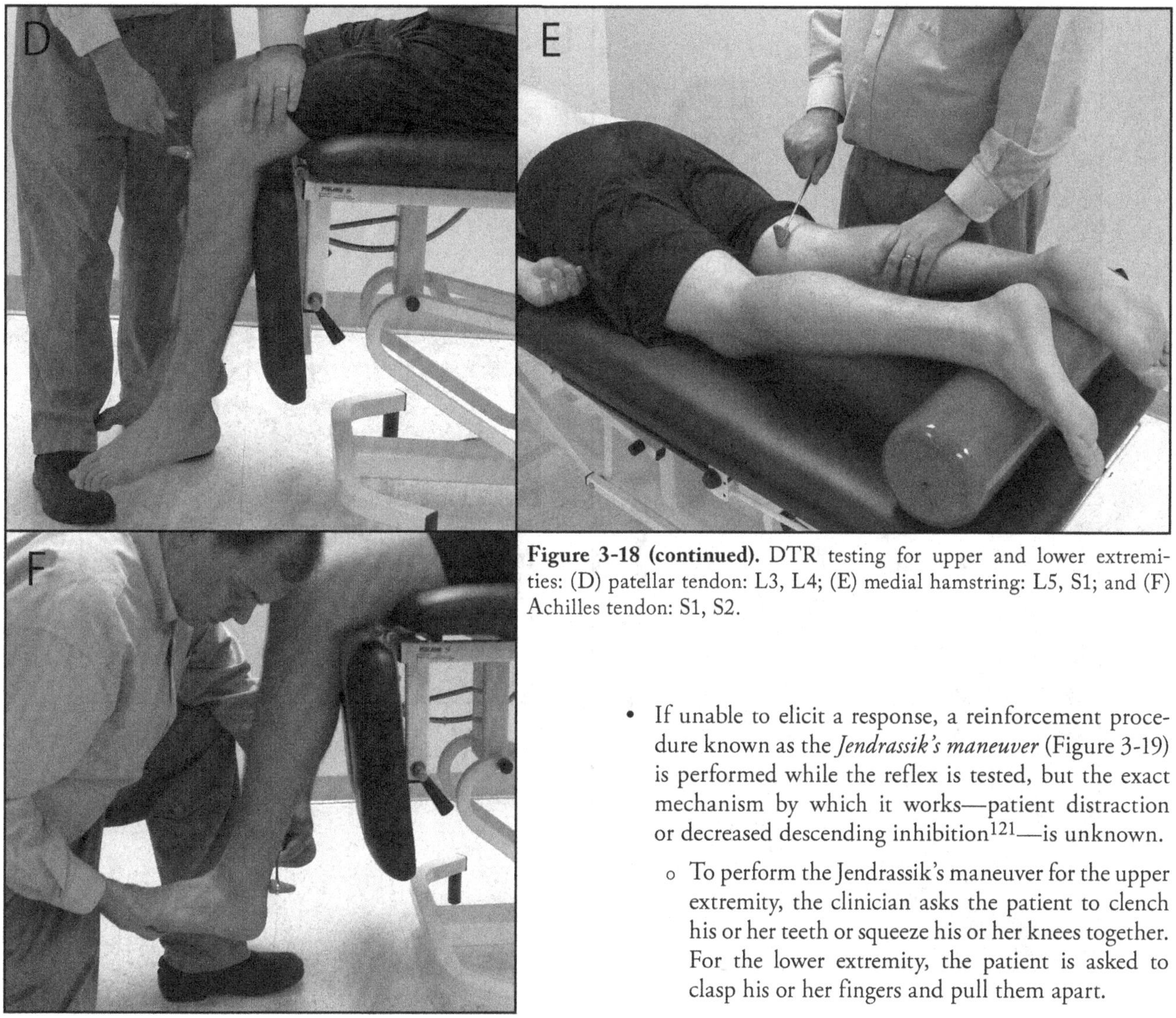

Figure 3-18 (continued). DTR testing for upper and lower extremities: (D) patellar tendon: L3, L4; (E) medial hamstring: L5, S1; and (F) Achilles tendon: S1, S2.

Deep Tendon Reflex Procedure

- Patient position is relaxed but varies among sitting, supine, or prone.
- Explain procedure and test uninvolved side first for comparison to the involved side.
- Palpate the tendon of interest.
- Use a consistent brisk tap to elicit an observable or palpable response. The tap may be repeated 3 to 6 times to obtain a consistent response.
    - o *Biceps reflex*: elbow flexion (see Figure 3-18A)
    - o *Brachioradialis reflex*: flexion and supination of the forearm (see Figure 3-18B)
    - o *Triceps reflex*: elbow extension (see Figure 3-18C)
    - o *Patellar tendon reflex*: knee extension (see Figure 3-18D)
    - o *Achilles tendon reflex*: ankle plantar flexion (see Figure 3-18F)
- If unable to elicit a response, a reinforcement procedure known as the *Jendrassik's maneuver* (Figure 3-19) is performed while the reflex is tested, but the exact mechanism by which it works—patient distraction or decreased descending inhibition[121]—is unknown.
    - o To perform the Jendrassik's maneuver for the upper extremity, the clinician asks the patient to clench his or her teeth or squeeze his or her knees together. For the lower extremity, the patient is asked to clasp his or her fingers and pull them apart.

Babinski's Sign

Babinski's sign[120] (Figure 3-20) is performed by running a sharp instrument across the plantar aspect of the foot from calcaneus to lateral border of forefoot. A positive or present Babinski's sign is extension of the great toe and splaying or abduction of the other toes. A negative or absent response is flexion of all toes. Prior to 6 months of age, Babinski's sign is present and considered normal. Though the time frame varies in some infants, after the age of 6 months, a positive or present Babinski's sign suggests a UMN problem. Babinski's sign has good sensitivity for testing UMN problems.[122]

Hoffmann's Sign

Hoffmann's sign or reflex[120] (Figure 3-21) is performed with the patient sitting or standing with the head in neutral. The therapist flicks the distal phalanx of the middle finger. A positive sign is flexion of the interphalangeal joint of the thumb with or without flexion of the index finger proximal or distal interphalangeal joints suggesting a UMN problem.[120] Evidence of neurological compromise

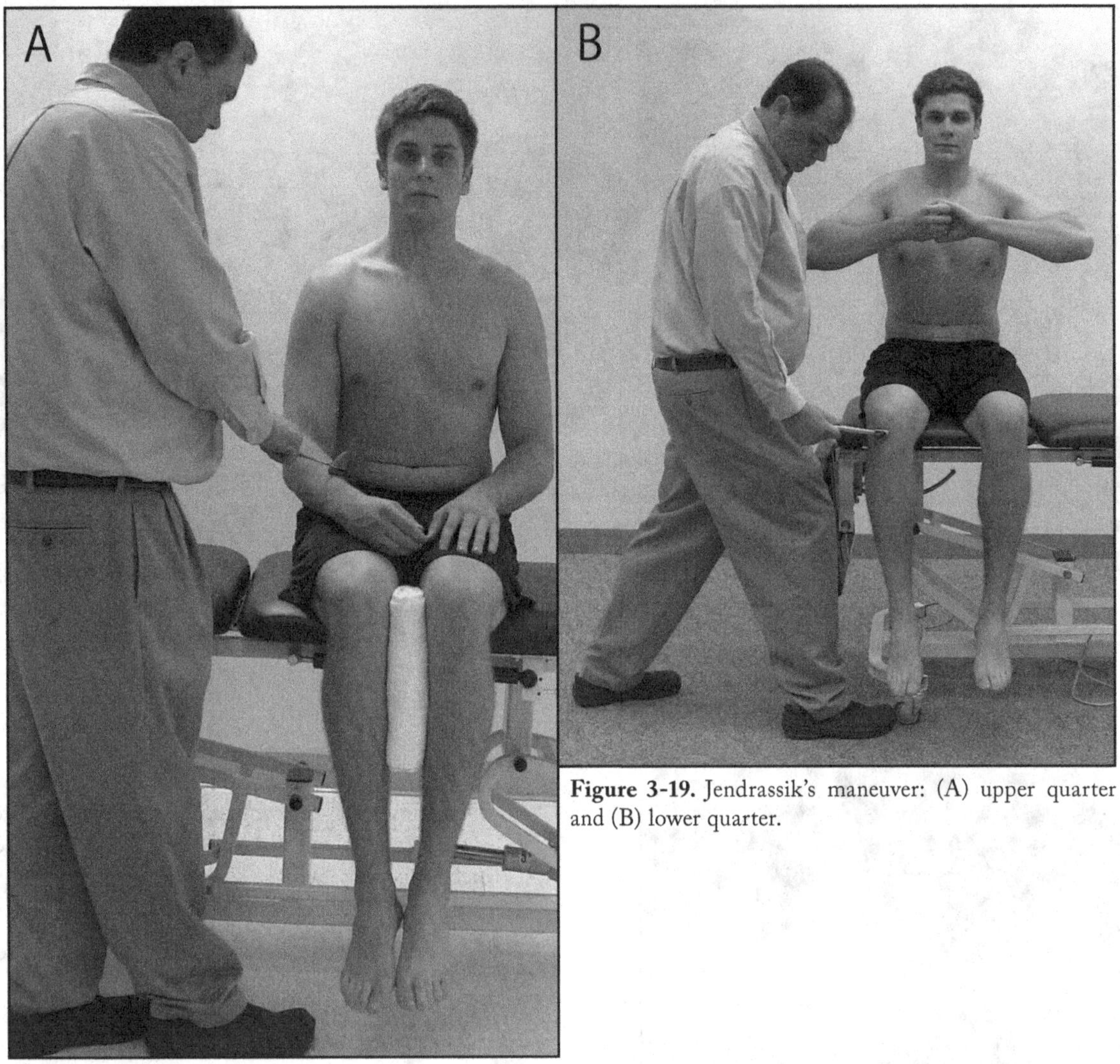

Figure 3-19. Jendrassik's maneuver: (A) upper quarter and (B) lower quarter.

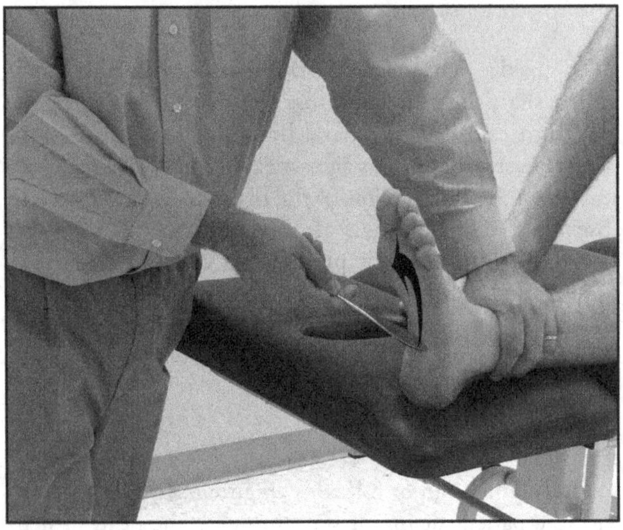

Figure 3-20. Babinski's sign.

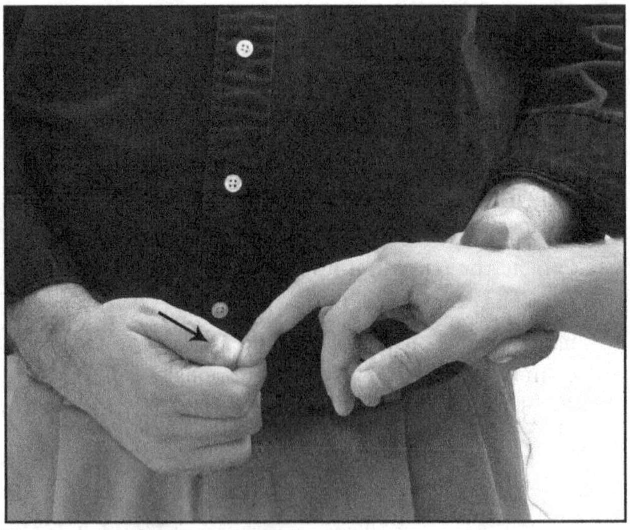

Figure 3-21. Hoffmann's sign.

such as spondylosis and cord compression on MRI in a group of 16 asymptomatic patients[123] was associated with a positive Hoffmann's sign, suggesting that the presence of this finding may be highly specific for neurologic compromise. A positive test in a patient combined with other UMN neurologic signs and symptoms warrants referral to a specialist for appropriate management.[123]

Diagnostic Accuracy for Radiculopathy

Using electrodiagnosis (EDx) as the diagnostic standard, 6 symptoms (weakness, numbness, arm pain, neck pain, tingling, and burning) and 3 exam findings (vibration/pinprick; reflexes of biceps, brachioradialis, and triceps; and manual muscle testing) were evaluated in patients referred for electrodiagnostic studies.[124] For persons diagnosed with a cervical radiculopathy, a complaint of numbness had the highest sensitivity (0.79); other symptoms were not helpful in this diagnosis (poor specificity 0.25 to 0.63). All exam findings had low sensitivities with weakness being the most sensitive (0.73) for radiculopathy. Reflexes changes (Sp 0.92 to 0.99) and combined exam findings were associated with high specificities: sensory and reflexes (Sp 0.97); sensory and weakness (Sp 0.74); and weakness and reflexes (Sp 0.98). Subjects with weakness and a reduced reflex were 9 times more likely to have a cervical radiculopathy. Having a normal examination and neck and upper extremity symptoms do not rule out the possibility of having an abnormal EDx.[124]

Using EDx as the diagnostic standard in the diagnosis of lumbosacral radiculopathy, radicular leg pain had the highest sensitivity (Sn 0.85, Sp 0.12) of the 6 symptoms (weakness, numbness, leg pain, back pain, tingling, and burning), but the specificities were low (Sp 0.12 to 0.60).[125] The OR indicated no significant association between components of the history and EDx to confirm lumbosacral radiculopathy. The physical exam findings sensation via vibration/pinprick, manual muscle testing, lower extremity reflexes, and ipsilateral SLR had low sensitivities. Patients referred with lower limb symptoms who presented with one abnormal physical exam finding had a 1.5 to 2.5 times greater chance of having a lumbosacral radiculopathy. If 2 or more physical exam findings were abnormal, patients had 2.0 to 4.5 times greater probability of having a lumbosacral radiculopathy. Combined exam findings were associated with high specificities: sensory and reflexes (Sp 0.93); sensory and weakness (Sp 0.77); weakness and reflexes (Sp 0.93); all 3 abnormal findings (Sp 0.97); and all 4 abnormal findings (Sp 0.99). In those subjects with normal physical examinations, 15% to 18% still had abnormal EDx findings.[125] In general, symptoms are more sensitive than specific and physical exam findings are more specific than sensitive for both cervical and lumbosacral radiculopathy.[126]

In a prospective cross-sectional study, Suri et al[127] examined the accuracy of the physical examination for the diagnosis of mid-lumbar (L2, 3, 4) nerve root impingement and low lumbar (L5 or S1) nerve root impingement using MRI as the reference standard. For mid-lumbar impingement, the femoral stretch test (FST), crossed FST, medial ankle pinprick sensation, and patellar reflex testing demonstrated +LRs ≥ 5.0. The FST combined with patellar reflex test or sit-to-stand test yielded +LR 7.0 (95% CI: 2.3 to 21) or LR infinity, respectively. The Achilles reflex demonstrated a +LR 7.1 (95% CI: 0.96 to 53) for the diagnosis of low lumbar nerve root impingement. Mid-level specific nerve root impingement observations included anterior thigh sensation at L2, a +LR 13 (95% CI: 1.8 to 87); FST at L3, a +LR 5.7 (95% CI 2.3 to 4.4); patellar reflex testing, a +LR 7.7 (95% CI: 1.7 to 35); medial ankle sensation (LR ∞) or crossed FST, a +LR 13 (95% CI: 1.8 to 87) at L4; and hip abductor strength at L5, a +LR 11 (95% CI: 1.3 to 84).[127]

Thoracic disc disease, fracture, thoracic herniated nucleus pulposus, and diabetes mellitus are common etiologies of thoracic pain, myelopathy, or radiculopathy.[128,129] In general, clinical presentations related to neurological compromise include spinal cord compression (ie, myelopathy) or nerve root compression (ie, radiculopathy). Myelopathic symptoms include increased muscle tone, hyperreflexia, gait ataxia, and urinary and bowel incontinence. Contralateral pain and temperature loss with ipsilateral spastic paresis below the level of the lesion and ipsilateral loss of tactile discrimination, vibration, and position sense below the level of the lesion are suggestive of Brown-Séquard syndrome or hemisection of the spinal cord. Hyperactive patellar or Achilles reflexes or clonus and Babinski's sign are usually present on exam.[128,129]

Thoracic radiculopathy may present with axial pain and intermittent or constant electric, burning, or shooting pains in a band-like distribution referred to the anterior thorax, chest, or abdomen.[128,129] Numbness or paresthesia in a dermatomal distribution is often reported. On physical exam, sensation to light touch and pinprick may be impaired in a dermatomal pattern (see Figures 2-4 and 2-5). T4 at the nipple line, T7 at the xiphoid process, and T10 for the umbilicus are commonly used landmarks. When absent, the superficial abdominal reflex suggests a UMN problem and, when absent unilaterally, suggests an LMN problem from T7 to T12 segmental levels. The superficial abdominal reflex (Figure 3-22) is tested using the end of a reflex hammer or tongue blade to stroke each quadrant of the abdomen in supine in a triangular fashion around the umbilicus and graded as present or absent. The stimulus is toward or away from the umbilicus. A normal response is abdominal contraction with movement of the umbilicus toward the quadrant of the stimulus.[8] T8 to T10 are tested above the umbilicus; T10 to T12 below the umbilicus. In normal young adults, superficial abdominal

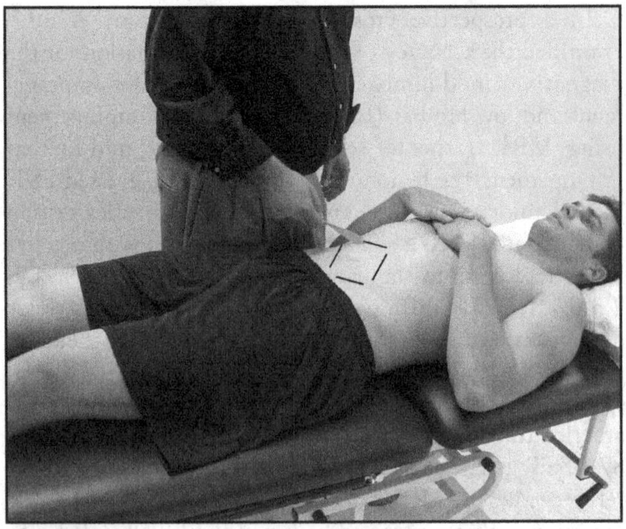

Figure 3-22. Superficial abdominal reflex.

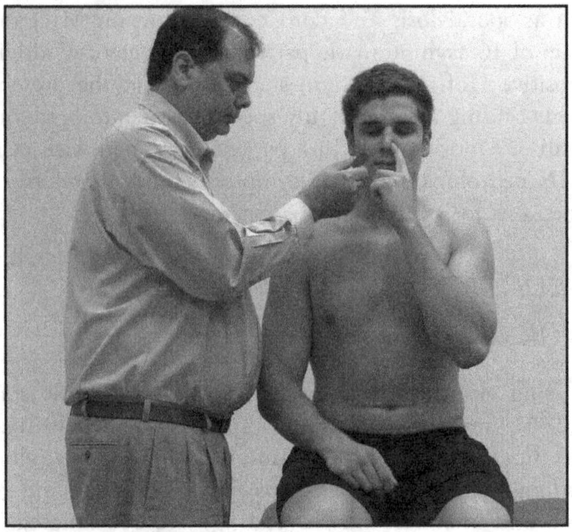

Figure 3-23. CN I—olfactory.

reflex test responses show wide variability such as asymmetry and absence in some or all quadrants.[130] Abdominal muscle strength tests can be tested through the use of standardized positions or observation of the umbilicus during a partial sit-up. The umbilicus normally does not change position. In the presence of lower abdominal weakness or paralysis, the upper rectus abdominis fibers are dominant and pull the umbilicus upward (a positive Beevor's sign).[131] Additional sources are available to review the diagnostic accuracy of tests for the neurological examination.[122,132]

Cranial Nerve Examination

Knowledge of the function of CNs provides many indications for performing a CN exam. CN dysfunction may affect vision, hearing, smell, chewing, swallowing, speaking, turning the head, and elevating the shoulder girdle. Some causes of CN dysfunction include tumors, inflammation, head trauma, and degenerative disorders resulting in vision loss, diplopia, ptosis, facial pain, neck pain, and headache. A limited examination is described as follows. Additional resources are available for review of a detailed neurological examination and interpretation of responses.

Cranial Nerve Test Procedures

- CN I—Olfactory (sense of smell; Figure 3-23)
  - o With EC, occlude one nostril and ask patient to smell orange, peppermint, chocolate, or coffee and report the odor. Repeat on the opposite side.
- CN II—Optic (sense of sight; Figure 3-24)
  - o Cover one eye and test visual acuity using a pocket visual acuity chart. Repeat on the opposite side.
  - o Cover one eye, ask the patient to look into examiner's eyes, and slowly present examiner's fingers or pen into his or her peripheral vision until visible. Repeat on each eye throughout the 360 degrees of peripheral vision.
- CN III, IV, VI—Oculomotor, trochlear, abducens (motor to extraocular muscles; Figure 3-25)
  - o Without moving the head, ask the patient to follow a penlight or pen using an H, X, and/or + pattern. Observe for conjugate eye movement.
- CN V—Trigeminal (motor to muscles of mastication and facial sensation; Figure 3-26)
  - o Assess light touch or sharp dull to the forehead, cheek, and jaw.
  - o Palpate the masseter and temporalis as the patient clenches teeth.
  - o Perform jaw jerk reflex—with patient's mouth slightly open, tap the mandible at the chin. A normal response is absence or slight elevation of the mandible.
- CN VII—Facial (motor to muscles of facial expression and sensory to anterior tongue; Figure 3-27)
  - o Ask the patient to raise eyebrows, close eyes tightly, frown, and smile.
  - o Note symmetry of motion.
- CN VIII—Vestibulocochlear (sense of hearing; Figure 3-28)
  - o The examiner rubs his or her fingers and thumb together at varying distances from the ear or whispers numbers in one ear with the opposite ear covered.
  - o Ask patient if he or she is able to hear the sound or repeat the numbers.

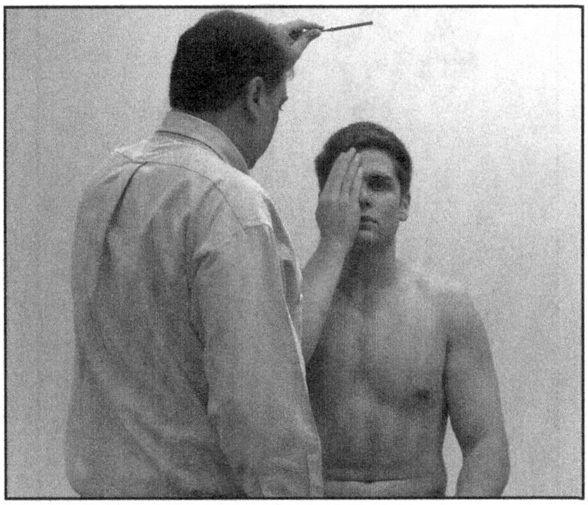

Figure 3-24. CN II—optic.

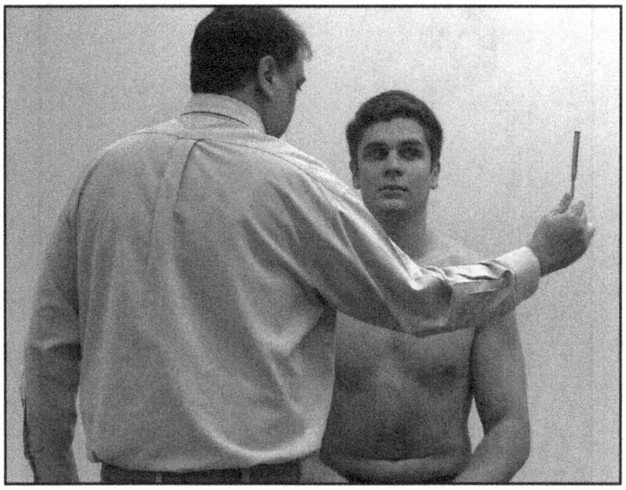

Figure 3-25. CNs III, IV, VI—oculomotor, trochlear, abducens.

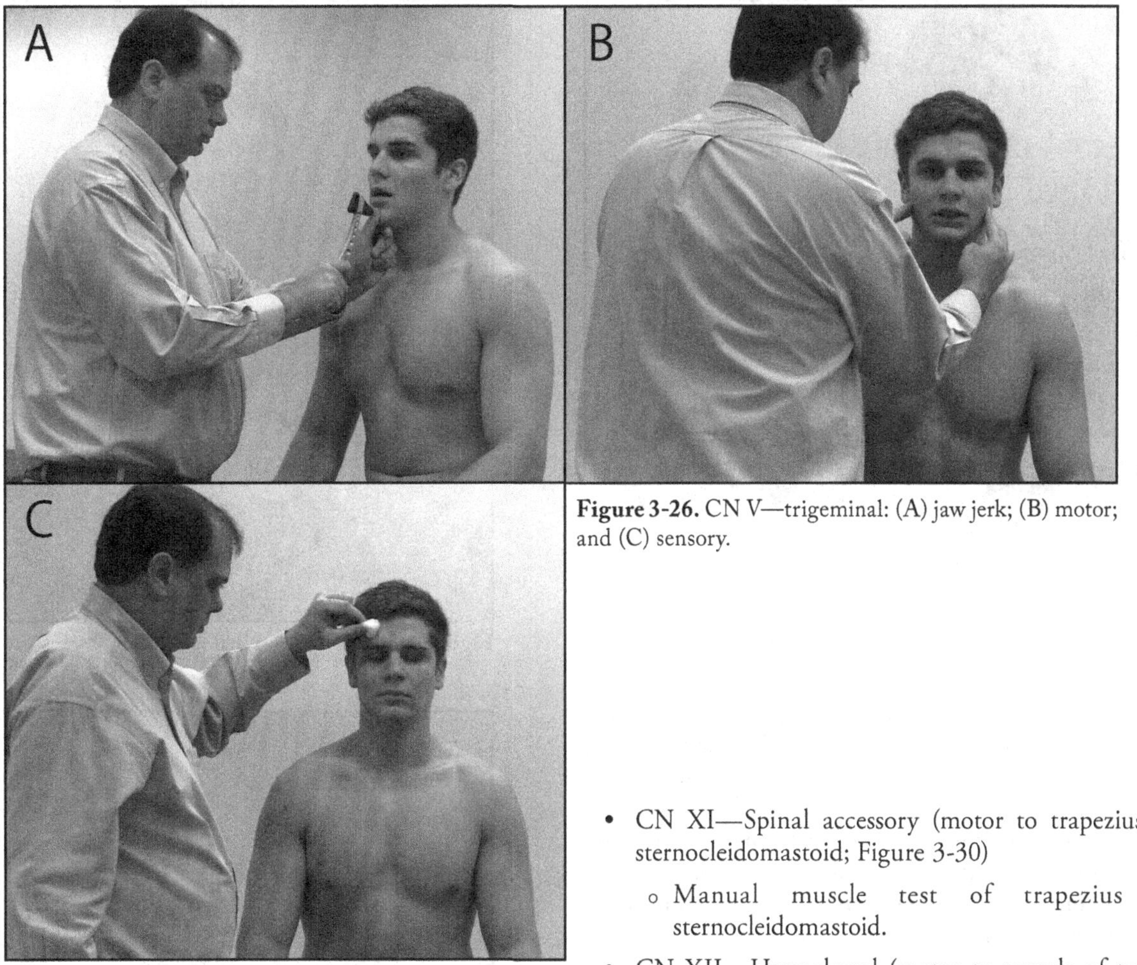

Figure 3-26. CN V—trigeminal: (A) jaw jerk; (B) motor; and (C) sensory.

- CN IX, X—Glossopharyngeal (sensory to palate) and vagus (motor to palate; Figure 3-29)
    - o Test gag reflex by touching the soft palate.
    - o Ask patient to say "ah." Observe the uvula for symmetrical elevation.
- CN XI—Spinal accessory (motor to trapezius and sternocleidomastoid; Figure 3-30)
    - o Manual muscle test of trapezius and sternocleidomastoid.
- CN XII—Hypoglossal (motor to muscle of tongue; Figure 3-31)
    - o Ask patient to protrude the tongue. Observe for movement to one side and atrophy.
    - o Ask the patient to push the tongue against the inside of the cheek. Resist the motion on each side and assess symmetry.

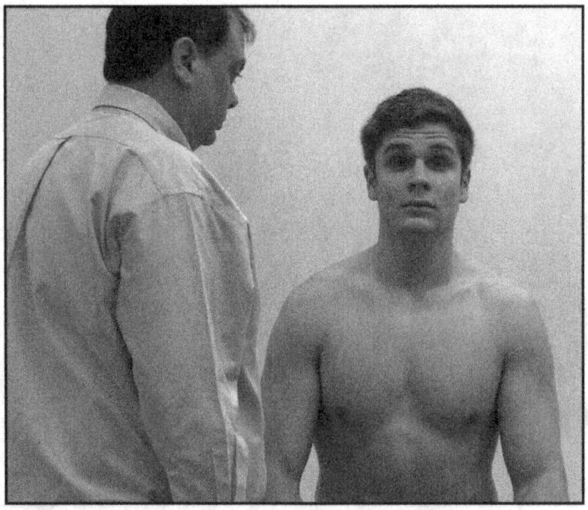

Figure 3-27. CN VII—facial.

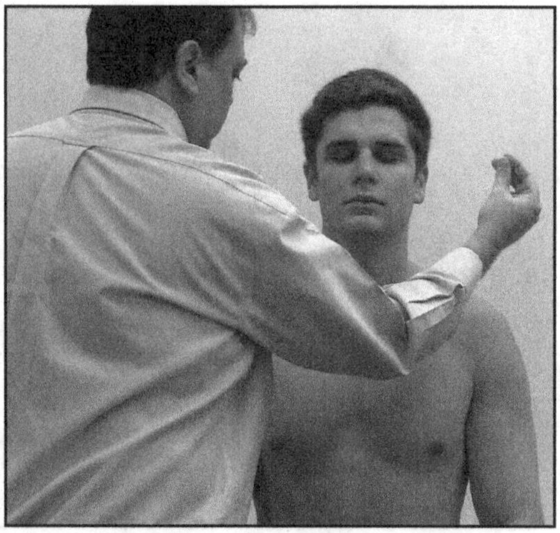

Figure 3-28. CN VIII—vestibulocochlear.

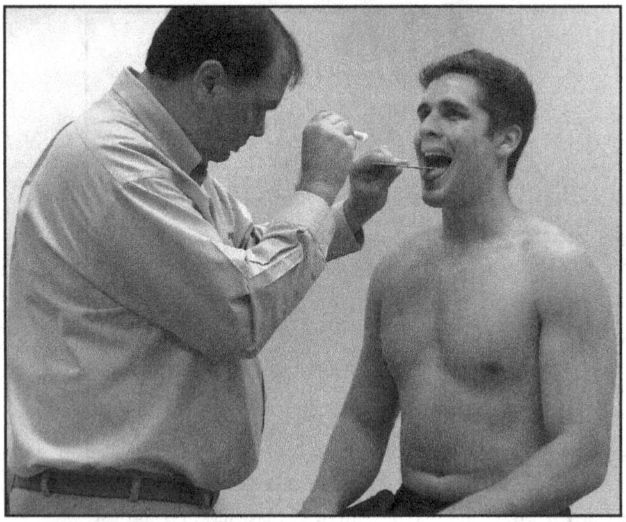

Figure 3-29. CNs IX, X—glossopharyngeal.

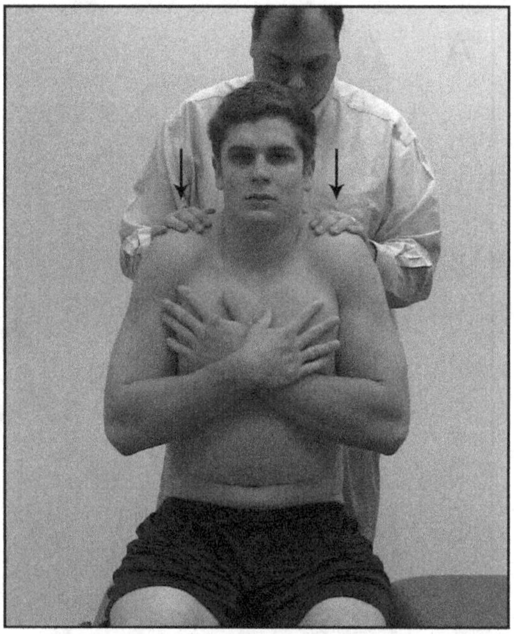

Figure 3-30. CN XI—spinal accessory.

Muscle Length Tests

Analysis of static and dynamic posture and various movements or activities lead the clinician to determine which muscle length tests should be performed. Theoretically, impairments in muscle length and strength may be either the cause or consequence of MS pain and altered movement patterns. The ability to detect and correct these impairments is viewed as a basic tenet of rehabilitation and prevention of reinjury.

Muscle length tests are used to determine whether muscle length is excessive or limited.[6] As previously discussed, certain muscle groups have a tendency to become short and strong, whereas others become long and weak. The purpose of muscle length tests is to determine whether (a) a muscle is too short to allow normal ROM or a desired activity, or (b) a muscle is too long, allowing too much ROM.[6] An increase or decrease in soft tissue length occurs

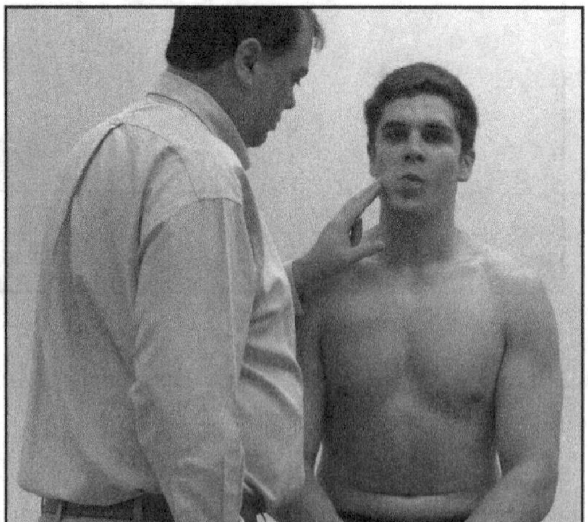

Figure 3-31. CN XII—hypoglossal.

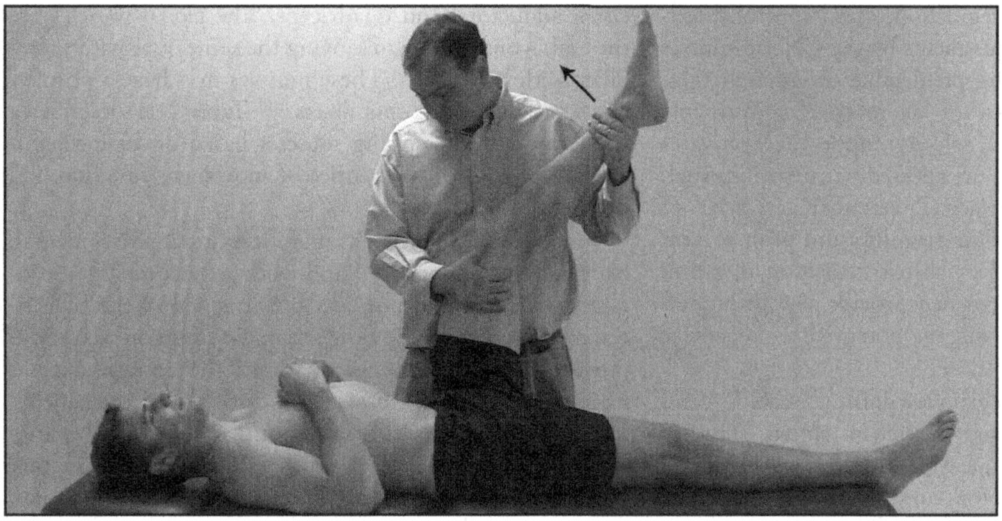

Figure 3-32. Hamstring length at 90/90 position.

commonly in postural syndromes, repetitive movement patterns, and as a result of trauma or prolonged immobilization. In patients with moderate to severe pain or presenting with high irritability, muscle shortness may be protective in nature due to actual tissue damage or neural tissue mechanosensitivity. Muscle length tests in these patients may be deferred to the point where pain is not a dominant feature.

Muscle length testing is a passive movement that involves lengthening the muscle in a motion that is directly opposite to its action. The technique (Figure 3-32) entails stabilizing one end of the muscle's attachment and passively moving the opposite end slowly to assess resistance through the range, available ROM, end feel, and symptom response.[133] The symptom response is usually felt in the muscle belly. If symptoms are felt over the joint or tendon, additional testing is required to determine the source of the symptoms. Results are often measured using a goniometer or inclinometer and compared to the uninvolved side. Abnormal or asymmetrical relevant findings are then used for reassessment and to guide intervention designed to correct the problem. For example, if a patient has short hamstring muscles that result in excessive lumbar flexion during flexion activities, intervention might include strategies to lengthen the hamstrings, shorten the lumbar extensors, and/or correct poor motor control patterns.

In prescribing an intervention, clinicians should determine the cause of the tightness or weakness. According to Janda et al,[134] muscles prone to weakness usually are stabilizers or tonic muscles, while muscles prone to shortness are movers or phasic muscles. Though there are likely many causes of muscle shortness such as static postures, emotional stress, or repetitive exercise patterns, another cause may be the result of a poor stabilization system resulting in prime mover or phasic muscles working as stabilizers. For example, short hamstrings may be the result of poor proximal trunk stabilization. Simply stretching the hamstrings is unlikely to adequately address the problem.

Tests for muscle length are based on knowledge of muscle structure and function. Antagonistic muscles demonstrate impaired function resulting in imbalances in muscle length and/or strength. The exact etiology of the muscle imbalance is unknown. However, both biomechanical factors such as tissue length and tension-generating ability and neurological factors such as timing, activation, and coordination factors are noted in clinical observations. The clinical literature describes standardized test positions, but many of these tests have not been validated or tested for their ability to distinguish between subjects or assess changes over time. Despite a lack of supportive evidence, clinicians continue to use muscle length tests as valued examination tools.[135] Many factors such as time of day, temperature, activity level, test positions and surfaces, and measurement tools may affect the results of a muscle length test. Clinicians are encouraged to control as many variables as possible to improve test-retest reliability and validity. Muscle length tests associated with each region are described in subsequent chapters.

Muscle Performance

The spine is naturally unstable and depends significantly on the performance of muscle for both static and dynamic stability. Panjabi[136] has described requirements for spinal stability through the interaction of 3 stabilization subsystems: (1) passive stability from the ligaments, discs, joint capsules, bones; (2) active stability from the muscles; and (3) control strategies guided by the nervous system. These systems respond to both expected and unexpected situations through the coordinated action of many muscles. A deficit in spinal stability may be caused by a problem in any 1 of the 3 subsystems.

Muscle activation levels, timing, and recruitment patterns are important in movement control and spinal stability. The CNS prepares the spine before, just prior to, and during movement to regulate postural control. Feed-forward or anticipatory adjustments by the CNS minimize postural disturbance during predictable or voluntary use of extremities. Feed-backward or reactive adjustments occur after movement via sensory input that activates automatic strategies during unexpected perturbations such as an unstable support surface. Preparatory activation of trunk muscles provides postural equilibrium prior to arm or leg movement. Delayed or absent activation of trunk muscles during daily activities may provide periods of inefficient spinal stabilization and the potential for repetitive microtrauma.

From a biomechanical viewpoint, McGill and Karpowicz[137] reported that sufficient spinal stability requires a balance of stiffness and force between many muscles, a responsive motor control system, muscular endurance, and sufficient tolerance of the spine to support loads. The amount of muscle activation for spinal stability is task dependent. In the healthy spine and for most daily activities, abdominal wall cocontraction with the extensors at about 10% of maximum voluntary contraction or less is sufficient.[137] Thus, a stable spine requires low, but continuous, muscle activation in all activities.

Altered Muscle Performance in Persons With Low Back Pain

Optimal sensorimotor control of the spine requires coordinated contributions from both global or superficial and local or deep muscles. Consequently, altered muscle performance can occur in the global or local muscles or, as is often seen clinically, in both muscle groups. In the presence of dysfunction and pain, some muscles lose extensibility and become overactive and excessively stiff, whereas others become excessively flexible, inhibited, or functionally weak. Daily activities and the requirements for muscle activation vary by posture, task, and environment. In persons with neck pain, thoracic pain, and LBP, muscle performance and control strategies are altered. Whether the altered motor control strategies are a cause or result of the spinal pain requires further study. Individuals with acute pain may adopt altered movement strategies to protect painful structures whereas long-term muscle performance deficits may result from altered neural input due to disuse or fear-avoidance behavior.

Muscle Classification Related to Function

As described by Bergmark,[138] superficial or global muscles such as abdominals and ES extend from the pelvis to the thoracic spine, rib cage, and/or the extremities. The primary muscles in this group include the ES, rectus abdominis, EO, hamstrings, gluteus maximus, latissimus dorsi, adductors, and quadriceps. The global muscles are the main contributors to moving the spine or providing stability with high loads. These muscles may have a primary role as stabilizers or mobilizers.[139] Table 3-11 describes a framework for classifying muscles based on biomechanical and physiological theories of movement function and dysfunction.[140-142]

Muscles that function as mobilizers are multisegmental, biarticular and superficial and work concentrically to produce movement and power. Cocontraction of the superficial muscles surrounding the trunk is a common strategy to provide the stiffness necessary for stability in tasks such as lifting. As mentioned previously, during gait, the superficial muscles act phasically in response to directional changes of the pelvis and at heel strike.[143] Muscles that function as stabilizers are primarily monoarticular or segmental, deep, and work tonically to control daily nonfatiguing functional movement. The deep or local system consists of muscles such as deep multifidus attaching directly to the lumbar vertebrae. Early low-load or tonic activation of the deep muscles presumed to control segmental movement has been observed during a variety of tasks involving upper and lower limb movement. This tonic activation is generally not direction specific and creates a stable foundation for movement of the extremities.[144-147] The diaphragm and pelvic floor muscles also aid in the control of the lumbar spine and pelvis in addition to their respective roles in respiration[148] and continence.[149]

Daily activities and occupations require a wide range of tasks involving a spectrum of muscle activation strategies to safely accomplish the demands of each task. The demands range from static to dynamic stability, low to high load, low movement to high movement, and low predictability to high predictability. Dynamic, low load, high movement, and high predictability activities require greater contributions from deep muscles. High-load, static, or unpredictable activities call for increased cocontraction of the superficial muscles.[31] Assessment of muscle performance during daily activities and occupations involve individual parameters of strength, endurance, and power and motor control of superficial and deep stabilizers. Assessment and motor control strategies for spinal pain are discussed in subsequent chapters.

Muscle Activation Patterns in Person With Low Back Pain

Muscle activation patterns exhibited by persons with LBP differ from healthy subjects. Van Dieën et al[150] suggested that altered muscle activity affecting movement and stability of the spine is task dependent, is related to the individual problem, and may be highly variable between and within individuals. Some individuals restrict movement while some move in a poorly controlled manner. No consistent pattern emerges, but the CNS generally adopts

TABLE 3-11. CLASSIFICATION OF MUSCLE RELATED TO FUNCTION AND DYSFUNCTION

MUSCLE	FUNCTION	DYSFUNCTION
GLOBAL MOBILIZERS		
• Rectus abdominis • Iliocostalis • Piriformis	• Generates torque to produce ROM • Contraction = concentric length change; therefore, concentric production of movement (rather than eccentric control) • Concentric acceleration of movement (especially sagittal plane: flexion/extension) • Shock absorption of load • Activity is direction dependent • Noncontinuous activity (on/off phasic pattern)	• Myofascial shortening—limits physiological and/or accessory motion (which must be compensated for elsewhere) • Overactive low threshold, low-load recruitment • Reacts to pain and pathology with spasm • Changes in muscle length and recruitment resulting in over-pull (short/overactive) at a motion segment • Global imbalance
GLOBAL STABILIZERS		
• Oblique abdominals • Spinalis • Gluteus medius	• Generates force to control or limit ROM • Contraction = eccentric length change; therefore, control throughout range especially inner range (muscle active = joint passive) and hypermobile outer range) • Low-load deceleration of momentum (especially axial plane rotation) • Noncontinuous activity Activity is direction dependent	• Muscle active shortening = joint passive) loss of inner range control: • If hypermobile, poor control of excessive range • Poor low threshold tonic recruitment • Poor eccentric control • Poor rotation dissociation • Changes in muscle length and recruitment resulting in under-pull (long/inhibited) at a motion segment • Global imbalance
LOCAL STABILIZERS		
• TrA • Deep multifidus • Psoas major (Posterior fascicles)	• ↑ Muscle stiffness to control segmental motion • Controls the neutral joint position • Contraction = no/minimal length change; therefore, does not produce ROM • Activity is independent of direction of movement • Continuous activity throughout movement • Proprioceptive input regarding joint position, range, and rate of movement	• Motor control deficit associated with delayed timing or recruitment deficiency • Reacts to pain and pathology with inhibition • ↓ Muscle stiffness and poor segmental control • Loss of control of joint neutral position • Changes in motor recruitment resulting in a loss of segmental control • Local inhibition

From Gibbons SGT, Comerford JM. Strength versus stability: part 1: concept and terms. *Orthop Div Rev.* 2001;March/April:21-27. Content reprinted with permission from KC International.

a strategy of increased stiffness or cocontraction of the superficial trunk muscles to adapt to pain or injury. This strategy normally reserved for high-load function, if not corrected, is used consistently for low-load postural control and normal functional movements.

Superficial Muscles

Trunk muscle recruitment patterns in persons with LBP compared to control subjects reflect a strategy that increases spinal stability.[151] The strategy might involve cocontraction of flexors and extensors or increased activity of either group alone and/or impaired activity of the deep muscles. A strategy of increased spinal stability may lead to a perceived decreased need for deep muscle activity, or impaired deep muscle activity may lead to a strategy of increased stiffness. These strategies are referred to as muscle imbalance, faulty movements, motor control impairments, and substitution or compensation strategies.

A strategy of increased stiffness or cocontraction of the superficial muscle systems is assumed to compensate for a loss of stability for the following reasons:

- Injury to the spine—either discs, ligaments, muscle—may result in reduced segmental stiffness requiring an increase in muscle activation to compensate.
- Muscle force or endurance may be reduced, resulting in limited ability to correct perturbations of equilibrium and prevent spinal instability.
- Sensorimotor integration is altered, limiting the ability to dynamically coordinate global and local muscles strategies for a variety of tasks. In persons with LBP, a static strategy of cocontraction, although not optimal, allows for movement control across a variety of conditions.[31,150]

Altered motor control strategies do not always resolve when the pain resolves. In some instances, continued use of a high-load strategy using dominant global mobilizers may have detrimental effects such as reduced motion, increased axial load, poor shock absorption, activity limitations, impaired respiration, and increased risk of recurrent LBP. Impairments of the superficial muscle system have been observed in a variety of disorders of the lumbopelvic complex.[152-154]

Deep Muscles

Feed-forward activation of the TrA is generally agreed upon, but simultaneous onset of TrA activation is not. In early studies with healthy subjects, the TrA, when tested unilaterally, was activated prior to use of the arms or legs independent of direction of movement to prepare the spine for contraction of the larger trunk muscles and for limb movement.[145,155] Allison et al[156] also reported feed-forward TrA activation in healthy subjects but examined bilateral TrA activation. In contrast to what was previously theorized, Allison et al[156] determined that both sides are activated before the arm moves but with contralateral TrA activation occurring prior to ipsilateral activation in a direction-specific manner. Despite this minor controversy, in submaximal tasks, the role of feed-forward TrA activation is believed to be enhanced stability as a strategy to improve trunk stiffness without a concurrent increase in activity of the torque producing trunk muscles.[157]

The TrA is thought to control segmental movement, particularly translation,[158] to aid in stability of the pelvic girdle[159] and to cocontract with the diaphragm,[160] the pelvic floor,[161] and the deep multifidus (DM).[144] In persons with LBP, activity of the TrA is delayed[162-164] or reduced[165,166] prior to arm or leg tasks. In these individuals, activity of the superficial abdominals (ie, rectus abdominis, EO) and ES is often increased,[167] but the pattern of activation in the superficial muscles is variable between individuals.[168,169] During experimentally induced LBP, at the L4 level, subjects had a decreased ability to contract the TrA during the abdominal drawing-in maneuver (ADIM; Figure 3-33).[170] In addition to the TrA, the internal oblique (IO), LM, ES, and contralateral EO muscles respond in a feed-forward manner during a unilateral upper extremity flexion task,[60,171,172] presumably to maintain trunk alignment and minimize center of mass displacement in all 3 planes at the same time.[172] These studies suggest that impairments in muscle recruitment and timing may be factors in chronic or recurrent LBP.

As evidenced by studies of heterogeneous samples of subjects with CLBP, altered muscle activity varies between individuals, yet only one study has examined for differences among subgroups. Silfies et al[172] investigated differences in muscle activation patterns among 3 subgroups of persons with mechanical LBP: an instability group, a noninstability group, and asymptomatic controls. Using a unilateral upper extremity flexion task, the study results generally agreed with previous reports that healthy subjects have a feed-forward response in certain muscles (TrA, IO, ES, LM, contralateral EO), although not all individuals used the same sequence of activations. Both the instability group and noninstability group had delayed onset of selected trunk muscles compared with the control group. The instability LBP group did not demonstrate feed-forward activity or individual muscle timing differences. Instead, this subgroup used a delayed general stiffening of the spine. The noninstability LBP subgroup was similar to the control group, activating trunk extensors in a feed-forward manner but significantly earlier than the instability group. Activation timing was more impaired in the instability group compared with the noninstability group. The authors concluded that not all subgroups of patients with LBP demonstrate the same postural response pattern and that both superficial and deep muscles are integrated into patterns for functional tasks.[172]

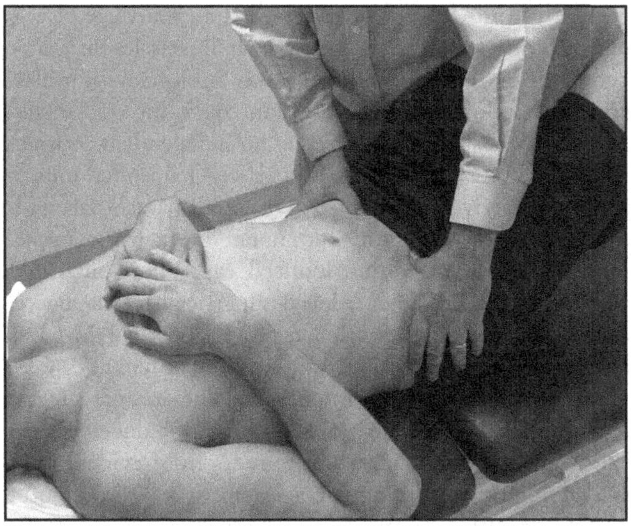

Figure 3-33. Abdominal drawing-in maneuver. Voluntary activation of the transversus abdominis by drawing the lower abdomen toward the spine performed in supine.

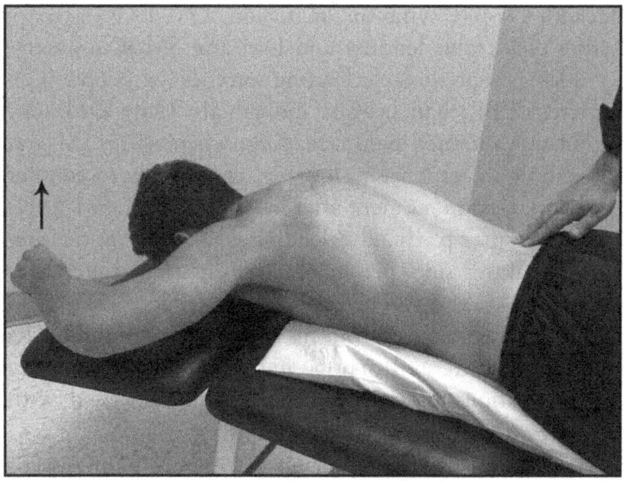

Figure 3-34. Multifidus activation with contralateral arm lift. The left arm is in 120 degrees of elevation with the elbow in 90 degrees of flexion and lifted 2 inches from the table.

The lumbar paraspinals consist of the deep lumbar multifidus (DM), superficial lumbar multifidus (SM), and the ES. Biomechanical models propose that the ES and SM produce extension of the lumbar spine and intervertebral compression.[173,174] The ES and SM, when cocontracted with the abdominals, also aid in segmental control.[175] The DM generate compressive forces with minimal torque,[174] do not rotate the lumbar vertebra,[176] and have the ability to control segmental motion.[175] The DM have the potential to control segmental motion without restricting movement of the spine.[175]

The ES, SM, and DM are differentially active in functional tasks. Unlike SM and ES, the DM is active in a non–direction-specific, feed-forward manner during rapid arm movements.[144] Differential activity of DM and SM has also been observed during expected trunk loading, but not in unexpected trunk loading.[177] Several studies have demonstrated abdominal and paraspinal muscle activity during the ADIM.[175,178-180] The DM[144] and TrA[181] are both active, although not simultaneously, in a non–direction-specific, feed-forward manner during unilateral arm movement.

In persons with LBP, changes in the LM are reflected in the DM more than the SM or ES.[180,182,183] The cross-sectional area of the multifidus is decreased on the painful side[184] and reduced as measured by computed tomography (CT).[185] Prevalence of asymmetrical LM atrophy is as high as 80% using MRI in persons with LBP.[186,187] Morphological changes in the deep back muscles in persons with LBP are more profound in the short fibers and on the painful side.[184,188]

Using rehabilitation ultrasound imaging, Kiesel et al[170] investigated the effect of experimentally induced pain on LM at the level and side of pain induction during a contralateral arm lifting task 2 inches from a table (Figure 3-34). Multifidus activation was reduced at the level and side of the pain induction, but no information was revealed about whether a more generalized response occurs. In acute LBP, altered activation of the LM has been reported as selective, reduced on the side of symptoms at the symptomatic level,[184,189,190] and in CLBP it has been found to be more generalized, reduced on both sides and at more than one level.[186,191,192] In 15 healthy subjects, Dickx et al[193] investigated the effect of unilaterally induced LBP on multifidus recruitment using a unilateral arm lifting task. These authors found a more generalized response in the LM where activity is reduced bilaterally and at multiple levels. Pain results in an immediate change in LM recruitment. Therefore, exercises that provoke pain are unlikely to aid in restoring control of the LM.[193]

MacDonald et al[194] concluded that onset of the DM and SM in persons with symptom-free recurrent unilateral LBP is different from healthy subjects during a rapid arm movement. Electromyography (EMG) recorded DM fiber onset occurred later in the LBP group. The observed delay was greater on the previously painful side than on the nonpainful side. The DM fiber contraction was active earlier than the SM on both sides in the healthy group and on the nonpainful side in the LBP group, but not on the painful side. The DM reportedly contributes up to two-thirds of lumbar segmental motion control.[195] Thus, abnormal control of the DM may result in altered joint loading and contribute to recurrent symptoms, but this association has not been determined. Resolution of LBP does not mean that normal control of the deep muscles has returned. On the contrary, motor control deficits continue to exist.[195]

MacDonald et al[196] investigated control of the DM and SM in symptom-free, recurrent unilateral LBP compared to healthy individuals in response to predictable and unpredictable trunk loading (ie, catching a 1-kg mass in a bucket). Despite symptom remission, DM EMG activity before predictable loading and DM and SM EMG activity during unpredictable loading were less in people with recurrent LBP than healthy individuals. Only DM activation was initiated before loading, whereas the SM was active only in response to loading, presumably to counter the trunk flexion moment after load onset. Peak SM EMG amplitude after predictable loading was earlier on the previously painful side, perhaps a compensation strategy for the reduced DM EMG before loading. Reduced DM EMG before loading may result in inadequate preparation of the spine for loading and may be important when retraining for occupations or daily tasks that are associated with trunk loading such as lifting.[196]

A person's beliefs[197] about his or her back pain and his or her anticipation of back pain[198] episodes also influence the motor control of back muscles. Spontaneous resolution of the changes in motor strategies did not occur in some people with unhelpful beliefs or the perception of threat to the back.[197] Continual unhelpful beliefs about back pain may lead to continued use of altered strategies to control movement. DM and abdominal muscle EMG are delayed in anticipation of experimentally induced LBP in healthy individuals.[198]

Altered Muscle Performance and Exercise Planning

An exercise plan appropriate to the individual patient is best determined through a thorough assessment. If osteoligamentous instability or poor load tolerance is present, maintaining or increasing the stability of the spine may be necessary. If deep muscle activity is impaired and normal and low-load activities are provocative, retraining the local stabilizers may take priority initially. Treatment effects of motor control exercise are greater in individuals with a poorer ability to recruit the TrA.[199] If a high-load strategy is responsible for persistent LBP, training to reduce the overactive superficial muscles and then training to coordinate the superficial and deep systems for dynamic stability may be most effective. The superficial and deep muscles should be assessed for specific impairments and training tailored to the nature of those deficits with the goal of restoring complex control strategies for multiple tasks. All trunk and associated pelvic and shoulder girdle muscles are considered important for optimal spinal stability.

Cognitive activation of specific trunk muscles such as repeated voluntary TrA contractions in isolation from other trunk muscles is often used in rehabilitation. This motor control training results in immediate[200] and persistent[201] improvement in coordination of the abdominal muscles in persons with recurrent LBP during arm movements and walking. These motor control changes were not replicated by bracing or generalized activation by all abdominal muscles during the curl-up, side bridge, or bird-dog.[200,202] Similarly, Tsao et al[203] investigated the immediate effects of 2 training strategies of the paraspinal muscles on motor coordination during untrained tasks. Subjects with unilateral LBP performed a single session consisting of 3 sets of 10 repetitions, 10-second holds of an independent contraction of the LM with minimal superficial paraspinal muscle activity or active extension to activate all paraspinals with a gentle lift of the head and upper body while prone. Independent LM training induced earlier and increased activity of the LM and reduced superficial trunk muscle activity during slow movements. EMG onset of LM was also earlier after extension training, but no changes were noted during slow trunk movement. The authors suggest that improved recruitment of the LM with reduced coactivation of the superficial trunk muscles most evident after skilled cognitive training is consistent with restoration of muscle activation toward levels observed in asymptomatic individuals.[203]

It is generally agreed that impairment in trunk muscle performance has a role as the cause, effect, contributor, or perpetuator of LBP in some individuals. Changes in structure such as cross-sectional area, fat infiltration, and altered motor control of various trunk muscles occur in acute, recurrent, and chronic or persistent LBP. A variety of movement control strategies exist for stabilization of the spine. Persons with LBP adopt unique strategies that are different than healthy controls and may require a corrective exercise program tailored to their specific impairments. Research findings continue to debate the most accurate clinical assessment of muscle performance and the most effective activation strategies and training programs. Specific assessment procedures and rehabilitation strategies are discussed in the chapters on LBP, thoracic pain, and cervical pain.

Altered Muscle Performance in Persons With Neck Pain

Neck pain is associated with deficits in isometric strength and endurance of craniocervical flexors,[204,205] cervical flexors,[206,207] and extensors.[207,208] Additional deficits in person with neck pain include precision during dynamic movement,[209] efficiency of contraction,[210] repositioning acuity,[211,212] and disturbed oculomotor control.[213,214] The deep cervical flexors, longus colli, longus capitis, and rectus capitis anterior show decreased activation and increased superficial flexor (sternocleidomastoid and scalene) activation during a low-load, craniocervical flexion test (Figure 3-35) compared to healthy controls.[215-221] A similar reorganization of motor control strategy has been observed during tasks of upper limb movement.[222,223] Reduced isometric endurance of the deep cervical flexors and a delay in the speed of activation when challenged by postural perturbations has been observed.[224] These impairments are common to individuals with a variety of neck disorders and

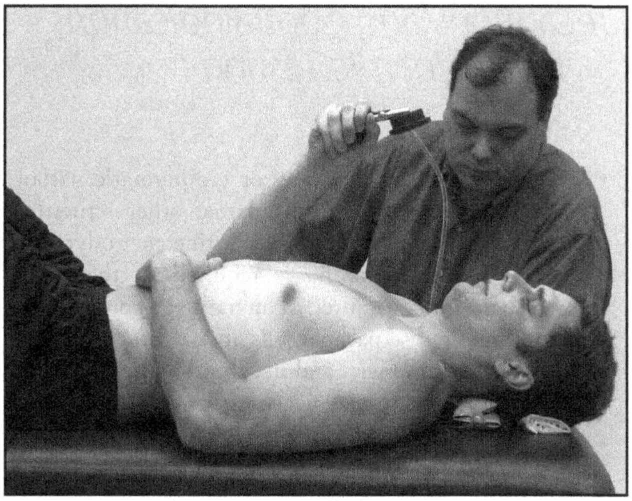

Figure 3-35. Craniocervical flexion test.

theorized to be linked with poor cervical spine orientation, support, and stability during functional activities.

Dysfunction of scapular muscles such as the trapezius and levator scapulae often result in altered scapular position and kinematics, but the association with neck pain is not clear. Because these muscles are capable of producing motion and axial load in the cervical spine, it is possible that altered patterns of activation may contribute to neck pain. During various occupational tasks, persons with neck pain show altered muscle control in the neck extensors, flexors, and UT[223,225]; difficulty relaxing the UT[226,227]; and higher levels of UT fatigue.[228] Research is lacking related to EMG studies comparing muscle activation patterns of the deep and superficial cervical extensors.

Motor control changes in the cervical spine occur quickly after the onset of neck pain.[229] Muscle pain causes instant inhibition of the cervical muscles when acting as agonists[230-232] suggesting a need for early pain-free intervention. Changes in muscle performance are present in persons with a history of neck pain or whiplash despite complete resolution of symptoms. Spontaneous recovery of muscle function does not appear to occur with relief of symptoms.[233] Continuation of altered strategies in this population is theorized to be an important factor associated with recurrent episodes. Because muscle performance deficits involve strength, endurance, and speed of activation, therapeutic exercise should involve low-load endurance and higher-load strength training. Specific assessment procedures and rehabilitation strategies are discussed in Chapter 6.

Special Tests

Clinical tests and measures, commonly referred to as *special tests*, are used to improve the accuracy and efficiency of the diagnostic process. However, as previously discussed at the start of this chapter, a systematic review identified only a few tests with acceptable accuracy for spinal conditions.[2] The difficulty in determining accuracy is that stress tests are unlikely to load only one specific structure. When a test provokes familiar pain, the clinician must consider whether the response is supportive of pathology in the targeted structure or supportive of another structure that is also stressed at the same time.

Clinicians are advised to carefully consider why a test is being performed and select special tests based on their psychometric properties and applicability to the individual patient. Before performing a diagnostic test, the clinician should establish in his or her mind the likelihood of the condition of interest as well as other conditions that are less likely. Because the patient's response typically impacts decision making related to intervention or prognosis, special tests should be analyzed on their accuracy to differentiate between persons who have a condition and those who do not.

Diagnostic accuracy studies vary based on the population studied, clinical environment, and interpretation of individual examiners. Therefore, decisions are rarely based on the findings from a single test. Information gleaned from clusters of tests appears to be more closely associated with clinical decision making.[2] Because many special tests demonstrate poor diagnostic accuracy, it is not necessary to learn or perform many or all of them. Overuse of special tests is likely to result in more diagnostic uncertainty and interfere with rather than assist in reaching a treatment threshold. Special tests related to each spinal region to include radiological imaging and laboratory assessment are discussed under the appropriate chapter.

Neurodynamic Tests

The word *neurodynamics*, previously termed *neural tension*, is now used to describe the biomechanical, physiological, and structural functions associated with the nervous system.[234,235] Nervous tissue needs the ability to slide, lengthen, and undergo compressive mechanical loads during functional activity. Inflammation, neural edema, reduced intraneural blood flow, or fibrosis associated with the nerve and/or the tissue it runs through may result in altered neurodynamics.[234,236] Neurodynamic test procedures such as the SLR, prone knee bend, slump test (Figure 3-36), and upper limb neurodynamic tests are designed to assess mobility and mechanically load parts of the nervous system.[236] The patient's response to the test procedure is compared with the uninvolved side, normative data, and standards of ROM. For example, the SLR assesses the ability of the sciatic nerve to move in relation to its surrounding tissues.[236] In surgical patients with LBP

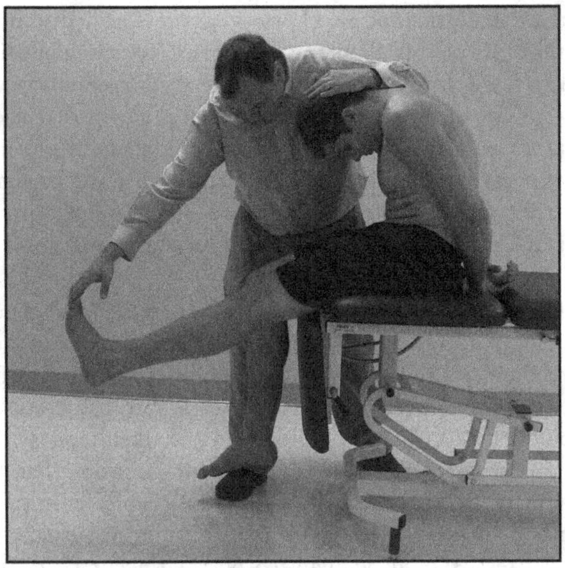

Figure 3-36. Slump test.

and sciatica, Kobayashi et al[237] showed that impairment in movement of the lumbosacral nerve roots correlated directly with both reduced intraneural blood flow and reduced ROM of the SLR at the exact position that the SLR was symptomatic. Surgical release of nerve root adhesions or disc protrusion produced simultaneous improvements in blood flow and ROM.

Special tests of nervous system mobility provide the clinician with a method of examining neural tissues for increased mechanosensitivity related to altered neurodynamics, a baseline movement for reassessment, and a potential intervention. Neurodynamic mobilization techniques aim to restore the movement of neural tissue relative to its anatomical surroundings.[238,239] General goals for managing pain related to increased mechanosensitivity of the nervous system are to reduce the mechanosensitivity and restore neural tissue mobility.[240] Theoretical benefits of neural mobilization include improved nerve gliding, increased neural vascularity, and improved axoplasmic flow.[235-239] Much research related to the validity and effectiveness of neurodynamic assessment and mobilization techniques is still needed.

Testing procedures are similar to those described for movement testing. Resting symptoms are established prior to starting the procedures. The clinician notes the quality, range of movement, resistance through the range and at the end of the range, and the symptom response. The test is considered positive if all or some of the patient's symptoms are reproduced, ROM is limited compared to the uninvolved side, and symptom reproduction occurs with a sensitizing maneuver. A sensitizing maneuver is necessary to differentiate between somatic versus a neural source of symptoms. Neurodynamic test procedures are discussed in subsequent chapters related to specific spinal regions.

Precautions and Contraindications to Neurodynamic Testing[241]

Precautions

- Aggravation of other tissues or symptomatic pathology. In addition to neural tissue, other structures are lengthened or compressed during neurodynamic tests. Clinical reasoning is required so that these structures are not injured or aggravated. For example, symptomatic disc pathology is at risk for aggravation during the slump test, and in symptomatic spinal stenosis, the response may occur earlier during testing.
- An irritable or worsening disorder
- Presence of neurological signs
- General health problems affecting the nervous system, such as diabetes
- Dizziness
- Circulatory symptoms
- Inexperience of the examiner

Contraindications

- Malignancy or acute inflammatory infection
- Recent onset of or worsening of neurological signs
- Cauda equina symptoms or syndrome
- Spinal cord injury or tethered cord syndrome
- Inexperience of the examiner

Screening Tests for Regions Above and Below the Area of Symptoms

Based on the concept of regional interdependence,[242] regions not under the primary area of complaint are examined as possible sources of or contributors to the problem. Within the first 2 to 3 sessions, the cervical/thoracic region is examined for all upper extremity complaints and the thoracolumbar region for all lower extremity complaints. Similarly, the cervical spine is examined for thoracic spine complaints and the thoracic spine is examined for lumbopelvic regional complaints. Through evidence-based clinical reasoning, examination findings are then prioritized to guide intervention and reassessment of potentially relevant relationships between regions. For example, patients with a chief complaint of LBP and knee pain receiving treatment directed at the hip experienced positive outcomes in randomized controlled trials.[243-245] Equally important to management of patients with primary knee[246] and hip[247] pain are interventions directed to the lumbar spine. Successful outcomes due to treatment directed to the thoracic spine and rib cage for patients with primary complaints of neck pain[248] and shoulder pain[249] have also been reported. Current evidence supports the use of a regionally interdependent examination model in MS management.[242]

Palpation

Palpation of the area of a patient's symptoms is considered a mandatory procedure. The extent, detail, and timing of palpation vary by clinician and are partly determined by the working hypothesis and the reason for performing palpation. Palpation should proceed in a systematic manner performed either statically or dynamically as in motion palpation during PAIVM or PPIVM. Findings must be correlated with the rest of the examination.

General palpation guidelines are as follows[8,250]:

- Explain the procedure and expose and support the area to be palpated.
- Use a gentle, layered approach, moving from superficial to deep.
- Palpate over the area of symptoms and tissue associated with the area of symptoms.
- Compare to the uninvolved side, noting location and nature of any abnormality.

Skin Mobility, Temperature, and Sweating

Use of the back of the hand is recommended for temperature, but occasionally, the palm may be used. Increased temperature suggests underlying inflammatory process, infection, or altered sympathetic activity. Decreased temperature suggests vascular insufficiency or altered sympathetic activity. Skin mobility relative to underlying tissue is also assessed.

Soft Tissue Mobility, Tenderness, Tissue Texture, Swelling, Edema, and Pulses

Clinicians should palpate the skin, subcutaneous tissues, muscle, and tendons. Soft tissue is normally supple and easily moved against underlying tissues and structures. Areas of decreased mobility, edema, nodules, lumps, gaps, thickening, or joint effusion are noted. Lumps or nodes more than 1.5 cm in diameter, tender or nontender, and immobile are considered abnormal and should be discussed with the patient, monitored, and followed up by a physician.[251] Tenderness is often unreliable because tissues can refer pain away from the site of the lesion, and referred tenderness is common. Muscle and tendon bulk or tones are examined for symmetry along with soft tissue or joint crepitus.

Palpation of muscle often reveals taut, linear bands called *myofascial trigger points* (MTrP). Travell and Simons[252] described an active MTrP as a focus of hyperirritability in a muscle or its fascia that refers a pattern of pain at rest and/or with motion and elicits a local muscle twitch response with direct stimulation.[252] A latent MTrP is similar to an active MTrP except it does not demonstrate pain at rest and is only painful with palpation.[252] Dysfunction attributed to MTrP presents as muscle shortening, muscle weakness, local or referred inhibition, poor coordination, fatigability, delayed recovery, rest pain, and pain on vigorous stretching and contraction.[253] Diagnosis of MTrP is usually based on physical examination. A systematic review[254] reports reliability for the following criteria: tenderness (κ range = 0.22 to 1.0), pain reproduction (κ range = 0.57 to 1.00), a taut band (κ range = –0.08 to 0.75), and local twitch response (κ range = 0.05 to 0.57).[254] Reliability of the physical examination for diagnosis of MTrP requires further investigation.

Joint and Bony Alignment Includes Ligament and Tendon Attachments

Bony asymmetry or structural malalignment may or may not be relevant. Bony enlargement may be noted at the site of a healing fracture or at joint margins in arthritic disease.

Additional Studies

Results of radiological studies such as x-ray, bone scan, MRI, or CT scan; laboratory tests such as urinalysis, complete blood count, or rheumatoid factor; or electrodiagnostic studies are reviewed or requested as needed. Referral or consultation with other health care providers is made when appropriate.

Evaluation

Evaluation is defined as the process of making clinical judgments based on the data gathered from the history and tests and measures.[255] At the end of initial data gathering, information is integrated to determine an overall assessment of the patient and the presenting problem. Reflection on the exam findings should reveal a relationship between the symptoms and signs that further develops the working hypothesis and establishes a functional baseline or outcome measures from which to evaluate and progress treatment.

Identification of relevant impairments, activity limitations, and participation restrictions should facilitate an understanding of the relationship among the patient's problem, impairments, and function. If the findings correlate with or confirm the initial hypothesis and a treatment threshold is reached, the clinician proceeds with management. If you are not able to reach a treatment threshold, further review of the history and physical examination and/or consultation with a colleague is required. If you suspect a non-MS or serious MS pathology, medical consultation is needed. Evaluation is then used to guide the diagnosis, prognosis, and overall patient management.

Diagnosis

The process of diagnosis is described as assigning a diagnostic classification, category, or syndrome based on clusters of signs and symptoms, which in turn guide the treatment.[255] Making a physical therapy diagnosis involves a combination of hypothesis testing, clinical pattern recognition, and evidence-based classification recognized by a cluster of signs and symptoms. The initial physical therapy classification or diagnosis is based on impairments of body structures, body functions, and activity limitations and with less emphasis on pathological entities of the biomedical model.[256,257] Patients often present with more than one problem and may have multiple or competing diagnoses. An evidence-based clinical reasoning process considers competing hypotheses that are defined through initial data collection and tested and clarified through further data collection and reassessment after intervention. Reassessment, subjectively and objectively, within and between intervention sessions either supports the diagnosis or suggests the need to modify. The diagnostic process (Figure 3-37) continues in this manner throughout each episode of care.

Each chapter on LBP, thoracic pain, and cervical pain begins with a brief introduction to diagnosis and diagnostic classification for that region. All patients do not fit into one classification system, and many patients have clinical findings that fit into more than one subgroup within a classification system. Key history and exam findings are used to place the patient into a diagnostic classification or impairment-based category of spinal pain that initially guides physical therapy intervention. The classification approach described in this text integrates current best evidence, clinical reasoning, and clinical practice guidelines to assist the clinician in arriving at an appropriate decision related to diagnosis and treatment. If unfamiliar with the classification approach to spinal pain and prior to reading the sections on history and tests and measures, students and clinicians should review the chapter sections on diagnostic classification for LBP, pelvic girdle pain, thoracic pain, and cervical pain.

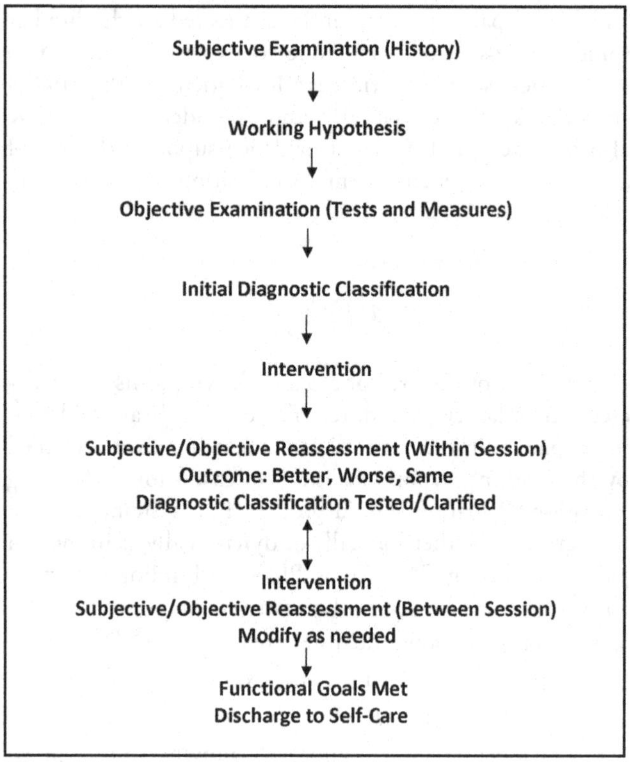

Figure 3-37. Diagnostic process.

Prognosis

Prognosis is explained as the process of making clinical judgments to determine the optimal level of improvement that might be attained through intervention and the amount of time required to reach that level.[255] Prognosis includes patient and clinician goals and an estimate of the sessions needed to meet functional expectations. Factors that will assist in prognosis and overall patient management are listed as follows[258]:

- Patient beliefs, attitudes, motivation, and understanding of the problem
- Self-efficacy and the ability and willingness to learn
- How the problem is affecting the patient's life in terms of anxiety, stress, financial burden
- Social, occupational, and economic status
- Patient perspectives and expectations
- Extent of impairments, activity limitations, or life participation restrictions
- Pain mechanisms of presenting symptoms
- Balance of mechanical versus inflammatory components
- Presence of pre-existing conditions and general health
- Length of history and progression of the disorder

Summary

The first goal of the physical examination is to reproduce the patient's complaint. The second goal is to determine the impact of posture, movement, work, and recreational factors as causes of, contributors to, or perpetuators of the patient's problem. Understanding the positive or negative effects of movement or activities on the patient's symptoms may assist in determining an appropriate diagnosis, intervention, and overall plan of care. The third goal is to establish the treatment threshold for a diagnosis or diagnostic classification. This process involves ruling out competing diagnoses, classifications, or sources of the patient's problem and confirming the diagnosis. The physical therapy diagnosis is linked to impairments of the articular, muscular, neural, and/or sensorimotor control systems and their relevance to the patient's symptoms and activity limitations. Establishing a diagnosis is an ongoing process that requires evaluation of the data from both the history and physical examination as well as following the model of assessment, intervention, and reassessment. Confirmation of the diagnosis is continued throughout the episode of care. The final goal is to establish an accurate baseline or outcome measures from which to evaluate and progress treatment. The outcome measures focus on identification of relevant impairments, activity limitations, and participation restrictions and facilitate an understanding of the relationship among symptoms, impairments, and function. Case studies with documentation of the history, planning the examination form, and physical examination findings are available related to LBP, thoracic pain, and cervical pain in Appendices C-I to aid in forming a diagnosis and planning the initial intervention.

References

1. American Academy of Orthopaedic Manual Physical Therapists. *Orthopaedic Manual Physical Therapy. Description of Advanced Clinical Practice.* Tallahassee, FL: Author; 2009.
2. Cook C, Hegedus E. Diagnostic utility of clinical tests for spinal dysfunction. *Man Ther.* 2011;16:21-25.
3. Jaeschke R, Guyatt GH, Sackett DL. User's guide to the medical literature. III. How to use an article about a diagnostic test. B. What are the results and will they help me in caring for my patients? The Evidence-Based Medicine Working Group. *JAMA.* 1994;271:703-707.
4. Jones MA, Jones HM. Principles of the physical examination. In: Grieve GP, ed. *Grieve's Modern Manual Therapy.* 2nd ed. London, England: Churchill Livingstone; 1994:491-501.
5. Janda V, Frank C, Liebenson C. Evaluation of muscular imbalance. In: Liebenson C, ed. *Rehabilitation of the Spine. A Practitioner's Manual.* 2nd ed. Philadelphia, PA: Lippincott Williams & Wilkins; 2007:203-225.
6. Kendall FP, McCreary EK, Provance PG, Rodgers MM, Romani WA. *Muscles Testing and Function With Posture and Pain.* 5th ed. Baltimore, MD: Lippincott Williams & Wilkins; 2005.
7. Kendall HO, Kendall FP, Boynton DA. *Posture and Pain.* Baltimore, MD: Williams & Wilkins; 1952.
8. Magee DJ. *Orthopedic Physical Assessment.* 5th ed. St Louis, MO: Saunders Elsevier; 2008.
9. Dutton M. *Orthopaedic Examination. Evaluation, and Intervention.* 2nd ed. New York, NY: McGraw Hill Medical; 2008:440-1012.
10. Kisner C, Colby LA. *Therapeutic Exercise.* 5th ed. Philadelphia, PA: FA Davis; 2007:383-404.
11. Hartvigsen J, Kyvik KO, Leboeuf-Yde C, et al. Ambiguous relation between physical workload and low back pain: a twin control study. *Occup Environ Med.* 2003;60:109-114.
12. Andersson GBJ. Epidemiology aspects on low-back pain in industry. *Spine.* 1981;6:53-60.
13. Kelsey JL, White AA III. Epidemiology and impact of low-back pain. *Spine.* 1980;5:133-142.
14. 14. Bakker EWP, Verhagen AP, van Trijffel E, Lucas C, Koes BW. Spinal mechanical load as a risk factor for low back pain. A systematic review of prospective cohort studies. *Spine.* 2009;34(8):E281-E293.
15. O'Sullivan P. Clinical instability of the lumbar spine: its pathological basis, diagnosis and conservative management. In: Boyling JD, Jull G, eds. *Grieve's Modern Manual Therapy.* 3rd ed. Amsterdam, The Netherlands: Elsevier; 2005:311-322.
16. Williams MM, Hawley JA, McKenzie RA, et al. A comparison of the effects of two sitting postures on back and referred pain. *Spine.* 1991;16:1185-1191.
17. O'Sullivan PB. Lumbar segmental "instability": clinical presentation and specific stabilizing exercise management. *Man Ther.* 2000;5:2-12.
18. Dankaerts W, O'Sullivan P, Burnett A, Straker L. Differences in sitting postures are associated with nonspecific chronic low back pain disorders when patients are subclassified. *Spine.* 2006;31:698-704.
19. Bell JA, Turton AK, Stigant M. Sitting postures at work are associated with current and future LBP. *J Bone Joint Surg Br.* 2009;91(suppl 3):486.
20. Griegel-Morris P, Larson K, Mueller-Klaus K, et al. Incidence of common postural abnormalities in the cervical, shoulder, and thoracic regions and their association with pain in two age groups of healthy subjects. *Phys Ther.* 1992;72:425-431.
21. Watson CH, Trott PH. Cervical headache: an investigation of natural head posture and upper cervical flexor muscle performance. *Cephalalgia.* 1993;13:272-284.
22. Dumas JP, Arsenault AB, Boudreau G, et al. Physical impairments in cervicogenic headache: traumatic versus nontraumatic onset. *Cephalalgia.* 2001;21:884-893.
23. Straker LM, O'Sullivan PB, Smith AJ, Perry MC. Relationships between prolonged neck/shoulder pain and sitting spinal posture in male and female adolescents. *Man Ther.* 2009;14:321-
24. Falla D, O'Leary S, Fagan A, Jull G. Recruitment of the deep cervical flexor muscles during a postural-correction exercise performed in sitting. *Man Ther.* 2007;12(2):139-143.
25. Yip CHT, Chiu TTW, Poon ATK. The relationship between head posture and severity and disability of patients with neck pain. *Man Ther.* 2008;13(2):148-154.
26. O'Sullivan PB, Dankaerts W, Burnett AF, et al. Effect of different upright sitting postures on spinal-pelvic curvature and trunk muscle activation in a pain-free population. *Spine.* 2006;31:E707-E712.
27. Caneiro JP, O'Sullivan P, Burnett A, et al. The influence of different sitting postures on head/neck posture and muscle activity. *Man Ther.* 2010;15:54-60.
28. Falla D, Jull G, Russell T, Vicenzino B, Hodges P. Effect of neck exercise on sitting posture in patients with chronic neck pain. *Phys Ther.* 2007;87:408-417.

29. Jull G, Sterling M, Falla D, Treleaven J, O'Leary S. *Whiplash, Headache, and Neck Pain. Research-Based Directions for Physical Therapies.* Philadelphia, PA: Churchill Livingstone Elsevier; 2008.
30. Claus AP, Hides JA, Moseley GL, Hodges PW. Is "ideal" sitting posture real?: measurement of spinal curves in four sitting postures. *Man Ther.* 2009;14:404-408.
31. Hodges PW, Ferreira PH, Ferreira ML. Lumbar spine: treatment of Instability and Disorders of movement control. In: Magee DJ, Zachazewski JE, Quillen WS, eds. *Pathology and Intervention in Musculoskeletal Rehabilitation.* St Louis, MO: Saunders Elsevier; 2009:389-425.
32. Harding VR, Williams AC, Richardson PH, et al. The development of a battery of measures for assessing physical functioning of chronic pain patients. *Pain.* 1994;58:367-375.
33. Simmonds MJ, Claveau Y. Measures of pain and physical function in patients with low back pain. *Physiother Theory Pract.* 1997;13:53-65.
34. Simmonds MJ, Olson SL, Jones S, et al. Psychometric characteristics and clinical usefulness of physical performance tests in patients with low back pain. *Spine.* 1998;23:2412-2421.
35. Keefe FJ, Hill RW. An objective approach to quantifying pain behavior and gait patterns in low back pain patients. *Pain.* 1985;21:153-161.
36. Hussein TM, Simmonds MJ, Olson SL, Jones S. Kinematics of gait in normal and low back pain subjects. *J Orthop Sports Phys Ther.* 1998;27:84.
37. Vogt L, Pfeifer K, Portscher M, et al. Influences of nonspecific low back pain on 3-dimensional lumbar spine kinematics in locomotion. *Spine.* 2001;26:1910-1919.
38. Murray MP, Kory RC, Clarkson BH, Sepic SB. Comparison of free and fast speed walking patterns of normal men. *Am J Phys Med.* 1966;45:8-23.
39. Murray MP, Kory RC, Sepic SB. Walking patterns of normal women. *Arch Phys Med Rehabil.* 1970;51:637-650.
40. Winter DA. Kinematic and kinetic patterns in human gait: variability and compensating effects. *Hum Mov Sci.* 1984;3:51-76.
41. Al-Obaidi SM, Al-Zoabi B, Al-Shuwaie N, et al. The influence of pain and pain-related fear and disability beliefs on walking velocity in chronic low back pain. *Int J Rehabil Res.* 2003;26:101-108.
42. Lee CE, Simmonds MJ, Etnyre BR, Morris GS. Influence of pain distribution on gait characteristics in patients with low back pain. Part 1: vertical ground reaction force. *Spine.* 32:1329-1336.
43. Brach JS, Van Swearingen JM, Newman AB, Kriska AM. Identifying early decline of physical function in community-dwelling older women: performance-based and self-report measures. *Phys Ther.* 2002;82:320-328.
44. Studenski S, Perera S, Wallace D, et al. Physical performance measures in the clinical setting. *J Am Geriatr Soc.* 2003;51:314-322.
45. Purser JL, Weinberger M, Cohen HJ, et al. Walking speed predicts health status and hospital costs for frail elderly male veterans. *J Rehabil Res Dev.* 2005;42:535-546.
46. Bohannon RW. Comfortable and maximum walking speed of adults aged 20-79 years: reference values and determinants. *Age Ageing.* 1997;26:15-19.
47. Lerner-Grankiel M, Varcas S, Brown M, Krusel L, Schoneberger W. Functional community ambulation: what are your criteria? *Clin Man Phys Ther.* 1986;6:12-15.
48. Perera S, Mody SH, Woodman RC, Studenski SA. Meaningful change and responsiveness in common physical performance measures in older adults. *J Am Geriatr Soc.* 2006;54:743-749.
49. Cesari M, Kritchevsky SB, Penninx BWHJ, et al. Prognostic value of usual gait speed in well-functional older people: results from the health, aging and body composition study. *J Am Geriatr Soc.* 2005;53:1675-1680.
50. Saunders SW, Coppeiters M, Magarey M, Hodges PW. Low back pain and associated changes in abdominal muscle activation during human locomotion. Paper presented at: Australian Conference of Science and Medicine in Sport; October 6-9, 2004; Alice Springs, Australia.
51. Saunders SW, Rath D, Hodges PW. Postural and respiratory activation of the trunk muscles varies with mode and speed of locomotion. *Gait Posture.* 2004;20:280-290.
52. Saunders SW, Schache AG, Rath D, Hodges PW. Changes in three dimensional lumbopelvic kinematics and trunk muscle activity with speed and mode of locomotion. *Clin Biomech.* 2005;20:784-793.
53. McGill S. *Low Back Disorders. Evidence-Based Prevention and Rehabilitation.* 2nd ed. Champaign, IL: Human Kinetics; 2007.
54. van der Hulst M, Vollenbroek-Hutten MM, Rietman JS, Hermens HJ. Lumbar and abdominal muscle activity during walking in subjects with chronic low back pain: support of the "guarding" hypothesis? *J Electromyogr Kinesiol.* 2010;20:31-38.
55. Horak FB. Postural orientation and equilibrium: what do we need to know about neural control of balance to prevent falls? *Age Ageing.* 2006;35 Suppl 2:ii7-ii11
56. Peterka R. Sensorimotor integration in human postural control. *J Neurophysiol.* 2002;88:1097-1118.
57. Byl NN, Sinnot PL. Variations in balance and body sway. *Spine.* 1991;16:325-330.
58. Louto S, Aalto H, Taimela S, et al. One-footed and externally disturbed two-footed postural control in chronic low back pain patients: a controlled follow-up study. *Spine.* 1996;21:2621-2627.
59. Mok NW, Brauer S, Hodges PW. Hip strategy for balance control in quiet standing is reduced in people with low back pain. *Spine.* 2004;29:E107-E112.
60. Mok NW, Brauer SG, Hodges PW. Failure to use movement in postural strategies leads to increased spinal displacement in low back pain. *Spine.* 2007;32:E537-E543.
61. Takala E, Viikari-Juntura E. Do functional tests predict low back pain? *Spine.* 2000;25:2126-2132.
62. Treleaven J, Jull G, Lowchoy N. Standing balance in persistent whiplash: a comparison between subjects with and without dizziness. *J Rehabil Med.* 2005;37:224-229.
63. Field S, Treleaven J, Jull G. Standing balance: a comparison between idiopathic and whiplash-induced neck pain. *Man Ther.* 2008;13:183-191.
64. Mok NW, Brauer SG, Hodges PW. Changes in lumbar movement in people with low back pain are related to compromised balance. *Spine.* 2010;36:E45-E52.
65. Radebold A, Cholewicki J, Polzhofer GK, et al. Impaired postural control of the lumbar spine is associated with delayed muscle response times in patients with chronic idiopathic low back pain. *Spine.* 2001;26:724-730.
66. della Volpe R, Popa T, Ginanneschi F, et al. Changes in coordination of postural control during dynamic stance in chronic low back pain patients. *Gait Posture.* 2006;24:349-355.
67. Henry SM, Hitt JR, Jones SL, et al. Decreased limits of stability in response to postural perturbations in subjects with low back pain. *Clin Biomech.* 2006;21:881-892.
68. Maribo T, Iversen E, Andersen NT, StengaardPedersen K, Schiøttz-Christensen B. Intra-observer and interobserver reliability of one leg stand test as a measure of postural balance in low back pain patients. *Int Musculoskelet Med.* 2009;31(4):172-177.

69. Bohannon RW, Larkin PA, Cook AC, Gear J, Singer J. Decrease in timed balance test scores with aging. *Phys Ther.* 1984;64:1067-1070.
70. Sung PS, Yoon B, Lee DC. Lumbar spine stability for subjects with and without low back pain during one-leg standing test. *Spine.* 2010;35:E753-E760.
71. Springer BA, Marin R, Cyhan T, Roberts H, Gill NW. Normative values for the unipedal stance test with eyes open and closed. *J Geriatric Phys Ther.* 2007;30:8-15.
72. Vellas BJ, Wayne SJ, Romero L, et al. One-leg balance is an important predictor of injurious falls in older persons. *J Am Geriatr Soc.* 1997;45:735-738.
73. Miur SW, Berg K, Chesworth B, et al. Balance impairment as a risk factor for falls in community-dwelling older adults who are high functioning: a prospective study. *Phys Ther.* 2010;90:338-347.
74. Jull G, Sterling M, Falla D, Treleaven J, O'Leary S. *Whiplash, Headache, and Neck Pain. Research-Based Directions for Physical Therapies.* Philadelphia, PA: Churchill Livingstone Elsevier; 2008.
75. Simmonds MJ. Measuring and managing pain and performance. *Man Ther.* 2006;11:175-179.
76. Van Dillen LR, Sahrmann SA, Norton BJ, et al. Reliability of physical examination items used for classification of patients with low back pain. *Phys Ther.* 1998;78:979-988.
77. Childs JD, Cleland JA, Elliott JM, et al. Neck pain: clinical practice guidelines linked to the International Classification of Functioning, Disability, and Health from the orthopaedic section of the American Physical Therapy Association. *J Orthop Sports Phys Ther.* 2008;38(9):A1-A34.
78. McCarthy CJ, Arnall FA, Strimpkos N, Freemont A, Oldham JA. The biopsychosocial classification of nonspecific low back pain: a systematic review. *Phys Ther Rev.* 2004;9:17-30.
79. Tuttle N. Do changes within a manual therapy treatment session predict between-session changes for patients with cervical spine pain? *Aust J Physiother.* 2005;51:43-48.
80. Tuttle N, Laasko L, Barrett R. Change in impairments in the first two treatments predicts outcome in impairments, but not in activity limitations, in subacute neck pain: an observational study. *Aust J Physiother.* 2006;52:281-285.
81. Chorti AG, Chortis AG, Strimpakos N, McCarthy CJ, Lamb SE. The prognostic value of symptom responses in the conservative management of spinal. A systematic review. *Spine.* 2009;34:2686-2699.
82. Wainner R, Fritz J, Irrgang J, Boninger M, Delitto A, Allison S. Reliability and diagnostic accuracy of the clinical examination and patient self-report measures for cervical radiculopathy. *Spine.* 2003;28:52-62.
83. Youdas J, Carey J, Garrett T. Reliability of measurements of cervical spine range of motion—comparison of three methods. *Phys Ther.* 1991;71:98-104.
84. Breum J, Wiberg J, Bolton J. Reliability and concurrent validity of the BROM II for measuring lumbar mobility. *J Manipulative Physiol Ther.* 1995;18:497-502.
85. Saur P, Ensink F, Frese K, Seegar D, Hildebrandt J. Lumbar range of motion: reliability and validity of the inclinometer technique in the clinical measurement of trunk flexibility. *Spine.* 1996;21:1332-1338.
86. Fritz JM, Piva S, Childs JD. Accuracy of the clinical examination to predict radiographic instability of the lumbar spine. *Eur Spine J.* 2005;14:743-750.
87. Hunt D, Zuberbier O, Kozlowski A, et al. Reliability of lumbar flexion, lumbar extension, and passive straight leg raise test in normal populations embedded within a complete physical examination. *Spine.* 2001;26:2714-2718.
88. McKenzie R, May S. *The Lumbar Spine Mechanical Diagnosis and Therapy.* Vols. 1 and 2. Raumatic Beach, New Zealand: Spinal Publications; 2003.
89. Hefford C. McKenzie classification of mechanical spinal pain: profile of syndromes and directions of preference. *Man Ther.* 2008;13:75-81.
90. Dionne C, Bybee RF, Tomaka J. Correspondence of diagnosis to initial treatment for neck pain. *Physiotherapy.* 2007;93:62-68.
91. Long A. The centralization phenomenon: its usefulness as a predictor of outcome in conservative treatment of chronic low back pain. *Spine.* 1995;20:2513-2521.
92. Karas R, McIntosh G, Hall H, Wilson L, Meles T. The relationship between non-organic signs and centralization of symptoms in the prediction of return to work for patients with low back pain. *Phys Ther.* 1997;77:354-360.
93. Werneke M, Hart DL. Centralization phenomenon as a prognostic factor for chronic low back pain and disability. *Spine.* 2001;26:758-765.
94. Skytte L, May S, Petersen P. Centralization: its prognostic value in patients with referred symptoms and sciatica. *Spine.* 2005;30:E293-E299.
95. Werneke M, Hart DL. Discriminant validity and relative precision for classifying patients with non-specific neck and back pain by anatomic pain patterns. *Spine.* 2003;28:161-166.
96. Abbott JH, Flynn TW, Fritz JM, Hing WA, Reid D, Whitman JM. Manual physical assessment of spinal segmental motion: intent and validity. *Man Ther.* 2009;14:36-44.
97. Wainner RS. Reliability of the clinical examination: how close is "close enough"? *J Orthop Sports Phys Ther.* 2003;33:488-491.
98. Landel R, Kulig K, Fredericson M, Li B, Powers CM. Intertester reliability and validity of motion assessments during lumbar spine accessory motion testing. *Phys Ther.* 2008;88:43-49.
99. Johansson F. Interexaminer reliability of lumbar segmental mobility tests. *Man Ther.* 2006;11:331-336.
100. van Trijffel E, Anderegg Q, Bossuyt PMMM, Lucas C. Interexaminer reliability of passive assessment of intervertebral motion in the cervical and lumbar spine: a systematic review. *Man Ther.* 2005;10:256-269.
101. Huijbregts PA. Spinal motion palpation: a review of reliability studies. *J Man Manip Ther.* 2002;19:24-39.
102. Cleland JA, Childs JD, Fritz JM, Whitman JM. Interrater reliability of the history and physical examination in patients with mechanical neck pain. *Arch Phys Med Rehabil.* 2006;7:1388-1395.
103. Fjellner A, Bexander C, Faleij R, Strender LE. Interexaminer reliability in physical examination of the neck. *J Manipulative Physiol Ther.* 1999;22:511-516.
104. Pool JJ, Hoving JL, de Vet HC, van Mameren H, Bouter LM. The interexaminer reproducibility of physical examination of the cervical spine. *J Manipulative Physiol Ther.* 2004;27:84-90.
105. Piva SR, Erhard RE, Childs JD, Browder DA. Inter-tester reliability of passive intervertebral and active movements of the cervical spine. *Man Ther.* 2006;11:321-330.
106. Jull G, Zito G, Trott P, Potter H, Shirley D. Inter-examiner reliability to detect painful upper cervical joint dysfunction. *Aust J Physiother.* 1997;43:125-129.
107. Brismée JM, Gipson D, Ivie D, et al. Interrater reliability of a passive physiological intervertebral motion test in the mid-thoracic spine. *J Manipulative Physiol Ther.* 2006;29:368-373.
108. Haas M, Raphael R, Panzer D. Reliability of manual end-play palpation of the thoracic spine. *Chiropr Tech.* 1995;76:786-792.
109. Abbott JH, Mercer SSR. Lumbar segmental hypomobility criterion-related validity of clinical examination items (a pilot study). *N Z J Physiother.* 2003;3:3-9.

110. Abbott JH, McCane B, Herbison P, Moginie G, Chapple C, Hogarty T. Lumbar segmental instability: a criterion-related validity study of manual therapy assessment. *BMC Musculoskelet Disord.* 2005;6:56.
111. Abbott JH, Fritz HM, McCane B, et al. Lumbar segmental mobility disorders: comparison of two methods of defining abnormal displacement kinematics in a cohort of patients with non-specific mechanical low back pain. *BMC Musculoskelet Disord.* 2006;7:45.
112. Schneider M, Erhard R, Brach J, Tellin W, Imbarlina F, Delitto A. Spinal palpation for lumbar segmental mobility and pain provocation: an interexaminer reliability study. *J Manipulative Physiol Ther.* 2008;31:465-473.
113. Flynn TW, Fritz JM, Whitman JM, et al. A clinical prediction rule for classifying patients with low back pain who demonstrate short-term improvement with spinal manipulation. *Spine.* 2002;27:2835-2843.
114. Fritz JM, Whitman JM, Childs JD. Lumbar spine segmental mobility assessment: an examination of validity for determining intervention strategies with low back pain. *Arch Phys Med Rehabil.* 2005;86:1745-1752.
115. Childs JD, Fritz JM, Flynn TW, et al. A clinical prediction rule to identify patients with low back pain most likely to benefit from spinal manipulation: a validation study. *Ann Int Med.* 2004;141:920-928.
116. Hicks GE, Fritz JM, Delitto A, McGill SM. Preliminary development of a clinical prediction rule for determining which patients with low back pain will respond to a stabilization exercise program. *Arch Phys Med Rehabil.* 2005;86:1753-1762.
117. Jull G, Bogduk N, Marsland A. The accuracy of manual diagnosis for cervical zygapophysial joint pain syndromes. *Med J Aust.* 1988;148:233-236.
118. Chou R, Qaseem A, Snow V, et al. Diagnosis and treatment of low back pain: a joint clinical practice guideline form the American College of Physicians and the American Pain Society. *Ann Intern Med.* 2007;147:478-491.
119. Lee MW, McPhee RW, Stringer MD. An evidence-based approach to human dermatomes. *Clin Anat.* 2008;21:363-373.
120. Scifers JR. *Special Tests for Neurologic Examination.* Thorofare, NJ: SLACK Incorporated; 2008.
121. Nardone A, Schieppati AM. Inhibitory effect of the Jendrassik maneuver on the stretch reflex. *Neuroscience.* 2008;156:607-617.
122. Cook CE, Hegedus EJ. *Orthopedic Physical Examination Tests. An Evidence-Based Approach.* Upper Saddle River, NJ: Pearson Prentice Hall; 2008.
123. Sung RD, Wang JC. Correlation between a positive Hoffmann's reflex and cervical pathology in asymptomatic individuals. *Spine.* 2001;26:67-70.
124. Lauder TD, Dillingham TR, Andary M, et al. Predicting electrodiagnostic outcomes in patients with upper limb symptoms: are the history and physical examination helpful? *Arch Phys Med Rehabil.* 2000;81:436-431.
125. Lauder TD, Dillingham TR, Andary M, et al. Effect of history and exam in predicting electrodiagnostic outcome among patients with suspected lumbosacral radiculopathy. *Amer J Phys Med Rehab.* 2000;79(10):60-68.
126. Lauder TD. Physical examination signs, clinical symptoms, and their relationship to electrodiagnostic findings and the presence of radiculopathy. *Phys Med Rehabil Clin N Am.* 2002;13:451-467.
127. Suri P, Rainville J, Katz JN, et al. The accuracy of the physical examination for the diagnosis of midlumbar and low lumbar nerve root impingement. *Spine.* 2011;36:63-73.
128. O'Connor RC, Andary MT, Russo RB, DeLano M. Thoracic radiculopathy. *Phys Med Rehabil Clin N Am.* 2002;13:623-644.
129. Malanga GA, McLean JP, Alladin I, Tai Q, Andrus SG, Smith R. Thoracic discogenic pain syndrome. *Medscape Reference.* http://emedicine.medscape.com/article/96284-overview. Updated December 14, 2011. Accessed July 29, 2010.
130. Yngve D. Abdominal reflexes. *J Pediatr Orthop.* 1997;17:105-108.
131. Pearce JM. Beevor's sign. *Eur Neurol.* 2005;53:208-209.
132. Cleland J, Koppenhaver S. *Orthopaedic Clinical Examination: An Evidence-Based Approach.* 2nd ed. Carlstadt, NJ: Icon Learning Systems; 2010.
133. Page P, Frank C, Lardner R. *Assessment and Treatment of Muscle Imbalance. The Janda Approach.* Champaign, IL: Human Kinetics; 2010.
134. Janda V, Frank C, Liebenson C. Evaluation of muscular imbalance. In: Liebenson C, ed. *Rehabilitation of the Spine. A Practitioner's Manual.* 2nd ed. Philadelphia, PA: Lippincott Williams & Wilkins; 2007:203-225.
135. Borstad JD, Briggs MS. Reproducibility of a measurement for latissimus dorsi muscle length. *Physiother Theor Pract.* 2010;26(3):195-203.
136. Panjabi MM. The stabilizing system of the spine. Part I. Function, dysfunction, adaptation, and enhancement. *J Spinal Disord.* 1992;5:383-389.
137. McGill SM, Karpowicz AK. Exercises for spine stabilization: motion/motor patterns, stability progressions, and clinical technique. *Arch Phys Med Rehabil.* 2009;90:118-126.
138. Bergmark A. Stability of the lumbar spine. A study in mechanical engineering, *Acta Orthop Scand.* 1989;60(suppl 230):1-54.
139. Comerford MJ, Mottram SL. Movement and stability dysfunction—contemporary developments. *Man Ther.* 2001;6:15-26.
140. Gibbons SGT, Comerford JM. Strength versus stability: part 1: concept and terms. *Orthop Div Rev.* 2001;March/April:21-27.
141. Comerford M, Mottram S. *Movement Dysfunction—Focus on Dynamic Stability and Muscle Balance: Kinetic Control Movement Dysfunction Course.* Southampton, England: Kinetic Control; 2000.
142. Gibbons SGT. Muscle function and a critical evaluation. Paper presented at: 2nd International Conference on Movement Dysfunction; September 23-25, 2005; Edinburgh, Scotland.
143. Saunders SW, Schache A, Rath D, Hodges PW. Changes in three dimensional lumbo-pelvic kinematics and trunk muscle activity with speed and mode of locomotion. *Clin Biomech.* 2005;20:784-793.
144. Moseley GL, Hodges PW, Gandevia SC. Deep and superficial fibers of lumbar multifidus are differentially active during voluntary arm movements. *Spine.* 2002;27:E29-E36.
145. Hodges PW, Richardson CA. Feedforward contraction of transversus abdominis is not influenced by the direction of arm movement. *Exp Brain Res.* 1997;114:362-370.
146. Hodges PW, Cresswell AG, Thorstensson A. Preparatory trunk motion accompanies rapid upper limb movement. *Exp Brain Res.* 1999;124:69-79.
147. Hodges PW, Eriksson AE, Shirley D, Gandevia SC. Intra-abdominal pressure increases stiffness of the lumbar spine. *J Biomech.* 2005;38:1873-1880.
148. Hodges P, Gurfinkel VS, Brumagne S, et al. Coexistence of stability and mobility in postural control: evidence from postural compensation for respiration. *Exp Brain Res.* 2002;144:293-302.
149. Pool-Goudzwaard A, van Dijke GH, van Gurp M, et al. Contribution of pelvic floor muscles to stiffness of the pelvic ring. *Clin Biomech.* 2004;19:564-571.
150. Van Dieën J, Selen L, Cholewicki J. Trunk muscle activation in low back pain patients, an analysis of the literature. *J Electromyogr Kinesiol.* 2003;13:333-351.

151. Van Dieën JH, Cholewicki J, Radebold A. Trunk muscle recruitment patterns in patients with low back pain enhance the stability of the lumbar spine. *Spine.* 2003;28:834-841.
152. Nadler SF, Malanga GA, DePrince M, Stitik TP, Feinberg JH. The relationship between lower extremity injury, low back pain, and hip muscle strength in male and female collegiate athletes. *Clin J Sport Med.* 2000;10:89-97.
153. Nadler SF, Malanga GA, Feinberg JH, Prybicien M, Stitik TP, DePrince MS. Relationship between hip muscle imbalance and occurrence of low back pain in collegiate athletes: a prospective study. *Am J Phys Med Rehabil.* 2001;80:572-577.
154. Nourbakhsh MR, Ara MM. Relationship between mechanical factors and incidence of low back pain. *J Orthop Sports Phys Ther.* 2002;32:447-460.
155. Cresswell A, Grundstrom H, Thorstensson A. The influence of sudden perturbations on trunk muscle activity and intra-abdominal pressure while standing. *Exp Brain Res.* 1994;98:336-341.
156. Allison GT, Morris SL, Lay B. Feedforward responses of transversus abdominis are directional specific and act asymmetrically—implications for core stablity theories. *J Orthop Sports Phys Ther.* 2008;38:228-237.
157. McCook D, Vicenzino B, Hodges P. Activity of deep abdominal muscles increases during submaximal flexion and extension efforts but antagonist co-contraction remains unchanged. *J Electromyogr Kinesiol.* 2009;19:754-762.
158. Hodges P, Eriksson A, Shirley D, et al. Intra-abdominal pressure increases stiffness of the lumbar spine. *J Biomech.* 2005;38:1873-1880.
159. Richardson C, Snijders C, Hides J, et al. The relation between the transversus abdominis muscles, sacroiliac joint mechanics, and low back pain. *Spine.* 2002;27:399-405.
160. Hodges PW, Richardson CA, Gandevia SC. Contractions of specific abdominal muscles in postural tasks are affected by respiratory maneuvers. *J Appl Physiol.* 1997;83:753-760.
161. Sapsford RR, Hodges PW, Richardson CA, Cooper DH, Markwell SJ, Jull GA. Co-activation of the abdominal and pelvic floor muscles during voluntary exercises. *Neurourol Urodyn.* 2001;20:31-42.
162. Hodges P, Richardson C. Inefficient muscular stabilization of the lumbar spine associated with low back pain. A motor control evaluation of transversus abdominis. *Spine.* 1996;21:2640-2650.
163. Hodges P, Richardson C. Delayed postural contraction of transversus abdominis in low back pain associated with movement of the lower limb. *J Spinal Disord.* 1998;11:46-56.
164. Hodges P, Richardson C. Altered trunk muscle recruitment in people with low back pain with upper limb movement at different speeds. *Arch Phys Med Rehabil.* 1999;80:1005-1012.
165. Hodges P, Moseley G, Gabrielsson A, et al. Experimental muscle pain changes feedforward postural responses of the trunk muscles. *Exp Brain Res.* 2003;151:262-271.
166. Ferreira P, Ferreira M, Hodges P. Changes in recruitment of the abdominal muscles in people with low back pain. Ultrasound measurement of muscle activity. *Spine.* 2004;29:2560-2566.
167. Teyhen DS, Gill NW, Whittaker JL, Henry SM, Hides JA, Hodges P. Rehabilitative ultrasound imaging of the abdominal muscles. *J Orthop Sports Phys Ther.* 2007;38:450-466.
168. Hodges PW, Cholewicki J, Coppieters M, MacDonald D. Trunk muscle activity is increased during experimental back pain, but the pattern varies between individuals. Paper presented at: XVI Congress of the International Society of Electrophysiology and Kinesiology Society; June 29-July 1, 2006; Torino, Italy.
169. Radebold A, Cholewicki J, Panjabi MM, Patel TC. Muscle response pattern to sudden trunk loading in healthy individuals and in patients with chronic low back pain. *Spine.* 2000;25:947-954.
170. Kiesel KB, Uhl T, Underwood FB, Nitz AJ. Rehabilitative ultrasound measurement of select trunk muscle activation during induced pain. *Man Ther.* 2008;13:132-138.
171. Hodges PW, Cresswell AG, Daggfeldt K, Thorstensson A. Three dimensional preparatory trunk motion precedes asymmetrical upper limb movement. *Gait Posture.* 2000;11(2):92-101.
172. Silfies SP, Mehta R, Smith SS, Karduna A. Differences in feedforward trunk muscle activity in subgroups of patients with mechanical low back pain. *Arch Phys Med Rehabil.* 2009;90:1159-1169.
173. Macintosh JE, Bogduk N. The biomechanics of the lumbar multifidus. *Clin Biomech.* 1986;1:205-213.
174. Bogduk N, Macintosh JE, Pearcy MJ. A universal model of the lumbar back muscles in the upright position. *Spine.* 1992;17:897-913.
175. MacDonald DA, Moseley GL, Hodges PW. The lumbar multifidus: does the evidence support clinical beliefs? *Man Ther.* 2006;11:254-263.
176. McGill SM. Kinetic potential of the lumbar trunk musculature about three orthogonal orthopaedic axes in extreme postures. *Spine.* 1991;16:809-815.
177. Moseley G, Hodges P, Gandevia S. External perturbation of the trunk in standing humans differentially activates components of the medial back muscles. *J Physiol.* 2003;547(Pt 2):581-587.
178. Richardson C, Toppenberg R, Jull G. An initial evaluation of eight abdominal exercises for their ability to provide stabilisation for the lumbar spine. *Aust J Physiol.* 1990;36(1):6-11.
179. Richardson C, Jull G, Toppenberg R, Comerford M. Techniques for active lumbar stabilisation for spinal protection: a pilot study. *Aust J Physiol.* 1992;38(2):105-112.
180. Arokoski JP, Valta T, Airaksinen O, Kankaanpaa M. Back and abdominal muscle function during stabilization exercises. *Arch Phys Med Rehabil.* 2001;82:1089-1098.
181. Hodges PW, Richardson CA. Feedforward contraction of transversus abdominis is not influenced by the direction of arm movement. *Exp Brain Res.* 1997;114:362-70.
182. Richardson C, Jull G, Hodges P, Hides J. Local muscle dysfunction in low back pain. In: Richardson C, Hodges P, Hides J, eds. *Therapeutic Exercise for Spinal Segmental Stabilization in Low Back Pain.* Sydney, Australia: Churchill Livingstone; 1999:61-76.
183. Hides J. Paraspinal mechanism in low back pain. In: Richardson C, Hodges P, Hides J, eds. *Therapeutic Exercise for Lumbopelvic Stabilization: A Motor Control Approach for the Treatment and Prevention of Low Back Pain.* 2nd ed. Edinburgh, Scotland: Churchill Livingstone; 2004:49-61.
184. Hides JA, Stokes MJ, Saide M, Jull GA, Cooper DH. Evidence of lumbar multifidus muscle wasting ipsilateral to symptoms in patients with acute/subacute low back pain. *Spine.* 1994;19:165-172.
185. Danneels LA, Vanderstraeten GG, Cambier DC, Witvrouw EE, DeCuyper HJ. CT imaging of trunk muscles in chronic low back pain patients and healthy control subjects. *Eur Spine J.* 2000;9:266-272.
186. Kader DF, Wardlaw D, Smith FW. Correlation between MRI changes in the lumbar multifidus muscles and leg pain. *Clin Radiol.* 2000;55:145-149.
187. Kjaer P, Bendix T, Sorensen JS, Korsholm L, Leboeuf-Yde D. Are MRI-defined fat infiltrations in the multifidus muscles associated with low back pain? *BMC Med.* 2007;25:2.

188. Zoidl G, Grifka J, Boluki D, et al. Molecular evidence for local denervation of paraspinal muscles in failed-back surgery/post discectomy syndrome. *Clin Neuropathol.* 2003;22:71-77.
189. Barker KL, Shamley DR, Jackson D. Changes in the cross-sectional area of multifidus and psoas in patients with unilateral back pain: the relationship to pain and disability. *Spine.* 2004;29:E515-E519.
190. Hodges P, Holm AK, Hansson T, Holm S. Rapid atrophy of the lumbar multifidus follows experimental disc or nerve root injury. *Spine.* 2006;31:2926-2933.
191. Cooper RG, St Clair Forbes W, Jayson MI. Radiographic demonstration of paraspinal muscle wasting in patients with chronic low back pain. *Br J Rheumatol.* 1992;31:389-394.
192. Parkkola R, Rytokoski U, Kormano M. Magnetic resonance imaging of the discs and trunk muscles in patients with chronic low back pain and healthy control subjects. *Spine.* 1993;18:830-836.
193. Dickx N, Cagnie B, Parlevliet T, Lavens A, Danneels L. The effect of unilateral muscle pain on recruitment of the lumbar multifidus during automatic contraction. An experimental pain study. *Man Ther.* 2010;15:364-369.
194. MacDonald D, Moseley GL, Hodges PW. Why do some patients keep hurting their back? Evidence of ongoing back muscle dysfunction during remission from recurrent back pain. *Pain.* 2009;124:183-188.
195. Wilke HJ, Wolf S, Claes LE, Arand M, Wiesend A. Stability increase of the lumbar spine with different muscle groups. A biomechanical in vitro study. *Spine.* 1995;20:192-198.
196. MacDonald D, Moseley GL, Hodges PW. People with recurrent low back pain respond differently to trunk loading despite remission from symptoms. *Spine.* 2010;35:818-824.
197. Moseley GL, Hodges PW. Reduced variability of postural strategy prevents normalization of motor changes induced by back pain: a risk factor for chronic trouble? *Behav Neurosci.* 2006;120:474-476.
198. Moseley GL, Nicholas MK, Hodges PW. Does anticipation of back pain predispose to back trouble? *Brain.* 2004.127:2339-2347.
199. Ferreira PH, Ferreira ML, Maher CG, Refshauge K, Herbert RD, Hodges PW. Changes in recruitment of transversus abdominis correlate with disability in people with chronic low back pain. *Br J Sports Med.* 2010;44(16):1166-1172. doi:10.1136/bjsm.2009.061515.
200. Tsao H, Hodges PW. Immediate changes in feedforward postural adjustments following voluntary motor training. *Exp Brain Res.* 2007;181:537-546.
201. Tsao H, Hodges PW. Persistence of improvements in postural strategies following motor control training in people with recurrent low back pain. *J Electromyogr Kinesiol.* 2008;18:559-567.
202. Hall L, Tsao H, MacDonald D, Coppieters MW, Hodges PW. Immediate effects of co-contraction training on motor control of the trunk muscles in people with recurrent low back pain. *J Electromyogr Kinesiol.* 2009;19:763-773.
203. Tsao H, Druitt TR, Schollum TM, Hodges PW. Motor training of the lumbar paraspinal muscles induces immediate changes in motor coordination in patients with recurrent low back pain. *J Pain.* 2010;11:1120-1128.
204. Watson DH, Trott PH, Cervical headache: an investigation of natural head posture and upper cervical flexor muscle performance. *Cephalalgia.* 1993;13:272-284.
205. O'Leary S, Jull G, Kim M, et al. Craniocervical flexor muscle impairment at maximal, moderate, and low loads is a feature of neck pain. *Man Ther.* 2007;12:34-39.
206. Silverman JL, Rodriquez AA, Agre JC. Quantitative cervical flexor strength in healthy subjects and in subjects with mechanical neck pain. *Arch Phys Med Rehabil.* 1991;72:679-681.
207. Barton PM, Hayes KC. Neck flexor muscle strength, efficiency, and relaxation times in normal subjects and subjects with unilateral neck pain and headache. *Arch Phys Med Rehabil.* 1996;77:680-687.
208. Placzek JD, Pagett BT, Roubal PJ, et al. The influence of the cervical spine on chronic headache in women: a pilot study. *J Man Manip Ther.* 1999;7:33-39.
209. Sjolander P, Michaelson P, Jaric S, Djupsjobacka M. Sensorimotor disturbances in chronic neck pain—range of motion, peak velocity, smoothness of movement, and repositioning acuity. *Man Ther.* 2008;13:122-131.
210. Falla D, Jull G, Edwards S, Koh K, Rainoldi A. Neuromuscular efficiency of the sternocleidomastoid and anterior scalene muscles in patients with chronic neck pain. *Disabil Rehabil.* 2004;26:712-717.
211. Kristjansson E, Dall'Alba P, Jull G. A study of five cervicocephalic relocation tests in three different subject groups. *Clin Rehabil.* 2003;17:768-774.
212. Treleaven J, Jull G, Lowchoy N. The relationship of cervical joint position error to balance and eye movement disturbances in persistent whiplash. *Man Ther.* 2006;11:99-106.
213. Treleaven J, Jull G, Lowchoy N. Smooth pursuit neck torsion test in whiplash-associated disorders: relationship to self-reports of neck pain and disability, dizziness and anxiety. *J Rehabil Med.* 2005;37:219-223.
214. Wenngren BI, Pettersson K, Lowenhielm G, Hildingsson C. Eye motility and auditory brainstem response dysfunction after whiplash injury. *Acta Otolaryngol.* 2002;122:276-283.
215. Jull G Kristjansson E, Dall'Alba P. Impairment in the cervical flexors: a comparison of whiplash and insidious onset neck pain patients. *Man Ther.* 2004;9:89-94.
216. Jull G, Sterling M, Kenardy J, Beller E. Does the presence of sensory hypersensitivity influences outcome of physical rehabilitation for chronic whiplash? A preliminary RCT. *Pain.* 2007;129:28-34.
217. Jull G, Barrett C, Magee R, Ho P. Further clinical clarification of the muscle dysfunction in cervical headache. *Cephalalgia.* 1999;19:179-185.
218. Sterling M, Jull G, Wright A. The effect of musculoskeletal pain on motor activity and control. *J Pain.* 2001;2:135-145.
219. Jull GA. Deep cervical flexor muscle dysfunction in whiplash. *J Musculoskelet Pain.* 2000;8;143-154.
220. Jull G, Amiri M, Bullock-Saxton J, Darnell R, Lander C. Cervical musculoskeletal impairment in frequent intermittent headache. Part 1: subjects with single headaches. *Cephalalgia.* 2007;27:793-802.
221. Chiu TT, Law E, Chiu TH. Performance of the craniocervical flexion test in subjects with and without chronic neck pain. *J Orthop Sports Phys Ther.* 2005;35:567-571.
222. Falla D, Bilenkij G, Jull G. Patients with chronic neck pain demonstrate altered patterns of muscle activation during performance of a functional upper limb task. *Spine.* 2004;29:1436-1440.
223. Johnston V, Jull G, Souvlis T, Jimmieson NL. Neck movement and muscle activity characteristics in female office workers with neck pain. *Spine.* 2008;33:555-563.
224. Falla D, Jull G, Hodges PW. Feedforward activity of the cervical flexor muscles during voluntary arm movements is delayed in chronic neck pain. *Exp Brain Res.* 2004;157:43-48.
225. Szeto G, Straker L, O'Sullivan P. A comparison of symptomatic and asymptomatic office workers performing monotonous keyboard work—1: neck and shoulder muscle recruitment patterns. *Man Ther.* 2005;10:270-280.
226. Veiersted K, Westgaard R, Andersen P. Electromyographic evaluation of muscular work patterns as a predictor of trapezius myalgia. *Scand J Work Environ Health.* 1993;10:284-290.

227. Fredin Y, Elert J, Britschgi N, Vaher A, Gerdle B. A decreased ability to relax between repetitive contractions in patients with chronic symptoms after trauma of the neck. *J Musculoskelet Pain.* 1997;5:55-70.
228. Falla D, Farina D. Muscle fiber conduction velocity of the upper trapezius muscle during dynamic contraction of the upper limb in patients with chronic neck pain. *Pain.* 2005;116:138-145.
229. Sterling M, Jull G, Vicenzino B, Kenardy J, Darnell R. Development of motor dysfunction following whiplash injury. *Pain.* 2003;103:65-73.
230. Madeleine P, Leclerc F, Arendt-Nielsen L, Ravier P, Farina D. Experimental muscle pain changes the spatial distribution of upper trapezius muscle activity during sustained contraction. *Clin Neurophysiol.* 2006;117:2436-2445.
231. Falla D, Farina D, Graven-Nielsen T. Experimental muscle pain results in reorganization of coordination among trapezius muscle subdivisions during repetitive shoulder flexion. *Exp Brain Res.* 2007;178:385-393.
232. Falla D, Farina D, Kanstrup Dahl M, et al. Muscle pain induces task-dependent changes in cervical agonist/antagonist activity. *J Appl Physiol.* 2007;102:601-609.
233. Sterling M, Jull G, Vicenzino B, Kenardy J, Darnell R. Physical and psychological factors predict outcome following whiplash injury. *Pain.* 2005;114:141-148.
234. Shacklock M. Neurodynamics. *Physiotherapy.* 1995;81:9-16.
235. Shacklock M. Improving application of neurodynamic (neural tension) testing and treatments: a message to researchers and clinicians. *Man Ther.* 2005;10:175-179.
236. Butler DS. *The Sensitive Nervous System.* Adelaide, Australia: NOI Publications; 2000.
237. Kobayashi S, Shizu N, Suzuki Y, Asai T, Yoshizawa H. Changes in nerve root motion and intraradicular blood flow during an intraoperative straight-leg-raising test. *Spine.* 2003;28:1427-1434.
238. Coppieters M, Stappaerts K, Wouters L, Janssens K. The immediate effects of a cervical lateral glide treatment technique in patients with neuropathic cervicobrachial pain. *J Orthop Sports Phys Ther.* 2003;33:369-378.
239. Rozmaryn L, Dovelle S, Rothman E, Gorman K, Olvey K, Bartko J. Nerve and tendon gliding exercises and the conservative management of carpal tunnel syndrome. *J Hand Ther.* 1998;11:171-179.
240. Nee RJ, Butler D. Management of peripheral neuropathic pain: integrating neurobiology, neurodynamics, and clinical evidence. *Phys Ther Sport.* 2006;7:36-49.
241. Butler DS. *Mobilisation of the Nervous System.* New York, NY: Churchill Livingstone; 1991.
242. Wainner RS, Whitman JM, Cleland JA, Flynn TW. Regional interdependence: a musculoskeletal examination model whose time has come. *J Orthop Sports Phys Ther.* 2007;37:658-660.
243. Deyle GD, Henderson NE, Matekel RL, Ryder MG, Garber MB, Allison SC. Effectiveness of manual physical therapy and exercise in osteoarthritis of the knee. A randomized, controlled trial. *Ann Intern Med.* 2000;132:173-181.
244. Deyle GD, Allison SC, Matekel RL, et al. Physical therapy treatment effectiveness for osteoarthritis of the knee: a randomized comparison of supervised clinical exercise and manual therapy procedures versus a home exercise program. *Phys Ther.* 2005;85:1301-1317.
245. Whitman JM, Flynn TW, Childs JD, et al. A comparison between two physical therapy treatment programs for patients with lumbar spinal stenosis: a randomized clinical trial. *Spine.* 2006;31:2541-2549.
246. Suter E, McMorland G, Herzog W, Bray R. Conservative lower back treatment reduces inhibition in knee-extensor muscles: a randomized controlled trial. *J Manipulative Physiol Ther.* 2000;23:76-80.
247. Cibulka MT, Delitto A. A comparison of two different methods to treat hip pain in runners. *J Orthop Sports Phys Ther.* 1993;17:172-176.
248. Cleland JA, Childs JD, Fritz JM, Whitman JM, Eberhart SL. Development of a clinical prediction rule for guiding treatment of a subgroup of patients with neck pain: use of thoracic spine manipulation, exercise, and patient education. *Phys Ther.* 2010;90:1239-1250.
249. Boyles RE, Ritland BM, Miracle BM, et al. The short-term effects of thoracic spine thrust manipulation on patients with shoulder impingement syndrome. *Man Ther.* 2009;14:375-380.
250. Maitland G, Hengeveld E, Banks K, English K. *Maitland's Vertebral Manipulation.* 6th ed. Woburn, MA: Butterworth Heinemann; 2002.
251. Boissonnault WG. *Primary Care for the Physical Therapist. Examination and Triage.* 2nd ed. Philadelphia, PA: Saunders; 2011.
252. Travell JG, Simons DG. *Myofascial Pain and Dysfunction: The Trigger Point Manual.* 2nd ed. Baltimore, MD: Williams & Wilkins; 1983.
253. Simons DJ. Diagnostic criteria of myofascial pain caused by trigger points. *J Musculoskelet Pain.* 1999;7:111-120.
254. Lucas N, Macaskill P, Irwig L, Moran R, Bogduk N. Reliability of physical examination for diagnosis of myofascial trigger points: a systematic review of the literature. *Clin J Pain.* 2009;25(1):80-89.
255. American Physical Therapy Association. The guide to physical therapist practice, 2nd edition. *Phys Ther.* 2001;81:9-746.
256. Jette AM. Diagnosis and classification by physical therapists: a special communication. *Phys Ther.* 1989;69:967-969.
257. Sahrmann SA. Diagnosis by the physical therapist—a prerequisite for treatment. *Phys Ther.* 1988;68:1703-1706.
258. Jones MA, Rivett DA. *Clinical Reasoning for Manual Therapists.* Philadelphia, PA: Butterworth-Heinemann; 2004.

Please visit www.routledge.com/9781556429323 to access additional material.

Chapter 4

Evidence-Based Physical Therapy Practice for Low Back Pain

Spine-related pain ranks among the most common problems reported by adults in the United States. In a 2002 survey, 26.4%—or an estimated 54 million American adults—experienced low back pain (LBP) and 14% reported neck pain in the previous 3 months.[1] From 1997 to 2006, national health care costs for spine problems increased 82% (7% per year on average), while general health status and physical functioning worsened.[2] Increasing total costs were largely accounted for by inpatient hospitalization, prescription medications, and emergency department visits. Outpatient visits were mainly a result of an increase in users of ambulatory services.[3] The prevalence of LBP and its persistent nature are some of the most costly problems in the United States health care system. Annual costs related to LBP and disability are estimated at $100 to $200 billion in health care and lost wages.[4] Considering the alarming increase in expenditures and no resultant improvement in health status, physical therapists along with insurers and other providers must contribute to slowing the growth of health care costs through increased adherence to evidence-based guidelines for managing spine-related pain.

One method to slow the growth of health care costs may relate to underutilization of physical therapy (PT) early after onset of LBP. In a cohort of 432 195 Medicare patients who received PT early after an acute LBP episode, Gellhorn et al[5] demonstrated a decreased use of medical services (ie, office visits, injections, or lumbar surgery) compared to PT that occurred at later times. Following the initial physician visit, only 16.2% received PT within 1 year. Of the patients receiving PT, 52.0% occurred within 4 weeks, 18.1% between 31 and 90 days, and 29.9% between 91 and 365 days. Patients evaluated by general practitioners were referred to PT least often.[5] Fritz et al[6] reported an association between use of PT within 90 days of onset of acute LBP and decreased use of medications, magnetic resonance imaging (MRI), and epidural injections in the year after discharge from PT. Similarly, Wand et al[7] showed that early PT (ie, within 6 weeks of onset of LBP) resulted in improved general health, disability, social function, anxiety, depression, and vitality when compared to advice to stay active. Delaying PT, defined as greater than 14 days after a new primary care LBP consultation, was associated with increased health care utilization and costs in the 18 months following the consultation. PT utilization was 7% with large geographic variability. Early PT was associated with a decreased risk of advanced imaging, added physician visits, surgery, injections, and opioid medications compared to delayed PT.[8] Considering that PT utilization was only 7%, the authors concluded that more research is needed to identify which patients with LBP should be referred to PT to decrease the risk of additional costs.[8]

Diagnosis

The medical diagnostic model has traditionally tried to classify persons with LBP based on a pathoanatomical source (ie, facet sprain, muscle strain, degenerative disc, herniated disc). However, in more than 85% of patients with LBP, a precise anatomical tissue cannot be reliably identified as the cause or pain generator.[9] Labeling most patients with LBP by using specific anatomical diagnoses

Stetts DM, Carpenter JG. *Physical Therapy Management of Patients With Spinal Pain: An Evidence-Based Approach (pp 113-341).*

has not been been validated in rigorous studies[10] or shown to improve outcomes.[11] However, specific anatomical diagnoses may be relevant in some instances such as cancer (0.7% of cases), compression fracture (4%), spinal infection (0.01%), ankylosing spondylitis (AS; 0.3%),[12] spinal stenosis (3%), and cauda equina syndrome (CES; 0.04%).[13] In the absence of red flags, current research supports a classification approach that reduces the focus on identifying anatomical lesions in favor of LBP subgroup classifications shown to improve outcomes.[14]

Limitations of the medical model for LBP have led to the diagnostic category of nonspecific LBP, often treated as a homogenous group that excludes medical disease and neurological compromise. Because all persons with nonspecific LBP are unlikely to benefit from a single intervention, the effectiveness of conservative management of LBP remains inconclusive, as shown in many clinical trials using this diagnostic category.[15,16] Inconclusive research findings offer no direction for informed decision making related to interventions and result in less than optimal outcomes, increased costs, and variations in PT practice patterns.[17,18]

In the development of an evidence-based approach to LBP management, the assumption that all persons with nonspecific LBP are equally likely to respond to a particular intervention is no longer valid. Most clinicians and researchers now recognize that persons with nonspecific LBP can be classified into subgroups based on patterns of signs and symptoms. Classifying persons with nonspecific LBP into subgroups with similar characteristics and matching those subgroups to the best management strategies results in improved PT outcomes when compared to an alternative approach.[19-21]

Classification Systems

Researchers and clinicians have described a variety of LBP classification approaches based on duration of symptoms; pathoanatomical sources; clinical patterns; movement impairments (MIs); health; work or functional status; biological, psychological, and social factors; and pain mechanisms.[22-24] Despite differences in methods of PT assessment, a common PT goal is "to identify a movement pattern related to a pain reduction strategy."[24(p1)] The best classification systems should meet criteria related to feasibility, reliability, validity, and generalizability[22] resulting in a best-evidence approach designed to assist the clinician with matching the patient's clinical presentation to the most suitable initial treatment. All patients do not fit into one classification system, and many patients have clinical findings that fit into more than one subgroup within a classification system. To inform clinical decision making, the classification approach described in this text integrates current best evidence, clinical reasoning, and clinical practice guidelines related to specific LBP, thoracic pain, and cervical pain subgroups, and the importance of characteristics that are likely to be most responsive to initial PT management strategies.

If unfamiliar with the classification approach to spinal pain and prior to reading the sections on history and tests and measures, students and clinicians should review the chapter sections on diagnostic classification for LBP, lumbopelvic pain, thoracic pain, and cervical pain. Key history and exam findings are used to place the patient into either a diagnostic classification and/or impairment-based category of LBP[14] that initially guides PT intervention. In a best-evidence approach, an LBP diagnostic classification assists the clinician with matching the patient's clinical presentation to the most suitable initial treatment. In an impairment-based approach, the clinician identifies relevant physical impairments such as limited range of motion (ROM), joint or muscle stiffness or hypermobility, and muscle coordination deficits. Evidence-based interventions are selected to target the prioritized impairments to address activity limitations or functional deficits important to the patient. For patients with LBP, the following evidence-based subgroups and key clinical characteristics are described:

- Mobilization/manipulation plus exercise also depicted as LBP mobility deficits (Table 4-1)
- Stabilization exercise classification also depicted as LBP with movement coordination impairments (Table 4-2)
- Direction-specific exercise (DSE) classification also depicted as LBP with lower extremity referred pain (Table 4-3)
- Mechanical traction classification for LBP with lower extremity-related pain (Table 4-4)
- Impairment-based classification for symptomatic lumbar spinal stenosis (LSS; Table 4-5)
- Impairment-based classification for LBP with altered neurodynamics
- Subclassification of low back-related leg pain (LBRLP) based on predominating pain mechanisms (ie, central sensitization, peripheral nerve sensitization, denervation, and musculoskeletal referred pain; Table 4-6)
- Chronic LBP (CLBP) or chronic, disabling lumbopelvic pain related to motor control impairments (MCIs) based on a biopsychosocial approach (Figures 4-1 and 4-2)
- Pelvic girdle pain (PGP) classification based on a biopsychosocial and neurophysiological pain mechanisms classification (Figures 4-3 and 4-4)
- Pregnancy-related PGP classification

The Natural Course of Low Back Pain

Nonspecific, mechanical LBP is also classified by the length of time that symptoms persist and is often described as acute, subacute, or CLBP. Commonly reported, although

TABLE 4-1. MANIPULATION AND MOBILIZATION PLUS EXERCISE LOW BACK PAIN SUBGROUP CLASSIFICATION SUMMARY

DIAGNOSTIC CLASSIFICATION	*KEY EXAM FINDINGS*	*FACTORS AGAINST*	*INTERVENTION*
• Manipulation and mobilization plus exercise LBP subgroup • International Classification of Functioning, Disability and Health category: o LBP with mobility deficits o Acute, sub-acute, chronic	• No symptoms distal to knee • Recent onset (< 16 days) • Low Fear-Avoidance Beliefs Questionnaire work scale (< 19) • Hypomobility of L-spine: o Lumbar AROM limited o End-range pain, increased but no worse with repeated movement o Passive accessory intervertebral movement or passive physiological intervertebral movement segmental hypomobility in the lower thoracic, lumbar, sacroiliac regions • Hip internal rotation ROM (> 35 degrees for at least 1 hip, measured prone) • Regional deficits: o Mobility o Muscle performance/length o Activity limitations	• Longer symptom duration • Symptoms below the knee • No lumbar hypomobility • (< 10 degrees) difference in left-to-right internal rotation ROM • Negative Gaenslen's sign • ↑ episode frequency • No pain with mobility testing • Peripheralization or centralization with motion testing • Acute, radicular pain • Signs and symptoms of nerve root compromise	• Lumbopelvic mobilization or manipulation • Muscle energy technique • Active ROM: anterior/posterior pelvic tilt (supine or quadruped, 10 reps, 3 to 4 times daily • AROM and stabilization exercises • Active/passive ROM to augment mobilization/manipulation • Address regional and functional deficits

not standardized, definitions include acute LBP up to 4 weeks, subacute LBP from 2 to 6 months, and CLBP starting at 3 to 6 months.[25-27] A *Joint Clinical Practice Guideline* from the American College of Physicians and the American Pain Society define acute LBP as less than 4 weeks, subacute LBP between 4 weeks and 3 months, and CLBP greater than 3 months.[11]

Understanding the course of LBP is important for clinicians, researchers, and patients because it provides information regarding expectations and the benefits of interventions. However, the recurrent and fluctuating nature of LBP challenges the use of symptom duration as a classification. According to a systematic review by Hestbaek and colleagues,[28] on average, the following occurs:

- 62% (range 42% to 75%) still have LBP after 12 months.
- 16% (range 3% to 40%) are sick-listed due to LBP at 6 months.
- 60% (range 44% to 78%) report relapses of pain.
- 33% (range 26% to 37%) report relapses of work absence at 6 months.
- The mean prevalence of LBP in persons with a previous history is 56% (range 14% to 93%) compared to 22% (range 7% to 39%) for persons without a prior history of LBP. The risk of LBP was twice as high for those with a history of LBP or recurrent episodes.

Similar to the variability in definitions of acute, subacute, and CLBP, the definitions of recurrent LBP are diverse, making interpretation of treatment outcomes difficult. A systematic review recommends authors of future research use the following features to describe recurrent LBP: include a start and end to define an episode of LBP (eg, a period of LBP lasting more than 24 hours preceded and separated by a period of at least 1 month without LBP) and consider the number of previous episodes of LBP and the time span over which they occurred (eg, at least 2 episodes in the past 12 months). When taking a history, clinicians should include specific questions to determine duration of symptoms as well as the details of previous episodes.[29] LBP is not a self-limiting condition with predictable recovery or outcomes during each phase.[29,30] Croft et al[31] demonstrated that 75% of LBP patients from a general practice still had pain 1 year later.

TABLE 4-2. STABILIZATION EXERCISE LOW BACK PAIN SUBGROUP CLASSIFICATION SUMMARY

DIAGNOSTIC CLASSIFICATION	KEY EXAM FINDINGS	FACTORS AGAINST	INTERVENTION
• Stabilization exercise LBP subgroup • International Classification of Functioning, Disability and Health: LBP with movement coordination impairments	• Younger age (<40) • 3 or more prior episodes • ↑ frequency of episodes • Generally > flexibility • Aberrant movement: Instability catch or thigh climbing, painful arc mid-range during lumbar flexion/extension • Average straight leg raise ROM >91 degrees • Lumbar (central posterior-to-anterior) passive accessory intervertebral movement hypermobility • No centralization or peripheralization • + prone instability test • For postpartum patients o + P4 test, active straight leg raise, Trendelenburg, pain with palpation of long dorsal sacroiliac ligament or pubic symphysis o Strength, endurance, coordination trunk deficits o Hip mobility deficits	• At least 3 of the following criteria: o Fear-Avoidance Beliefs Questionnaire with physical activity <9 o Negative prone instability test o No aberrant movements o No lumbar hypermobility o >10 degrees difference between right and left straight leg raise ROM	• Promote isolated contraction and cocontraction (endurance) of the deep trunk muscles • Generalized strengthening of the superficial trunk muscles • Manual therapy and exercise for thoracic/hip mobility, motor control, and strength deficits

Evaluation

History and Diagnostic Triage

As discussed in Chapter 2, most diagnoses or diagnostic hypotheses emerge during the patient history, and the rest during the physical examination.[32] Clinicians agree that 80% of the information needed to explain the cause of a patient's problem is extracted during the interview.[33] Optimal PT management depends on an accurate classification-based diagnosis. Current recommendations suggest that clinicians conduct a focused history and physical examination to classify patients into 1 of 3 categories: nonspecific LBP; LBP with potential radiculopathy or spinal stenosis; or LBP potentially due to serious spinal pathology such as tumor, infection, or AS.[11]

The process of classifying persons with LBP is also called *diagnostic triage* and begins with ruling out serious underlying disease such as metastatic disease; inflammatory arthritis; infection; or nonspinal pathology such as endometriosis, kidney disease, abdominal aortic aneurysm (AAA), or gastrointestinal disease through screening for medical red flags. This step determines whether the patient is appropriate for PT services or if a medical referral is needed. Refer to Chapter 2 to review details of the components of the subjective examination (Table 4-7) regarding medical screening to re-examine clinical features that will assist in identifying systemic disease or illness that can mimic neuromusculoskeletal symptoms or conditions.

The likelihood of serious spinal pathology as indicated in the next section is low, but a missed or delayed diagnosis is costly, often resulting in prolonged illness and sometimes death. Most medical red flags are symptoms and can be obtained prior to the physical examination, but key clinical signs may add to the diagnostic accuracy for identifying serious pathology associated with LBP and are presented here as part of the differential diagnosis.

TABLE 4-3. DIRECTION-SPECIFIC EXERCISE LOW BACK PAIN SUBGROUP CLASSIFICATION SUMMARY

DIRECTION-SPECIFIC EXERCISE LOW BACK PAIN CLASSIFICATION SUBGROUPS INTERNATIONAL CLASSIFICATION OF FUNCTIONING, DISABILITY AND HEALTH: LOW BACK PAIN WITH RELATED (REFERRED) LOWER EXTREMITY PAIN	*KEY EXAMINATION FINDINGS*	*INTERVENTION GUIDELINES*
Extension subgroup	• Symptoms distal to knee • Symptoms centralize with extension • Symptoms peripheralize with flexion • Signs and symptoms of nerve root compression may be present • + straight leg raise may be present	• Extension exercises • Mobilization to promote extension • Temporarily avoid flexion activities • Address neurodynamics and other deficits as needed
Flexion subgroup	• Directional preference for extension • Nerve mobility deficits possible • Older age (> 65) • Imaging evidence of LSS • Symptoms distal to knee • Signs and symptoms of nerve root compression may be present • + straight leg raise may be present	• Flexion exercises • Mobilization to promote flexion • Imaging evidence of central spinal stenosis • Unweighted ambulation • Temporarily avoid extension • Address neurodynamics and other deficits as needed
Lateral shift subgroup	• Symptoms peripheralize with extension • Symptoms centralize with flexion or directional preference for flexion • Symptoms of neurogenic claudication may be present • Nerve mobility deficits possible • Visible frontal plane deviation of the shoulders relative to the pelvis • Asymmetrical side-bending active ROM • Gross limitation of side-bending ROM in the direction opposite the lateral shift • Painful and restricted extension active ROM • Signs and symptoms of nerve root compression may be present • + straight leg raise may be present • Nerve mobility deficits possible	• Lateral shift correction • Manual or self-correction in standing • Nonweightbearing shift correction exercises: repeated extension in lying with hips off center • Address neurodynamics and other deficits as needed

TABLE 4-4. TRACTION LOW BACK PAIN DIAGNOSTIC CLASSIFICATION SUMMARY

DIAGNOSTIC CLASSIFICATION	KEY EXAMINATION FINDINGS	INTERVENTION GUIDELINES
Traction	• + leg symptoms (below the buttock), pain, and/or paresthesia • Signs and symptoms of nerve root compression • Peripheralization with extension • Inability to centralize symptoms • Peripheralization with crossed straight leg raise	• Parameters highly variable based largely on expert opinion • Extension-oriented treatment approach • Mechanical traction, 3-dimensional, prone, static for 12 minutes at 40% to 60% body weight • Mechanical traction, static, supine with hips and knees flexion to 90 degrees supported on stool, 5 to 60 kg, 10 to 20 minutes • Manual traction • Optimal dosage parameters for mechanical traction are unknown

Screening for Red Flags: Clinical Signs and Symptoms of Serious Spinal Pathology

Screening for Cancer (Table 4-8)

The most common cancers that may result in metastases to the spine (Figure 4-5) are breast, lung, and prostate.[12] Prevalence of cancer in persons with LBP ranges from 0.1% to 3.5%.[34] Deyo and Diehl[35] reported 4 clinical findings with the highest positive likelihood ratios (+LR) for detecting the presence of metastatic cancer in LBP:

1. Previous history of non-skin cancer (+LR 14.7)
2. Failure of conservative management in the past month (+LR 3.0)
3. Age > 50 years (+LR 2.7)
4. Unexplained weight loss of more than 4.5 kg in 6 months (+LR 2.7)

The absence of all 4 of these clinical findings essentially rules out cancer (Sn 1.0, Sp 0.6). Of these 4 red flags, the most useful is a previous history of cancer, with a pooled +LR of 23.7, while the other 3 had +LRs of 3.[34] The following laboratory test results had significant LRs:

- Erythrocyte sedimentation rate (ESR) > 50 mm/hr (+LR 18.0, –LR 0.46)
- Presence of anemia (+LR 3.9, –LR 0.53)
- Hematocrit < 30% (+LR 18.2)
- White blood cell count > 12 000 (+LR 4.1)[35]

Providing LRs on the diagnostic accuracy of clinical features assists clinicians in determining the need for referral and further testing. Henschke and colleagues[34] concluded that only 4 features, when used alone, significantly raise the posttest probability of cancer: a previous history of cancer (+LR 23.7), an elevated ESR (+LR 18.0), low hematocrit (+LR 18.2), and clinician judgment (+LR 12.1). Other symptoms suggestive of cancer include constant pain not affected by position or activity, worse at night and with weightbearing, no relief with bed rest, insidious onset of symptoms, and constitutional symptoms.[33]

Screening for Spinal Fracture (Table 4-9)

In primary care centers, the prevalence of vertebral fractures in persons presenting with acute LBP is between 0.5%[36] and 4%, specifically compression fractures (Figure 4-6).[37] Age < 50 years lowers the odds of compression fracture (–LR 0.26, +LR 2.2).[12] Fractures in young people are rare unless major trauma is the cause.[38] Stress fractures related to repetitive microtrauma are potential causes of LBP in gymnasts[39] and fast bowlers in cricket.[40] Two studies reported age > 70 increases the odds of compression fracture (+LR 5.5, –LR 0.81[11] and +LR 4.4[41]). Corticosteroid use is a specific clinical feature that significantly raises the suspicion of a compression fracture (+LR 12).[12] Compression fractures usually occur in older adults as a result of osteoporosis in the absence of significant trauma. Eighty percent of osteoporosis cases are women and 20% are men. With a history of compression fractures, the risk of subsequent fracture is greatly increased.[42] Significant risk has been reported in all ethnic backgrounds.[43]

Accurate clinical diagnosis of compression fracture is vital for proper management because patients with this diagnosis present similarly to nonspecific LBP. In fact, in the absence of major trauma, vertebral fractures present

TABLE 4-5. SELECTED MANUAL THERAPY TECHNIQUES AND EXERCISES FOR CONSIDERATION IN MANAGING PERSONS WITH SYMPTOMATIC LUMBAR SPINAL STENOSIS

POTENTIAL IMPAIRMENTS BASED ON EXAMINATION	*POTENTIAL INTERVENTIONS*
Lumbar active ROM mobility deficits	• Side-lying rotational mobilization or manipulation in neutral • Central or unilateral posterior-to-anterior passive accessory intervertebral movement • Thoracic spine as needed • Single and double knee to chest • Home rotational exercise to augment manual therapy
Decreased walking tolerance	• Body weight-supported treadmill, walking, cycling, aquatics therapy, mall walking • Body weight-supported treadmill: o Use minimum (20% to 40% body weight) needed to eliminate buttock/thigh/leg symptoms; if unable to eliminate symptoms, use 50% body weight o Self-selected, regular, comfortable pace, not to exceed 7 on 10-point perceived exertion scale o To tolerance, max 45 minutes; each visit ↑ by 10% body weight • Daily walking: o Distance and pace that does not aggravate lower extremity symptoms using similar parameters as for body weight-supported treadmill
Hip ROM mobility deficits—priority to extension Daily muscle lengthening: three 30-second bouts	• Supine inferior glide to hip in flexion • Supine iliacus/psoas lengthening • Prone posterior-to-anterior glide • Prone rectus femoris lengthening • Other lower extremity (knee, ankle/foot) as needed • Home exercise to augment the manual therapy
Decreased hip muscle performance—priority to hip extension and abduction Dosage: individualized to patient needs	• Clamshell, bridging, side-lying abduction • Bilateral squat, sit-to-stand, step up • Leg press • Home exercise • Aquatic therapy
Decreased trunk muscle performance—priority to poor abdominal activation	• Stabilization exercise • Abdominal drawing-in maneuver/abdominal brace (sit/stand), heel slides, wall slides, bridging, quadruped (single leg lifts), side bridge
Altered neurodynamics	• Neurodynamic mobilization

so similarly to acute nonspecific LBP that only 30% are identified in clinical practice.[44] In a review of 12 studies and 9 categories of clinical features, Henschke et al[44] identified 5 features that can raise or lower the probability of vertebral fracture:

1. Age > 50 years (+LR 2.2, –LR 0.34)
2. Female gender (+LR 2.3, –LR 0.67)
3. Major trauma (+LR 12.8, –LR 0.37)
4. Pain and tenderness (+LR 6.7, –LR 0.44)
5. A distracting painful injury (+LR 1.7, –LR 0.78)

Table 4-6. Predominating Mechanisms for Low Back-Related Leg Pain

DIAGNOSTIC GROUP	*CENTRAL SENSITIZATION*	*DENERVATION*	*PERIPHERAL NERVE SENSITIZATION*	*MUSCULOSKELETAL*
Classification	Neuropathic	Neuropathic	Neuropathic or nociceptive	Nociceptive
Symptomatic structure	Neural	Neural	Neural	Musculoskeletal
Mechanisms	• Sensitization of wide dynamic range neurons • Disinhibition • Forebrain-mediated central sensitization	• Wallerian degeneration • Demyelination	• Inflammation • Increased sodium channel and mechanosensitive channel expression and conductance	• Convergence
Effect	• Enhanced processing of peripheral input	• Conduction block • Deafferentation	• Enhanced nerve trunk mechanosensitivity	• Mental projection of pain to the limb
Symptoms	• Distal pain • Hyperaesthesia • Hyperalgesia • Paraesthesia • Allodynia	• Segmentally distributed distal pain • Hypoesthesia • Weakness • Palsy	• Pain anywhere in the leg • Pain associated with movements that elongate the nerve trunk	• Referred leg pain • Pain tends to be worse proximally • Normal neurological function
Signs	• LANSS score P12 • May have features of the diagnostic group's denervation and peripheral sensitization	• Diminished light touch and pinprick • Diminished or absent reflexes • Muscle weakness • Minimal features of peripheral sensitization • LANSS score < 12	• Nerve is sensitive to elongation and pressure • Reduced active movements corresponding to nerve mechanosensitivity • LANSS score < 12	• None of the signs shown left • LANSS score < 12

LANSS indicates Leeds Assessment of Neuropathic Symptoms and Signs

Reprinted from *Man Ther*, 14(2), Schäfer A, Hall T, Briffa K, Classification of low back related leg pain—a proposed patho-mechanism-based approach, 222-230, Copyright 2009, with permission from Elsevier.

Trauma with neurological signs and structural deformity or neurological deficit are also significant features (+LR 14.4 and +LR 46.4), though corticosteroid use and altered consciousness do not significantly alter the probability of fracture.[44] Deyo et al[13] reported from unpublished data that LBP and long-term corticosteroid therapy has a specificity of 0.995 and, thus, a compression fracture is considered likely until proven otherwise. A limited number of studies and poor methodological quality provide limited support for these commonly used red flags to screen for vertebral fracture.

Screening for Infection

Spinal infections are commonly acquired from other sites but are often related to specific risk factors: intravenous drug abuse, urinary tract infection, indwelling urinary catheters, or skin infection with a sensitivity of about 0.4; specificity is unknown.[12,45,46] In a primary care

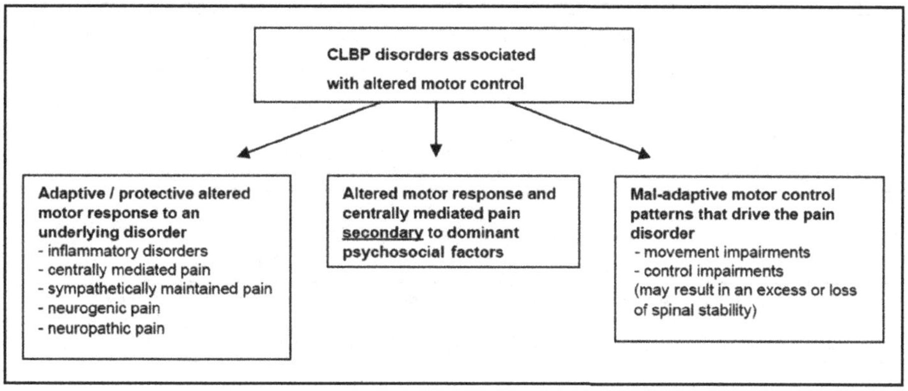

Figure 4-1. Altered motor responses in the 3 subgroups of a CLBP classification. (Reprinted from *Man Ther,* 10, O'Sullivan P, Diagnosis and classification of chronic low back pain disorders: maladaptive movement and motor control impairments as underlying mechanisms, 242-255, Copyright 2005, with permission from Elsevier.)

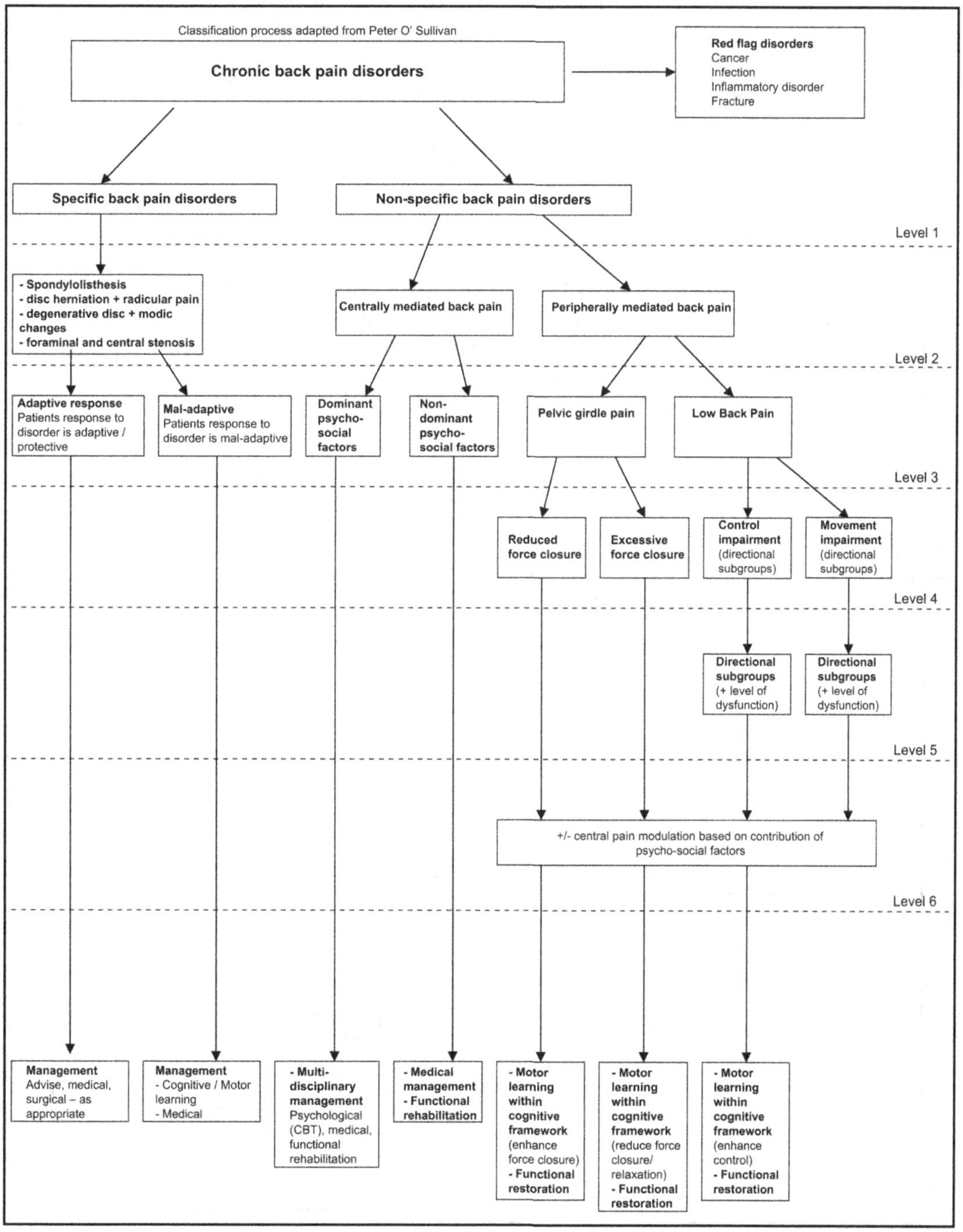

Figure 4-2. Overview of the classification for CLBP. (Reprinted from *Man Ther,* 14, Fersum KV, O'Sullivan PB, Kvåle A, Skouen JS, Inter-examiner reliability of a classification system for patients with non-specific low back pain, 555-561, Copyright 2009, with permission from Elsevier.)

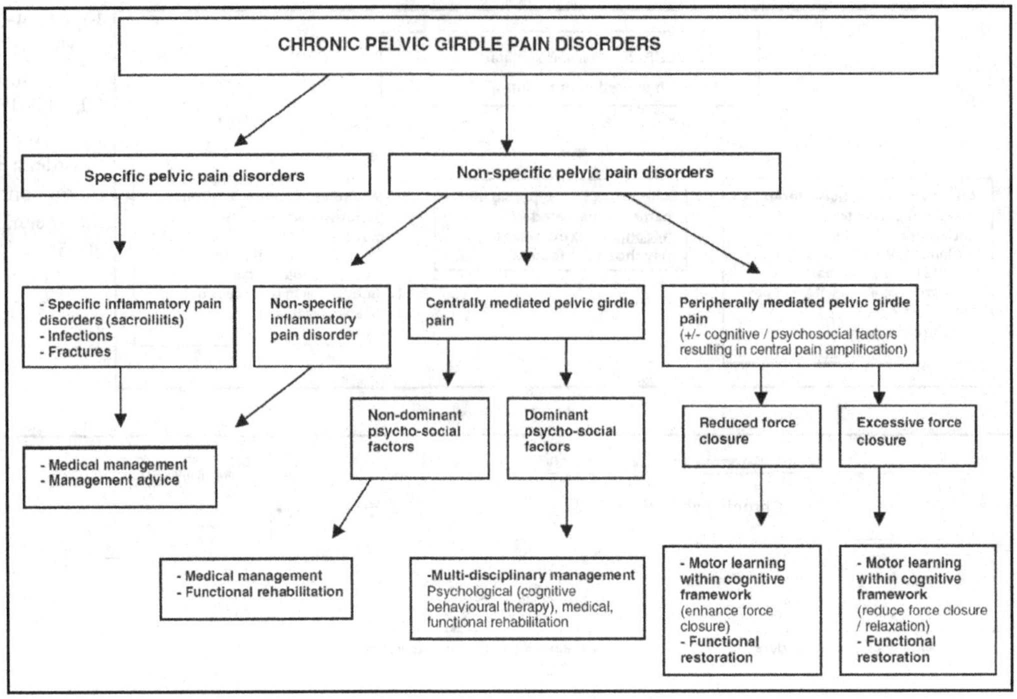

Figure 4-3. Classification of chronic pelvic pain disorders. (Reprinted from *Man Ther,* 12, O'Sullivan PB, Beales DJ. Diagnosis and classification of pelvic girdle pain disorders—part 1: a mechanism based approach within a biopsychosocial framework, 86-97, Copyright 2007, with permission from Elsevier.)

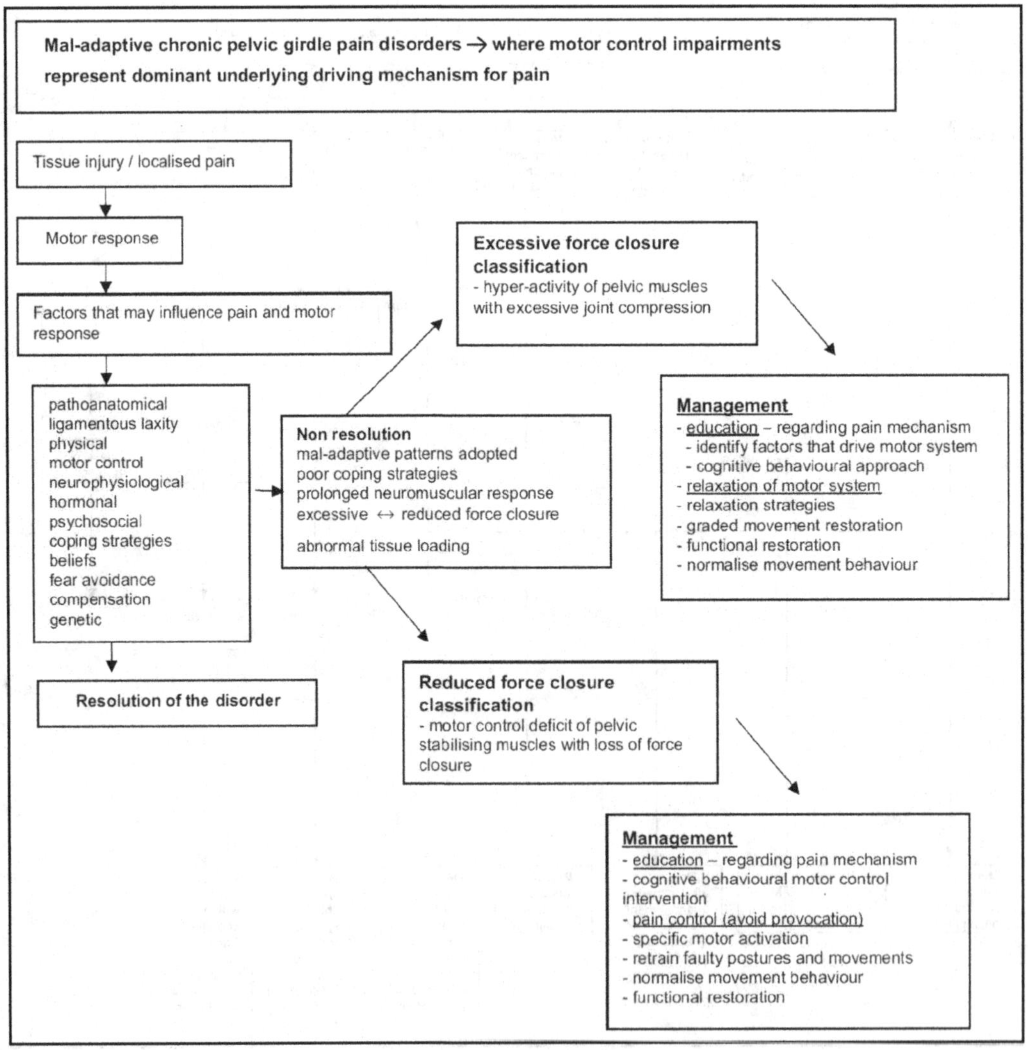

Figure 4-4. Peripherally mediated pelvic girdle pain disorders. (Reprinted from *Man Ther,* 12, O'Sullivan PB, Beales DJ. Diagnosis and classification of pelvic girdle pain disorders—part 1: a mechanism based approach within a bio-psychosocial framework, 86-97, Copyright 2007, with permission from Elsevier.)

TABLE 4-7. COMPONENTS OF THE SUBJECTIVE EXAMINATION

- Administer self-report outcome measures
- Patient profile or general demographics
- Chief complaint
- Description of symptoms, assessment of pain, completing body chart
- History of present episode
- History of previous episodes of similar problem
- Symptom behavior (aggravating factors, easing factors, and 24-hour behavior)
- Review of Medical Screening Questionnaire
- General health, systems review, past medical history, past surgical history
- Medication use
- Imaging
- Patient expectations
- Interview summary
- Review for red flags, yellow flags, predictors of chronicity
- Review baseline self-report outcome measures
- Establish working diagnostic hypotheses, classification, pretest probability
- Plan tests and measures

TABLE 4-8. SCREENING FOR CANCER

CLINICAL FINDINGS	*SN*	*SP*	*+LR*	*−LR*
1. Previous history of non-skin cancer[35]			14.7*	
2. Failure of conservative management in past month[35]			3.0	
3. Age ≥ 50 years[35]			2.7	
4. Unexplained weight loss > 4.5 kg 6 months[35]			2.7	
5. Absence of 1 through 4 above[35]	1.0	0.6		
6. Previous history cancer (pooled data)[34]			23.7	
7. ESR ≥ 50 mm/h[34]			18.0*	0.46
8. Presence of anemia[34]			3.9	0.53
9. Hematocrit < 30%[34]			18.2*	
10. White blood cell count > 12 000[34]			4.1	
11. Clinician judgment[34]			12.1*	

*When used alone, raises the posttest probability of cancer to a clinically significant level.

setting, infection accounts for about 0.01% of cases presenting with LBP. The specificity of fever for infection is 98% (+LR 25); however, the sensitivity of fever for different diagnoses varies from 27% for tuberculosis osteomyelitis to 50% for pyogenic osteomyelitis[47] and 83% for spinal epidural abscess.[48] For that reason, the presence of fever increases the suspicion of infection as a cause of the LBP, but the absence of fever does not significantly decrease the odds of infection.[46] Other risk factors that may raise the index of suspicion for infection are recent bacterial infection; pneumonia; and immunocompromised states such as corticosteroid therapy, organ transplants, or diabetes.

Screening for Abdominal Aortic Aneurysm

An AAA (Figure 4-7) is defined as an infrarenal aortic artery whose diameter exceeds 3.0 cm.[49] The risk of AAA rupture increases with diameters of 5.5 cm or greater. Rates of rupture are 9% for 5.5 to 5.9 cm, 10% for 6.0 to 6.9 cm, and 33% for 7.0 or more.[50] Prevalence of AAA from population-based ultrasonography screening studies is 4% to 9% in men and 0.5% to 1.5% in women.[51,52] The prevalence in older adults aged 65 to 80 years is 7.6% in men and 1.3% in women.[53] Sparse evidence of AAA as a cause of LBP is available only in the form of published case reports.[54,55]

TABLE 4-9. SCREENING FOR SPINAL FRACTURE

CLINICAL FINDINGS[44]	+LR	–LR
1. Age > 50 years	2.2	0.34
2. Female gender	2.3	0.67
3. Major trauma	12.8	0.37
4. Pain and tenderness	6.77	0.44
5. Distracting painful injury	1.7	0.78
6. Trauma with neurological signs	14.4	
7. Structural deformity or neurological deficit	46.4	

Note: Corticosteroid use and altered consciousness did not alter the probability of fracture.

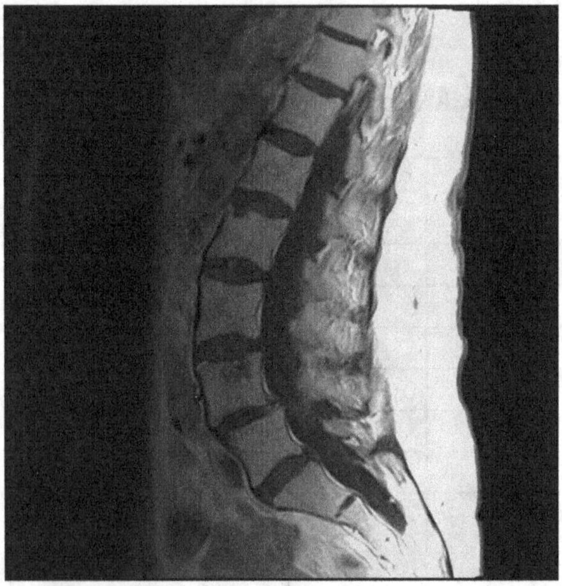

Figure 4-5. MRI lumbar spine with metastasis.

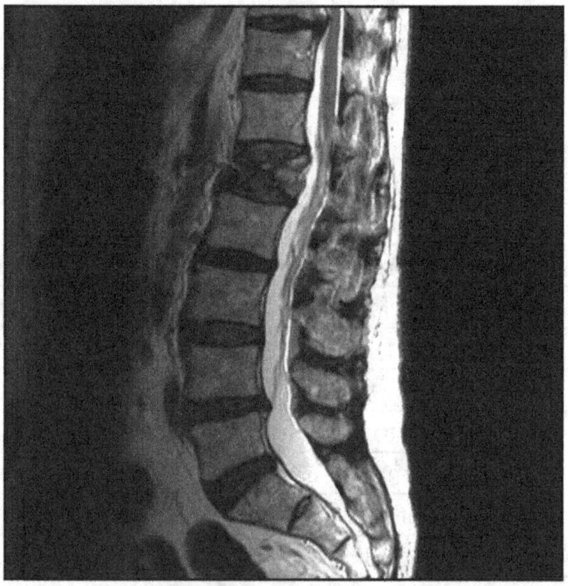

Figure 4-6. MRI lumbar spine compression fracture (L1).

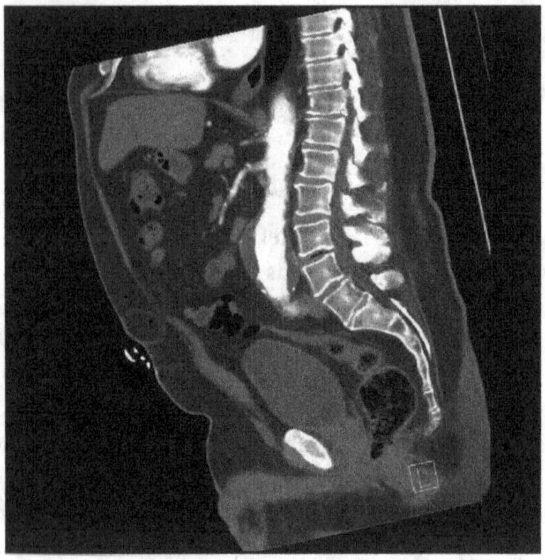

Figure 4-7. MRI of AAA.

The presentation of AAA is highly variable. Some patients may report lower thoracic or lumbar back pain and abdominal pain or hip, groin and buttock pain. However, 75% of persons with AAA are asymptomatic. The diagnosis is often an incidental radiological finding. Some patients report nausea, early satiety, and weight loss.[54,56] Symptom descriptors and behavior may also include a constant, deep, boring pain occasionally described as throbbing or pulsating, and absence of aggravating factors related to movement. Major risk factors for AAA include male gender, a history of smoking (100 cigarettes in a person's lifetime), and age 65 years or older.[57] Additional risk factors include family history, coronary heart disease, claudication, hypercholesterolemia, hypertension, cerebrovascular disease, and increased height.[57] Female gender, diabetes mellitus, and African American race are associated with a decreased risk.

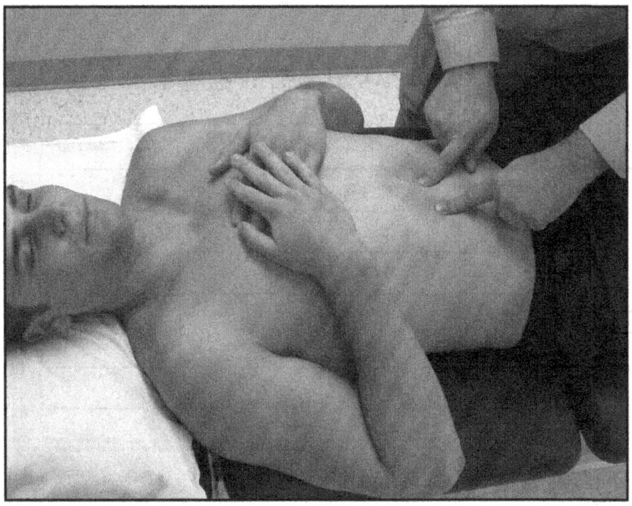

Figure 4-8. Palpation of abdominal aorta. The pulse is located along the left parasternal line and assessed for intensity using a 0 to 4+ scale (0 = absent; 2+ = normal; 4+ = bounding). Both index fingers are placed side by side over the pulse and then slowly separated to locate the borders of palpation to assess the width.

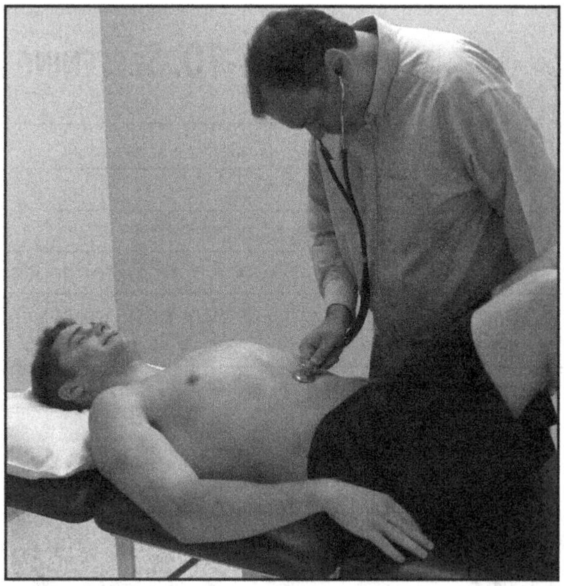

Figure 4-9. Abdominal auscultation. Auscultation begins in midline about 2 inches superior to the umbilicus and progresses distally. Right and left upper and lower quadrants are also assessed. Presence of a pulse (bruit) is considered abnormal.

Abdominal palpation to identify aortic pulsation and to measure its width is warranted for screening suspected AAA in persons with LBP. Fink and colleagues[58] reported the following overall diagnostic accuracy of AAA detection through abdominal palpation:

- Sn 68% (60% to 76%), Sp 75% (68% to 82%)
- +LR 2.7 (2.0 to 3.6), –LR 0.43 (0.33 to 0.56)

The ability to detect an AAA by palpation is associated with the patient's girth, with the obese abdomen being more difficult to palpate. Sensitivity is significantly higher (91%) when abdominal girth is less than 100 cm or the abdomen is rated as not obese (85%). Sensitivity is 100% when girth is less than 100 cm and the AAA diameter measured 5.0 cm or greater—the diameter of AAA most likely to undergo elective surgery.[58] The presence of an abdominal (Sn 11%, Sp 95%)[59] or femoral (Sn 17%, Sp 87%)[59] bruit using auscultation may be a useful clinical finding, but the absence of a bruit is not helpful for ruling out the possibility of an AAA.[55] In persons with LBP and/or at high risk for developing an AAA, clinicians should consider abdominal palpation (Figure 4-8) and auscultation (Figure 4-9) where appropriate in the differential diagnosis of persons presenting with LBP, realizing that a smaller diameter AAA may be missed with palpation.[55] A referral for radiological studies is necessary for this potentially life-threatening cause of LBP.

Screening for Kidney or Urinary Disorders

Some urological disorders are asymptomatic until the disease progresses, such as chronic kidney failure or tumors. Unilateral flank, lower abdominal pain above the pubic bone, LBP with or without radiation to the groin, difficulty initiating urination, painful urination, or blood in the urine should raise suspicion of a urological condition. Additional questions related to a history of urinary tract infections or past episodes of similar symptoms may assist with the differential diagnosis. Bilateral swelling of the lower extremities is suggestive of a kidney problem but may also be related to other diseases such as heart failure or liver disease.[33]

Screening for Cauda Equina Syndrome (Table 4-10)

CES is a rare neurological emergency with 0.04% prevalence in patients presenting with LBP.[11,13] The most common cause for CES is a large, midline posterior disc herniation (Figure 4-10), commonly at L4-5, L5-S1, or L3-4, that compresses the nerve roots in the spinal canal below the level of the spinal cord. CES occurs in 1% to 2% of all disc herniations requiring surgery.[13,60-63] Other causes of CES such as spinal stenosis, spinal tumor, infection, or fracture have been reported. CES onset may be sudden or progress quickly over a few hours to 1 to 2 days. A high index of suspicion or an obvious diagnosis of CES requires immediate referral to an orthopedic surgeon or neurosurgeon. Definitive surgical treatment should occur within 48 hours due to increased risk of permanent neurological deficit with delays of 72 hours and longer.[60,63] Poor outcome is identified with a history of CLBP, preoperative rectal dysfunction (ie, impaired motor or sensory function), and surgical intervention greater than 48 hours after CES onset.[60]

TABLE 4-10. SCREENING FOR CAUDA EQUINA SYNDROME

CLINICAL FINDINGS	SN	SP	+LR	-LR
1. Urinary retention[13,65-67]	0.90	0.95	18	0.01
2. Unilateral or bilateral sciatica[13,67]	>0.80			
3. Unilateral or bilateral sensory and motor deficits[13,67]	>0.90			
4. Sensory deficit: buttock, posterior-superior thigh, and perianal region[13,67]	0.75			
5. Positive straight leg raise[65,66,68]	>0.80			

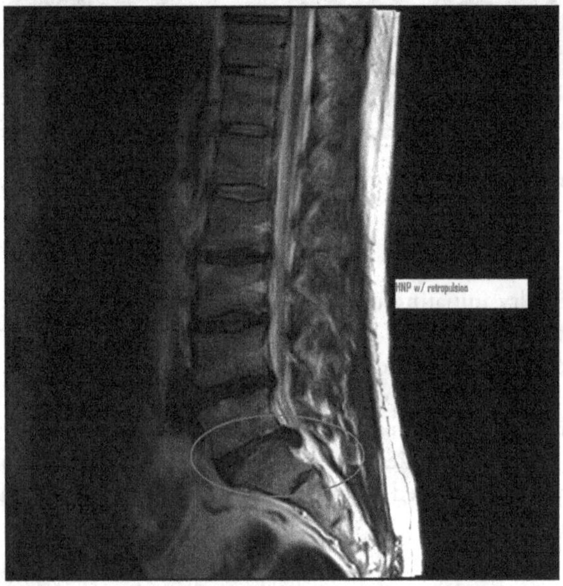

Figure 4-10. MRI of disc herniation causing CES.

In addition to the screening questions for LBP, unilateral or bilateral sciatica, and unilateral or bilateral motor and sensory signs and symptoms, screening questions for CES are related to changes in bowel and bladder such as incontinence or retention or changes in sensation in the genital and perianal regions.[64] Urination retention is the most consistent finding (Sn 0.90, Sp 0.95; +LR 18, –LR 0.01).[13,65-67] In patients without urinary retention, the probability of CES is approximately 1 in 10000.[11] Unilateral or bilateral sciatica (Sn >0.90), sensory and motor deficits (Sn >0.90), and abnormal passive straight leg raise (SLR) tests are common findings.[13,67] Sensory deficits most commonly occur over the buttocks, posterior-superior thighs, and perineal regions (ie, saddle anesthesia; Sn 0.75). Fecal incontinence due to diminished or loss of anal sphincter muscle tone occurs in 60% to 80% of cases.[65,66,68]

Screening for Vascular Claudication (Table 4-11)

Intermittent vascular claudication is usually a symptom of peripheral arterial disease (PAD) commonly at the aortoiliac junction. Claudication is often described as a crampy, achy, tired leg pain that occurs with exertion, especially walking, due to insufficient blood flow to the lower extremity. Symptoms can be unilateral or bilateral, most commonly in the calf, but also occur in the feet, thighs, buttocks, and low back region[69,70] and therefore can mimic neurogenic claudication. Patients with vascular claudication report that symptoms typically come on with walking the same distance each time; increase with walking uphill or stairs; and resolve promptly by standing still, sitting down, or resting for 1 to 10 minutes regardless of spinal position.[69-71] In contrast, neurogenic claudication is increased with walking and spinal extension; less painful when walking uphill; and decreased by sitting, lying down, bending forward, or flexed spinal positions, and the pain may persist for hours.[70] Risk factors associated with PAD include age greater than 40 years, cigarette smoking, diabetes mellitus, hypercholesterolemia, hypertension, obesity, sedentary lifestyle, and a family history of coronary heart disease.[71,72]

In addition to an accurate history, physical examination with exercise-associated leg pain should include palpation of the abdominal aorta, bilateral femoral, popliteal, dorsalis pedis, and popliteal pulses, which are graded absent, diminished, or normal. Documentation of bruits, inspection of the peripheral skin, and the ankle-brachial index assist in determining whether a patient should be referred for diagnostic testing. The ankle-brachial index (Sn 0.95, Sp 1.00) is the reference standard for diagnosing PAD compared to angiography.[70] In a review by Khan,[73] the diagnostic accuracy of the clinical examination to predict PAD revealed the following. For patients with leg symptoms, the most useful findings are the following:

- Presence of cool skin (+LR 5.90 [4.10 to 8.60])

TABLE 4-11. SCREENING FOR VASCULAR CLAUDICATION

CLINICAL FINDINGS[73]	+LR	-LR
1. Presence of cool skin	5.90	
2. Presence of at least one bruit (iliac, femoral, popliteal)	5.60	0.39
3. Any palpable pulse abnormality	4.70	0.38

Combinations of findings did not increase the likelihood of PAD. When all findings are normal, the likelihood of PAD is lower.

TABLE 4-12. SCREENING FOR ANKYLOSING SPONDYLITIS (INFLAMMATORY LOW BACK PAIN)

CLINICAL FINDINGS[80]	SN	SP	+LR	-LR
1. Morning stiffness >30 minutes duration				
2. Improvement in back pain with exercise but not rest				
3. Nocturnal awakening (second half of the night only)				
4. Alternating buttock pain				
If 2 of 4 criteria are present	0.70	0.81	3.7	
If 3 of 4 criteria are present			12.4	

- Presence of at least one bruit (+LR, 5.60 [4.70 to 6.70])
- Palpable pulse abnormality (+LR, 4.70 [2.20 to 9.90])

The absence of any bruits (iliac, femoral, or popliteal; –LR, 0.39 [0.34 to 0.45]) or pulse abnormality (–LR, 0.38 [0.23 to 0.64]) reduces the likelihood of PAD. Combining physical examination findings does not increase the likelihood of PAD. However, when combinations of clinical findings are all normal, the likelihood of disease is lower than when individual symptoms or signs are normal. The pooled LR of the individual finding must be used in context with pretest probability. Independent exam findings cannot rule in or rule out PAD with certainty.[73]

Screening for Ankylosing Spondylitis (Table 4-12)

AS is part of a family of disorders, spondyloarthropathies, or chronic, systemic inflammatory diseases leading to fibrosis and ossification (Figure 4-11) and involving the sacroiliac joints; axial skeleton; and, to a smaller degree, peripheral joints, eyes, skin, and cardiovascular systems. A specific etiology is unknown but involves environmental and genetic factors that are strongly associated with the HlA-B27 gene.[73] Prevalence of AS is 0.1% to 0.2% overall, more common in Caucasians, lower in African Americans, and higher in the specific Native American populations. Age of onset is from late teens to 40 years, with a more frequent diagnosis in males than females (3:1).[74] Onset often occurs insidiously over months or years with complaints of LBP and diffuse radiation into both buttocks. Morning stiffness is characteristic and fatigue is common. The diagnosis of AS is often delayed in primary care partly due to difficulty in differentiating it from nonspecific, mechanical LBP.[75] Earlier diagnosis may be possible with increased use of clinical information with the highest diagnostic accuracy.

The early diagnosis of AS is usually based on a history of LBP. Until recently, the criteria of Calin et al[76] have been supported to define inflammatory LBP. If 4 of 5 criteria—age at onset <40 years, duration of back pain >3 months, insidious onset, morning stiffness, and improvement with exercise—were present, inflammatory LBP was considered to be present (Sn 95%, Sp 76%). Subsequent studies reported Calin et al's screening criteria[76] at 75% sensitivity[77,78] but low specificity (23% to 38%).[77,79] Rudwaleit et al[80] proposed a new set of criteria for inflammatory LBP: morning stiffness of >30 minutes' duration, improvement in back pain with exercise but not with rest, nocturnal awakening in the second half of the night only, and alternating buttock pain. The sensitivity is 70.3%, specificity 81.2%, and +LR for disease presence is 3.7 if 2 of the 4 criteria are fulfilled. If 3 of the 4 criteria are present, the +LR increased to 12.4.[80] Further studies are needed to validate these criteria.

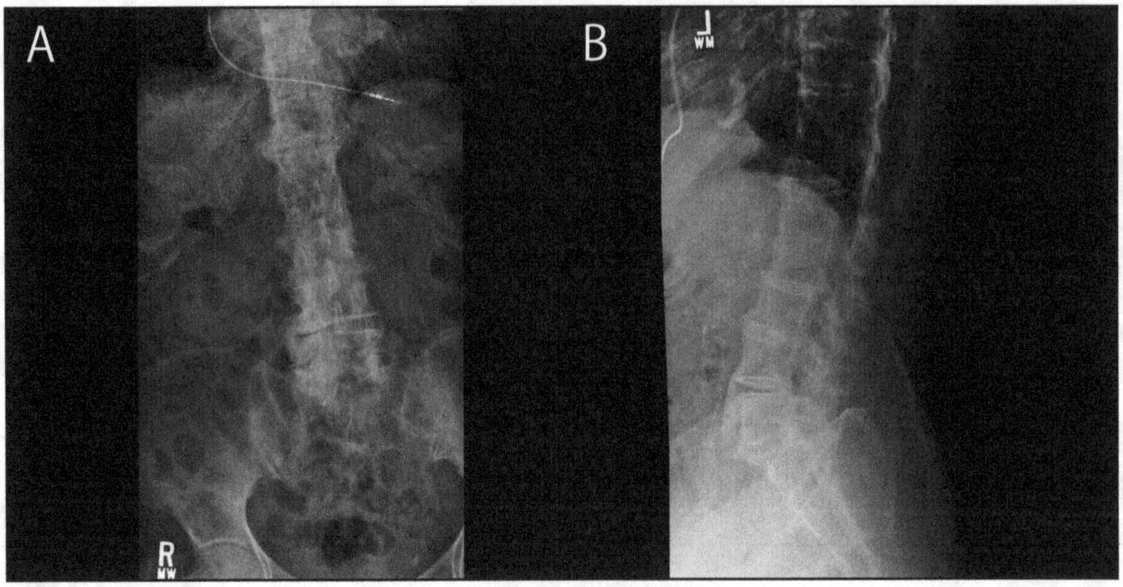

Figure 4-11. Radiograph of AS: (A) anterior-posterior view and (B) lateral view.

Physical examination findings such as Schober's mobility (lumbar flexion) test < 4 cm, chest expansion < 2.5 cm, reduced lateral mobility, and lumbar or sacral provocative tests demonstrate poor sensitivity in early AS. Reduced chest expansion, Schober's test < 4 cm, restricted anteroposterior pelvic compression, lateral pelvic compression, or reduced hip extension demonstrate relatively high specificities (> 0.80)[11,13,81-86] but are typically found only in late-stage disease, are common with CLBP, and are generally not helpful in diagnosis. The diagnostic accuracy of history and physical examination for early diagnosis of AS before radiographic abnormalities is still evolving.

Clinical Signs and Symptoms of Low Back Pain Associated With Neurological Involvement

Screening for Neurological Impairment

Persons with LBP and neurological impairment are more likely to have slower recovery rates, more recurrent episodes, and an increased risk for surgery than individuals without neurological involvement. For those reasons, accurate and timely identification of neurological involvement are critical. Classifications of neurological involvement include CES, lumbar radiculopathy, and symptomatic LSS.

Screening for Lumbosacral Radiculopathy (Table 4-13)

The term *radiculopathy* refers to the signs and symptoms associated with nerve root pathology (Figure 4-12) including paresthesia, hypoesthesia, anesthesia, motor loss, and pain.[87] Lifetime prevalence of radiculopathy is 4% in females and 5% in males.[88,89] An estimated 5% to 10% of patients with LBP have sciatica.[90] Lateral canal stenosis and herniated disk are the 2 most common causes of radiculopathy.[91,92] More than 90% of clinically important lumbar disc herniations occur at the 2 lowest levels (L4-5 and L5-S1) and involve the L5 or S1 nerve roots.[13] Thus, common physical examination findings are weakness of the ankle (Sn 0.35, Sp 0.7; +LR 1.17, –LR 0.93) and great toe dorsiflexors (Sn 0.50 to 0.61, Sp 0.55 to 0.70; +LR 1.36 to 1.67, –LR 0.71) and sensory loss along the dorsum of the foot (L5); or weakness of ankle plantar flexors (Sn 0.47 to 0.60, Sp 0.76 to 0.95; +LR 1.96 to 12.0, –LR 0.42 to 0.70), diminished ankle reflex (Sn 0.47 to 0.50, Sp 0.6 to 0.90; +LR 1.25 to 4.70, –LR 0.83), and sensory loss along the lateral aspect of the foot (S1).[12,13,67,93] Involvement of the higher lumbar nerve roots is associated with about 2% of disc herniations.[13] Signs and symptoms often involve pain and/or numbness in the anterior thigh more prominently than the lower leg, quadriceps (Sn 0.01 to 0.40, Sp 0.89 to 0.99; +LR 1.00 to 3.64, –LR 0.67 to 1.00), and/or psoas weakness and absent patellar tendon reflex (Sn 0.14, Sp 0.93; +LR 4.11, –LR 0.78).[13,93] Sensory impairment is considered abnormal when either vibration or pinprick is diminished (Sn 0.50, Sp 0.62; +LR 1.32, –LR 0.81).[94] If all 3 clinical findings of reflexes, weakness, and sensation are impaired, the sensitivity is decreased and specificity is increased (Sn 0.12, Sp 0.97; +LR 4.0, –LR 0.90).[94] If all 3 findings and the SLR are abnormal (Sn 0.60, Sp 0.99; +LR 6.00, –LR 0.95), the likelihood of radiculopathy increases.[94]

The diagnostic value of history and physical examination factors to classify persons with neurological impairment has not been thoroughly investigated.[93] The first clinical finding of radiculopathy usually comes from the history—a complaint of a sharp pain radiating down the posterior or lateral aspect of the leg, commonly called

TABLE 4-13. SCREENING FOR LUMBAR RADICULOPATHY

CLINICAL FINDINGS	SN	SP	+LR	–LR
1. Ankle dorsiflexion weakness[12,13,67,93]	0.35	0.7	1.17	0.93
2. Great toe extensor weakness[12,13,67,93]	0.5 to 0.61	0.55 to 0.70	1.36 to 1.67	0.71
3. Sensory loss dorsum of foot (L5) or plantarflexion weakness[12,13,67,93]	0.47 to 0.60	0.76 to 0.95	1.96 to 12.0	0.42 to 0.70
4. Diminished ankle reflex[12,13,67,93]	0.47 to 0.50	0.60 to 0.90	1.25 to 4.70	0.83
5. Quadriceps or psoas weakness[12,13,67,93]	0.01 to 0.40	0.89 to 0.99	1.00 to 3.64	0.67 to 1.00
6. Absent patellar tendon reflex[12,13,67,93]	0.14	0.93	4.11	0.78
7. Vibration or pinprick diminished[94]	0.50	0.62	1.32	0.81
8. Weakness, diminished reflexes and sensation[94]	0.12	0.97	4.0	0.90
9. Reflexes, strength, sensation, SLR; all 4 findings abnormal[94]	0.60	0.99	6.00	0.95
10. Complaint of sciatica[94]	0.95			
11. S1 dermatomal pattern of pain[95,96]	0.65	0.80		
12. Pain worse in leg than the back[93]	0.82	0.54	1.74	0.33
13. Focal muscle weakness[93]	0.27	0.93	4.11	0.78

sciatica (Sn 0.95, Sp undetermined)[95,96] and often associated with numbness or paresthesia.[13] Radicular pain is commonly expected to follow a dermatomal pattern, but little evidence supports this assertion. In a review of 226 nerve roots in 169 patients, just under two-thirds (64.1%) of cases in the lumbar spine were nondermatomal.[97] The sensitivity and specificity for a dermatomal pattern of pain are low with the exception of the S1 nerve root (Sn 0.65, Sp 0.80).[97] Pain radiating below the knee rather than pain limited to the buttocks or thigh is more likely to represent true radiculopathy. Pain is sometimes aggravated by coughing, sneezing, or the Valsalva maneuver.[12]

Vroomen and colleagues[93] have identified the following significant independent predictors of nerve root compression:

- Two patient characteristics (age 51 to 81 and duration of disease 15 to 30 days)
- Four symptoms from the history (pain worse in the leg than the back [Sn 0.82, Sp 0.54; +LR 1.74, –LR 0.33]; a dermatomal distribution of pain [Sn 0.89, Sp 0.31; +LR 1.3, –LR 0.34]; paroxysmal pain; and pain worse on coughing, sneezing, or straining
- Two signs from the physical examination (focal muscle weakness [Sn 0.27, Sp 0.93; +LR 4.11, –LR 0.78] and increased finger to floor distance >25 cm [Sn 0.45, Sp 0.74; +LR 1.71, –LR 0.75])

The SLR test was not a significant predictor. Evidence also suggests that reproduction of symptoms on crossed SLR (pooled Sn 0.29, Sp 0.88)[98] and absent reflexes (Sn 0.14, Sp 0.93; +LR 2.21, –LR 0.78)[93] rule in nerve root syndrome, while the absence of symptoms on SLR (pooled Sn 0.91, Sp 0.26)[98] can be used to rule out the diagnosis. Selected aspects of the patient history appear to be better for ruling out nerve root compression, and the physical examination appears better for ruling in.[64]

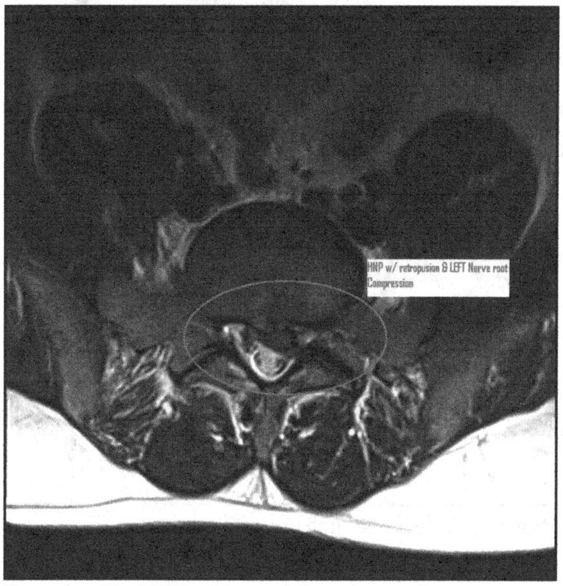

Figure 4-12. MRI of herniated nucleus pulposus causing symptomatic left nerve root compression (radiculopathy).

TABLE 4-14. SCREENING FOR SYMPTOMATIC LUMBAR SPINAL STENOSIS

CLINICAL FINDINGS	SN	SP	+LR	−LR
1. Absence of pain while seated[101]	0.46	0.93	6.6	0.58
2. Pain below buttocks[101]	0.88	0.34	1.3	0.35
3. Pain below knees	0.56	0.63	1.5	0.70
4. Age >65[101]	0.77	0.69	2.5	0.33
5. No pain with flexion[101]	0.79	0.44	1.4	0.48
6. Best posture sitting[102]	0.89	0.33	1.5	0.28
7. Worst posture standing or walking[102]	0.89	0.33	1.3	0.33
8. 2-stage treadmill test[102]:				
a. Longer total walking time inclined	0.50	0.92	6.49	0.54
b. Earlier symptom onset with level walking	0.68	0.83	4.07	0.39
c. Prolonged recovery after level walking	0.82	0.68	2.59	0.26
d. Earlier symptom onset and prolonged recovery with level walking		0.947	14.51	

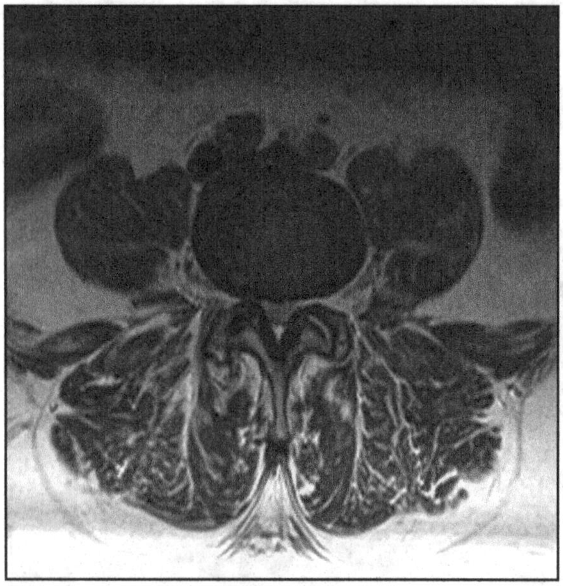

Figure 4-13. MRI of lumbar central canal stenosis.

Screening for Symptomatic Lumbar Spinal Stenosis (Table 4-14)

LSS (Figure 4-13), a narrowing of the spinal canal or lateral recess, is usually a result of degenerative (most common), developmental, or congenital disorders. A narrow canal in radiographic imaging is not a definitive diagnosis. LSS is defined by symptoms and clinical findings combined with radiographic evidence. Lateral recess or foraminal stenosis generally results in spinal nerve or nerve root compression. In central canal stenosis, the cauda equina is compressed unless the stenosis occurs at the upper lumbar (L1-L2) vertebral levels. Since the spinal cord ends at the L1-L2 vertebral levels, narrowing the spinal canal in this location may result in myelopathy and the signs and symptoms of an upper motor neuron disorder. Myelopathy is discussed in Chapter 6 on neck pain.

Evidence on the diagnostic utility of the history and physical examination for detecting LSS is scarce.[99] Reported symptoms are variable, but patients classically complain of neurogenic claudication with or without LBP. Neurogenic claudication, characterized by pain referred into the legs that may persist for hours, weakness, numbness, and tingling, is increased with walking and spinal extension but less painful when walking uphill and decreased by sitting, lying down, bending forward, or in a flexed spinal position.[33]

Konno et al[100] used a self-reported history questionnaire as a tool to assess the diagnostic value of the history in patients with LSS and cauda equina or nerve root compression. The key predictive factors between the 2 categories of LSS were age >50, lower extremity pain or numbness, increased pain when walking and standing, and relief of symptoms on bending forward (odds ratio [OR] ≥2). The key predictive factors for cauda equina symptoms were numbness or burning sensation around the buttocks, walking almost causing urination, numbness in the soles of both feet and legs, and numbness without pain (OR ≥ 2).[100]

A systematic review of diagnostic tests for LSS concluded that tests, study population, and reference standards prohibited statistical pooling.[99] Absence of pain while seated (Sn 0.46, Sp 0.93; +LR 6.6, –LR 0.58) is a highly specific finding[101] useful to ruling in a diagnosis of LSS. Additional findings from Katz et al[101] are as follows:

- Pain below buttocks (Sn 0.88, Sp 0.34; +LR 1.3, –LR 0.35)
- Age > 65 (Sn 0.77, Sp 0.69; +LR 2.5, –LR 0.33)
- No pain with flexion (Sn 0.79, Sp 0.44)

Patient ranking of sitting as the best posture (Sn 0.89, Sp 0.39; +LR 1.5, –LR 0.28) and standing or walking as the worst posture (Sn 0.89, Sp 0.33; +LR 1.3, –LR 0.33) are highly sensitive or useful for ruling out a diagnosis of LSS.[102] The absence of reporting sitting as the best posture and standing or walking as the worst posture decreases the likelihood of LSS. Fritz and colleagues[102] also reported on the usefulness of the 2-stage treadmill test (TSTT) in determining the presence of LSS. The TSTT compares the results of a patient's walking tolerance with no incline and a 15% inclined setting at a self-selected comfortable pace. The presence of a longer total walking time during inclined walking is predictive of LSS (Sn 0.50, Sp 0.923; +LR 6.49, –LR 0.54). Using a radiological reference standard, the best classification of LSS was associated with the findings of an earlier onset of symptoms and prolonged recovery time with level treadmill walking (Sp 0.947; +LR 14.51).[102] A summary with additional factors is provided in Table 4-14.

Clinical Signs and Symptoms of Low Back Pain Associated With Psychological Involvement

Diagnostic Triage: Screening for Yellow Flags

A risk factor is a feature related to a higher rate of back pain onset. In addition to medical red flag screening, the clinician should also assess for the presence of yellow flags or psychosocial risk factors predictive for chronic disability and pain.[11] A yellow flag is a psychosocial risk factor that may serve as a barrier to recovery leading to a poorer prognosis. A prognostic indicator is used to predict the outcome after back pain has started. In some individuals, a poor prognostic indicator such as depression may suggest that the episode of LBP is likely to be prolonged. Yellow flags raise the index of suspicion for the potential to develop a chronic problem that may require appropriate cognitive and behavioral management strategies. In some instances, a yellow flag such as severe clinical depression may warrant immediate referral for intervention. Accurate identification of patients with risk factors that interfere with the normal recovery process is necessary to provide appropriate interventions that prevent acute problems from becoming chronic.

Psychosocial factors can potentially influence LBP during various stages: prior to the onset of any back pain; during the acute onset of LBP when seeking health care; and during the transition to or maintenance of chronicity.[103] Factors related to the maintenance or chronicity of LBP have been more thoroughly investigated than the other 2 stages and are discussed under a separate section on chronic or persistent LBP. This section discusses the complexity of transitioning from acute nonspecific LBP to CLBP with a focus on identifying modifiable risk factors associated with the individual, provider, health care system, and workplace or home environment that could prevent acute nonspecific LBP from becoming chronic.

Though not all research provides a consensus, several studies[104-111] indicate that depression and distress, pain-related fear, and fear of movement or reinjury are strong predictors of observable physical performance and are highly associated with self-reported disability levels in chronic as well as in subacute pain. In a systematic review, Linton[110] consistently identified a significant relationship between stress distress, anxiety, mood, and depression and the development of back or neck pain. This relationship existed independently of other variables. Cognitive factors such as fear-avoidance beliefs and passive coping strategies were also related to the development of pain and disability.

A systematic review of prospective cohort studies of acute or subacute LBP concluded that robust evidence existed for distress or depressed mood and, to a lesser degree, somatization[112] (ie, when symptoms present in more than one part of the body with no known cause) as significant predictors of an unfavorable outcome. Work-related variables were not included. The role for other factors such as fear-avoidance beliefs and catastrophizing, which is exaggeration toward painful stimuli, was not confirmed by the available evidence in this review.[112]

A prospective study of acute LBP without neurologic deficits assessed prognostic factors for nonrecovery over 12 weeks.[113] In this sample of 91 patients with acute LBP for < 3 weeks, only a small number (8.7%) were at risk for chronicity. A comparison between recovery and nonrecovery groups revealed that pain, physical mobility, emotional reactions, sleep, energy level, and distress subgroups, as measured by the Roland-Morris Disability Questionnaire (RMDQ) and Nottingham Health Profile (NHP), were statistically significantly lower in the recovery group. Recovery was defined as resolution of pain and < 4 on RMDQ. Additionally, NHP-pain score (recovery, 52.3 ± 31.9 versus nonrecovery, 73.8 ± 22.3) was the best prognostic factor for nonrecovery in the short term.[113]

A prospective cohort study[114] of 66 patients with acute or subacute LBP seeking PT in primary care also concluded pain at baseline as a significant predictor on the subscale of the Acute Low Back Pain Screening Questionnaire (ALBPSQ). The ALBPSQ correctly identified 80% of nonrecovered patients at 12 weeks with a relative risk of not being recovered of 3.75 (1.63 to 8.52). Using multiple regression analyses, baseline scores on the ALBPSQ, Pain Coping Inventory, Fear-Avoidance Beliefs Questionnaire (FABQ), and Tampa Scale for Kinesiophobia were not associated with nonrecovery at 3 months.[114] Pain scores and scores on the psychosocial variables were not associated at 12 weeks. These conclusions[113,114] contrast with 2 earlier systematic reviews that report psychosocial factors such as fear of movement or reinjury, poor job satisfaction, and emotional distress as stronger predictors of LBP outcomes than either physical examination findings or pain severity and duration.[111,112]

High pain intensity is a threatening experience that often results in escape and avoidance,[115] but fear of pain is often more disabling than pain itself.[116] In the Fear-Avoidance Model of Exaggerated Pain Perception (FAMEPP), fear of pain and resultant fear-avoidance beliefs and behaviors (see Table 2-7) are theorized to be important factors in determining whether a person with acute nonspecific LBP recovers in the short term or transitions to CLBP.[117,118]

In the FAMEPP model, a person's fear-avoidance response to acute nonspecific LBP rests somewhere along a continuum of confrontation to avoidance.[117,118] Confronters are patients with low levels of fear-avoidance who are associated with a normal recovery process and gradual return to prior functional levels. Avoiders have a higher level of fear-avoidance usually associated with a maladaptive response to LBP and the potential to develop chronic pain and disability. The FAMEPP model describes a specific psychosocial factor relevant to the development of chronic disability from LBP.[119]

Other factors that influence the outcome in patients with acute LBP include patient expectations and satisfaction. In a secondary analysis of a randomized trial comparing usual care alone to usual care plus choice of chiropractic, acupuncture, or massage, Myers et al[120] concluded that higher patient expectations for recovery are associated with greater functional improvement. Several patient expectations of treatment for LBP have been reported and include a clear diagnosis of cause of his or her pain, instructions, pain relief, a physical examination, and confirmation that the pain is real, along with understanding, listening, respect, and being part of the decision-making process.[121] Other expectations are more diagnostic tests, other therapy, specialist referrals, and sickness certification. In a prospective cohort study of 544 working adults with acute LBP, Shaw et al[122] reported that positive provider communication such as explaining the problem clearly, trying to understand the patient's job, and advice to prevent reinjury accounted for more variation in patient satisfaction at 1 month than was explained by clinical improvements in pain and function. At 3 months, clinical improvement was the strongest predictor of patient satisfaction. Provider counseling and education are highly valued and important for patient satisfaction for patients with work-related LBP.[122]

The ability to predict a failure to return to work due to nonspecific LBP lasting less than 3 months is an area of interest because of personal, social, and economic costs. Once again, positive expectations of recovery are associated with better work outcomes in LBP, but it is unclear how strong a predictor recovery expectation is and the best method to measure it. A person who indicates low expectations for recovery raises the index of suspicion that psychosocial factors are present. Iles et al[123] reported that there is moderate evidence that fear-avoidance beliefs are predictive of work outcome. Fear-avoidance beliefs and behaviors are related to concern of how much pain will be caused by performing work activities. Pain-related fear can lead to an enhanced perception of disability, deconditioning, and diminished functional participation.[124-127] The best method to measure fear-avoidance is unclear, but the FABQ[128] was the most common tool in this review.

Pincus et al[129] suggested that the current state of knowledge clearly indicates 2 factors appropriate for screening at primary care: depression/distress and fear-avoidance in the early stages of LBP. Depression is a predictor of developing LBP and also a response to the experience of LBP. In the acute phase of back pain, anxiety and worry are natural reactions, but the lack of an exact cause and inadequate pain relief may result in helplessness, anger, and depression. An underlying depression often impairs the ability to cope with pain, potentially leading to an increased perception or experience of pain. Individuals with self-reported depression are twice as likely to develop back pain.[130,131] Individuals who have more severe pain have a higher likelihood of depression.[132] Screening questions for identifying individuals at high risk for depression are discussed in Chapter 2 and should be included on the medical screening questionnaire.

According to Iles et al,[123] depression is not predictive of work outcome in nonchronic, nonspecific LBP. This conclusion is not in agreement with the review by Pincus et al,[112] which did not include work outcomes. Depression is known to adversely impact rehabilitation outcomes and contribute to work-related disability,[133-136] and it is likely to be an unintended consequence of work disability, but depression does not predict ongoing work disability.[123] Stress, anxiety, and level of job satisfaction are not predictive of work outcomes in nonchronic, nonspecific LBP. The evidence related to compensation status was insufficient.[123]

The role and interaction of psychosocial factors (ie, fear-avoidance, depression, patient expectations) in the transition from acute LBP to CLBP is not fully understood or agreed upon. Despite a lack of consensus regarding the role of risk factors associated with the transition of acute LBP to CLBP, the evidence supports screening for yellow flags, provision of appropriate PT management strategies, and/or referral to speciality services as part of the management of acute LBP. Research is needed to comprehensively

TABLE 4-15. SELF-REPORT OUTCOME MEASURES

OUTCOME MEASURE	RELIABILITY AND VALIDITY	RESPONSIVENESS
RMDQ v 2.0[148,149]	Valid; good test-retest reliability at initial evaluation and up to 6 weeks	• MCID = 2 to 3 points for baseline RMDQ <9 • MCID = 5 to 9 points for baseline RMDQ 9 to 16 • MCID 8 to 13 points for those with baseline RMDQ 17 to 24 points[153] • MCID range = 2 to 13, absolute 5, or 30% improvement from baseline[154]
Oswestry LBP Disability Index v 2.0[149]	Valid; good retest reliability at initial visit and 2 or 4 weeks or discharge	• MCID range = 9 to 16[152] • MCID range = 4 to 15[154] • Absolute MCID = 10[154] • 30% improvement from baseline[154]
Modified Oswestry LBP Disability Questionnaire[157]	Nonsurgical rehabilitation; ICC 0.90 (95% CI = 0.78 to 0.96) across 4 weeks	• MCID = 6[157] • MCID = 10.66 (ages 62 or older)[160] • 50% improvement[159]
Patient-Specific Functional Scale[162]	Reliable and valid in patients with LBP	• MDC for average score = 2 • MDC for single activity = 3
Global Rate of Change Scale	Test-retest reliability CLBP is high; face validity is high	• MCID 15-point scale[165]: o ±3 to ±1 a small change o ±4 to ±5 a moderate change o ±6 to ±7 a large change o +5 or more[169]

MCID indicates minimal clinically important difference; MDC, minimal detectable change.

determine which factors constitute increased risk, the best screening instruments to identify them, and what to do when they have been identified.

Standardized Self-Report Outcome Measures

Standardized instruments measure various factors related to current level of pain, function, activities, participation, quality of life, or health status (Table 4-15). Outcome measures use closed-ended questions or specific procedures to provide a baseline quantitative assessment of a patient's perceived activity limitations and participation in life restrictions.[137] These same outcome measures are then repeated at intervals following intervention and used to verify whether clinically meaningful change has occurred. In addition to providing objective data related to meaningful change, outcome measures are used to identify patients at risk for poor outcomes,[138] to assess clinician and clinic performance,[139] to ascertain the most effective interventions,[140,141] and to set therapeutic goals. As discussed in Chapter 2, specific self-report outcome measures should possess the properties of reliability, validity, and responsiveness.

Reliability describes the consistency with which a self-report instrument measures the variable of interest such as pain, health status, ROM, function, and work status.[142] Reliability ranges from –1 to 1 when measured by kappa values and from 0 to 1 when measured by intraclass correlation coefficients (ICCs). Reliability coefficients below 0.50, between 0.50 and 0.75, or above 0.75 have poor, moderate, and good reliability, respectively.[142] Although reliability scores of 0.90 or more are deemed optimal for use in clinical decision making, others consider values over 0.70 as acceptable.[143]

Validity describes the extent that the self-report instrument accurately quantifies what it intended to measure.[142] Relative to clinical tests and measures, the test is valid if the conclusions made from it are appropriate, useful, and meaningful. Responsiveness is the ability to accurately detect whether a true or clinically meaningful change in a patient's health status has occurred over time.[143,144] One way of determining when meaningful change in an outcome measure has occurred is the minimal detectable change (MDC), the amount of change necessary to exceed measurement error.[144] From a statistical perspective, if the MDC for a specific self-report measure is 5, any change score below a 5 is attributed to measurement error and not a true change in patient status. However, statistically significant change is not always clinically meaningful. Another method of determining whether change is clinically relevant is the minimal clinically important difference (MCID) or change (MCIC). The MCID was initially defined by Jaeschke et al[145] as the smallest difference in score in the domain of interest such as pain or function that a patient perceives as beneficial. Knowledge of the MCID allows clinicians to compare baseline and postintervention scores to determine whether a patient has improved and if the amount is perceived as beneficial or important to the patient.

While the concept of MCID seems relatively simple, the methods for determining MCID are not. Different methods used to determine MCID or MCIC result in different values.[146] Clinicians should be familiar with these methods and other factors such as floor and ceiling effects, baseline scores, stage (ie, acute, subacute, or chronic) of the patient's problem, cultural settings, or whether the patient has only nonspecific LBP or LBP and leg pain that may result in a range of MCID values.

Longo et al[147] listed 28 rating scales for LBP. No gold standard exists for the use of self-report outcome assessment in the management of LBP. Each self-report tool has advantages and disadvantages. Commonly used self-report outcome measures for LBP are discussed next.

Functional Status Questionnaires

Roland-Morris Disability Questionnaire

The original version of the RMDQ (Figure 4-14) contains 24 "yes" or "no" items that focus on a limited range of physical functions, but no psychosocial items related to LBP.[148,149] Patients respond to each item as the statements apply to them over the past 24 hours. Each item is scored (yes = 1 point or agree with statement; no = 0 points or disagree with statement) and summed to equal a potential range of 0 (no disability) to 24 (maximum disability). Higher scores are reported for acute LBP and LBP with radiculopathy. RMDQ completion and scoring take about 6 minutes. Modifications of the RMDQ involve shortened versions, but recommendations continue for use of the original version.[146,147,150] Reliability and validity are well-established for patients with LBP.[146,151,152] The RMDQ has good reliability when used at initial evaluation and up to 6 weeks after intervention with a recommended MCID cutoff of 5.2.[152]

Stratford et al[153] suggested that a clinically meaningful change varies depending upon the patient's initial RMDQ score as follows:

- MCID 2 to 3 points for baseline RMDQ <9
- MCID 5 to 9 points for baseline RMDQ 9 to 16
- MCID 8 to 13 points for baseline RMDQ 17 to 24

Consistent with the above MCIDs, Ostelo et al[154] reported a range of MCID values (2.0 to 13) based on empirical evidence and recommended an absolute MCID of 5 and a 30% improvement from baseline as a guide.

Oswestry Low Back Pain Disability Index

The Oswestry Disability Index (ODI) Version 2.0 (Figure 4-15) is a self-administered, reliable, and valid questionnaire that takes about 6 minutes to complete and score.[152,155-158] Version 2.0 is recommended for use.[146,149] The questionnaire contains 10 sections related to activities of daily living and pain designed to describe the patient on the day of the visit. Each section has 6 statements related to severity and is scored from 0 to 5 points.[149] If the first statement in each section is marked, the score is 0. If the last statement is marked, the score is 5 with the other statements ranked 1, 2, 3, or 4 accordingly. If more than one box is marked in each section, the highest score is used. If all 10 sections are completed, calculate the score as follows: a total score of 16 out of 50 × 100 = 32%. If one section is not scored, the final score is: total score/(5 × number of questions answered) × 100%.[145] A higher percentage suggests a greater perceived level of disability by the patient:

- 0 to 30: minimal disability
- 20 to 40: moderate disability
- 40 to 60: severe disability
- 60 to 80: crippled
- 80 to 100: bed-bound or symptom magnifier[156]

Similar to the RMDQ, the ODI has good test-retest reliability and can be given on the initial visit and then re-evaluated at 2 or 4 weeks or at discharge.[152] Davies and Nitz[152] concluded in a systematic review that the MCID is between 9 and 16. For the ODI, Ostelo et al[154] reported a range of MCID values (4.0 to 15) based on empirical evidence and recommended an absolute MCID of 10 and a 30% improvement from baseline as a guide.

Fritz and colleagues[159] suggested that the MCID on a modified version of the ODI may not sufficiently discriminate a successful treatment outcome from the favorable natural history of LBP. Instead of using the MCID, which has a range of values and the 30% baseline suggested by Ostelo et al,[154] Fritz et al[159] proposed using a threshold of 50% improvement on the ODI for individual patients as a valid measure of a successful outcome. Percent improvement on the ODI is calculated as follows: (initial ODI – ODI @ # weeks)/initial ODI × 100.[159]

Modified Oswestry Low Back Pain Disability Questionnaire

Several versions of the ODI have been reported in the literature.[147] The measurement characteristics for a common modification used by physical therapists were first reported in 2001.[157] These authors substituted a section on

The Roland-Morris Disability Questionnaire

When your back hurts, you may find it difficult to do some of the things you normally do.
This list contains sentences that people have used to describe themselves when they have back pain.
When you read them, you may find that some stand out because they describe you *today*.
As you read the list, think of yourself *today*. When you read a sentence that describes you today, put a tick against it. If the sentence does not describe you, then leave the space blank and go on to the next one. Remember, only tick the sentence if you are sure it describes you today.

1. I stay at home most of the time because of my back.
2. I change position frequently to try and get my back comfortable.
3. I walk more slowly than usual because of my back.
4. Because of my back I am not doing any of the jobs that I usually do around the house.
5. Because of my back, I use a handrail to get upstairs.
6. Because of my back, I lie down to rest more often.
7. Because of my back, I have to hold on to something to get out of an easy chair.
8. Because of my back, I try to get other people to do things for me.
9. I get dressed more slowly than usual because of my back.
10. I only stand for short periods of time because of my back.
11. Because of my back, I try not to bend or kneel down.
12. I find it difficult to get out of a chair because of my back.
13. My back is painful almost all the time.
14. I find it difficult to turn over in bed because of my back.
15. My appetite is not very good because of my back pain.
16. I have trouble putting on my socks (or stockings) because of the pain in my back.
17. I only walk short distances because of my back.
18. I sleep less well because of my back.
19. Because of my back pain, I get dressed with help from someone else.
20. I sit down for most of the day because of my back.
21. I avoid heavy jobs around the house because of my back.
22. Because of my back pain, I am more irritable and bad tempered with people than usual.
23. Because of my back, I go upstairs more slowly than usual.
24. I stay in bed most of the time because of my back.

The score of the RDQ is the total number of items checked – i.e. from a minimum of 0 to maximum of 24

Figure 4-14. The RMDQ. (Reprinted from Roland M, Fairbank J. The Roland-Morris Disability Questionnaire and the Oswestry Disability Questionnaire. *Spine*. 2000;25:3115-3124.)

employment and home-making activities for the section related to sex life because the sex life section was often left blank. This version was originally called the Oswestry Low Back Pain Disability Questionnaire and later revised as the Modified Low Back Pain Disability Questionnaire.[157] For this ODI modification and patients undergoing nonsurgical rehabilitation, Fritz and Irrgang[157] reported an ICC of 0.90 (95% confidence interval [CI]: 0.78 to 0.96) across 4 weeks, and an MCID of 6 points. The modified ODI, MDC 10.66 points, is recommended for use among geriatric patients with LBP who are ages 62 or older.[160]

A comparison of the RMDQ and ODI suggests that both tools similarly measure a patient's perceived level of disability associated with LBP.[152] Reliability and validity are high for both instruments. The RMDQ is most sensitive and appropriate for patients with mild to moderate disability (ie, low severity and irritability), while the ODI may be more appropriate for persistent severe disability or symptoms of high severity and irritability.[152] The RMDQ is appropriate for patients with LBP only who are more acute and who have had LBP for less than or equal to 30 days, whereas both the RMDQ and ODI are appropriate for patients with LBP and related leg pain to include

Could you please complete this questionnaire. It is designed to give us information as to how your back (or leg) trouble has affected your ability to manage in everyday life. Please answer *every section*. Mark *one box only* in each section that most closely describes you *today*.

Section 1: Pain intensity

□ I have no pain at the moment.
□ The pain is very mild at the moment.
□ The pain is moderate at the moment.
□ The pain is fairly severe at the moment.
□ The pain is very severe at the moment.
□ The pain is the worst imaginable at the moment

Section 2: Personal care (washing, dressing, *etc.*)

□ I can look after myself normally without causing extra pain.
□ I can look after myself normally but it is very painful.
□ It is painful to look after myself and I am slow and careful.
□ I need some help but manage most of my personal care.
□ I need help every day in most aspects of self care.
□ I do not get dressed, wash with difficulty, and stay in bed.

Section 3: Lifting

□ I can lift heavy weights without extra pain.
□ I can lift heavy weights but it gives extra pain.
□ Pain prevents me from lifting heavy weights off the floor but I can manage if they are conveniently positioned, *e.g.*, on a table.
□ Pain prevents me from lifting heavy weights but I can manage light to medium weights if they are conveniently positioned.
□ I can lift only very light weights.
□ I cannot lift or carry anything at all.

Section 4: Walking

□ Pain does not prevent me walking any distance.
□ Pain prevents me walking more than 1 mile.
□ Pain prevents me walking more than a quarter of
□ Pain prevents me walking more than 100 yards.
□ I can only walk using a stick or crutches.
□ I am in bed most of the time and have to crawl to the toilet.

Section 5: Sitting

□ I can sit in any chair as long as I like.
□ I can sit in my favorite chair as long as I like.
□ Pain prevents me from sitting for more than 1 hour.
□ Pain prevents me from sitting for more than half an hour.
□ Pain prevents me from sitting for more than 10 minutes.
□ Pain prevents me from sitting at all.

Section 6: Standing

□ I can stand as long as I want without extra pain.
□ I can stand as long as I want but it gives me extra pain.
□ Pain prevents me from standing for more than 1 hour..
□ Pain prevents me from standing for more than half an hour.
□ Pain prevents me from standing for more than 10 minutes.
□ Pain prevents me from standing at all.

Section 7: Sleeping

□ My sleep is never disturbed by pain.
□ My sleep is occasionally disturbed by pain.
□ Because of pain I have less than 6 hours' sleep.
□ Because of pain I have less than 4 hours' sleep.
□ Because of pain I have less than 2 hours' sleep.
□ Pain prevents me from sleeping at all.

Section 8: Sex life (if applicable)

□ My sex life is normal and causes no extra pain.
□ My sex life is normal but causes some extra pain.
□ My sex life is nearly normal but is very painful.
□ My sex life is severely restricted by pain.
□ My sex life is nearly absent because of pain.
□ Pain prevents any sex life at all.

Section 9: Social life

□ My social life is normal and causes me no extra pain.
□ My social life is normal but increases the degree of pain.
□ Pain has no significant effect on my social life apart from limiting my more energetic interests, *e.g.*,sport, *etc.*
□ Pain has restricted my social life and I do not go out as often.
□ Pain has restricted social life to my home.
□ I have no social life because of pain.

Section 10: Traveling

□ I can travel anywhere without pain.
□ I can travel anywhere but it gives extra pain.
□ Pain is bad but I manage journeys over 2 hours.
□ Pain restricts me to journeys of less than 1 hour.
□ Pain restricts me to short necessary journeys under 30 minutes.
□ Pain prevents me from traveling except to receive treatment.

Figure 4-15. Oswestry Disability Index Version 2.0. (Reprinted from Roland M, Fairbank J. The Roland-Morris Disability Questionnaire and the Oswestry Disability Questionnaire. *Spine.* 2000;25:3115-3124.)

more chronic pain lasting longer than 30 days regardless of patient's stage (ie, acute or chronic) at entry.[161]

Patient-Specific Functional and Pain Scale

The Patient-Specific Functional and Pain Scale (PSFS; Figure 4-16)[162] is patient-specific, as opposed to condition- or region-specific fixed-item questionnaires such as the RMDQ and ODI. The PSFS allows the patient to identify up to 5 important activities that they are having difficulty with or unable to perform and rate the difficulty level of each activity on an 11-point scale (0 = unable to perform activity; 10 = able to perform activity at same level as before injury or problem). At follow-up sessions, patients are informed of their initial activities and scores prior to reassessment. The PSFS can be administered in about 4 minutes as the clinician reads the instructions and records the activities and ratings. Reliability and validity have been established for patients with LBP.[162] The total score equals the sum of the activity scores divided by the number of activities. MDC for an average score is 2 points; MDC for a single activity score is 3 points.[162] The PSFS average and individual activity scores correlate moderately to highly (*r* range, 0.59 to 0.74) with the RMDQ.[162] Some research in patients with LBP suggests that scales such as the PSFS are more responsive to clinical change than questionnaires with predefined items.[163]

PATIENT SPECIFIC FUNCTIONAL AND PAIN SCALES (PSFS)

Clinicians to read and fill in *Functional Goal and Outcome Worksheet.*
Note: Complete at the end of the history and prior to the physical examination.

Read at Baseline Assessment

I'm going to ask you to identify 3 to 5 important activities that you are unable to do or are having difficulty with as a result of your____________ problem. Today, are there any activities that you are unable to do or have difficulty with because of your __________problem? (Clinician: show scale)

Supplement: Are there any other activities that you are having just a little bit of difficulty with? For examples, activities that you might assign a score of 6 or more to. List up to 2 activities. (record as Supplementary 1 and 2 (S1 and S2).

Read at Follow-up Visits

When I assessed you on (state previous assessment date), you told me that you had difficulty with (read all activities from list one at a time).

Today, do you still have difficulty with 1 (have patient score each item); 2(have patient score each item); 3 (have patient score each item); etc.

Patient Specific Activity Scoring scheme (Point to one number):

0 1 2 3 4 5 6 7 8 9 10

Unable to perform activity (0) — Able to perform activity at same level as before injury or problem (10)

Date/Score

ACTIVITY						
1.						
2.						
3.						
4.						
5.						
Additional						

(233)

Figure 4-16. PSFS. (Reprinted with permission from Stratford PW, Gill C, Westaway M, Binkley JM. Assessing disability and change on individual patients: a report of a patient-specific measure. *Physiother Can.* 1995;47:258-263.)

Global Rate of Change Scales

The Global Rate of Change (GRC) scale (Figure 4-17) is a commonly used self-perceived outcome measure. The scale consists of one question that quantifies a patient's improvement or deterioration over a period of time and, along with other outcomes, assists in establishing the effect of an intervention in clinical practice or research.[164] The question asks the patient to rate the change in his or her health status related to a specific condition over a period of time. The person's ability to recall and quantify overall status at a previous date and time is required for proper use of the GRC. A sample question might be, "With respect to your LBP, overall, how would you describe yourself now as compared to when you first came to physical therapy for treatment?" The patient then recalls his or her status at initial PT visit and assesses the difference between the 2 points in time to rate the amount of change.[164]

The design and title of GRC scales vary widely with commonly used scales of 7, 11, or 15 points. A 15-point scale as described by Jaeschke et al[165] ranges from –7 (a very great deal worse) to 0 (about the same) to +7 (a very great deal better). Additional descriptors (see Figure 4-17) are attached to the other values on the scale (–1 to –6 and +1 to +6). In a cohort of subjects with CLBP, test-retest reliability on an 11-point scale is high (ICC 0.90; 95% CI: 0.884 to 0.93).[166] Face validity or whether the measure makes sense to the patient is also high.[167] Strong correlations (Pearson's r = 0.50) exist on the GRC 7-point scale between GRC scores and change in the ODQ[163] and the modified ODI (r = 0.78).[157] Agreement of 87% accuracy between patient and clinician GRC scores is acceptable.[168]

The MCID varies in some studies due to arbitrary cutoff scores. On a 15-point scale, clinically important improvement was defined as +5 or more and deterioration as –5 or less because patients with lesser change scores sought further

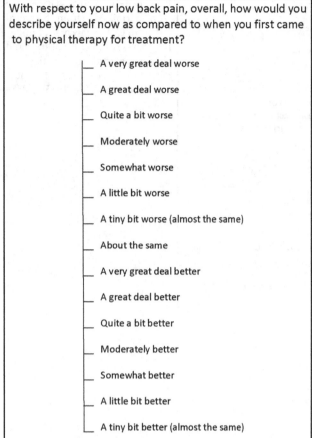

With respect to your low back pain, overall, how would you describe yourself now as compared to when you first came to physical therapy for treatment?

- ___ A very great deal worse
- ___ A great deal worse
- ___ Quite a bit worse
- ___ Moderately worse
- ___ Somewhat worse
- ___ A little bit worse
- ___ A tiny bit worse (almost the same)
- ___ About the same
- ___ A very great deal better
- ___ A great deal better
- ___ Quite a bit better
- ___ Moderately better
- ___ Somewhat better
- ___ A little bit better
- ___ A tiny bit better (almost the same)

Figure 4-17. Example of a 15-point GRC.

treatment.[169] Using a 15-point scale, Childs et al[170] used a rating of +3 or higher, meaning at least "somewhat better," as clinically relevant improvement. Lauridsen et al[171] reported no significant difference in responsiveness in a head-to-head comparison of 7-point and 15-point scales. An MCID for the GRC between +3 and +1 represents a small change; scores between +4 and +5 represent a moderate change; and scores of +6 or +7 represent a large change.[165]

Ferreira et al[172] tried to answer the question, "How much of an effect do common PT interventions need to have for patients with LBP to perceive they are worth the cost, discomfort, risk, and inconvenience?" In 77 patients with nonspecific LBP, the authors measured the smallest worthwhile effect in terms of global perceived change on a 5-point scale and visual analogue scale (VAS) percentage (0% = no better; 100% = fully recovered) of perceived change. An example of a global perceived change question is, "I would see a physiotherapist for spinal manipulation: 0 = even if it made me no better; 1 = only if it made me a little better; 2 = only if it made me much better; 3 = only if it made me very much better; and 4 = only it made me fully recover." Subjects perceived that a PT intervention would have to make them "much better" or 1.7 ± 0.7 on the 5-point scale or reduce their symptoms by 42% to consider it worthwhile. These estimates are baseline reductions in symptoms and not the difference in outcome between the 2 interventions.[172]

The GRC is simple to score and administer and allows the patient to decide what aspects of pain, disability, or function are most important when deciding about his or her health status. Kamper et al[164] concluded that sufficient evidence exists to support the use of a balanced 7- or 11-point numerical scale. For all outcome measures in all settings, administration of the GRC should be standardized. If rehabilitation occurs over several months, GRC serial measures are preferred due to the potential affect on validity of an increasing length of recall time.[164]

Pain-Related Fear Questionnaires

The fear-avoidance model attempts to explain the role of pain-related fear in the development and maintenance of chronic disability from LBP. Pain-related fear often results in psychophysiological responses such as heightened muscle reactivity, escape and avoidance behavior, and cognitive responses such as catastrophizing thoughts.[173] In patients with acute LBP, pain-related fear is associated with decreased participation in activities of daily living,[174] a higher perceived disability,[175] and repeated sick leave.[176] In several studies, pain-related fear was predictive of subsequent higher disability,[177] decreased probability of return to work, and greater probability of being on sick leave.[104,178,179] In CLBP patients, pain-related fear results in either complete avoidance of specific activity or reduced performance through the use of safety behavior or submaximal effort.[180,181] Avoidance behaviors tend to advance disability and disuse; however, Pincus et al[182] concluded that studies measuring fear-avoidance did not provide convincing evidence that fear-avoidance beliefs are a risk factor for poor outcomes, stating that 6 of 9 studies did not show a statistically significant association or only a weak association. Fear of pain, work-related activities, movement, and reinjury are often described in some patients with LBP and measured by validated self-report questionnaires.[173]

Fear-Avoidance Beliefs Questionnaire

The FABQ (Figure 4-18) developed by Waddell et al[128] contains a work scale (FABQW) and a physical activity scale (FABQPA) totaling 16 items. However, not all 16 items are used for screening purposes. The FABQW has 7 items (items 6, 7, 9, 10, 11, 12, and 15; score range 0 to 42) to assess fear-avoidance beliefs about work. FABQPA has 4 items (items 2, 3, 4, and 5; score range 0 to 24) to assess fear-avoidance beliefs about general activity.

The FABQ has high test-retest reliability.[183,184] The FABQ subscale scores demonstrate a strong relationship to disability due to LBP[128,185,186] and have predictive validity for future disability for patients in general settings[178,187-189] and those receiving PT.[104,190,191] Higher scores on either the work or physical activity scale indicate elevated fear-avoidance beliefs. Therefore, the FABQ is

Name: ______________________ Date: ______________

Here are some of the things which other patients have told us about their pain. For each statement please circle any number from 0 to 6 to say how much physical activities such as bending, lifting, walking or driving affect or would affect your back pain.

	COMPLETELY DISAGREE			UNSURE			COMPLETELY AGREE
1. My pain was caused by physical activity	0	1	2	3	4	5	6
2. Physical activity makes my pain worse	0	1	2	3	4	5	6
3. Physical activity might harm my back	0	1	2	3	4	5	6
4. I should not do physical activities which (might) make my pain worse	0	1	2	3	4	5	6
5. I cannot do physical activities which (might) make my pain worse	0	1	2	3	4	5	6

The following statements are about how your normal work affects or would affect your back pain.

	COMPLETELY DISAGREE			UNSURE			COMPLETELY AGREE
6. My pain was caused by my work or by an accident at work	0	1	2	3	4	5	6
7. My work aggravated my pain	0	1	2	3	4	5	6
8. I have a claim for compensation for my pain	0	1	2	3	4	5	6
9. My work is too heavy for me	0	1	2	3	4	5	6
10. My work makes or would make my pain worse	0	1	2	3	4	5	6
11. My work might harm my back	0	1	2	3	4	5	6
12. I should not do my normal work with my present pain	0	1	2	3	4	5	6
13. I cannot do my normal work with my present pain	0	1	2	3	4	5	6
14. I cannot do my normal work until my pain is treated	0	1	2	3	4	5	6
15. I do not think that I will be back to my normal work within 3 months	0	1	2	3	4	5	6
16. I do not think that I will ever be able to go back to that work	0	1	2	3	4	5	6

Figure 4-18. FABQ. (Reprinted with permission from Waddell G, Newton M, Henderson I, et al. A Fear-Avoidance Beliefs Questionnaire (FABQ) and the role of fear-avoidance beliefs in CLBP and disability. *Pain.* 1993;52:157-168. This questionnaire has been reproduced with permission of the International Association for the Study of Pain [IASP]. The questionnaire may not be reproduced for any other purpose without permission.)

believed to be a useful screening tool to identify patients with elevated fear-avoidance beliefs who may be at risk for a poor outcome. However, a cutoff score that consistently identifies patients who may be at risk has not been defined. In a cohort of patients with acute LBP, the MDC for the FABQPA = 9 points and for the FABQW = 12 points.[192]

Several authors have proposed various cutoff scores in working with the FABQ. Burton et al[193] reported an elevated FABQPA score as > 14, defined as a score greater than the median for patients seeking treatment from primary care physicians, but this score does not represent an increased probability of a poor outcome. In a population of patients seeking PT for acute, work-related LBP, Fritz et al[104] proposed a cutoff for elevated FABQW scores as > 29 (–LR 0.08) based on an external criterion of return to work as the strongest predictor of return to work after 4 weeks of PT. Al-Obaidi et al[190] reported a FABQPA score of > 29 (+LR 3.78) at baseline as predictive of not having a clinically meaningful improvement after a 10-week exercise program. In that study, patients had more than 2 months of LBP and were not receiving worker's compensation. However, this score is not easy to interpret because it was derived by using all 5 of the FABQPA items instead of the recommended 4 items.[190]

In a retrospective review, Cleland et al[194] examined the usefulness of the FABQ in a typical PT practice. These authors concluded that the FABQW and FABQPA baseline scores did not demonstrate predictive validity for patients with private insurance. A previously used cut-off score[195] for the FABQPA of > 13 did not result in significant improvement in prediction of a poor outcome for patients with private insurance or those receiving worker's

TABLE 4-16. PAIN-RELATED FEAR QUESTIONNAIRE

QUESTIONNAIRE	OUTCOME	PROPERTIES MDC IN CLBP[198]
FABQ	Fear-avoidance influence on pain, physical impairment, and disability	FABQW = 6.8 FABQPA = 5.4
Fear of Pain Questionnaire	Fear of pain influence on specific activities	5.6
Tampa Scale for Kinesiophobia	Fear of movement and reinjury	4.8
Pain Catastrophizing Scales	Extent of cognitions (helplessness, magnification) related to pain catastrophizing	9.1

compensation. Only the FABQW used with patients receiving worker's compensation had sufficient predictive validity to guide clinical decision making in this population. In this study, the sample consisted of privately insured, subacute and chronic patients only 35% who had symptoms <3 weeks and those receiving workers' compensation, of whom 54% had symptoms <3 weeks. This study[194] agreed with the previously reported initial FABQW cutoff score >29 for predicting return to work at 4 weeks[104] but only in patients receiving worker's compensation. These authors recommend caution when interpreting FABQ scores in non–work-related LBP, because it has poor discriminative ability to identify patients at risk for poor outcome in PT. The results of this study indicate more research is needed to determine the usefulness of the FABQ for patients with LBP who do not have work-related LBP.[194]

In contrast to the conclusions of Cleland et al,[194] a secondary analysis of 2 randomized clinical trials in a cohort of patients without work-related LBP found that the FABQW is a better predictor of 6-month outcomes in comparison to the FABQPA scale. George et al[138] reported FABQW scale scores >20 (+LR 2.3 to 5.1) were associated with an increased risk of reporting no improvement in 6-month ODI scores. The FABQW is not a definitive screening tool for predicting poor outcome and should be used with other examination findings.[138] In patients with high fear-avoidance based on FABQPA scores and centralization with repeated movements, Werneke et al[196] suggested that formal intervention using cognitive-behavioral techniques may not be necessary. However, the presence of high fear and noncentralization of symptoms is an indication to consider a cognitive-behavioral approach to optimize outcomes.[196]

A FABQW score of <19 has been identified as one factor in a 5-factor clinical prediction rule (CPR) for a manipulation classification used to identify patients with LBP who are likely to respond to manipulation as a treatment strategy.[140,141] In the preliminary development of a CPR for a stabilization classification, a FABQPA score of <9 is 1 of 4 factors predictive of failure, identifying patients who were not likely to receive even minimal benefit from a stabilization treatment strategy.[197]

In a PT outpatient setting, George et al[198] investigated the psychometric properties of 4 fear-avoidance measures (Table 4-16): FABQ, Fear of Pain Questionnaire (FPQ), Tampa Scale for Kinesiophobia (TSK-11), and the Pain Catastrophizing Scale (PCS) in a cohort of patients with CLBP of more than 3 months. The FPQ[199,200] assesses fear of pain to specific activities. The TSK-11[201,202] assesses kinesiophobia or fear of movement and reinjury. The PCS[203,204] measures the extent of cognitions such as rumination, helplessness, and magnification related to pain catastrophizing. Higher scores on the TSK-11 and PCS indicate higher amounts of fear of movement and pain catastrophizing, respectively. For all questionnaires, test-retest ICC coefficients ranged from 0.90 to 0.96 with the MDC (ie, amount of change needed to exceed measurement error) for FABQW = 6.8, FABQPA = 5.4, FPQ = 5.6, TSK-11 = 4.8, and PCS = 9.1. Due to construct redundancy and similar stability estimates in the 4 measures, the results suggest that assessment of fear-avoidance for patients with CLBP should include only the PCS and the FABQ. The PCS, which is associated with depression, is useful in determining the fear-avoidance influence on emotional function, and the FABQ is useful in determining the fear-avoidance influence on pain intensity, physical impairment, and disability.[198]

Components of the Patient's History (Subjective Examination)

A patient's experience of LBP is multifactorial, consisting of individual, occupational, and psychosocial factors. The relative contribution of each of these factors varies with each patient as they relate to the development and persistence of LBP. However, the goals related to obtaining a relevant history during the patient interview are consistent. During the interview, the clinician reflects on the patient responses and the context in which the patient presents as potential key factors to developing a preliminary PT diagnosis, prognosis, and plan for the physical examination. The information obtained through the interview guides decision making throughout the episode of care. Readers are encouraged to review basic questions and concepts related to the subjective examination. Patients vary in their ability to accurately recall events and understand and answer questions. Patience, care, and good listening technique in the patient-therapist relationship are important to obtain accurate information. The goals as discussed in Chapter 2 are listed as follows:

- Obtain a patient demographic profile.
- Make a preliminary decision regarding whether the patient is appropriate for PT.
- Obtain a detailed description of all of the patient's symptoms and determine if a link exists between the presenting symptoms.
- Determine the aggravating factors, easing factors, and 24-hour behavior of each symptom.
- Determine contraindications or precautions to examination and treatment.
- Obtain a sequential history (present and past episodes) of the patient's problem.
- Determine patient expectations.
- Develop a diagnostic hypothesis, classification, or pretest probability of the disorder.
- Evaluate the data from the patient history.
- Establish a baseline level of symptoms, activity limitations, and participation restrictions from which progress is measured.
- Establish a basis for planning the physical examination and selecting appropriate diagnostic tests—determine what should be examined and in what detail.

Demographic Profile Considerations for Patients With Low Back Pain

Age, Gender, Race, Ethnicity Considerations

Age, gender, race, and ethnicity considerations related to medical (red flag) and psychosocial (yellow flag) screening have been described in the previous sections. Most studies related to LBP focus on adults and working populations. However, LBP is a problem in all age groups. LBP begins early in life with a steady increase in lifetime prevalence of 1% at 7 years of age to 17% at 12 years of age and 17% at 12 years to 53% at 15 years.[205] The increase around 15 years is associated with the age of rapid growth spurt in adolescents, which for males is 10.3 to 14.3 years and for females is 13.5 to 17.5, and plateaus in later teens.[206] Despite inconsistent reports, factors such as increased height, scoliosis, genetic predisposition, socioeconomic status, and athletic activities may increase the risk for back pain in children.[207,208] LBP in adolescence is likely a risk factor for the development of LBP in adulthood.[209] For adults, 15% to 20% experience back pain during a single year and 50% to 80% experience at least one episode of back pain during an individual lifetime.[209,210] The highest rates of back pain are found in adults during the third to sixth decades, with the likelihood of new onset in the third decade.[211-213] Prevalence rates are lower in ages 20 to 35 with rates increasing with age until ages 60 to 65.[210-214]

Studies show that the prevalence rates of LBP for men and women are similar, although some differences may exist regarding outcomes. Though further studies are required, George et al,[215] in a cohort of patients with acute LBP receiving PT over 4 weeks, reported that men and women have similar reports of pain-related disability, and men and women have similar reports of reductions in pain intensity and pain-related disability in response to standardized treatments of manipulation, lumbar stabilization, and directional preference (DP). In contrast, several studies suggest that women with LBP are more likely to use health care, take more days off from work, have a poor outcome after a single episode, and develop persistent, chronic pain for longer than 3 months.[216-218]

LBP is a frequently reported musculoskeletal problem among older adults[219] and is potentially related to poor physical mobility and psychosocial outcomes.[220] LBP in older adults is likely intermittent or persistent in nature rather than new onset.[212] Back pain appears to be more frequent in older women than men, possibly due to a higher risk for osteoporosis.[213,221,222] Hicks et al[223] have reported that moderate to severe LBP is associated with functional decline in older adults.

The relationship between age and the development of LBP is not clear. The increased prevalence rates of LBP in young adults may be due to increased physical activity in this population or a more pronounced impact on their daily lives, resulting in a need for health care. With increasing age, anatomic changes may play a role in predisposing some individuals to persistent or CLBP.[224]

Occupational Considerations

A patient's occupation and leisure activities involve various risks for LBP. Static postures and various work-related activities produce biomechanical loads that may predispose to LBP. Some of these risks may be potential barriers to a successful outcome in terms of work demands or pain-related fear.

The relationship between LBP and the physical demands of work is both inconsistent and complex. Jobs with more physical demands commonly have higher reports of LBP, but most reports are related to normal everyday activities such as bending and lifting.[225] In a retrospective study, both heavy physical workload and sedentary work were predictors for LBP among both genders with a slightly stronger association for women.[226] A systematic review concluded that moderate evidence supports a relationship between heavy physical work and manual handling techniques and pain, but there was no evidence for an association with prolonged standing or sitting.[37] The amount and type of physical work performed regularly may affect the development of LBP, but studies reporting on the level of physical work as a predictor of LBP demonstrate conflicting results.[224]

Occupational and recreational activities that include material handling, heavy lifting, moving, carrying, bending, or twisting and static positions such as prolonged sitting and high exposure to low-frequency whole-body vibration such as driving are risk factors for LBP.[227,228] Sales, clerical work, repair, and transportation positions are more likely associated with LBP than other occupations.[229] Occupations classified as low risk for stress on the back include managers, professionals, and clerical or sales workers, whereas operators, service workers, and farmers are at higher risk.[230] The degree of acute physical load applied to the back and the cumulative or long-term load to the back may play a role in the development of pain.[227] Individuals with jobs requiring standing or walking for more than 2 hours per shift or women who lift > 25 pounds are more than twice as likely to seek care for back pain than individuals with a sedentary job without lifting requirements.[231]

Epidemiological evidence related to LBP is often linked to the physical demands of work, but the work is not necessarily the cause of the LBP. Heavy manual laborers report more LBP, but individuals not working or with lighter jobs have similar symptoms. People with more physically demanding jobs have a harder time returning to work if their back hurts, so they may take more time off work, a potential effect of LBP rather than the cause.[225] Physical stresses may overload certain anatomical structures in some individuals. However, in general, little evidence supports that the demands of physical work cause permanent damage.[225] A systematic review by Lis et al[232] concluded that sitting by itself does not increase the risk of LBP, but combinations of sitting greater than half a workday, whole-body vibrations, and/or awkward postures greatly increases the likelihood of LBP and/or sciatica. Certain individuals in certain jobs are at higher risk for LBP, but the physical demands of work account for only a small amount of the total impact of work-related LBP.[225] Chronic disability and care-seeking due to LBP depends more on complex individual and psychosocial factors than on clinical factors or demands of work.[233-234]

Over 100 risk factors have been identified in previous research related to spinal mechanical load and LBP.[235] In a review of prospective cohort studies, Bakker et al[235] evaluated exposures of spinal mechanical load as related to adults with LBP. Findings of this systematic review converge with previous studies and conclude as follows:

- Conflicting evidence exists for heavy physical work as a risk factor for LBP.
- Strong evidence exists that prolonged standing, walking, and sitting at work is not associated with LBP.
- Conflicting evidence exists for whole-body vibration as a risk factor for LBP.
- Conflicting evidence exists for the association between work in a bent or twisted position of the trunk and the development of LBP.
- Conflicting evidence exists for nursing tasks as a risk factor for LBP.
- No evidence exists related to sleeping as a risk factor for LBP.[235]

A cross-sectional study of school-age (11 to 14) children examined the role of both mechanical and psychological factors.[236] A summary of the findings is as follows:

- One-month prevalence was 23.9% (330/1446).
- An association between body mass index (BMI) and LBP was not observed.
- Carrying a rucksack or shoulder backpack (mean load 9.7% of body weight, BW) was not associated with LBP.
- LBP was strongly associated with emotional problems, behavioral conduct problems, headache, abdominal pain, and sore throats.[236]

The relationship between spinal loading and individuals with LBP is inconsistent and complex. Nonspecific LBP likely has multiple causative factors. Therefore, for most individuals, the impact of one independent risk factor is likely to be small. Clinicians should know and understand the individual's occupation and associated postural stresses and whether the patient is off work at present or remaining at work. Physical activities or postures that produce physical stresses associated with the occurrence of back pain across the various studies include heavy or frequent lifting, whole body vibration (driving), prolonged or frequent bending or twisting, and postural stresses (ie, high spinal loads or awkward postures). Although no studies suggest that particular occupations or positions cause LBP, a clinician needs to consider the individual risk factors of all work and recreational activities of a patient with LBP because returning to work and recreational activities is frequently a primary rehabilitation outcome.

Leisure and Sport Activity Considerations

In addition to work and daily activities, leisure and sports may contribute to a predisposition or persistence for LBP. In adolescents, computer use greater than 15 hours per week is a risk factor for LBP.[237] Children 9 years of age who played video games >2 hours per day had significantly more LBP.[238] In a national survey of 14- to 18-year-olds, Hakala and colleagues[239] asked the question, "Have you had LBP during the last 6 months?" The results demonstrated a higher prevalence of LBP among girls that increased with age. More time was spent by boys on computers, the Internet, and gaming; girls spent more time on mobile phones. Equal time viewing TV, videos, or DVDs was reported by both boys and girls. Greater than 42 hours per week and >5 hours per day of computer use, >42 hours per week of Internet use, and >5 hours per day of digital gaming significantly increased risk of LBP. Hakala et al[239] concluded that increased computer usage is an independent risk factor for LBP in adolescents.

The relationship between level of physical activity and LBP is thought to follow a U-shaped curve where too little or too much activity equally increases the risk of LBP.[240,241] Physical activity is not associated with CLBP examined by type (eg, daily, leisure, or sport activities), intensity, or duration. However, extremes of the total physical activity pattern are associated with CLBP. A moderate increased risk for CLBP was noted for persons with a sedentary lifestyle (OR 1.31: 95% CI: 1.08 to 1.58) and for persons involved in strenuous physical activities (OR 1.22: 95% CI: 1.00 to 1.49) especially for women, providing some evidence for a U-shaped relationship between physical activity and CLBP.[241] From a systematic review, Bakker et al[235] concluded that conflicting evidence exists for leisure time activities such as do-it-yourself home repair, gardening, or yardwork as risk factors for LBP.

No evidence exists for professional-level sports as a risk factor for LBP.[235] A cross-sectional survey of adults aged 22 to 70 within a defined community revealed high-demand occupational activities contributed to increased LBP prevalence, but high sporting activities contributed to a decline.[242] LBP prevalence or severity is not associated with certain types of sporting activities: low-level activity such as yoga and calisthenics, moderate-level activity such as walking and swimming, or high-level activities of cycling or jogging. Persons without LBP reported a higher perception of general health.[242] Engaging in sport activity is associated with less CLBP (OR 0.78; 95% CI: 0.66 to 0.93)[241] but does not contribute independently to a lower prevalence of LBP.[242] Encouraging persons with LBP to participate in appropriate levels of leisure and sport activities may promote a healthier lifestyle.[242]

Socioeconomic Considerations

A systematic review by Dionne et al[243] found that low educational status is consistently associated with increased prevalence of LBP with a strong effect on duration, persistence, and poorer outcomes rather than onset of LBP. According to Goubert et al,[244] a lower educational level is not a risk factor of LBP but is a risk factor of LBP disability. Patients with LBP and a low level of education have more misconceptions about LBP that result in poor adjustment to chronic pain.[244] Misconceptions such as the need for a medical diagnosis, treatment, and cure may play a role in delaying the recovery process. The study by Dionne et al[243] highlighted an important relationship between low educational level, socioeconomic status, and LBP that is not completely understood.

Chief Complaint

Eliciting the chief complaint usually begins with an open-ended question such as, "In your own words, please tell me about your problem," that gives the patient a chance to express immediate concerns and reasons for seeking treatment. The primary problem usually includes a report of pain, but some patients have no pain and instead report symptoms of weakness, stiffness, balance, dizziness, or numbness and tingling sensations. Documentation of the chief complaint using a body diagram includes recording the exact location and pattern of symptoms as well as the quality, depth (ie, superficial or deep), variability (ie, constant/varying, constant/nonvarying, or intermittent), worst area, intensity, and any relationship among or between symptoms. Chapter 2 discusses the process of obtaining a detailed description of patient symptoms.

Description and Assessment of Symptoms for Patients Presenting With Low Back Pain

The patient should be adequately undressed so that the clinician is able to precisely note the area and extent of symptoms—usually pain. When the patient points to the area of pain, the clinician confirms an understanding of the location by placing a hand on the patient and tracing the distribution. In persons presenting with a primary complaint of LBP, the clinician should question or screen areas that the patient has not reported as symptomatic such as the following:

- Lower thoracic spine and lumbosacral spine (unilaterally and centrally)
- Bilateral buttocks and both lower extremities (circumferentially)
- Abdomen and groin (anteriorly)

If not offered by the patient, specifically ask for numbness and tingling or other sensations or areas that do not feel normal.

Pain patterns may be classified as nonmusculoskeletal, musculoskeletal, or have components of both disorders. The patient's description and pattern of pain or other symptoms often form the initial impression or working diagnosis, which in turn focuses the rest of the history and identifies areas for further questioning and clarification.

Nonmusculoskeletal Pain or Visceral Referred Pain

Visceral referred LBP is most likely to be the result of gastrointestinal, pulmonary, urologic/kidney, or gynecological disease. In addition to LBP, pain from these visceral structures could be located in the abdomen or chest wall and tends to be diffuse and poorly localized. Visceral referred pain patterns that may mimic musculoskeletal patterns in persons with LBP are depicted in Chapter 2 (see Figure 2-3). If the pain pattern generates an initial hypothesis for a nonmusculoskeletal disorder, clinicians should question for clusters of symptoms and signs that may suggest which body system is involved.

Musculoskeletal Pain (Somatic Referred Pain)

Persons with LBP report a wide array of symptoms generally from the 12th rib to the inferior gluteal folds with or without referral to the abdomen and/or lower extremities. Pain from the somatic structures (eg, ligament, facet, muscle, intervertebral disc) of the lumbar spine or pelvic girdle can be local LBP or referred into the lower extremity.[245-259] Somatic referred pain is perceived in an area that shares the same segmental innervation as its source.

Many studies have demonstrated local pain and somatic referred pain patterns from the experimental stimulation of muscle,[249] interspinous ligaments,[250] facet joints,[252,255] dura,[258] and the intervertebral disc.[260-262] Patients describe somatic referred pain as deep,[245,249,250,252] dull,[245,253,257,263] aching,[247,250,252,253,255] gnawing, and expanding into wide areas that are difficult to localize,[250-253,255,264] usually focused in the gluteal region and proximal thigh,[252,254] but can extend as far as the foot. Somatic referred pain patterns are not dermatomal and are not consistently segmental among subjects or between studies.[265,266] Somatic referred pain does not involve spinal nerve or nerve roots, so neurological signs are absent.[266] A review of the current literature does not support the theory of sclerotomal patterns nor does it support consistently identifying segmental level of the spine based on the location of pain of somatic origin.[265]

Radicular Pain

Radicular pain is associated with damage or injury to or inflammation of the spinal nerve, nerve roots, or dorsal root ganglion and is clinically believed to be consistently located in the corresponding dermatome.[266-269] Radicular pain is consistently described as well localized,[270] intense,[271] severe,[272] sharp,[272] and lancinating.[272] In a study that directly stimulated the nerve roots on awake patients,[272] the resultant pain was a lancinating, 2- to 3-inch-wide band that traveled the length of the lower limb. However, pain may be distributed anywhere along the dermatome or in specific locations within the dermatome and not always a continuous line traveling the length of the lower limb. Waddell[273] reported that motor and sensory impairments are not always present. Tension signs such as SLR occur earlier and are more common than motor and sensory changes.[273]

Based on a current review of the literature,[265] the patterns of segmental radicular pain are not easily distinguished from one another. General agreement exists for a consistent dermatomal pattern for L5 and S1 radicular pain, specifically if the pain extends into the foot. L5 radicular pain most likely extends in the anterolateral aspect of the leg into the dorsum of the foot and big toe, while S1 reaches into the heel and lateral aspect of the foot.[265] L4, L5, and S1 radicular pain above the ankle is difficult to differentiate.[265,271] Limited evidence supports a consistent dermatomal pattern into the lower extremity for L1, L2, L3, L4, and S2 nerve roots. More research is needed.[265] Bogduk[266] concluded that a segmental origin of radicular pain can only be estimated when radiculopathy and radicular pain occur together with the dermatomal distribution of numbness, not pain, identifying the segmental origin.

Completion of the body diagram and patient's description of symptoms provide information to initiate and/or continue the process of diagnostic triage, hypothesis generation, and classification. The pain pattern may be either nonspecific LBP of somatic or somatic referred pain; LBP with radiculopathy or neurological involvement with somatic, somatic referred, and/or radicular pain; serious spinal pathology with nonmusculoskeletal pain; or a combination. The body chart may also demonstrate a pattern that suggests the patient has more than one problem (eg, a complaint of right-sided LBP and right anterior hip pain reported as 2 distinct areas of pain with each pain being present independent of the other). This presentation suggests that the patient may have 2 problems: LBP and hip pain rather than LBP with referred pain to the right hip. Further questions related to onset and behavior of symptoms will increase or decrease the likelihood of 2 separate musculoskeletal problems and identify where to place emphasis throughout the interview.

Accurate documentation of the patient's pain experience helps to establish a baseline of symptoms for use as an outcome measure, as a prognosis, or for classification. "No symptoms distal to the knee" has been identified as one factor in a 5-factor CPR for a manipulation classification used to identify patients with LBP who are likely to respond to manipulation as a treatment strategy.[140,141] In contrast, symptoms distal to the knee that tend to change location such as moving from distal to proximal or from proximal to distal may generate a hypothesis for a DSE classification.[274] Patients who present with a pattern of back and unilateral, dominant leg pain may generate a hypothesis of nerve root irritation.[275] A presentation of bilateral leg pain should raise suspicion for symptomatic spinal pathology such as central canal stenosis, a central disc herniation,

PAD, bilateral lateral canal stenosis, or metastatic disease. Widespread pain is associated with a worse prognosis compared to localized LBP.[276] Careful and unbiased attention to patient's descriptions of symptoms quickly reveals that spinal musculoskeletal pain presents in a highly variable form but provides valuable information to assist with diagnostic triage, classification, and intervention.

Paresthesia or Anesthesia

Complaints of numbness and tingling or other concerns of altered sensation are usually associated with neurological or vascular impairment and are possibly a result of compression, constriction, or frictional forces.

Pain Intensity Outcomes

Pain, a highly subjective and multidimensional experience, is one of the main reasons patients seek PT services. High pain intensity, a unidimensional measure, is perceived as a threatening experience and can substantially contribute to a patient's account of disability.[119] During the acute stage of LBP, pain intensity is strongly related to functional disability.[127,277,278] The best predictors of future chronicity are pain intensity and previous episodes of LBP.[278] Therefore, self-report questionnaires of pain are important outcomes when measuring meaningful change in clinical practice as well as for future studies related to intervention.

Numeric Pain Rating Scale

A numeric pain rating scale (NPRS; see Figure 2-6) usually has an 11-point scale from 0 (no pain) to 10 (the worst imaginable pain) and results in a self-report measure of pain intensity. Test-retest reliability of the NPRS varies from moderate (0.67) to high (0.96).[279,280] The instrument has predictive and concurrent validity.[281-283] Jensen et al[282] concluded that composite NPRS scores of the average current level, worst level, and best pain level may be more useful than individual ratings where maximal reliability is needed, such as in small samples or clinical settings, to monitor change in individuals. Childs et al,[170] in a cohort of patients with LBP and an ODI of at least 30% and receiving PT, concluded that a 2-point change at 1- and 4-week follow-up on the NPRS signifies a clinically meaningful change that exceeds the bounds of measurement error. Patients rated the level of their current, best, and worst pain during the past 24 hours. The 3 ratings were averaged to determine an overall pain intensity. An MCID of 2-points is consistent with findings of the Farrar et al[284] study that included patients with a variety of chronic pain conditions including LBP. Similar findings were reported by van der Roer and colleagues[285] where the MCIC on the NPRS ranged from 3.5 to 4.7 in subacute patients with LBP and 2.5 to 4.5 in chronic patients with LBP. Ostelo and de Vet[146] suggested that the MCIC for acute LBP and CLBP should be 3.5 and 2.5, respectively. Systematic review[154] concluded that empirical values for the minimally important change (MIC) on the NPRS are 1.0 to 4.5 points, representing a 30% improvement from baseline. An absolute cutoff of the MIC proposed by consensus is 2 on the NPRS.[154]

Visual Analog Scale

The VAS (see Figure 2-7), a self-reported measure of pain intensity, consists of a 10-cm horizontal or vertical line with extreme anchors of "no pain" to "worst imaginable pain."[286,287] A patient marks his or her perceived level of pain for a specific period of time. The examiner scores the VAS by measuring the distance in millimeters from the "no pain anchor" to the patient's mark. Higher scores represent more pain. A score of >30 mm suggests $\geq$ "moderate" pain; a score of >54 suggests $\geq$ "severe" pain.[288] Fifteen-minute test-retest reliability in postoperative pain patients on days 1 and 2 is acceptable (ICC = 0.73 to 0.882).[279] The VAS demonstrates high correlation with the NPRS.[279] The VAS exhibits moderate validity (0.71 to 0.78) when compared with the NPRS.[289]

A prospective descriptive study of adults presenting to the emergency department categorized VAS pain scores of 30 mm or less as mild pain, 31 to 69 mm as moderate pain, and 70 mm or more as severe pain.[290] The MCID for the overall group was 12 mm (95% CI: 9 to 15) with no statistical difference between groups. At 20-minute intervals, the MCID was defined as a patient report of "a little better" or "a little worse." In a cohort of 81 patients with nonspecific LBP for greater than or equal to 6 weeks who were assessed before and after 5 weeks of treatment, Beurskens et al[155] reported a clinically important change for the VAS as 10 to 18 mm on a 100-mm scale. A similar MCID of 18 to 19 mm for the VAS was reported in a cohort of patients with severe CLBP of at least 2 years' duration.[291] Ostelo and de Vet[146] suggested that the MCIC should not be a fixed value. For the VAS and patients with acute LBP, subacute LBP, and CLBP, the MCIC should be at least 35, 20, and 20 mm, respectively. The proposed consensus of empirical values for the MIC for the 0- to 100-mm VAS pain scores were reported as 2 to 29 points with an absolute cutoff of 15.[154]

Current research supports the use of the NPRS and VAS as reliable and valid clinical measures of pain intensity. Grotle et al[292] reported that both the NPRS and VAS are comparable in a sample of patients with acute LBP. However, the NPRS is more responsive than the VAS in a sample of patients with CLBP.[292-294] When considering ease of use, format, and administrative properties, the RMDQ, ODI, and NPRS can be recommended as appropriate functional and pain assessment measures for patients with acute and CLBP.[292]

History of the Current Episode

Details of the current episode should establish the manner in which the present symptoms started, the progression of those symptoms, and the stage and stability of the problem.[295] The clinician should elicit chronological details about the mode of onset (eg, macro- or microtraumatic versus nontraumatic), date of onset, progression of each symptom, all treatments to date and their effects, and the overall progression of the problem. Details of the current episode help to determine the nature (ie, musculoskeletal or nonmusculoskeletal), stage (ie, acute, subacute, chronic), and stability (ie, getting better, worse, or staying the same) of the problem. When the most recent episode of symptoms is not the patient's first episode, the quickest way to obtain relevant data is to start with the present episode.

Mode and Date of Onset

Careful inquiry by the clinician often reveals the cause of the patient's problem. Asking the question, "How or when did the problem begin?" allows the clinician to explore the exact mechanism of injury or nature of the onset. If the onset is sudden or related to a specific event such as a fall, the clinician should determine the activity, position, and direction and magnitude of forces related to the injury. Injury related to lifting or a motor vehicle accident (MVA) may provide information related to potential or extent of injured structures, severity of onset, and intervention. With an acute condition or recent onset, a full examination may not be possible due to severity or irritability. The clinician performs a limited examination with test procedures that provide the most information and minimize stress to the patient.

If the onset is gradual or insidious (ie, occurred for no apparent reason), the clinician must ask about predisposing factors such as unusual activity, repetitive activities, changes in work, training, recent illness, or stress. "Gradual" may mean over one day or over weeks to months. Spinal loads with cumulative or repetitive stress and biomechanical creep loading may subject some tissues to fatigue damage. A truly insidious onset merits concern about the underlying cause of the condition and raises the suspicion of a nonmusculoskeletal problem.

Progression of Symptoms

Using the completed body diagram, the clinician asks for the progression of each symptom since onset. Changes in area and severity of symptoms provide clues to the relationship and stability of the problem. For example, if a patient reports the onset of right-sided LBP 3 days ago and now has lateral calf pain radiating to the right foot and numbness and tingling, the clinician may infer the condition is worsening. A condition may worsen if the pain or symptom distribution becomes more widespread and distal (ie, peripheralization). Likewise, the patient whose lower extremity symptoms have resolved over the past week and now reports only right-sided LBP describes a condition that is likely improving with time. A condition in which the symptom distribution moves proximally toward the midline of the low back and becomes more localized normally indicates improvement (ie, centralization).

Treatments and Effects

To determine the effects of current or previous treatment, the clinician asks, "Have you had any treatment? Did it help?" If yes, "In what way?" Specific details of the previous exact treatment and patient response help with treatment planning. Treatment that has worked in the past may again be appropriate; however, treatment that was unsuccessful is unlikely to be recommended. Symptoms unchanged, worsened, or improved and then get worse again despite appropriate PT intervention are considered a red flag.

Stability (Getting Better, Worse, Staying the Same?)

Determining the stability of the problem is established by asking, "Compared to when this first started, is the pain or other symptoms getting better, worse, or staying the same?" If better or worse, the clinician should then ask, "In what way?" Changes in the intensity, severity, duration, and location of symptoms reveal the stability of the problem and assist with prognosis and the rate and level of recovery. When a patient reports worsening symptoms, clinicians should look for red flags or lifestyle risk factors such as mechanical factors or yellow flags, which may be delaying recovery. When symptoms are improving, contributing risk factors are addressed to prevent recurrence.

History of Previous Episode(s) of a Similar Problem

Risk of LBP is about twice as high for persons with a history of LBP.[28] Due to the recurrent nature of LBP, a previous history is the best predictor of future LBP.[225] The history of previous episodes begins with the question, "Have you had this problem before?" If the patient is not sure, the clinician may clarify, "Is it similar to what you are feeling now?" With a long history of recurrence, chronologically determine the initial manner of onset, severity, previous treatment and effects, frequency of recurrences, time to recover, level of recovery, and status between episodes.

The initial onset and mechanism of injury should be described in detail. Frequency and duration of episodes and level of recovery from the last episode or between episodes may affect the potential for recovery. Is there a pattern to the manner of onset? For example, if each episode of LBP is associated with prolonged sitting during business travel, an important aspect of intervention and recurrence involves addressing the activity of sitting in this environment. Previous treatment and effects and level of recovery put the present injury in perspective, help to establish reasonable goals for treatment and likelihood of recurrence, and provide data on the stability of the problem over time.[265] If the symptoms are easier to provoke and last longer with each episode, and full recovery does not occur between episodes, then the clinician infers that over time the problem is getting worse.

Symptom Behavior (Aggravating Factors, Easing Factors, and 24-Hour Behavior)

The purpose of determining the symptom behavior is to understand how the symptoms respond to activity, postures, movement, and the time of day. Some musculoskeletal problems get better with certain positions or movements while others get worse. In-depth questioning regarding which postures or movements result in a change in the location, intensity, or quality of a patient's symptoms helps to determine the mechanical nature of the problem, activity limitations, the severity or impact on function, irritability or ease of symptom provocation, and alleviation of the problem. A consistent pattern of aggravating and easing factors guides the classification, prognosis, and intervention. For example, a patient whose symptoms get worse with walking and completely relieved by sitting has an increased likelihood of responding to specific flexion exercises. Details related to obtaining specific symptom behavior are discussed in Chapter 2.

Aggravating Factors

Everyday activities, postures, and movements require use of the low back with mechanical LBP often varying according to the patient's daily activity. The patient identifies the exact movement or posture and amount of time, distance, or repetitions it takes to produce or increase each symptom and how long it takes for the provoked symptom or symptoms to ease. Common aggravating factors for LBP include the following:

- Static postures of sitting, standing, or bending, and travel (eg, vibration)
- Movements or activities such as walking, transfers of sit to stand and stand to sit, bending, repeated bending, running, or climbing stairs
- Specific work such as repetitive lifting, bending, twisting, or reaching, and recreational activities
- Daily care activities such as dressing, bathing, sleeping, or doing laundry

Aggravating factors may also be obtained from self-report measures such as the RMDQ or ODQ.

Activities should be analyzed to determine the general requirements for motion and stability of the lumbar spine and associated regions such as the cervical spine, thoracic spine, hip, knee, or ankle. For example, standing and walking are activities requiring mostly lumbar extension, lower extremity loading and balance, hip stability and mobility; relaxed sitting involves mostly lumbar flexion and adequate hip mobility. Bending produces more flexion of the lumbar spine than squatting. Lying in bed depends on many factors, but also upon position—supine, prone, or side-lying. Daily activity limitations and participation restrictions associated with a person's LBP should be documented at baseline. The baseline aggravating factors are then used to set functional goals and reassessed to evaluate intervention effectiveness over the episode of care. Analysis of the aggravating movements or posture also provides guidance for the selection of specific tests and measures or interventions.

Easing Factors

Easing factors such as movement, positions, medication, or other treatments should be sought for all symptoms and may serve as a factor in the initial intervention or the overall management of a patient's problem. Similar to the analysis of aggravating factors, lumbar spine and associated regions should be considered for requirements of movement or postural control that result in a decrease or elimination of the patient's symptoms. For example, a patient who reports walking as an easing factor for LBP may require a specific dosage of walking as a therapeutic exercise intervention. A clinician should ask patients if they have good and bad days. Finding out what movements or positions create good days is equally as important as determining the aggravators on bad days. The patient with a chronic problem and a central sensitization component may require a multidisciplinary approach with a focus on resolving activity limitations rather than resolution of pain.

24-Hour Behavior

Clinicians must inquire about the behavior of symptoms over a 24-hour period with specific emphasis on a patient's ability to sleep through the night. The quality of sleep is important for restoration of body function. With a disruptive sleep pattern, the body and mind are not capable of optimal function. In addition to pain, medication side effects, increased urination, and night sweats are a few factors related to sleep deprivation that can interfere with the rehabilitation process.[296]

Night

Pain at night is often deemed a red flag suggestive of cancer, but further clarification is needed when a patient answers "yes" to the question, "Does it wake you at night?" The clinician should follow-up by asking, "What is it that wakes you?" Pain at night is typical of mechanical problems when the patient reports an inability to lie on the involved side or reports waking with symptoms that are simply relieved by a change of position and return to sleep. If the pain is the most intense at night and the patient is unsure of what wakes him or her, reports that he or she must get up and walk around, and has difficulty returning to sleep, the clinician should consider the possibility of an active inflammatory component or more serious pathology such as neoplasm.[297] If night pain is a primary mechanical complaint, the clinician should determine the frequency, provocative position, and symptoms produced. This information is helpful to reassess at subsequent visits as one way to determine treatment effectiveness.

Morning

Most musculoskeletal problems are better in the morning eased by rest. Some degenerative joint disorders are better or less painful in the morning, but patients often report stiffness that is eased with movement within 30 to 60 minutes. Systemic inflammatory disorders such as AS are usually better with rest but present with the greatest stiffness first thing in the morning, usually lasting longer than 60 minutes.[298] Symptoms that are worse in the morning may be due to poor sleeping posture. Symptoms that are unchanged in the morning may be nonmechanical or minor mechanical problems.

Evening

Clinicians should ask patients how symptoms change throughout the day or vary with work days versus nonwork days. Symptoms that are improved in the morning and remain better with movement throughout the day are likely mechanical in nature and a good prognostic indicator. Symptoms that are improved in the morning but worsen with activities of the day are mechanical and may have a limited prognosis. Follow-up questions should identify those activities for intervention and as potential barriers to recovery. Symptoms that do not vary with daily activities are minor mechanical problems or suggestive of a more serious pathology.

Review of Medical Screening Questionnaire/General Medical History

Review of the medical screening questionnaire is a limited discussion of general health; a systems review; and an evaluation of past medical, surgical, medication, and diagnostic test histories. This review screens for systemic disease that may mimic musculoskeletal conditions and requires referral to another medical provider or may identify precautions or contraindications related to PT intervention. Synthesis of this information helps the clinician formulate a diagnosis, prognosis, plan of care, and select direct interventions.

The clinician must be alert for the presence of red or yellow flags during the history and physical examination. Screening for red flags such as cancer, infection, AAA, fracture, kidney disorder, CES, or neurological involvement was discussed earlier. Please see Chapter 2 (see Tables 2-7 and 2-8) to review fear-avoidance beliefs/behaviors and the characteristics of systemic disease. The following discussion is a brief review of general health factors that may influence the examination or management of patients with LBP.

General Health Status Considerations Related to Low Back Pain

Clinicians frequently ask, "In general, how would you rate your health?" Most patients respond with excellent, very good, good, fair, or poor. Self-assessment of general health is a complex process related to patient experience with and knowledge of diseases. Health status rated as poor is predictive of future mortality,[299] functional limitations,[300] and the development of chronic conditions.[213] The patient's response to the general health question is a potential warning signal, but—as with all risk factors or red flags—should be considered in the context of the whole person and the clinical presentation. Exploring general health status gives insight into the patient's clinical presentation and the prognosis for rehabilitation.

Persons with a perception of poor health status are more likely to have back pain.[213,301] These same individuals have a variety of health problems including headaches; respiratory, cardiac, or gastrointestinal diseases; and other joint diseases such that the presence of back pain is only one factor related to a perception of poor health rather than the cause of perceived poor health.[224] Persons with poor general health due to comorbidities are likely to progress slowly with rehab and are at risk for delay in the normal healing process.

Smoking

Smoking is related to increased degenerative spinal changes, increased risk for osteoporosis, and decreasing bone density, but a direct link for smoking as a cause of LBP is not strong.[224] A modest association between LBP and smoking was recently described through meta-analysis,[302] where the authors found that both current and former smokers have a higher prevalence and incidence of LBP than persons who never smoked. In current smokers, the association and incidence of LBP is stronger in adolescents than adults.[302] Regular smoking of 9 or more cigarettes daily in adolescents between ages 16 and 18 is associated with LBP in young adults.[303] Smoking may also be an indicator of other health risk factors such as cardiovascular disease (CVD).

Obesity

The obesity factor, when patients have a BMI greater than 30, is believed to be an independent predictor for the development of LBP and chronic disability with a stronger association in women.[304,305] Compared to non-overweight people, obese and overweight people have a higher prevalence of LBP and the strongest association with seeking care for LBP and CLBP.[306]

Obesity is recognized as a major public health problem associated with musculoskeletal problems and is only a weak risk factor for back pain. In a study of 23 healthy, obese individuals with and without CLBP, obesity in CLBP was characterized by a generally reduced ROM of the spine, specifically reduced pelvic and thoracic levels with a static postural adaptation of an increased anterior pelvic tilt or lumbar lordosis, and reduced lateral bending when compared to obese patients without LBP and healthy, nonobese women.[307] Subjects with CLBP showed a significant reduction in thoracic and shoulder movements as compared to the obese and control groups. Specifically, thoracic ROM was significantly lower in obese women without LBP. In this group, forward flexion was performed mainly by the lumbar spine. The authors concluded that thoracic stiffness with normal lumbar ROM appears to be a feature of obesity and may predispose to the development of LBP. Hypothetically, reduced thoracic ROM may pose additional demands for mobility on both the cervical and lumbar spine, suggesting the need for assessment of these regions in subjects presenting with LBP. However, additional studies are needed to determine a cause and effect relationship.

Cardiovascular Considerations

Billek-Sawhney and Sawhney[308] reported that 62% of patients examined in an orthopedic PT have CVD. To minimize the risk of an adverse cardiac event related to physical activity or exercise, baseline screening should determine whether CVD exists or whether CVD risk factors are present.[309] Screening is generally accomplished during the interview process. The American College of Sports Medicine[310] (ACSM) presents guidelines for screening for risk of CVD. These risk factors include age, family history, cigarette smoking, sedentary lifestyle, obesity, hypertension, dyslipidemia, and prediabetes.[310] Individuals are stratified according to risk based on the presence or absence of CVD factors.

The ACSM[310] risk stratification is described as low, moderate, or high. Low-risk persons have no signs, symptoms, or diagnosis of CVD, pulmonary, and/or metabolic disease and have less than or equal to one CVD risk factor. Moderate-risk persons have no signs or symptoms of or no diagnosis of CVD, pulmonary, and/or metabolic disease, but have at least 2 CVD risk factors. Persons at high risk have one or more signs or symptoms of or have a diagnosis of CVD, pulmonary, and/or metabolic disease.[310] Recommendations for both low- and moderate-risk individuals allow engagement in low (<3 muscle energy techniques [MET]) to moderate (3 to 6 MET) intensity physical activities without a clearance medical examination. Medical clearance for vigorous intensity exercise (>6 MET) is recommended for moderate risk and for any intensity activity or exercise in high-risk individuals. No standard of CVD screening exists in the PT literature. Cardiovascular screening is recommended to identify individuals with medical precautions or contraindications to physical activity and exercise.

Medication Usage

Chou and Huffman[311] summarized the benefits and risks of the most common medications used to treat acute and CLBP. These medications include acetaminophen, nonsteroidal anti-inflammatory drugs (NSAIDs), antidepressants, benzodiazepines, antiepileptic drugs, skeletal muscle relaxants, opioid analgesics, tramadol, and systemic corticosteroids for acute or CLBP with or without leg pain. Of these medications, the most commonly prescribed are NSAIDs, skeletal muscle relaxants, and opioid analgesics.[312-314]

Any person who seeks medical care for LBP is likely to receive pharmacological therapy. Clinicians should inquire about all types of medication and the purpose, duration of use, dosage, tolerance, adherence, and effectiveness. Since these medications may hide symptoms, documentation of any medication and its effectiveness prior to the visit is important.

Recommendations for first-line medications for LBP are acetaminophen or NSAIDs.[11] Side effects of common medications include the following:

- *NSAIDs*: Back and/or shoulder pain due to retroperitoneal bleeding, gastrointestinal symptoms, kidney, liver problems, or myocardial infarction
- *Corticosteroids*: Avascular necrosis femoral head, osteoporosis, immunosuppression, or steroid-induced myopathy
- *Antidepressants*: Movement disorders
- *Skeletal muscle relaxants*: Sedation
- *Statin-related drugs*: Musculoskeletal pain
- *Opioids*: Nausea, constipation, dry mouth, dizziness, or addiction[11,33]

Imaging or Other Diagnostic Test Results

The traditional role of imaging has been to provide accurate diagnostic anatomic information that guides the treatment decision-making process. However, even with extensive testing, a pathological cause for LBP cannot be reliably identified in at least 85% of cases because many structural abnormalities are common in persons with and without LBP.[315] The inability to identify a specific cause of LBP has lead to the recommendation that expensive investigations such as radiography, MRI, computed tomography (CT), nerve conduction tests, and myelography are only indicated when the clinical examination suggests an increased likelihood of serious pathology or progressive neurological deficit.[11] In these cases, a delay of diagnosis and treatment may result in poorer outcomes.

Diagnostic imaging is often a common procedure for most patients with LBP presenting in a primary care setting. In the absence of a clear indication, radiography is done to reassure patients, to meet patient expectations, or for financial reimbursement purposes.[316,317] However, imaging is associated with a potential negative effect of labeling a patient with a diagnosis based on irrelevant imaging findings[318] and risks of gonadal radiation in women from radiography and CT[12] with doses equivalent to a daily chest radiograph over 6 years.[319,320] Imaging may not affect treatment, may increase direct costs,[321-323] and may lead to increased use of expensive unnecessary invasive procedures.[324] Patients who receive early MRI compared to early plain radiography and receive similar treatment report similar reductions in symptoms. A higher frequency of lumbar MRI is associated with increased rates of spine surgery without the clear benefit of improved outcomes.[321-325]

Radiographic imaging may not be helpful because imaging findings are poorly associated with symptoms and important causes of LBP cannot be identified with plain radiographs.[37] The prevalence of disk degeneration, vertebral osteophytes, and facet arthritis increase with age and are common in patients without LBP.[326] Spondylolysis occurs equally in symptomatic and asymptomatic subjects.[326] Spondylolisthesis occurs in 1% to 5% of asymptomatic subjects. Higher grades of spondylolisthesis (ie, greater than 25% slippage of vertebral width) are more likely associated with symptoms but rare, and less than 25% slippage is common in individuals with and without LBP. Spina bifida, transitional vertebra, and Scheuermann's disease do not appear to be associated with LBP and are found in both symptomatic and asymptomatic individuals.[326] However, more recent studies report that transitional vertebrae may account for some LBP.[327,328] A herniated intervertebral disk and spinal stenosis, common causes of nerve root compression, cannot be diagnosed from plain lumbosacral radiographs[329]; advanced imaging, CT, or MRI is required to make those diagnoses.[37]

The association between disk abnormalities and spinal stenosis and LBP is controversial. Several studies report that lumbar disk abnormalities are seen in asymptomatic persons and are not predictive of LBP.[326,330,331] Jensen et al[330] observed in subjects without a history of LBP that 40% to 50% had a bulging disk and 20% to 30% had a herniated disc with both findings common in older adults. In subjects over 60 years of age, spinal stenosis is noted in more than 20% of subjects without LBP or leg pain.[330-332] Beattie et al[332] concluded that the presence on MRI of disc extrusion or severe nerve root compression is strongly associated with distal leg pain. Videman et al[333] concluded that, in clinical practice, MRI findings of annular tears and disc height alone have limited value.

Routine laboratory tests such as ESR, urinalysis, or complete blood count are not needed for a person with LBP unless the history or examination suggests serious pathology as a cause. ESR may be helpful to screen for cancer or infection because this test, although nonspecific, is more sensitive than plain radiographs.[334] In suspected cases of bladder or kidney infection, a urinalysis is a useful test.[37]

Routine imaging or other diagnostic tests in patients with acute, nonspecific LBP of less than 6 weeks' duration is not recommended because it does not improve clinical outcomes when compared with usual clinical care without immediate imaging.[11,37,335] Anatomic abnormalities are easily identified by imaging, but most of these abnormalities are found even in asymptomatic subjects. Therefore, imaging may result in irrelevant findings and is unlikely to result in finding a specific cause for a patient's LBP.

The recommendations for CLBP are not as clear due to insufficient research. Routine CT or MRI for CLBP might not be indicated because of small or uncertain benefits.[321] For persistent LBP lasting longer than 6 weeks, MRI and CT offer comparable results, but the frequency of abnormalities in normal adults limits the specificity of these tests.[336] For radicular pain possibly caused by herniated disk or spinal stenosis, early imaging is unnecessary unless major neurological impairments are noted because most patients improve with conservative care. However, careful observation of neurological status is warranted.[337,338] According to Kleinstück et al,[336] an MRI has the greatest sensitivity and specificity for suspicion of systemic disease.

Clinicians should carefully consider the role and relative impact of imaging on the overall management of individual patients with LBP. Serious pathology can present as LBP, and clinicians should perform adequate screening to recognize these presentations with re-evaluation on a frequent basis. For individuals who do not respond quickly within 4 to 6 weeks of onset, selective investigations may be warranted.[339]

Patient Expectations or Goals

Clinicians generally ask patients to describe their functional goals or expectations from PT treatment. Previous research has documented an association between positive patient expectations and improved health outcomes.[340] In a secondary analysis, Myers et al[341] investigated the association between patients' general expectations for recovery from acute LBP and their functional outcomes. Patients were asked to rate on a 0 to 10 scale (where 0 = no improvement and 10 = complete recovery) the amount of improvement they expected in 6 weeks. The mean expectation for recovery was 8.8 (SD 1.7). The patient's response appears to have some predictive value. Based on their findings, patients with higher expectations for a speedy recovery are likely to show more improvement. Establishing patient goals provides an opportunity to listen to patient concerns and assists with tailoring interventions to recovery of specific functional needs.[342]

Interview Summary

At the end of the formal interview, the clinician should ask, "Are there any other problems or concerns that you would like to tell me about or that we have not discussed?" The clinician should then present a brief summary of the key findings from the interview and discuss the plan for the physical examination.

Clinical Reasoning Guide to Plan the Tests and Measures

At the end of the formal interview, clinicians should briefly review the subjective data and begin planning the physical examination. This reflection challenges both the novice and experienced clinician to identify anatomical and biomechanical relationships, MIs, pain patterns, activity limitations, risks, and prognostic factors that direct the search for further information and might influence the rehabilitation process. This deliberate approach allows for a systematic review of the important points of the history and provides a database that initially dictates the focus and depth of the physical examination and provides a baseline that can be used in the reassessment of the patient's progress. As a clinician gains experience and more easily recognizes patterns emerging from the history, this process occurs with less deliberation; however, a reflective process is always useful with any patient especially the complex patient or a patient that is not responding as expected.

The process of planning the examination was discussed in Chapter 2 using a planning the examination form (see Table 2-9) to assist the clinician with analyzing the information gained from the history, plan the appropriate tests and measures, and increase the probability of performing an efficient and appropriate examination. To plan the extent and vigor of the physical examination, the clinician considers the severity, irritability, nature, stage, and stability of the patient's symptoms or complaints.[343] The clinician also considers risk factors associated with the development of persistent LBP or other factors contributing to the condition such as ergonomics, conditioning, depression, job requirements, body awareness and sensorimotor integrity, trauma, previous episodes, and other medical problems. The end result of this process is to generate a working diagnostic classification or working hypothesis(es) of the patient's LBP and a plan to test the working hypothesis(es) through the physical examination and continued reassessment. The clinician should establish a clear plan of what needs to be examined on the first day and over the next 1 to 2 visits. Two sample case studies (Appendices A and B) using the clinical reasoning guide to plan the examination form are provided in Appendix section. Another case study (Appendix C) provides an example of using the clinical reasoning guide to plan the tests and measure portion of the examination.

Summary of Diagnostic Triage and Subjective Examination

Considering the emerging evidence that acute LBP is not a benign and self-limiting problem, the importance of the data gained from the subjective examination cannot be underestimated. An accurate report from the patient may assist in identifying individuals more likely to develop chronic and disabling LBP. Recurrence is common. A large percentage of persons with LBP experience low intensity pain and disability but continue to work. A pooled cumulative risk of at least 1 recurrence within 12 months varies from 66% to 84% and is 84% at 3 years.[339] A variety of factors (ie, psychological, work-related, and a previous history of LBP) easily identified in the interview are thought to contribute to a poor outcome after an episode of LBP or to prolong recovery. The chronicity of a problem has implications related to mechanism of pain, management, and prognosis.

The subjective examination reveals both risk and prognostic factors related to the onset or persistence of LBP. Review of studies of risk factors is important because of the potential link to etiology of LBP, but no single factor seems to have a strong effect. Risk factors associated with the development and persistence of LBP are multidimensional, poorly understood, and not necessarily the cause of a person's LBP. Several systematic reviews have reported conflicting results regarding the impact of individual risk factors. Physical attributes, socioeconomic status, general medical and psychological health, and occupational factors all interact and contribute in varying amounts to an individual's risk or predisposition for experiencing LBP.[227] Therefore, individual risk factors such as health status, occupation, lifestyle, and leisure or sport should be investigated to determine current functional limitations and to determine which factors may interfere with recovery or contribute to recurrence. Any predisposing risk can be a contributing factor to the development or maintenance of a person's problem. Clinicians should recognize the potential impact of risk factors and address as needed through ongoing management.

A history of LBP is the strongest predictor of future LBP. Leg pain is associated with poorer outcomes and an increased chance of developing chronic symptoms. Centralization of leg symptoms is linked to good outcomes, while failure to centralize symptoms is considered a strong predictor of chronicity. Psychosocial risk factors known as yellow flags also play a role in the transition to chronic persistent LBP and failure to return to work. The transition from acute to CLBP may be predicted more by psychosocial factors than clinical factors in some individuals. Similar to risk factors, prognostic factors are complex and contribute in varying amounts among individuals. Early identification may prevent the transition to the chronic stage.

Table 4-17. Components of the Physical Examination

- Observation (anthropometric: height, weight, body fat composition, girth)
- Gait
- Posture
- Functional tests
- Active ROM
- Passive ROM (physiological, accessory, segmental motion testing)
- Resisted tests
- Neurological screening examination
- Muscle length/flexibility tests
- Muscle performance (strength/power/endurance)
- Screen region/joints above and below
- Special tests
- Palpation

The subjective examination seeks to identify key information from all patients with the context and details specific to the patient's presenting problems. This early information provides the basis to form initial diagnostic hypotheses or classifications, which then guide the focus and comprehensiveness of the physical examination. Obtaining accurate, relevant data from the patient aids in diagnostic triage, planning the physical examination, and implementing an effective management strategy.

Components of the Physical Examination

The physical examination continues the process of diagnostic triage and diagnostic classification of nonspecific LBP, which seeks to rule in or rule out an underlying seriously pathological condition, any condition resulting in neurological compromise or other competing medical disease.[344] Basic components and general procedures of the physical examination are discussed in Chapter 3. Initially, the history assists with prioritizing the tests and measures that are conducted at the first session.

In addition to pain and disability in patients with LBP, physical impairments of body structure and function are routinely used by physical therapists to assess progress and treatment effectiveness. Common impairment measurements include lumbar spine ROM, SLR ROM, and muscle strength and endurance. However, not all measurements used in the clinic are equally useful in the diagnosis and management of nonspecific LBP. In general, impairment measurements have uncertain convergent validity with patient satisfaction, pain, or disability measures and have poor ability to distinguish between symptomatic and asymptomatic individuals.[345,346]

In patients with LBP physical impairments, loss or abnormality of physiologic or anatomic structure or function generally do not correlate well with pain, disability, and work status.[168,347,348] Furthermore, the responsiveness of physical impairments for patients with LBP has not been sufficiently investigated.[163] After 6 weeks of treatment, Pengel et al[163] compared self-report pain and disability measures and physical impairment measures (ie, ROM and SLR) in a cohort of subjects with LBP of 6 weeks' to 3 months' duration. The PSFS was the most responsive outcome followed by the NPRS and RMDQ, both the 18- and 24-item versions. Physical impairment measures were less responsive than self-report pain and disability measures. Due to the lower responsiveness of physical impairments, their routine use to monitor recovery in individual patients may not be the best way to determine if meaningful change has occurred. Pengel et al[163] proposed that clinicians place more emphasis on meaningful change in pain and disability scores rather than on physical impairment. Using a less responsive outcome measure increases the risk of falsely concluding a change has occurred.[163] Further study is recommended to determine whether painful and restricted movements are more responsive outcome measures than a standardized set of self-report disability measures.

Fritz and Piva,[349] in a cohort of 68 patients with acute LBP of less than 3 weeks, reported that a group of physical impairment measures was more responsive than the individual impairment measures but less responsive than the ODI. The authors theorize that measures of strength and motion, though important to the patient, are not necessarily linked to the patient's concerns about functional activities such as walking or lifting.[349]

A basic premise of diagnostic triage and classification of individuals with LBP is that subgroups can be identified from key history and clinical examination findings. Not all of the tests and measures discussed in this section should be performed on every patient. The physical examination is a continuation of the history designed to test hypotheses generated by the subjective examination. As the clinician proceeds through the physical examination toward establishing a diagnostic classification, multiple measures from the history and physical examination are identified to place a patient with LBP into a specific subgroup or subgroups designed to guide and initiate intervention. Table 4-17 lists the basic components for the physical examination. Table 4-18 outlines commonly used tests and measures

TABLE 4-18. EXAMINATION OUTLINE LUMBOPELVIC REGION (INCLUDES LOWER THORACIC) T10-T12 SPINE

STANDING	• General observation and baseline vital signs • Functional activity such as squatting, putting on shoes and socks • Gait • Balance • Neurological exam: manual muscle test (MMT) toe/heel walk L4-5; L1-S2	• Posture (iliac crest, posterior-superior iliac spine, anterior-superior iliac spine, etc; leg length; lordosis, kyphosis, lateral shift, scoliosis, atrophy, skin inspection) • Lateral shift correction • Active ROM (flexion/extension, side-bend) overpressure as needed • Repeated movements as needed: repeated extension in standing/repeated flexion in standing, side glide in standing as needed • Combined movement testing, lumbar quadrant as needed
SITTING	• Sitting posture • Active ROM: rotation as indicated with overpressure • Neurological screening (L2-S2)	• MMT, deep tendon reflexes (DTRs): knee jerk, ankle jerk, hamstrings (prone); sensation as needed • Slump test
SUPINE	• Observe ability to transition to supine • Repeated movements—repeated flexion in lying • SLR: plus sensitizing maneuvers dorsiflexion, adduction, internal rotation • Palpation: iliac crest, anterior-superior iliac spine, pubic tubercle symmetry; hip, abdomen as needed • Screen hip: flexion/internal rotation (also prone)/external rotation, overpressure; abduction/adduction, overpressure, flexion, abduction, external rotation	• Screen knee: flexion/extension, overpressure • Muscle length: piriformis, hamstring, (SLR or 90/90), latissimus; Thomas test (iliopsoas, rectus femoris, iliotibial band) • Transverse abdominis/multifidus: palpation/ biofeedback cuff/rehabilitative ultrasound imaging • SIJ distraction/compression, thigh thrust, Gaenslen's test, sacral thrust
PRONE	• Repeated movements: (sustain or repeated 10x, assess response) • Prone on pillow, prone, prone on elbows • Repeated extension in lying (REIL) • REIL with sag • REIL with mobilization belt • REIL with hips offset	• Prone knee bend/femoral nerve stretch test • Hip extension: MMT (gluteus maximus, hamstrings), hamstrings (DTR) • Hip internal rotation ROM: bilaterally • Palpation/passive accessory intervertebral movement: central and unilateral (sacrum to T10) • Prone instability test • Passive lumbar extension test
SIDE-LYING	• Passive physiological intervertebral movements—flexion/extension/ side-bend/rotation • Ober's test	• Hip abduction/adduction: strength

sequenced by patient position such as standing, sitting, supine, prone, and side-lying to assist with organization of the physical examination. The sequence is varied according to patient and condition, and not all tests and measures are performed on every patient. Key findings for diagnostic classification are highlighted under the appropriate test or

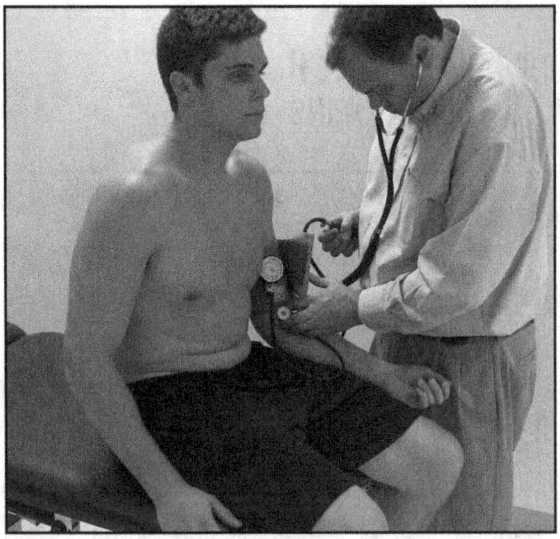

Figure 4-19. Vital signs—blood pressure.

measure. For purposes of discussion, the tests and measures are presented by patient position (ie, standing, sitting, supine, prone, and side-lying).

Goals of the Physical Examination

Appropriate selection of examination procedures should result in the data to support or negate working hypotheses by altering the pretest probability beyond the treatment threshold or the point where the examination ends and treatment begins. The goals of the physical examination are to do the following:

- Reproduce the patient's symptoms in patterns consistent with the information obtained in the patient interview.
- Determine the impact of posture, movement, work, recreational psychosocial factors as causes of, contributors to, or perpetuator's of the patient's problem.
- Establish the treatment threshold for a diagnostic classification.
- Establish an accurate data baseline or outcome measures from which to evaluate and progress treatment.

Physical Examination of the Lumbopelvic Region (Includes Lower Thoracic Spine)

Examination Procedures in Standing

- General observation and vital signs
- Functional activity such as hopping, squatting, putting on shoes and socks
- Gait and balance
- Neurological exam
- Posture
- Lateral shift correction
- Active ROM (AROM), with overpressure (OP) as needed
- Repeated movements
- Combined movement testing

General Observation and Vital Signs

Observation begins when first meeting the patient and continues throughout the examination. Initial observations include facial expression, postural characteristics, general fitness and well-being, quality of movement, rising from the waiting room chair, transitions of supine to sitting, sitting, walking, and willingness to move. A patient's unwillingness to move is related to poor outcomes[349,350] and may be a behavior related to fear of pain or reinjury that should be addressed. Prior to the interview or formal observation, baseline data such as height, weight, pulse, respiration, or blood pressure (Figure 4-19) are collected. Detailed assessment of respiratory patterns is discussed in Chapter 5. At the start of the physical examination, baseline symptoms should be documented and monitored as the examination continues. Establishing resting symptoms prior to each test and during each test or measure enables the clinician to ensure the symptoms are not worsening during testing and ensures documentation of an accurate response to posture, movement, and activity. Observation requires adequate exposure of the region or areas of interest.

Functional Activity

During all tests and measures, the clinician observes the quality and quantity of motion involved and asks the patient what the effect was in order to determine the symptom response. If appropriate, the clinician asks the patient to perform a functional activity or movement from the history that reproduces or increases the patient's symptoms. The therapist may select a specific movement from the history for further analysis or allow the patient to select one. Not all functional movements that are aggravating factors should be tested due to the potential for cumulative stresses that may make the patient's symptoms worse. In Chapter 2, the concepts of severity, irritability, nature, stage, and stability were used as a guide to determine the amount of examination at the first session. For example, some patients may only be able to walk a few feet because of pain, whereas others may need to walk for 5 minutes in order to produce or increase symptoms. The instructions to the patient and the amount of examination of walking will be markedly different for these 2 patients. Functional activities should be important to the patient and may include walking, moving from sitting to standing, putting on socks and shoes, bending, reaching, lifting, stair climbing, stepping up and down (Figure 4-20), getting into and out of the car, hopping, or squatting. Squatting also serves as an initial screen of hip, knee, and ankle mobility. In addition to qualitative analysis of the motion and postural control, functional movements are often baseline provocative measures and indicators of motor control strategies.

Analysis of functional movement requires development of observational and palpation skills. A framework for qualitative assessment of optimal movement strategies includes observation for the following:

- Joint control in the kinetic chain while allowing sufficient motion to accomplish the task
- Maintenance of posture within and between regions of the lumbar, pelvic girdle, thoracic spine, and cervical spine
- Maintenance of postural equilibrium
- Continued respiration, continence, and internal organ support[351]

All 4 components are necessary for control in varying degrees for varying tasks, both predictable and unpredictable. Failure to demonstrate any of these components suggests a nonoptimal altered motor control strategy.[351] Clinicians should utilize this context to qualitatively assess all tests and measures that require movement to generate hypotheses about why the motor control strategy is altered.

Squat

During a functional squat such as sit-to-stand from a chair, the thoracic and pelvic spine alignment of a neutral pelvis and spinal curves should not change. Keeping the trunk over the base of support forward movement of the trunk occurs as the hips and pelvis move posteriorly. The pelvic girdle anteriorly tilts on the femoral heads; the hips, knees, and ankle flex. The knees remain centered over the foot without varus, valgus, or rotational movements.[351] Alterations from these positions suggest altered motor control strategies. For example, an increase in lumbar lordosis may suggest overactivation of the erector spinae (ES). A loss of lumbar lordosis may suggest hip mobility deficits.

Gait

Walking—a complex functional activity—is difficult for many individuals with LBP. Clinicians almost universally observe gait in anterior, posterior, and lateral views in persons with LBP and often recommend walking as regular exercise. Individuals with LBP walk slower and take shorter asymmetrical steps in comparison to age-matched asymptomatic controls.[352-356] When asked to walk faster, individuals with LBP increase their cadence,[357] whereas pain-free individuals increase stride length.[358]

Furthermore, individuals with LBP and leg pain walk slower than controls and those with LBP only[359] and tend to use strategies such as an asymmetrical gait[352,359] to reduce vertical ground reaction force by slowing the affected extremity or by taking a shorter step on the opposite side.[360] The use of viscoelastic insoles or walking on a BW-supported treadmill (BWST) results in less pain and improved functional ability because of reduced axial loads during walking.[361,362] Fear-avoidance belief about physical activity is a strong predictor of gait velocity and must be considered when assessing individuals with LBP.[363] Research has defined some of the gait characteristics associated with LBP but is limited with respect to the mechanisms of how LBP affects walking.

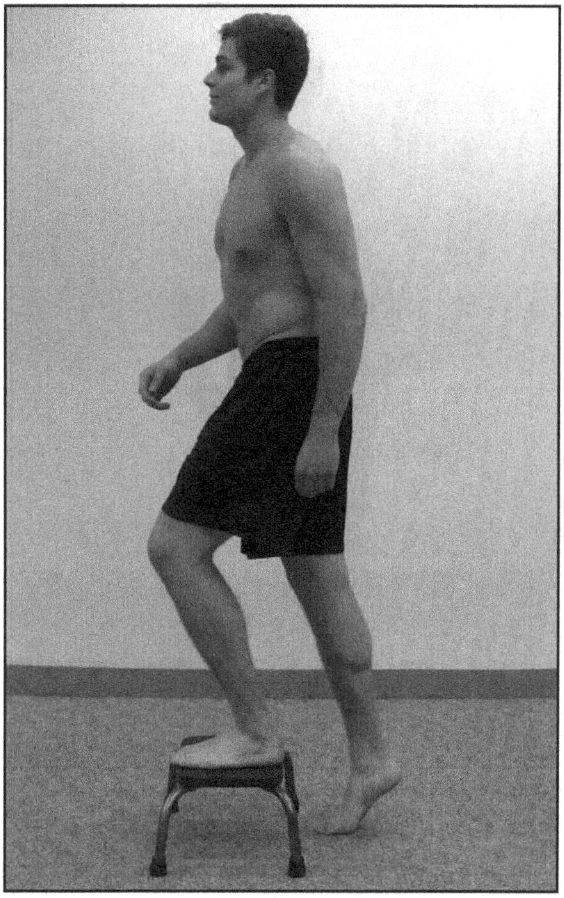

Figure 4-20. Functional activity—step up.

Observation of trunk motion may be important in patients with LBP. Trunk muscle activation patterns in patients with LBP differ from controls. Comparing healthy individuals and those with LBP, Lamoth et al[364,365] examined pelvic-thoracic rotation in treadmill walking at speeds of 1.4 to 5.4 km/h. At 3.0 km/h or 1.86 miles/h or higher, patients with LBP demonstrated reduced coordination between the transverse plane rotations of the pelvis and thorax but not the amplitudes of the motions. The authors agreed with previous studies[352,366,367] that the control of trunk muscle activity is affected and is often visualized clinically as trunk rigidity. In subjects with CLBP, van der Hulst and colleagues[368] demonstrated increased superficial muscle activity of the ES and rectus abdominis (RA), but not of the external oblique abdominals. These differences

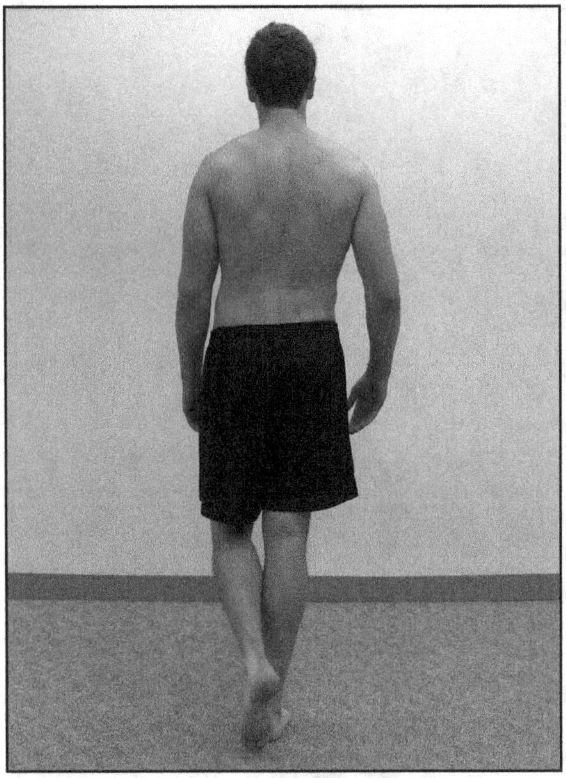

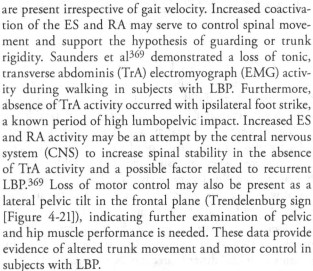

Figure 4-21. Gait posterior view. Trendelenburg sign.

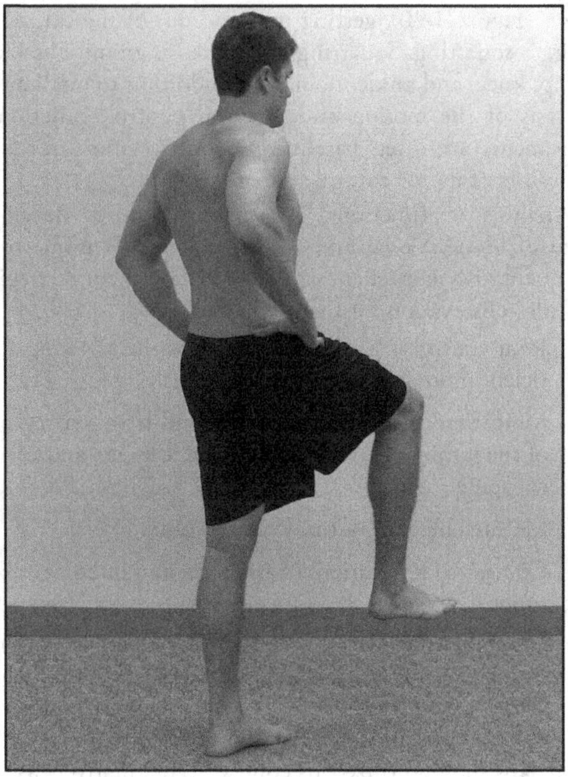

Figure 4-22. Unilateral standing posture.

are present irrespective of gait velocity. Increased coactivation of the ES and RA may serve to control spinal movement and support the hypothesis of guarding or trunk rigidity. Saunders et al[369] demonstrated a loss of tonic, transverse abdominis (TrA) electromyograph (EMG) activity during walking in subjects with LBP. Furthermore, absence of TrA activity occurred with ipsilateral foot strike, a known period of high lumbopelvic impact. Increased ES and RA activity may be an attempt by the central nervous system (CNS) to increase spinal stability in the absence of TrA activity and a possible factor related to recurrent LBP.[369] Loss of motor control may also be present as a lateral pelvic tilt in the frontal plane (Trendelenburg sign [Figure 4-21]), indicating further examination of pelvic and hip muscle performance is needed. These data provide evidence of altered trunk movement and motor control in subjects with LBP.

Patients with LBP who have difficulty walking should be assessed for altered motor control of the lumbopelvic hip complex. The relationship between walking and LBP is complex and should be considered in the context of whole body due to the interdependence of the spine, pelvis, and lower extremities.[370] Walking may need to be broken down into specific kinematic components such as heel strike and toe off to determine why walking has become provocative. Posture and balance are dynamic processes with many factors interacting at one time as they relate to the onset and recurrence of LBP. See Chapter 3 for further interpretations of abnormal gait.

Balance

Postural control is a requirement for all activities of daily living. An optimal balance strategy should result in maintenance of the normal standing posture on the weightbearing side with minimum effort and normal breathing (Figure 4-22). Qualitatively, the spinal curves, pelvis, and lower extremities should remain stable in all planes. Loss of control in any plane or region indicates the need for further examination of the neuromuscular system.

Balance impairments have been demonstrated in individuals with LBP.[371-373] Byl and Sinnot[371] showed that LBP subjects have significantly increased postural sway, keep their center of force significantly more posterior, and are significantly less likely to be able to balance on one foot with eyes closed. Mok et al[373] found that, when compared with age- and gender-matched controls, individuals with LBP had poorer standing balance with altered postural adjustment strategies such as reduced hip strategy and increased visual dependence. Takala and Viikari-Juntara[374] correlated future LBP with poor balance in asymptomatic subjects with less than 8 days LBP over the last 12 months and symptomatic subjects with more than 30 days of LBP over the last 12 months. Standing and single limb balance tests as described in Chapter 2 should be examined at some

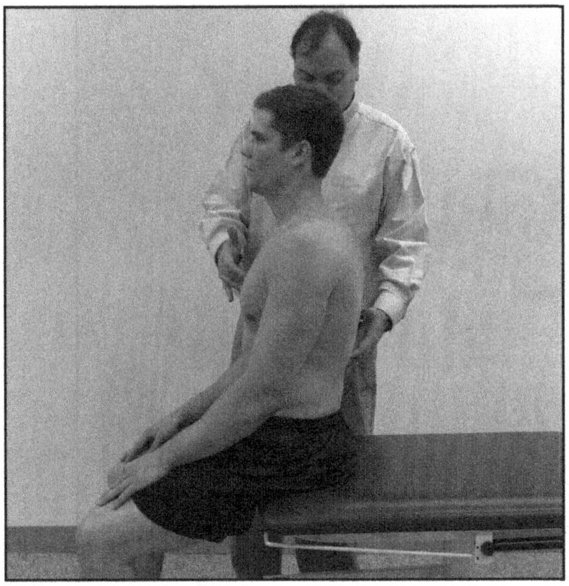

Figure 4-23. Posture—manubriosternal junction in line with the pubic symphysis.

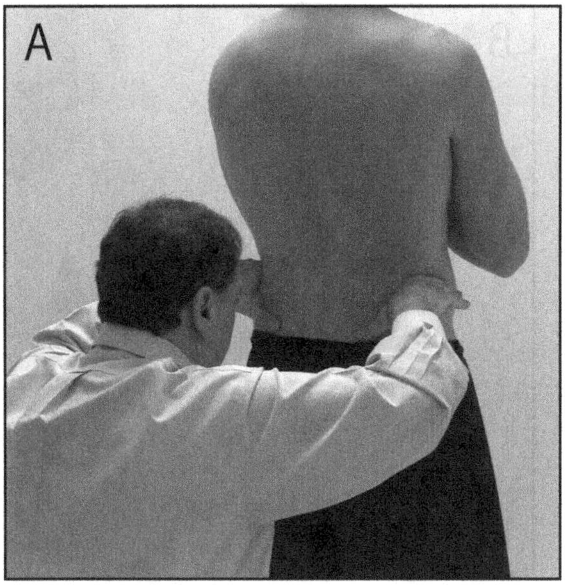

Figure 4-24. Pelvic landmarks: (A) iliac crests. *(continued)*

point throughout the examination process, but it may not be appropriate if weightbearing is painful (ie, severe and irritable). These tests may be useful as baseline provocative measures if LBP is nonsevere and nonirritable when viewed as important functional activities for the individual patient or for individuals who are at risk for falls. Normative values for single limb stance time were provided in Table 3-5 in Chapter 3.

Neurological Exam

Toe and heel walk are quick functional tests for the L5-S1 and L4-5 myotomes, respectively. S1-2 may also be tested and graded in the manual muscle test (MMT) position for the gastroc-soleus complex in standing.

Posture

The history suggests which posture(s) to emphasize initially. For example, if sitting is a primary aggravating factor and standing and walking are not related to the patient's symptoms, more time may be spent analyzing a sitting posture described in Chapter 3. Formal examination usually begins with observation of the patient's posture in standing with specific emphasis on the spine, pelvis, and lower extremities using anterior, lateral, and posterior views. Generally, the patient wears appropriate clothing to provide adequate exposure, removes his or her shoes, faces away from the examiner, and stands with the legs comfortably apart in a relaxed standing position. The clinician initially observes global posture from all views, gradually focusing on the lumbopelvic and lower extremity regions for the presence of scoliosis, lordosis, kyphosis, lateral shift, or patterns suggestive of muscle imbalance. See Chapter 3 for further description.

In the neutral position of the pelvis with anterior-superior iliac spine (ASIS) and posterior-superior iliac spine (PSIS) relatively in the same planes, a normal anterior curve (ie, lordosis) is present in the low back. Excessive anterior tilt of the pelvis results in an increased lordosis or increased anterior curve, and excessive posterior tilt of the pelvis results in a flat back or decreased anterior curve. The thorax, using the manubriosternal junction as a landmark, should be in line with pubic symphysis (PS) and the ASIS (Figure 4-23). The femoral heads should be centered in the acetabulum without excessive femoral internal rotation (IR) or external rotation (ER). Because standardized definitions for good or ideal posture do not exist, the presence or absence and/or degree of these postures are based on clinical opinion.

Pelvic Landmark Assessment

Assessment of pelvic bony landmarks for positional asymmetry is commonly used to screen for leg length discrepancies or PGP. Iliac crests and the PSIS are observed and palpated posteriorly and the ASIS anteriorly (Figure 4-24). A systematic review[375] of 10 articles reported that average interexaminer reliability for bony anatomical landmark positional asymmetry assessment of the lumbar spine and pelvis was slightly above chance for all landmarks except the medial malleolus. On average, interexaminer reliability was less than intraexaminer reliability and too low to be clinically useful.[375] Despite limitations, observation of pelvic symmetry is still accepted as useful by some clinicians.

The clinician judges symmetry of the pelvic landmarks at eye level. To compare PSIS levels, the PSIS bony landmarks are palpated using the thumbs directly under the most inferior aspect of the bony landmark on each side and

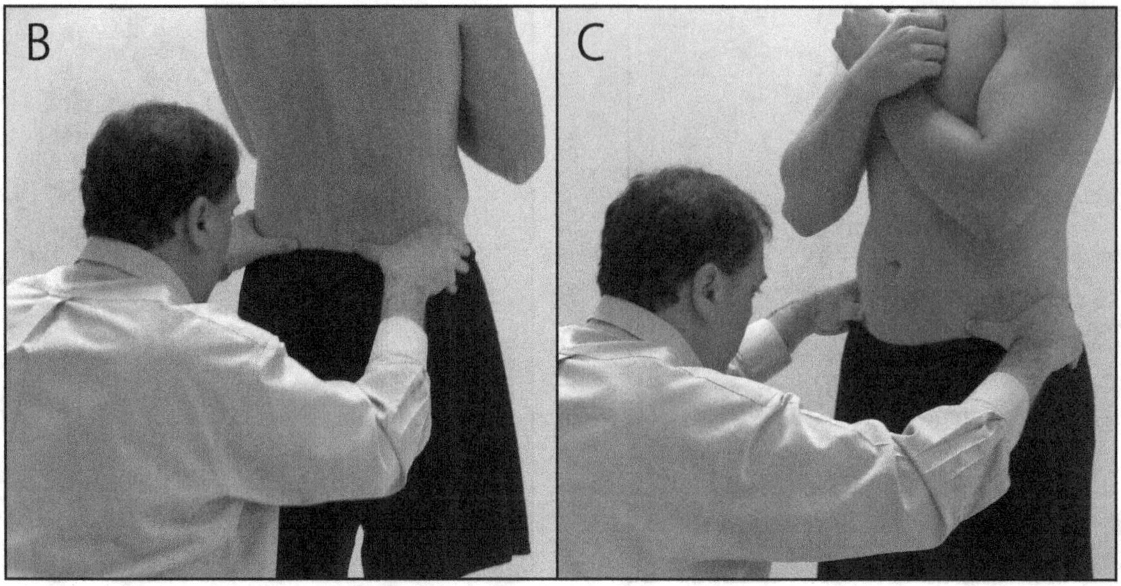

Figure 4-24 (continued). Pelvic landmarks: (B) PSIS and (C) ASIS.

the rest of the hand gently encompassing the ilium. ASIS levels are palpated in a similar manner. Palpation results include the following possibilities:

- Symmetrical pelvic landmarks in standing—normal
- Increased height of the ASIS, PSIS and iliac crest on the same side suggests an apparent leg length discrepancy
- Asymmetrical heights of ASIS, PSIS and iliac crests (eg, low PSIS on left, high iliac crest on left, and high ASIS on left) suggests apparent pelvic girdle asymmetry

The presence of apparent asymmetries or leg length discrepancy requires further examination of the lumbopelvic and lower extremity regions to determine if the findings are relevant, incidental, or simply bony asymmetry. The height of lower extremity landmarks such as ischial tuberosities, greater trochanters, fibular heads, and medial malleoli are also palpated. If an apparent leg length discrepancy is identified, a standing block to level the pelvis may be tried and symptom response assessed. Measurement of leg length using the tape measure or standing blocks (ie, placing a shim under the foot) may be useful, but it is not as reliable or accurate as imaging modalities.[376] Radiography is the gold standard for true length discrepancy. Little consistency exists relative to the amount of leg length discrepancy that is clinically meaningful as well as the reliability and validity of assessment methods.[377]

Saulicz et al[378] demonstrated that pelvic asymmetry is present in healthy, asymptomatic subjects ages 18 to 39 without a history of pelvic or LBP. Gnat et al[379] concluded that pelvic asymmetry is a frequent occurrence in response to mechanical loading. In response to a 60-cm jump-down landing on one foot, all subjects demonstrated asymptomatic pelvic asymmetry that resolved immediately with manual stretching and mobilizing techniques. The authors described 2 types of pelvic asymmetry as an adaptive response to the transmission of asymmetrical mechanical loads such jumping on one foot or asymmetrical exercise for the biceps femoris or piriformis:

1. *Fresh* asymmetry in response to daily asymmetrical activities
2. *Cemented* asymmetry, which is resistant to correction and could produce symptoms within the lumbopelvic hip region[379]

Pelvic asymmetry alone appears to have little to no clinical value.

Lumbar Lordosis

The range of lordosis varies in symptomatic and asymptomatic individuals (Figure 4-25). Systematic review[380] determined that the intertester and intratester reliability of visual observation is low in terms of describing lumbar lordosis as increased, decreased, or normal.[381,382] Fedorak et al[382] demonstrated fair intrarater reliability and poor interrater reliability for visual assessment of lumbar lordosis. In addition to observing the lumbar region, clinicians should also palpate the spinous processes (SPs) for alignment to compare with visual assessment. The use of electronic inclinometers[383] or radiography[384] enhances the reliability of measuring lordosis, but may not be useful for clinical purposes.

No clear relationship between posture and LBP has been established. In vivo research both supports[385,386] and refutes[387,388] a relationship between posture and LBP. However, Scannell and McGill[389] suggested that a 12-week PT training program for individuals quantified

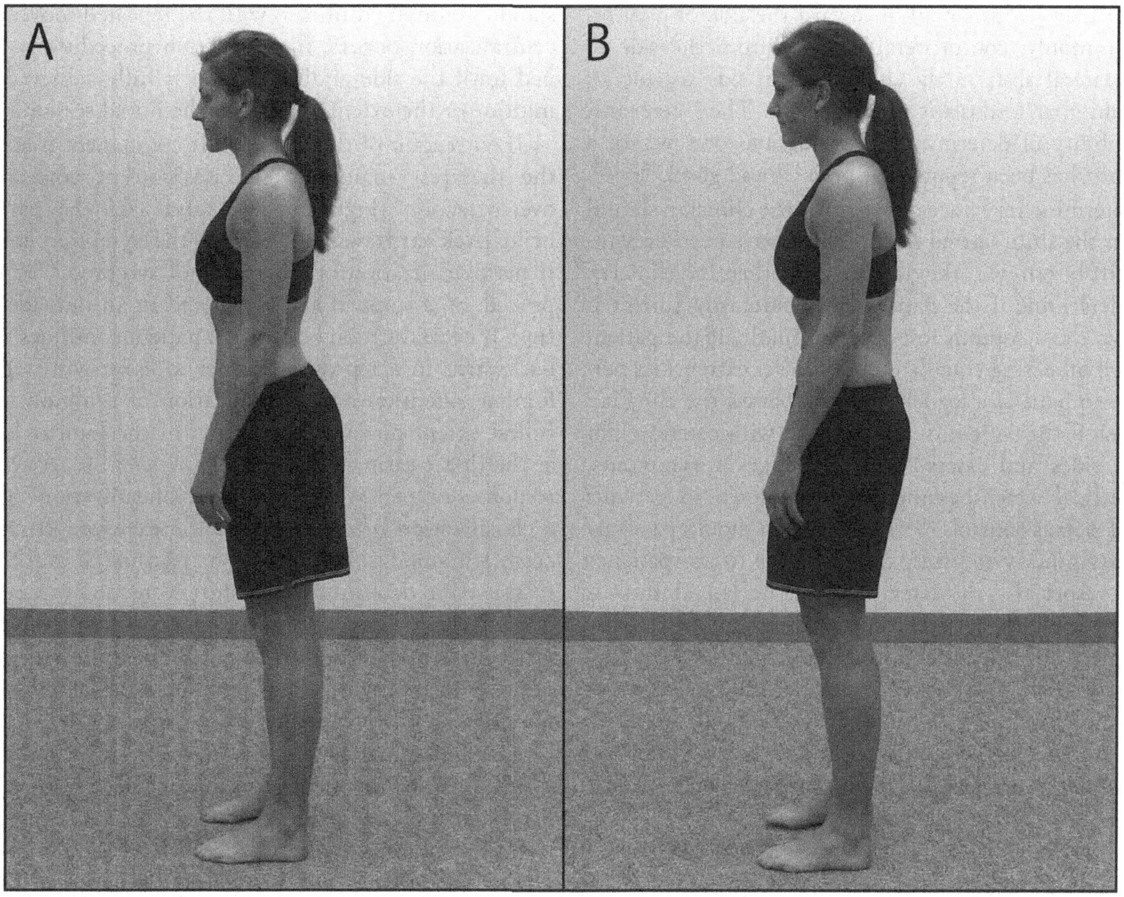

Figure 4-25. Lumbar lordosis: (A) increased and (B) reduced.

as having hyperlordosis or hypolordosis may potentially benefit individuals with LBP by altering lumbar strain during various activities of daily living. Minor deviations from ideal posture are unlikely to be relevant. However, extreme deviations such as a lateral shift or lumbar kyphosis warrant investigation. In an acute presentation of lumbar kyphosis, the patient may have extreme difficulty maintaining an upright position. To determine relevance of an exaggerated posture, passive correction of the posture or asking the patient to alter it to assess symptom response provides information to support the posture as habitual or related to the patient's problem. The clinician wants to know, "Does altering the posture make the symptoms better, worse, or result in no change?" as well as, "Does altering the posture affect other regions of the spine or extremities?"

Lateral Shift Correction

A lateral shift, also called *sciatic scoliosis*, occurs in individuals with LBP with or without leg pain and is observed by looking at the frontal and sagittal plane alignment of the lumbar and thoracic spines. A right lateral shift (Figure 4-26) involves a nonstructural shift of the upper body or thoracic spine to the right relative to the lower body or lumbar spine and pelvis.[390] A left lateral shift is the reverse.

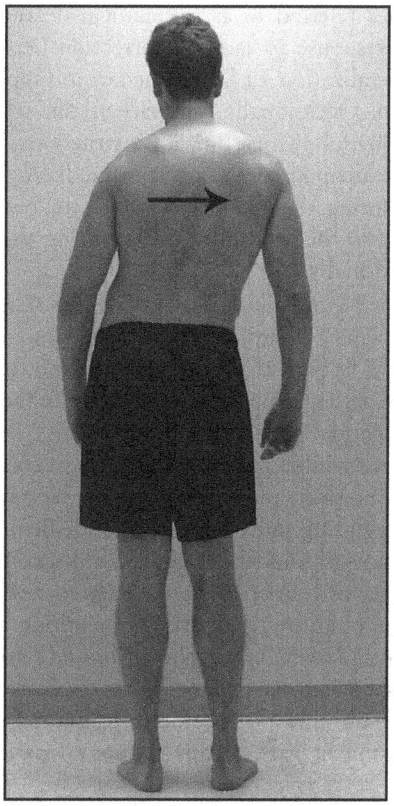

Figure 4-26. Right lateral shift.

The shift may be ipsilateral or toward the side of pain or, more commonly, contralateral or away from the side of pain. A lateral shift rarely changes from side to side. A reduced lumbar lordosis is often present. The interexaminer reliability of determining the side and presence of a lateral shift has been reported as poor[391] and good.[392,393]

To determine relevance of the shift, the clinician should ask when the shift started or if it has always been present. If the shift began with the onset of LBP, then the clinician should determine if the patient can voluntarily correct it and assess the symptom response. Similarly, if the patient is not weightbearing equally on both lower extremities perhaps due to pain or a leg length discrepancy, the clinician should ask if the patient is able to stand with equal weight on both sides and assess for any change in symptoms. Asymmetrical weightbearing has been noted in patients with LBP versus controls.[394] The clinician should passively correct asymmetry to assess the relevance to the patient's problem, especially the lateral shift. The lateral shift is widely believed to be associated with symptomatic disc pathology,[395-398] but the exact mechanism of shift production is unknown.[399] Theories include a disc protrusion or space occupying lesion or tumor that results in the trunk moving away from the painful mass[395,396] or an active or reflex avoidance of a painful nerve compression.[400]

Manual Lateral Shift Correction in Standing

Presence of a lateral shift may be a key finding for a provisional diagnosis of DSE classification (see Table 4-3) or sometimes referred to as mechanical derangement.[390] The initial response to manual correction (ie, centralization, peripheralization, or DP) is the key to supporting this classification. Occasionally, the patient can self-correct a lateral shift by following clinician instructions. If self-correction fails, manual correction is immediately attempted while monitoring the patient's response (ie, better, worse, or the same) to the procedure and ensuring the patient is breathing normally.

To perform a manual lateral shift correction in standing, the therapist stands or sits on the same side as the lateral shift. The patient flexes the elbow and the therapist encircles the patient's hips while placing his or her shoulder against the patient's shoulder (Figure 4-27A). After establishing resting symptoms and maintaining a constant pressure at the shoulder, the therapist pulls the patient's hips using a side-gliding movement, not a side-bending movement. The side-gliding movement is performed in an oscillatory manner with brief holds to gently correct the lateral shift while monitoring the patient's breathing and symptoms for centralization or peripheralization (Figure 4-27B). If peripheralization occurs, the procedure is stopped and attempted in an unloaded position. Resistance to the side-gliding movement varies from patient to patient, but it should gradually diminish with the repeated movement. If centralization occurs, the correction procedure is continued until the side-gliding motion is fully achieved across midline or the extent possible at the initial session.

If correction of the lateral shift component is achieved, the therapist maintains the position of correction or overcorrection (Figure 4-27C) and asks the patient to bend backwards while assessing the symptom response. If peripheralization or worsening of symptoms occur, the procedure is stopped and attempted in an unloaded position. If centralization occurs, the patient continues to bend backwards in a repeated manner to assist with regaining lumbar extension and centralization of symptoms to the fullest extent possible (restoration of the lumbar lordosis) at the first treatment session (Figure 4-27D). A symptom response of centralization or peripheralization supports a classification of direction-specific exercise. After a successful manual shift correction, posture or walking are reassessed to determine if the shift correction can be maintained. Patient education and additional shift correction procedures may also be required in an unloaded position or prone to assist with self-correction of the lateral shift and maintaining the lumbar lordosis.

The desired patient response or outcome from the lateral shift correction is a centralization or DP. DP for postures or movements in one direction decreases, abolishes, or centralizes symptoms and results in an increase of movement; DP for postures or movements in the opposite direction causes symptoms to worsen.[401] Centralization is a progressive abolition of pain that is retained over time in a distal-proximal direction in response to repeated end-range movement or static end-range loading and corrective postures; sometimes the proximal pain increases as the distal pain resolves. With LBP only, the pain becomes more local centrally and is abolished.[402] If the response is positive, the patient is classified under the DSE classification (see Table 4-3) for lateral shift or derangement and instructed in self-correction and maintenance of the lateral shift correction. These procedures are discussed in this chapter in the section on intervention.

Laslett[399] presents several points of clinical observation for safety during the procedure, including the following:

- Progressive worsening of pain or peripheralization or pain that refers or radiates distally into the lower extremity indicates that the shift correction should be stopped and repeated in a nonweightbearing position, usually prone.
- Signs and symptoms of radiculopathy or CES are reasons to abandon the process.
- If the shift cannot be corrected across midline after 1 to 2 days, the condition is likely irreversible.
- Nausea or faintness indicates trial of an alternative management procedure.

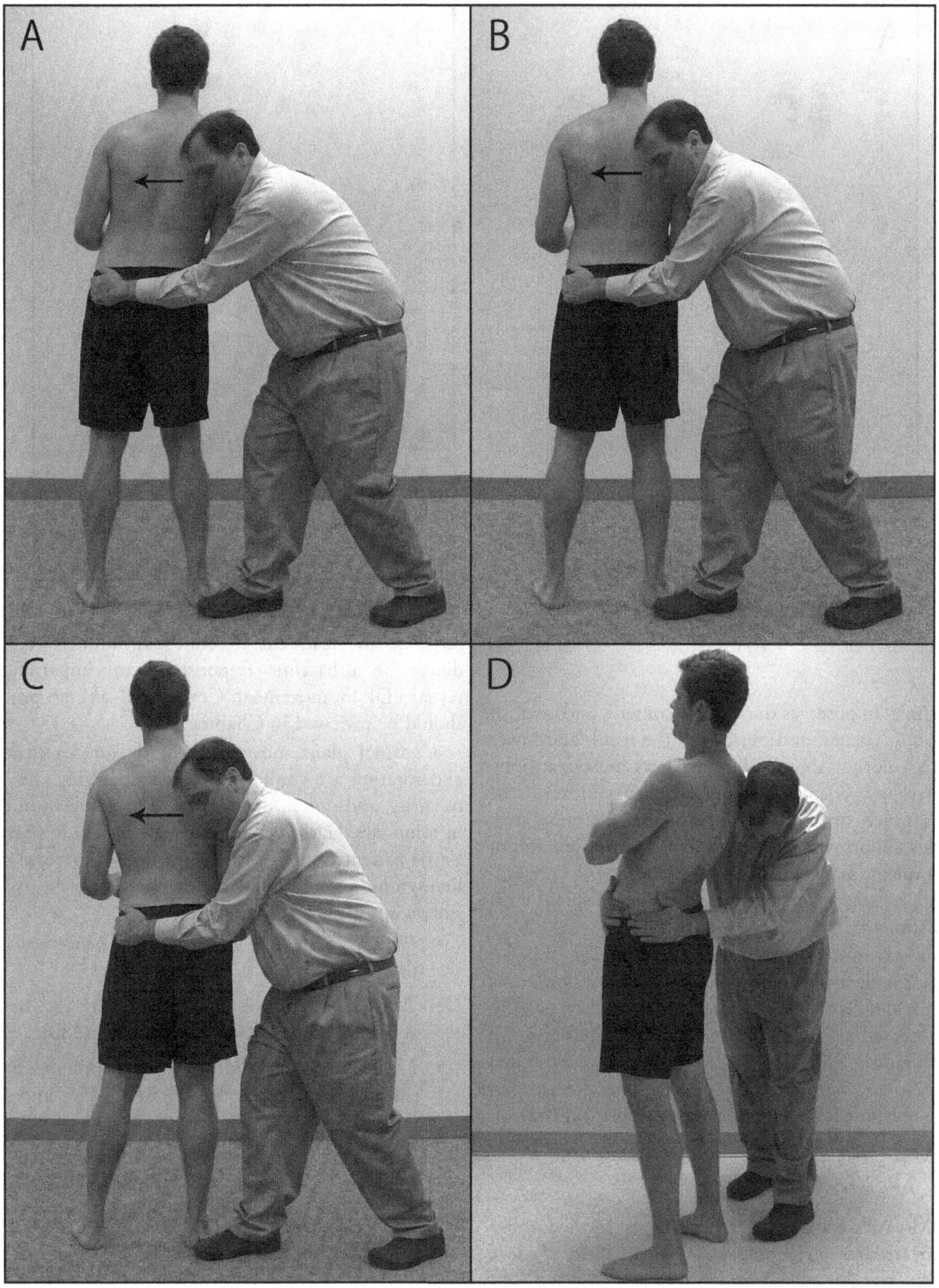

Figure 4-27. Manual shift correction right lateral shift: (A) part 1—start position; (B) correction; (C) overcorrection; and (D) part 2—restoration of lumbar lordosis.

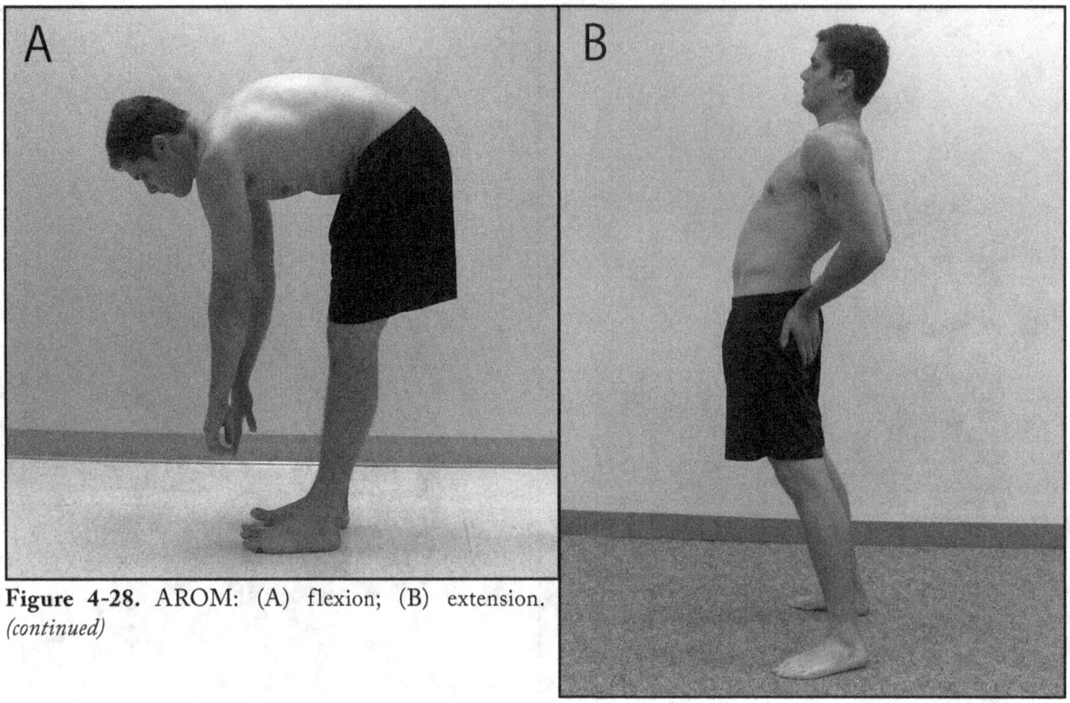

Figure 4-28. AROM: (A) flexion; (B) extension. *(continued)*

Additional Observations Related to Posture

The clinician observes the quality, contour, and color of the skin, soft tissues, and muscles of the trunk and lower extremities, noting abnormalities such as muscle atrophy or hypertrophy, edema, scarring, signs of infection, or the appearance of moles or other skin discolorations. Cutaneous abnormalities, birth marks, or hairy patches of skin over the lumbar spine may be associated with congenital anomalies such as spina bifida occulta or spinal cord malformations.[403]

Because asymmetry in posture is common, the clinician must link the postural findings to the patient's symptoms on an individual basis. As indicated by the history, posture can be observed in both static and dynamic positions and its contribution individually determined by continued examination and noting the symptom response to altering the observed posture or the demands of postural control. See Chapter 3 for further analysis of posture.

Active Range of Motion

AROM varies widely among individuals. In the lumbar region, mean values in degrees ± SD are 51 ± 12 for flexion, 25 ± 15 for extension, 49 ± 3 for left rotation, 9 ± 4 for right rotation, 19 ± 5 for left LF, and 20 ± 45 for right LF for healthy men with a mean age 31 years ranging from 24 to 36.[404] Therefore, the quality and symptom response may be more important than the gross available range. Though nonpainful, AROM measures do not correlate highly with function or disability. A gain or loss from baseline in pain-limited AROM often indicates a positive or negative response to treatment. Record pain-limited AROM to determine a baseline response, reveal impairments, or reveal a DP for movement. General AROM test procedures should be reviewed in Chapter 3.

Cardinal plane movements of flexion, extension, LF, and rotation are commonly tested observing the quality, quantity, and symptom response. The clinician must keep in mind whether he or she wants the patient to move as far as the patient can or only to the onset or increase of baseline symptoms. The following commands to the patient are simple but variable:

- *Flexion*: With your knees straight, bend forward as if to touch the floor (Figure 4-28A).
- *Extension*: With your knees straight and hands on your hips, bend backwards (Figure 4-28B).
- *Left and right LF*: Slide your left/right hand down the side of your right/left leg (Figures 4-28C and 4-28D).
- *Left and right rotation*: Turn your body to the left/right while standing or seated (Figures 4-28E and 4-28F).

Observations of Active Range of Motion

During AROM testing, the clinician should observe quantity of movement (ie, gross range of movement), quality of movement (ie, ease and control and quality of the curve), and symptom response. During movement and at end-range, clinicians should observe the behavior of symptoms as any change in pain intensity or location from the rest position and where in the range the symptoms change. The clinician should watch for deviations from

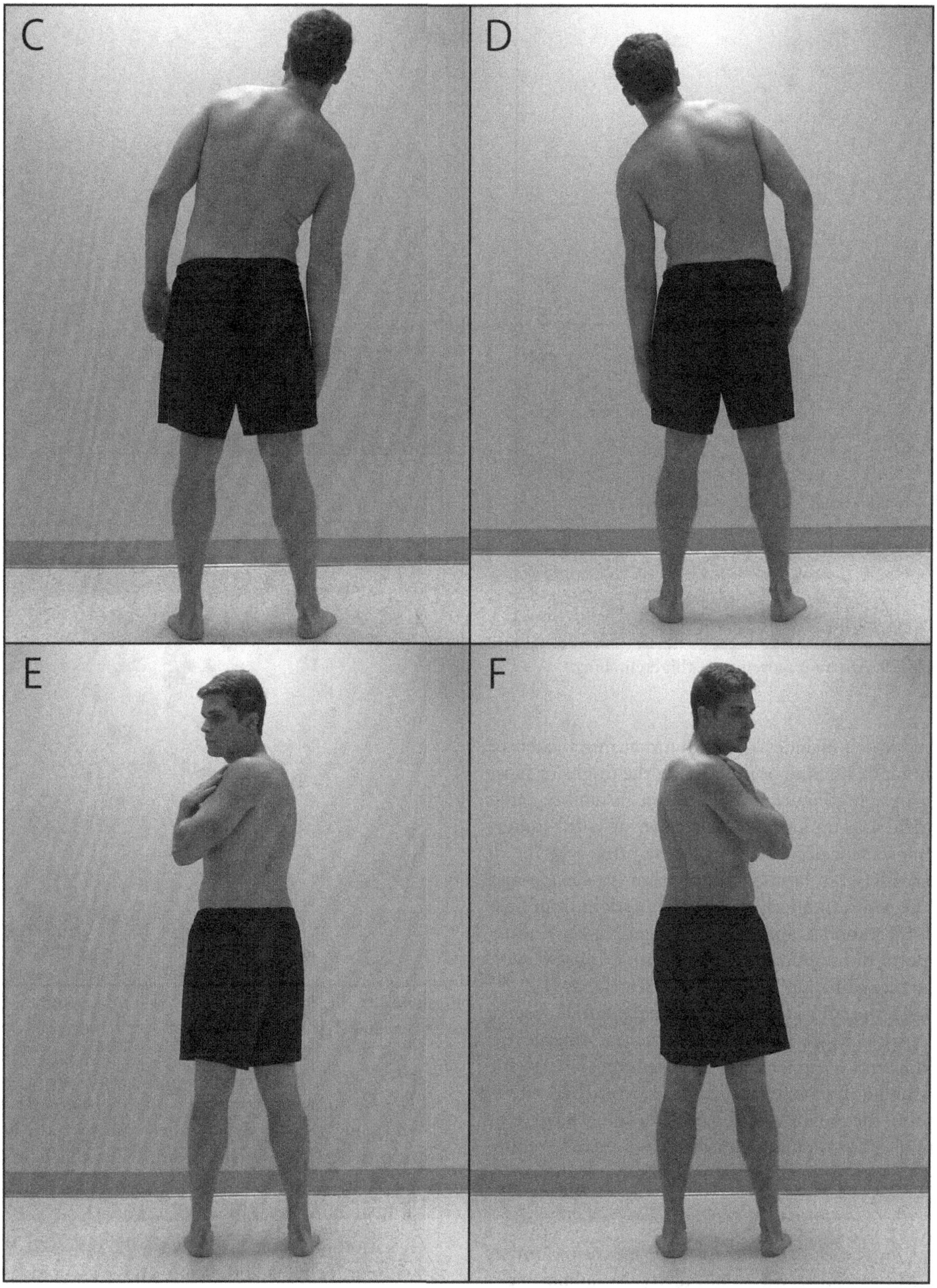

Figure 4-28 (continued). AROM: (C) LF right; (D) LF left; (E) rotation in standing left; and (F) rotation in standing right.

the requested plane of motion. For instance, rotation of the pelvic girdle or thorax in the transverse plane should not occur during flexion, extension, or LF. The clinician should correct deviations from the expected movement plane either during or at the end of range to determine relevance of the deviation. If correction alters the patient's symptoms, then relevance is established. Another common deviation from normal motion is the presence of aberrant

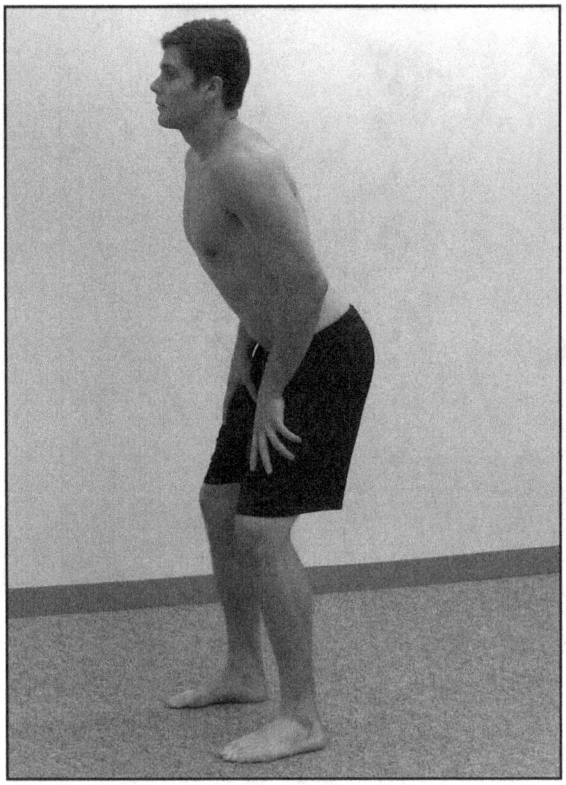

Figure 4-29. Aberrant movement—thigh climbing.

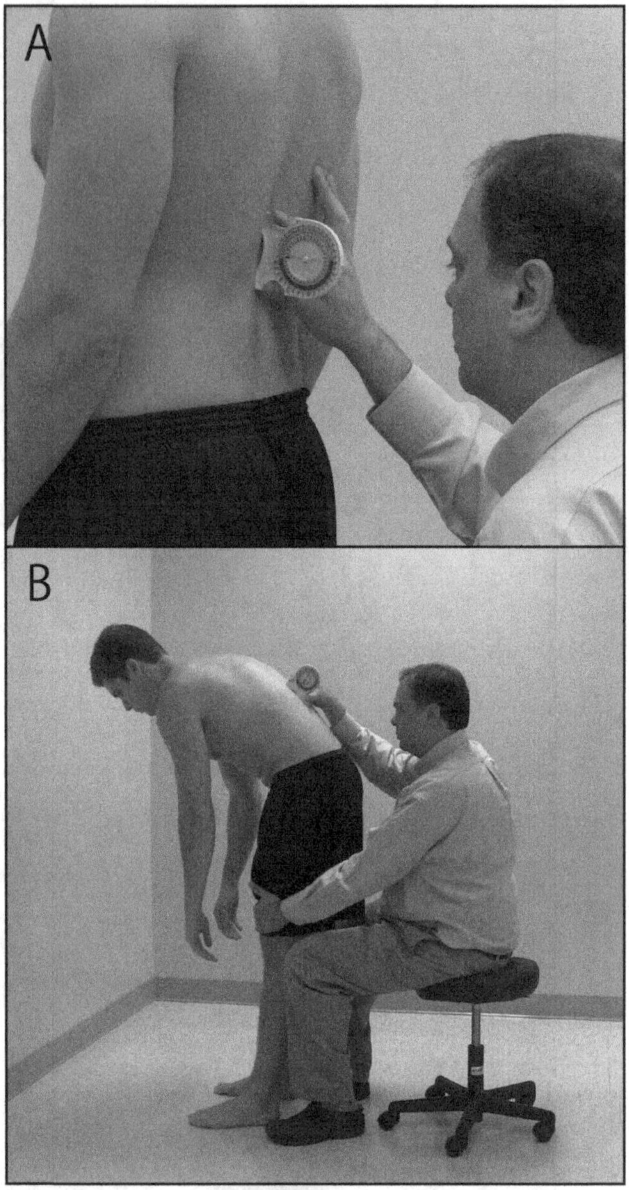

Figure 4-30. Single inclinometry: (A) starting position flexion/extension and (B) flexion. *(continued)*

movement, which includes a painful arc during flexion or on return; high climbing or pushing on the thighs to assist return to upright (Figure 4-29); and an instability catch or a sudden acceleration or deceleration of trunk movement or movement occurring out of the primary plane of motion or reversal of lumbopelvic rhythm (ie, flexion and shifting the pelvis anteriorly to return to upright from flexion).[405] Observation of aberrant movement is a key finding that supports the stabilization classification or LBP with movement coordination impairment (see Table 4-2).[405] Additionally, the clinician should both palpate and observe for symmetrical pelvic girdle motion such as anterior tilt with flexion and posterior tilt with extension. Finally, the clinician should observe segmental or intervertebral movement, noting the presence or absence of a smooth curve or a fulcrum or sharp angulation that suggests altered—either reduced or excessive—segmental mobility.

Active Range of Motion Measurement

Several methods are available to measure lumbar AROM. Measurement with the gravity or bubble inclinometer has acceptable reliability for LBP.[406-409] The use of an inclinometer is used for flexion, extension, and LF:

- *Single inclinometry* (Figures 4-30 and 4-31): One inclinometer placed at the T12 SP provides a measure in degrees of total flexion, extension, or LF. The amount measured combines motion available at the lumbopelvic and hip regions.
- *Double inclinometry*: Place one inclinometer at T12 and one at the S2 SP, then subtract the amount recorded at the sacrum from T12, which provides a measure of lumbar spine motion only. S2 – T12 = lumbar spine AROM.
- Rotation in standing is visually observed with or without pelvic stabilization and with a side-to-side comparison.

Visual estimates of AROM can be documented as follows (Figure 4-32): Each line represents the full ROM or 100% of expected AROM. The clinician records the visual estimate representing a percentage of the range, quality, and symptom response as noted in the example shown previously.

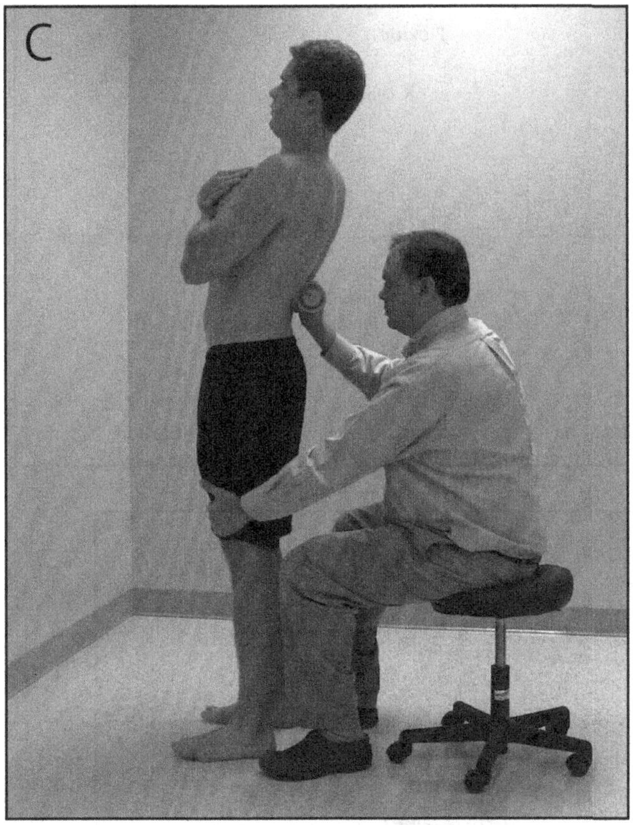

Figure 4-30 (continued). Single inclinometry: (C) extension.

Active Range of Motion With Overpressure (Figure 4-33)

If indicated and safe for the patient and if AROM is full range and painless, passive OP is performed in an oscillatory manner and the limit of the movement confirms the end feel and effect on symptoms. For flexion, the clinician stabilizes the pelvis and applies passive OP with the forearm across the lower thoracic spine into flexion. For extension, the clinician steps behind the patient, whose arms are crossed, and places one hand at the lower lumbar region while the other hand reaches across the upper body to provide OP into extension. For LF, the clinician stabilizes the pelvis on the side opposite the LF and applies OP through the opposite shoulder into LF. AROM with OP for rotation is performed in sitting. If AROM with OP is normal, the clinician should try repeated movements, sustained movements, or combined movements to reproduce or alter the patient's symptoms.

Repeated Movements

The response to repeated movements is important for classifying patients with LBP into subgroups.[401,402,410,411] When a patient's symptoms centralize during repeated movements such as flexion, extension, or lateral shift (ie, side glide), the direction that produces the centralization suggests a subgroup classification within the direction-specific classification or derangement syndrome (see Table 4-3). The direction of the repeated movement (ie, flexion, extension, or lateral shift) that results in centralization indicates that repeated exercise in that direction is an appropriate initial intervention. For example, if centralization occurs with repeated extension, then repeated extension is the recommended intervention. In a large subgroup of LBP patients with a DP for repeated movements,

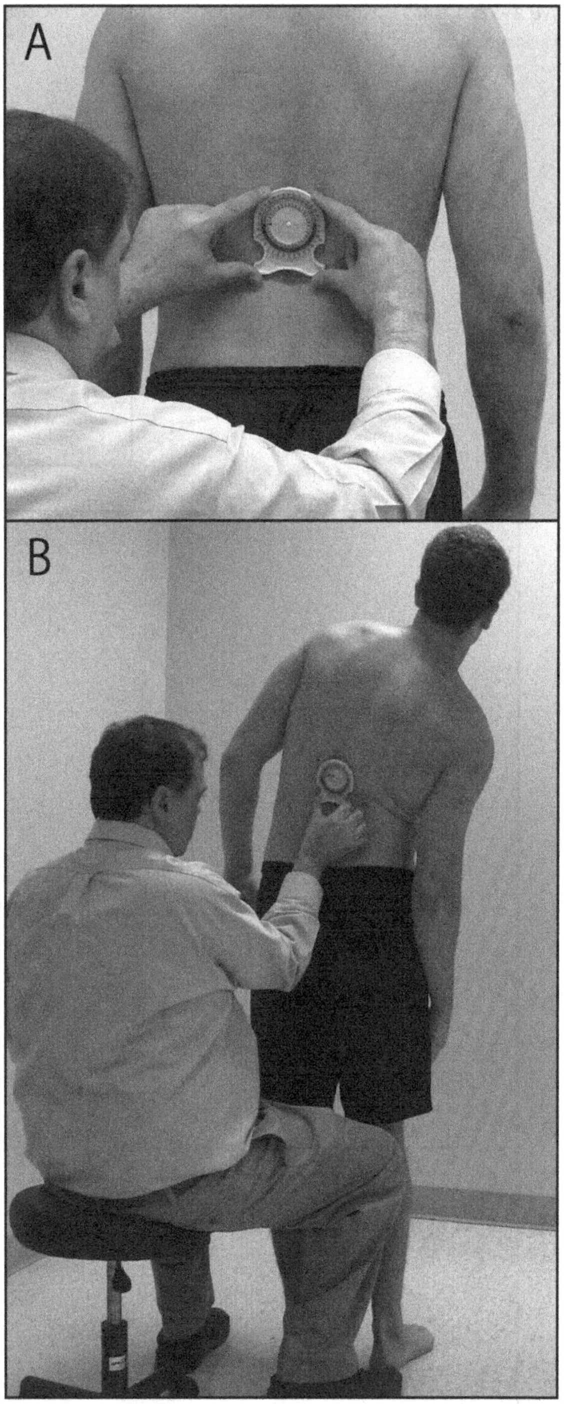

Figure 4-31. Single inclinometry: (A) starting position LF and (B) LF right.

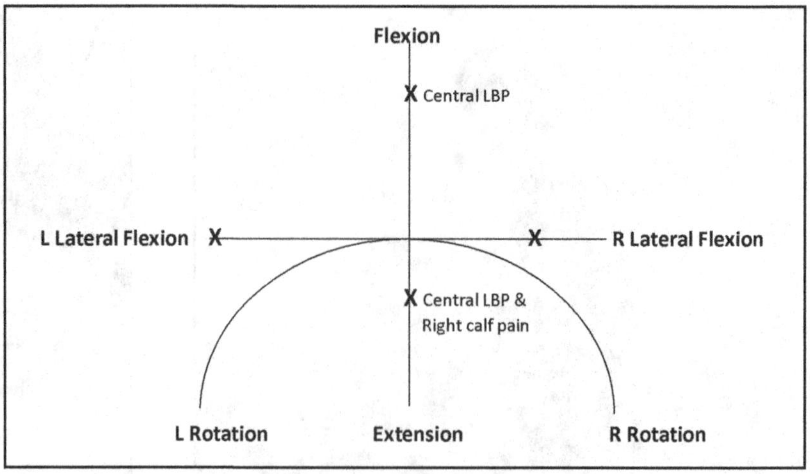

Figure 4-32. Visual estimate of AROM documentation diagram.

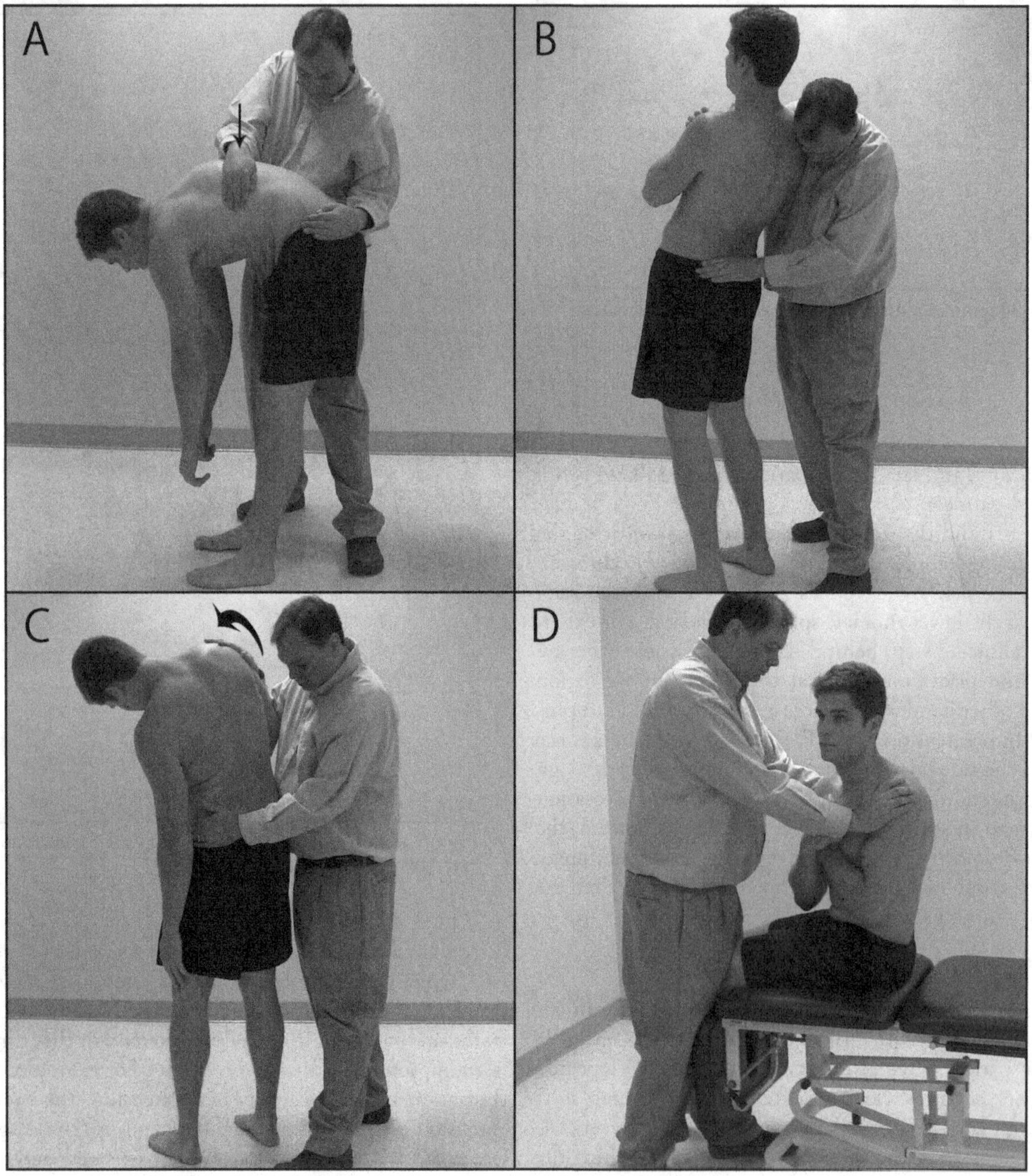

Figure 4-33. AROM with OP: (A) flexion; (B) extension; (C) LF; and (D) rotation.

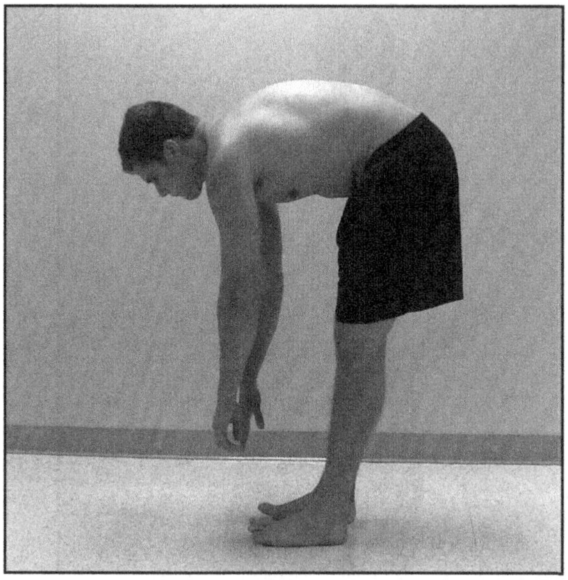

Figure 4-34. RFIS.

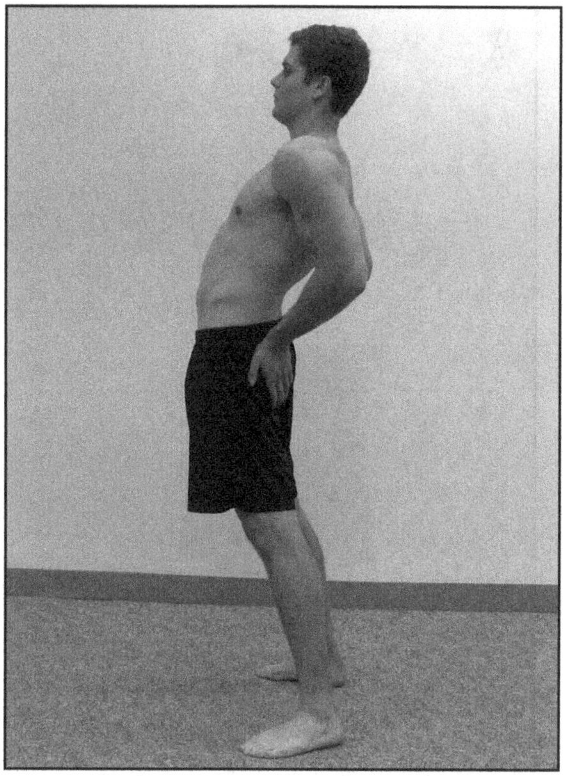

Figure 4-35. REIS.

exercise matching the DP resulted in significant and rapid decreased pain, medication use, disability, depression, and work interference when compared to exercise matching a direction opposite to the subjects' DP or nondirectional exercises.[411]

Centralization is a clinical phenomenon that can be reliably detected[412-414] and appears to identify a substantial subgroup of spinal patients. Werneke and Hart[415] reported that complete centralization occurred in only 3.2% of an acute-subacute LBP population in the initial evaluation, and over several days, 68% had complete centralization in response to intervention. In a chronic pain sample, prevalence of centralization was 32% at initial evaluation.[416] When centralization is noted on initial examination in the absence of severe disability or psychosocial distress, positive provocation discography is highly likely and a diagnosis of discogenic pain is reasonable (Sn 0.40 [0.28 to 0.54], Sp 0.94 [0.73 to 0.99]; +LR 6.9 [1.0 to 47.3], –LR 0.63 [0.49 to 0.82]), but a diagnosis of discogenic pain does not explain all cases of the centralization phenomenon. The sensitivity of centralization does not allow its use as a screening tool to select patients for discography, but its high specificity enables a diagnosis of discogenic pain without the need for invasive discography.[416]

Centralization is associated with a good prognosis and good outcomes of reduced pain, greater functional improvement return to work, and decreased health care usage, and failure to centralize is associated with a poor outcome at 1 year. Patients who fail to centralize are classified as noncentralizers and at higher risk for delayed recovery, chronic disability, and greater health care usage.[412,417] Alternatively, failure to centralize may mean these persons are nonresponders to this approach and may need a different intervention.

Sagittal plane movements, flexion or extension, are usually tested first because of the higher prevalence of these subgroups. Frontal plane or horizontal plane movements such as repeated side glide in standing (RSGIS) are tested as needed, such as when the response to sagittal plane movement is inconclusive or with unilateral or asymmetrical symptoms. Clear communication is necessary to correctly note the patient's response. Baseline symptoms are established and, based on the history and response to one repetition of AROM, the clinician decides which end-range movements are to be tested and explains the process to the patient. Not all procedures are performed on every patient. The patient's response guides the extent of repeated movement testing. General concepts of repeated end-range movement testing are discussed as follows, with recommendations to study the works of McKenzie and May.[401,402]

- Repeated flexion in standing (RFIS; Figure 4-34)
- Repeated extension in standing (REIS; Figure 4-35)
- RSGIS to the right and left performed by the patient:
    - The response to RSGIS may be assessed when a lateral shift is present, sagittal plane movements are inconclusive, or with asymmetrical or unilateral symptoms.
    - The first movement is hips away from the painful side. For left RSGIS (Figure 4-36), the trunk moves to the left, hips to the right, and shoulders

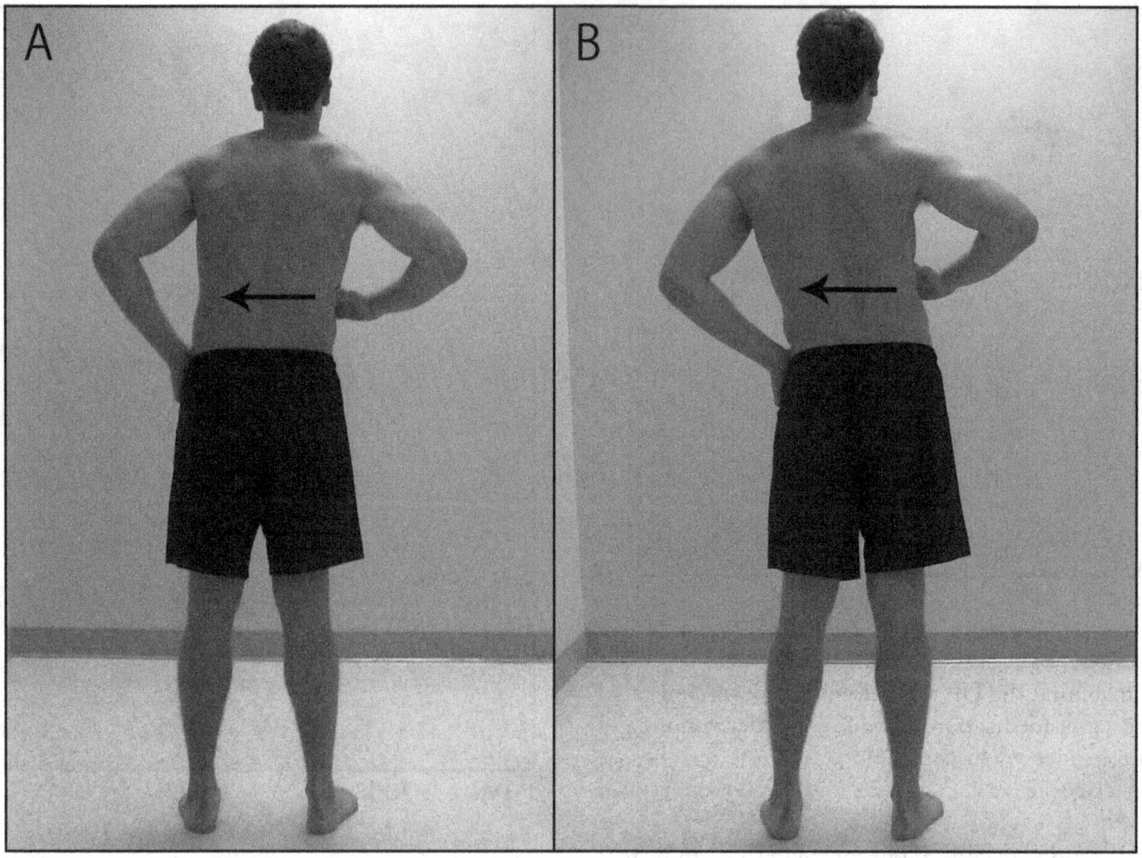

Figure 4-36. Left RSGIS: (A) starting position and (B) overcorrection.

are parallel to the ground. Similar to the manual shift correction process, if centralization occurs, the patient is instructed to bend backwards to restore extension while the side glide is maintained.

- During the repeated end-range movements of 10 to 15 repetitions, continually ask the patient about any change in symptom behavior, location, or intensity during movement or at end-range and note any change in quantity of movement.
- Record the response about 1 to 2 minutes after the movements.
- Responses (see Chapter 3 for definitions): centralized, peripheralized, better, no better, worse, no worse, or no effect.
  - If possible, appropriately classify the patient at this time as DSE classification (ie, extension, flexion, or lateral shift subgroup; see Table 4-3).
- If repeated movements decrease, abolish, or centralize symptoms or a DP is obtained, further testing may be unnecessary.[401,402]
  - If centralized or DP, proceed with matched intervention of REIS, RFIS, or lateral shift.
  - If peripheralized or partially centralized in weight-bearing, the clinician attempts to obtain centralization through repeated movements in unloaded positions (ie, repeated flexion in lying [RFIL], repeated extension in lying [REIL]).
  - If the response is limited motion and end-range pain (ie, produced, increased, or no worse) with no centralization or peripheralization, further examination is needed. The clinician considers a classification of LBP with mobility deficits (see Table 4-1).

Combined Movement Testing

If AROM and repeated movements are full range and do not provoke a patient's symptoms or are inconclusive, combined movements may be used. Introduced by Edwards,[418] this concept combines movements of either flexion or extension with LF. For example, extension and LF to the left are thought to produce maximal compression forces to the spinal structures on the left. Flexion and LF to the left are thought to produce maximal tensile stresses to the spinal structures on the right. In addition to being used as a provocative test, combined movements may help to direct positioning during treatment. Intraexaminer reliability has been reported as high (ICC 0.79 to 0.93).[419] Interexaminer reliability and validity are unknown. Rotation can be added to the combined movements, but reliability is generally poor.[420] A detailed review of examination and intervention using combined movement in the lumbar spine is available by McCarthy.[421]

Lumbar Quadrant

The lumbar quadrant, a combined movement of extension, LF, and rotation to the same side (right and left compared) is theorized to result in maximal loading of spinal structures and narrowing of the intervertebral foramen on the side of LF and rotation and may be useful in ruling out pain originating from the lumbar spine. After establishing resting symptoms, the patient is instructed to first reach behind the uninvolved knee followed by comparison to the opposite side. OP may also be used. This test is considered very provocative (Sn 0.70)[422] but not specific (ie, unable to identify a specific structure).[423] In patients with symptomatic degenerative LBP, the quadrant was a strong predictor of clinically meaningful low back symptom severity, but not predictive of impaired function.[422]

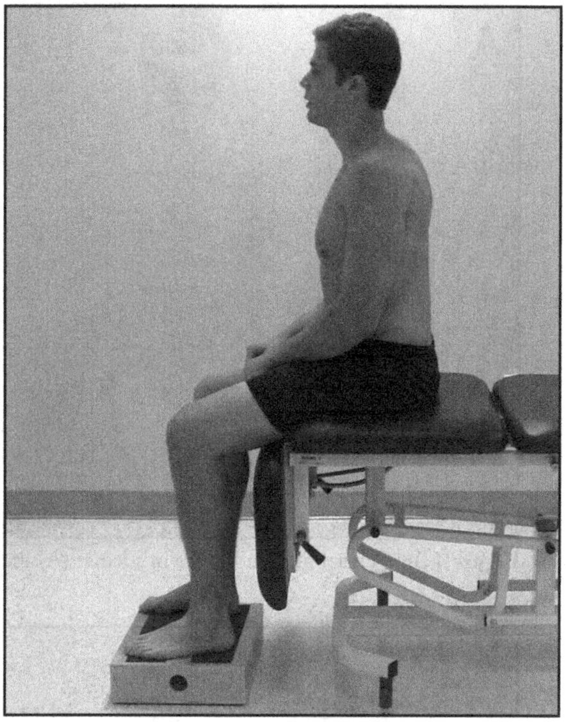

Figure 4-37. Sitting posture assessment—lateral view.

Examination Procedures in Sitting

- Sitting posture
- AROM: rotation as indicated with OP
- Neurological screening exam
- Slump test

Sitting Posture (Figure 4-37)

Observe the patient's ability to transition to sitting. The process of assessing sitting posture and the analysis of lumbopelvic upright, thoracic upright, and slump sitting postures on muscle activation patterns is detailed in Chapter 3. Support the patient's feet with hips at 80 degrees flexion. Note posture in anterior, posterior, and lateral views; correct if needed; and assess corrective effect on symptoms and determine the patient's ability to find neutral.

If asymmetry of pelvic bony landmarks is noted in standing, reassessment in sitting (Figure 4-38) may provide additional information since any contributions from a leg length discrepancy or lower extremity muscle length are lessened in the seated position. Asymmetry in standing that is no longer present in sitting may be related to the lower extremity or clinician error. Asymmetry in standing that remains in sitting may be structural or related to impairments in the lumbopelvic hip complex or clinician error.

Active Range of Motion: Rotation as Indicated With Overpressure (Figure 4-39)

Because a small amount of rotation is available in the lumbar spine, the need to assess rotation is often determined by the history or specific needs of the individual patient. A patient's report that activities involving rotation are provocative is an indication to assess rotation AROM. However, some clinicians routinely assess rotation. In comparison to rotation in standing, testing rotation in sitting serves to stabilize the pelvic girdle and lower extremities, but manual stabilization of the lower extremities may still be necessary. AROM is generally viewed posteriorly and anteriorly. OP is added if AROM is full range and symptom-free. With the patient's arms crossed, OP is provided by placing one hand on the posterior thorax and one hand on the anterior opposite shoulder.

Neurological Screening Exam

A neurological examination is required for all patients who exhibit LBP with symptoms extending below the gluteal folds, weakness, numbness, paresthesia, anesthesia, radicular pain, referred pain, a history of neurological deficit, or lower quarter symptoms of an unknown origin. Details from the history should indicate the need for an upper motor neuron, lower motor neuron, or cranial nerve examination. Procedures for testing sensation, MMTs, and deep tendon reflexes (DTRs) for the lower extremity are discussed in Chapter 3.

Slump Test

The purpose of the slump test[424,425] is to test neurodynamics of neuromeningeal structures in the vertebral canal and intervertebral foramina[426,427] and mobility of the peripheral nervous system of the lower extremity in subjects with spinal and lower limb pain.[425] Philip et al[428]

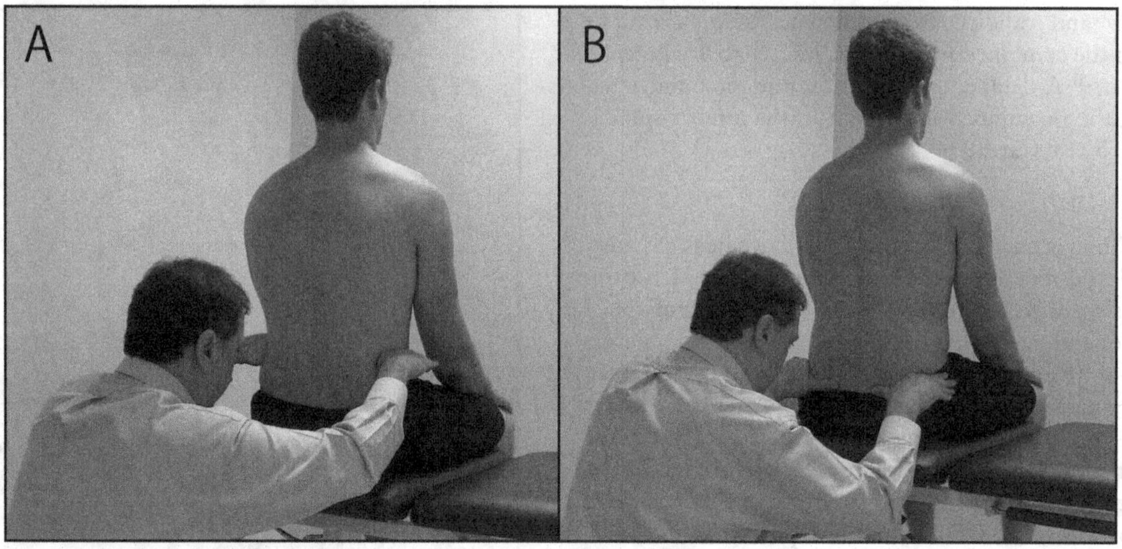

Figure 4-38. Pelvic bony landmarks in sitting: (A) iliac crest and (B) PSIS.

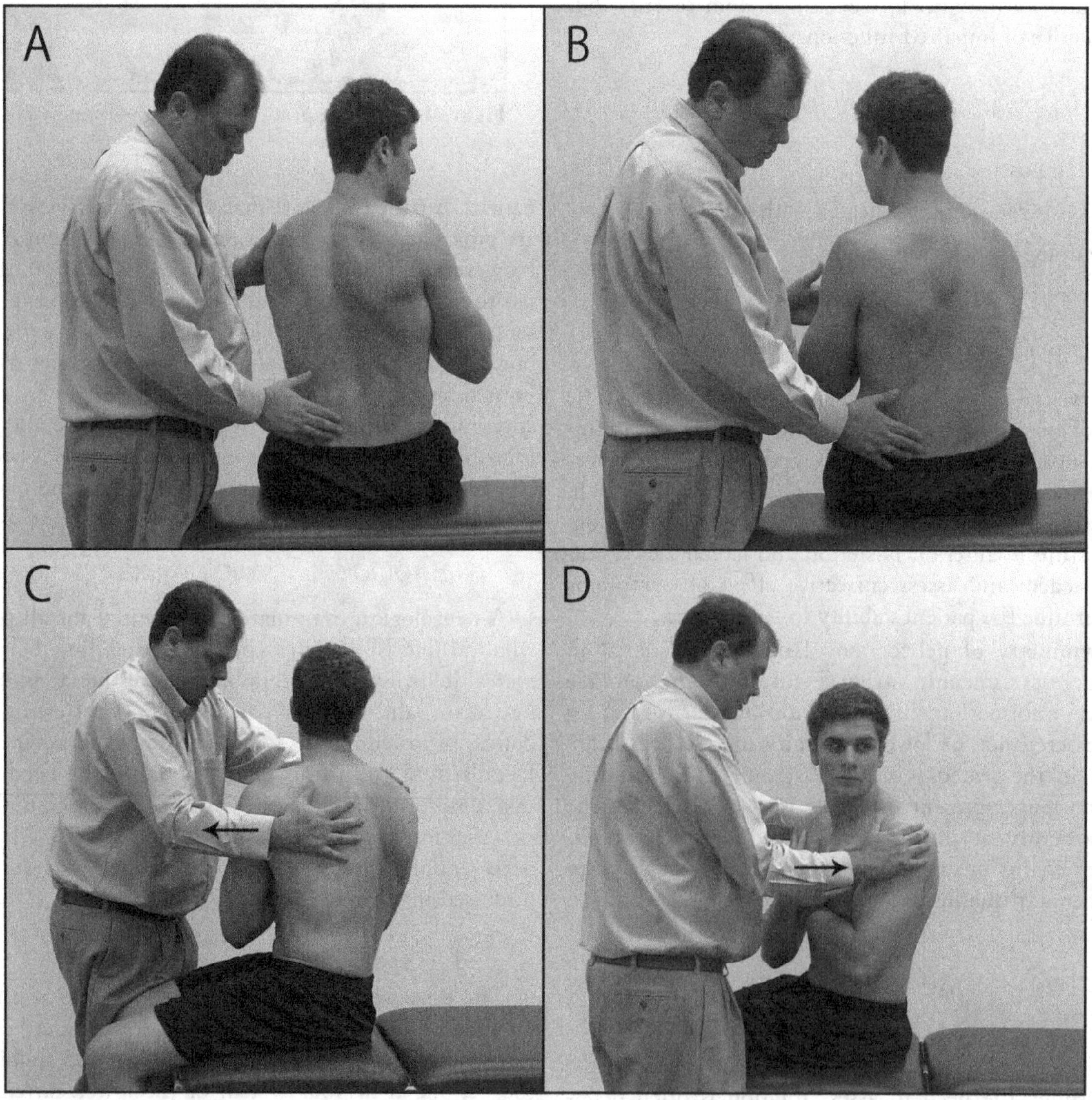

Figure 4-39. AROM—rotation in sitting. (A) right rotation; (B) left rotation; (C) right rotation with OP; and (D) left rotation with OP.

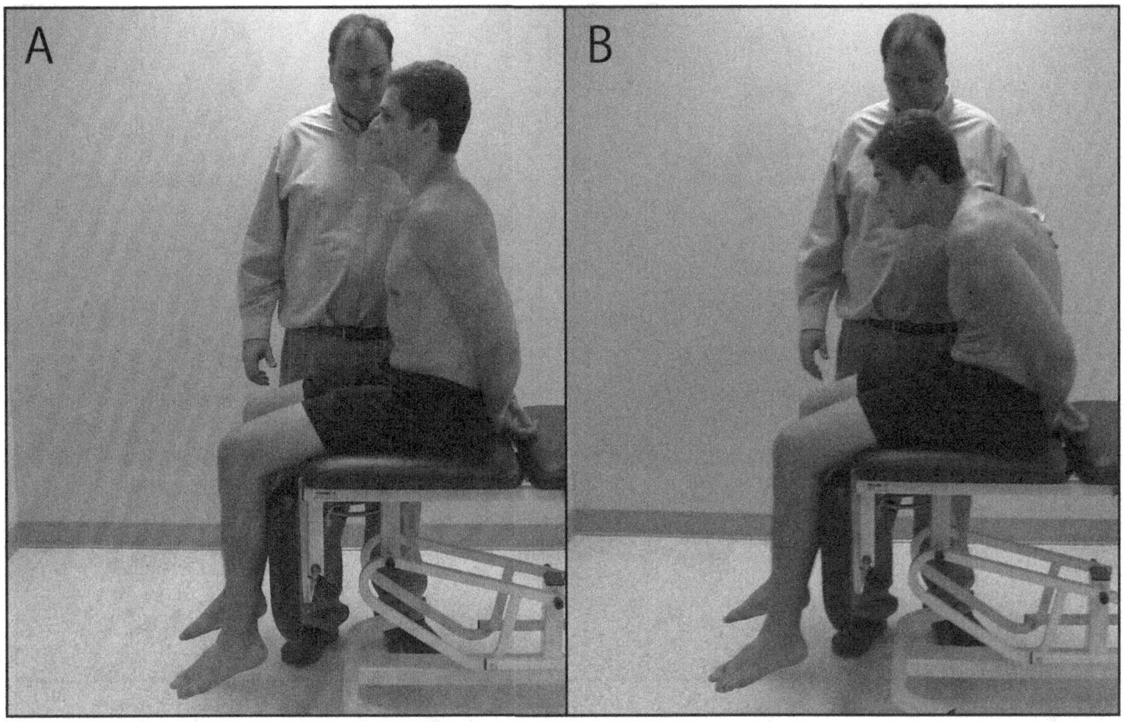

Figure 4-40. Slump test. (A) Patient sitting with thighs fully supported, knees together, and hands linked behind back. Establish resting symptoms. Begin with uninvolved side. (B) Ask the patient to slump, but do not allow neck flexion; assess response. *(continued)*

found that the slump test demonstrated high interrater reliability (κ = 0.83) among physical therapists with varied experience. Coppieters et al[429] demonstrated that pain of nonneural origin (ie, experimentally induced) was not exacerbated by the slump tests. The authors suggest that the results of their study support the use of neurodynamic tests (NDT) including slump in the identification of altered neurodynamics. Majlesi et al[430] reported good diagnostic accuracy for the slump test: Sn 0.84 (0.74 to 0.90), Sp 0.83 (0.73 to 0.90), +LR 4.94, –LR 0.19 in patients with and without lumbar disc herniations on MRI. Evidence for diagnostic utility in the differentiation between neural and nonneural structures is limited.

Test Procedure

Care is required at each step to assess the range of movement, quality of movement, and symptom response. The sequence of test procedures is generally standardized as described next, but may vary.[424,425] If symptoms are produced at any step in the procedure, the clinician attempts to differentiate between neural and nonneural structures by assessing the patient's response to the release of neck flexion (Figure 4-40).

- *Patient position*: Patient is sitting with thighs fully supported, knees together, and hands behind back.
- *Therapist position*: Therapist is standing beside patient and begins with uninvolved side.
- *Step 1*: Explain procedure and establish resting symptoms.
- *Step 2*: Ask patient to slump, but do not allow neck flexion; assess response.
- *Step 3*: Gently overpress thoracic/lumbar spine maintaining sacrum vertical; assess response.
- *Step 4*: Add active neck flexion, then OP; assess response.
- *Step 5*: Add active left knee extension; assess response of uninvolved side.
- *Step 6*: Add active left ankle dorsiflexion (DF); assess response. If no response at this step, add hip flexion, which is generally not required; assess response.
- *Step 7*: Repeat steps 5 and 6 with right leg (involved side).
- *Step 8*: Repeat steps 5 and 6 with both legs as needed.
- *Step 9*: When symptoms are reproduced, release neck flexion; assess response. If symptoms decrease or disappear, increase the range of the limited side until symptoms are once again reproduced.

Positive Slump Test

A positive slump test[424,425] occurs when the test results in 3 responses:

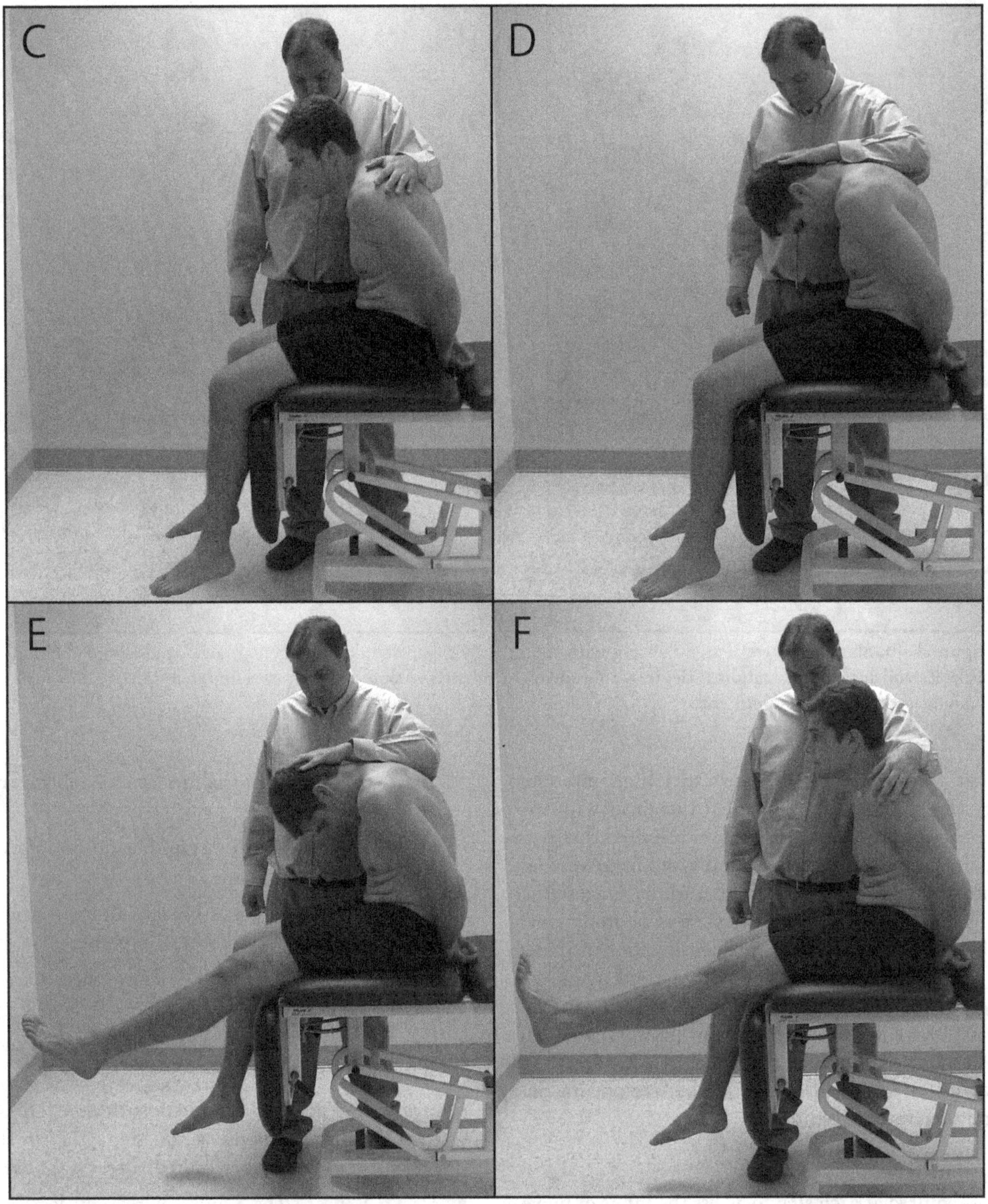

Figure 4-40 (continued). Slump test. (C) Gently overpress thoracic/lumbar spine, maintaining sacrum vertical; assess response. (D) Add active neck flexion, then OP; assess response. (E) Add active left knee extension; assess response of uninvolved side. Add active left ankle DF; assess response. If no response at this step, add hip flexion, which is generally not required; assess response. Repeat from knee extension with the involved side. (F) When symptoms are reproduced, release neck flexion; assess response.

1. Reproduction of the patient's symptoms
2. Asymmetry between uninvolved to involved sides
3. A positive sensitizing maneuver (ie, release of neck flexion) altering symptoms helps to differentiate between neural and nonneural structures. A sensitizing maneuver is movement at a site distant to the location of symptoms that attempts to preferentially load neural tissue without placing stress on other tissues that could be related to the production of symptoms.

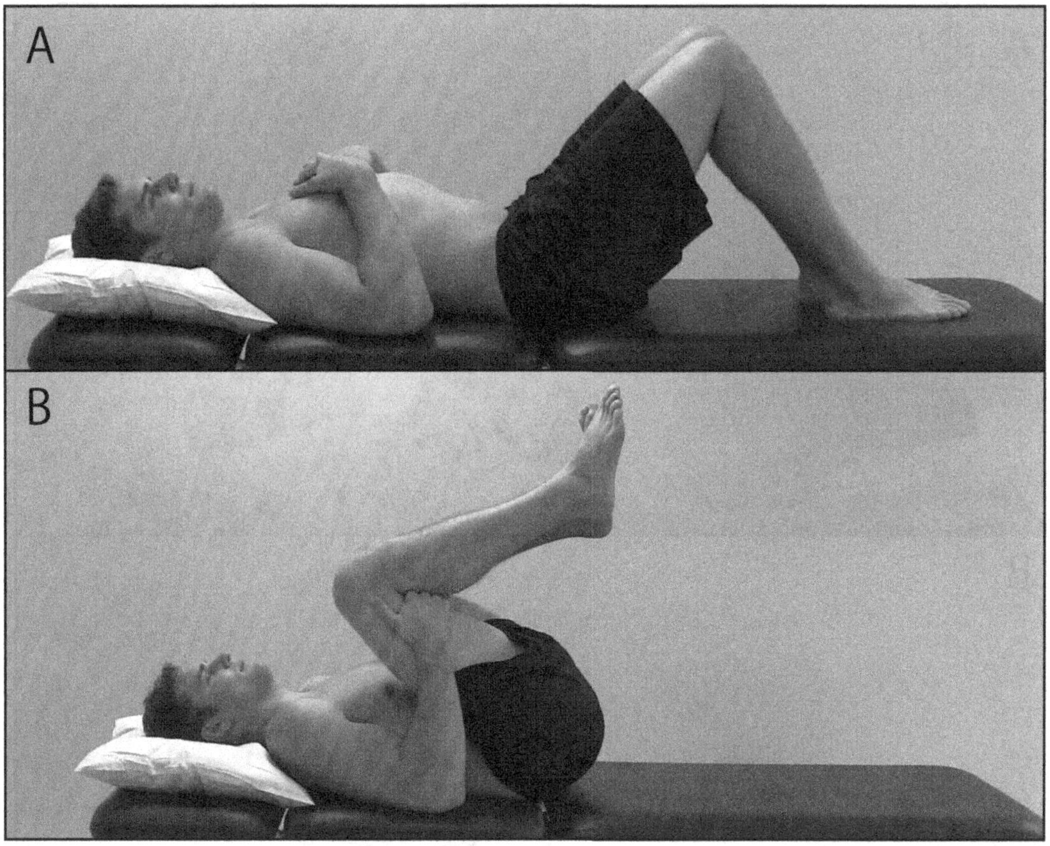

Figure 4-41. RFIL: (A) Start position and (B) flexion in lying.

Normal Responses to the Slump Test in Asymptomatic Subjects[425,426]

- Pain or discomfort in the mid-thoracic area on trunk and neck flexion
- Pain or discomfort behind knees in hamstrings in the trunk/neck flexion/knee extension position increased with the addition of ankle DF
- Some restriction of ankle DF in the trunk/neck flexion position
- Some restriction of ankle DF in the trunk/neck flexion/knee extension position; the restriction should be symmetrical
- A decrease in pain other than the patient's symptoms in one or more areas with release of neck flexion
- An increase in range of knee extension and/or ankle DF with release of neck flexion

Examination Procedures in Supine

Observe the ability to transition to supine and resting posture in supine:

- RFIL
- SLR
- Active SLR (ASLR)
- Palpation: iliac crest, ASIS, pubic tubercle symmetry; hip, abdomen as needed
- Hip, knee, and ankle examination for LBP as indicated by the history
- Muscle length tests
- Trunk muscle performance
- Special tests: sacroiliac joint (SIJ) provocation tests

Repeated Flexion in Lying[401,402]

The clinician should observe the patient's transition to supine and note the symptom response. Resting posture in supine is also observed for provocative and easing positions. If RFIL is tested, resting symptoms are obtained first. In supine hook-lying with the feet flat on the table, the patient grasps and pulls both knees to produce maximum lumbar flexion and then returns to the start position (Figure 4-41).[401,402]

Some differences are noted between RFIS and RFIL.[401,402] In severe cases, RFIS may be more difficult, possibly due to the effects of gravity. Segmental lumbar motion during RFIS occurs from proximal to distal, whereas in RFIL, the motion occurs from distal to proximal, possibly causing increased tension of lower lumbar segments more quickly than RFIS. RFIS where knees are extended places more tension on the lumbosacral nerve roots than RFIL where the knees are flexed. Symptoms

Figure 4-42. SLR. (A) SLR without sensitization and (B) SLR plus DF. *(continued)*

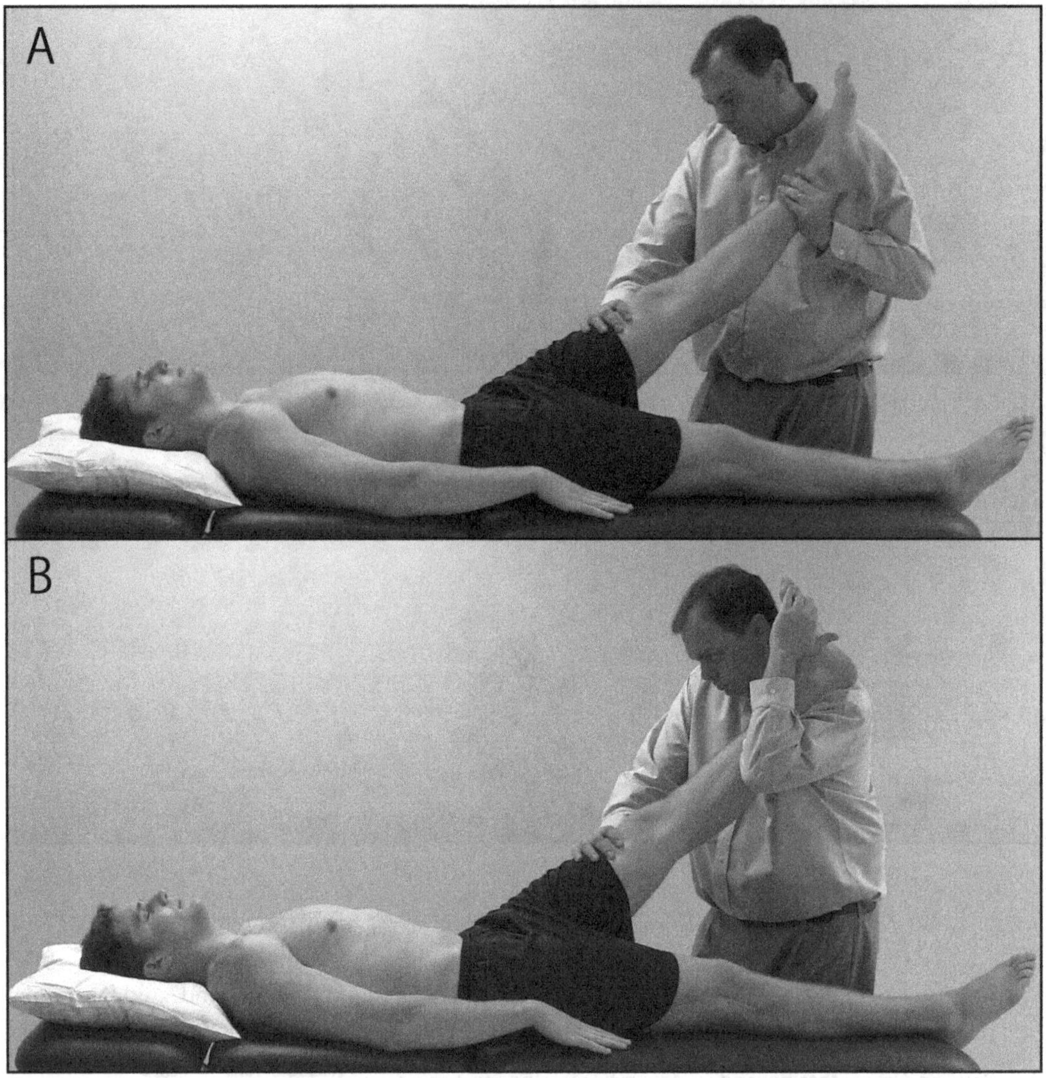

aggravated by RFIS may be caused by stress to both non-neural structures or neural neurodynamics, but symptoms aggravated by RFIL are most likely caused only by nonneural structures because the neural structures are on slack (ie, the hips and knees are flexed).[401,402] The repeated movements are tested as described under RFIS with potential responses listed as follows[401,402]:

- If centralization or DP, classify as DSE (ie flexion subgroup) and proceed to matched intervention (ie, RFIL).
- If peripheralization, examine with repeated extension in attempts to centralize.
- If failure to centralize, additional testing is necessary.
- If the response is limited motion and end-range pain (ie, produced, increased, or no worse) with RFIL and no centralization or peripheralization occur, further examination is needed. The clinician considers a classification of LBP with mobility deficits (see Table 4-1).

Straight Leg Raise

The passive SLR (Figure 4-42) is the most widely used NDT indicated for patients presenting with LBP and LBP-related leg pain. The test is traditionally performed to tension the sciatic nerve to aid in the diagnosis of nerve root compression of the lower lumbar (L4 to S1) nerve roots due to lumbar disc herniation, or to determine if there is mechanosensitivity of nerve roots or the sciatic nerve. The test causes traction on the sciatic nerve, lumbosacral nerve roots (primarily L4 to S1), and dura mater.[431,432] The reliability of ROM measurements during SLR testing is high with ICC values between 0.87 to 0.96 when an inclinometer is used.[348] Kappa values for a dichotomous judgment of the SLR as either positive or negative is high (κ = 0.66 to 0.83).[433,434]

The ipsilateral SLR test is reported to be highly sensitive with a low –LR. The contralateral SLR is reported to be highly specific with a larger +LR, but lower sensitivity values. A systematic review[435] of the accuracy of the

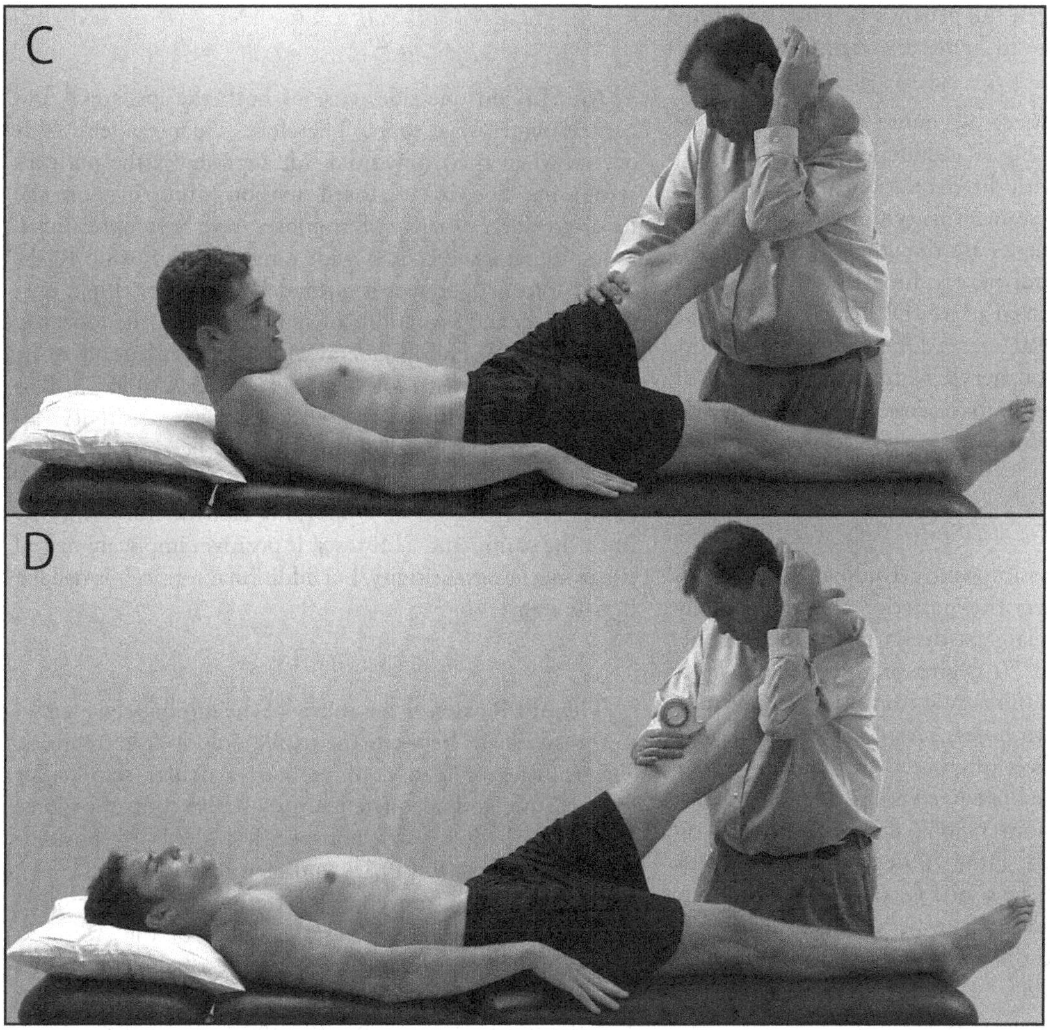

Figure 4-42 (continued). SLR. (C) SLR plus DF and neck flexion and (D) SLR plus DF with inclinometer.

ipsilateral SLR test in diagnosing herniated disks reveals a pooled estimate of Sn 0.91 (0.82, 0.94), Sp 0.26 (0.16, 0.38), +LR 1.23, and –LR 0.35. The pooled estimate for the contralateral SLR reveals Sn 0.29 (0.24, 0.34), Sp 0.88 (0.86, 0.90), +LR 2.42, and –LR 0.81. The absence of an ipsilateral SLR is, therefore, useful for ruling out a diagnosis of disc herniation, while a positive contralateral SLR is supportive of a diagnosis related to disc herniation.

Poor diagnostic accuracy of the SLR test is because the SLR could be positive for reasons other than mechanical effects of disk herniation or nerve compression. Many structures such as the lumbar spine, hip joints, muscles, and neural tissue are moved with the passive SLR. Though a positive SLR finding of pain and limitation of movement theoretically may be caused by the presence of a symptomatic disc, the mechanosensitivity of neural tissue may be due to inflammatory chemicals leaking from the disk rather than direct nerve root compression. Pain responses may be due to increased sensitivity rather than nerve compression. However, research into the use of the SLR as a test of neural tissue mechanosensitivity is lacking.

Test Procedure

The uninvolved side is tested first.

- Position the patient supine, pillow under head only if necessary.
- PT places one hand under ankle and other hand above knee.
- Passively lift into hip flexion, maintaining hip-neutral knee extension, until symptoms are produced or significant resistance, whichever comes first, is reached.
- Note onset of resistance, hip flexion angle, and symptoms. An inclinometer may be zeroed on the proximal tibial crest to measure hip flexion angle (see Figure 4-42). Average ROM of the left and right sides exceeding 91 degrees is a key factor in a preliminary CPR to determine whether a patient will benefit from a lumbopelvic stabilization program (see Table 4-2).[405] The SLR demonstrated good interrater reliability (ICC 0.87 to 0.96).[436]

- Distinguish between the patient's familiar symptoms and symptoms due to hamstring tightness, which is not a positive test.
- The SLR is sensitized (ie, more tension added) by adding ankle DF, hip IR, adduction (ADD), or neck flexion to assist with differentiation between somatic versus a neural source of symptoms. Additional sensitizing movements are thought to bias the lower extremity peripheral nerves: hip IR adds tension to the common peroneal nerve; DF with eversion adds tension to the tibial nerve; DF with inversion adds tension to the sural nerve; plantarflexion (PF) with inversion adds tension to the common peroneal nerve; and PF with eversion adds tension to the saphenous nerve.[437,438]

Ipsilateral Straight Leg Raise Positive Test

Historically, the classic positive finding is a response of radicular pain down the posterior thigh below the knee when the clinician passively raises the straight leg to between 30 and 70 degrees of hip flexion. From 0 to 35 degrees, dural and sciatic nerve slack is taken up and usually not positive unless severe acute pathology is present. Clinically, this is often seen in a patient who is unable to straighten the knee in standing or supine due to LBP-related leg pain. From 35 to 70 degrees, tension in the sciatic nerve is increased. From 70 degrees and higher, no further deformation of the sciatic nerve occurs. Symptoms after 70+ degrees are thought to be related to loading of other structures such as the hamstrings, gluteals, hip, lumbar spine, or pelvic girdle.

A positive test is described as follows:

- Reproduction of the patient's familiar symptoms reproduced between 30 and 70 degrees or less of hip flexion
- Limited motion compared to the uninvolved side
- Altered symptoms with a sensitizing maneuver

A sensitizing maneuver is movement at a site distant to the location of symptoms that attempts to preferentially load neural tissue without placing stress on other tissues that could be related to the production of symptoms. For example (see Figure 4-42), a positive SLR at 45 degrees that produces buttock and mid-posterior thigh pain is sensitized by adding ankle DF. If the symptoms are increased, neural tissue mechanosensitivity is implicated. If the symptoms do not change, neural tissue mechanosensitivity is excluded. A positive SLR may support a hypothesis of LBP with lower extremity referred pain (see Table 4-3) and a subclassification of LBP-related leg pain (see Table 4-6) due to lumbosacral, neural tissue mechanosensitivity. A negative test may exclude mechanosensitivity and implicate somatic referred leg pain.[439]

Contralateral, Crossed, or Well-Leg Straight Leg Raise Positive Test

An SLR on one side tensions both the ipsilateral and contralateral nerve roots. Therefore, a contralateral SLR occurs when the uninvolved side reproduces the patient's symptoms due to increased tension occurring on the involved side. A variety of responses have been observed in asymptomatic subjects. A wide range of hip flexion ROM from 50 to 120 degrees is normal.[440] Posterior thigh, posterior knee, and posterior calf symptoms into the foot may be normal.[441] The ipsilateral SLR has been found to be highly sensitive with low –LRs. The contralateral SLR is highly specific with a larger +LR but lower sensitivity values. The absence of an ipsilateral SLR is therefore useful for excluding a diagnosis of disk herniation, while a positive contralateral SLR is an important confirmatory finding. Both the slump and SLR tests, if positive, implicate neural tissue mechanosensitivity, but additional research is needed in this area.[439]

Active Straight Leg Raise

The ASLR assesses the ability of the lumbopelvic region to transfer loads between the trunk and lower extremities. The transfer of load requires both articular stability or form closure and adequate neuromuscular control or force closure.[442] Patients with nonspecific LBP,[443-447] postpartum pelvic pain (PPPP),[448] and sacroiliac disorders[442,449] show changes in movement patterns and force closure during the ASLR. Test-retest reliability of the ASLR in women with PPPP is ICC 0.83. The best balance between specificity (0.94) and sensitivity (0.87) occurs when scores 1 to 10 are designated as positive and 0 as negative.[450] The ASLR is able to discriminate between patients who are disabled by PPPP and healthy subjects. The ASLR test is also reliable in patients with nonspecific LBP.[451] The ASLR test has good predictive validity for identifying patients with PPPP associated with asymmetric SIJ laxity.[452]

Test Procedure

The ASLR test (Figure 4-43)[450] is performed in supine with the legs straight and feet 20 cm apart. The patient is asked to raise one leg at a time 20 cm (7.9 inches) above the table without bending the knee and asked to score the amount of effort needed to raise the leg on a 6-point scale: not difficult at all = 0; minimally difficult = 1; somewhat difficult = 2; fairly difficult = 3; very difficult = 4; unable to do = 5. The scores of both sides are added, resulting in a summed score from 0 to 10. A score of 1 or higher reported by the patient is considered a positive test. The ASLR is then repeated with manual or belt compression through the ilia, and any change in effort or pain is noted. The clinician observes for poor motor control strategies such as breath holding, thoracolumbar rotation, and pelvic rotation to stabilize the thorax, low back, and pelvis. A positive test suggests a lack of dynamic stabilization and impaired load transfer.[351,450]

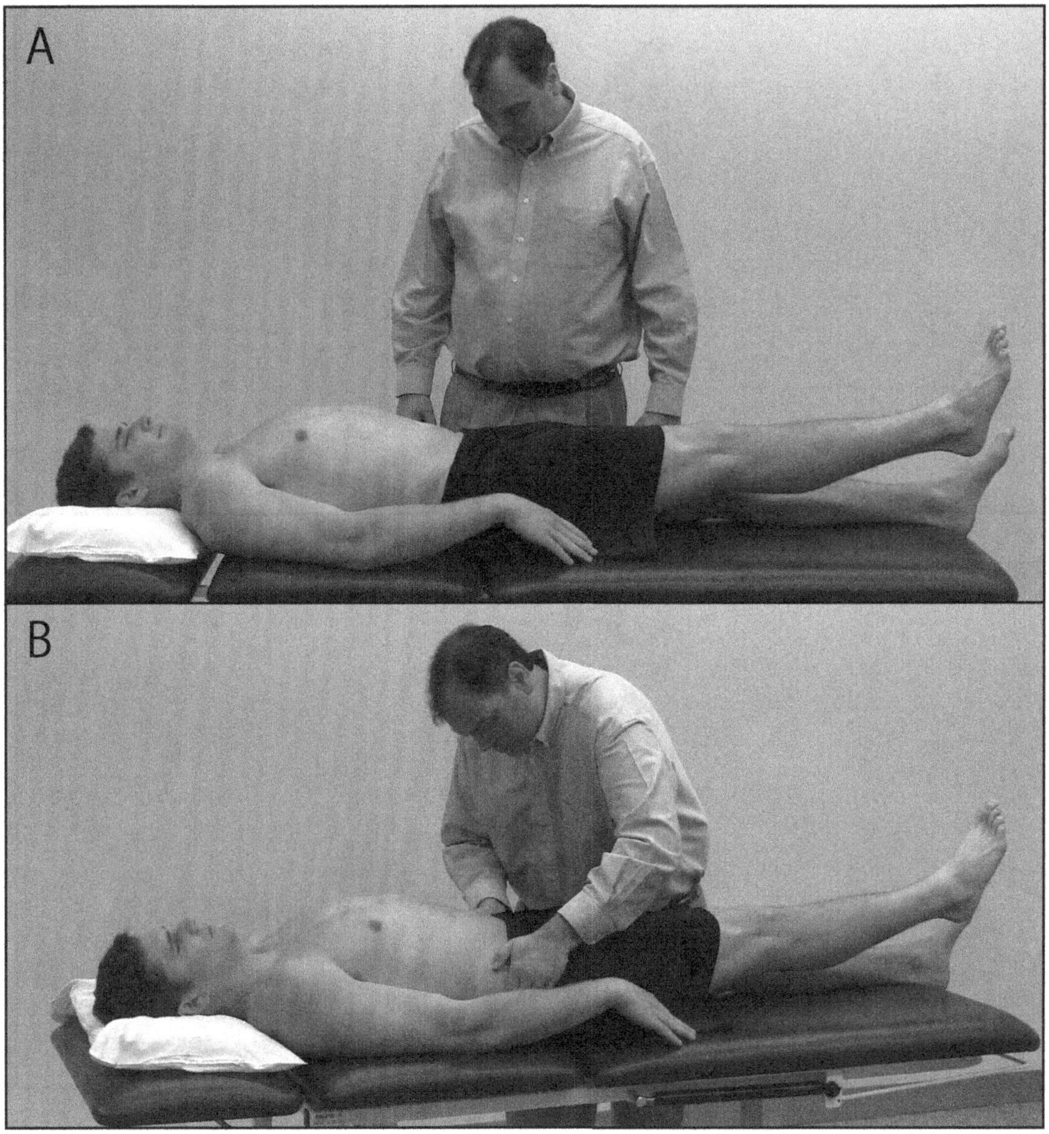

Figure 4-43. ASLR: (A) observation without pelvic compression and (B) with manual pelvic compression at the ASIS bilaterally.

Positive Test

Using both global and local muscles, healthy subjects should be able to lift a straight leg in nonweightbearing without effort, without movement of the pelvis, without pain, and with a normal breathing pattern.[453] During the ASLR, the pelvis should not move (ie, no flexion, extension, LF, or rotation should occur) relative to the lumbar spine, thorax, and/or lower extremity. Breathing should remain normal. The rib cage should not move in or out excessively, suggesting overactive external obliques or internal obliques, respectively, that may limit lateral rib cage expansion with inspiration. If the thoracic spine extends, overactivation or stabilization using the ES is suspected.[453] The use of a pelvic belt has been shown to reduce the effort needed to lift the leg for patients with PGP.[448] In some patients, anterior rotation of the ilium on the side of the raised leg is observed.[448] Altered kinematics of the diaphragm and pelvic floor area has been noted during the ASLR compared to healthy subjects.[449] Diaphragmatic motion is decreased during the ASLR, suggesting a splinting or bracing action. A significant drop of the PF indicates reduced tension in the PF muscles (PFM). Manual iliac compression has been shown to normalized diaphragmatic and PF motion.[449] In subjects with a positive ASLR, de Groot et al[454] demonstrated significantly more muscle activity in the hip flexors, hip adductors, and external oblique but a reduced force output compared to controls, suggesting that the ASLR is related to muscle function for load transfer over the pelvic region.

In some patients, manual compression may make it harder to lift the leg, suggesting that excessive compression may be present.[351] Additional examination may be needed to determine the cause of the excessive compression and whether it is related to an overactivation of the superficial system or excessive form closure (ie, mobility deficits), suggesting that stabilization exercise is most likely not

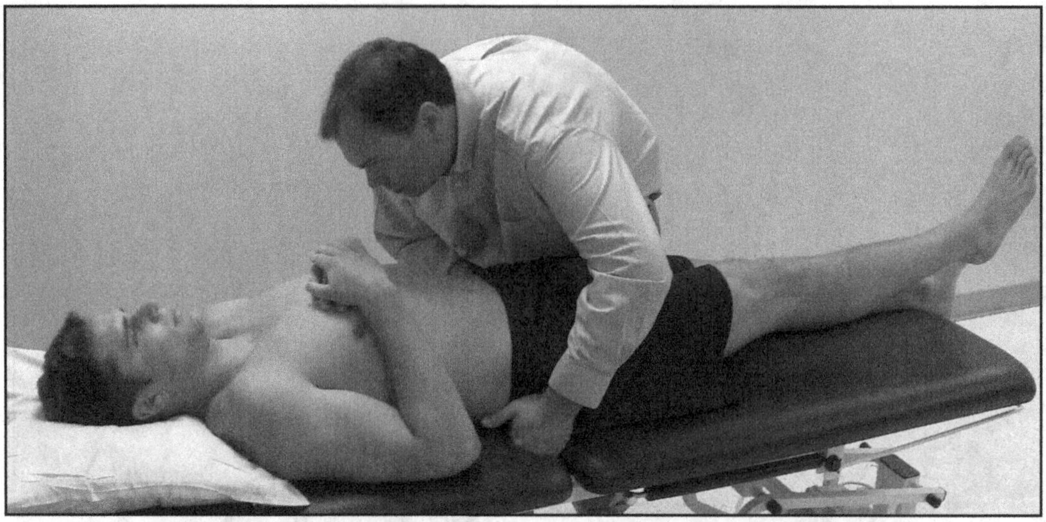

Figure 4-44. ASLR with posterior compression at the level of the PSIS bilaterally.

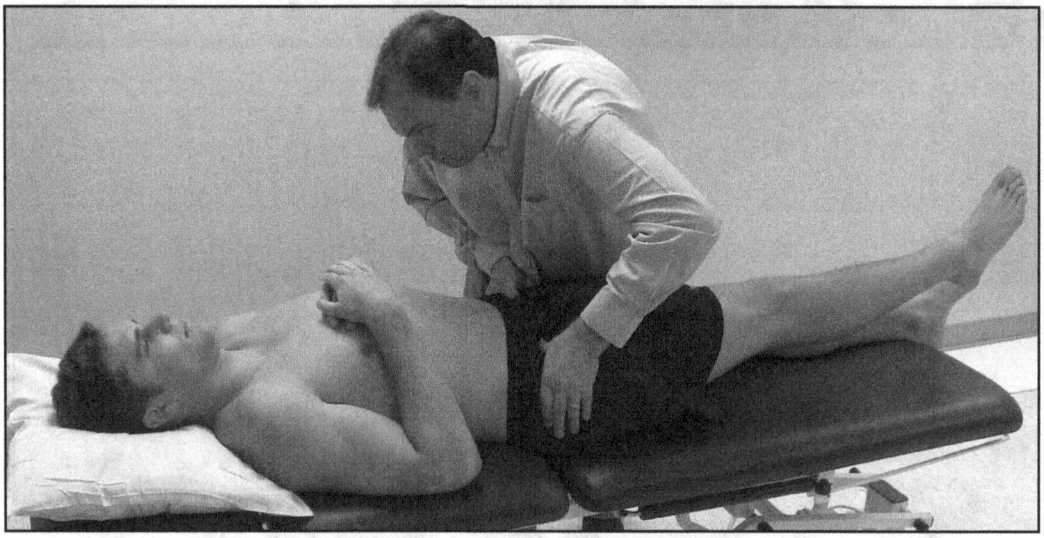

Figure 4-45. ASLR with anterior compression at the level of the PS bilaterally.

appropriate under these circumstances. Reassessment of the ASLR should occur after intervention (ie, mobilization, manipulation or relaxation of the superficial system) for the excessive compression.[351]

Theoretically, the site of manual compression can be varied to guide further examination of the trunk muscles and determine which muscles require training to provide optimal stabilization.[351,453] As an example, if compression anteriorly at the level of the ASISs (see Figure 4-43B) reduces the effort required to lift the leg, then the patient is asked to activate the TrA prior to performing the ASLR. If the effort to lift the leg is reduced, the hypothesis of impairment in TrA activation is supported and specific TrA training is indicated.[453] Theoretically, anterior compression of the pelvis at the level of the ASISs simulates the force produced by contraction of TrA, anterior abdominal fascia, and internal oblique; compression of the posterior pelvis at the level of the PSISs (Figure 4-44) simulates that of the sacral multifidus (MF) and thoracodorsal fascia; and anterior compression at the level of the PS (Figure 4-45) simulates the action of the anterior PF, TrA, and internal oblique.[351] Simultaneous compression can be applied to one side anteriorly and the opposite side posteriorly for further analysis.[351,454]

Teyhen et al[455] compared bilateral ultrasound images of the TrA and internal oblique during an ASLR in subjects with unilateral lumbopelvic pain and age-matched controls. The control group demonstrated a 23.7% increase in the TrA width and 11.2% increase in the internal oblique width of muscle thickness, while the unilateral lumbopelvic pain group demonstrated only a 6.4% increase in the TrA and a 5.7% increase in the internal oblique. During the ASLR, both the TrA and the internal oblique respond symmetrically regardless of which lower extremity is lifted or if there is unilateral pain. These results provide potential construct validity of the ASLR to assess varying motor control strategies of the TrA and internal oblique in subjects with unilateral lumbopelvic pain. Training of the TrA has been shown to enhance the functional stability of the pelvis.[446]

Palpation

Palpation in supine includes any area of the patient's symptoms and varies from patient to patient. These areas or structures might include the iliac crest, ASIS, PS, anterior hip or groin, and abdomen. For the abdominal area, general inspection, observation of breathing patterns, palpation, percussion, and auscultation procedures may be needed.[456] Abdominal musculature is generally palpable through overlying soft tissue.

Begin at the iliac crests and move anteriorly to the ASIS, looking for symmetry. By flexing and abducting the hip, attachments of the rectus femoris and tensor fascia lata to the ASIS become easily palpable. With the thumbs on the ASIS, the fingers will reach to the lateral aspect of the thigh for palpation of the greater trochanter and gluteus medius. From the ASIS to the pubic tubercle on each side, palpate the inguinal ligament and PS. The superior border of the femoral triangle is the inguinal ligament. Below the inguinal ligament is medial border of the adductor longus and lateral border of the sartorius. Within the femoral triangle, from lateral to medial, are the femoral nerve, femoral artery with a palpable pulse, femoral vein, and lymph nodes.

Hip, Knee, and Ankle Examination for Low Back Pain as Indicated by the History

The history and working diagnoses dictate the extent and need for examination of the hip, knee, or ankle and foot. For example, a hip examination is needed to aid in differentiating a primary hip problem from nonspecific LBP or to determine the presence of problems in both regions. Common pain patterns for hip joint problems include anterior, lateral, or posterior hip pain and groin pain with referral down the anterior medial thigh to the medial knee. The hip must be examined because of overlap in referral patterns from the lumbar spine, pelvic girdle, and hip regions.

Given the anatomical and biomechanical relationships, the hip joint is a possible contributor to LBP and should be assessed in all patients presenting with LBP. In comparing subjects with and without LBP, several studies[457-461] reported deficits in hip ROM, hip extensor strength in female athletes,[462] and hip adductor or hip flexor endurance[463] in subjects with LBP. Additionally, emerging evidence supports a regional interdependence relationship between impairments at the hip and persons with LBP.[457-466] In the diagnostic classification of patients with LBP, the presence of IR greater than 35 degrees in 1 or both hips increased the likelihood of benefiting from manipulation of the lumbopelvic region (see Table 4-1).[140,141] Patients with an average SLR > 91 degrees are more likely to experience reduced disability at 8 weeks from a lumbar stabilization program (see Table 4-2).[197]

Given the current evidence, a detailed hip examination should be considered within the first 3 sessions for patients with LBP. Identifying potential impairments local to the low back or remote such as hip, knee, ankle or foot that may contribute or perpetuate a patient's primary concern of LBP are important. In the absence of research identifying a subgroup of patients with LBP who might benefit from treatment aimed at the hip and lower extremity, clinicians must utilize clinical reasoning, clinical expertise, and current best evidence to make decisions to prioritize an impairment-based approach to treatment of the lower extremity.

The following section does not include a comprehensive examination of the hip, knee, and ankle/foot. The clinician must decide on the level of examination for the first session as a means to implicate or rule out each region. The patient's response to selected procedures dictates the need for a more detailed examination at subsequent visits. Clinical practice guidelines related to hip pain and mobility deficits provide detailed evidence-based information related to examination and intervention.[466]

Hip Region Examination

The initial examination of the hip, knee, and ankle/foot varies based on the subjective findings for each person. A screening examination may include functional tests, AROM/PROM with OP, passive accessory movement tests, muscle performance tests, and certain special tests to assist in implicating the lower extremity as a contributor to the patient's main LBP problem. For example, a preliminary study[467] revealed 5 predictors of hip osteoarthritis (OA):

1. Pain aggravated with squatting
2. Lateral or anterior hip pain with the scour test
3. Active hip flexion causing lateral hip pain
4. Pain with active hip extension
5. Passive range of hip IR less than 25 degrees

The diagnostic utility for hip OA when all 5 variables were present was Sn 0.14 (0.04, 0.37), Sp 0.98 (0.88, 1.0), +LR 7.3 (1.1, 49.1), –LR 0.87 (0.73, 1.1).[467] Additional studies are needed to validate these results. Similarly, the American College of Rheumatology classified persons with symptomatic hip OA by: hip IR < 15 degrees, hip flexion < 115 degrees and age > 50; or hip IR > 15 degrees, pain with IR, morning stiffness < 60 minutes, and age > 50.[468] When compared to radiographs, the following properties were reported: Sn 0.86, Sp 0.75, +LR 3.44, and –LR 0.19.[468] Other diagnostic classifications are considered for examination findings that do not fit these criteria.

- **Functional tests of the hip:** Squat, step-up, lunge (Figure 4-46), stair climbing, and sit-to-stand are the common functional tests discussed previously. Activities that are important to the patient should be assessed when appropriate.

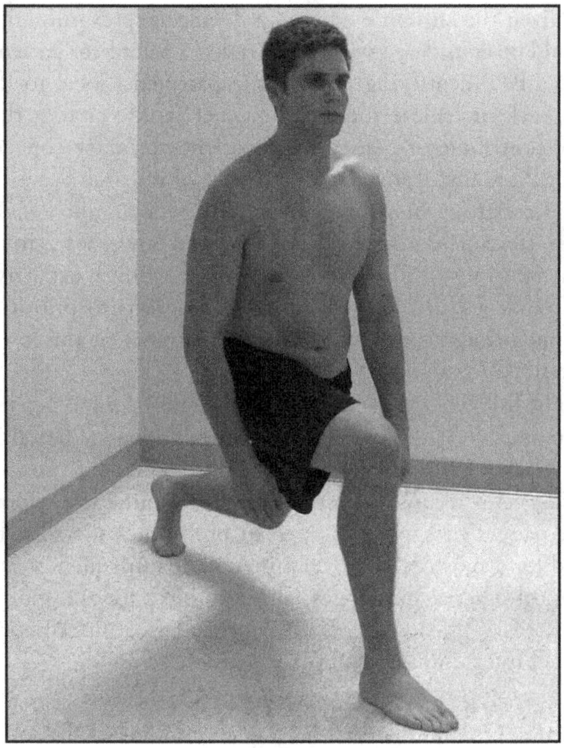

Figure 4-46. Functional tests: lunge.

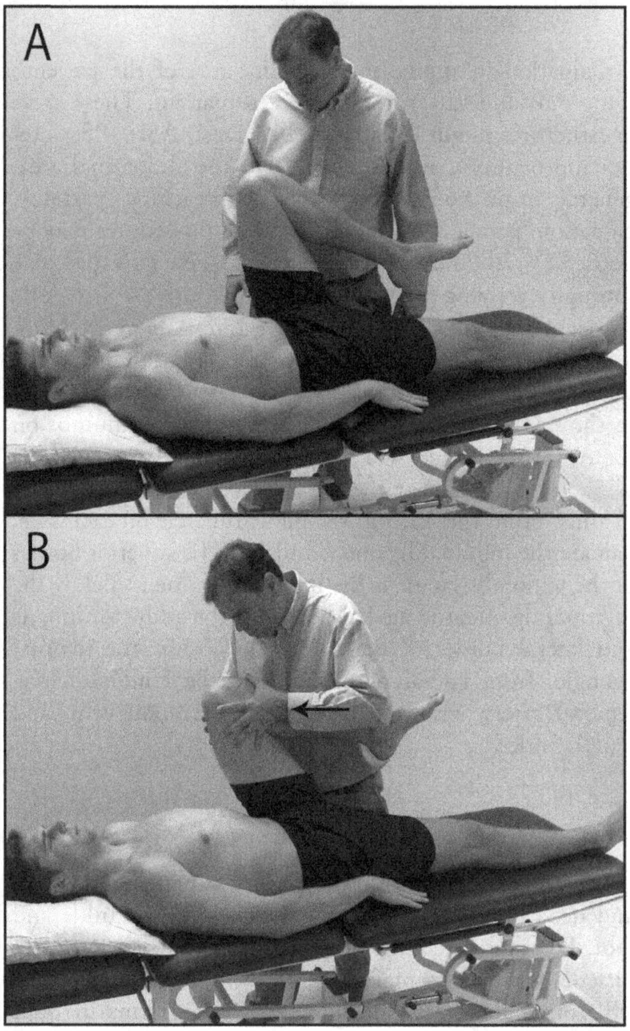

Figure 4-47. AROM: (A) hip flexion and (B) hip flexion with OP.

- **Hip AROM and PROM with OP:** Cardinal plane movements of flexion, extension, IR, ER, abduction (ABD), and ADD are commonly tested, observing the quality, quantity, and symptom response. All movements should be qualitatively assessed for optimal trunk control strategies. Nonoptimal trunk and pelvic control may result in an apparent weakness. Optimal trunk and pelvic control is generally demonstrated by maintenance of a neutral lumbar spine and pelvis and no breath holding. Loss of spinal segmental control such as hinging into extension or flexion or loss of pelvic control on either side should not occur. When performing OP, the clinician stabilizes the pelvis appropriately to prevent unwanted motion of the spine. Keeping in mind whether the patient should move as far as he or she can or only to the onset or increase of baseline symptoms, AROM or PROM instructions to the patient are simple, but variable:
  - *Flexion* (supine; Figure 4-47): Ask the patient to bring the knee up toward the chest; if full range and no symptoms, add OP; or the clinician passively performs hip flexion.
  - *IR* (sitting, supine, prone; Figure 4-48): In sitting with the hip in 90 degrees of flexion and 0 degrees ABD or ADD, ask the patient to bring the foot up and out; OP is applied as indicated. With the hip in the same position in supine, ask the patient to turn the foot out toward the side; or the clinician passively performs IR with OP. Alternatively, IR and ER can be assessed in prone with the hip in neutral flexion, ABD, and ADD.
  - *ER* (sitting, supine, or prone; Figure 4-49): In sitting with the hip in 90 degrees of flexion and 0 degrees ABD or ADD, ask the patient to bring the foot up and in; OP is applied as indicated. With the hip in the same position in supine, ask the patient to turn the foot in toward the midline; or the clinician passively performs ER with OP.
  - *ABD/ADD* (supine; Figure 4-50): The patient actively abducts or slides the leg away or adducts toward midline. With the pelvis stabilized, the clinician passively moves through the range of ABD or ADD; OP is applied as indicated.
  - *Extension* (prone; Figure 4-51): With the knee extended, the patient raises the leg off the table; OP may be applied if the lumbar spine, pelvis,

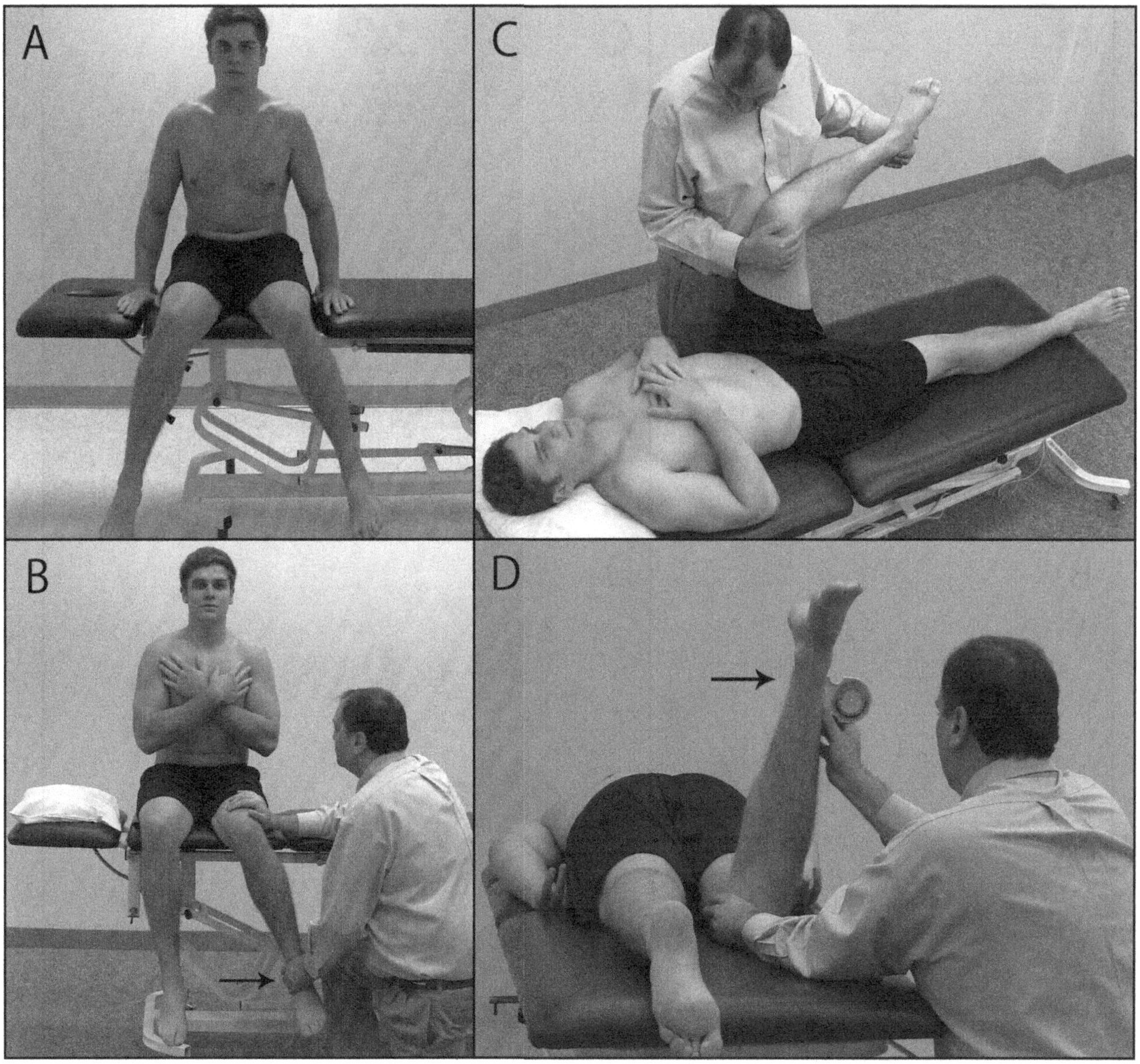

Figure 4-48. AROM hip IR: (A) sitting: AROM IR bilaterally; (B) sitting: IR with OP; (C) supine: IR with OP; and (D) prone: IR with inclinometer.

and hip are controlled. The clinician stabilizes the pelvis at the PSIS or ischial tuberosity, grasps the distal thigh with the knee extended or flexed, and passively moves the hip into extension; OP is added as indicated.

- **ROM measurement of the hip (Figure 4-52):** Measurements of hip ROM using a goniometer[467,469] or inclinometer[467] have sufficient reliability in persons with hip OA. Pua et al[469] reported the following for ROM measurements: ICC from 0.86 to 0.97 and standard error of the mean (SEM) from 3.1 to 4.7 degrees. Hip flexion ROM showed the highest ICC (0.97) and SEM (3.5 degrees). Hip extension ROM showed the lowest ICC (0.86) and the highest SEM (4.7 degrees).
- **Hip muscle performance:** Considering the potential impact of deficits in hip muscle force production in persons with LBP with or without hip pain, baseline muscle performance measures (MMTs) or hand-held dynamometry are indicated along with noting symptom response in addition to strength. MMT for the hip extensors (82% interrater agreement)[470] and hip flexors ($\kappa = 0.67$)[471] have good reliability. Using a hand-held dynamometer, Pua et al[469] reported the following for measurement of hip muscle strength, ICC ranged from 0.84 to 0.97, and the coefficient of variation (CV) ranged from 8% to 15.7%. Hip extensors and internal/external rotators showed high ICC (<0.96) and low CV ($<9.8\%$). Hip abductors showed the lowest ICC (0.84) and the highest CV (15.7%).[469]

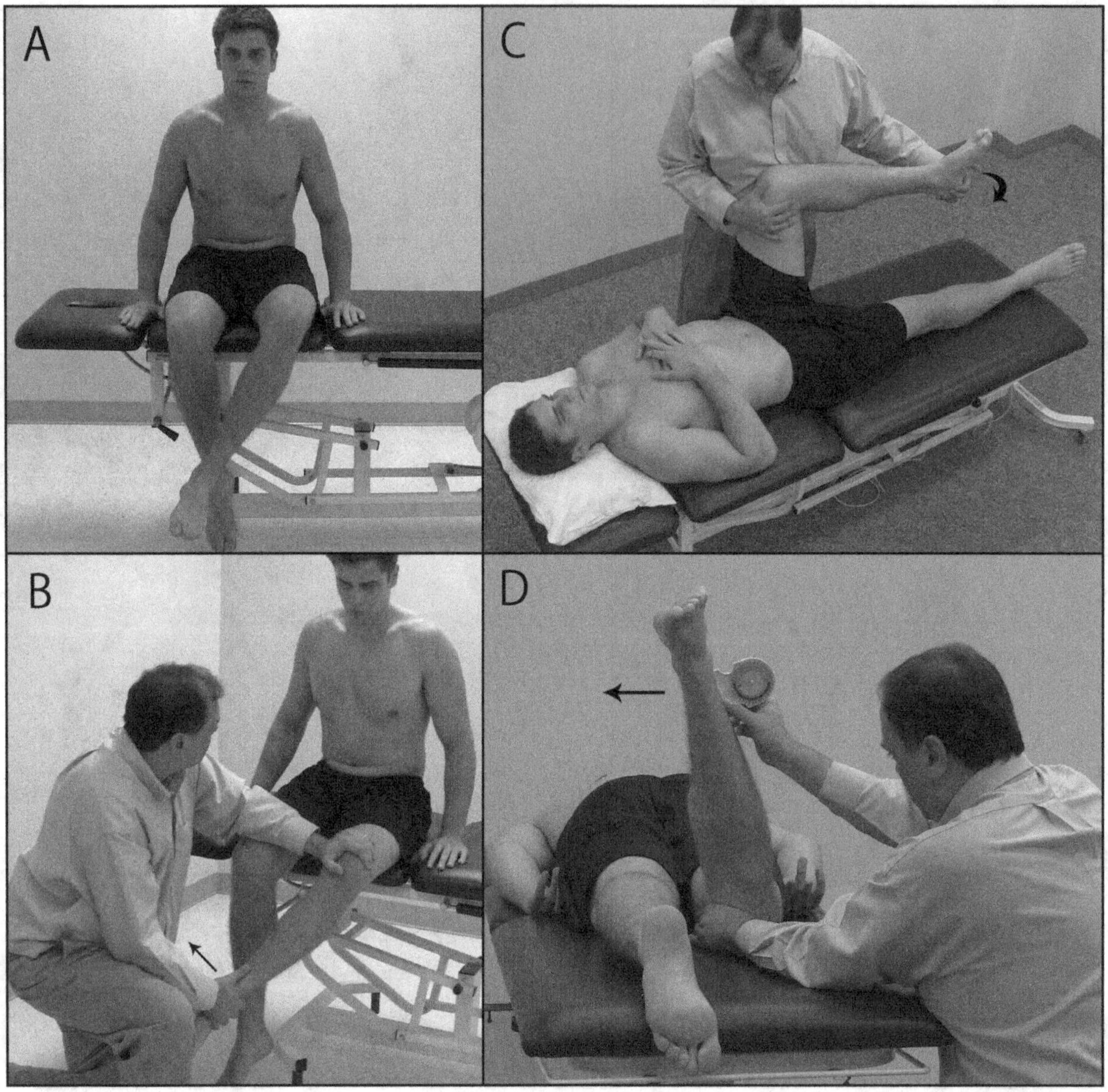

Figure 4-49. AROM hip ER: (A) sitting: ER; (B) sitting: ER with OP; (C) supine: ER with OP; and (D) prone: ER with inclinometer.

Figure 4-50. AROM hip ABD/ADD with and without OP: (A) ABD side-lying. *(continued)*

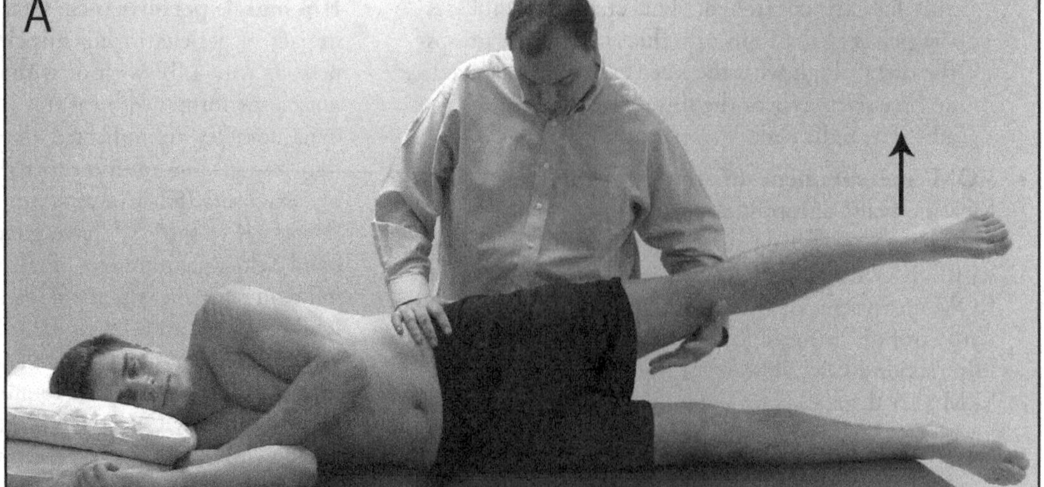

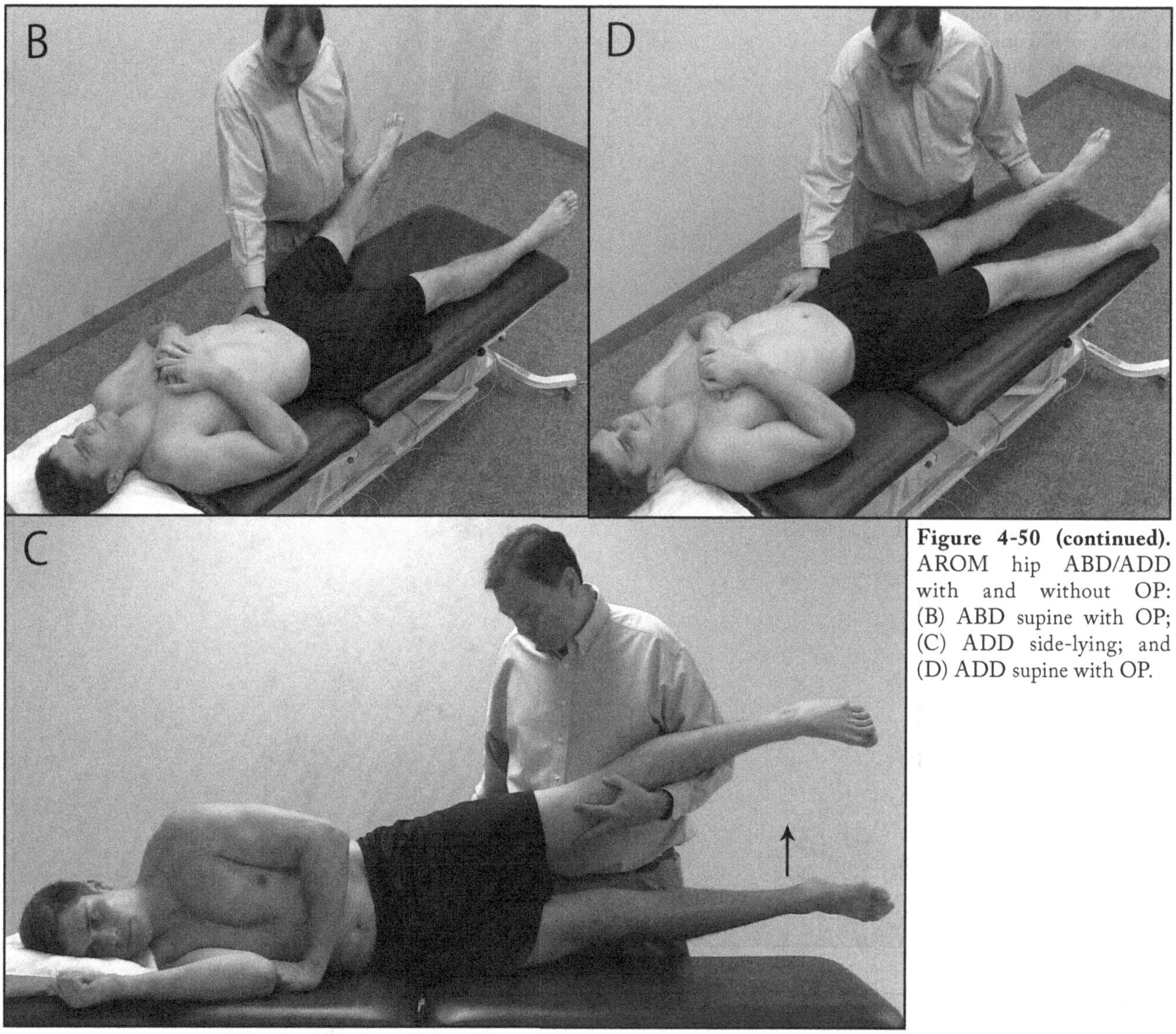

Figure 4-50 (continued). AROM hip ABD/ADD with and without OP: (B) ABD supine with OP; (C) ADD side-lying; and (D) ADD supine with OP.

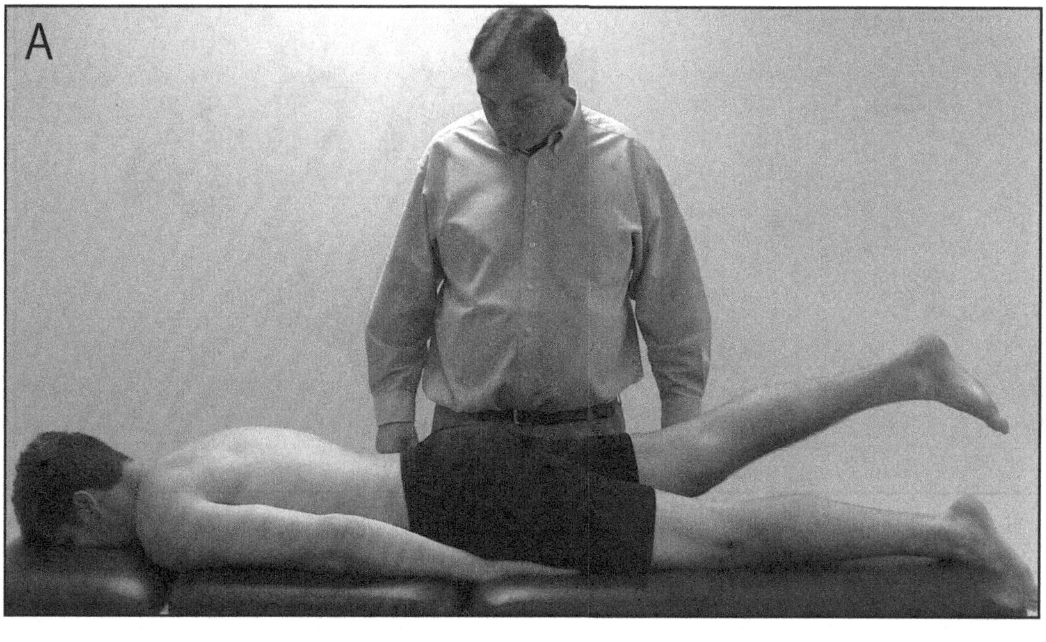

Figure 4-51. AROM hip extension: (A) hip extension with knee extended. *(continued)*

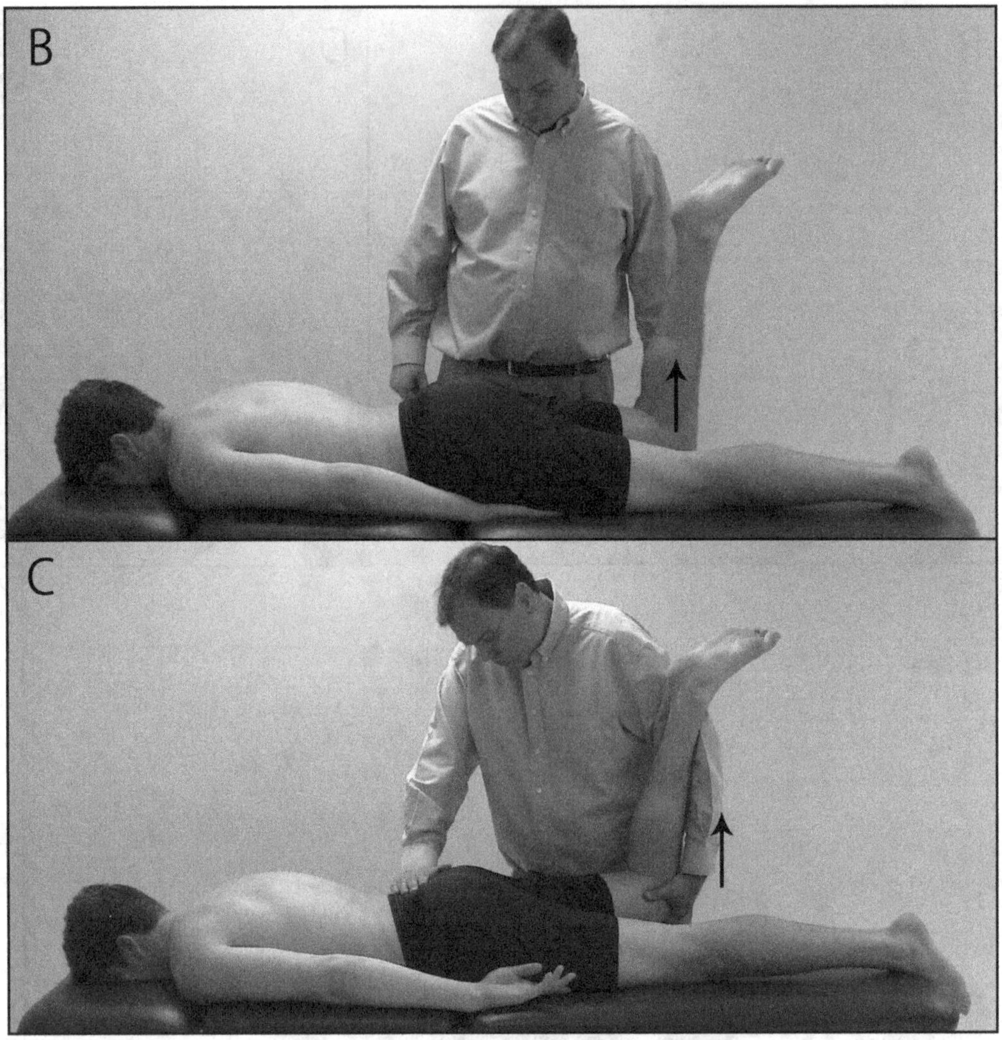

Figure 4-51 (continued). AROM hip extension: (B) hip extension with knee flexed; and (C) hip extension OP with knee flexed.

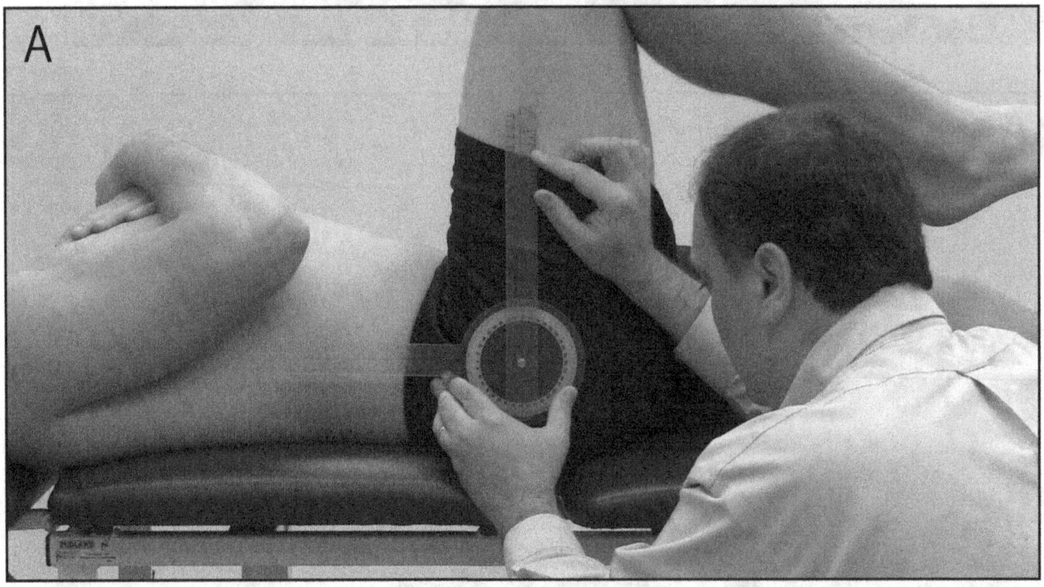

Figure 4-52. Hip AROM measurement: (A) hip flexion supine. *(continued)*

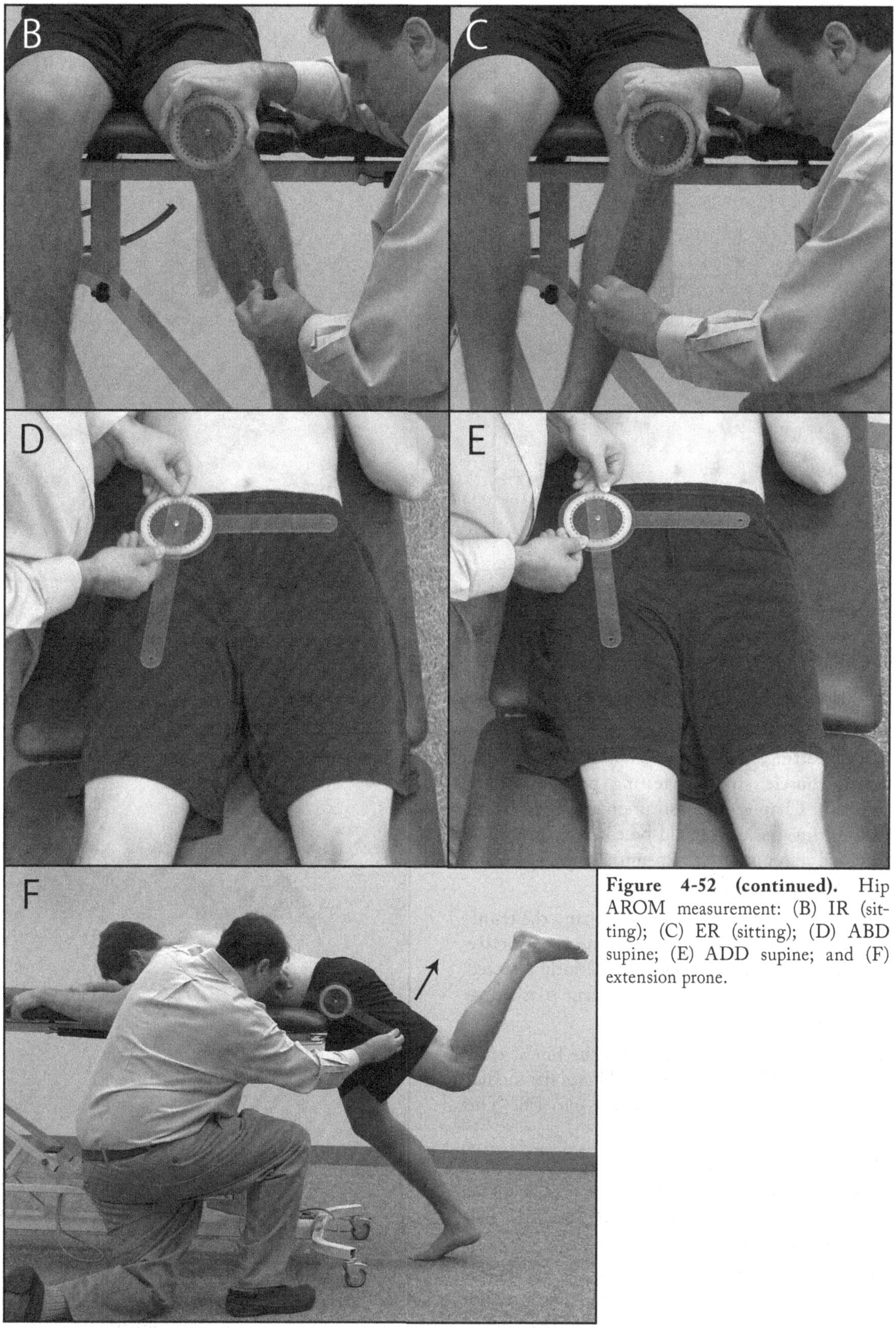

Figure 4-52 (continued). Hip AROM measurement: (B) IR (sitting); (C) ER (sitting); (D) ABD supine; (E) ADD supine; and (F) extension prone.

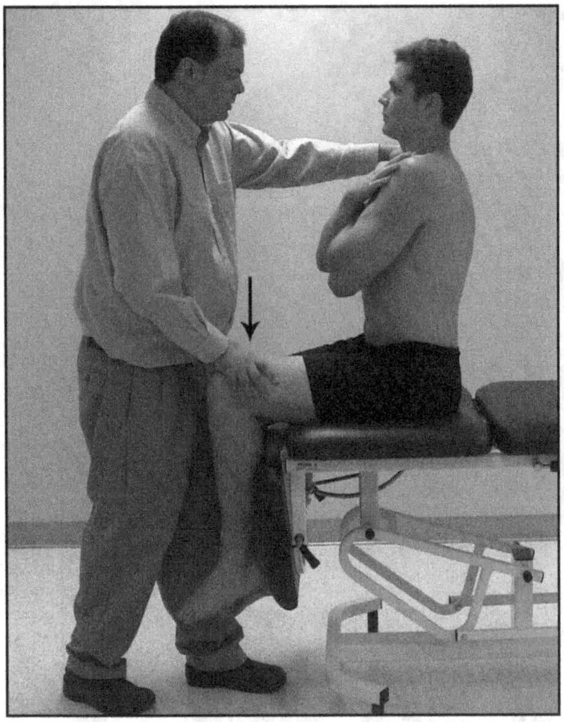

Figure 4-53. Hip flexion MMT.

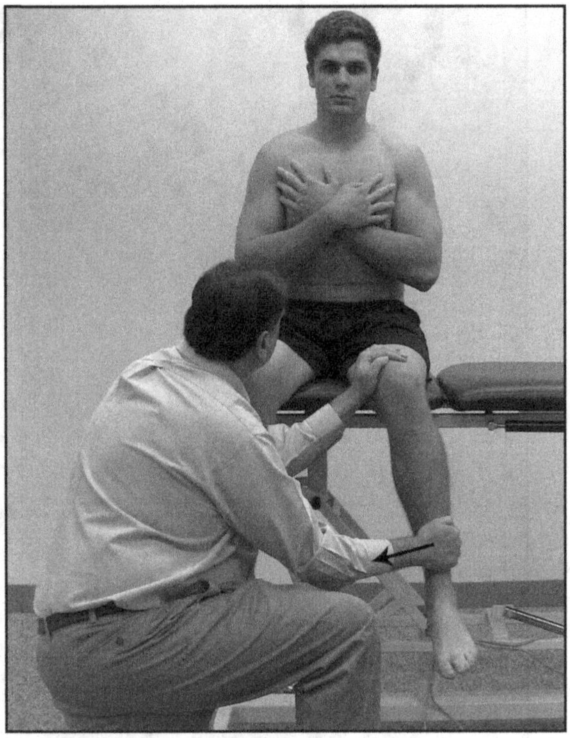

Figure 4-54. Hip IR MMT.

Reliability and a variety of test procedures for assessing hip muscle force production are reported in Cleland and Koppenhaver.[472] Hip ABD and ADD can be assessed in supine or side lying, flexion and IR/ER in sitting, and extension usually in prone. Standard muscle strength testing procedures are described in Chapter 3. Substitution and poor trunk control during the test should be corrected or noted and graded appropriately. Hip muscles groups commonly tested are as follows:

- *Flexion* (Figure 4-53): While stabilizing the trunk in neutral sitting and the hip at end-range active flexion, the clinician applies an inferiorly directed force on the distal thigh. The patient is asked to resist this force.
- *IR* (Figure 4-54): In sitting with the hip at end-range active IR, the clinician stabilizes the medial knee and applies a force directed into ER. The patient is asked to resist this force.
- *ER* (Figure 4-55): In sitting with the hip at end-range active ER, the clinician stabilizes the lateral knee and applies a force directed into IR. The patient is asked to resist this force.
- *ABD* (Figure 4-56): While stabilizing the pelvis in side lying or supine with the hip at end-range active ABD, the clinician provides a force directed into ADD. The patient is asked to resist this force.

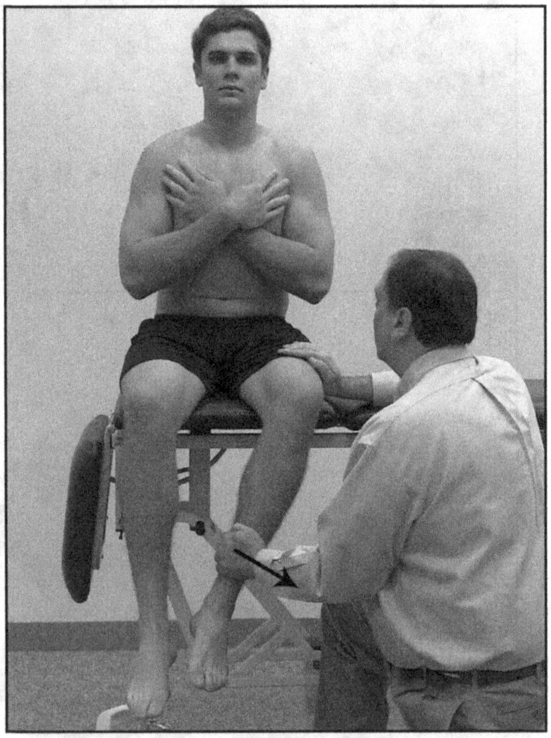

Figure 4-55. Hip ER MMT.

- *ADD* (Figure 4-57): While stabilizing the pelvis in side lying or supine with the hip at end-range active ADD, the clinician provides a force directed into ABD. The patient is asked to resist this force.

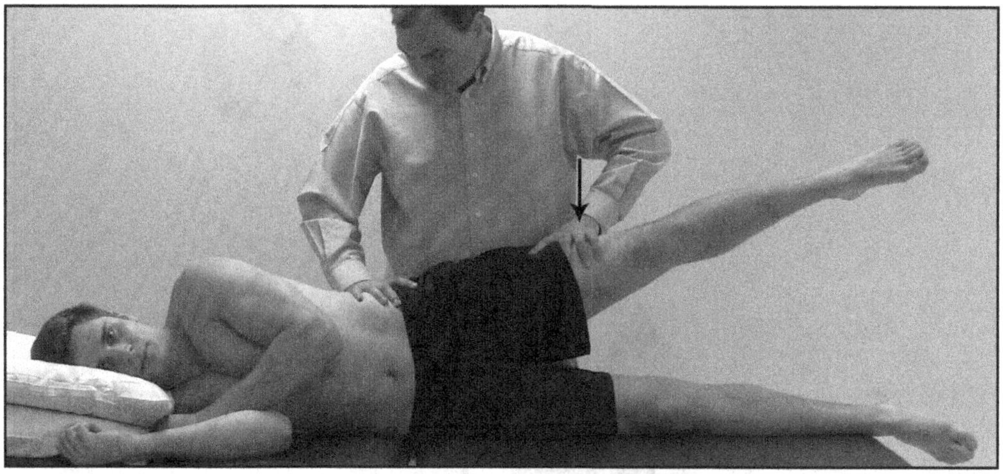

Figure 4-56. Hip ABD MMT.

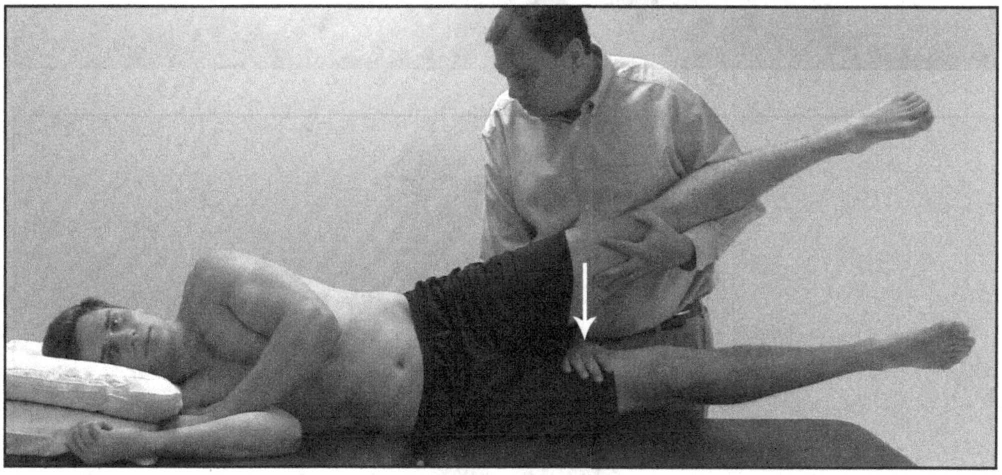

Figure 4-57. Hip ADD MMT.

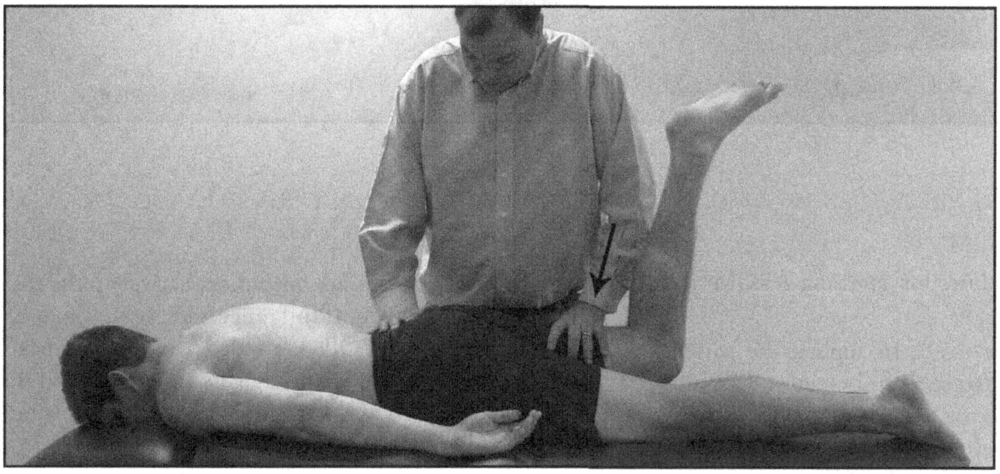

Figure 4-58. Hip extension MMT.

- *Extension* (Figure 4-58): While stabilizing the pelvis in prone with the hip at end-range active extension, the clinician provides a force directed into flexion. The patient is asked to resist this force. If poor trunk control is noted and to enhance the control of prone extension, performance of the abdominal drawing-in maneuver (ADIM) is advised to limit excessive anterior pelvic tilt and minimize overactivity of the superficial spinal extensors.[473]

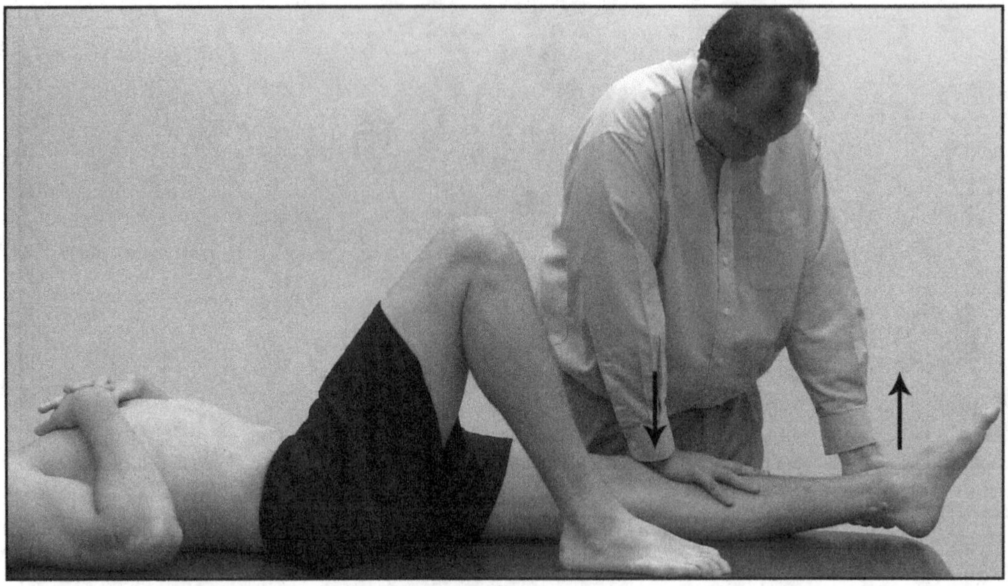

Figure 4-59. AROM knee extension with OP.

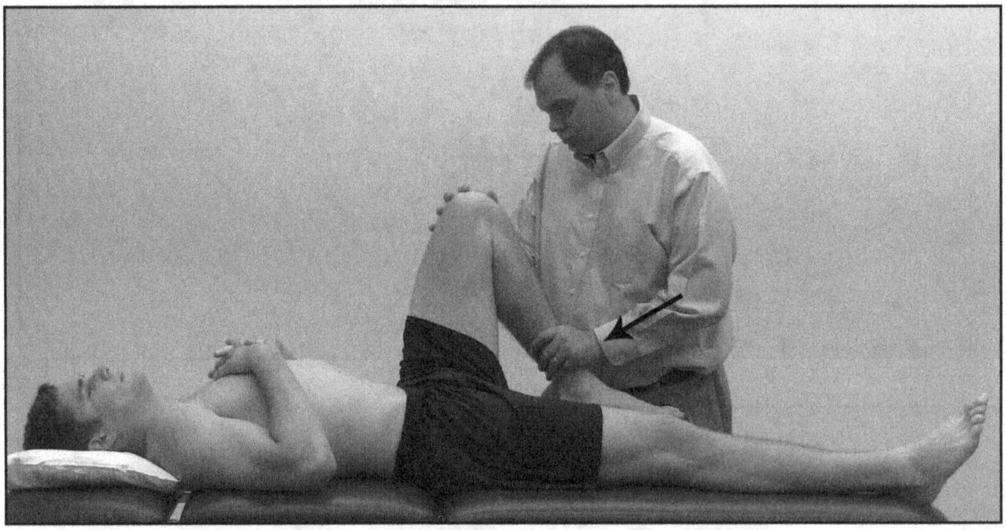

Figure 4-60. AROM knee flexion with OP.

Knee Active and Passive Range of Motion With Overpressure

Refer to standard procedures for assessing AROM and PROM in Chapter 3.

- *Knee extension* (Figure 4-59): In supine, the patient actively straightens the knee. If full range and asymptomatic, OP is applied. As needed, the clinician passively moves the knee through its full range of extension and applies OP. AROM or PROM is measured using a goniometer or inclinometer.
- *Knee flexion* (Figure 4-60): In supine, the patient actively bends the knee. If full range and asymptomatic, the clinician applies OP. As needed, the clinician passively moves the knee through its full range of flexion and applies OP. AROM or PROM is measured using a standard goniometer.

Ankle Active and Passive Range of Motion With Overpressure

- *DF*: In sitting or supine, the patient actively pulls the foot and toes upward. If full range and asymptomatic, the clinician applies OP. As needed, the clinician passively moves the ankle through its full range of DF and applies OP. AROM or PROM is measured using a standard goniometer.
- *Plantarflexion*: In sitting or supine, the patient actively points the foot and toes down. If full range and asymptomatic, the clinician applies OP. As needed, the clinician passively moves the ankle through its full range of plantarflexion and applies OP. AROM or PROM is measured using a standard goniometer.

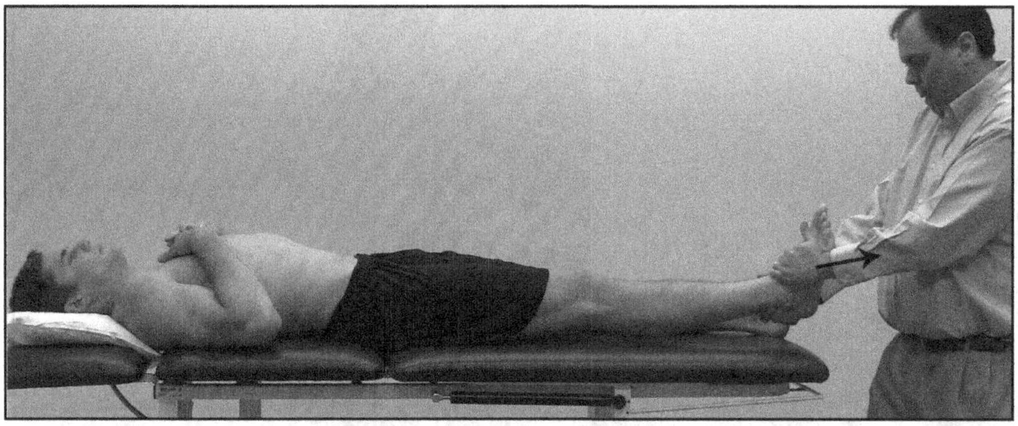

Figure 4-61. Hip passive accessory movement tests—long-axis distraction.

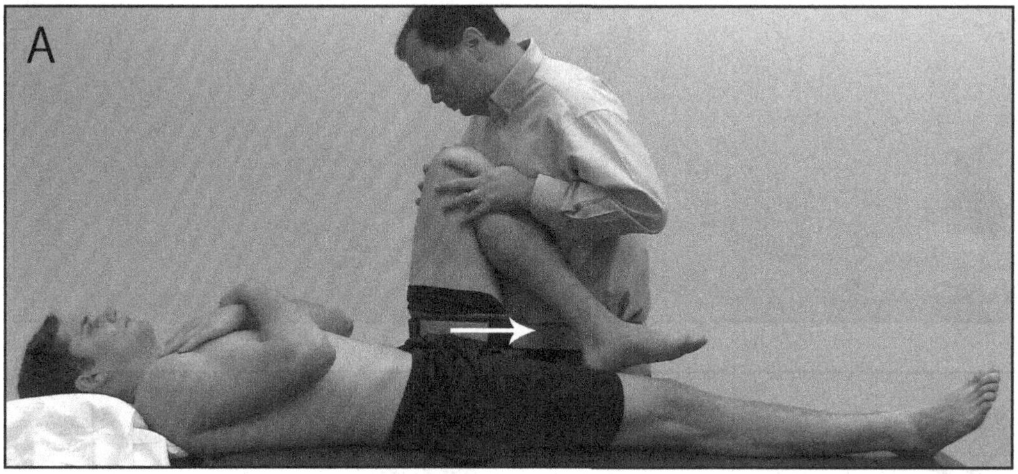

Figure 4-62. Hip passive accessory movement tests: (A) inferior glide with belt. *(continued)*

Passive Accessory Movements of the Hip

Passive accessory movements are necessary for normal physiological movement at any joint. These movements occur at the joint surfaces and usually cannot be performed actively by the patient, but they can be performed by the clinician.[269] The term *arthrokinematics* is used to describe motions of the bone at the joint surfaces such as gliding, sliding, translation, distraction, rolling, or spinning. Standardized test procedures for assessing passive accessory movements are discussed in Chapter 3.

Passive accessory movements of the hip joint are tested in supine or prone to assist with identifying mobility impairments and to guide intervention. As always, quality, quantity, and symptom response are identified. Mobility is judged as hypomobile, normal, or hypermobile. Reliability of passive accessory movements at the hip is unknown. All passive accessory movements are described as being applied on the proximal femur in an oscillatory manner to assess onset of symptoms, stiffness through range, and end feel to assess a pain and stiffness relationship. The following passive accessory movements are tested at the hip:

- *Long-axis distraction* (Figure 4-61): In supine, the clinician grasps the patient's ankle, passively moving the hip into 20 to 30 degrees of hip flexion and 30 degrees of ABD. A longitudinal distraction force is applied.
- *Inferior glide* (Figure 4-62): In supine with the hip passively held at 90 degrees flexion, the clinician grasps the proximal thigh as close to the hip joint as possible and applies an inferiorly directed force. In side-lying with the lower leg in 45 degrees of hip flexion, an inferior or medial glide is performed through the greater trochanter while supporting the leg in ABD.
- *Lateral glide* (Figure 4-63): In supine with the hip passively held at 90 degrees flexion, the clinician grasps the proximal thigh as close to the hip joint as possible and applies a laterally directed force.
- *Posterior glide* (Figure 4-64): In supine with the hip passively flexed to 90 degrees and internally rotated and adducted to tolerance, the clinician applies a posteriorly directed force in line with the long axis of the femur.
- *Anterior glide* (Figure 4-65): In prone with the hip extended to neutral or near end-range, the clinician applies an anteriorly directed force over the posterior aspect of the greater trochanter or over the proximal femur just distal to the ischial tuberosity. The knee may be flexed or extended.

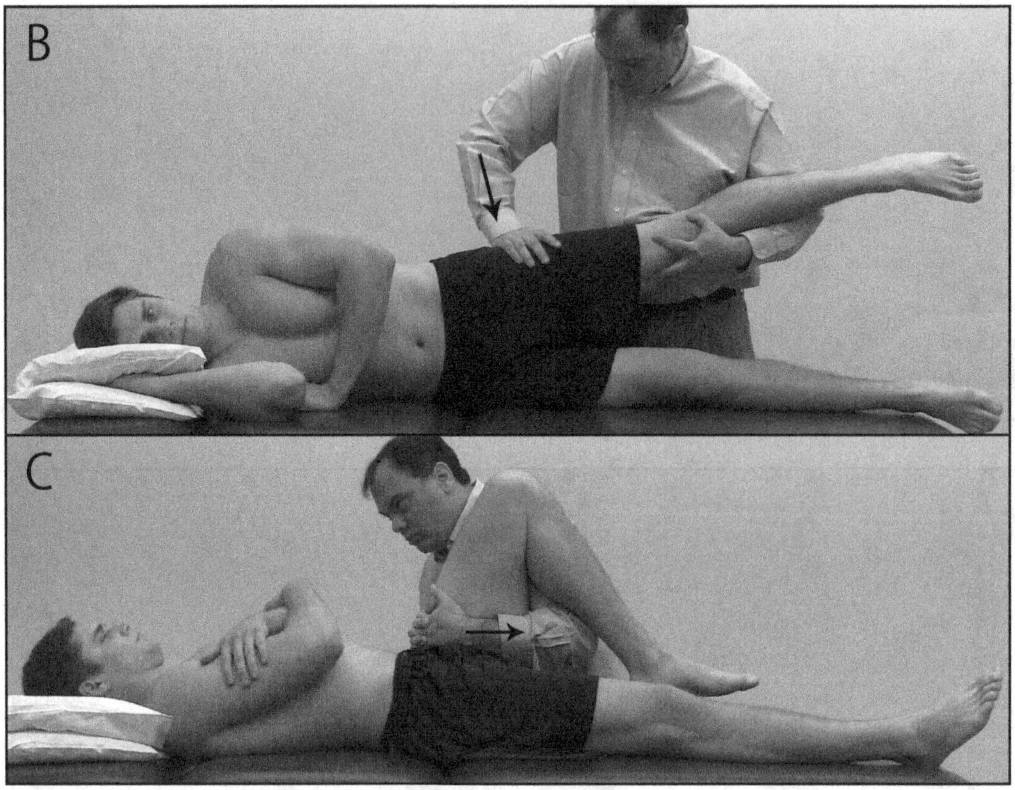

Figure 4-62 (continued). Hip passive accessory movement tests: (B) inferior/medial glide and (C) manual inferior glide.

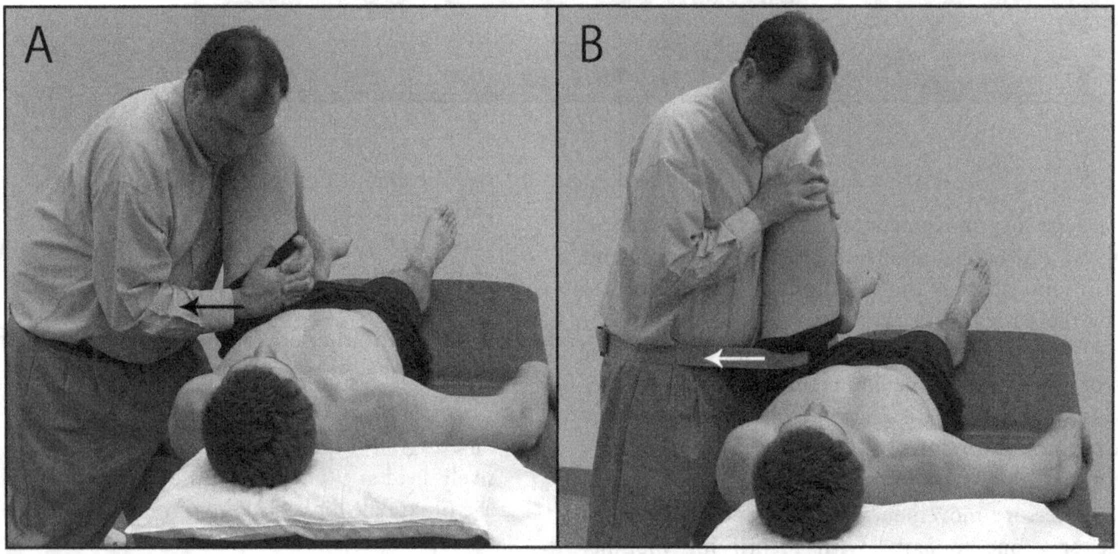

Figure 4-63. Hip passive accessory movement tests: (A) lateral glide manual and (B) lateral glide with belt.

Flexion, Internal Rotation, Adduction Impingement Test

This test is essentially a combined movement test. Several variations of performing this test are available in the literature. The description provided here is described by Martin and Sekiya[474] to assess for intra-articular hip pathology. In patients with hip pain, interrater reliability for reproduction of symptoms is moderate, $\kappa = 0.58$ (95% CI: 0.29 to 0.87).[474] Using intra-articular hip pain as defined by >50% relief with intra-articular anesthetic-steroid, diagnostic accuracy is Sn 0.78 (0.59 to 0.89), Sp 0.10 (0.03 to 0.29), +LR 0.86 (0.67 to 1.1), and –LR 2.3 (0.52 to 10.4).[475] The same study showed that the diagnostic accuracy of the flexion, abduction, external rotation (FABER) test (discussed next) is Sn 0.6 (0.41 to 0.77), Sp 0.18 (0.07 to 0.39), +LR 0.73 (0.5 to 1.1), and –LR 2.2 (0.8 to 6). Candidates for hip arthroscopy with a labral tear on MRI arthrogram had varied responses to

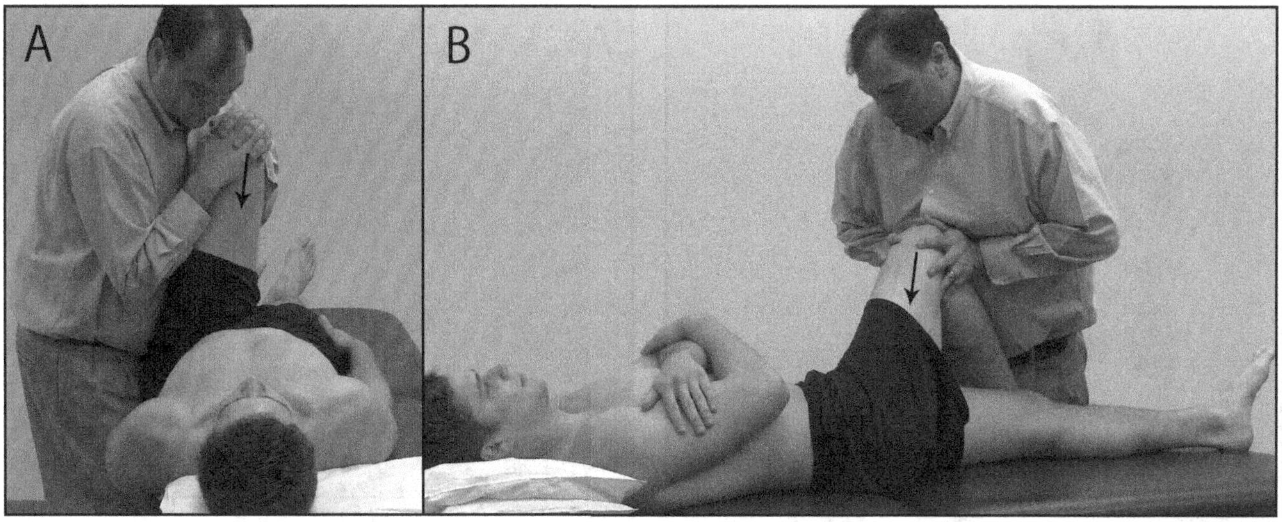

Figure 4-64. Hip passive accessory movement tests: (A) posterior glide at 90 degrees flexion and (B) posterior glide in flexion/ADD below 90 degrees.

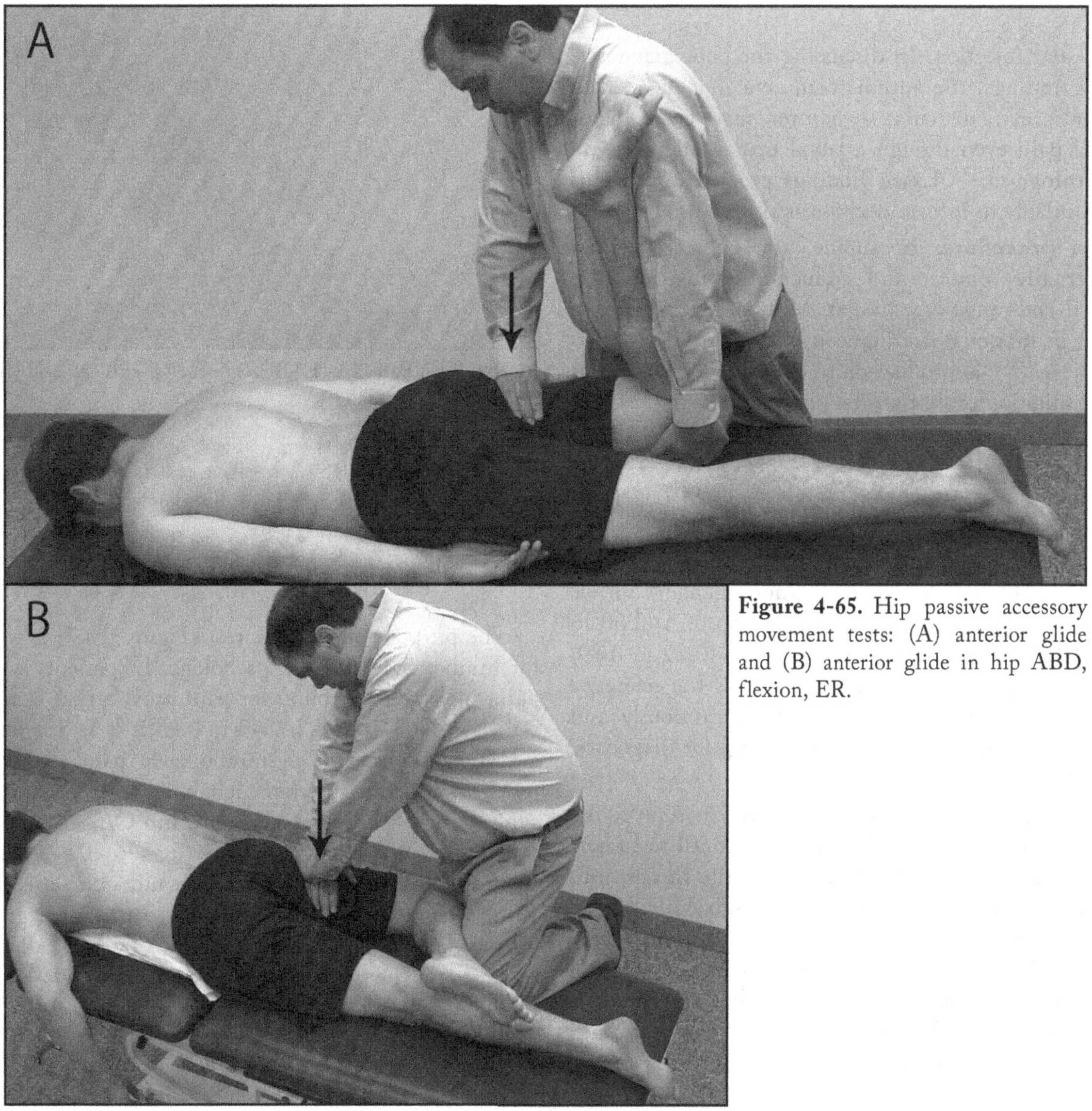

Figure 4-65. Hip passive accessory movement tests: (A) anterior glide and (B) anterior glide in hip ABD, flexion, ER.

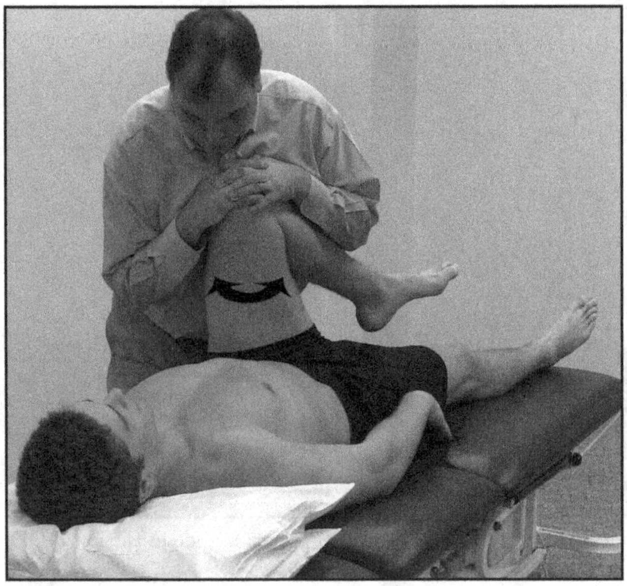

Figure 4-66. Scour test.

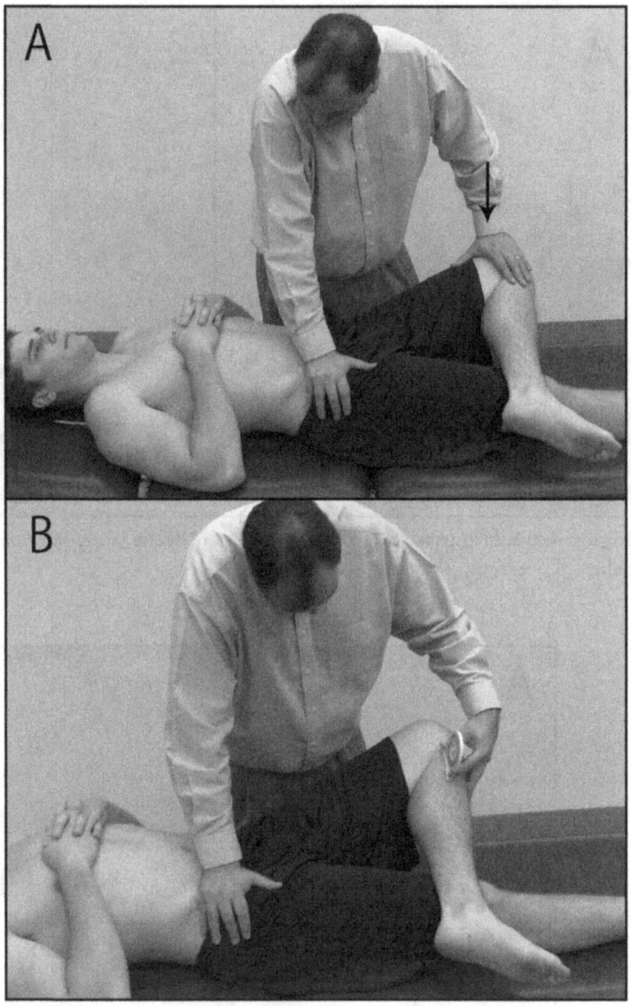

Figure 4-67. Patrick's (FABER) test: (A) with OP and (B) inclinometer measurement.

intraarticular injection. In discussing the poor diagnostic accuracy findings, the authors comment that in 43% of individuals, extra-articular structures may be a major source of pain even though a labral tear is suggested on MRI arthrogram.[475] Exam findings produced with this test are unlikely to inform decision making.

- **Test procedure**: In supine, the clinician flexes, internally rotates, and adducts the involved hip until end-range is achieved. Motion continues with the 3 motions simultaneously until end-range is achieved.[474] Reproduction of the patient's symptoms or limitation of motion is a positive test.

Scour Test

The purpose of the Scour test (Figure 4-66) is to assess for hip OA[467] or to determine irritability of the hip joint.[476] Reliability for capsular versus noncapsular end feel is κ = 0.52 (0.08 to 0.96) and 86.7% agreement.[467] Sutlive et al[467] reported Sn 0.62 (0.39 to 0.81), Sp 0.75 (0.60 to 0.85), +LR 2.4 (1.4 to 4.3), and –LR 0.51 (0.29 to 0.89) using radiographic findings for hip OA as the reference standard. Findings should be considered cautiously and combined with other examination findings for diagnostic purposes.

- **Test procedure**[476]: With the patient in supine, the examiner flexes and adducts the hip until resistance to movement is noted. Maintaining the flexion into resistance, the hip is gently moved into ABD, bringing the hip through 2 full arcs of motion. If the patient has no pain, the test is repeated while applying long-axis compression through the femur. The test is administered with good communication so as to not exacerbate symptoms. The patient rates the pain on a 1 to 10 NPRS. A positive test is provocation of the patient's symptoms laterally or in the groin.

Patrick's Test or Flexion, Abduction, External Rotation Test

The purpose of Patrick's test (Figure 4-67) is to assess for lumbopelvic and hip pathology. In patients with hip pain, interrater reliability for pain provocation is substantial (κ = 0.63 [95% CI: 0.43 to 0.83]).[474] In persons with a primary complaint of lumbopelvic pain, the FABER test has moderate interrater reliability for reproduction of symptoms.[140,477] In subjects with hip OA on radiograph, Sutlive et al[467] report Sn 0.57 (0.34 to 0.77), Sp 0.71 (0.56 to 0.82), +LR 1.9 (1.1 to 3.4), and –LR 0.61 (0.36 to 1.00) when the FABER test ROM was <60 degrees. In 40 subjects with CLBP and sacroiliitis by MRI, diagnostic accuracy for the right/left sides is Sn = .66 (0.30, 0.90)/0.54 (0.24, 0.81), Sp = 0.51(0.33, 0.69)/0.62 (0.42, 0.78); +LR = 1.37 (0.76, 2.48)/1.43 (0.70, 2.93), and –LR = .64 (0.24, 1.72)/0.73 (0.36, 1.45).[478]

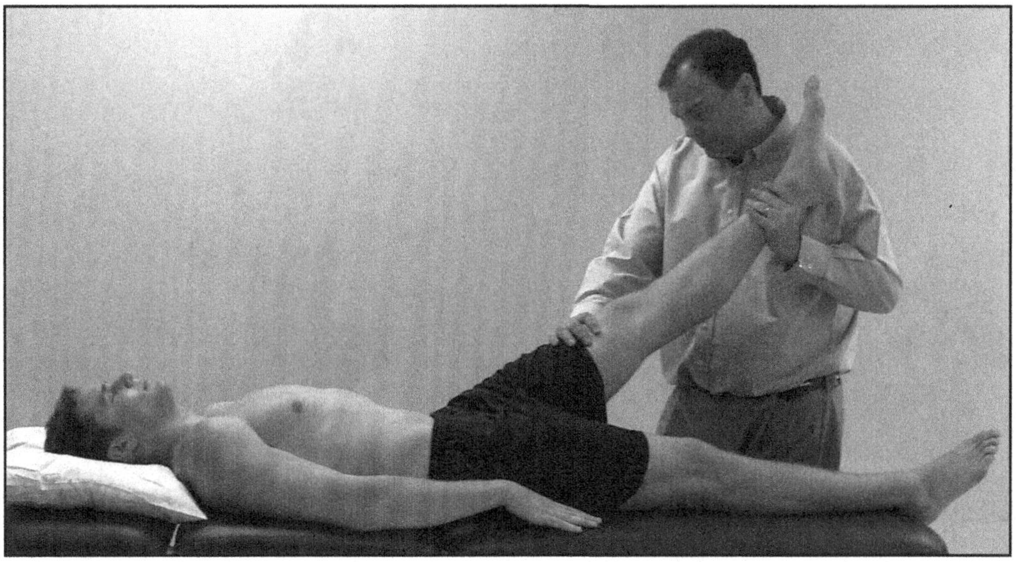

Figure 4-68. Hamstring muscle length: SLR test position.

- **Test procedure**: With the patient in supine, the clinician flexes, abducts, and externally rotates the hip such that the lateral ankle rests on the opposite thigh just above the knee. While stabilizing the opposite side of the pelvis at the ASIS, the knee of the involved side is lowered toward the table until end-range is reached. If no symptoms, OP is added in an oscillatory manner. With the inclinometer zeroed against a wall, ROM is measured with the inclinometer placed 2.5 cm distal to the patient's flexed knee (Figure 4-67B). A positive test is reproduction of the patient's symptoms or limitation of motion.[467]

Muscle Length Tests

Muscle imbalance during specific functional movements implies that a person has an inadequate balance of mobility and stability. A postural and movement analysis may suggest a pattern of muscle imbalance that requires muscle length testing. However, a stiff muscle is most likely only one component of a dysfunctional movement pattern. For example, excessive lumbar extension during walking may be related to stiff hip flexors, weak trunk stabilizers, weak hip extensors, or stiff lumbar extensors. All factors related to creating a balance of mobility and stability during walking must be examined.

Hamstring Muscle Length Test

The hamstrings may act as primary hip extensors in the presence of a weak gluteus maximus. The altered recruitment pattern often results in short hamstrings.[479] For the SLR test position, interexaminer reliability is ICC = 0.92 (0.82, 0.96).[480] The knee extension (90/90) test demonstrates substantial intratester and intertester reliability.[481,482]

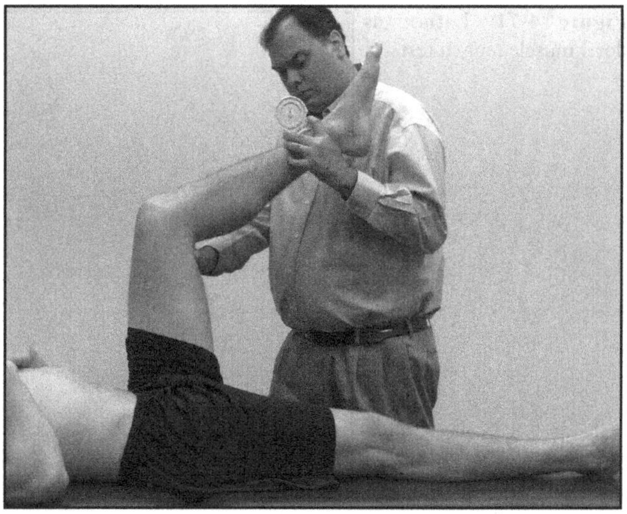

Figure 4-69. Hamstring muscle length: knee extension at 90/90 with inclinometer.

- **Hamstring test position using the SLR** (Figure 4-68): The inclinometer is zeroed on the upper anterior border of the tibia. In supine, the tested knee is passively extended while the other leg is stabilized flat on the table to prevent posterior pelvic tilt. Measurement is taken at the end-range with a firm end feel while preventing posterior pelvic tilt.
- **Hamstring test position using knee extension at 90/90 with inclinometer** (Figure 4-69): In supine, the untested lower extremity is stabilized on table with the knee extended. The clinician holds the tested lower extremity in 90 degrees of hip flexion and passively extends the knee to end-range of hamstring length. A positive test is asymmetry from side to side. Relevance is based on clinical experience. Normative data are not available for either test position.

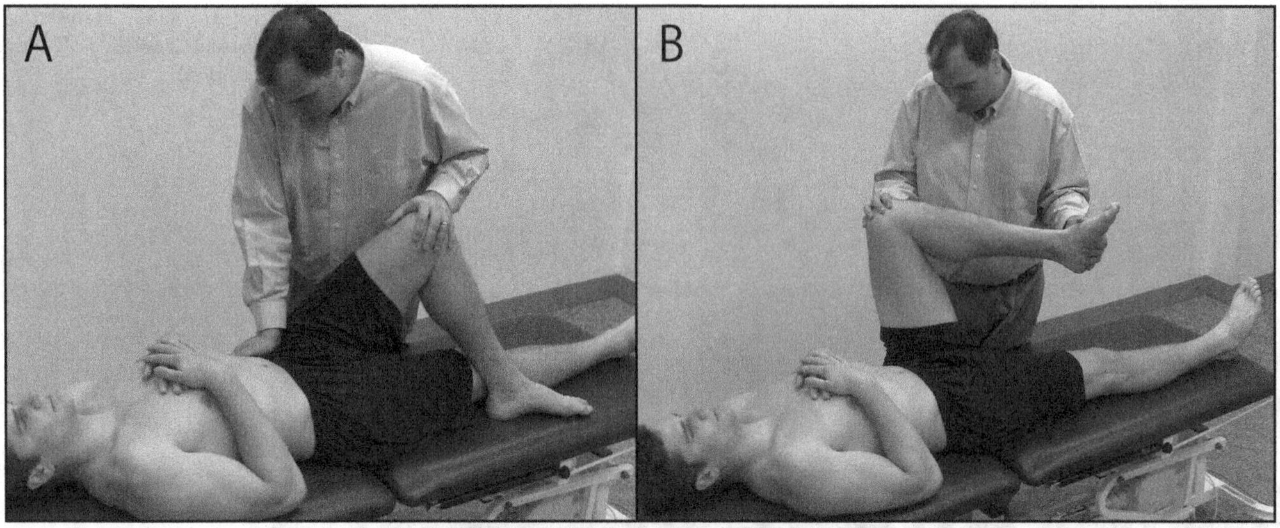

Figure 4-70. Piriformis muscle length: (A) below 90 degrees hip flexion and (B) above 90 degrees hip flexion.

Figure 4-71. Latissimus dorsi muscle length test.

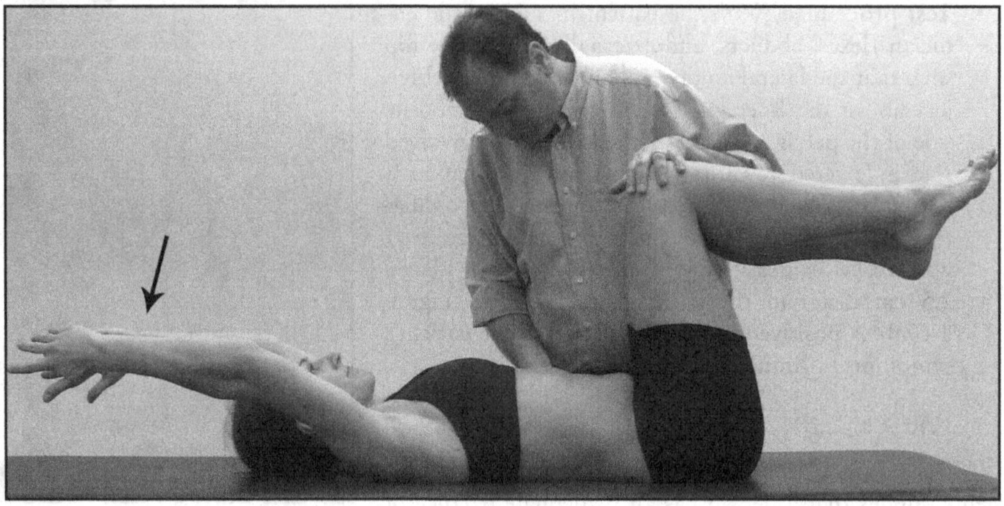

Piriformis (Hip External Rotator) Muscle Length Test

The piriformis muscle length test also assesses the other hip external rotators, but it is commonly known as the *piriformis muscle length test*. The piriformis is primarily an external rotator of the hip and assists with ABD and extension. When the gluteal muscles are weak or inhibited, the piriformis may overwork to assist hip extension and ABD, resulting in a short muscle. With the hip above 60 degrees of flexion, the piriformis acts a hip internal rotator.[479] The diagnostic utility is unknown.

- **Test procedure with the piriformis below 90 degrees of hip flexion** (Figure 4-70A): In supine place the foot of the tested lower extremity just lateral to the untested knee if the pelvis remains in neutral; or if the pelvis elevates from the table place the foot of the tested lower extremity just medial to the untested knee. While manually stabilizing the pelvis on the tested side, passively move the hip into ADD and IR by moving the knee toward midline. A positive test is side-to-side asymmetry. Relevance is based on clinical experience. A normal test response is unknown.
- **Test procedure with the piriformis above 90 degrees of hip flexion** (Figure 4-70B): In supine, flex the hip to 90 and add ER. While maintaining flexion and ER, adduct the hip toward the opposite shoulder.

Latissimus Dorsi Muscle Length Test

In subjects with neck pain interrater reliability during a single session latissimus dorsi muscle length test (Figure 4-71) is right side κ = 0.80 (0.53, 1.0) and left side κ = 0.69 (0.30, 1.0).[483] Using a similar test procedure in healthy subjects, Borstad and Briggs[484] reported on 6-week between-session measurements in healthy subjects. ICCs for all raters, novice and experienced, were poor. These authors did not recommend this technique to assess within-subject change over time.[484]

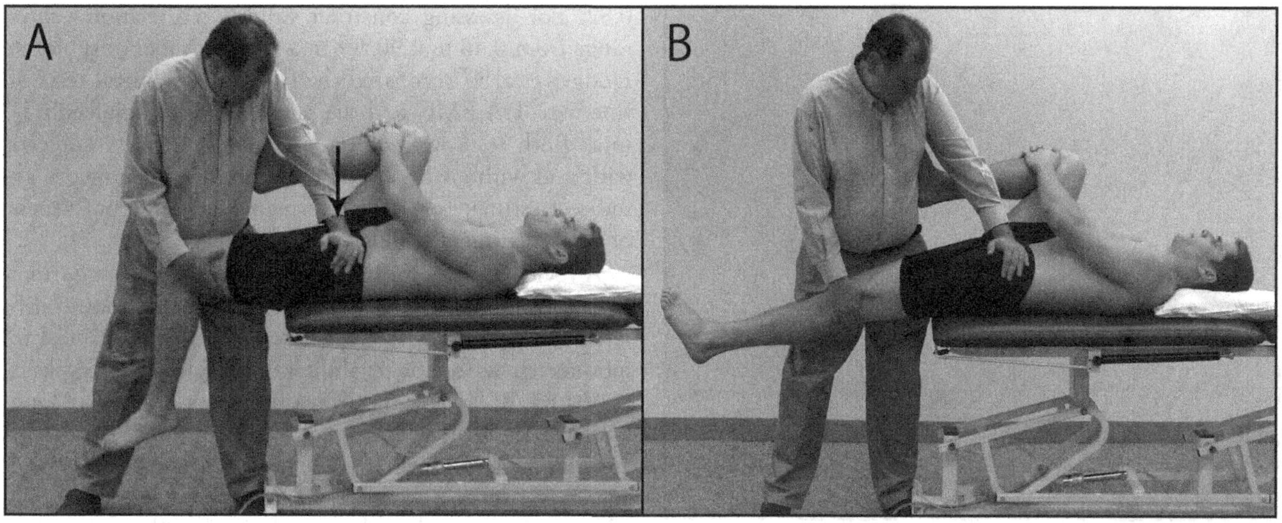

Figure 4-72. Modified Thomas test: (A) observe hip and knee position and (B) adding knee extension allows further hip extension implicating 2-joint hip flexors.

- **Test procedure**: Patient is supine with hips and knees flexed with or without feet flat on the table. With the patient maintaining a posterior pelvic tilt, the shoulder is passively or actively flexed in the sagittal plane. At the end of passive or active flexion, a ROM measurement is taken with a standard goniometer. The arms should be able to lie flat on the table. In the description by Borstad and Briggs,[484] medial and lateral humeral epicondyles were palpated to determine onset of passive IR, suggesting the end of latissimus dorsi length. Either a firm end feel or IR marked the end of the test procedure. A positive test is side-to-side asymmetry. Relevance is based on clinical experience, the patient's examination, and quality of movement. Bilaterally, a dominant or stiff latissimus dorsi facilitates a lumbopelvic lordosis, thoracic kyphosis, altered scapular, and shoulder girdle movement; increased glenohumeral IR, extension, and ADD; and lateral trunk flexion on one side. Normative data are not available.

Modified Thomas Test

The modified Thomas test is used to assess the length of the iliacus and psoas major (ie, 1-joint hip flexors) and the rectus femoris (ie, a 2-joint hip flexors) and tensor fascia latae (TFL). The inclinometer and goniometer are reliable instruments for measuring hip extension.[485] Harvey[486] reported ICCs of 0.91 to 0.94 for goniometric measurements of hip extension, knee flexion, and hip ABD. In this study of 117 elite athletes, hip extension measured –12 degrees from the horizontal, knee flexion at 52 degrees, and hip ABD at 15 degrees relative to the pelvis. Flexibility varied with the individual sport. The nondominant limb was generally more flexible than the dominant limb. Harvey[486] recommended that flexibility should be sufficient to allow performance of the desired sporting activity and that asymmetries are addressed.

- **Modified Thomas test procedure** (Figure 4-72): The patient sits at end of table and lies down while bringing both knees to the chest. The patient maintains one limb in hip flexion, keeping the lumbar spine and sacrum flat to table. The clinician passively lowers the tested limb over the end of the bed toward the floor. The clinician observes to see if the hip is in neutral or flexed in the sagittal plane and whether neutral or abducted in the frontal plane. The lower leg should be in neutral rotation with the knee flexed. Compare both sides and observe asymmetry.
- **Positive test**: To differentiate between the 1- and 2-joint hip flexors when the thigh does not touch the table, the clinician extends the knee to place the 2-joint hip flexors on slack. If hip extension increases, the 2-joint hip flexors are implicated (see Figure 4-72B). If there is no change in hip extension, the 1-joint hip flexors are implicated. ABD or ER of the thigh suggests tightness of the TFL. If the thigh is abducted, the clinician brings the patient's thigh to neutral. If hip flexion increases, the TFL-iliotibial band complex is short.[479] If knee flexion is less than 80 degrees, a short rectus femoris is suggested.[479]
- **Normal response**: Hip extension, ABD, ER, and/or knee flexion are measured by goniometer or inclinometer. A normal length of the 1-joint hip flexors is identified by 0 degrees of hip extension with the thigh resting on the table and 80 degrees of knee flexion with no ABD or ADD and neutral hip rotation. With slight OP, the hip should extend 10 to 15 degrees further.[479] Harvey[486] questioned the proposed normal range as discussed previously. The nondominant limb was generally more flexible than the dominant limb. Criteria are arbitrary and vary between genders and limb dominance and depend on the types and level of activity undertaken by the individual.

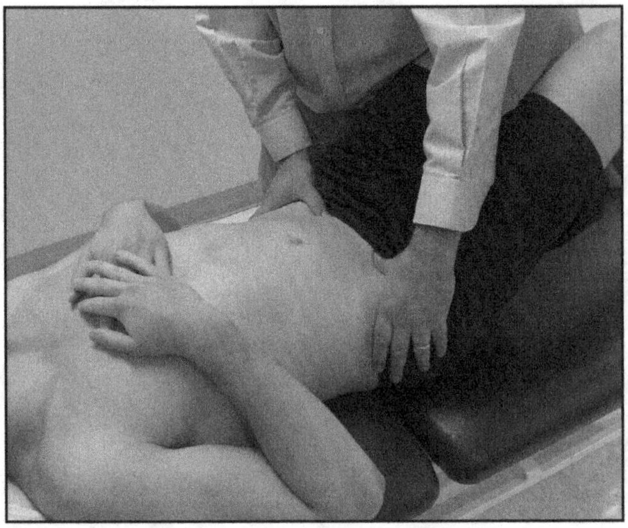

Figure 4-73. TrA palpation in hook-lying.

Trunk Muscle Performance

Identification of specific impairments in motor control or muscle performance is necessary to aid in selecting those patients most likely to benefit from stabilization exercise programs (see Table 4-2). As discussed in Chapter 3, changes in trunk muscle performance in persons with LBP include strength, endurance, and motor control issues such as correct timing, amplitude, and coordination. These changes are complex and somewhat variable, affecting both the superficial and deep trunk muscles. Keep in mind that all muscles are important in spinal stability with no one muscle being more important than another. Clinical assessment of the deep muscles is discussed first. Assessment of the superficial or global muscles requires a higher level of performance that may not be appropriate for the painful patient during the first session. These tests are discussed at the end of the examination.

Deep Trunk Muscle Clinical Tests

Three methods of assessment are used to assess the deep muscles: palpation, biofeedback, or rehabilitative ultrasound imaging (RUSI). RUSI, when available, is the most objective method for assessing the deep muscles. All methods can be used for assessment or training. The tests can be performed in a variety of positions. The purpose is to assess if the patient is able to preferentially activate the TrA and MF. Fine-wire EMG and MRI are the gold standard measures of deep muscle performance. However, those tests are expensive, invasive, and not suited for clinical assessment. Costa et al[487] reports moderate reliability for supine palpation of the TrA (κ = 0.52, 95% CI: 0.29 to 0.75) and for prone use of the biofeedback cuff, ICC 0.58 (95% CI: 0.28 to 0.78). A systematic review[488] of the clinimetric properties of the biofeedback unit to assess the TrA reveals ICC values for intraexaminer reliability from 0.50 to 0.81. ICC values for interexaminer reliability range from 0.47 to 0.82. For assessing construct validity, correlation values range from 0.48 to 0.90.[488] In a small number of subjects, Hodges et al[489] compared the findings of clinical tests of fine wire TrA EMG and the prone use of the biofeedback unit. Both tests were able to accurately identify subjects with and without LBP. The biofeedback unit provides an indirect estimate of TrA performance. The responsiveness of this instrument is unknown.

A review by Ghamkhar et al[490] concluded that current research supports RUSI as a reliable and valid tool to differentiate patients with LBP from normal subjects and to monitor the effect of rehabilitation programs. In subjects with LBP RUSI thickness measurements of the TrA and lumbar MF (LM) when based on the mean of 2 measures are highly reliable when taken by a single examiner and adequately reliable when taken by different examiners.[491] All baseline tests should be performed with the lumbar spine in neutral.

TrA Palpation Test Procedure

In supine, hook-lying, and neutral spine posture (Figure 4-73),[492,493] the clinician gently palpates a point 2 cm medial and inferior to the ASIS. During relaxed breathing and at the end of breathing out, the clinician asks the patient to perform a slow, gentle TrA contraction (ie, 15% of maximum) by drawing the navel in toward the spine and up toward the chest, which is also known as the ADIM or abdominal hollowing. The patient should hold the contraction for 10 seconds while continuing to breathe normally. Alternate cues for women are to gently lift your pelvic floor; men are asked to imagine gently lifting the testicles. When the muscle contracts properly, an increase in deep tension can be palpated. If a bulging or quick contraction is felt, the internal oblique is palpated/contracted rather than the TrA. The patient's head and upper trunk must remain stable with relaxed breathing. Breath holding is not allowed. The lumbar spine and pelvis should not move in any way (ie, no tilting, flexing forward or backward, or rotating). The rib cage should not depress or flare, nor should the patient push with the feet. Any of these abnormal responses suggest the patient is unable to preferentially activate the TrA, may be compensating with excessive superficial muscle activation, and should be corrected. If performed correctly, the procedure can be repeated for 10 repetitions of 10-second holds to assess endurance. Correct performance includes evidence of deep muscle activity; minimal superficial muscle activity; a smooth, slow contraction; and normal breathing. Palpation of the TrA during the ADIM may also be done in quadruped, side-lying, standing, or using arm or leg-loading tasks.

Supine TrA Test Using a Biofeedback Pressure Unit or Blood Pressure Cuff

In hook-lying, the cuff is placed under the lumbar spine and inflated to 40 mm Hg (Figure 4-74). The procedure for TrA activation is the same as for palpation. A successful

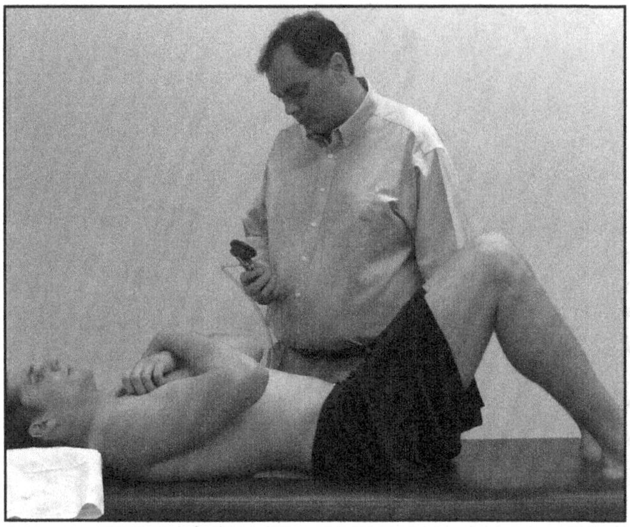

Figure 4-74. Supine TrA test using biofeedback pressure unit.

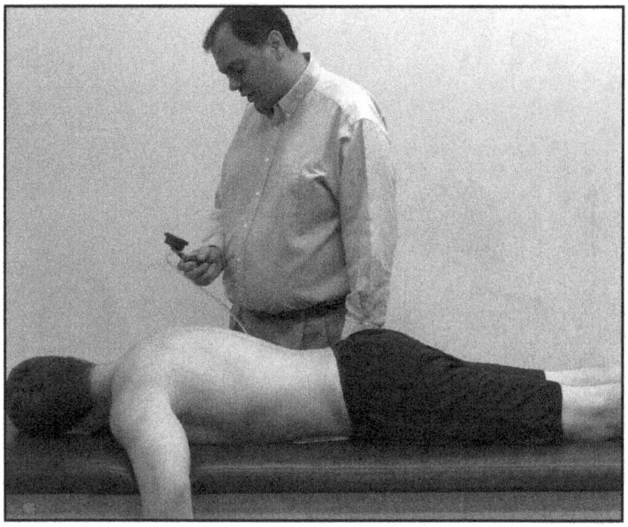

Figure 4-75. Prone TrA test using biofeedback pressure unit.

contraction is an increase of 0 to 5 mm Hg and the ability to maintain the change in pressure. A firm or hard surface is recommended to minimize measurement error. The addition of a series of leg-loading activities such as unilateral heel slides may be used as a progression.

Prone TrA Test Using a Biofeedback Pressure Unit or Blood Pressure Cuff

The cuff is placed under the abdomen with the navel in the center and the distal edge of pad in line with the ASIS on both sides (Figure 4-75). Inflate the cuff to 70 mm Hg and allow the reading to stabilize. The dial will move with normal respiration. The procedure for TrA activation is the same as for palpation. A successful contraction lowers the reading by 6 to 10 mm Hg. A change of <2 mm Hg, no change, or an increase suggests the person is unable to correctly contract the TrA.

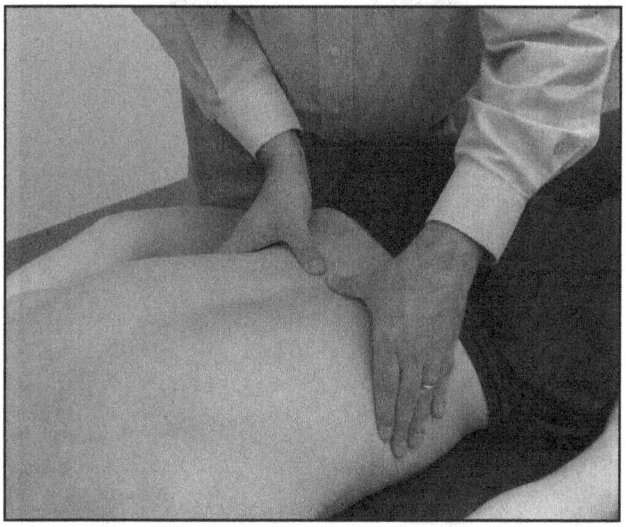

Figure 4-76. MF palpation in prone.

Palpation of the Multifidus in Prone

Palpation may be done in prone, side-lying, quadruped, or standing using the same procedures. Palpation is described in Figure 4-76 for the prone position. Palpation is performed at each segment adjacent to the SP with the patient relaxed. A side-to-side comparison is made with focus at the symptomatic, segmental level because segmental atrophy has been noted on MRI at the symptomatic segment.[494] The procedure is similar to TrA palpation relative to breathing. To preferentially activate the MF at the end of exhalation, the patient is asked to gently and slowly contract and swell out the muscles under the clinician's fingers without moving the spine or pelvis. The clinician feels for deep tension in the muscle. The goal is to hold the contraction for 10 seconds while breathing naturally. If able to perform correctly, a test of 10 repetitions with 10-second holds is performed. Incorrect activation occurs if no tension is palpated, rapid superficial tension develops, or superficial thoracic ES are activated and palpable, resulting in stiffness or arching of the spine. Additional cues for MF activation are asking the patient to draw the PSISs together, gently lift the pelvic floor, or perform the ADIM.

The MF can be activated and palpated in prone through a contralateral, upper extremity lift of 5 cm (2 inches) with the shoulder abducted to 120 degrees and the elbow flexed to 90 degrees (Figure 4-77). A small hand weight is normalized to the patient's body mass. During fine-wire EMG, this process engages about 30% of the maximum voluntary isometric contraction of the MF.[495]

Rehabilitative Ultrasound Imaging

Used as a clinical test, RUSI provides quantitative data related to muscle structure and activation for assessment and training of the TrA and MF. Current research supports the reliability and validity of using RUSI in the

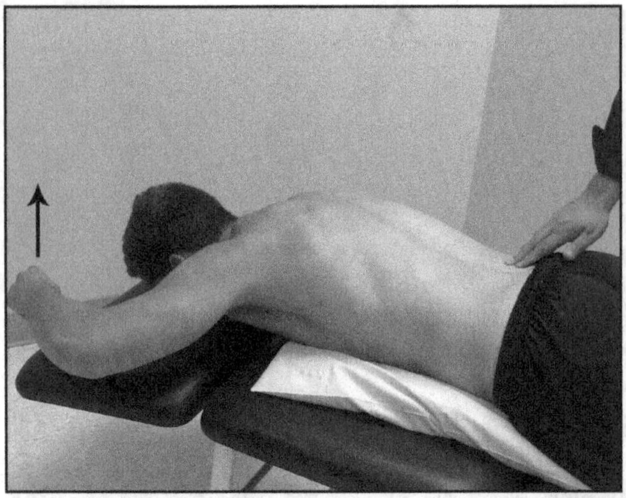

Figure 4-77. MF activation with contralateral upper extremity lift.

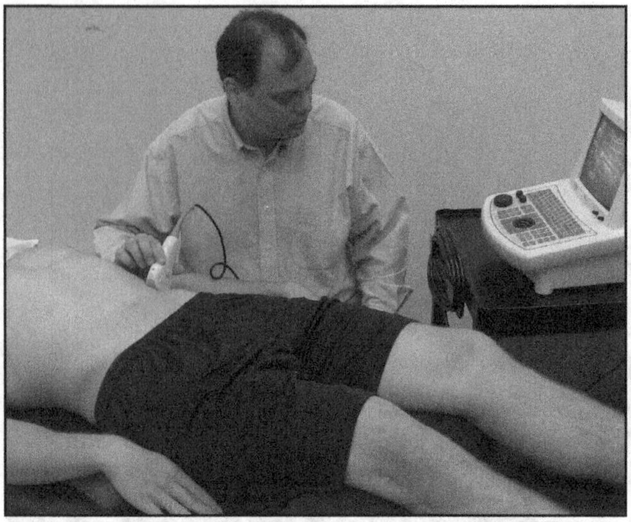

Figure 4-78. Ultrasound imaging of lateral abdominal muscles

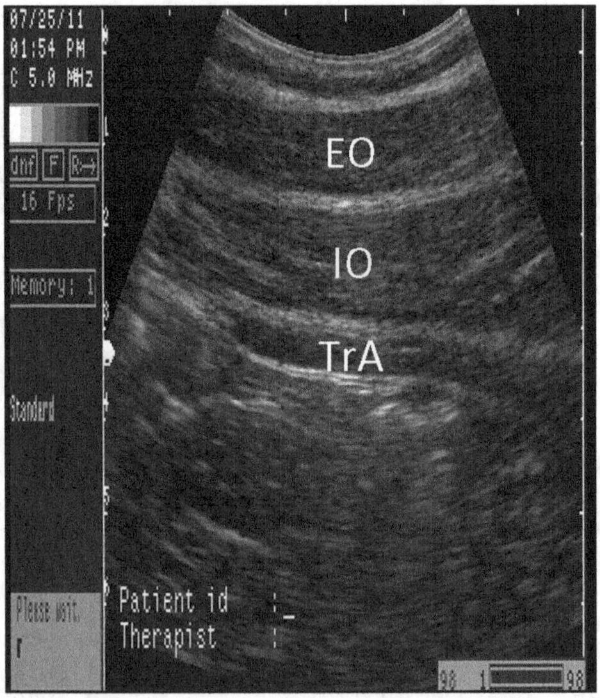

Figure 4-79. Ultrasound image of the lateral abdominal wall.

measurement of trunk muscle geometry through comparisons with MRI and fine wire EMG.[496,497] Changes in ultrasound measurements of muscle thickness of the lateral abdominal muscles including the TrA[498] and MF[495] have been correlated with increased EMG values during activity. The performance of RUSI is beyond the scope of this book. Several authors describe the process in detail.[495,497]

- **RUSI of the lateral abdominal muscles** (Figures 4-78 and 4-79): To obtain an image of the TrA, the ultrasound transducer is placed halfway between the ASIS and the lower rib cage along the anterior axillary line. Images are taken at rest and during TrA contraction. The TrA, internal oblique, and external oblique are identified and measured at rest and during contraction.[492]
- **RUSI of the MF** (Figure 4-80): To obtain an image of the MF muscle, the ultrasound transducer is placed horizontally over the SP (as pictured) or longitudinally along the spine with the mid-point over the SP of interest and then moved laterally and angled slightly medially until the zygapophyseal joint is identified. The LM is identified and measured from the zygapophyseal joint to the subcutaneous tissue at rest and during contraction with the transducer oriented longitudinally.[492]

Assessment of Abdominal Bracing Versus Abdominal Drawing-In Maneuver

In contrast to the ADIM, the abdominal brace (AB) is a low-level (5% to 10% maximum voluntary isometric contraction) stiffening or isometric cocontraction of the muscles around the trunk (ie, abdominals, paraspinals, and TrA) with no attempt to preferentially activate the TrA. The spine or pelvis should not move and the abdominal wall is not sucked in or pushed out. According to McGill,[499] the AB stabilizes the spine in bending and twisting perturbations whereas the ADIM does not.

Grenier and McGill[500] provided support that suggests the AB is an optimal method for activating spinal musculature. From a mechanical perspective, bracing appears to provide patterns of greater stability, while the ADIM does not appear to enhance stability.[500] Training of the TrA and MF are related to motor control aspects of segmental spinal stability, initially de-emphasizing the use of the global stabilizers. AB appears to function by providing dynamic spinal stability through all muscles of the trunk, both deep

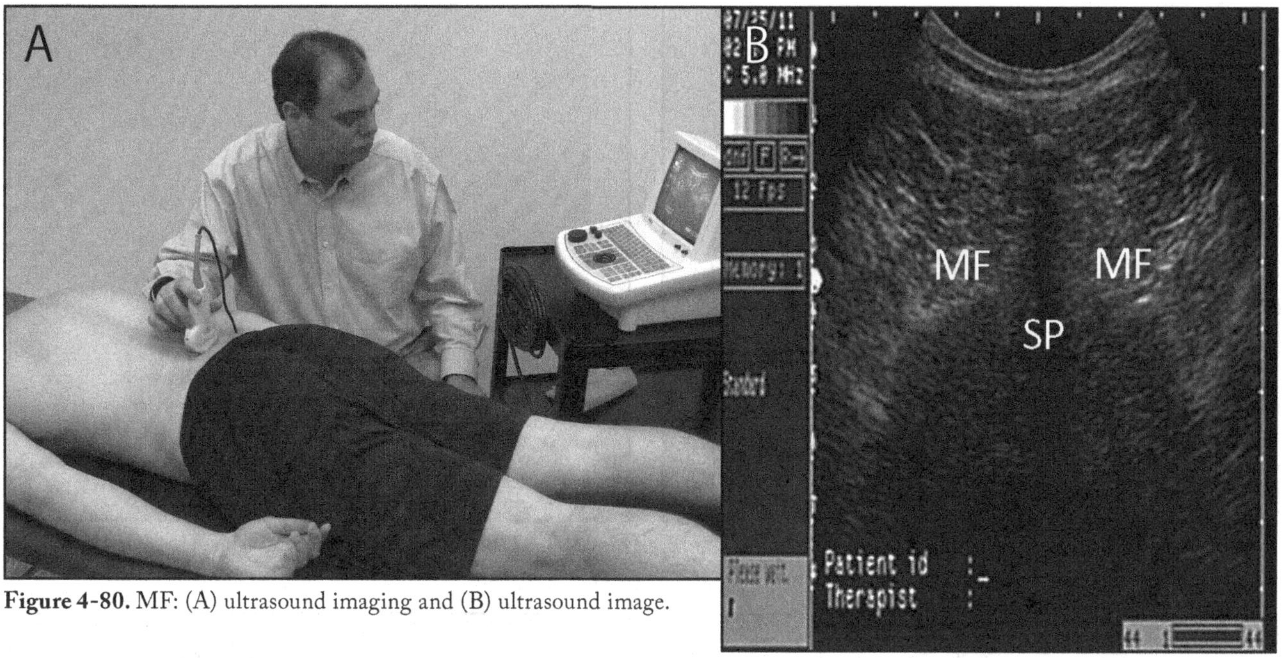

Figure 4-80. MF: (A) ultrasound imaging and (B) ultrasound image.

and superficial. Examination of the patient, the amount of load his or her spine will tolerate, and the specific tasks he or she needs or desires to perform will help the clinician determine whether to start with AB or ADIM.

Sacroiliac Joint Provocation Tests

This cluster of tests includes distraction, compression, thigh thrust, Gaenslen's, and sacral thrust[501,502] performed to reproduce or increase a patient's familiar symptoms in the SIJ in an attempt to implicate or rule out a symptomatic SIJ. The tests have good to excellent interrater reliability (kappa): distraction (0.69), compression (0.73), thigh thrust (0.88), Gaenslen's (0.76), and sacral thrust (0.56).[503] Laslett et al[501,502] reported the following statistics to suggest a symptomatic SIJ in patients having positive SIJ diagnostic injections and no centralization or peripheralization based on a repeated movement examination. If 3 or more of the above are positive, Sn is 0.91 (95% CI: 0.62 to 0.98), Sp is 0.87 (95% CI: 0.68 to 0.96), +LR is 6.97 (95% CI: 2.70 to 20.27), and –LR is 0.11 (95% CI: 0.02 to 0.44). Using only 4 tests of distraction, thigh thrust, sacral thrust, and compression, only 2 of the 4 tests need to be positive for a diagnosis of SIJ-related pain: Sn 0.88 (0.64, 0.97), Sp 0.78 (0.61, 0.89), +LR 4.0 (2.13, 8.08), and –LR (0.04, 0.47). If all 6 tests do not produce familiar pain, the SIJ can be ruled out. Each test position is held 7 to 10 seconds and performed as follows.[501,502]

Distraction

In supine, the clinician applies a posteriorly directed force through both ASISs purported to distract the anterior aspect of the SIJ (Figure 4-81).

Compression (Side-Lying)

In side-lying with hips and knees flexed to about 90 degrees, the clinician applies a downward vertical force through the upper iliac crest, purported to compress both SIJs anteriorly (Figure 4-82).

Thigh Thrust

In supine with hip flexed to 90 degrees and knee comfortably flexed, the clinician applies a downward vertical force through the femur (Figure 4-83). The clinician stabilizes the sacrum with one hand and encircles the flexed knee. The force is purported to provide a posterior shearing force to the SIJ on that side.

Gaenslen's Test

In supine with one hip flexed toward the patient's chest and the other extended over the edge of the table, the clinician applies OP to both sides at the same time (Figure 4-84). The test is performed on both sides and purported to create a posterior rotational load to the SIJ of the flexed hip and an anterior rotational load to the SIJ of the extended hip side.

Sacral Thrust

In prone, the clinician applies a posterior-to-anterior (PA) force to the center of the sacrum purported to produce an anterior shearing force of the sacrum on both ilia (Figure 4-85).

Positive Sacroiliac Joint Provocation Tests

A positive test occurs when the patient's familiar symptoms are reproduced or increased, but the test does not indicate a specific pathology or help direct treatment.

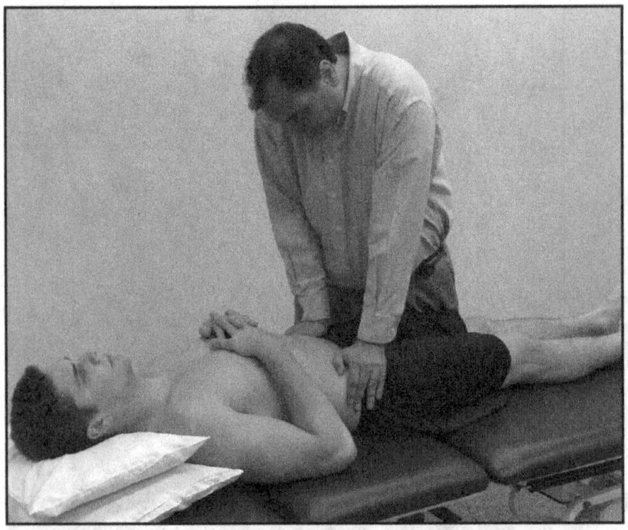

Figure 4-81. SIJ provocation—distraction.

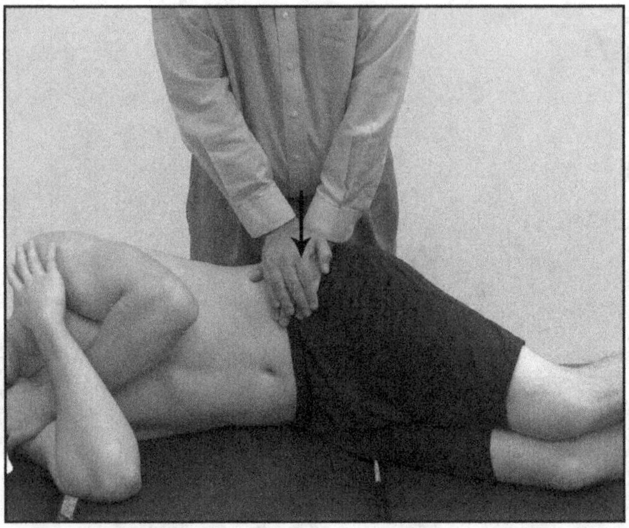

Figure 4-82. SIJ provocation—compression (side-lying).

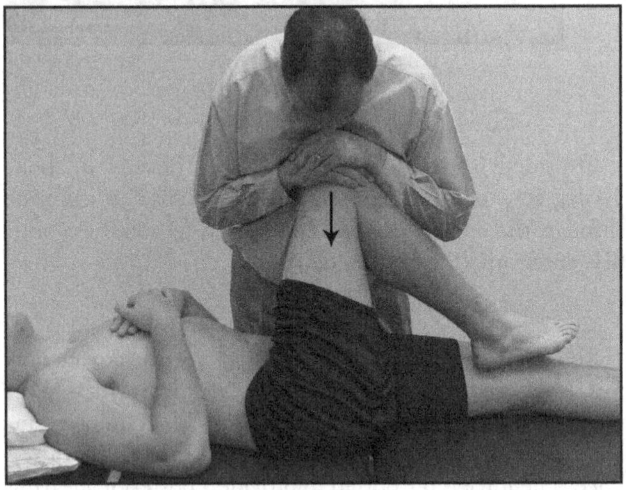

Figure 4-83. SIJ provocation—thigh thrust.

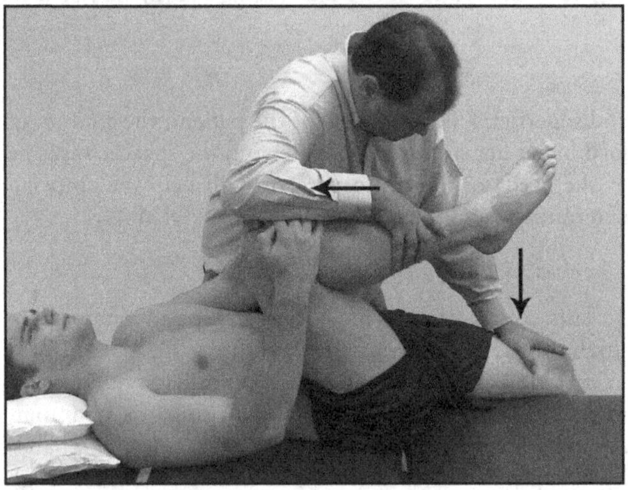

Figure 4-84. SIJ provocation—Gaenslen's test.

Figure 4-85. SIJ provocation—sacral thrust.

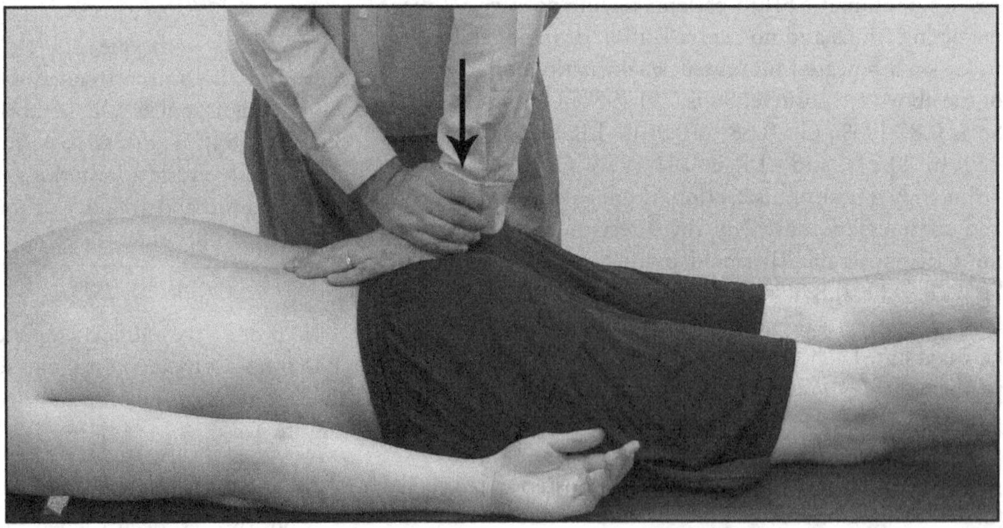

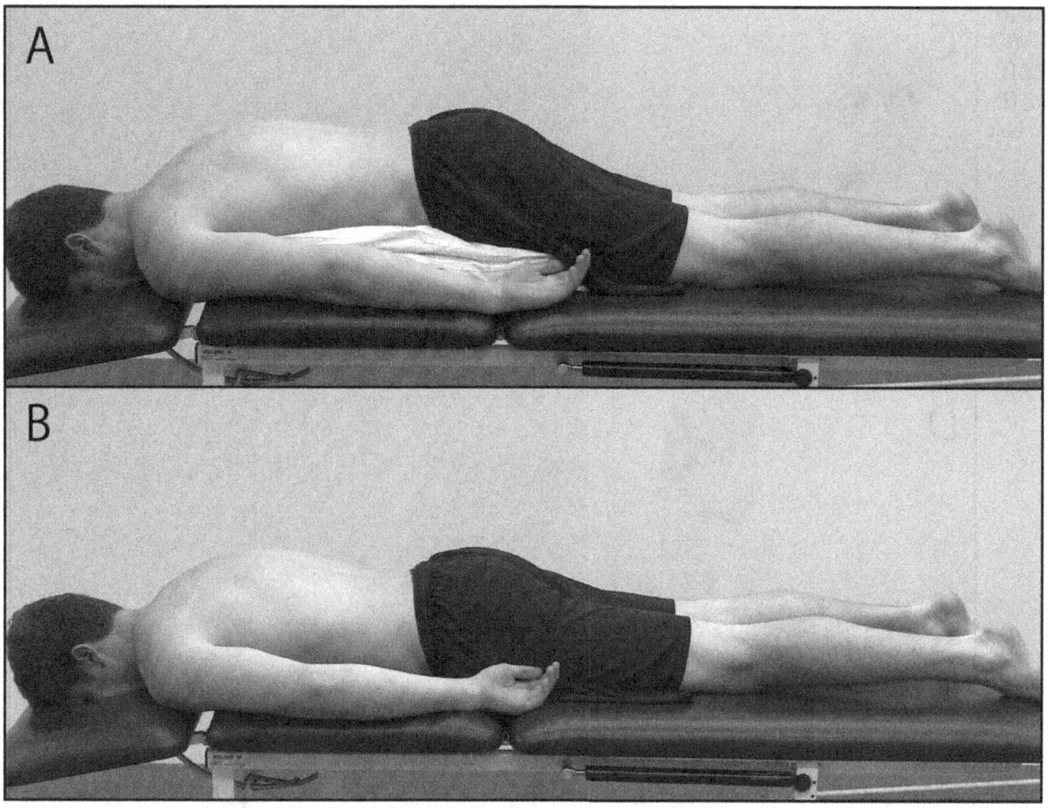

Figure 4-86. Repeated movements: (A) prone on pillows sustained and (B) prone sustained. *(continued)*

Examination Procedures in Prone

- Repeated movements
  - Prone on pillow, prone, prone on elbows
  - REIL
  - REIL with sag, REIL with mobilization belt, REIL with clinician OP, REIL with hips offset
- Prone knee bend (PKB)/femoral nerve stretch test/ quadriceps length.
- Hip extension: MMT (GMax, HS), HS (DTR)
- Hip IR ROM: bilaterally
- Palpation/passive accessory intervertebral movement (PAIVM): central and unilateral
- Prone instability test (PIT)
- Passive lumbar extension (PLE) test

Repeated Movements[401,402]

The clinician should observe the patient transition to prone and note symptom response. Resting posture in prone is also observed for provocative and easing positions. If peripheralization or partial centralization occurs in weightbearing during REIS or manual lateral shift correction, continuation of the repeated movement examination occurs in prone in an attempt to obtain centralization. On occasion, the patient presents with a kyphotic lumbar spine and major loss of extension that is not amenable to REIS or, if the patient is unable to lie prone for a continued examination, a progressive examination sequence is necessary to obtain centralization and regain the lumbar lordosis. As symptoms centralize, patients may experience a temporary increase centrally in LBP, which should gradually decrease as the process of centralization continues. Additional resources are available for an in-depth discussion on the use of repeated movement test procedures.[401,402] A common sequence of test procedures—although not all-inclusive of procedures—is performed as needed[401,402]:

- **Prone on pillow or pillows** (sustained; Figure 4-86A): Position is sustained for 5 to 10 minutes. As centralization occurs, the pillow(s) are gradually removed.
- **Prone** (sustained; Figure 4-86B): Position is sustained for 5 to 10 minutes. Progression is to prone on elbows or REIL if indicated.
- **Prone on elbows** (sustained; Figure 4-86C): Progression is to REIL as indicated.
- **REIL** (Figure 4-86D): A patient who peripheralizes with REIS may be able to centralize with REIL. REIL produces a greater mechanical effect than REIS. In prone with hands under the shoulders, the patient raises the upper half of the body by gradually straightening the arms. The pelvis and thigh remain relaxed and allow the abdomen to sag. Initially, the response to 10 to 15 repetitions is observed.

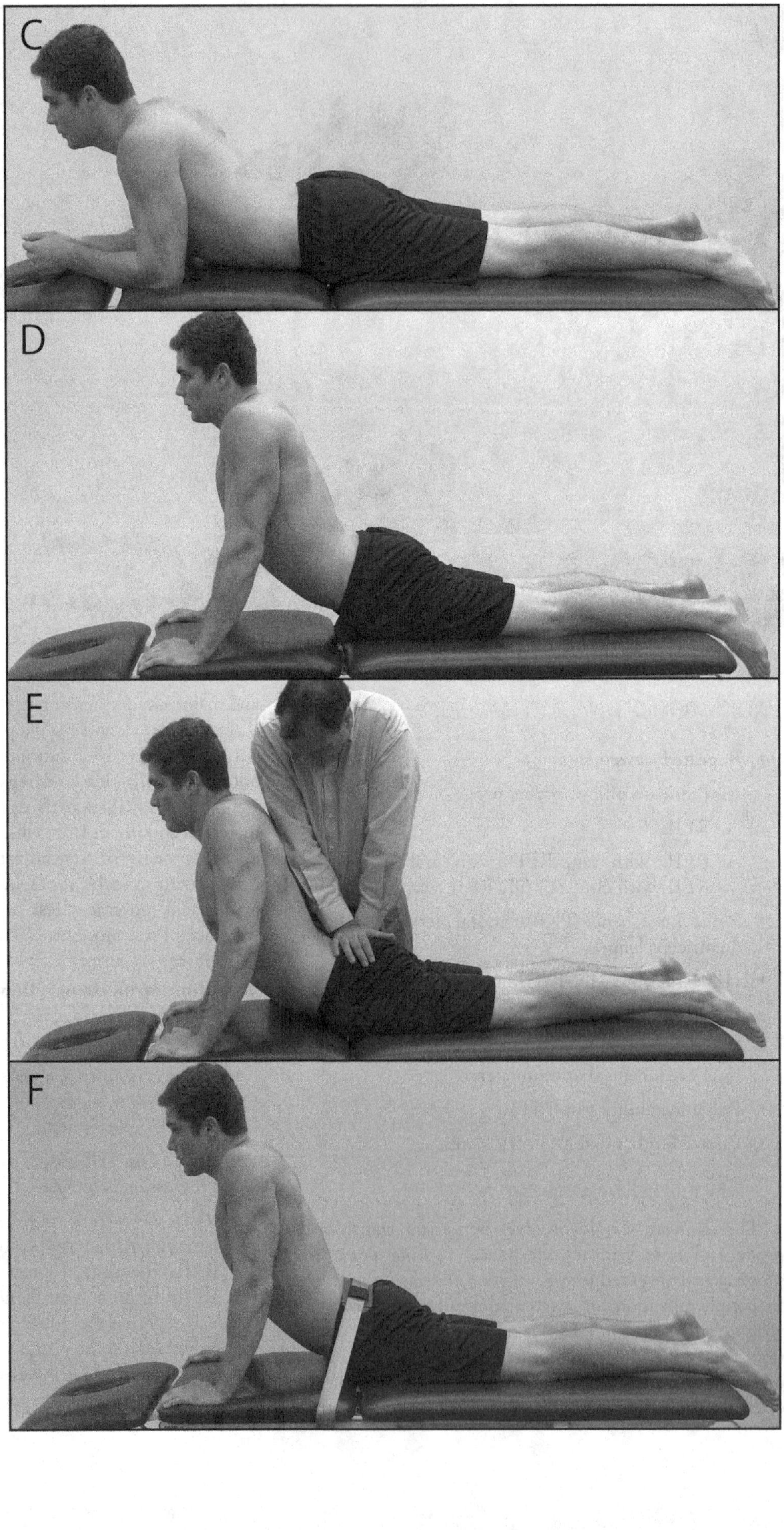

Figure 4-86 (continued). Repeated movements: (C) prone on elbows; (D) REIL; (E) REIL with OP; and (F) REIL with mobilization belt fixation. *(continued)*

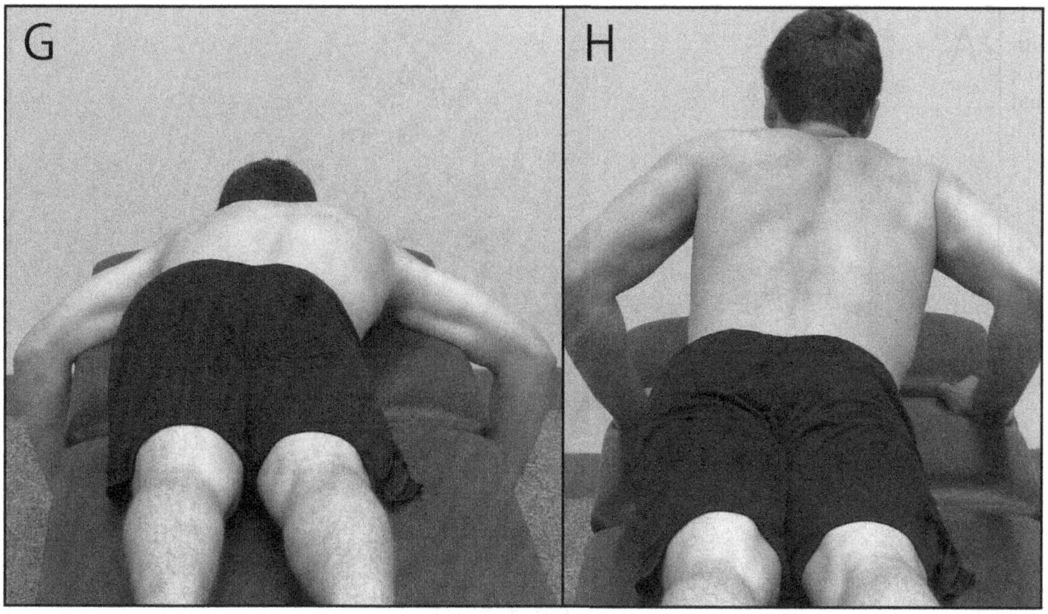

Figure 4-86 (continued). Repeated movements: (G) REIL with hips off center to the left starting position and (H) REIL with hips shifted to the left.

- **REIL with sag**: As patients attain the full range of REIL with arms extended, additional lumbar extension force may be gained if needed by exhaling at the end-range.
- **REIL with clinician OP** (Figure 4-86E): The clinician uses a cross-arm technique to place one hypothenar eminence of each hand over the transverse process of the same segment. By leaning forward, a gentle, symmetrical pressure is performed as the patient performs REIL. The clinician allows the motion to occur. If the pressure produces more pain, derangement (direction-specific) or dysfunction (mobility deficit) classification may be present. If the pressure decreases symptoms or creates centralization, a DSE classification (see Table 4-3) is likely.
- **REIL with mobilization belt fixation** (Figure 4-86F): This procedure is used only if indicated by an appropriate response to REIL with clinician OP. The fixation belt is used as part of a home exercise program or when indicated as treatment for an extension dysfunction (ie, mobility deficit). The belt is applied around the pelvis and table to provide additional extension force to the lumbar spine.
- **REIL with hips off center**: This procedure is indicated when unilateral symptoms worsen or do not respond to sagittal plane movements of REIS or REIL. The procedure is the same as for REIL except for the starting position with the hips off center (Figure 4-86G), creating a lateral force in an extension procedure. The hips are usually shifted away from the painful side and REIL is performed (Figure 4-86H). If worse or no effect, assess the response with the hips shifted to the painful side.[401,402]

Test Procedure

The procedure is the same as listed under movement testing for repeated movements in standing and the response is recorded. If centralization or DP occurs, classify as DSE (extension or lateral shift; see Table 4-3) or derangement and proceed to matched intervention. If peripheralization occurs and attempts to centralize the symptoms fail, the clinician must consider an alternative classification such as mechanical traction (see Table 4-4). If the response to REIL is limited motion and end-range pain (ie, produced, increased, or no worse) and no centralization or peripheralization occur, further examination such as passive segmental mobility testing is needed. The clinician considers a classification of LBP with mobility deficits (see Table 4-1).

Prone Knee Bend—Neurodynamic Test

As an NDT,[424,425] the PKB places a tension load on the upper- and mid-lumbar nerve roots (L2 to L4) through tension of the femoral nerve during knee flexion.[504] The test is indicated for patients with hip, knee, thigh, or upper lumbar (L2 to L4) symptoms and is suggested to aid in the diagnosis of lumbar radicular symptoms at these levels.[424] The prevalence of upper lumbar radiculopathies is 3% to 5%, which adds to the difficulty of diagnostic accuracy research on this population. Intertester reliability of the PKB is low, κ = 0.38 (0.19, 0.56).[505] In a sample of 16 patients with lumbar radicular pain and MRI as the reference standard, intertester reliability for the slump knee bend test—a side-lying version of the PKB test is κ = 0.71 (95% CI: 0.33 to 1.0). Diagnostic accuracy is Sn 1.00 (0.40 to 1.00), Sp 0.83 (0.52 to 0.98), +LR 6.0 (1.58 to 19.4), and –LR 0 (0 to 0.6).[506]

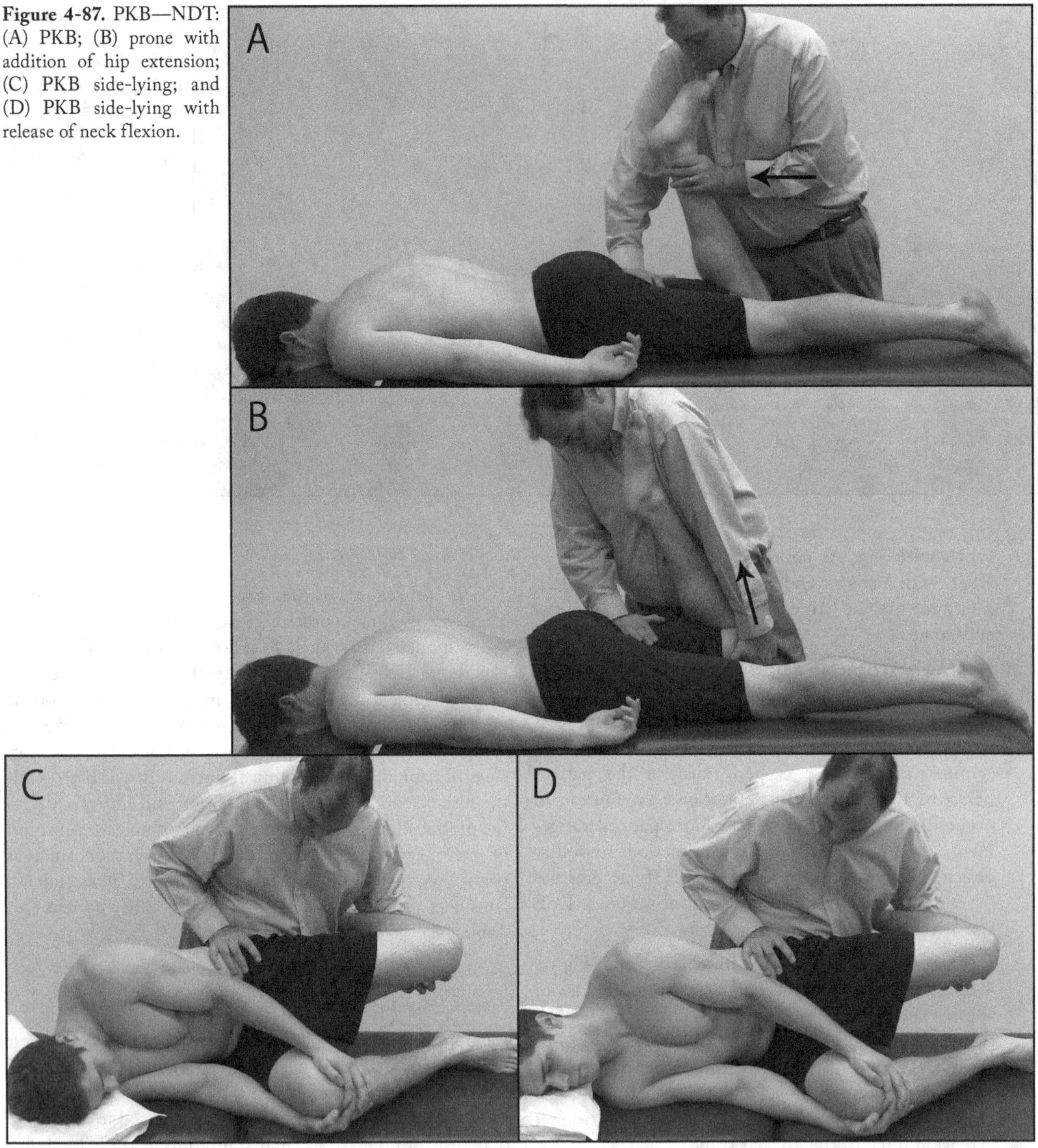

Figure 4-87. PKB—NDT: (A) PKB; (B) prone with addition of hip extension; (C) PKB side-lying; and (D) PKB side-lying with release of neck flexion.

Test Procedure

The PKB test (Figures 4-87A and 4-87B) can be performed in prone or side-lying, which is known as the *slump knee bend test*. In prone with the hip in neutral and the pelvis stabilized, the clinician passively flexes the knee, attempting to differentiate symptoms from the lumbar spine, hip, knee, quadriceps or neural tissue mechanosensitivity. The addition of hip extension may be used as sensitizing maneuver, but still allows movement of various somatic structures.[424,425]

The slump knee bend test (Figure 4-87C) allows for differentiation of neural mechanosensitivity and symptomatic somatic structures. In side-lying, the patient positions the head and trunk in flexion while grasping the knee of the untested side and pulling it toward the chest, creating trunk and neck flexion. While maintaining trunk and neck flexion, the clinician stabilizes the pelvis and supports the weight of the upper leg in neutral with the knee flexed to 90 degrees. Hip extension is then added slowly to the point of symptom reproduction. If no symptoms occur with hip extension, knee flexion may be added. When symptoms are reproduced, the patient is asked to extend the neck. If symptoms are changed, neural mechanosensitivity is implicated. If symptoms do not change, somatic-related symptoms are implicated.[424,425] For both the prone and side-lying versions of this test, an increase or reproduction of the patient's familiar symptoms, asymmetry between uninvolved to involved sides, and a positive sensitizing maneuver describe a positive test. Symptoms of pulling or pain related to tension on the rectus femoris or quadriceps or hip or knee somatic structures are normal responses. Symptoms may also refer from the lumbar spine or hip.

Prone Knee Bend—Quadriceps Length Test

In patients with patellofemoral pain, interexaminer reliability is ICC = 0.91 (0.80, 0.96) using an inclinometer.[480] The quadriceps length test is performed in prone. While preventing anterior pelvic tilt and lumbar spine extension, the clinician passively flexes the patient's knee. Knee flexion is measured with a bubble inclinometer placed over the distal tibia and zeroed to the horizontal (Figure 4-88). A positive test is side-to-side asymmetry. Relevance is based on clinical experience. Normative data are not available.

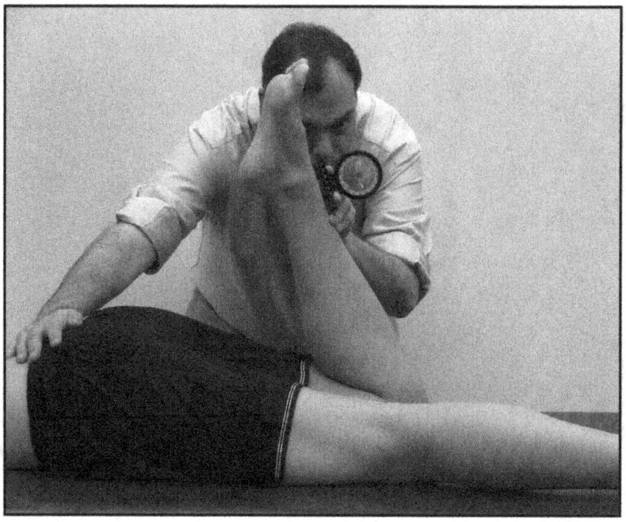

Figure 4-88. PKB—quadriceps length test.

Hip Extension and Knee Flexion

MMT procedures are discussed in Chapter 3.

Hip Internal Rotation Active and Passive Range of Motion

Hip IR AROM and PROM are measured bilaterally in prone (see Figure 4-48D). At least one hip with > 35 degrees of IR measured with an inclinometer in prone is a key factor in a validated CPR that identifies patients with LBP who may benefit from manipulation (see Table 4-1).[140,141] This ROM procedure has excellent interrater reliability (ICC 0.95 to 0.97). In prone with the cervical spine in midline, the leg opposite the one to be measured is placed in 30 degrees of ABD. The hip on the side to be tested is in line with the body with the knee flexed to 90 degrees. The gravity inclinometer is zeroed on the distal aspect of the fibula in line with the bone. IR is measured at the point when the pelvis first begins to move.[141]

Lumbopelvic Hip Palpation in Prone

Palpation in prone should include any area of the patient's symptoms. An approach to palpation of this area is discussed below, but not all areas are palpated on every patient. General guidelines are to begin with palpation for changes in temperature and sweating with progression in a layered manner to assess tone and mobility of skin and soft tissue structures and bony symmetry. The skin and muscles should be soft and easy to move. Areas of tenderness are noted in a side-to-side comparison. Final palpation involves segmental passive movement tests to assess PAIVM. Palpation procedures are not standardized in the literature.

General Palpation Scheme

The index fingers are used to locate the iliac crests bilaterally. The L4-5 interspace generally bisects an imaginary line connecting the iliac crests. The clinician should verify the level of the SP by palpating the SPs and supraspinous ligament from L4 to T10 and the SPs from L4 to S5 and the coccyx. The lumbar SPs are broad and flat except for L5, which is pointed. In locating 3 spinal levels by palpation (C5, T6, L5), Billis et al[507] reported poor intertester reliability at these spinal levels but good intratester reliability. LM are located immediately adjacent to the SPs. The lateral border of the MF begins at L1 SP and descends on a diagonal to the PSIS bilaterally. The lumbar facet joints are not palpable but are generally located 2 to 3 cm (0.8 to 1.0 inches) lateral to the SPs. The PSISs are located approximately at the level of S2 SP. Immediately distal to the PSIS, the long dorsal sacroiliac ligament (LDL) is palpable. Lateral to the PSISs, the clinician palpates the gluteal muscles moving toward the greater trochanter. The clinician locates the greater trochanter and the gluteus medius attaching to its superior aspect. The piriformis and other ERs are palpated from the inferior and lateral border of the sacrum to the greater trochanter. In the center of the gluteal fold, the clinician palpates the ischial tuberosity and the attachment of the hamstrings. Halfway between ischial tuberosity and the greater trochanter, the sciatic nerve is often palpable as it emerges under the gluteus maximus. The lateral border of the quadratus lumborum is palpated from the tip of the 12th rib to the iliac crest.

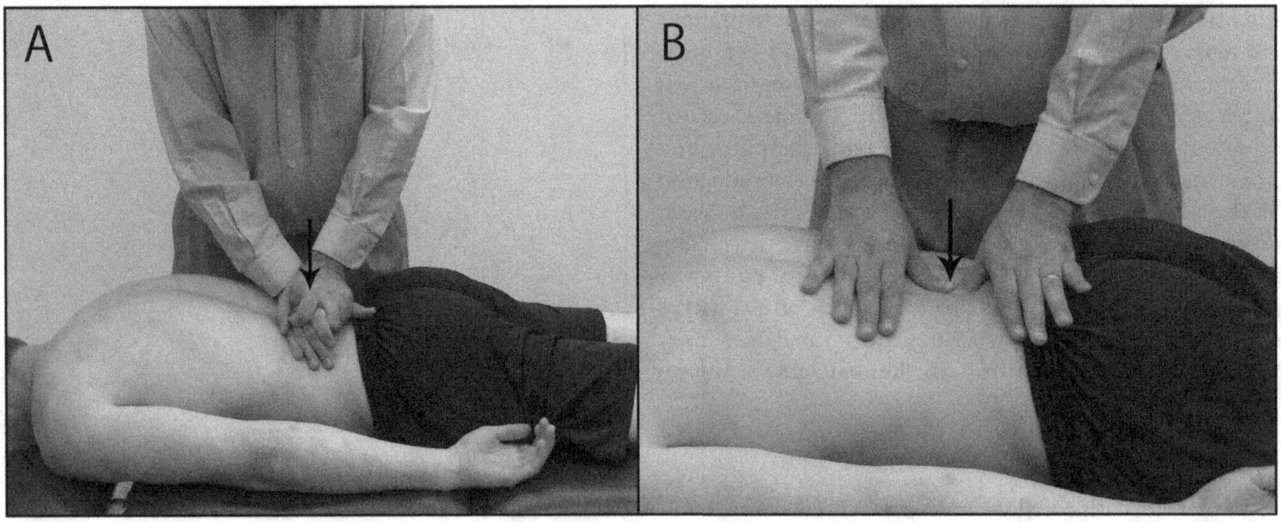

Figure 4-89. PAIVM lumbar spine: (A) central PA PAIVM and (B) unilateral PA PAIVM.

Passive Accessory Intervertebral Movement Assessment[269]

Segmental motion tests used in combination with other clinical findings demonstrate predictive validity and usefulness for determining treatment and outcome.[140,141,197,508] Lumbar hypomobility identified with a central PAIVM combined with key history and physical exam findings is useful in predicting which patients are most likely to improve with manipulation.[140,141] Lumbar hypermobility assessed with a central PAIVM, a factor in a multivariate CPR, is predictive of a successful outcome with a stabilization program.[197] Fritz et al[508] concluded that persons with LBP judged by a central PAIVM to have lumbar hypomobility experienced greater benefit from an intervention including manipulation, while those with hypermobility were more likely to benefit from a stabilization exercise program. Despite the low reliability associated with PAIVM tests, judgments of hypomobility or hypermobility provide useful and valid information for clinical decision making when combined with other examination findings.[508]

The purpose of PAIVM is to determine whether movement at an appropriate spinal segment reproduces the patient's symptoms and which segments are normal, hypomobile, or hypermobile for purposes of diagnostic classification and guiding intervention. For assessment, central PA (CPA) and unilateral PA (UPA) PAIVMs are performed over the sacrum (S1-5) and the SP of the vertebrae from L5 through T10 or higher. PAIVM are both provocation and mobility tests of the lumbar segments. Reproduction of lumbar symptoms with PAIVM in the lower thoracic spine requires a detailed examination of the thoracic spine. Diagnostic utility is discussed in Chapter 3. Hicks et al[436] defined segmental mobility associated with PAIVM as follows:

- *Hypermobility*: More motion than normally expected between the tested segment and the adjacent segments
- *Normal mobility*: Motion at the segmental level is within normally expected limits
- *Hypomobility*: Less motion than normally expected between the tested segment and the adjacent segments

Central Posterior-to-Anterior Passive Accessory Intervertebral Movement[269]

With the patient in prone with arms at the side, the clinician places the hypothenar eminence just distal to the pisiform over the SP of the vertebra (Figure 4-89A). The other hand is gently placed on top of this hand and assists in keeping the wrist extended. The elbows are straight, allowing the clinician's sternum to be directly over the SP. Assessment is performed superficial to deep in a progressive oscillatory manner to assess symptom response and quality of movement through range and at end-range. The clinician does not push on the spine but instead leans forward, translating the weight of the trunk through the arms to the spine.

Unilateral Posterior-to-Anterior Passive Accessory Intervertebral Movement[269]

In the same position as described for CPA PAIVM, the clinician uses both thumbs to produce the passive accessory movement (Figure 4-89B). The thumbs are placed in the area of the zygapophyseal joints, 2 to 3 cm lateral to the SP, beginning on the uninvolved side, making a side-to-side comparison.

- Explain the procedure and establish resting symptoms.
- Ask the patient for symptoms produced during the movement test.
- Perform CPA or UPA PAIVM at each level of interest.

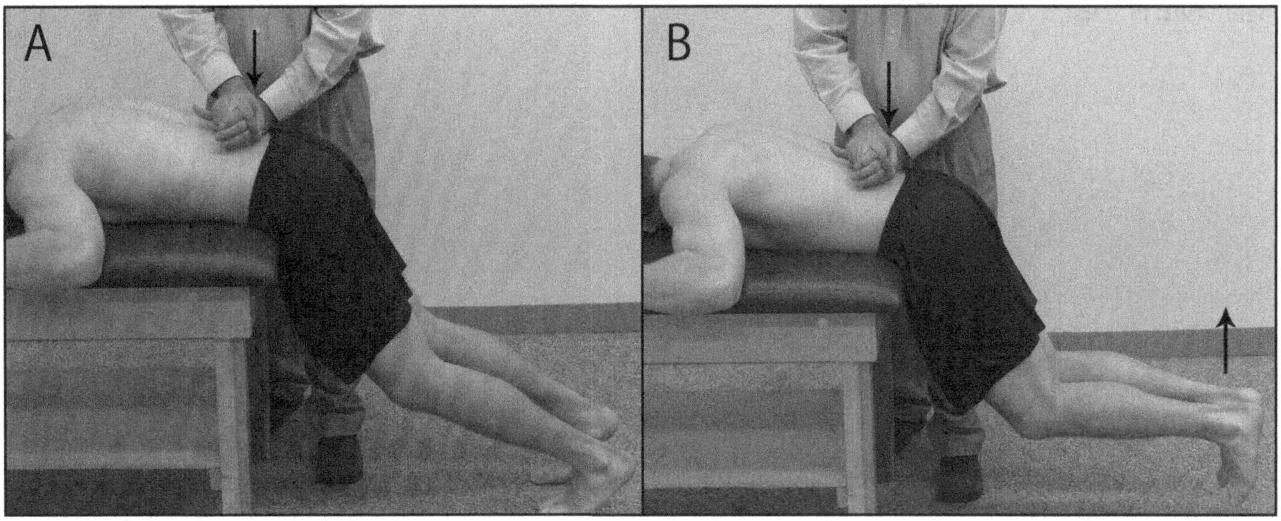

Figure 4-90. PIT: (A) step 1 and (B) step 2.

- Determine which movements produce or increase the patient's familiar or local symptoms.
- Assess the relationship between pain and resistance.
- Determine if movement is normal, hypomobile, or hypermobile.
- Compare findings with levels above and below and on the opposite side for UPA.

Prone Instability Test

The purpose of the PIT is to aid in the diagnosis of lumbar segmental instability. Interrater reliability is excellent (κ = 0.87 [0.80 to 0.94]).[436] A positive or negative PIT is a key variable in a preliminary CPR important for identifying persons with LBP who are likely or unlikely to benefit from a stabilization training program.[197]

The test (Figure 4-90) is performed with the patient in prone with the trunk supported on the table and feet resting on the floor.[197] In this position, the clinician performs a CPA PAIVM on the symptomatic segment. The patient is asked to lift the legs off the floor less than 6 inches while holding onto the table and the CPA PAIVM is repeated. The patient is asked to report any change in symptoms comparing the test with feet on the floor versus with the feet lifted. The test is positive if the symptoms reported on the first part of the test disappear on the second part of the test. If pain is present with the initial CPA PAIVM but is not present with the CPA PAVIM and lifting the legs, which activates spinal extensors, the theory is that force closure or muscle activation is capable of stabilizing the symptomatic segment.

Passive Lumbar Extension Test[509]

The purpose of the PLE test is to aid in the diagnosis of lumbar segmental instability.[509] Sensitivity (0.84), specificity (0.90), and +LR (8.84 [4.51 to 17.33]) were determined by comparing a positive or negative PLE test in 122 subjects ages 39 to 88 years with degenerative lumbar disease using the gold standard of flexion-extension radiographs.[509]

The test is performed (Figure 4-91) with the patient in prone; the clinician elevates both lower extremities at the same time approximately 30 cm (11.8 inches) from the table while keeping the knees straight and gently pulling the legs. The response is assessed during elevation of both legs and then on return of both legs to the table. During elevation of both legs, the test is considered positive if the patient complains of strong pain in the lumbar region or LBP, a very heavy feeling on the low back, or a feeling as if the low back is coming off, and if the pain goes away when the legs are lowered to the table. Complaints such as mild numbness or a prickling sensation do not indicate a positive test.[509]

Examination Procedures in Side-Lying

- Passive physiological intervertebral movements (PPIVMs): flexion, extension, LF, rotation
- Ober's test
- Hip ABD/ADD strength test

Passive Physiological Intervertebral Movement Test[269]

The PPIVM tests are performed to assess passive physiological flexion, extension, LF, and rotation segmental motion of L5-S1 through T10-12 and determine whether movement at an appropriate spinal segment reproduces the patient's symptoms and whether the segmental motion is normal, hypomobile, or hypermobile for purposes of diagnostic classification and guiding intervention. Diagnostic utility is discussed in Chapter 3. The following PPIVM tests[269] may be performed on the lumbar spine.

Figure 4-91. PLE test.

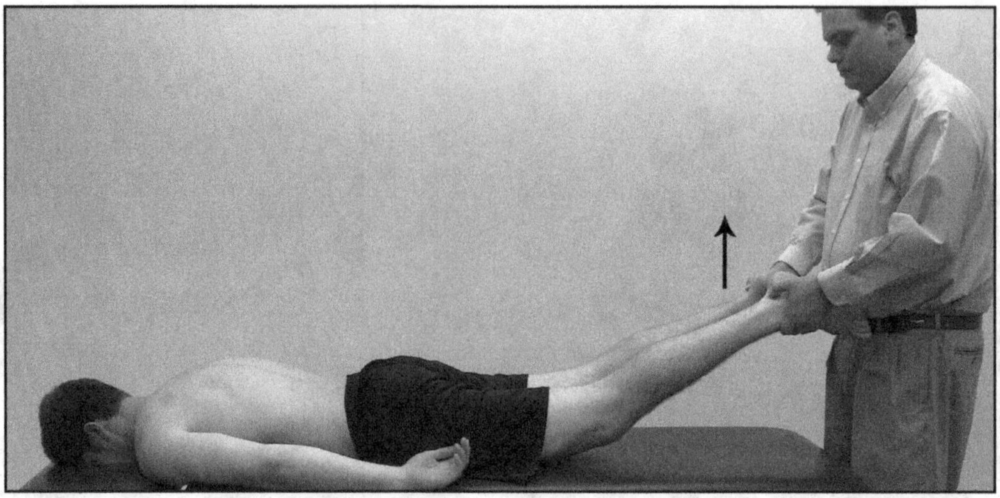

Flexion

Patient is in side-lying in neutral lumbar spine with the knees flexed (Figure 4-92A). The clinician is facing the patient, supporting the uppermost leg or both legs at the ankle with the knees resting on the clinician's thigh. The other hand palpates starting at the L5-S1 interspace using the middle or index finger. A neutral position for each segment should be the starting position for assessment. As the clinician slowly brings the hips into flexion, motion is recruited at each spinal motion segment. The clinician assesses the amount of opening at the interspinous space.

Extension

Patient is in side-lying in neutral lumbar spine with hips and knees flexed (Figure 4-92B). The clinician is facing the patient, supporting the uppermost leg or both legs at the ankle with the knees resting on the clinician's thigh. The other hand palpates starting at the L5-S1 interspace using the middle or index finger. A neutral position for each segment should be the starting position for assessment. As the clinician slowly brings the hip or hips into extension, motion is recruited at each spinal motion segment. The clinician assesses the amount of closing at the interspinous space.

Lateral Flexion Left

Patient is in right side-lying in neutral lumbar spine (Figure 4-92C). The clinician is in a walk stance position facing the patient's feet while supporting the uppermost leg or both legs at the ankle with the patient's knees resting on the clinician's thigh. A neutral position for each segment should be the starting position for assessment. The other hand palpates between the SPs on the left side or uppermost side. The clinician creates LF by shifting weight onto the back foot and bringing the patient's legs with him or her. A closing motion at the interspinous space (eg, L4-5) is felt as the L5 SP moves toward the L4 SP into the palpating finger. For LF right, the patient is side-lying left.

Rotation Left

The patient is side-lying on the right in a neutral spine position with hips and knees flexed to about 45 degrees (Figure 4-92D). The clinician faces the patient and stabilizes the pelvis with his or her trunk, placing the right forearm along the spine with the middle finger of the hand at the underside of the interspinous space at the level for motion palpation starting at L1-2. The clinician places the left forearm alongside the patient's rib cage and gently imparts a left rotation force through the patient's lower rib cage. A neutral position for each segment should be the starting position for assessment. The palpating finger at the interspinous space of L1-2 will feel the SP of L1 move into the pad of the middle finger. When L2 SP starts to move, the end of segmental rotation is reached. The process continues distally to L5-S1.

Ober's Test[510]

Ober's test (Figure 4-93) assesses TFL and iliotibial band tightness. Using an inclinometer placed at the distal thigh over the lateral epicondyle, Reese and Bandy[510] reported intrarater reliability of the repeated measurements on separate days as 0.90 for the Ober's test and 0.91 for the modified Ober's test. Validity of this test is unknown.

In side-lying with the lower leg flexed at the hip and knee for stability, the clinician stabilizes the pelvis and passively places the upper hip in ABD and extension. The knee can be flexed to 90 degrees or extended (modified Ober's test). With the hip in line with the trunk, the thigh is lowered into ADD. A positive test result is if the hip does not adduct past the horizontal or when symptoms or complaints of tightness are reproduced. If the thigh is at horizontal, 0 degrees is recorded. If below horizontal, a positive number is recorded. If above horizontal, a negative number is recorded. Given that the modified Ober's test allows significantly greater hip ADD than the original Ober's test, the 2 examination procedures should not be used interchangeably.[510]

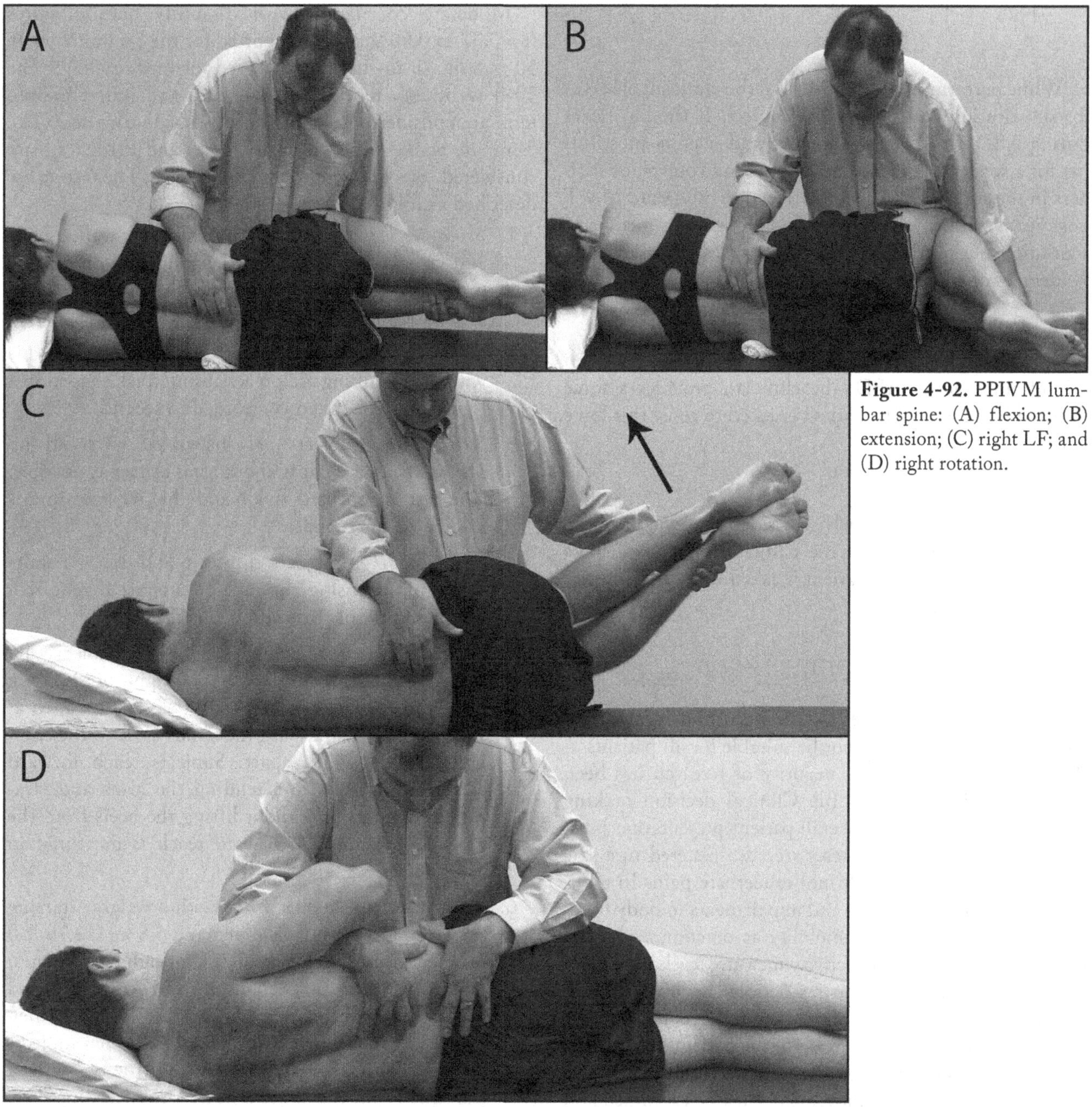

Figure 4-92. PPIVM lumbar spine: (A) flexion; (B) extension; (C) right LF; and (D) right rotation.

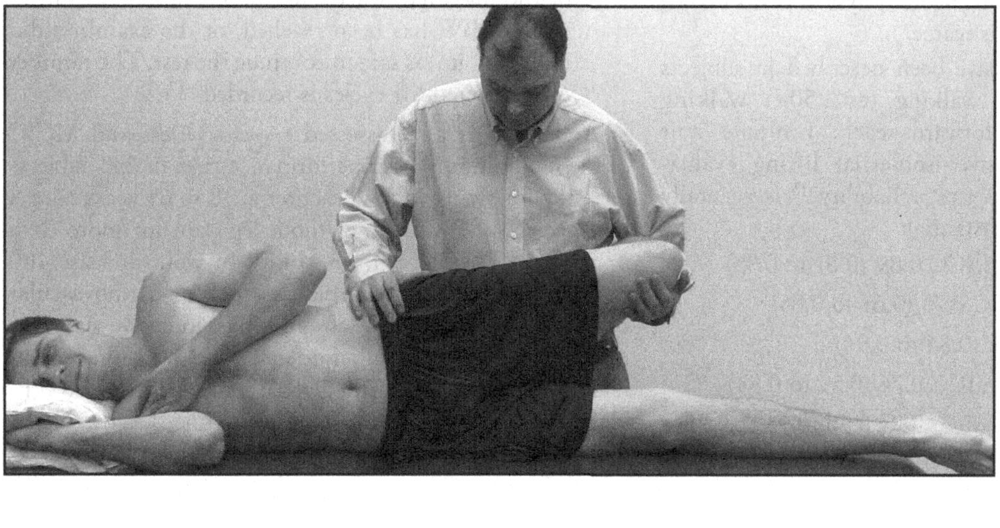

Figure 4-93. Ober's test knee flexed.

Hip Abduction/Adduction Manual Muscle Tests

While performing the hip MMTs, the clinician observes for substitution and poor trunk control. If the hip flexes during ABD, the TFL is overactive and may be substituting for a weak gluteus medius, poor trunk control, or stiffness in the adductors. An alternative to the standard MMT position is performing an MMT of the gluteus medius in a position of 35 degrees ABD, 10 degrees extension, and 10 degrees of ER.[511]

Abduction

While stabilizing the pelvis in side-lying with the hip at end-range active ABD, the clinician provides a force directed into ADD. The patient is asked to resist this force (see Figure 4-56).

Adduction

While stabilizing the pelvis in side-lying with the hip at end-range active ADD, the clinician provides a force directed into ABD. The patient is asked to resist this force (see Figure 4-57).

Physical Performance Tests

These tests are described at the end of the examination section because they may not be suitable for all patients at the initial evaluation. The majority of research has been done on subjects with CLBP. Clinical decision making based on the SINSS and overall patient presentation must be considered so that the tests are administered in a safe manner. These tests should not exacerbate pain. In addition to self-report measures and impairments in body function such as strength and mobility as outcomes, physical performance tests that objectively measure levels of activity limitation and participation restrictions are often recommended. Functional tests should be tailored to activities that are necessary and important to the patient. In addition to parameters such as time, distance, or number of steps, quality and efficiency of movement must be examined and trained. However, research related to physical performance tests in patients with LBP is scarce.

Six performance tests have been described in subjects with CLBP: a 5-minute walking test, 50-ft walking test, sit-to-stand, loaded forward reach, 1-minute stair climbing, and a progressive isoinertial lifting evaluation (PILE).[354,512-514] Test-retest reliability[515] is generally reported as moderate to substantial:

- 5-minute walking test: ICC 0.89 (0.81 to 0.93)
- 50-ft walking test: ICC 0.76 (0.61 to 0.85)
- Sit-to-stand: ICC 0.91 (0.84 to 0.94)
- Loaded forward reach: ICC 0.74 (0.59 to 0.84)
- One-minute stair climbing: ICC 0.96 (0.93 to 0.98)
- PILE: ICC 0.92 (0.87 to 0.96)

Moderate correlation with disability questionnaires (r = 0.37 to 0.60) has been reported for the 5-minute walk, 50-ft walk, sit-to-stand, and loaded forward reach.[354] The 50-ft walk test, repeated sit-to-stand, and stair climbing tests are considered tests of speed and coordination. The 5-minute walk, loaded forward reach, and PILE tests are considered tests of strength and endurance. The 6 tests are described as follows:

1. *5-minute walk*: For 5 minutes, subjects walk as fast and far as possible without a walking aid on a 30-m walking track shaped in a figure 8. Distance walked is recorded in meters.[354]
2. *50-ft walk*: Subjects walk 50 feet as fast as possible without a walking aid on a walking track shaped in a figure 8. Time taken is recorded in seconds.[354]
3. *Sit-to-stand*: Subjects are instructed to stand up 5 times from a chair without arms as fast as possible. The test is repeated twice and the average time is calculated in seconds.[354]
4. *Stair climbing*: Subjects climb up and down 5 stairs for 1 minute using the rail for support if required. Total amount of steps climbed is recorded.[516]
5. *Loaded forward reach* (Figure 4-94): Subjects are asked to hold a stick with a weight of 2.25 kg (4.96 lbs) for women or 4.5 kg (9.92 lbs) for men at shoulder height and with the hands close to the chest and shoulder-width apart. Subjects reach forward as far as possible by extending the arms and flexing the trunk but without lifting the heels from the ground. Distance of forward reach is measured in centimeters.[354]
6. *PILE test*: Subjects lift a box with a weight, starting at 3.6 kg (7.94 lbs) for women and 5.8 kg (12.79 lbs) for men, from the floor to a 75-cm-high (29.5 inches) table 4 times in 20 seconds. After every completed cycle, the weight is increased by 2.25 kg for women and 4.5 kg for men. The test is stopped when subjects decide to quit, they are unable to lift the box within the time limit, they have a heart rate exceeding 85% of the maximal heart rate, the maximum weight of 60% of BW has been reached, or the examiner did not think it was safe to continue the test. The number of completed lift cycles is recorded.[517,518]

Andersson et al[519] assessed responsiveness and MCIC of the 6 commonly used performance tests in 233 subjects with the following inclusion criteria: 18 to 65 years of age, nonspecific LBP with or without leg pain for more than 3 months, RMDQ >3, an ability to walk at least 100 m, and no medical comorbidities such as cardiovascular or metabolic disease which prohibits intensive exercise. Assessments were made before and after a 10-week treatment program. A 7-point global perceived effect (GPE) scale was used to assess change over time. Of the 6 performance tests, only the sit-to-stand and the stair climbing

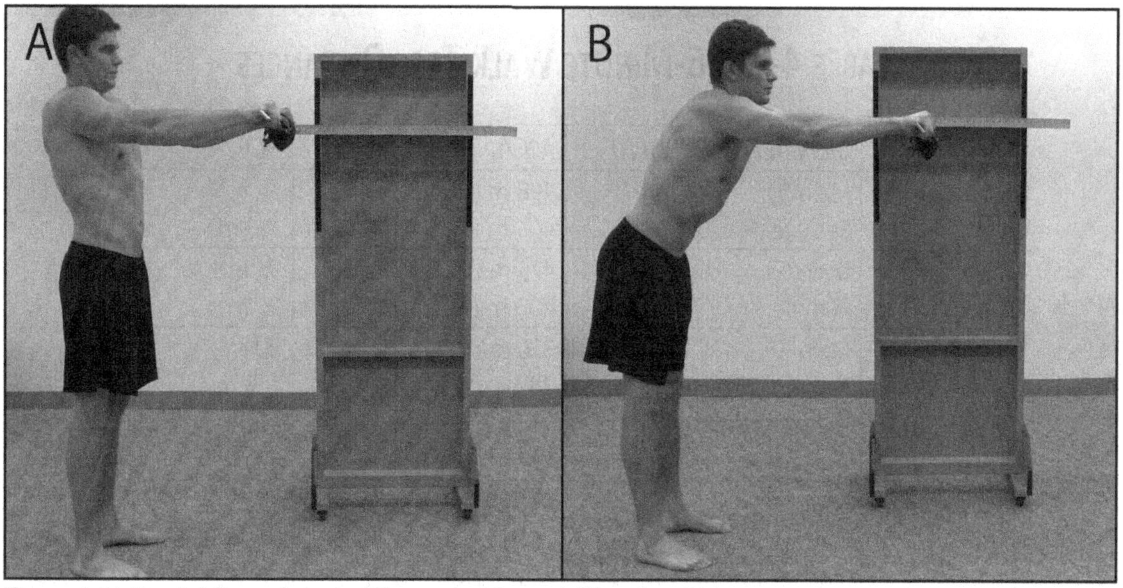

Figure 4-94. Loaded forward reach: (A) start position and (B) end position.

tests demonstrate adequate responsiveness. For sit-to-stand, the MCIC ranged from 4.1 to 9.8 seconds. For stair climbing, the MCIC ranged from 14.5 to 23.9 steps. The authors suggest that future research should define a battery of tests with multiple attributes, which should be tested on subgroups of persons with LBP who report similar levels of limitation.[519] Additional tests discussed next are the timed up and go test and the 6-minute walk test (6-MWT).

Timed Up and Go Test

The Timed Up and Go test correlates with gait speed, balance, and functional level and is used to assess change over time. The test measures the time needed to go from sit-to-stand, walk 3 m (9.84 ft), turn around, walk 3 m, and return to the seated position safely. A score of < 10 seconds is normal. A score > 14 is associated with a high fall risk in community-dwelling frail older adults.[520,521] A score > 24 at time of discharge is predictive of falls within 6 months after hip fracture.[521] In frail older adults, a score of > 30 is predictive of being dependent in ADLs and requiring an assistive device for ambulation. Normative values by age[522] are as follows: at least 60 years of age, 9.4 (8.9 to 9.9); 60 to 69 years, 8.1 seconds (7.1 to 9.0); 70 to 79 years, 9.2 seconds (8.2 to 102); and (e) 80 to 99 years, 11.3 (10.0 to 12.7).

6-Minute Walk Test

The 6-MWT measures the self-paced distance walked in 6 minutes on a level surface safely. The original purpose was to test exercise tolerance in patients with moderate to severe heart or lung disease. The test is used as a performance-based measure in other populations that includes, but is not limited to, healthy older adults,[523,524] persons with hip or knee OA,[525] and persons with fibromyalgia. Refer to the American Thoracic Society statement[526] for guidelines on safely administering this test. In community dwelling older adults, Lusardi et al[527] published normative values (Table 4-19) for the 6-MWT distances in 76 male and female subjects with a mean age of 83 ± 8. Exclusion criteria were unstable angina, cardiac event or cardiac surgery in the last 6 months, use of oxygen or inhalers, and neurological disease. Normative data vary based on medical history and test conditions. MCID also varies with no standard of change widely applicable to all populations.[528] For people with COPD, the MCID is reported as 54 to 82 m (229.6 to 269 ft).[526,528,529]

Trunk Muscle Endurance Tests

Muscle imbalance is a common theme associated with musculoskeletal rehabilitation of persons with LBP. McGill et al[530] suggested that a prior history of LBP appears to be linked to imbalance of the flexion to extension endurance ratios, where extensor endurance is diminished relative to both the flexors and the lateral musculature. Other studies have demonstrated a decrease in back extensor muscle endurance in subjects with LBP.[531-534] Abdominal muscular endurance in subjects with LBP is less when compared to healthy subjects.[535-538]

Normative values have been established for trunk endurance among young, healthy subjects (Table 4-20) without a history of LBP[535,539] and older adults[540,541] (Tables 4-21 and 4-22). These procedures have demonstrated excellent reliability,[539] but diagnostic accuracy and MCID are unknown. This research suggests that assessment of trunk muscle endurance deficits resulting in fatigue and potential loss of motor control during various tasks may be an important variable in persons with recurrent LBP. McGill et al[530] compared subjects with no history of LBP to subjects with a history of LBP who were asymptomatic at the

Table 4-19. 6-Minute Walk Test Distances

AGE	GENDER (NUMBER)	MEAN	SD
60 to 69	Male (1)	498 m (1634 ft)	-
	Female (5)	405 m (1329 ft)	110 m
70 to 79	Male (9)	475 m (1558 ft)	93 m
	Female (10)	406 m (1332 ft)	95 m
80 to 89	Male (9)	320 m (1050 ft)	80 m
	Female (24)	282 m (922 ft)	123 m
	No assist device (24)	328 m (1076 ft)	102 m
	Assist device (9)	197 m (646 ft)	82 m
90 to 101	Male (2)	296 m (971 ft)	15 m
	Female (15)	261 m (856 ft)	81 m
	No assist device (7)	324 m (1063 ft)	70 m
	Assist device (10)	224 m (735 ft)	51 m

Data extracted from Lusardi MM, Pellecchia GL, Schulman PT. Functional performance in community living older adults. *J Geriatr Phys Ther.* 2003;26(3):14-22.

Table 4-20. Mean Trunk Endurance Scores (Seconds) and SD of Normal, Young Healthy Subjects (Mean Age 21; n = 137)

TEST	MEN (SECONDS), (SD)	WOMEN (SECONDS), (SD)
Extension	161 (61)	185 (60)
Flexion	136 (66)	134 (81)
Right side bridge	95 (32)	75 (32)
Left side bridge	99 (37)	78 (32)

Data extracted from McGill S. *Low Back Disorders. Evidence-Based Prevention and Rehabilitation.* 2nd ed. Champaign, IL: Human Kinetics; 2007.

Table 4-21. Mean Trunk Extensor Endurance Scores (Seconds) and SD (n = 475; Men 242; Women 233) in Older Adults

AGE	MEN (SECONDS), (SD)	WOMEN (SECONDS), (SD)
35 to 39	97 (43)	93 (55)
40 to 44	101 (57)	80 (55)
45 to 49	99 (58)	102 (64)
50 to 54	89 (55)	69 (60)

Data extracted from Alaranta H, Hurri H, Heliovaara M, Sonkka A, Harju R. Nondynamometric trunk performance tests: reliability and normative data. *Scand J Rehabil Med.* 1994;26:211-215.

Table 4-22. Normative Trunk Flexor (Partial Curl-Up) Endurance Scores (Seconds) Are Presented in Percentiles (N = 548)

AGE	MEN (25TH TO 75TH PERCENTILE)	WOMEN (25TH TO 75TH PERCENTILE)
19 to 29	30 to 81	36 to 78
30 to 39	28 to 84	25 to 84
40 to 49	30 to 85	18 to 73
50 to 59	27 to 120	15 to 85
60+	18 to 60	1 to 62

Data extracted from McIntosh G, Wilson L, Affleck M, Hall H. Tunk and lower extremity muscle endurance: normative data for adults. *J Rehabil Outcomes Meas.* 1998;2(4):20-39.

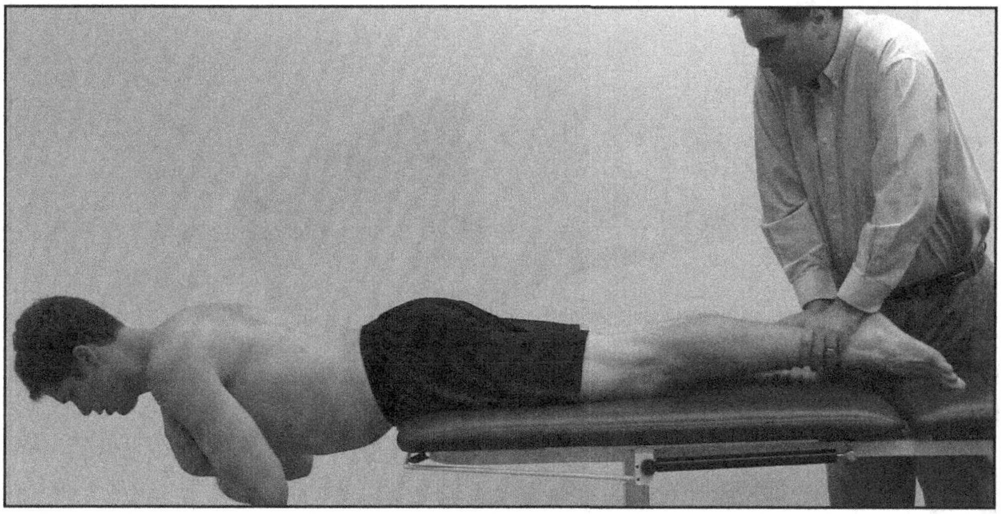

Figure 4-95. Extensor endurance test.

time of testing and found that a history of LBP is associated with a larger waist girth, a greater potential for CLBP from psychosocial questionnaires, unbalanced flexion to extension strength and endurance ratios, and motor control deficits across a variety of tasks. The flexor to extensor strength ratio was different in those with a history of LBP. Additionally, muscle endurance seems to be more affected in those with a history of LBP, specifically the ratio between flexion and extension endurance and the ratio between left and right side bridge positions and extension, suggesting unbalanced endurance in the trunk muscles.[530] The following ratios suggest trunk muscle imbalance:

- Flexion:extension endurance >1.0. Values <1.0 are desirable with 0.84 normal for healthy young males.
- Right side bridge:left side bridge endurance >0.05.
- Side bridge (either side):extension endurance >0.75.

The 3 trunk endurance tests as described by McGill[499] are the extensor endurance test, flexor endurance test, and the side bridge test or lateral musculature test.

Extensor Endurance Test

Subjects are prone with the lower body fixed to the table at the ankles, knees, and hips and the upper body extended over the edge of the table (Figure 4-95). The table surface is 25 cm (9.8 inches) above the surface of the floor. Subjects rest their upper bodies on the floor or chair before the extension. Upper extremities are held across the chest with the hands resting on the opposite shoulders as the upper body is lifted off the floor until the upper torso is horizontal to the floor. Subjects maintain the horizontal position as long as possible. The endurance time is recorded in seconds from the point at which the subject assumes the horizontal position until the upper body drops from horizontal.[499]

Flexor Endurance Test

Subjects sit on the table and place the upper body against a support with an angle of 55 degrees from the horizontal (Figure 4-96). Both the knees and hips are flexed to

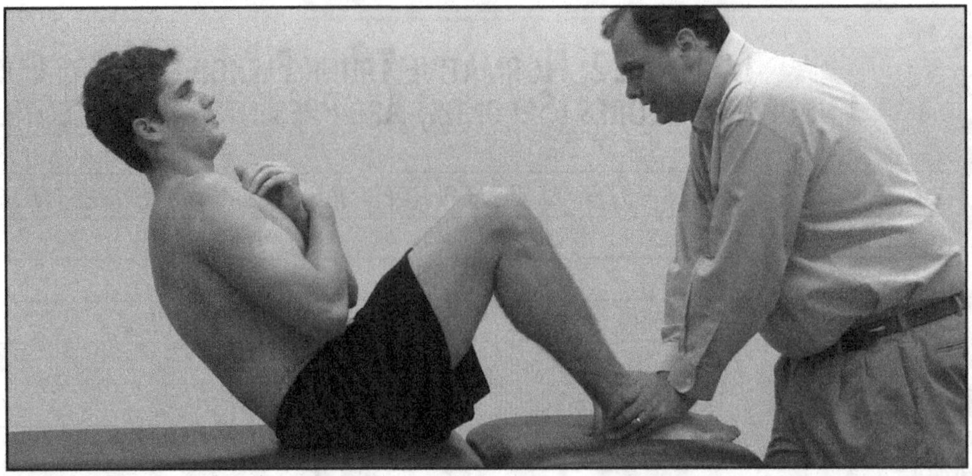

Figure 4-96. Flexor endurance test.

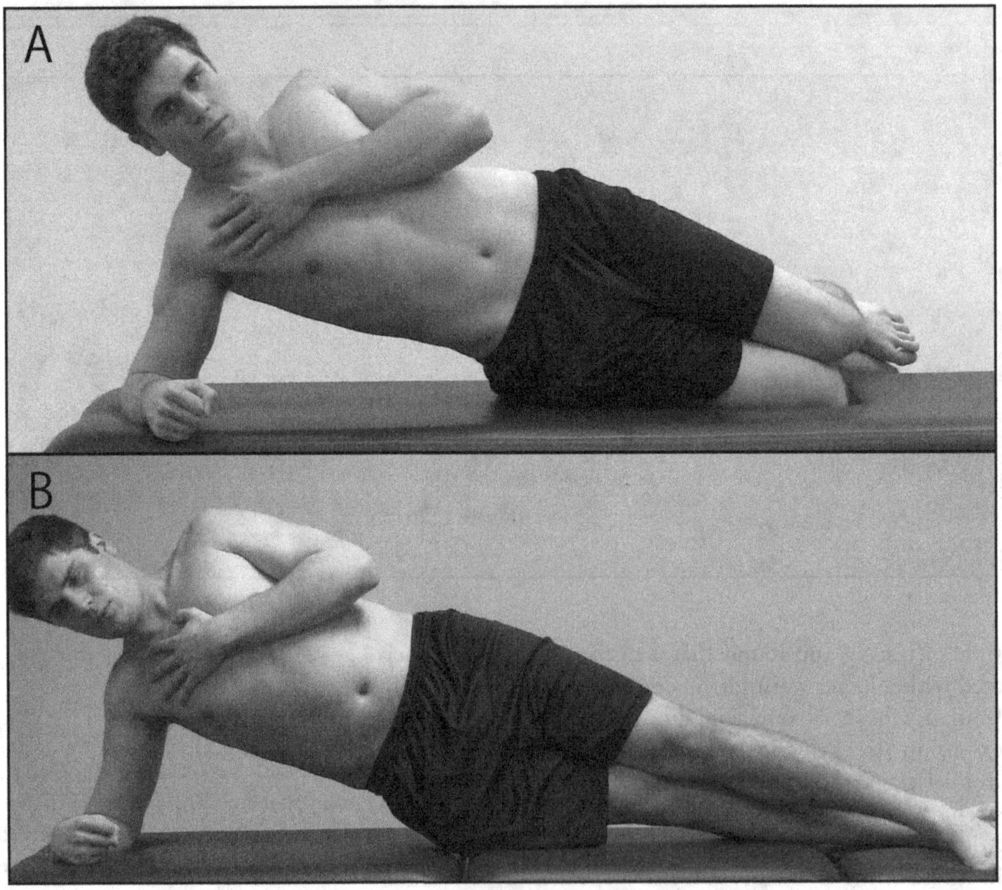

Figure 4-97. Side bridge test: (A) knees flexed and (B) full knees extended.

90 degrees with arms folded across the chest, hands placed on the opposite shoulder, and feet stabilized manually or under straps. Subjects are to maintain the body position while the supporting wedge is pulled back 10 cm to begin the test. The test ends when the upper body falls below the 55-degree angle.[499]

Side Bridge Test or Lateral Musculature Test

Subjects are in full side bridge with knees and hips extended and the top foot in front of the lower foot (Figure 4-97). If subjects cannot maintain the neutral hip and extended knee position, they may flex the hips and knees. Subjects support themselves on one elbow and both feet, lifting their hips off the mat to maintain a straight line over their full body length. The uninvolved arm is held across the chest with the hand on the opposite shoulder. The test is timed and ends with loss of the straight back posture and the hips returned to the table.[499]

Two-Stage Treadmill Test

Fritz and colleagues[102] reported on another diagnostic tool, the TSTT, for determining the presence of symptomatic LSS. The TSTT compares the results of a patient's walking tolerance with a level and a 15% inclined setting at a self-selected comfortable pace. The presence of a longer total walking time during inclined walking is predictive of LSS (Sn 0.50, Sp 0.923; +LR 6.49, –LR 0.54). Using a radiological reference standard, the best classification of those with LSS (see Table 4-5) is associated with the findings of an earlier onset of symptoms and prolonged recovery time with level treadmill walking (Sp 0.947; +LR 14.51).[102]

The TSTT assists in differentiating between neurogenic and vascular claudication. The test is begun by the patient walking on a level treadmill for up to 10 minutes followed by a 10-minute rest in sitting. The test continues with walking on the treadmill at a 15-degree incline for up to 10 minutes. The speed is gradually adjusted to a comfortable pace for the patient. The patient reports on any change in symptoms from baseline and has the opportunity to stop if symptoms are not tolerable. At the end of the test, the clinician notes the time for recovery of symptoms to baseline. A positive test is associated with an earlier onset of symptoms and prolonged recovery time with level treadmill walking. The patient exhibits a greater tolerance for walking on an incline, which places the lumbar spine in a more flexed posture.[102]

Imaging Guidelines

At this point in the examination, the clinician may consider whether to recommend diagnostic imaging and/or refer to a medical colleague or subspecialist. The index of suspicion for recommending diagnostic imaging should be high enough that it is likely to change the intervention or alter the treatment threshold. Clinical decision making to use diagnostic imaging requires careful consideration of the history, the physical examination, and, if initiated, the response to intervention.

The American College of Radiology (ACR) has established appropriateness criteria to assist providers in making the most appropriate imaging decisions.[542] The ACR[542] recommends radiographs for acute LBP when any of the following red flags are present: recent significant trauma, milder trauma with age >50, unexplained weight loss or fever, immunosuppression, history of cancer, IV drug use, prolonged use of corticosteroids, osteoporosis, age >70, focal neurologic deficit with progressive or disabling symptoms, and duration longer than 6 weeks.

For LBP associated with low velocity trauma, osteoporosis, and/or age >70, MRI without contrast is usually appropriate. Lumbar spine MRI without and with contrast is usually appropriate for suspicion of cancer, infection, or immunosuppression. For a surgical or intervention candidate with LBP and/or radiculopathy, MRI without contrast is usually appropriate. A CT is useful if MRI is contraindicated or unavailable and/or for problem solving.[542] For postsurgical patients with LBP, MRI is usually appropriate to differentiate disc versus scar tissue extending beyond the interspace.[542]

The bone scan is moderately sensitive for detecting tumor, infection, or occult fractures of the vertebrae, but has poor specificity. For imaging for spondylolysis or stress fracture in athletes, bone scintigraphy with CT, followed by limited CT if scintigraphy is positive, is more sensitive than MRI.[543] Plain and contrast-enhanced MRI reveal inflammatory, neoplastic, and most traumatic lesions not available on isotope studies.[544] Gadolinium-enhanced MRI reliably shows the presence and extent of spinal infection.[545] Bone scan is indicated to survey the entire skeleton for metastatic disease.

MRI, CT, myelography, or myelography and CT are not recommended for uncomplicated acute LBP with or without radiculopathy and no red flags.[542] LBP complicated by radiculopathy or CES are common indications for MRI. However, a randomized controlled trial (RCT) depicting stenosis or nerve root compression on MRI in the first 48 hours after acute LBP or radiculopathy onset did not affect the outcome after 6 weeks of conservative intervention.[546] For suspicion of CES, MRI without or with contrast is usually appropriate. CT scans provide superior bone detail when compared to MRI but are not as useful to demonstrate disk herniations. Indications for CT scan include spondylolysis; pseudarthrosis; scoliosis; and postsurgical evaluation of bone graft, fusion, and instrumentation.[547]

Clinical practice guidelines provide 3 strong recommendations related to diagnostic imaging.[11] Imaging or other diagnostic tests such as electrophysiologic evaluation should not be routinely ordered in patients with nonspecific LBP. For patients with severe LBP or progressive neurologic deficits or when serious underlying conditions are suspected, diagnostic imaging is recommended. Persons with persistent LBP and signs or symptoms of radiculopathy or spinal stenosis should be evaluated with MRI or CT only if they are potential candidates for surgery or epidural steroid injection (ESI).

Concluding the Physical Examination

At the conclusion of the physical examination, the clinician briefly reflects on whether the goals of the examination have been met. The physical examination should do the following:

- Reproduce the patient's symptoms in patterns consistent with the information obtained in the patient interview

Figure 4-98. Clinical decision-making process.

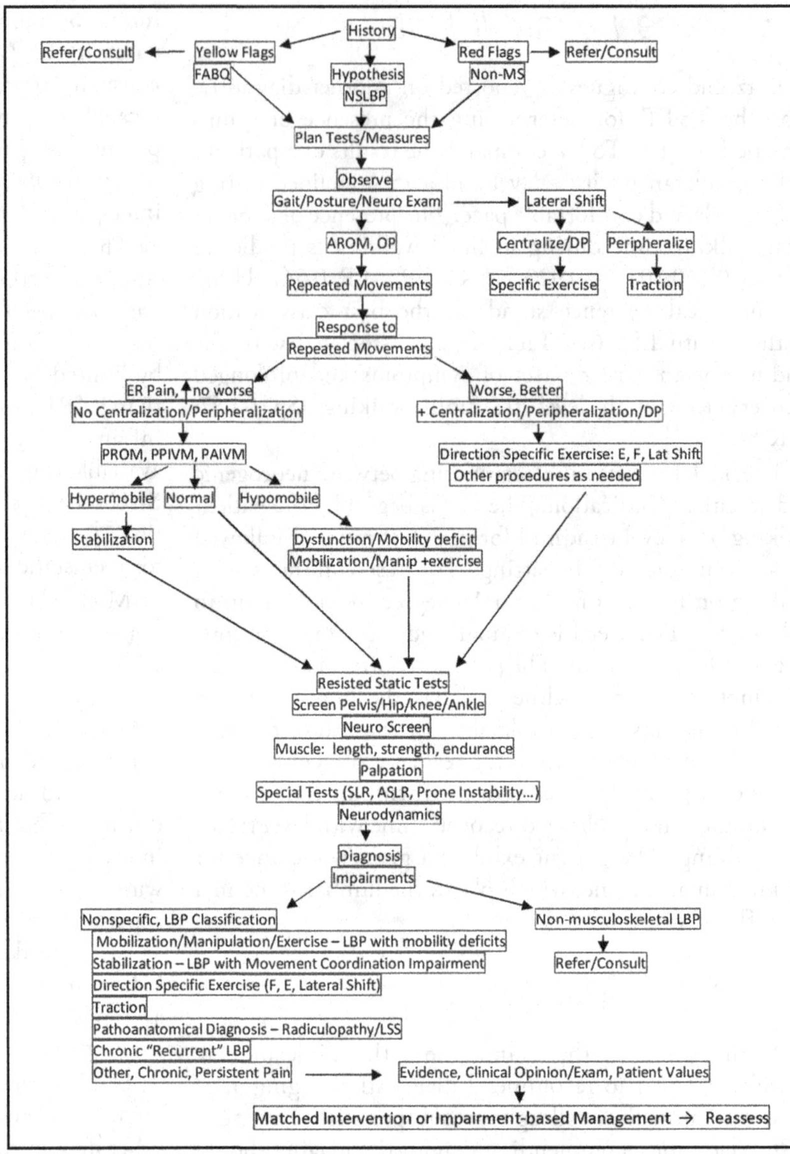

- Result in a determination of the impact of posture, movement, work, recreational and psychosocial factors as causes of, contributors to, or perpetuator's of the problem
- Establish the treatment threshold for a diagnostic classification
- Establish an accurate, data baseline or outcome measures from which to evaluate and progress treatment

Review of examination findings should provide data to enhance, support, or negate competing hypotheses to the point where the examination ends and treatment begins. Key history and exam findings are used to place the patient into a diagnostic classification or impairment-based category of LBP that initially guides PT intervention. An algorithm of the clinical decision-making process is shown in Figure 4-98.

Diagnostic Classification and Matched Intervention

At this point in the evaluation, the clinician has taken into account the presence and importance of red and yellow flags, designated a baseline diagnostic classification, and decided to proceed with PT intervention. With little evidence to support classification based on a pathoanatomical source, current evidence suggests use of a classification system that identifies subgroups of patients who are most likely to respond to specific interventions with the potential to maximize outcomes. Many classifications for LBP exist with no one classification system known to be superior to another.[548] In the absence of red flags, current research supports a classification approach that reduces the focus on identifying anatomical lesion in favor of LBP subgroup classifications shown to improve outcomes.[410]

Low Back Pain Classification Systems

Researchers and clinicians have described several LBP classification approaches based on duration of symptoms; pathoanatomical sources; clinical patterns; MIs; health; work or functional status; biological, psychological, and social factors; and pain mechanisms.[22-24] Despite differences in methods of assessment, a common PT goal is "to identify a movement pattern related to a pain reduction strategy."[24(p1)] All patients do not fit into one classification system; many patients have clinical findings that fit into more than one subgroup within a classification system. To inform clinical decision making, the classification approach described in this text integrates current best evidence, clinical reasoning, and clinical practice guidelines related to specific LBP, thoracic pain, and cervical pain subgroups and the importance of the characteristics that are likely to be most responsive to initial PT management strategies.

Key history and exam findings are used to place the patient into a diagnostic classification[274,410] and/or impairment-based category of LBP[14] that initially guides PT intervention. In a best-evidence approach, a LBP diagnostic classification assists the clinician with matching the patient's clinical presentation to the most suitable initial treatment. In an impairment-based LBP category[14] approach, the clinician identifies relevant physical impairments such as limited ROM, joint or muscle stiffness or hypermobility, and/or muscle coordination deficits. Evidence-based interventions are selected to target the prioritized impairments to address activity limitations or functional deficits important to the patient. For patients with LBP, the following subgroups describe a synthesis of evidence-based key clinical characteristics described as the following:

- A manipulation and mobilization plus exercise LBP subgroup also depicted as LBP mobility deficits (see Table 4-1)
- A stabilization exercise LBP subgroup also depicted as LBP with movement coordination impairments (see Table 4-2)
- A DSE classification also depicted as LBP with lower extremity referred pain (see Table 4-3)
- A traction classification for LBP with lower extremity radiating or related pain (see Table 4-4)
- An impairment-based classification for symptomatic LSS (see Table 4-5)
- An impairment-based classification for LBP with altered neurodynamics
- A subclassification of LBRLP based on predominating pain mechanisms (ie, central sensitization, peripheral nerve sensitization, denervation, and musculoskeletal referred pain; see Table 4-6)
- A CLBP or chronic, disabling lumbopelvic pain classification related to MCIs based on a biopsychosocial approach (see Figure 4-1)
- A PGP classification based on a biopsychosocial and neurophysiological pain mechanisms classification (see Figures 4-3 and 4-4)
- A pregnancy-related PGP classification

Treatment-Based Classification for Low Back Pain

A treatment-based classification (TBC), originally proposed by Delitto et al,[410] unrelated to pathoanatomical labels, distinguishes subgroups based on key clinical findings to inform and prioritize treatment decision making. The original system was described for patients with acute LBP or acute exacerbations of LBP. Some validation reports have included persons with subacute and CLBP,[20,141,411,549] but no validation studies have been conducted for persons with CLBP.

TBC consists of 4 subgroups: manipulation, stabilization, DSE (flexion, extension, lateral shift groups), and traction.[274] Intrarater reliability has been reported as acceptable (κ = 0.49 to 0.65) in clinicians familiar with the system.[550-552] Validity of the TBC system has been investigated by Fritz et al,[19] who compared TBC to clinical practice guidelines that recommend advice to remain active and performance of low-level aerobics for patients with acute work-related LBP of less than 3 weeks duration. Patients treated using a TBC approach to PT showed greater improvement in disability at 4 weeks, were more satisfied, and were more likely to return to unrestricted work within the first 4 weeks of treatment. In another study of TBC based on clinical presentation, Brennan et al[20] compared outcomes of 123 patients with LBP of less than 90 days duration receiving treatment matched or unmatched to the baseline classification. Patients receiving treatment matched to their subgroups had better outcomes and greater short-term (4 weeks) and long-term (52 weeks) reduction in disability. The authors concluded that subgrouping for the purpose of guiding PT treatment can improve outcomes.

Apeldoorn et al[553] attempted to determine the effectiveness of the TBC in patients with subacute or CLBP for current episodes > 12 weeks with a mean ODI = 20 at baseline. The TBC was slightly modified substituting DP for centralization and eliminating the traction subgroup. The comparison treatment group was also different from the study by Fritz et al,[19] where the TBC was compared to advice to remain active, low-stress aerobic exercises, and general muscle reconditioning. In the Apeldoorn et al[553] study, patients received personalized, individually tailored PT sessions. The results suggest that the TBC approach used in this study did not improve outcomes in this population over usual PT care. No statistically significant differences between treatment groups were found at 8, 26, and 52 weeks.[553] Findings that warrant additional study include GPE and dichotomized ODI scores improved over the 52 weeks in the TBC group but deteriorated in the last 26 weeks in the usual care group, and GPE and dichotomized ODI scores slightly favored subjects with an initial clear classification in the TBC group compared to the usual PT care group at 52 weeks. The authors offer the following recommendations to improve the use of the TBC classification in CLBP: centralization rather than a DP should be used for classification; the use of key psychological factors may be need to be explored for the TBC classification; and criteria for the stabilization classification needs to be validated.[553]

Even though research suggests classification systems result in improved outcomes when compared to use of no classification,[19,411] evidence for its clinical usefulness is still limited.[553] However, the goal of initiating the earliest effective management based on subgroups and matched intervention to facilitate a quick recovery and prevent a progression to chronic, persistent LBP is still supported.[5,8] The TBC system is continually changing based on emerging evidence. Considering the complex nature of LBP, patients often present with criteria from more than one subgroup and most require multimodal treatment. In this situation, clinicians use clinical reasoning to prioritize key criteria for initial classification when deciding on the best initial treatment. Continued assessment and reassessment of the patient's response to treatment provide additional criteria for reclassification and progression of treatment.

The classification subgroups and matched interventions are presented in the order listed above. Key characteristics from the TBC, clinical practice guidelines, clinical reasoning, and additional sources are combined to support the subgroup classifications and current evidence-based management strategies.

Manipulation and Mobilization or Low Back Pain With Mobility Deficits Subgroup

A mobilization/manipulation procedure is defined as a continuum of skilled passive movements to the joints and/or related soft tissues applied at varying speeds and amplitudes, including a small amplitude, high-velocity thrust manipulation within or at end-range of joint motion.[554] Manual therapy (MT) techniques, including mobilization or manipulation of soft tissue and joints, are defined as skilled hand movements used to improve tissue extensibility; increase ROM; induce relaxation; modulate pain; or reduce soft tissue swelling, inflammation, or restriction.[554] Variations in these definitions exist based on legal, professional, and state practice acts and policies.

Many variations of mobilization and manipulation have been described. The superiority of manipulation over mobilization or one manipulation technique versus another has not been proven. One reason is that current evidence suggests that mobilization and manipulation procedures are not as precise as traditionally believed. For example, descriptive studies of segmental lumbar spine mobility reveal that a central PAIVM on the lumbar spine causes extension at the target segment and the entire lumbar spine. The magnitude and direction of the segmental motion varies depending on the segmental level.[555,556] Similarly, a central, grade III PA central mobilization directed to C5 is not specific to that segment.[557] While tradition and biomechanical theories support the need for precision in spinal manipulative therapy (SMT), current evidence suggests that SMT is not precise, causing motion to occur at levels other than the targeted segment. Ross et al[558] reported that lumbar and thoracic spine manipulation is accurate only 46% and 53% of the time, respectively. An investigation into the cavitation sounds of a technique directed at L5 and one directed at the SIJ revealed no correlation between the spinal levels producing cavitation and the levels targeted by the techniques.[559] Additionally, an audible pop during a thrust manipulation in patients with LBP is not related to the patient's outcome.[560] Similar findings have been reported for the cervical spine. In subjects with neck pain, a comparison of a randomly assigned level for thrust manipulation versus a clinician-selected level based on end feel assessment resulted in both groups achieving an equally significant reduction in pain and stiffness.[561,562] In the lumbar spine, Chiradejnant et al[562] found no difference in short-term outcomes of pain and ROM between a therapist-determined level for lumbar mobilization or a randomly selected technique. However, mobilization to the lower lumbar levels resulted in better outcomes than mobilization to the upper lumbar levels. A specific technique may not be as important as identifying the person who benefits the most.[562]

Contraindications

Contraindications to manipulation are generally characterized as absolute, meaning extremely high risk of harm to the patient if manipulation is performed, or relative, meaning high risk of harm requiring considerable thought in weighing benefits versus risks prior to use. A list of recommended absolute and relative contraindications for manipulation and mobilization compiled from several sources is listed next.[274,563,564] Absolute and relative contraindications to manipulation and mobilization are not agreed upon, are not standardized, and may change based on emerging evidence, or they vary with individual patient presentation, clinical reasoning, and clinician experience. Prior to the selection and use of application of a mobilization or manipulation procedures, clinicians should conduct a careful examination and adhere to sound clinical reasoning, economy of vigor in technique, an evidence-based approach with treatment guided by assessment and reassessment throughout the plan of care, and careful analysis in the presence of a deterioration of signs and symptoms.[563]

Absolute Contraindications to Mobilization and Manipulation[274,563,564]

Contraindications marked with an asterisk (*) are considered absolute for both mobilization and manipulation. If no asterisk is marked, the absolute contraindication is only for manipulation.

- Malignancy of the region of interest; metastasis must be ruled out*
- Red flags such as signs and symptoms of cancer, fracture, systemic disease*
- Rheumatoid collagen necrosis*
- Unstable upper cervical spine*
- Vertebrobasilar insufficiency, which may be indicated by drop attacks, blackouts, loss of consciousness, nausea, vomiting, poor general health, dizziness, vertigo, disturbance of vision including diplopia, unsteady gait and general feeling of weakness, dysarthria or swallowing difficulty, hearing disturbances, headache of undetermined origin, facial numbness or tingling*
- Frank spinal deformity due to old pathology such as adolescent osteochondrosis
- Bone disease such as osteoporosis, osteomyelitis, tuberculosis, Paget's disease*
- Inflammatory arthritis such as rheumatoid or septic arthritis, AS, gout*
- CES, transverse myelitis, demyelinating conditions*
- Myelopathy with signs and symptoms of spinal cord involvement*
- Radiculopathy involving more than one nerve root on one side*
- Spinal fusion*
- Congenital hypomobility
- Spondylolisthesis or other segmental instability*
- Advanced diabetes
- Medically unstable*
- Advanced degenerative changes such as severe foraminal encroachment
- Severe nerve root pain or acute radiculopathy
- Deteriorating CNS pathology*
- Undiagnosed pain*
- Anticoagulant medications, vascular disorders in the region, blood clotting disorders*
- Irritable disorder and protective guarding
- Pregnancy and immediately postpartum
- Children/teenagers
- Clinician lack of ability*

Relative Contraindications to Mobilizations and Manipulation

- Active, acute inflammatory condition
- Significant segmental stiffness
- Systemic disease
- Rheumatoid arthritis if there is no acute inflammation except in the cervical spine, which is an absolute contradiction whether acute inflammation is present or not
- Neurological deterioration
- Irritable disorder
- Osteoporosis depending on intent and direction of movement
- Condition is worsening with present treatment
- Acute nerve root irritation or irritability
- When history and exam findings do not make sense
- Use of oral contraceptives must be considered if the cervical spine is the region of interest
- Long-term oral corticosteroid use must be considered if cervical spine is the region of interest
- Immediately postpartum, may be contraindicated in the lumbar spine, pelvic girdle, and/or thoracic spine

Adverse Events

CES is the most serious complication associated with lumbar spine manipulation. Review of the literature over a 77-year period found only 10 reports of CES after lumbar manipulation.[565] Other reports estimate the risk of CES at less than 1 out of 100 million manipulations.[566,567] Minor side effects of lumbar manipulation were reported from a survey of 1058 patients over 4712 treatments, approximately 75% of which included lumbar manipulation. About 55% reported at least one minor side effect that included radiating discomfort (10%), fatigue (11%), headache (12%), and local discomfort (53%). No severe side effects were noted, but 64% of minor side effects began within 4 hours after treatment and 74% disappeared within 24 hours.[567]

Adverse effects from cervical spine manipulation vary from mild soreness to serious neurovascular compromise. Adverse effects of cervical manipulation from a survey of 280 subjects 2 weeks after participating in a cervical spine clinical trial included headache, dizziness, a temporary increase in neck pain, ringing in the ears, or impaired vision.[568] Increased neck pain and stiffness lasting less than 24 hours after the manipulation was reported by 25% of the subjects. Subjects more likely to report minor adverse effects had pain ratings of 8+ out of 10, neck disability index scores > 16, a history of trauma, worsening of symptoms since onset, pain less than 1 year, moderate or severe headache, nausea during the past month, and lack of confidence in the treatment.[568] Subjects treated with nonthrust cervical techniques reported significantly less adverse effects.

In a survey of 465 patients after the first session of spinal manipulation, Caigne et al[569] reported that 60% had at least one adverse event with onset within 4 hours and resolution within 24 hours. Subjects, women more likely than men, reported radiating discomfort (12.1%), fatigue (12.1%), local discomfort (15.2%), stiffness (19.5), and headache (19%). Upper cervical manipulation was 3.17 times more likely to cause headache than lower cervical spine manipulation, with age (ie, for every 1 year increase of age risk of headache decreases by 2.4%), regular medication use (ie, 2.2 times more likely to get a headache than those who do not), and gender (ie, women have 1.66 times more risk than men) identified as independent predictors of headache.

Though minor side effects are fairly common, the most serious adverse event related to cervical spinal manipulation is cervical artery dysfunction (CAD) related to vertebral basilar or internal carotid artery insufficiency rarely resulting in stroke or death. The proposed underlying pathology is atherosclerosis, which may predispose the arteries to dissection linked with mechanical forces. Mechanisms of CAD or dissection include a spontaneous event such as turning the head to reverse the car; a traumatic event such as whiplash, intubation, or MT; or endothelial inflammatory disease such as temporal arteritis.[570] Consensus is lacking on the best way to assess for the possibility of CAD as a result of cervical manipulation. The ability to predict patients who may suffer CAD after cervical manipulation is difficult. Further discussion of assessment of CAD is located in the cervical spine chapter. Readers are encouraged to review additional articles.[570-573]

Estimates of a serious adverse event related to cervical manipulation vary considerably: 1 out of 50 000 manipulations to 1 out of 15 million with the risk of death 3 in 10 million manipulations.[574] In a literature review of 177 patients (1925 to 1997) reported in the literature, Di Fabio[575] determined the primary adverse event was arterial dissection and brain stem lesions, with 32 cases (18%) resulting in death. Physical therapists were involved in less than 2% of cases with no associated deaths. Even though the potential risk is low, the adverse event is catastrophic. When reported, most cases involved a manipulation that included rotation with 10% reporting the adverse event after the first manipulation. Di Fabio[575] recommended the use of nonthrust mobilization or manipulation techniques when treating the cervical spine. In a review 367 cases of CAD from 1966 to 1993, Haldeman et al[576] concluded that vertebral artery dissection should be considered a rare, random, and unpredictable complication associated with activities such as daily neck movement (43%), trauma (16% sudden neck movement), MVA (10%), and manipulation (31%).

The systematic review and meta-analysis by Carnes et al[577] was in line with earlier reports. Approximately 50% of people treated with MT may experience minor to moderate adverse events after treatment. The incidence of major adverse events is small. The relative risk of minor or moderate adverse events is similar for MT, exercise treatments, and sham or passive control interventions. The meta-analysis revealed that the relative risk of having a minor or moderate adverse event with MT, meaning high velocity thrust, is significantly less than the risk of taking medication. Estimated risk of death from using NSAIDS for OA is 100 to 400 times the risk of death from cervical manipulation.[578] Lumbar manipulation is 37 000 to 148 000 times safer than NSAIDs and 55 000 to 444 000 times safer than surgery for lumbar disc herniation, and CES is 7400 to 37 000 times more likely to occur from surgery than manipulation.[579] Carnes et al[577] concluded with the suggestion that all health care interventions have inherent risk that should be weighed against patient-perceived outcomes and available alternatives.

Effects of Manual Therapy/Manipulation

Even with evidence supporting its effectiveness, the mechanisms by which MT works (ie, joint manipulation/mobilization, soft tissue mobilization, neurodynamic mobilization) have not been established. Two categories of mechanism, biomechanical and neurophysiological, dominate the theoretical debate. Evidence is lacking to support traditional, widely accepted theories of treating specific biomechanical dysfunctions, hypomobilities, or joint signs. Reliability in identifying joint signs, positional asymmetry, or segmental dysfunction is low. MT techniques are not as precise as once thought. An MT technique applied to a randomly selected segment or a therapist-selected segment results in similar outcomes in subjects with neck and LBP. Improvement in signs and symptoms often occur away from the site of MT. For example, treatment directed to the thoracic spine and rib cage for patients with primary complaints of neck pain can result in successful outcomes.[580] The current evidence to support a manipulation classification suggests that a successful outcome is linked to correctly identifying individuals who are responders to manipulation rather than a clinician's ability to accurately localize a dysfunctional segment, localize a technique to a specific level, or use a specific manipulation technique.[581]

While the evidence supporting an independent biomechanical mechanism is lacking, a model proposed by Bialosky et al[582] suggested that a mechanical stimulus is required to initiate the potential neurophysiological mechanisms that deliver the beneficial outcomes associated with MT. MT works, but the mechanisms that predominate may not be biomechanical. Hypomobility, a biomechanical concept, is one variable in the manipulation classification. The authors propose a model with supporting research that accounts for the complex interaction of the peripheral and CNSs that may be linked to pain relief from all forms of MT. Nonspecific neurophysiological effects related to patient expectations and placebo must also be accounted for due to the possible influence on pain perception and clinical outcomes.[582-583]

In addition to a biomechanical influence, the neurophysiological effects model includes peripheral, spinal, and supraspinal mechanisms.[584] During the acute inflammatory response to tissue injury, pain usually comes from nociceptors in the injured tissues. Over time, if the nociceptors continue firing, the dorsal horn may become hypersensitive due to the presence of increased neurotransmitters. MT may directly affect this response by altering chemical mediators in the peripheral nervous system.[585-588] MT effects related to increased sensory input from joint and muscle mechanoreceptors are thought to modulate pain at the spinal cord level or act as a counterirritant.[589-592] Bialosky et al[584] identified several potential mechanisms that result in decreased activation of supraspinal regions responsible for central pain processing. Finally, placebo, patient expectations,[592,593] effects on the sympathetic nervous system, and psychological factors[594] are considered important links to neurophysiological mechanisms and the effectiveness of MT. For instance, negative expectations for SMT may increase pain perception after treatment,[582,593] and MT may improve psychological factors.[594] Placebo is estimated to account for 10% to 25% of the benefits of spinal manipulation.[595]

SMT often has an immediate analgesic effect on pain. Immediately after manipulation, this effect called *hypoalgesia* is evident as a reduced pain response from an average of 7/10 to 4/10 or reduced pain sensitivity to external pressure or heat stimuli.[592,596] A similar effect is noted during lumbar mobilization, but an optimum treatment dose has not been found. Krouwel et al[597] investigated the potential hypoalgesic effects of PA lumbar spine mobilization with large amplitude, small amplitude, and sustained oscillations as measured by pressure pain thresholds. In asymptomatic subjects a systemic hypoalgesic response was noted for all amplitudes of mobilization with no significant difference between amplitudes. Chiradejnant et al[598] reported an immediate analgesic effect of CPA mobilization treatment in subjects with LBP. The authors compared treatment delivered to the painful or dysfunctional level identified by the clinician versus treatment delivered to a randomly selected level. Significantly greater reduction in current pain intensity was observed when 1-minute repetitions of CPA mobilization were applied twice to the symptomatic level rather than to a randomly assigned level. Systematic review supports involvement of supraspinal systems in mediating the effects of passive cervical joint mobilization.[599] The authors concluded that cervical PAIVM produces hypoalgesia that extends beyond the specific body segment receiving treatment and lasts up to 24 hours. Therefore, the CNS is involved in mediating reduced pain responses to passive joint mobilization and manipulation.

In some persons with chronic or persistent LBP, central sensitization is associated with the progression of acute pain to chronic pain and in the maintenance of chronic pain.[600,601] Acute pain from peripheral mediators may provoke neuroplastic changes or produce altered sensory processing within the CNS, leading to a heightened pain response, and result in a move to centrally maintained pain perception.[600,601] SMT results in hypoalgesia and is theorized to alter neuroplastic changes associated with central sensitization.[591] Immediate hypoalgesia may be an indicator of change in central sensitization. Therefore, SMT interventions that prevent or alter central sensitization may be useful in the management of persons with cervical or LBP. Bialosky et al[584] provided an in-depth discussion of potential neurophysiological mechanisms important to understanding the effects of SMT.

The effect of SMT on the motor control system is unclear, with some studies reporting inhibition and others facilitation, which increases muscle tone or muscle performance. In 18 subjects with anterior knee pain, Suter et al[602] observed a significant increase in knee extension torque on the involved side after a side-lying, SIJ manipulation with contact point and direction of thrust at the clinician's discretion. Subjects receiving thrust manipulation[603] or Grade IV mobilization which is a nonthrust manipulation,[604] to the thoracic spine demonstrated significant increase in lower trapezius strength. In 16 subjects with chronic neck pain, a thrust manipulation to C5-C6 and C6-C7 resulted in improved biceps muscle strength.[605] A potential effect of CPA nonthrust manipulation was observed as a decrease of the superficial cervical muscles during the craniocervical flexion test, possibly indicating facilitation of the deep cervical muscles.[606] In another example of a manual technique to one region affecting other regions, thrust manipulation to the thoracic and lumbar spine reduces paraspinal EMG activity when compared to controls.[607] A case report[608] and a case series[609] have demonstrated TrA muscular thickness changes during the ADIM in persons with LBP immediately after a lumbar thrust manipulation. These reports suggest that the TrA muscle thickness changes due to descending pain-inhibitory influences might result in TrA relaxation or decreased thickness at rest and increased thickness during ADIM contraction. A report in 35 healthy subjects revealed no change in TrA resting or contraction thickness after a side-lying lumbar spine thrust manipulation (Figure 4-99) compared to a sham procedure, indicating that the proposed changes in TrA thickness after manipulation may only occur in subjects with pain.[610]

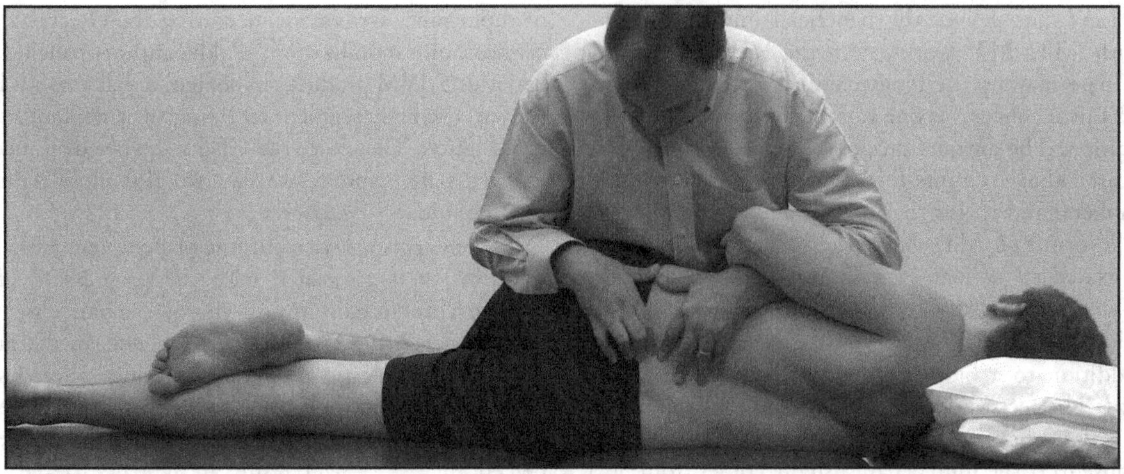

Figure 4-99. Right side-lying lumbar spine thrust manipulation or mobilization targeting L4-L5 segment. The patient is in side-lying with the painful side up. The clinician flexes the top hip until motion is felt at the interspinous space (L4-L5) and places the patient's foot in the popliteal fossa. Maintaining this position, the clinician gently grasps the lower shoulder and arm to introduce side-bending and rotation until motion is felt at the L4-L5 interspinous space. While maintaining the setup, position the patient's arms around the clinician's arm and log roll toward the clinician. A high-velocity, low-amplitude thrust manipulation is applied to the pelvis using the right arm in an anterior direction. The more symptomatic side is selected for manipulation. If one side is not more symptomatic, the clinician selects the side to be manipulated. In the Cleland et al[595] study, the therapist selected the level to be manipulated or chose the L4-L5 segment because previous research suggested that procedures directed toward the lower lumbar region were more effective.[572] Using the same setup, this technique may also be used as a rotational mobilization.[574]

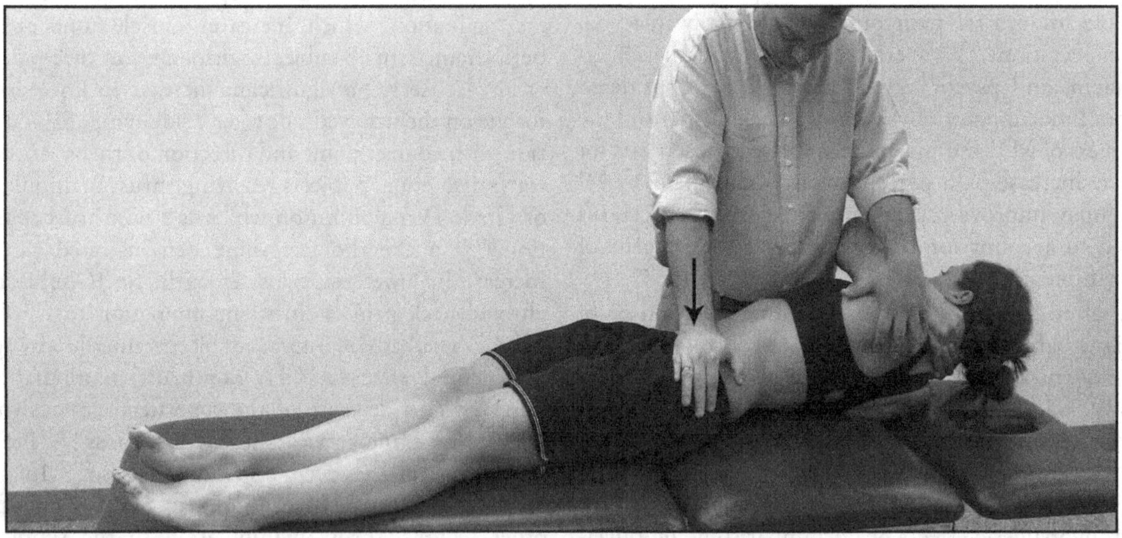

Figure 4-100. Right supine lumbopelvic regional thrust manipulation. This technique was used in the development and validation of the manipulation CPR.[136,137] The patient is supine with fingers interlocked behind his or her head. The clinician stands opposite the side to be manipulated and passively moves the patient into LF toward the side to be manipulated. Maintaining the laterally flexed position, the therapist places the thrust hand on the ASIS and passively rotates the patient toward him or her and then performs a high-velocity, low-amplitude thrust to the ASIS in a posterior and inferior direction. Based on patient self-report, the more symptomatic side is manipulated. Otherwise, the clinician selects the side to be manipulated.

In a preliminary investigation, Fritz et al[611] examined the immediate and short-term effects of SMT (Figure 4-100) on spinal stiffness, MF recruitment, and status on the manipulation CPR and related observed changes to clinical outcomes. Regardless of outcome on the ODI, significant immediate decreases in global and terminal stiffness occur after SMT. ODI improvement is related to a greater immediate decrease in global stiffness (P = .025) and less initial terminal stiffness (P = .01). Further analysis suggests that clinical outcome of SMT is mediated by improvements in MF recruitment and immediate decrease in global stiffness. The authors concluded that the underlying mechanisms supporting SMT appear to be multifactorial and include changes in spinal stiffness characteristics and MF recruitment.[611]

Similarly, Koppenhaver et al[612] examined the relationship between improved disability and changes in abdominal and MF thickness using ultrasound imaging following SMT in subjects with LBP. The preliminary findings suggest that contracted thickness of the MF, not the TrA or internal oblique, are associated with improvement after SMT, supporting the importance of the MF in persons with LBP. Immediate changes in the TrA and internal oblique thickness appear transient and unrelated to improved disability after SMT.[612] Though the feed-forward activation of the TrA and internal oblique was not measured in this study, Marshall and Murphy[613] have reported on improved feed-forward activation immediately after SMT. Motor control of the deep muscle system is complex, but preliminary findings suggest a relationship between activation of this system and SMT.

When a patient asks how or why SMT works, Bialosky et al[614] suggested informing the patient that the SMT causes short-term and widespread forces to be absorbed through the treated area. These forces produce a large input into the nervous system, sending responses between the spinal cord and the brain and possibly resulting in pain inhibition and/or improved muscle performance. A strictly biomechanical or neurophysiological explanation may be incorrect. Persons with LBP with or without a heightened pain response such as central sensitization due to centrally mediated mechanisms may respond to MT techniques.

Evidence for Manipulation and Mobilization

A systematic review by Bronfort et al[615] concluded that recommendations can be made with some confidence regarding the use of SMT and/or mobilization as a viable option for the treatment of both LBP and neck pain. High-quality studies are limited when distinguishing between acute and chronic patients and limited to short-term follow-up. A review of RCTs from January 2000 to January 2008 concluded that SMT is preferred for short-term relief of LBP when compared with general exercise and dynamic strengthening exercises. SMT plus exercise is more effective than exercise alone.[616]

A synthesis of clinical practice guideline recommendations[617] for acute LBP management includes short-term use of SMT, acetaminophen, and NSAIDS. For CLBP, back exercises, behavioral therapy, and short-term opioid analgesics are additional recommendations. Similar suggestions are made for the management of LBP with neurological compromise with consideration for imaging studies for those who do not respond to conservative management and desire ESI or decompressive surgery. In a retrospective review of 1190 patients with acute LBP receiving PT, adherence to clinical practice guideline for active treatment was associated with better clinical outcomes and reduced cost.[618]

A systematic review[617] of RCTs related to SMT for acute LBP concluded that SMT is either superior or equivalent to many commonly used interventions including education, mobilization, modalities, or medication for 5 to 10 sessions over 2 to 4 weeks in improvement in pain and function for short-, intermediate-, and long-term follow-up. No harms were reported in these studies. They recommend SMT as a treatment option for patients with acute LBP who do not find adequate symptomatic relief with self-care and education alone. Emerging evidence continues to support the inclusion of manipulation and mobilization in the management of persons with acute LBP.[619]

Manipulation and Mobilization Plus Exercise Low Back Pain Subgroup or Low Back Pain With Mobility Deficits and Matched Interventions

A CPR was developed by Flynn et al[140] to assist clinicians in identifying patients who fit a manipulation classification. The associated International Classification of Functioning, Disability and Health (ICF) impairment-based category is LBP with mobility deficits.[14] The CPR consists of 5 factors:

1. Duration of symptoms less than 16 days (ie, acute LBP)
2. FABQW subscale 18 or less (ie, low fear-avoidance)
3. No symptoms distal to the knee
4. At least one hip IR PROM greater than 35 degrees, measured prone
5. Hypomobility at one or more lumbar levels assessed with CPA PAIVM or spring testing. Improvement over 2 treatment sessions was defined as a 50% or greater reduction in self-reported disability on the modified ODI.

A supine lumbopelvic regional (see Figure 4-100) high-velocity, low-amplitude (HVLA) manipulation was initially directed to the most painful side or at the therapist's discretion. A successful manipulation was determined by an audible pop or cavitation. A maximum of 2 manipulations to each side were allowed. In addition to manipulation, each subject performed supine pelvic tilt ROM exercise (Figure 4-101) and was instructed to maintain usual activity within limits of pain. In this study, random manipulation of subjects resulted in about a 45% chance of success. If 4 of the 5 factors were present, the probability of improvement with manipulation plus exercise rose to 95% (+LR 24.38; 95% CI: 4.6, 139.4). If 2 or 3 out of 5 factors were present, the likelihood of improvement decreases to 49% (+LR 1.18 [1.09, 1.42]) and 68% (+LR 2.61 [1.78, 4.15]), respectively, and an alternative treatment is considered. Subjects included in the study were 18 to 60 years of age with a primary symptom of LBP with or without

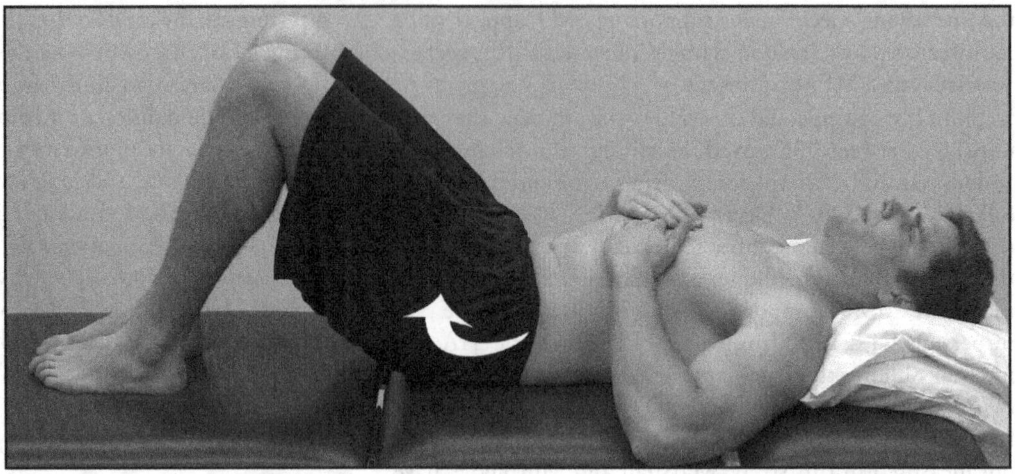

Figure 4-101. Supine pelvic tilt ROM exercise. In supine with hips and knees bent and feet flat on the floor, the patient slowly flattens the low back by gently drawing in the stomach and rotating the pelvis backwards without breath holding. The ROM exercise is pain-free and performed 10 times, 3 to 4 times per day.

referral into the lower extremity and a modified ODI >30%. Subjects excluded from the study were patients who were over 60, had signs of nerve root compression such as diminished DTRs, had strength and/or sensory deficits (+SLR <45), had spondylolisthesis, had osteoporosis, had bony abnormality or weakness, were pregnant, had previous surgery to lumbar spine or buttocks, or had the presence of red flags.[140]

Some individuals with acute LBP should not be managed with manipulation. In subjects who did not improve or worsened with manipulation (see Table 4-1) in the Flynn et al[140] study, 6 characteristics were identified: longer symptom duration, having symptoms in the buttock or leg, absence of lumbar hypomobility, less average total hip rotation ROM, less discrepancy between left and right IR ROM, and a negative Gaenslen's sign, explaining 64% of the variance in manipulation outcome.[620]

Childs et al[141] validated the CPR in a separate trial of 131 patients who were examined and classified as positive (ie, 4 out of 5 criteria met) or negative (ie, 3 or less out of 5 criteria met) on the CPR and then randomized to receive manipulation plus exercise (ie, a standardized exercise program of trunk strengthening [Figure 4-102] and 10-minute treadmill or bicycle) or exercise alone for a total of 5 treatment sessions over 4 weeks. Patients who were + on the CPR and manipulated had greater improvement at 1 week, 4 weeks, and 6 months than patients who were – on the CPR and manipulated. Patients who were + on the CPR and manipulated had greater improvement at 1 week, 4 weeks, and 6 months than patients who were + on the CPR and received only exercise. If the patient received manipulation, improvements in disability and pain were greater whether the patient was + or – on the CPR. A patient who was positive on the rule and received the matched intervention of manipulation experienced significantly more change than the other groups. At 6-month follow-up, patients in the exercise group had significantly more medication, health care utilization, and lost time from work than patients in the manipulation group. Positive on the CPR and receiving manipulation resulted in a +LR 13.2 (3.4, 52.1). Less than 3 criteria on the CPR were associated with a –LR 0.10 (0.03, 0.41).[141]

Hancock et al[621] investigated whether the manipulation CPR by Childs et al[141] generalized and identified responders to SMT. Subjects (n = 239) were randomized to 4 groups: placebo SMT and placebo NSAID of diclofenac, placebo SMT and active diclofenac, active SMT and placebo diclofenac, and active SMT and active diclofenac. The results suggested that the CPR was no better for pain and disability than chance in identifying patients with acute, nonspecific LBP most likely to respond to SMT at 1, 2, 4, and 12 weeks. The authors concluded that the manipulation CPR did not generalize to patients with acute LBP. However, many variations between the studies could explain the different results. The authors report that most subjects (97%) received a variety of low-velocity mobilization techniques and only 5% received HVLA techniques.[621] In the Childs et al[141] study, all clinicians used the same HVLA technique for all patients randomized to receive HVLA manipulation. Hancock et al[622] did suggest that the CPR may not generalize to low-velocity techniques. The results of another study by Cleland et al[581] supported this assertion.

To determine generalizability of the spinal manipulation CPR to alternative manual techniques, Cleland et al[581] compared 3 different techniques in patients with LBP who fit the CPR with 4/5 factors present. In this study, mean duration of symptoms was 50 days with only 14% satisfying the less-than-16-day criteria. Subjects were 18 to 60 years of age, scored greater than 25% on the modified ODQ, and were randomly assigned to receive 1 of 3 MT treatments for 2 sessions followed by 3 sessions of strengthening exercises. The exercise program (see Figure 4-102) targeted trunk stabilizing musculature, including abdominal hollowing for TrA, bridging and quadruped arm and leg extensions for MF/ES, and side-support exercises (see Figure 4-97B) for oblique abdominals as performed in the Childs et al[141] validation study. The 3 MT techniques

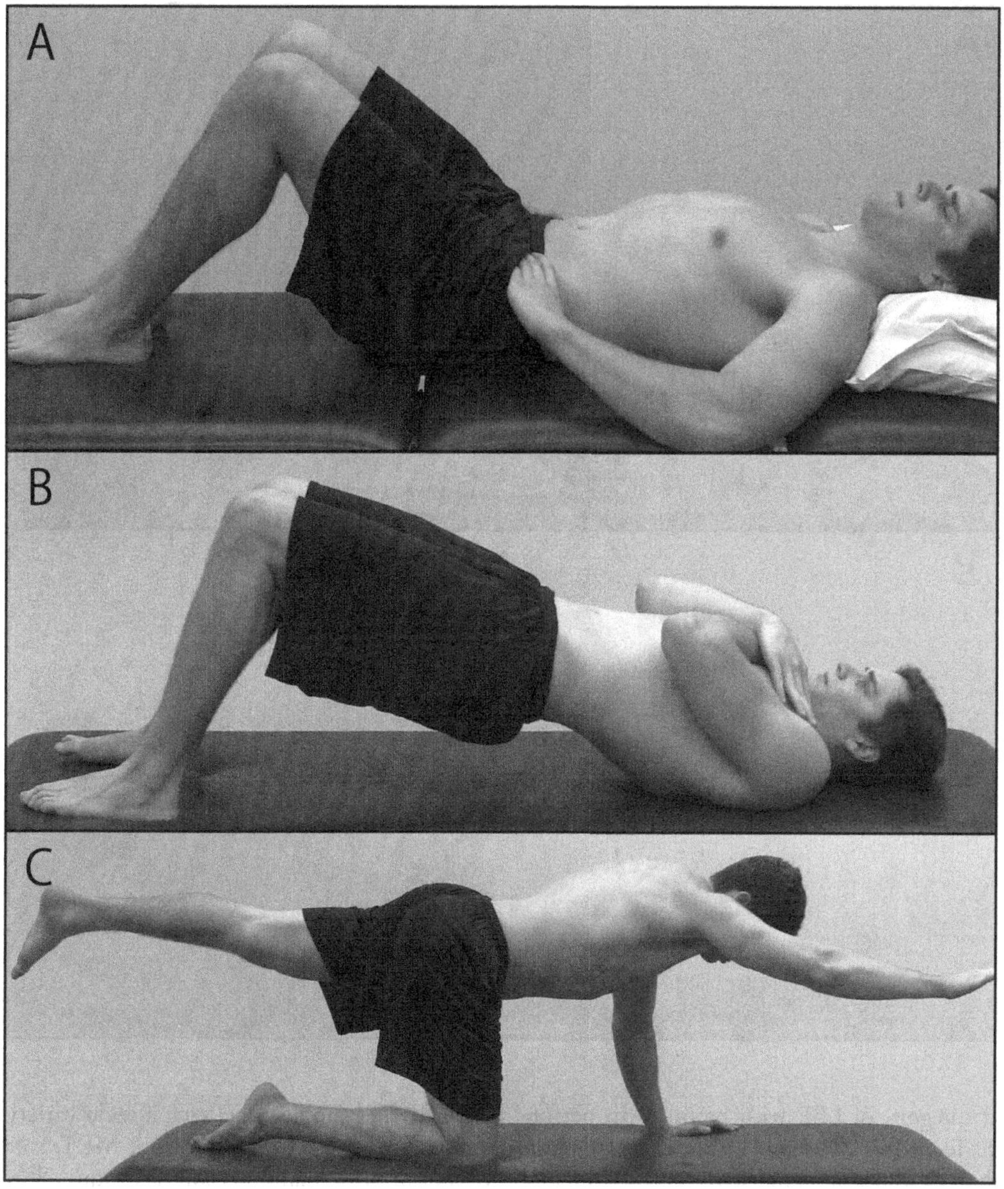

Figure 4-102. Trunk strengthening exercises: (A) abdominal hollowing for TrA; (B) bridging for the MF/ES; and (C) quadruped arm and leg extensions for the MF/ES.

were a supine lumbopelvic thrust manipulation (see Figure 4-100), a side-lying lumbar thrust manipulation (see Figure 4-99), and a nonthrust manipulation of CPA mobilization (Figure 4-103). The results revealed no differences between the supine thrust manipulation and the side-lying thrust manipulation at 1 week, 4 weeks, or 6 months. A significant difference was observed between the thrust manipulation and nonthrust manipulation groups in ODQ and pain scores at 1 and 4 weeks and for ODQ at 6 months in favor of the thrust manipulation groups. At the 6-month follow-up, 91.9% (supine thrust), 89.5% (side-lying thrust), and 67.6% (nonthrust) of subjects achieved a successful outcome of at least 50% reduction in ODQ. This study did not include a control or placebo group and was unable to account for variables of spontaneous recovery, patient expectations, or placebo, but did support the generalizability of the CPR to another thrust manipulation technique and not the nonthrust technique and provided support for generalization to different settings. Future research is still required to examine these findings.[581]

An intervention based on the manipulation CPR diagnostic classification may be effective for some patients, but may not always be effective or indicated for others for several reasons including patient expectations, patient preference or previous negative or positive experience, clinician experience, contraindications, or, in some cases, state practice acts that prohibit manipulation by physical therapists. Additionally, in some patients, the research will not apply or not apply clearly. Initially these individuals would fit into a similar ICF classification, LBP with mobility deficits. In this instance, an evidence-based approach that matches these individuals to intervention strategies such as joint mobilization, soft tissue mobilization, or MET and exercise to improve mobility still applies.

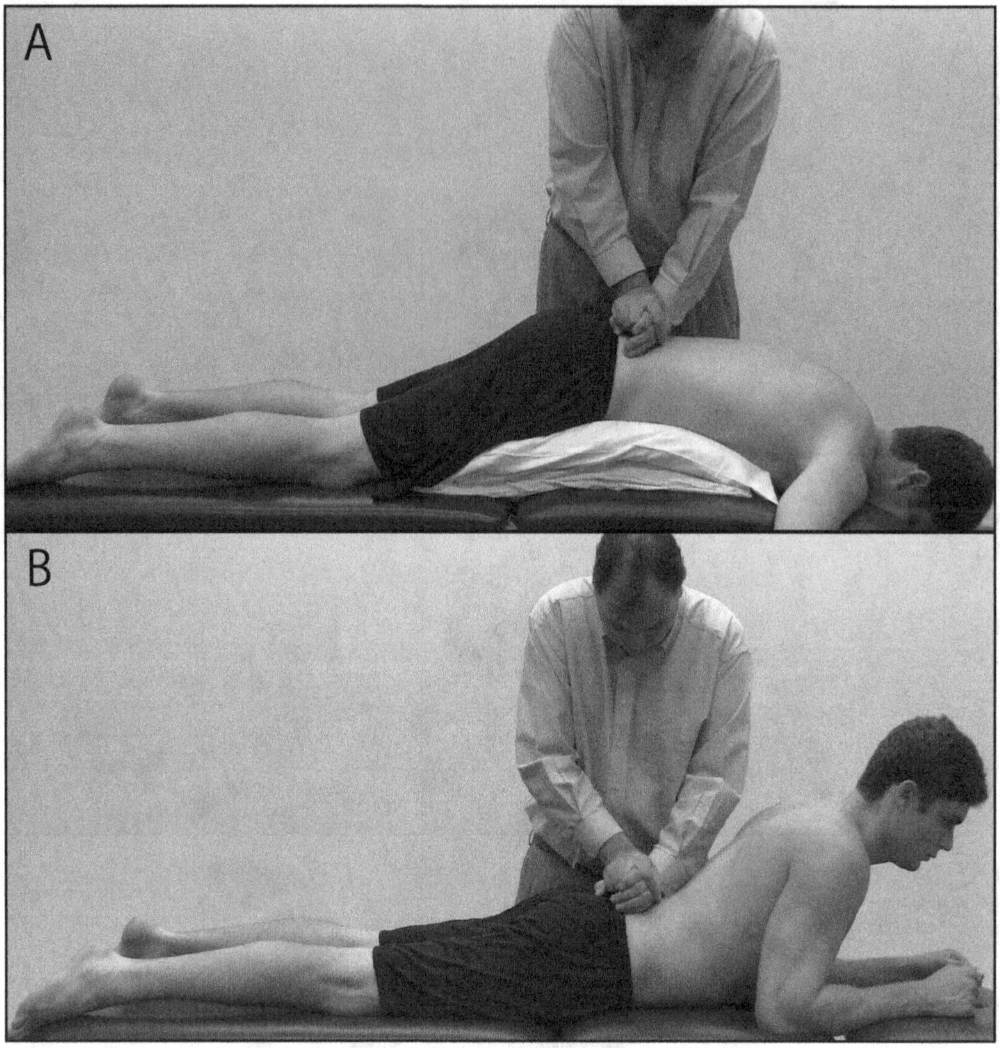

Figure 4-103. Nonthrust manipulation: prone, lumbar CPA mobilization. The CPA mobilization is performed in a similar manner to CPA PAIVM assessment (see Figure 4-85A) described earlier in this chapter. In the Cleland et al[595] study, the CPA was directed at L4-L5 using an HVLA oscillatory force at 2 Hz for a total of 60 seconds for 2 sets with 30 seconds of rest between sets. The therapist selected the level to be manipulated or chose the L4-L5 segment because previous research suggested that procedures directed toward the lower lumbar region were more effective.[572] Variations or progressions of this technique include positioning the patient in flexion over a pillow, extension, or LF. (A) CPA in flexion and (B) CPA in extension.

In an impairment-based category of LBP with mobility deficits, the clinician identifies relevant physical impairments such as lumbar or thoracic spine and hip ROM impairments related to joint or muscle stiffness. Intervention, then, is directed toward prioritized impairments linked to activity limitations or performance deficits important to the patient. Using exam findings such as hypomobility from CPA PAIVM or PPIVM testing to guide clinical decision making for selecting an intervention is one example of an impairment-based approach. The presence of segmental hypomobility suggests that a patient may benefit from an interventions such as MET, mobilization, or manipulation and exercise.[508] Though research is scarce, both CPA (see Figure 4-103) and UPA PAIVM (Figure 4-104) and PPIVM may be used as mobilization techniques to decrease pain and improve mobility. Powers et al[623] demonstrated an immediate increase in lumbar extension and decreased pain after a single session of CPA PAIVM mobilization of 3 bouts of 40 seconds to the most painful segment followed by 2 bouts of 40 seconds to each of the other lumbar levels in persons with LBP.[623] In persons with LBP and mobility deficits, a wide variety of manual interventions such as mobilization, MET, soft tissue mobilization, or other manipulation techniques plus exercise could be appropriate.

Muscle Energy Technique

Many MT approaches and techniques, including MET, have limited research related to clinical outcomes. MET is based on biomechanical models and assessment of coupled spinal motion, but reproducibility and validity of the tests are in doubt.[624] MET uses muscle contraction[625] (Figure 4-105) to mobilize joints and soft tissues in the management of stiff muscles, weak muscles, joint hypomobility, and pain. The exact mechanism by which MET works is unclear, but it is likely to be biomechanical and neurophysiological in nature.

Several studies showed improvements in cervical,[626,627] thoracic,[628] and lumbar spinal ROM supporting the use of MET for mobility deficits.[628-630] Schenk et al[629] used a side-lying MET technique for 5 minutes 2 times per week over 4 weeks compared to a control group to improve

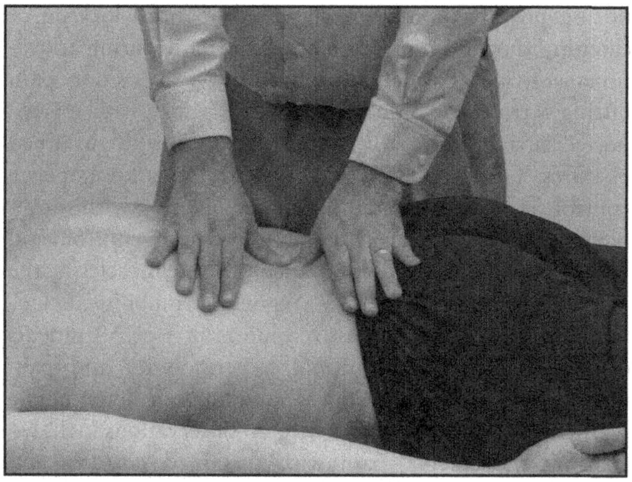

Figure 4-104. Nonthrust manipulation: prone, lumbar UPA mobilization. Technique performance is the same as for assessment. Treatment of the painful level and dysfunctional level is more effective in pain reduction than a randomly selected level.[608] In asymptomatic subjects, no difference was found between amplitudes or grades of mobilization as measured by pressure pain thresholds.[607] Variations or progressions of this technique include positioning the patient in flexion, extension, or LF.

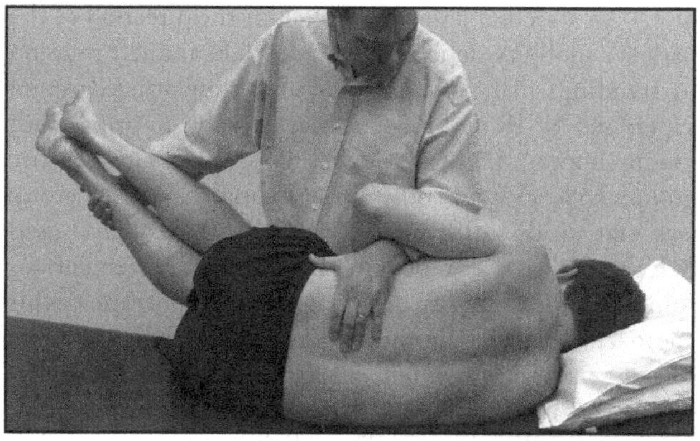

Figure 4-106. MET for lumbar flexion mobility deficit: flexion, right LF, right rotation mobility deficit at L4-L5.[635] In right side-lying, the clinician palpates the L4-L5 interspinous space and flexes the patient's legs until motion is palpated at L5. The clinician then introduces flexion from above until motion is palpated at L4 and then left rotation. The clinician introduces left LF by lifting both feet toward the ceiling. Maintaining the position of flexion, left LF, and left rotation, the clinician asks the patient to pull both feet toward the floor for a 5-second isometric contraction for 4 repetitions. After each repetition, motion is introduced further into flexion, right LF, and right rotation.

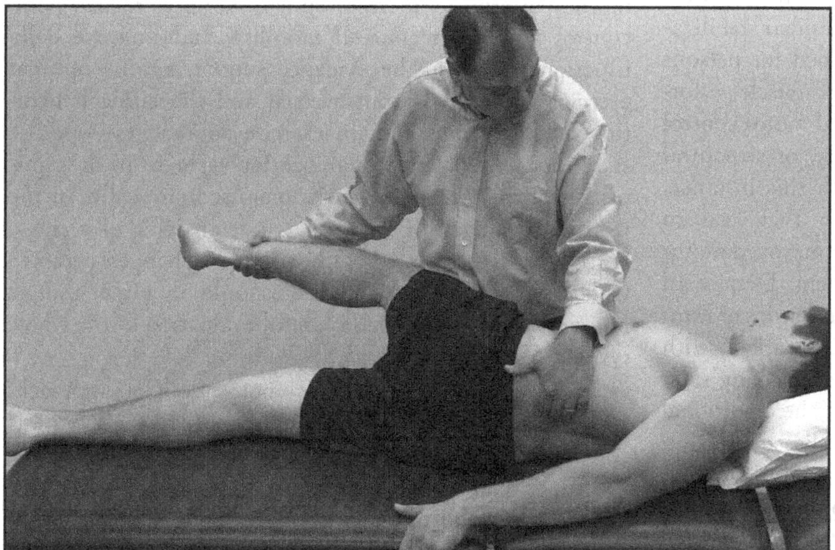

Figure 4-105. MET for lumbar extension mobility deficit: extension, left LF, left rotation mobility deficit at L4-L5.[635] In right side-lying, the clinician introduces extension at L4-L5 by translating the trunk from PA and fine tunes extension from above at the shoulder, monitoring for movement up to L5 as needed. Both shoulders remain perpendicular to the table. Left rotation is introduced by rotating the left shoulder posteriorly until motion is felt at L4. The patient grasps the edge of the table to maintain this position. The clinician's right hand lifts the left leg to introduce left LF to L4-L5. Maintaining this position, the patient pulls the left knee toward the table for a 5-second isometric contraction for 4 repetitions. After each repetition, motion is introduced further into the range for extension and left LF.

lumbar extension. Fryer and Ruszkowski[627] examined the effect of duration of 5 seconds, 20 seconds, and a sham control group of MET isometric contractions on active atlantoaxial rotation ROM. A significant difference in the mean change of axial rotation was revealed between the 5-second MET and control, but not between the 20-second MET and control. The 5-second isometric contraction was more effective for increasing cervical rotation with MET than a longer contraction time.[627]

In a prospective pilot clinical trial, Wilson et al[630] compared MET treatment coupled with supervised neuromuscular re-education (NMR) and resistance training (RT) to NMR and RT alone. Subjects were 18 to 65 years old, ODI 20% to 60%, with acute LBP without referral to the buttocks or lower extremity, and a lumbar flexion mobility deficit (physiological and segmental) as determined by motion palpation of the lumbar spine in flexion. MET was performed in side-lying (Figure 4-106) 2 times per week over 4 weeks. Following the MET procedure, the patient's ROM and positional segmental mobility were reassessed. The MET procedure was a success if the positional asymmetry and the ROM limitation in flexion and asymmetry in side-bending were no longer observed. A home exercise program was prescribed to augment the MET consisting of a 5- to 7-second pain-free stretch in the direction of the patient's mobility deficit (flexion, left LF, and left rotation in standing). All patients received a standardized set of supervised NMR and RT exercises available in print. Both groups improved in ODI score (85% MET plus exercise group; 65% exercise only group), but the MET group was statistically different.[630] Several studies have used MET[631-634] as a component of overall management for spinal pain, lending further evidence to support use of this approach. Table 4-1 summarizes key exam findings of, factors against, and potential intervention for the manipulation and mobilization plus exercise LBP subgroup and ICF category of LBP with mobility deficits.

Stabilization Exercise Low Back Pain Subgroup or Low Back Pain With Movement Coordination Impairments and Matched Intervention

Common alterations in both structure and function of the superficial and deep trunk muscles in persons with LBP are discussed in Chapter 3. Theoretically, lumbar stabilization exercises are most commonly prescribed for persons with LBP who demonstrate deficits in trunk muscle performance thought to be associated with altered motor control strategies resulting in segmental instability, or structural changes resulting in clinical instability. In this instance, improvements in trunk muscle function that lead to reduced pain and disability are credited to improved motor control of spinal segments during movement. Despite an abundance of research related to the biomechanics of lumbar instability, a gold standard for identifying patients with lumbar instability has not been established, making such a diagnosis difficult and poorly defined. The traditional medical diagnosis of lumbar instability relies on flexion and extension radiographs, which unfortunately have high false-positive rates and significant variation in asymptomatic subjects.[635] Additionally, radiographs do not provide information about neuromuscular control. A patient's need for stabilization exercises is necessarily based on clinical examination findings with or without radiographic images. The associated ICF category of LBP that fits the stabilization exercise classification is LBP with movement coordination deficits,[14] which could include, but does not require, a medical diagnosis of lumbar instability.

Subjective and objective descriptors of clinical lumbar spine instability have been identified based on clinical expert consensus.[636] Subjective descriptors aiding in the differential diagnosis of clinical lumbar instability include giving way and giving out, frequent episodes of LBP, a condition that is progressively getting worse, and a frequent need to manipulate the spine. Common complaints during posture or movement include painful locking or catching during twisting or bending, pain during transitional activities, pain on return from a flexed position, pain during a trivial or sudden activity, difficulty with unsupported sitting, and pain that is worsened with sustained postures. Objective descriptors include poor lumbopelvic control such as segmental hinging or pivoting with movement, poor coordination or neuromuscular control, and decreased strength and endurance of local muscles at the level of segmental instability. Segmental mobility including pain provocation, excessive motion of 1 or 2 segments during flexion and extension, hypermobility and pain provocation with CPA PAIVM, and adjacent hypomobile segments were also reported. Motion observations included aberrant movements, pain with sustained postures and positions, Gower's sign (ie, thigh climbing), and poor posture and postural deviations such as the lateral shift. The authors concluded that these descriptors are similar to those reported in spine-related instability literature and may aid clinical differential diagnosis.[636]

Stabilization Exercise Approaches

The goals of stabilization exercise are to train muscular motor patterns to increase spinal stability, reduce pain, control aberrant segmental mobility, and improve daily functional ability. The evidence supporting the optimal exercise approach is controversial and the clinical literature extensive, but 2 main exercise approaches—specific stabilization and general stabilization—persist in the clinical literature with many variations used clinically. In the words of Hodges, "Back pain is not an issue of a single muscle, it is associated with complex changes across a whole system" and "rehabilitation should not target a single muscle, but instead include careful evaluation of the whole system."[637(p942)]

In the specific exercise or motor control approach, activation of the deep trunk muscles (TrA and MF) is consistently observed as delayed or reduced in LBP, while the superficial muscles are often overactive.[638] In these individuals, stabilization exercise involving an early motor control intervention targeting the deep muscles of the TrA and MF may be needed, but this is unlikely to be the only target of trunk muscle performance in the exercise program. One misconception about this approach is that the only focus is preferential activation of the TrA and MF. Posture, muscle activation, and functional movement patterns are also addressed. The goal of this approach aims to retrain normal stabilizing motor patterns of coordination between the superficial and deep trunk muscles, which are often compromised in persons with LBP.

In contrast, biomechanical models involving EMG and stiffness analyses provide a different view. Cholewicki and McGill[639] state that sufficient spine stability depends on the task and requires involvement of all trunk muscles.

For most daily activities, a 10% abdominal wall cocontraction or abdominal bracing along with the extensors and quadratus lumborum is sufficient to maintain stability.[640] All muscles are important, especially their endurance component, and clinical focus on one muscle does not ensure stability. According to McGill,[640] all muscles are important to quantify stabilization, thus a classification of superficial and deep muscles offers no benefit for clinical decision making. With regard to the importance of the TrA, Grenier and McGill[641] concluded that no mechanical rationale exists for using the ADIM to enhance stability. Abdominal bracing improved stability by 35% with a 15% increase in lumbar compression versus 0.14% for the TrA with a less than 0.1% decrease in lumbar compression. In this view, any benefit of TrA activation appears not related to its ability to provide stability. McGill[640] described stability as a moving target with constantly changing function in 3 planes of motion needed to support daily postures and movements. Activity requires complex interaction of many muscles, a responsive motor system, muscular endurance, and a spine that tolerates loads. The general exercise approach places greater emphasis on exercises designed to improve the endurance and stabilizing function of the superficial trunk muscles (ie, ES, oblique abdominals, quadratus lumborum) without regard to preferential activation of the deep muscles. Research[642-644] comparing specific stabilization exercise (SSE) and a more general exercise approach has shown no differences favoring one approach over the other. Of more importance is the fact that an active exercise approach is beneficial in reducing pain and disability in some individuals with LBP.[642-644]

Evidence for Stabilization Exercise

In persons with LBP, trunk muscle function[645,646] and structure[642,647,648] can be improved with stabilization exercise. However, controversy exists regarding whether stabilization exercise and improvements in trunk muscle performance represent improvements in functional outcomes. Several studies support the effectiveness of stabilization exercise for LBP.[643,649-651] Other reports showed no difference between stabilization and conventional rehabilitation or MT.[644,652,653] In addition to controversy regarding whether stabilization exercise results in improved clinical outcomes, no consensus exists for an optimal evidence-based lumbar stabilization exercise approach with known mechanisms of effectiveness.

Ferreira et al[654] conducted a systematic review from 1966 to 2004 of the efficacy of SSE for spinal and pelvic pain after pregnancy. The authors concluded that SSE of preferential deep muscle activation and use of a motor control approach produces modest beneficial effects for persons with spinal and pelvic pain. Benefits were observed for treatment of cervicogenic headache, neck pain, and pelvic pain, and for decreasing recurrence of LBP after an acute episode. In general, SSE was superior to no treatment, usual care, or education, but no greater than the effects of SMT or conventional physiotherapy. A brief period of SSE combined with education offered similar effects to spinal fusion surgery for patients with disc degeneration. SSE reduced pain and disability in chronic LBP, but not in acute LBP. The underlying mechanisms for SSE are unknown. Preliminary evidence suggests that cognitive activation of the deep muscles can immediately influence the manner in which these muscles are recruited in untrained functional movements. Theoretically, SSE induces changes in motor patterns that may alter spinal loading and improve symptoms.[655]

A systematic review[656] through October 2005 suggested that moderate evidence exists for improved pain and disability levels, increased MF muscle cross-sectional area, and limited evidence for improved quality of life for SSE. Hides et al[648] demonstrated in acute LBP patients that the MF cross-sectional area increased in the intervention group at 4 and 10 weeks but not in the control group. Long-term follow-up by the same authors[650] showed that the patients in the intervention group had fewer recurrences of LBP at both 1-year and 3-year follow-up. Recurrences for the intervention group were 30% and 35%, and for the control group 84% and 75%, respectively. O'Sullivan et al[649] compared an SSE program to a general exercise approach for patients with LBP with or without radiating pain into the lower extremity and a radiological diagnosis of spondylolysis. The specific exercise group had a significant reduction in pain intensity and disability maintained at the 30-month follow-up. The control group had no significant change from baseline.[649]

May and Johnson[657] reviewed 21 studies from 1982 to October 2006, reporting similar findings to the previous reviews. SSE may reduce pain and disability in chronic but not acute LBP. SSE was superior to no treatment, usual care, or minimal intervention. For the first time, authors stated that SSE may be more effective in certain subgroups rather than nonspecific LBP groups. A systematic review[658] provides evidence that SSE alone or as part of another therapy is effective in reducing pain and disability in patients with persistent LBP. The authors found no convincing evidence that SSE is superior to other forms of exercise, MT, or surgery.[658] Kriese et al[659] reported that SSE is as effective as treatment by a general practitioner in reducing short-term pain or disability. After an acute episode of LBP, SSE is more effective in reducing recurrence. For CLBP, SSE is more effective than minimal intervention and as effective as other PT interventions in reducing pain and disability. SSE and a general exercise approach are usually not recommended for nonspecific acute LBP and appear equally effective for nonspecific CLBP. A general consensus supports the need for active exercise in LBP, but no agreement exists on which exercises are most effective, the optimal method for implementation, and who is most likely to benefit.

TABLE 4-23. STABILIZATION EXERCISES AND PROGRESSION

EXERCISES—WITH ABDOMINAL BRACING	PROGRESSION CRITERIA
Supine abdominal bracing	30 reps, 8-second hold
Supine heel slides	20 reps per leg, 4-second hold
Supine leg lifts	20 reps per leg, 4-second hold
Supine bridging	30 reps, 8-second hold, progress to 1 leg
Standing	30 reps, 8-second hold
Standing row	20 reps per side, 6-second hold
Walking	30 reps with 8-second hold on each side
Quadruped arm lifts bracing	30 reps with 8-second hold on each side
Quadruped leg lifts	30 reps with 8-second hold on each side
Quadruped alternate arm and leg lifts	30 reps with 8-second hold on each side
Side support with knees flexed	30 reps with 8-second hold on each side
Side support with knees extended	30 reps with 8-second hold on each side

Data extracted from Hicks GE, Fritz JM, Delitto A, McGill SM. Preliminary development of a clinical prediction rule for determining which patients with low back pain will respond to a stabilization exercise program. *Arch Phys Med Rehabil.* 2005;86:1753-1762.

Stabilization Exercise Classification and Matched Intervention

To assist in identifying a subgroup of patients likely to respond to stabilization training, a preliminary CPR was developed by Hicks et al.[197] All subjects received the same stabilization program 2 times per week with a daily home program over 8 weeks. The exercise program favored a general approach based on biomechanical and EMG studies[660-666] focusing on repeated submaximal efforts to encourage stabilizing motor patterns for cocontraction of the large, superficial trunk muscles.[660-666] Exercise progression was based on specific criteria at the discretion of the therapist (Table 4-23). Subjects not included in this study had previous spinal fusion surgery; LBP as a result of current pregnancy; acute fracture, tumor, or infection; and the presence of 2 or more signs of nerve root compression (diminished lower-extremity strength, sensation, or reflexes).

The following 4 variables were identified as most predictive of success with stabilization exercise:

1. Age less than 40
2. Aberrant movement during AROM
3. Maximum tolerated average SLR of greater than 91 degrees as calculated by right + left/2
4. A positive PIT[197]

The best rule for predicting success was 3 or 4 of the variables with a +LR 4.0 (1.6 to 10.0). Assuming a 33% chance of success, the probability increased to 67%. Although not part of the CPR, other variables predictive of success include previous episodes of LBP with increasing frequency and CPA PAIVM hypermobility.[197] Hebert et al[667] examined the relationship between the prognostic factors for success with stabilization exercise and TrA and MF activation using ultrasound imaging. The authors found decreased MF muscle activation but not TrA is associated with the presence of factors predicting success with a stabilization program and cited the potential clinical importance of targeting the MF during stabilization training.[667]

From the Hicks et al[197] study, 4 factors were identified as predictive of failure of stabilization exercise as an intervention, meaning less than 6 points improvement on the modified ODQ:

1. Less than 9 on the FABQPA scale
2. Absence of CPA PAIVM hypermobility
3. Absence of aberrant movements during sagittal plane AROM
4. A negative PIT

The presence of at least 3 of these findings suggests failure with stabilization is likely (+LR 18.8). A 25% pretest probability of failure and at least 3 of these factors increases the probability of failure to 86%. More research is needed to validate this CPR. Preliminary research supports that it is possible to identify individuals who are likely to benefit most from stabilization exercise and those who are unlikely to benefit.[197]

Alqarni et al[668] conducted a systematic review of clinical utility tests that aid in the diagnosis of lumbar segmental instability. In 42 patients with CLBP sensitivity, specificity, and +LRs were as follows:

- PAIVM (0.46, 0.49, 2.4)
- Posterior shear test (0.57, 0.48, 1.1)
- Beighton hypermobility scale (0.36, 0.86, 2.5)
- Aberrant motions (0.18, 0.90, 1.90)
- PIT (0.61, 0.57, 1.4)[408]

In subjects with CLBP, Abbott et al[669] reported the diagnostic accuracy for PAIVM to diagnose lumbar spine instability as specificity (0.89), sensitivity (0.29), and +LR 2.5. Similarly, PPIVMs in flexion and extension respectively demonstrated low sensitivity (0.05, 0.16), high specificity (0.99, 0.98), and +LRs (8.7, 7.1). The PLE test demonstrated sensitivity (0.84), specificity (0.90), +LR 8.8 (4.5 to 17.3), and –LR 0.2 in 122 elderly patients with mixed lumbar degenerative diseases.[670] Further studies are needed to determine the validity of the PLE test and combinations of factors to assist in diagnosing and managing patients with clinical lumbar segmental instability.[668]

Postpartum women with posterior PGP, discussed later in this chapter, are another subgroup of LBP that may benefit from stabilization exercise. A composite of clinical findings and tests for this subgroup of women were used as inclusion criteria to evaluate the effects of SSE after pregnancy compared to stabilization exercise plus PT on pain, function, and quality of life.[671] Location of the PGP was distal and/or lateral to the L5-S1 area in the buttocks and/or in the PS with onset during pregnancy or within 3 weeks. The posterior pelvic pain provocation (also known as the P4 or thigh thrust test),[672] ASLR test,[450] palpation provocation of the long dorsal sacroiliac ligament and PS,[673] and a modified Trendelenburg test[674] were also positive tests. The P4 test or the ASLR test has to be positive on the right and/or left side, and at least one of the other 3 tests had to be positive. No statistical properties have been reported for this composite of tests. Although both groups improved, SSE was more effective for postpartum women with PGP than PT without SSE across all outcomes after 20 weeks and 1 year.[671] Table 4-2 summarizes key findings, factors against, and potential interventions for the stabilization exercise LBP subgroup and the ICF category of LBP with movement coordination impairment.

Specific Stabilization Exercise Approach Guidelines

The guidelines discussed next are a brief overview of SSE for dynamic control of the spine from a motor control training perspective based on extensive research.[675] Many exercise variations tailored to the patient's needs are used in this approach. The goal of any stabilization program is optimum control of the spine to meet the patient's functional demands. Rehabilitation of motor control of the spine using a specific approach begins with assessment of posture, movement patterns, breathing, and activation of the deep and superficial muscles, as previously discussed in the section on examination. Mobility and motor deficits of the hips, knees, ankles, or thoracic spine may impact the ability to control the spine as well as the presence of fear-avoidance beliefs. When the patient is identified as one who will benefit from stabilization exercise or transitions to a stabilization classification, assessment identifies the deficits that must be addressed. Not all patients with LBP have the same deficits or start at the same level.

The SSE approach uses principles of motor learning for skill acquisition. Generally, 3 phases are involved: cognitive (ie, learning what to do), associative (ie, refining the movement pattern), and automatic phases (ie, developing skill).[676] As an example, phase 1 begins with specific low-level cocontraction of the TrA and MF with minimal superficial activation. Feedback about movement sequence and quality of performance is important as the patient learns what to do. Phase 2 encourages the pain-free, cocontraction strategy in a variety of positions—sitting, standing, walking, or transitions. Consistency in movement develops with less cognitive demand as the movement pattern is refined and previously painful activities are practiced. Finally, in phase 3, the low-level cocontraction becomes automatic while performing functional daily activities or performing under altered environments of speed, accuracy, or loads.[493,676]

The SSE approach begins with preferential, low-level coactivation of the local muscle system with minimized activity of the global systems. The motor pattern of activation of the local system must be learned with precision and normal breathing and facilitated in a variety of postures such as sitting, standing, prone, quadruped, or side-lying. Cues and techniques such as palpation, RUSI, and pressure biofeedback for facilitating the TrA and MF are the same as those used for assessment. As discussed in postural assessment, posture should be comfortable with a neutral, flexible spine, but not rigid. A rigid posture implies an overactive superficial system. Training control in sitting and standing postures is also recommended. When coactivation can be performed without feedback for 10 repetitions, 10-second holds, and normal breathing, coordination training between the deep and superficial systems begins for static control and then dynamic control.[493,675]

Static control involves activation using ADIM or whatever strategy works for the patient, first holding the deep muscles and then imposing resistance in a variety of ways (Figure 4-107) to superimpose superficial muscle activity. When load is added, the superficial system is needed to maintain neutral, lumbopelvic alignment. Training in and out of daily postures, sitting, standing, and transitional postures such as sit to stand is also needed.[493,675]

Dynamic control involves activating the deep muscles first, holding the contraction while movement is performed, and breathing normally. Some activities include balancing on an unstable surface or wobble board or sitting on a ball while incorporating arm or leg movement.

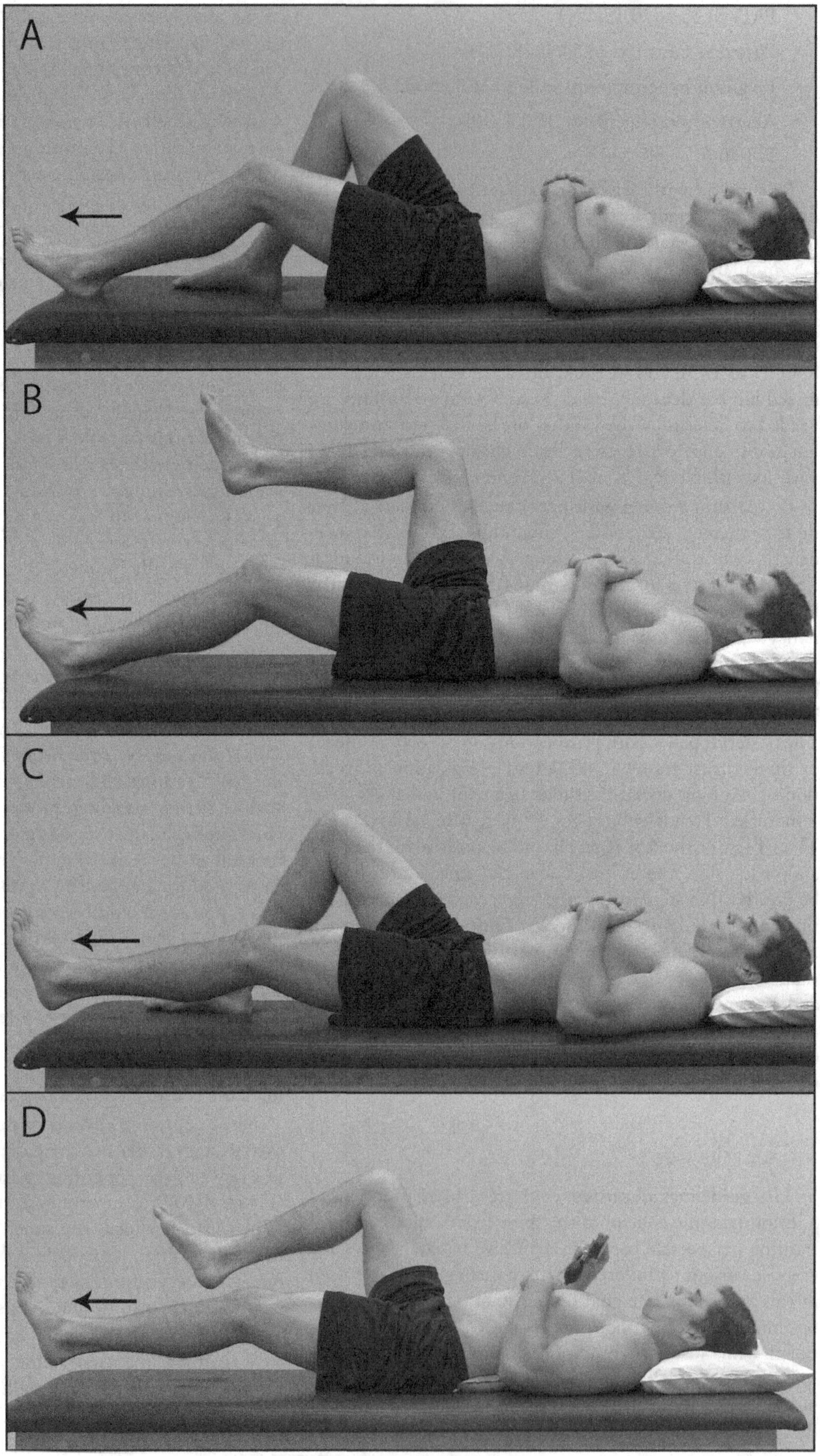

Figure 4-107. Static coordination training of the deep and superficial systems through upper and lower limb loading in supine and quadruped prone: (A) single-leg heel slide, opposite leg supported; (B) single-leg heel slide, opposite leg unsupported; (C) single-leg slide, opposite leg supported; and (D) single-leg slide, opposite leg unsupported using biofeedback pressure. *(continued)*

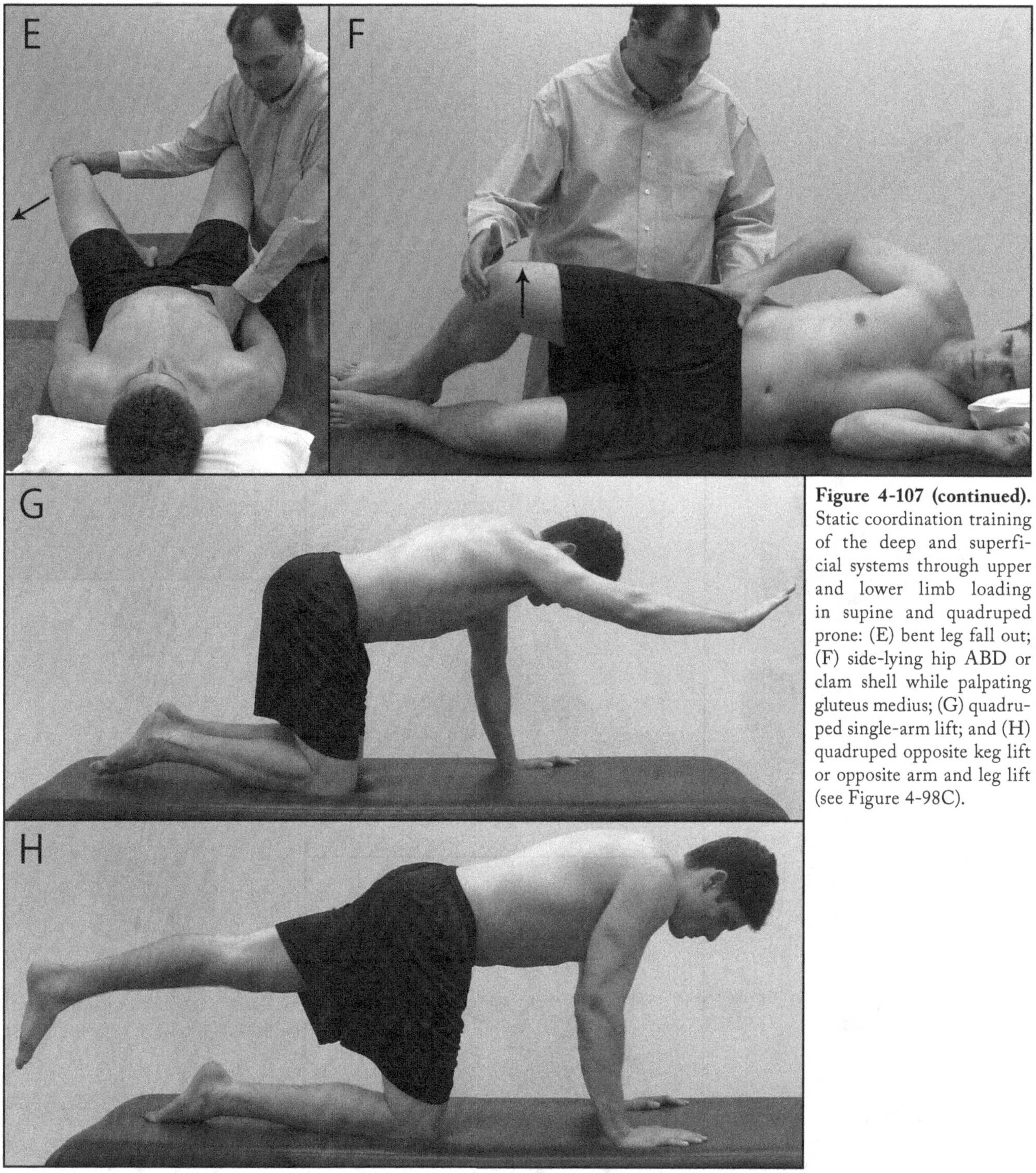

Figure 4-107 (continued). Static coordination training of the deep and superficial systems through upper and lower limb loading in supine and quadruped prone: (E) bent leg fall out; (F) side-lying hip ABD or clam shell while palpating gluteus medius; (G) quadruped single-arm lift; and (H) quadruped opposite keg lift or opposite arm and leg lift (see Figure 4-98C).

Balancing on an unstable surface requires movement and dynamic control of the spine. The spine is not static (Figure 4-108). Progression of activities involves analysis of the patient's daily functional requirements related to position, load, and movement such as standing, reaching overhead, lifting, pushing, or pulling (Figure 4-109). Activities important to the patient and previously painful to the patient should be relearned. Activities are often broken into parts before practicing the entire movement. This progression leads to the final phase centering on performance of functional tasks at home, at work, or in community environments. The goal of the final phase is automatic activation of the deep muscles first, holding the contraction while movement is performed, and breathing normally. Extensive details of the motor control approach are found in other resources.[493,675,677]

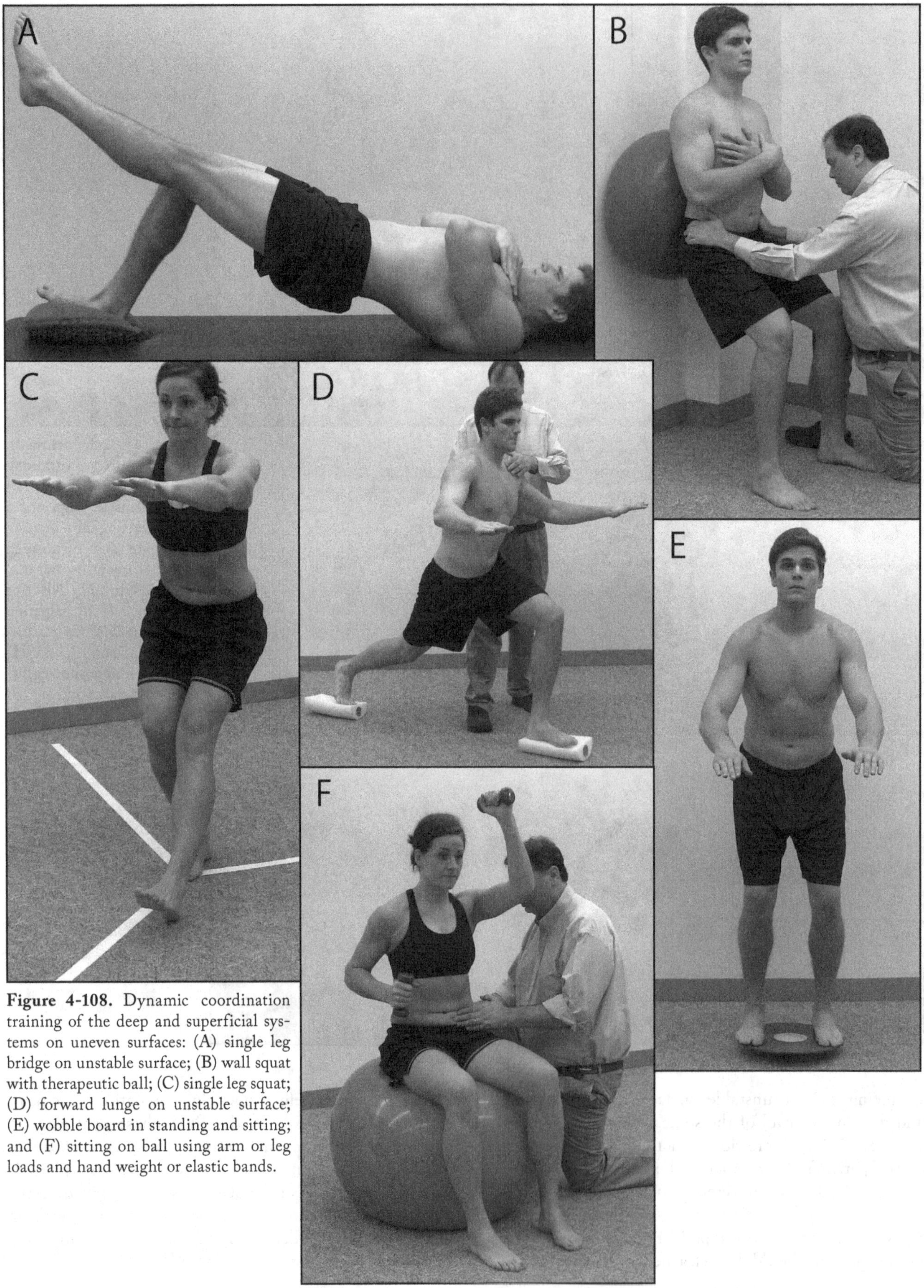

Figure 4-108. Dynamic coordination training of the deep and superficial systems on uneven surfaces: (A) single leg bridge on unstable surface; (B) wall squat with therapeutic ball; (C) single leg squat; (D) forward lunge on unstable surface; (E) wobble board in standing and sitting; and (F) sitting on ball using arm or leg loads and hand weight or elastic bands.

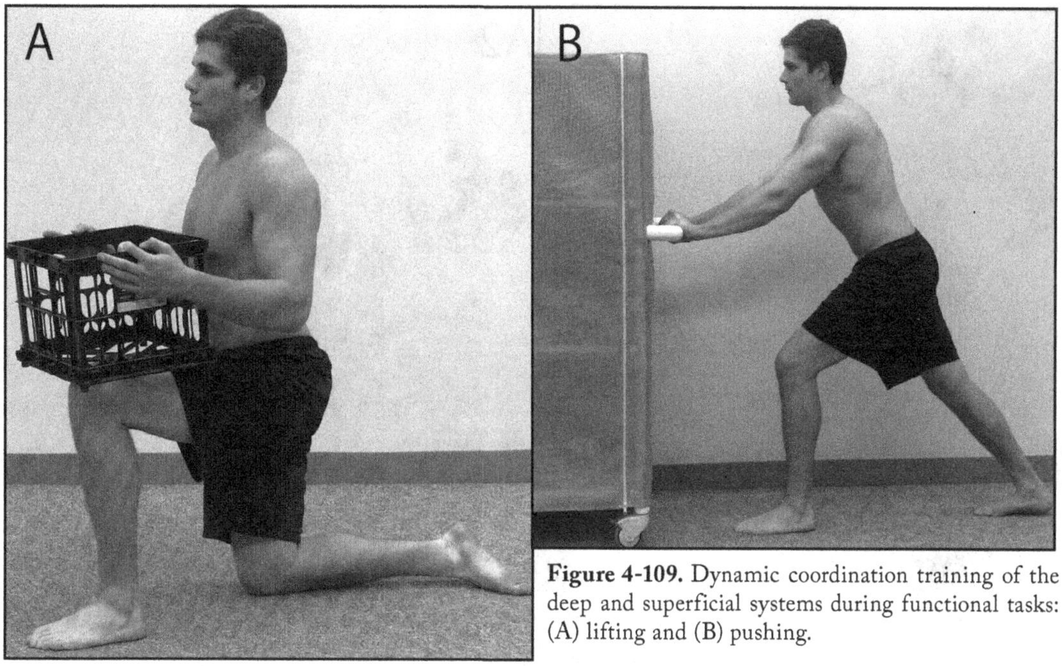

Figure 4-109. Dynamic coordination training of the deep and superficial systems during functional tasks: (A) lifting and (B) pushing.

General Stabilization Exercise Guidelines

Many general exercise programs exist with wide variation in clinical practice. A brief overview of rehabilitation guidelines for dynamic control of the spine are presented based on biomechanical modeling studies that quantify stability and tissue loading resulting from muscle activation patterns.[499,678,679] The stabilization exercises used in the Hicks et al[197] study were based on these principles. As opposed to the ADIM, the AB, meaning isometric or stiffening cocontraction in neutral spine, is used in this approach for reasons previously discussed. Exercise dosage favors muscular endurance for protection of spinal health and recovery rather than strength with emphasis on good form and normal breathing patterns. Exercises such as the sit-up and lumbar extension against gravity are not recommended due to excessive spinal compression loads.

In the early stages, the "big 3" are recommended to challenge trunk muscles, spare the spine of high compressive loads, and ensure sufficient stability.[499] The big 3 include the curl-up for the rectus abdominis; the side bridge for the obliques, TrA, and quadratus lumborum; and the bird dog in quadruped for the back extensors. Five stages are associated with this approach.[499] The first 3 stages are used in rehabilitation to identify and correct abnormal motion and motor patterns, build whole body and joint stability related and transferred to daily activities, and increase endurance. Abdominal bracing with the big 3 is held no longer than 7 to 8 seconds with endurance building through repetitions rather than duration. Stages 4 and 5 involve the development of strength, speed, power, and agility necessary for athletic performance.[499]

McGill[499] provided a potential list of exercises for stages 1, 2, and 3 that might include a warm-up activity such as a 5-minute walk or cycle; basic AROM exercises such as cat and camel (Figure 4-110A); teaching abdominal bracing with neutral spine; and assessing and training gluteal activation using the clam shell, back bridge, double-legged squat, single legged squat, transitions, rising from sit to stand, pushing, pulling, and lifting activities (Figure 4-110D). The exercises and teaching cues are discussed next as described by McGill.[499]

Teaching Abdominal Bracing

The patient is asked to contract the muscles to make them stiff. The abdominal wall is not drawn in or pushed out. Bracing is used to encourage cocontraction of the abdominal wall and paraspinals at low levels (ie, 10% to 15% of maximum voluntary isometric contraction) in supine and then used in functional activities such as getting into and out of car and getting on and off the toilet.[499]

Gluteal Activation Using the Clam Shell

Accurate gluteal activation is necessary for a healthy spine, especially during squatting activities such as getting into and out of a chair or car (see Figure 107F). Substitution by the hamstrings and ES produce excessive load on the spine in the presence of weak gluteals. To perform gluteal activation in side-lying with knees and hips flexed, the patient palpates the gluteus medius with the fingers posteriorly and thumb on the ASIS. Keeping the heels together, the knees are separated. Assess for neutral spine, good trunk stabilization, and motion through the range. Training may start here or progress to more advanced gluteal activation patterns such as hip ABD in side-lying or standing.[499]

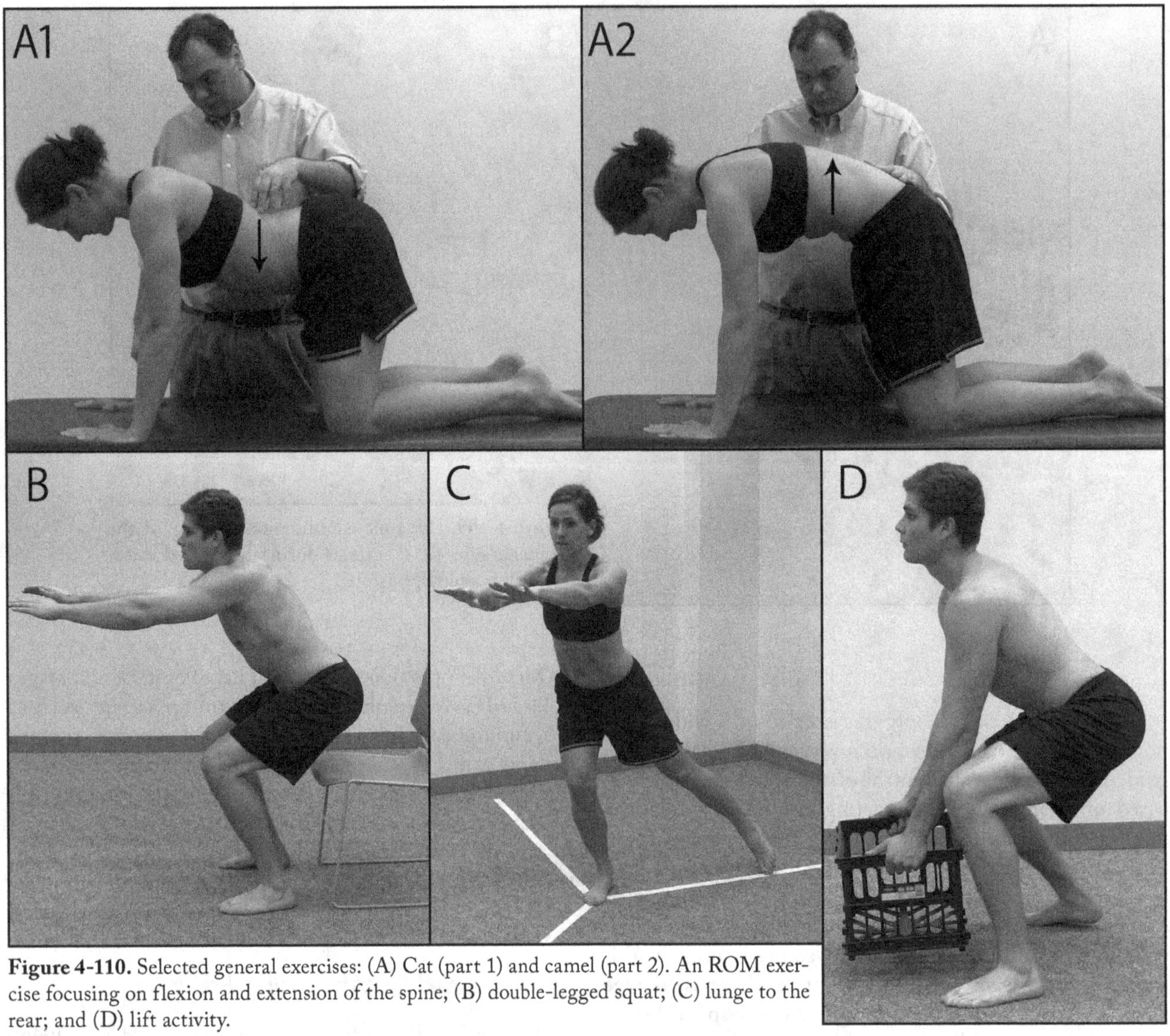

Figure 4-110. Selected general exercises: (A) Cat (part 1) and camel (part 2). An ROM exercise focusing on flexion and extension of the spine; (B) double-legged squat; (C) lunge to the rear; and (D) lift activity.

Gluteus Maximus Using the Back Bridge

In supine, hook-lying with a neutral, braced lumbar spine (see Figure 4-102B), the patient uses imagery for gluteal activation (ie, gluteal squeeze). Keeping the spine in neutral, the patient initiates a gluteal squeeze, which raises the trunk to form a bridge, and maintains the gluteal squeeze throughout trunk elevation and lowering to the rest position. Hamstrings are minimized by beginning with a gluteal squeeze or blocking the feet and asking for slight knee extension.[499]

Double-Legged Squat

This exercise (Figure 4-110B) is a daily activity that many patients with LBP perform incorrectly. Begin in standing or sitting and the spine braced in neutral. The motion requires the hips to move along a 45-degree angle from the vertical, moving the buttocks back and not down in order to sit down. The legs are shoulder width apart with the hips externally rotating to engage the gluteus maximus. Initial practice may be done to surfaces higher than normal chair height, but progression to rising to and from a chair follows. The spine remains in neutral. The arms may be placed in front of the body for balance.[499]

Single-Legged Squat or Lunge

Performance is the same as for the double-legged squat except that the nonweightbearing leg is extended in varying directions to the back, side, or front (Figure 4-110C). The forward angles are difficult because they promote lumbar flexion. The spine is neutral and braced with normal breathing.[499]

All exercises are performed with abdominal bracing, neutral spine, normal breathing, and adherence to perfect technique. All exercises should be done in a pain-free manner. Observation of poor movement and correction of the motion and motor patterns by the clinician should eliminate pain. If not, the activity may be too advanced.[499]

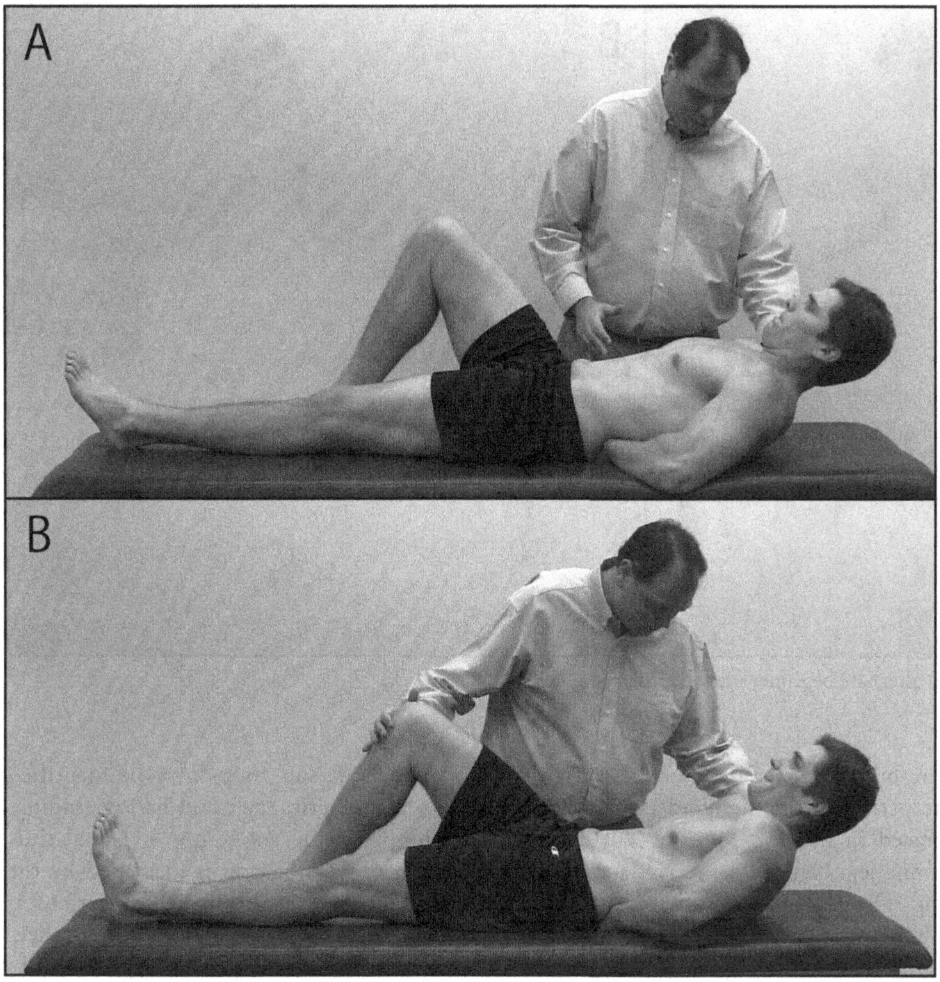

Figure 4-111. Beginner and intermediate curl-up. (A) Beginner: in supine with one knee flexed, the other leg extended, the hands are supporting under the lumbar spine with elbows on the mat. The spine remains in neutral. The head and neck are stabilized on the trunk and move as a unit. Rotation occurs about the thorax by activating the rectus abdominis and obliques without any lumbar spine motion. The head and shoulders are raised slightly off the table. Breathing is normal. The neck should not flex. (B) Intermediate: performance is exactly as for the beginner except that the elbows are lifted slightly off the table. Adding prebracing and deep breathing becomes the advanced curl-up.

The curl-up (Figure 4-111), side bridge (Figure 4-112), and bird dog (Figure 4-113) exercises are depicted in beginner and intermediate stages as described by McGill.[499] The beginner level 1 side bridge (see Figure 4-112) is performed against the wall with the elbows flexed and feet close together. With the spine braced, the patient pivots on the balls of the feet from the left side bridge position to the front plank position and then to the right plank position in a slow, controlled manner with no motion in any plan occurring in the spine and normal breathing. Beginner level 2 side bridge (see Figure 4-97A) and intermediate level side bridge (see Figure 4-97B) are described as follows. In right side-lying with knees flexed and hips in neutral, the left hand grasps the right shoulder. The right hip and right elbow support the side-flexed trunk. With the spine braced, the trunk is straightened until the body is supported on the elbow and knee in line with the hips and shoulders. The intermediate side bridge is performed the same as beginner except now the lower extremities are extended. The upper leg is slightly in front of the lower leg. The trunk is straightened until the body is supported on the elbow and feet and in line with the hips and shoulder.[499]

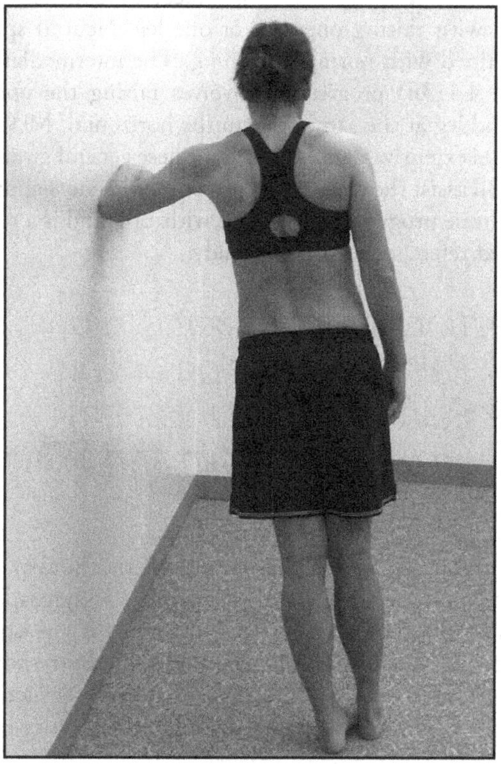

Figure 4-112. Beginner level 1 side bridge.

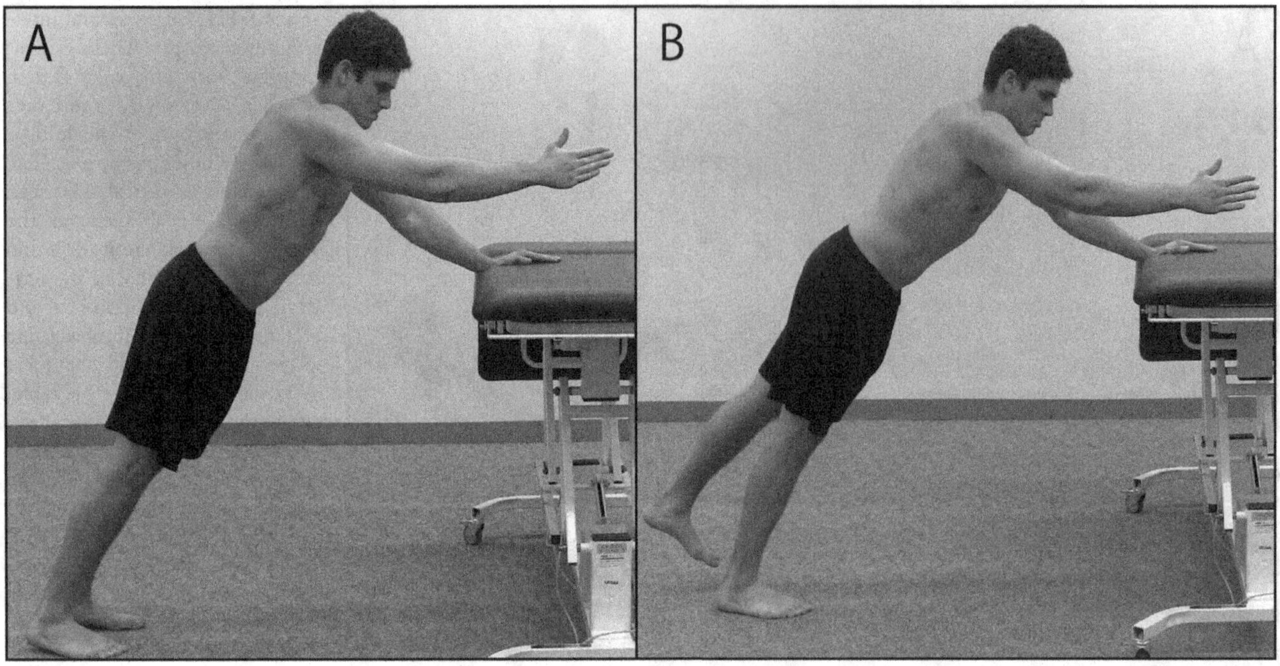

Figure 4-113. Bird dog exercise: (A) alternate beginner and (B) intermediate.

The beginner and intermediate bird dog exercises (see Figures 4-107G and 4-107H) are performed in the quadruped position and the spine braced in neutral. Motion begins with raising one hand or one leg. Neutral spine is maintained with normal breathing. The goal is to raise the arm or leg to the horizontal. An alternate beginner bird dog exercise (see Figure 4-113A) begins in standing, leaning against a counter top, and spine braced in neutral. Motion begins with raising one arm or one leg. Neutral spine is maintained with normal breathing. The intermediate (see Figure 4-113B) progression involves raising the opposite arm and leg at the same time to the horizontal. McGill[499] provides extensive details related to these general guidelines that will assist the clinician in providing the most appropriate exercise programs for persons with LBP and is a recommended reference for further study.

Direction-Specific Exercise Low Back Pain Classification or Low Back Pain With Lower Extremity-Related (Referred) Pain and Matched Intervention

As discussed in Chapter 3 and in the lumbar spine examination section in this chapter, a symptomatic response to repeated end-range movements is a reasonable method to classify patients who preferentially respond to exercises in a specific direction.[390] The associated ICF category corresponds to LBP with lower extremity-related (referred) pain. Three DSE subgroups may be identified using centralization as the primary examination finding: an extension subgroup, flexion subgroup, or lateral shift subgroup.[274,390,401,402] The subgroup is identified by the direction of movement that results in centralization. If a repeated movement decreases, abolishes, or centralizes symptoms or a DP is obtained, further examination may not be required since a treatment threshold is reached. The matched intervention for a DSE subgroup is the use of repeated or sustained end-range movements such as flexion, extension, or lateral shift (ie, side-glide) in the direction that causes centralization during the examination. If peripheralization or partial centralization occurs in weightbearing, assessment continues in unloaded positions such as RFIL or REIL in an attempt to obtain maximum centralization. Based on a centralization response to repeated movements in unloaded positions, matched intervention begins in unloaded positions such as RFIL or REIL. If no centralization or peripheralization occurs and the response is limited mobility with end-range pain that is no worse or no better, a classification of LBP with mobility deficits is considered. With additional examination (ie, segmental mobility tests) to confirm the classification, a matched intervention includes an MT and exercise approach to improve mobility in the direction of the motion limitation or movement dysfunction. A response of status quo to all repeated movements is a factor against a DSE classification. When a patient is classified as DSE and all attempts to obtain centralization fail initially, mechanical traction may be considered.

Evidence for Direction-Specific Exercise Classification

An RCT examined the short-term effects of adding a repeated movement approach[390,401,402] to primary care of advice, assurance, and acetaminophen for patients with acute LBP.[680] The addition of the mechanical diagnosis and therapy[390,401,402] or repeated movements method added to first-line care of patients with acute LBP produced statistically, but not clinically, significant reductions in pain and no additional effects on GPE, disability, or function. The repeated movements approach reduced health utilization but did not reduce the risk of persistent symptoms. Meta-analysis concludes that a repeated movement approach[390,401,402] is more effective than educational booklets, ice packs, massage, and advice to stay active for acute LBP.[681] However, the small effect size is not considered clinically worthwhile. The authors suggested classifying patients with LBP before assigning them to treatment.

Cook et al[682] performed a systematic literature review rating only articles with homogeneous samples of LBP using the patient response method and physical therapist-directed exercises. The patient response method as described by Cook et al[682] assessed the patient's response to single or repeated movements or positions. Both the TBC method[410] and the mechanical diagnosis and therapy method[390,401,402] are considered patient response methods. Intervention techniques are similar to the assessment methods or based on the movements that reproduce the patient's primary complaint. Only 5 trials were included in the review, 4 of which included components of the response to repeated movements and centralization as assessment. The authors concluded that a PT-directed exercise program using the patient's response was significantly better than control or comparison groups. Only one of the articles showed that classification exercise was less effective than manipulation.[683] The authors cautiously stated that patient response methods may lead to improved outcomes.[682]

Miller et al[684] randomized 30 subjects with CLBP of more than 7 weeks to compare the effectiveness of a repeated movement approach versus an SSE approach. Both management approaches were effective for pain levels and function with no significant difference noted between the groups. Peterson et al[685] compared the effectiveness of a repeated movement approach versus an intensive strength training program over 8 weeks with a maximum of 15 sessions. Both approaches were deemed equally effective at 2 and 8 months in a group of subjects with CLBP of at least 8 weeks' duration. Lack of a treatment effect between groups is possibly due to an incorrect assumption that subjects with CLBP are a homogenous group.[685]

Long et al[411] compared the response of 230 patients with acute, subacute, or CLBP, or LBP and related lower extremity pain who were classified into subgroups with an established DP. The subjects were randomized to 3 subgroups: exercises matching the DP, exercises opposite to the DP, or a nondirectional exercise group for 3 to 6 sessions over 2 weeks. Significantly greater improvements occurred in matched subjects compared to the other 2 groups, including a 3-fold decrease in medication use.[411] From within this population and similar to previous studies, the most common DP was extension (83%) with flexion (7%) and lateral shift (10%).[411] In a retrospective analysis of Long et al,[411] subjects who received matched treatment had a 7.8 times greater likelihood of a good outcome defined by at least 30% improvement in the RMDQ.[686] Matching subjects to their DP is a stronger predictor of outcome than other biopsychosocial factors. Outcome and lower leg pain scores were negatively correlated, meaning patients with higher scores of lower leg pain had a poorer outcome.[686] Subjects who had a DP, but received unmatched exercises were negatively associated with a good outcome meaning an incorrect exercise prescription may be detrimental to the outcome.[411]

In a sample of 48 subjects with LBP who centralized with repeated extension, subjects were randomly assigned to an extension-oriented treatment approach (EOTA) or a strengthening exercise program over 8 sessions with 1-, 4-, and 24-week follow-up.[549] The EOTA group received a progression of extension exercises from static in prone to end-range repeated movements in standing and CPA PAIVM lumbar mobilization. The strengthening group followed the Hicks et al[197] program. The EOTA group had significantly greater improvement in disability at all follow-ups, but only greater change in pain at 1 week.[549] Research is somewhat limited but is evolving to support a classification that suggests some patients respond best to repeated movements in a specific direction.

Gillan et al[687] examined 40 patients with a lateral shift randomized to receive repeated lateral shift exercises compared to massage and nonspecific advice. The repeated end-range movement group had quick resolution of the shift, but no differences in disability were noted between groups. In a non-RCT, Harrison et al[688] compared a novel method of mechanical traction and mirror image shift correction exercises with a self-management group over 12 weeks of care and an average of 36 visits. Fifty percent of the treatment group had statistically significant changes of 50% in all radiographic measurements of the shift and a decrease in pain from 3.0 to 0.8 on a 10-point scale. No significant changes were noted in the self-treatment group. Laslett[399] presented a case report on the successful treatment of a patient with acute LBP and a right lateral shift deformity using manual and self-correction procedures followed by a core endurance training program based on the principles of McGill.[499]

Extension Subgroup of the Direction-Specific Exercise Low Back Pain Classification and Matched Intervention

This discussion represents a brief overview of the clinical picture of the 3 subgroups (ie, extension, flexion, and lateral shift) and intervention strategies based on the response to repeated movements. For extensive details related to the management of persons with LBP using repeated movements, additional resources are recommended.[401,402]

The extension subgroup of the DSE LBP classification presents in persons with acute, subacute, or CLBP with or without varying degrees of related lower extremity pain and with or without signs and symptoms of nerve root compression. The onset is often related to flexion movements and flexion activities such as sitting or bending that produce or worsen symptoms, and extension activities such as standing or walking decrease or abolish symptoms. Reversal of the lumbar curve after prolonged sitting or bending is challenging and provocative. Exam findings include a slumped sitting posture, reduced lordosis, pain, and extension AROM deficit greater than flexion. Repeated flexion produces, worsens, or peripheralizes symptoms, and PAIVM are hypomobile and painful. SLR may or may not be positive. Repeated extension abolishes, reduces, or centralizes symptoms and increases extension ROM. Therefore, the specific exercise prescription is repeated extension. The home exercise program includes maintenance of the lumbar lordosis via temporary avoidance of flexion activities, posture correction, and the appropriate level of extension exercise repeated 10 times every 2 to 3 hours.[401,402]

Matched intervention strategies are based on examination findings and the specific movements or positions, loaded or unloaded, that cause symptoms to abolish, reduce, or centralize. Based on the patient's response to repeated extension movements, the following is a list of extension exercises that may be prescribed, progressing from unloaded to positions:

- Prone on 1 or 2 pillows (see Figure 4-86A)
- Prone lying without pillows (see Figure 4-86B)
- Prone lying on elbows (see Figure 4-86C)
- Prone press-up or REIL (see Figure 4-86D)
- Prone press up with exhalation at the end of extension
- REIL with belt fixation (see Figure 4-86F)
- REIL with therapist OP (see Figure 4-86E)
- Extension mobilization (ie, CPA PAIVM; see Figure 4-89A)
- REIS (see Figure 4-35)[401,402]

Not all patients start at the lowest level. All patients do not progress through each level. The starting point is determined by the clinician. The progression is determined by patient response. In the presence of unilateral symptoms that worsen, temporarily centralize, or do not change with sagittal plane extension movements, a trial of extension in lying with hips off center (see Figure 4-86H) is recommended. The hips are usually shifted away from the painful side (see Figure 4-86G).[401,402]

If the response to repeated extension is limited mobility with end-range pain that is increased but no worse with no centralization or peripheralization, the clinician considers the manipulation or mobilization classification or the ICF category of LBP with mobility deficits. Further examination is warranted to assign a diagnostic classification.

Flexion Subgroup of the Direction-Specific Exercise Low Back Pain Classification and Matched Intervention

A flexion subgroup is much less common than an extension subgroup. The clinical presentation is not well defined. Patients generally prefer flexion activities such as sitting to extension activities such as standing and walking. Flexion AROM may be limited with extension AROM full range. PAIVM may be provocative. SLR may or may not be positive. Repeated extension produces, worsens or peripheralizes symptoms, and repeated flexion abolishes, reduces, or centralizes symptoms and may increase flexion ROM. Therefore, the specific exercise prescription is repeated flexion performed 10 times every 2 to 3 hours.[401,402] Commonly prescribed flexion exercises are RFIS (see Figure 4-34), RFIL (see Figure 4-40B), and repeated flexion in sitting (Figure 4-114).[401,402]

If the response to repeated flexion is limited mobility with end-range pain that is increased but no worse with no centralization or peripheralization, the clinician considers the manipulation or mobilization classification or the ICF category of LBP with mobility deficit. Further examination is warranted to assign a diagnostic classification.

Patients with symptomatic LSS who are over age 65 and have radiographic imaging evidence of stenosis may benefit from flexion exercise as part of an overall management strategy. Signs and symptoms of nerve root compression and neurogenic claudication may be present. Patients with symptomatic LSS may also benefit from impairment-based management, which may include mobilization or manipulation for the lumbar spine and hip, lower extremity strengthening, neural mobilizations, and a walking program with BWST ambulation. Management strategies for patients with symptomatic LSS are discussed later under the DSE classification.

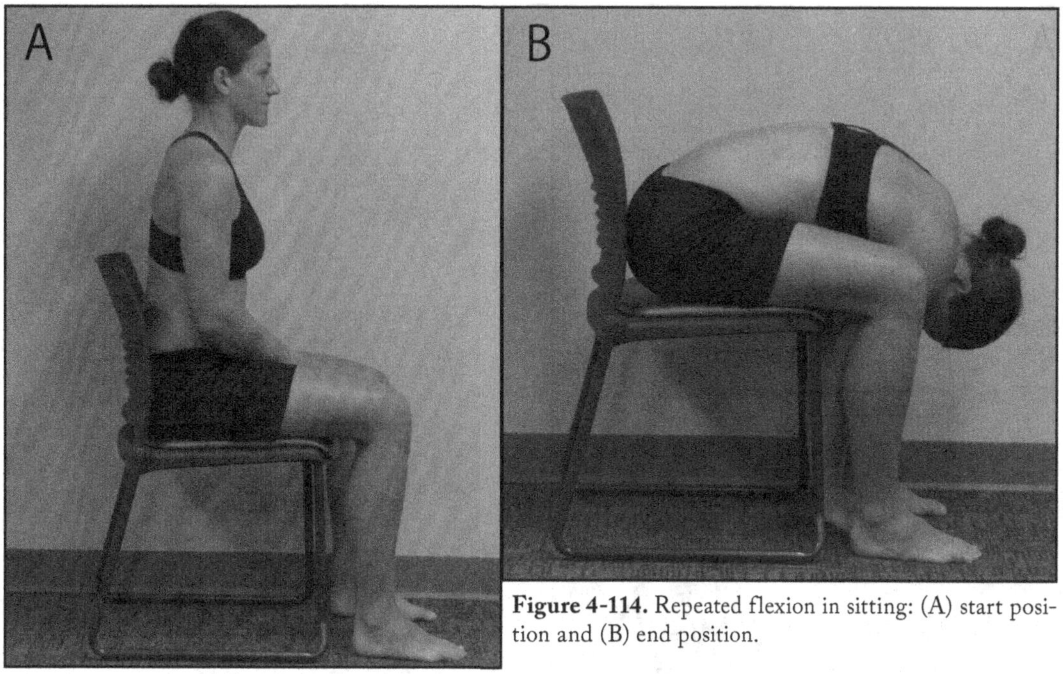

Figure 4-114. Repeated flexion in sitting: (A) start position and (B) end position.

Lateral Shift Subgroup of the Direction-Specific Exercise Low Back Pain Classification and Matched Intervention

Key findings for the lateral shift subgroup include unilateral or asymmetrical symptoms, a sudden or recent postural change, flexion and extension activities aggravate, standing and walking aggravate, and side-lying may be an easing position. Signs and symptoms of nerve root compression may be present. Exam findings include a visible lateral shift or frontal plane deviation of the shoulders relative to the pelvis, reduced lumbar lordosis, asymmetrical LF AROM, reduced LF in the direction opposite the lateral shift, and painful and restricted extension AROM. PAIVM may be hypomobile and provocative. SLR may or may not be positive. Symptoms centralize or get better with lateral movements such as manual lateral shift correction or self-lateral shift correction in loaded (standing) or unloaded (prone) positions. Symptoms peripheralize with attempts at sagittal plane movements without shift correction. A right lateral shift is visualized by a shift to the right of the trunk and shoulders. A contralateral shift means the shift is away from the side of the patient's symptoms. An ipsilateral shift means the shift is toward the side of the patient's symptoms.[401,402]

A lateral shift correction or side glide procedure involves moving the hips away from the pain. The clinician should have the patient attempt self-correction of a lateral shift in standing (see Figures 4-36A and 4-36B) or against the wall first (Figure 4-115). If unsuccessful, a manual shift correction in standing (see Figure 4-27) is tried. If the procedures in standing are successful and centralization occurs, the patient is instructed in self-correction in prone with REIL, hips off center as needed (see Figure 4-86H), as well as procedures in standing (see Figure 4-115). The exact progression depends on the patient's response. In prone, the hips may be shifted off center by the patient (see Figure 4-86G) before beginning extension in lying or assisted manually by the therapist to maintain the hips offset position (Figure 4-116). Figure 4-86H shows the self-correction of a lateral shift or side glide and extension in lying with hips off center. A manual shift correction was previously described in the examination section and demonstrated in Figure 4-27. The same principles apply to self-correction. The home exercise program includes self-correction of the lateral shift and REIL with hips off center repeated 10 to 15 times every 2 to 3 hours, maintenance of lordosis if attained, and postural correction.[401,402] Patients in this classification who fail to centralize are assessed for the mechanical traction classification.

For all persons in the DSE classification, overall management focuses on self-treatment through education of posture, activities, and movement that centralize symptoms. In the early stages, movements that cause peripheralization should be avoided. Often, prescribed exercise may cause an increase in LBP as the leg pain improves or goes away (a common response). The exercises should be continued and discontinued only if peripheralization occurs. When a patient is asymptomatic for a period of several days, recovery of function begins. The patient begins exercise in the direction that has been avoided or that has produced peripheralization.[401,402] For example, in the extension subgroup category, RFIL exercises at the rate of 5 to 6 reps 5 to 6 times per day are initiated, followed by

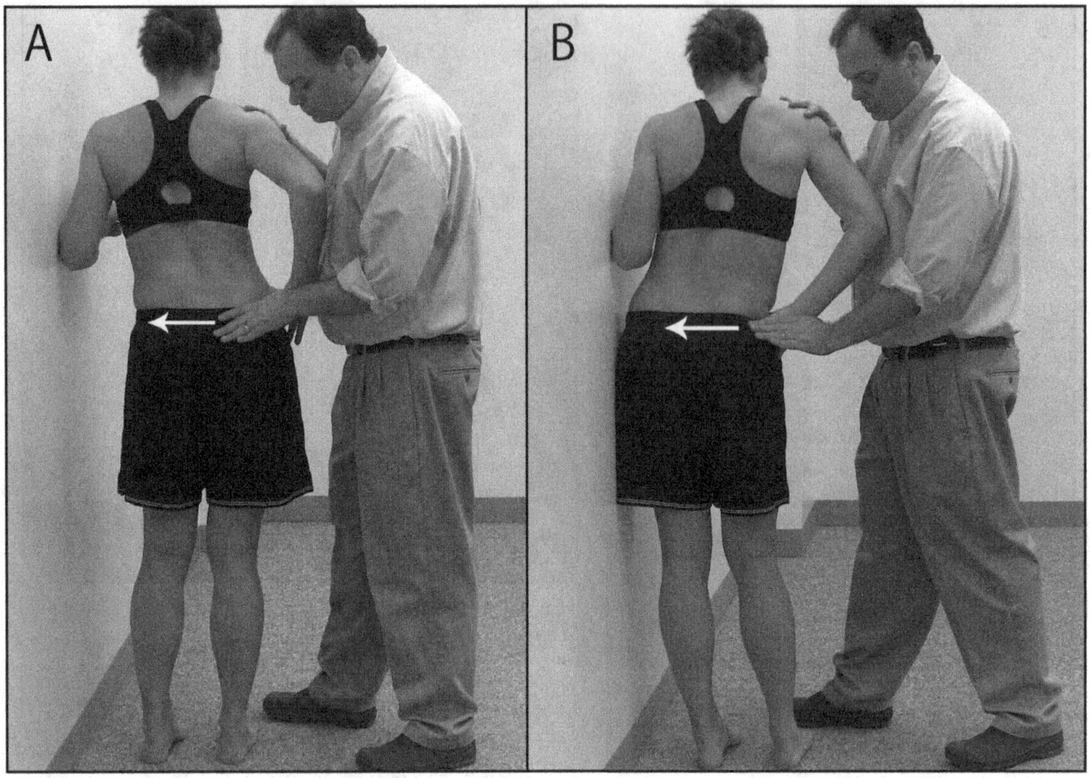

Figure 4-115. Self-correction of left lateral shift[409,410]: (A) start position and (B) self-correction of lateral shift in standing against wall with therapist assist.

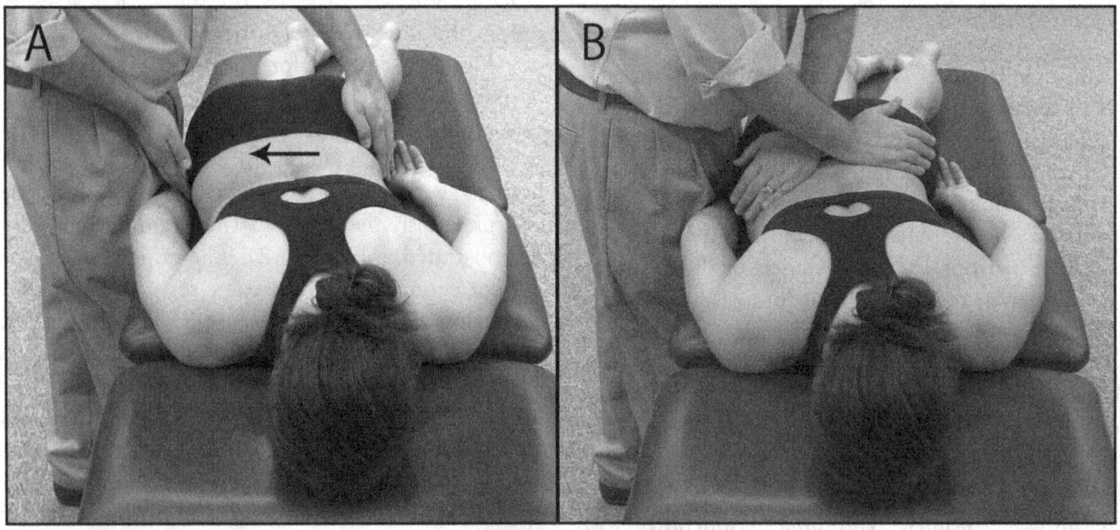

Figure 4-116. Extension in lying with hips offset[409,410]: (A) therapist assist to shift hips to the right in attempt to correct left lateral shift and (B) therapist maintains hips off center prior to extension in lying.

repeated extension over 1 to 2 days. If no return of symptoms, flexion may progress slowly to sitting and standing, always followed by repeated extension exercises. Education on the recurrent nature of LBP is important as well as what to do if symptoms return.[401,402] Reassessment through the episode of care and further examination may result in reclassification or identification of additional impairments for intervention. The majority of persons with LBP require multimodal treatment.

Impairment-Based Classification for Symptomatic Lumbar Spinal Stenosis

The clinical presentation of persons with symptomatic LSS is discussed early in this chapter under diagnostic triage and under the flexion subgroup of the DSE LBP classification. The main complaints are LBP with related lower extremity symptoms and diminished walking tolerance.

LSS is described as a relatively stable disorder in which severe disability and neurological deficits may develop over time, but not usually in a rapid manner. In fact, some persons with LSS remain the same or improve over time. Johnsson et al[689] reported on 32 individuals not considered for surgery. At 4-year follow-up, 85% were improved or had no change in symptoms while 75% increased walking tolerance or reported no change. In a retrospective analysis of 49 individuals with varied conservative treatment over 3 years, more than half improved in symptoms and walking tolerance.[690] The long-term picture is not one of expected deterioration, but it is unknown who may improve over time.[691] Rather than a wait-and-see approach, surgical or conservative management strategies are recommended for symptomatic LSS. Although a trial of conservative care is recommended prior to surgical intervention,[692] the duration and the description of conservative care are highly variable. The therapeutic effectiveness of conservative and surgical approaches needs further evaluation.

Two trials evaluated surgery versus nonsurgery for LSS with[693] or without degenerative spondylolisthesis.[694] The results in these trials are difficult to interpret because nearly half of the patients did not adhere to the assigned treatment group. Based on intention-to-treat analysis, physical function as measured by Short Form-36 (SF-36) and ODI were not significantly different at 2 years, but pain as measured by SF-36 significantly favored surgery. In the as-treated analysis, surgery was moderately superior (ie, 16 to 18 points on ODI) to nonsurgical therapy on the ODI and SF-36 pain and functional scores at 2 years for LSS with degenerative spondylolisthesis,[693] and slightly to moderately superior (8 to 12 points on ODI) to nonsurgical therapy for LSS without degenerative spondylolisthesis.[694] In both trials, mean ODI and SF-36 improvements from baseline in patients who did not have surgery were 10 points. Both groups improved, and the nonsurgery groups received usual care of active PT, home exercise, counseling or education, and NSAIDs as tolerated.

In another study, Weinstein et al[695] presented the 4-year outcomes for LSS without spondylolisthesis. The as-treated analysis showed that the clinically significant advantages for surgery reported at 2 years were maintained through 4 years. Both groups were stable between 2 and 4 years. Results of a higher quality study of surgery versus nonsurgery for LSS reported benefits favoring surgery were statistically significant through 4 years, but lessened or were not present after 8 to 10 years.[696] A similar study at 6-year follow-up reported a mean ODI difference of 9.5 (0.9 to 18.1). Intensity of leg or back pain did not differ at the time. Walking ability did not differ between the groups at any time.[697]

Relative to improved outcomes from surgery, guidelines of the North American Spine Society (NASS)[691] concluded that in severe LSS, surgery is effective 80% of the time; in moderate to severe LSS, surgery is more effective than medical intervention treatment; in mild to moderate LSS, medical intervention treatment is effective about 70% of the time; and placement of a small spacer device without surgical fusion is more effective than medical interventional treatment. The long-term results of surgical management are good to excellent in 50% to 79% of patients. Patients and physicians appear to prefer a surgical approach. The outcome of surgery depends on several factors. Strong predictors of unsuccessful outcome include lower self-rated preoperative health status, comorbidity, depression, and limited presurgical walking ability.[698]

NASS guidelines[691] suggest that a single radiographically guided, transforaminal, ESI has short-term benefits of 2 to 3 weeks for radiculopathy, but long-term effectiveness is inconclusive. Multiple injections can produce long-term relief through transforaminal or caudal ESI for LSS or radiculopathy. Koc et al[699] compared inpatient PT of ultrasound, moist heat, transcutaneous electrical nerve stimulation (TENS) for 2 weeks, ESI, and a control group. All groups received diclofenac and a stretching and strengthening program for the trunk and lower extremities. Both PT and ESI groups demonstrated significant improvements in pain and function, with no differences between groups at 2 weeks and 1, 3, and 6 months. The control group also noted significant improvements from baseline.[699]

In a comparative study of two 6-week PT programs, Whitman et al[457] included patients with pain in the lumbopelvic region and lower extremities, 50 years of age or older, MRI findings consistent with LSS, and reports of sitting as a better position for symptom severity than standing or walking. One group—manual physical therapy exercise and walking group (MPTE × WG)—received impairment-based PT of MT, exercise, and BWST walking including mobilization/manipulation to the thoracic, lumbopelvic, and lower extremity regions; home exercise program; lower extremity stretching and strengthening; and lumbar stabilization exercises.[457,700] MT and exercise interventions were performed at the discretion of the therapist based on examination findings. The overall impairment-based program was prescribed individually to restore upright posture, increase thoracic and lumbar extension, increase hip extension, and strengthen the lower extremities. Also, included were intentional walking, core stabilization exercises, and a home exercise to augment the in-clinic program. Selected manual procedures targeting the spine were lumbar side-lying rotational mobilization/manipulation (see Figure 4-99), CPA or UPA lumbar mobilization (see Figures 4-103 and 4-104), and thoracic mobilization or manipulation (Figure 4-117A) described in Chapter 5. Additional manual techniques included hip mobilization, inferior glide (see Figure 4-62) and anterior glide (see Figure 4-65), MET for hip flexor (Figure 4-117B) and rectus femoris (Figure 4-117C) lengthening, and knee mobilization augmented with quadriceps activation (see Figure 4-59) and ankle DF mobilization. To augment the

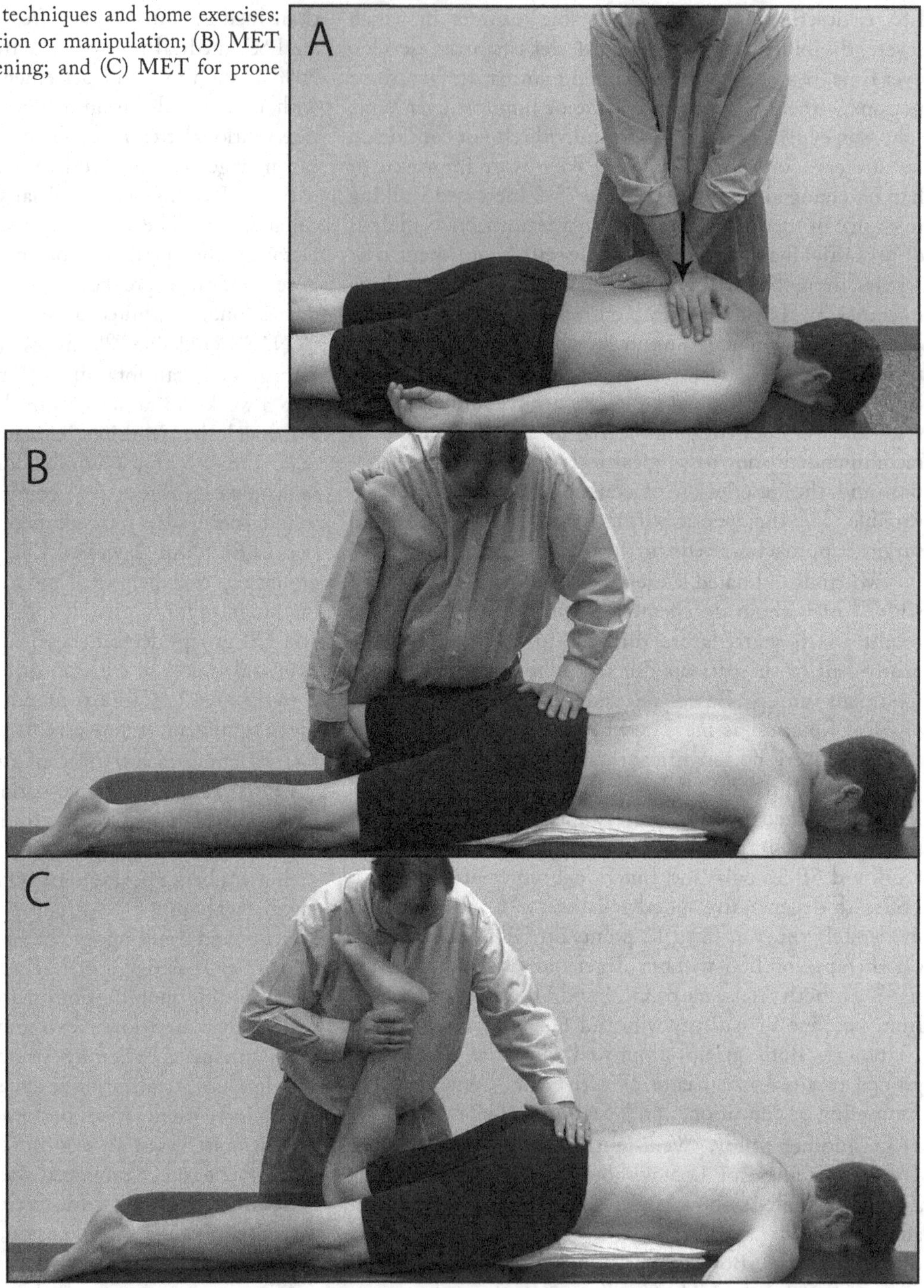

Figure 4-117. Selected MT techniques and home exercises: (A) prone thoracic mobilization or manipulation; (B) MET for prone hip flexor lengthening; and (C) MET for prone rectus femoris lengthening.

MT, home exercises included hip flexor stretch in supine or standing, quadriceps activation, knee flexion mobilization, and ankle DF stretch. BWST walking (Figure 4-118) used the minimum amount of unloading needed to minimize or alleviate the patient's symptoms and allow walking as comfortably as possible. As tolerated, the overall goal was to gradually increase walking pace and distance while decreasing the amount of BW support.[457] The other group—lumbar flexion exercise and walking group (FE × WG)—received lumbar flexion exercise of single and double knee to chest exercise, a treadmill walking program, and 10 minutes of subtherapeutic ultrasound. Both groups had clinically meaningful outcomes. A greater proportion of patients in the MPTE × WG (79%) reported recovery at 6 weeks compared to the FE × WG (41%). At 1 year, 62% of the MPTE × WG and 41% of the FE × WG still reported recovery. All of the secondary outcomes, NPRS, modified ODQ, walking tolerance test, and satisfaction favored the MPTE × WG group at 6 weeks and 1 year. About 3 patients need to be treated (NNT = 2.6) with the MPTE × WG program to prevent 1 patient from not achieving perceived recovery at 6 weeks.[457]

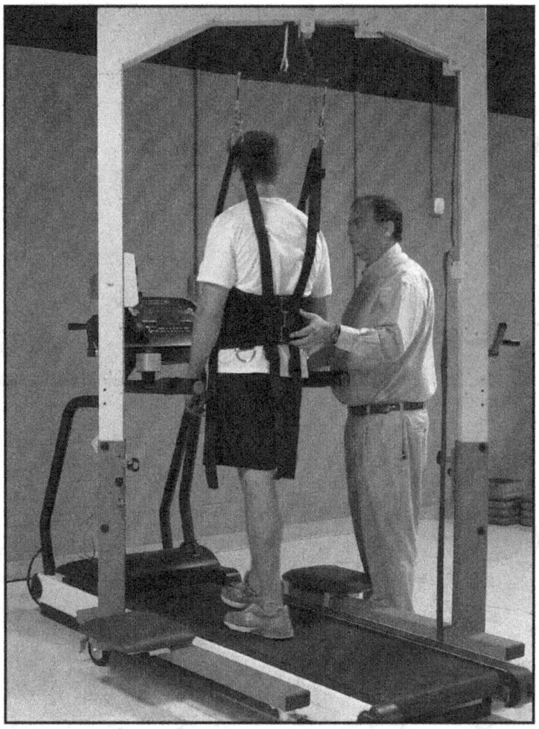

Figure 4-118. BWST walking using the Biodex Unweighing System (Biodex Medical Systems, Inc).

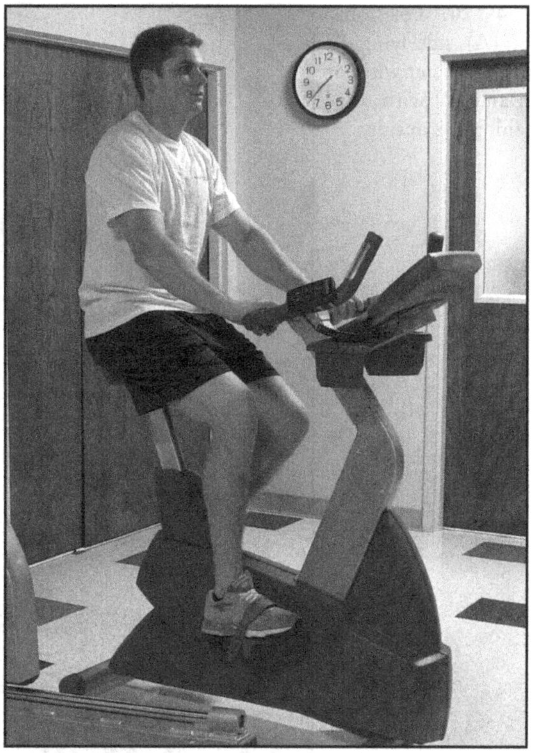

Figure 4-119. Upright stationary cycling.

Pua et al[701] investigated the effectiveness of 12 sessions in 6 weeks of a BWST program compared to upright cycling (Figure 4-119) in subjects with LSS. The BWST group walked at a comfortable pace with a pain-free gait (30% to 40% of BW) for the first 2 weeks. Treadmill was performed to tolerance or maximum of 30 minutes from weeks 3 to 6. The upright cycle group began at 50 to 60 rpm in a flexed posture and a comfortable pace and progressed to moderate intensity for a maximum of 30 minutes or to tolerance. Both groups also received 20 minutes of shortwave diathermy, intermittent lumbar traction (15 minutes in supine with hips and knees flexed to 90 degrees supported on a stool, 30 seconds:10 seconds [on:off cycle], 30 to 40% BW:on/10% BW:off) and 3 flexion neurodynamic mobilization exercises performed daily. Both groups improved, but no difference was observed between groups. Limitations of this study were the absence of a control group and short-term follow-up.[701]

A systematic review concluded that there is insufficient high-quality evidence regarding the effectiveness of MT for patients with LSS.[702] Further research is needed, but patients with LSS can benefit from PT interventions. Backstrom et al[703] recommended patient education, MT, mobility and strengthening exercises, and aerobic training (ie, BWST, inclined treadmill, cycling, or aquatic therapy) as the standard of conservative care. Table 4-5 describes guidelines and selected exercises for consideration in the management of persons with symptomatic LSS.[457,700,704] In most comparative studies and systematic reviews, the nonsurgical approach is poorly described. A "usual care" comparison to surgical intervention does not assist the physical therapist in the management of patients with symptomatic LSS. Insufficient data exist on when to recommend surgery or nonsurgical care and who is most likely to respond to PT intervention. Key findings and potential intervention strategies for the DSE LBP classification subgroups and associated ICF category of LBP with lower extremity-related pain are summarized in Table 4-3.

Traction Low Back Pain Diagnostic Classification or Low Back Pain With Lower Extremity Radiating or Related Pain and Matched Intervention

Traction is commonly used as an intervention for patients with LBP and related lower extremity pain or lumbar radiculopathy, but its effectiveness is unclear.[705-708] Contraindications and precautions for lumbar traction include any condition for which movement is contraindicated, acute strains or sprains, inflammatory processes, hypermobility or instability, rheumatoid arthritis, respiratory problems, cancer, metastases, osteoporosis, infection, current pregnancy, uncontrolled hypertension, aortic aneurysm, severe hemorrhoids, abdominal hernia, and hiatal hernia.[511,709] Traction is classified as positional (Figure 4-120), manual (Figure 4-121), or mechanical (Figures 4-122 and 4-123) and may be performed in a sustained or intermittent manner, most commonly in supine or

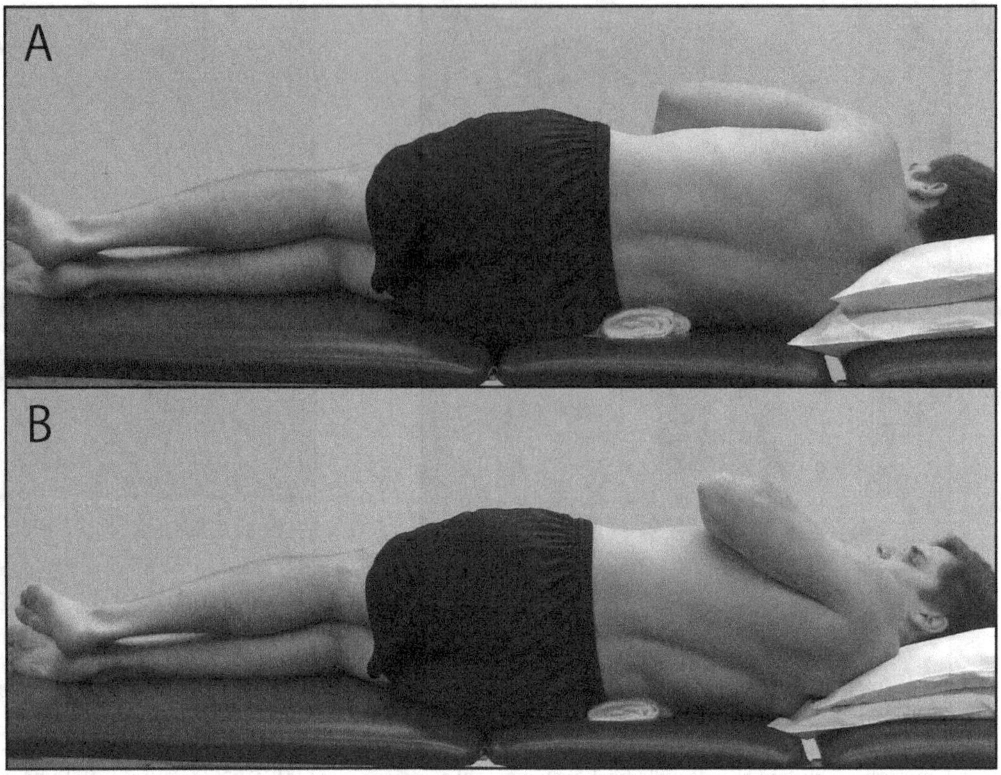

Figure 4-120. Positional traction: (A) side-lying in flexion with bolster without rotation and (B) with rotation opening the upside.

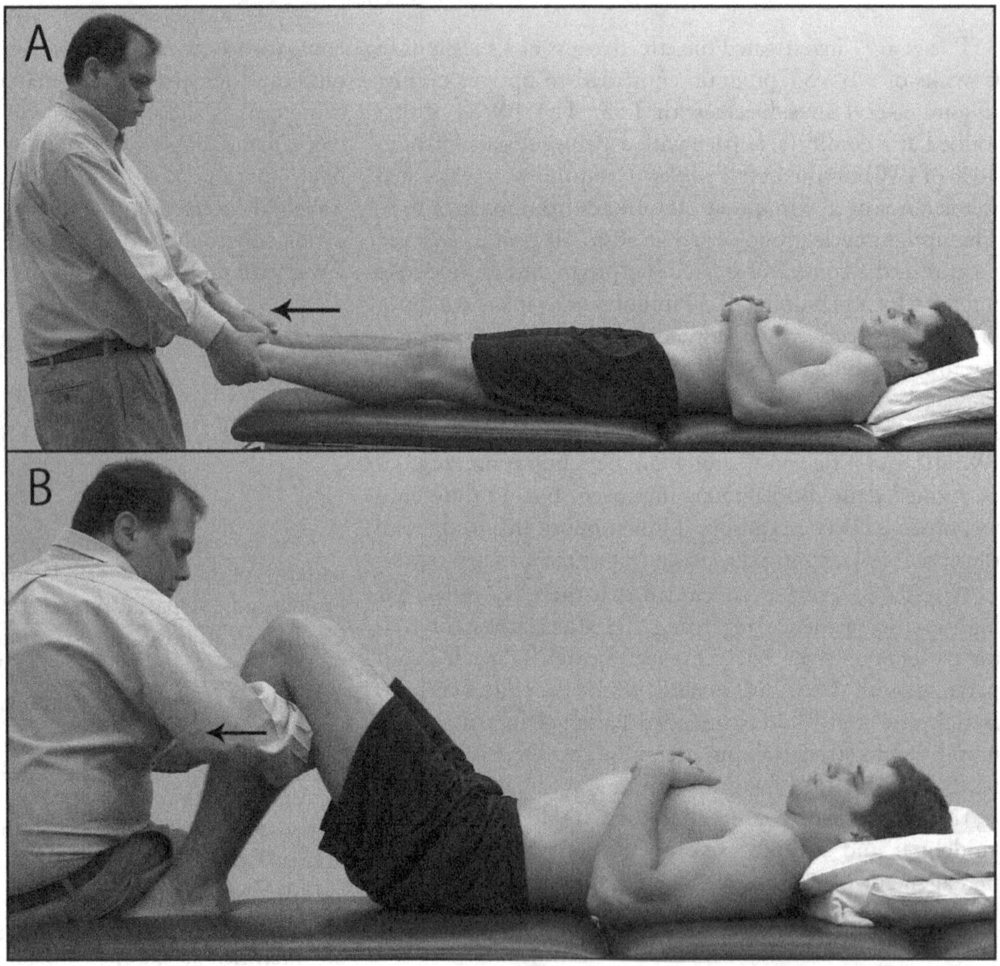

Figure 4-121. Manual traction: (A) in supine bilaterally or unilaterally through the legs and (B) in hook-lying bilaterally.

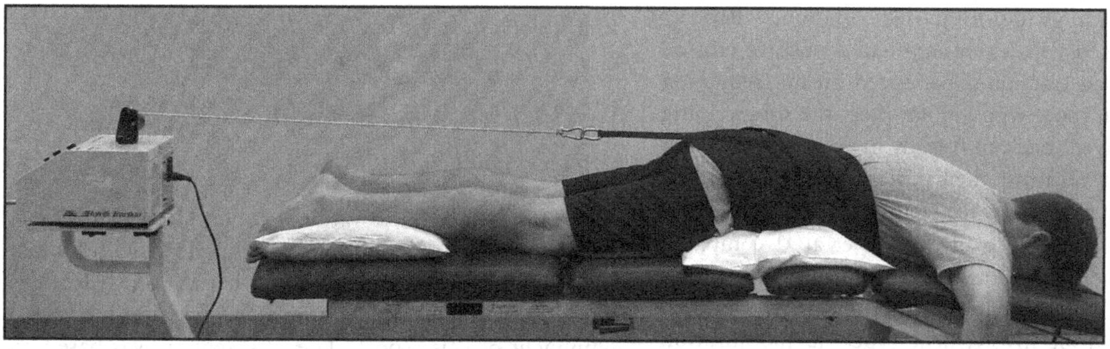

Figure 4-122. Prone mechanical traction.

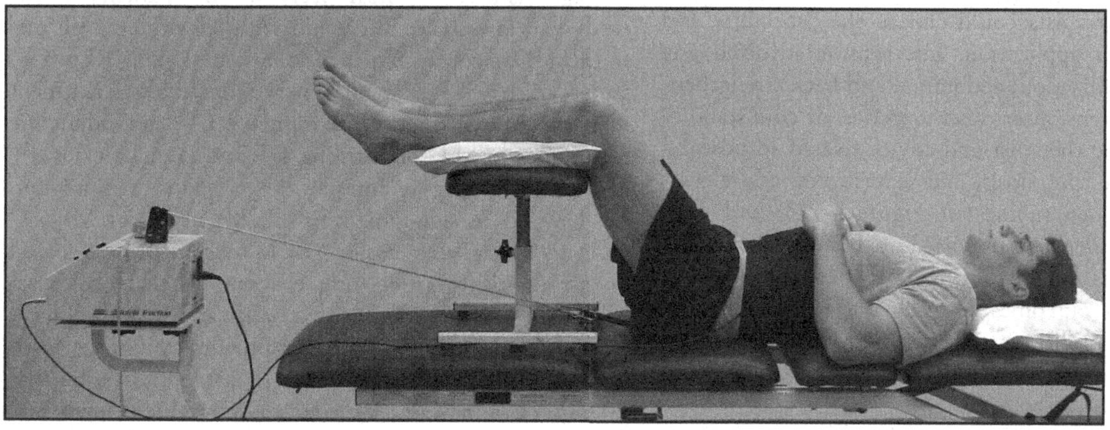

Figure 4-123. Supine mechanical traction.

prone. Optimal dosage, position, and type of traction are unknown and largely based on clinical opinion. Additional resources are available for discussion of mechanical and physiological effects and prescription parameters.[710,711] Manual traction may be tried to determine the response before application of mechanical traction. Traction is commonly used for patients with LBP and nerve root compression or radiculopathy or for patients with LBP and related lower extremity pain who fail to centralize with repeated or sustained end-range movements. A goal of traction is centralization with progression to another classification and matched or impairment-based intervention. If signs and symptoms of radiculopathy worsen, referral for medical intervention is warranted.

Evidence for Traction Diagnostic Classification

Intermittent or continuous traction as a single treatment for LBP cannot be recommended for mixed groups of patients with or without sciatica.[707] When applied across all LBP patients, mechanical lumbar traction is no more effective than no treatment, sham, or placebo. For persons with LBP and sciatica, results are inconsistent.[707] Little evidence is available to support the use of mechanical lumbar traction or to assist the clinician in determining who is most likely to benefit from traction intervention.

Preliminary research has identified a subgroup of patients with LBP who might benefit from traction. In an RCT over 6 weeks, Fritz et al[712] examined subjects from 18 to 60 years with symptoms distal to the buttock in the past 24 hours; Oswestry scores of >30%; reflex, sensory, or muscle strength deficit; and positive SLR at less than 45 degrees. Patients were randomized to 2 groups: an EOTA group and a traction plus EOTA group. The EOTA group received sustained and repeated end-range extension exercise of 3 sets of 10 every 4 to 5 hours, CPA PAIVM mobilization of Grade 3 or 4, 10 to 20 oscillations, maintenance of lordosis education, and avoidance of activities that cause peripheralization. Intervention was initiated and progressed at the clinician's discretion for 2 times per week for weeks 1 to 3, and 1 time per week for weeks 4 to 6. The traction plus EOTA group received the same EOTA intervention with the addition of prone mechanical traction during the first 2 weeks. Mechanical traction was provided using a 3-dimensional, adjustable table to maximize centralization before beginning the exercise. Traction was applied statically for 12 minutes with a 1-minute ramp up and 1-minute ramp down at 40% to 60% BW. After the traction, subjects remained prone for 2 minutes and then performed a set of prone press-up extension exercises. A maximum of 4 traction sessions for weeks 1 and 2 were allowed, followed by only EOTA intervention 1 time per week for weeks 3 to 6. The study found greater reductions in disability and fear-avoidance beliefs for the traction plus EOTA group at 2 weeks, but no difference between groups at 6 weeks. The authors reported on additional examination findings defining this subgroup. Patients who peripheralized with extension, had a positive crossed SLR, and received traction experienced greater reduction in disability than those who did not meet the subgrouping criteria and received traction. A study in progress may assist in validating or refuting these criteria for subgrouping patients as likely responders to traction.[713]

In a similar feasibility study, Harte et al[714] compared the differences between 2 treatment protocols—MT, exercise, and advice with or without traction in persons with LBP and nerve root involvement. Specific mobilization or manipulation procedures were defined by 2 approaches,[715,716] but therapists could choose the procedure and spinal region for application. Intervention involved any appropriate mobilization, abdominal and back strengthening exercises, extension or other exercises, or core stability prescribed by the therapist and advice related to posture, remaining active, prognosis, and recurrences. Static traction was performed supine (see Figure 4-123) with hips and knees at 90 degrees supported on a stool, 5 to 60 kg, 10 to 20 minutes for 2 to 3 times per week. Both groups improved in all outcomes at discharge, 3 months, and 6 months with no difference between groups. Differences between groups at baseline and a natural progression could partially account for the results.[714]

Gagne and Hasson[717] presented a case report on a patient with a medical diagnosis of a lumbar herniated disc at L5-S1 with compression of the L5 nerve root confirmed by MRI. The first 5 sessions of intervention consisted of repeated lumbar extension exercises based on the centralization phenomenon. At the end of the first 2 weeks, clinically significant outcomes were not achieved; therefore, static, supine traction for 20 minutes at 38.4 to 40.9 kg (85 to 90 lbs) was added to the extension exercise prescription for the next 3 weeks for a total of 9 sessions. At discharge, patient goals had been met and clinically meaningful changes in pain and function were observed.[717]

Current evidence suggests that traction should not be widely used for persons with nonspecific LBP without related lower extremity pain, but in patients with LBP with radiating or related lower extremity pain, inability to centralize with repeated end-range loading techniques and the presence of nerve root involvement may prove to be key factors in defining a subgroup likely to respond favorably to mechanical lumbar traction. No consensus is available for optimal traction treatment parameters for position, duration, type, or force. The LBP traction classification is summarized in Table 4-4. If patients are not appropriate for the LBP traction classification and matched intervention and are considering the limited evidence to support a traction intervention for this LBP subgroup, nonsurgical approaches for persons with the ICF category of LBP with lower extremity-related pain with or without nerve root involvement show promise as effective treatment strategies and are discussed next.

Manual Therapy and Exercise Evidence for Conservative Management of Radiculopathy Without Traction

In a prospective observational cohort study, Murphy et al[718] reported on the outcomes of 49 patients with lumbar radiculopathy secondary to disk herniation (LRSDH) treated with a nonsurgical approach. Traction was not a component of this report. The intervention was based on a diagnosis-based clinical decision rule. Patients in the study had lower extremity pain with or without LBP due to LRSHD, a confirmatory disk herniation on MRI or CT, and a positive SLR or femoral nerve stretch test. Treatment focused on a distraction manipulation,[719] neurodynamic techniques in SLR performing DF and plantarflexion,[424] end-range loading techniques,[401,402] joint manipulation (ie, HVLA) in side-lying painful side up,[720] or MET[721] and myofascial techniques.[722] Management was based on an algorithm combining elements of the TBC classification, impairment-based classification, and clinical reasoning. If centralization was present, end-range loading techniques were used first. If no centralization was present, examination proceeded to determine if segmental joint signs, neurodynamic signs, or muscle signs were present. Manipulation was implemented for segmental signs, neurodynamic techniques for neurodynamic signs, and myofascial therapy of trigger point and muscle lengthening for muscle signs. Perpetuating factors such as altered motor control, fear, or catastrophizing behaviors were treated with stabilization exercise, graded exposure, and education to focus on function rather than pain. With a favorable prognosis for most patients, exercise was provided early with advice to remain active. Treatment was managed on an individual basis initially for 2 to 3 times per week for 3 weeks and then 1 to 2 times per week as needed. Mean duration of symptoms was 60.5 weeks over a mean 13.2 sessions. Postdischarge improvement was described as good or excellent by 90% of patients. Clinically meaningful improvements in pain and disability were seen in 79% and 70% of patients, respectively. Average long-term follow-up of 14.5 months noted good or excellent improvement by 80% of patients.[718] The observational design prohibits conclusions related to efficacy, but the examination and clinical reasoning process are similar to the TBC approach and impairment-based management.

Treatment-Based Classification Summary

The TBC is constantly being refined based on current research. Stanton et al[723] described the prevalence and reliability of a classification algorithm,[19,274,551] previously

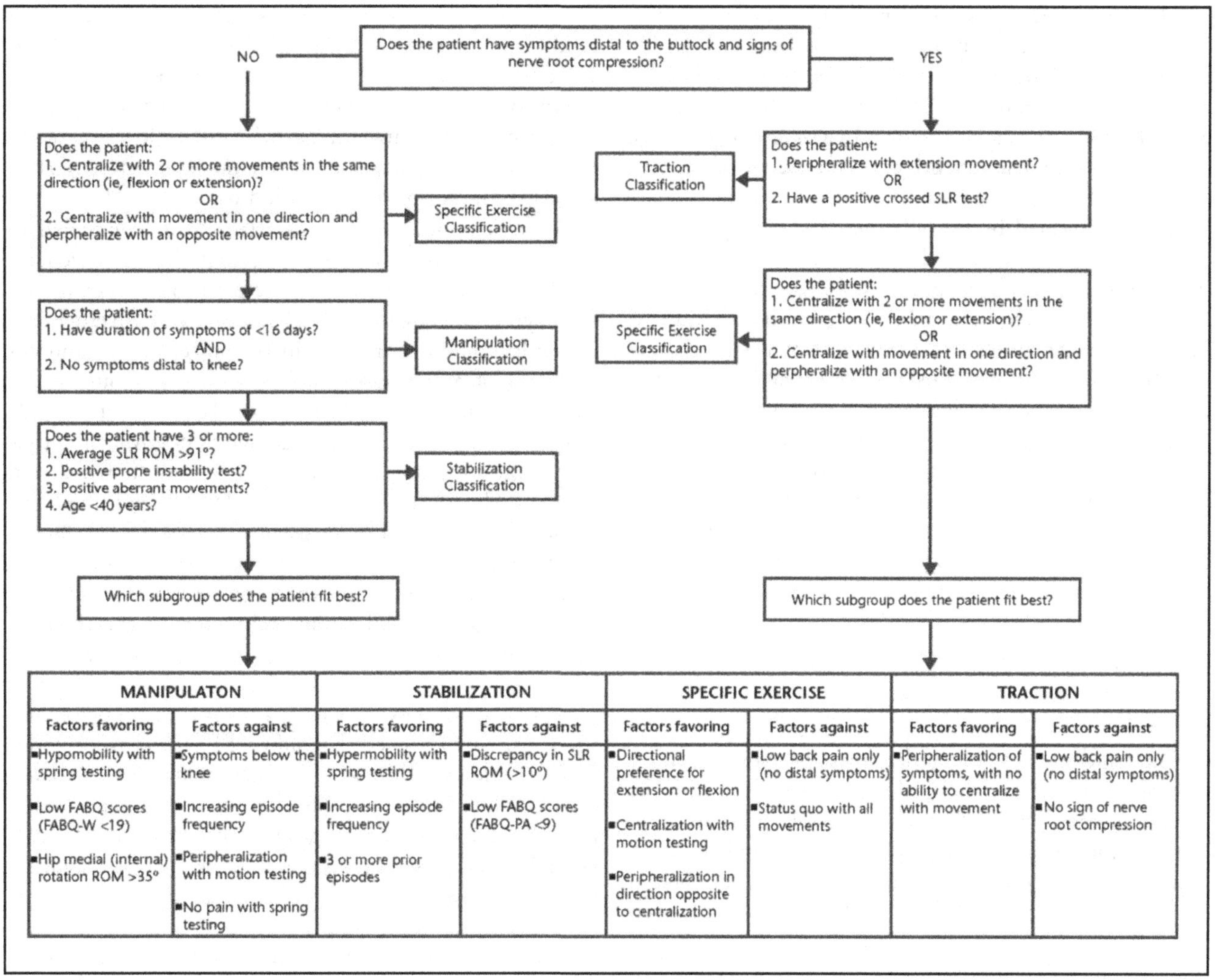

Figure 4-124. Comprehensive algorithm for LBP. (Reprinted from Stanton TR, Fritz JM, Hancock MJ, et al. Evaluation of a treatment based classification algorithm for low back pain: a cross-sectional study. *Phys Ther.* 2011;91:496-509, with permission of the American Physical Therapy Association. This material is copyrighted, and any further reproduction or distribution requires written permission from the APTA.)

known as TBC and now termed a comprehensive algorithm for LBP (Figure 4-124). The comprehensive algorithm for LBP translates the individual criteria for the 4 subgroups of manipulation, specific exercise, stabilization, and traction into a clinical reasoning strategy. A group of 250 patients with acute or subacute LBP with or without leg pain for more than 24 hours, but less than 90 days, ages 18 to 65, and ODQ greater than or equal to 20% were included. Exclusions were made for patients whose most prominent symptoms were other than LBP or leg pain (eg, pain in lumbar, thoracic, and cervical spine, where cervical pain is the worst); pregnancy; lumbar surgery in the previous 6 months; previous spinal fusion or scoliosis hardware; any known or suspected serious pathology such as fracture; tumor; spinal steroid injections within the last month; previous sclerosing injections; botulinum toxin injections in the low back, abdominal, or pelvic area; or denervation procedures.[723]

The prevalence rates for each subgroup based on meeting criteria for more than one subgroup were: specific exercise (48%), manipulation (35.2%), stabilization (12.8%), and traction (9.6%). Based on individual subgroup criteria, 25.2% (95% CI: 19.8% to 30.6%) of subjects did not meet the criteria for any subgroup; 49.6% (95% CI: 43.4% to 55.8%) met the criteria for only one subgroup; and 25.2% (95% CI: 19.8% to 30.6%) met the criteria for more than one subgroup. The most common combination of subgroups was manipulation and specific exercise accounting for 68.4% of the subjects who met the criteria for 2 subgroups. Algorithm decision reliability was moderate (κ = 0.52, 95% CI: 0.27 to 0.77, percentage agreement = 67%) and acceptable for clinical use.[723] The authors concluded that the decision-making strategy fit about one-half of patients seeking PT care for LBP in 2 settings: Australia and the United States.[723]

The Stanton et al[723] study demonstrated everyday clinical reality such that about half of the patients seeking PT fall into one subgroup, another 25% meet the criteria for more than one subgroup, and the rest cannot be classified using the TBC. If a patient belongs in a subgroup, evidence supports a matched intervention to improve outcomes over an unmatched intervention. Clinicians should initiate treatment indicated by the subgroup and closely monitor the patient's response, specifically for those patients who fit more than one subgroup. For those who do not clearly fit a particular subgroup, an impairment-based strategy, clinical practice guidelines, clinical reasoning, or other classification systems are considered. Current best evidence is necessary to guide further research to improve the comprehensive algorithm and clinical decision making. With the emergence of new evidence, subgroup criteria may be refined, additional subgroups or treatments added, and/or the hierarchical ordering of the algorithm altered with ultimate goal of improving patient outcomes.[723] Other classifications are discussed next.

Neurodynamic Diagnostic Classification Evidence

The word *neurodynamics* describes the biomechanical, physiological, and structural functions associated with the nervous system,[424,425,724] which needs the ability to adapt to mechanical loads (ie, elongation, sliding, and compression) during functional activity. Inflammation, neural edema, reduced intraneural blood flow, or fibrosis associated with the nerve and/or the tissues it runs through may result in altered neurodynamics.[424,425,724] Theoretically, the benefits of neural mobilization include improved nerve gliding, reduced nerve adherence, increased neural vascularity, and improved axoplasmic flow. When altered neurodynamics are identified on examination, neural mobilization is one intervention with goals to reduce neural tissue mechanosensitivity and restore its movement capabilities.[424,425,438,725]

Ellis and Hing[726] completed a systematic review to assess the therapeutic efficacy of neural mobilization for treatment of altered neurodynamics. The authors concluded that only limited evidence exists to support the use of neural mobilization. Future research is warranted. Eleven studies met minimal inclusion criteria. Three of the 11 studies were related to spinal pain, neuropathic cervicobrachial pain,[727] nonradicular LBP,[728] and postoperative spinal pain.[729] Brief summaries of the 3 studies are described next.

Scrimshaw and Maher[729] investigated 81 persons after lumbar discectomy, fusion, or laminectomy randomized to standard postoperative care (SPOC) or SPOC plus neural mobilization. The neural mobilization exercises included active and passive variations of neck flexion, SLR, and SLR with plantarflexion and DF, designed to mobilize the lumbosacral nerve roots and sciatic tract. At 12-month follow-up, no statistically significant benefits were provided by the addition of neural mobilization based on pain, disability, and GPE.[729] The presence of a heterogeneous patient population may account for the lack of treatment effect. Nerve mobilization appears no more effective than standard care for patients after lumbar surgery.[14]

A single-blind, randomized trial[727] was conducted to determine the effects of 2 MT interventions on cervicobrachial pain syndrome. Subjects were 18 to 75 years of age with symptoms greater than 3 months and altered upper extremity neurodynamics. Thirty subjects were randomized to 1 of 3 groups—2 MT plus exercise groups and a control. Group 1 received contralateral cervical lateral glide mobilization in a pain-free range, shoulder girdle mobilization prone with hand behind back over acromial area, and contract-relax techniques into shoulder ABD and ER. The home exercise program consisted of cervical LF exercises away from the painful side of 10 repetitions 1 to 3 times daily and active shoulder ABD and ER exercises. Group 2 received joint mobilization techniques to the shoulder in supine PA glides in neutral progressing through ABD and thoracic spine UPA PAIVM on the painful side from T2-T5. The home exercise program consisted of pendulum exercises, AAROM wand shoulder ER in supine, anterior and posterior shoulder girdle stretches, and resistive band exercises into ABD and ER. Group 3 was the control. After 8 weeks, the control group crossed over to group 1. Both MT plus exercise groups were effective at reducing pain and improving pain quality and disability scores. At 8 weeks, group 1 had a significantly lower pain score, indicating the positive treatment effects of neurodynamic mobilization.[727]

In a case series of 6 patients with nonradicular LBP, George[730] reported successful outcomes in response to slump stretching. Based on the case series by George,[730] 30 subjects who were hypothesized to benefit from slump stretching were randomized into 2 treatment groups. Subjects had symptoms distal to the buttocks, no change in symptoms with flexion or extension (ie, no centralization), and a baseline ODI greater than 10%. Subjects who had signs or symptoms of nerve root involvement or a +SLR less than 45 degrees were excluded.[728] Group 1 received lumbar mobilization of CPA PAIVM mobilization, grades III to IV to hypomobile joints, exercise of pelvic tilts, bridging, wall squats, quadruped alternate arms and legs for 2 sets of 10 reps as described by Childs et al,[141] and slump stretching. Slump stretching (Figure 4-125) was performed in the long sit position and ankles in 0 degrees DF with feet against the wall. The clinician applied OP to the cervical spine, held for 30 seconds and 5 repetitions at the point where the patient's symptoms were reproduced. The exercise was repeated at home for 2 repetitions with a 30-second hold. Group 2 received only mobilization and exercise. Short-term results after 6 sessions over 3 weeks favored patients receiving slump stretching. Significantly greater improvements in disability, pain, and centralization were observed in group 1.[728]

Melbye[731] presented a case report on a patient with a diagnosis of an adherent nerve root (ANR), a clinical presentation characterized by adherent connective tissue around the nerve root thought to cause symptoms associated with altered mobility. The clinical presentation for ANR is a recent history of sciatica, symptoms for at least 6 to 8 weeks, a major limitation of flexion in standing, and intermittent leg symptoms consistently produced with repeated end-range movements that ease immediately after each repetition. Centralization or peripheralization does not occur. The patient met all of the criteria: an 18-month history of sciatica plus a decreased Achilles reflex, decreased sensation over the lateral border of the left foot, a positive left SLR at 20 degrees, and fear related to bending. After ruling out the presence of centralization or peripheralization, the patient was started on RFIL plus left leg neural mobilization. With the hip at 90 degrees flexion, the knee was actively extended with the ankle in neutral to symptom onset (Figure 4-126) for 6 to 8 repetitions 5 to 6 times per day followed by 10 repetitions of REIL. The exercises were progressed to repeated flexion in sitting with the left knee extended and then RFIS. After 6 sessions and a 5-month follow-up, the patient was asymptomatic for 4 weeks. Flexion AROM significantly improved, sensation was normal, and left SLR was 80 degrees with hamstring tightness only, but the left Achilles reflex was still diminished.[731]

Neurodynamic Mobilization Intervention

In the presence of limited evidence to support the use of neurodynamic mobilization, Nee and Butler[725] proposed that conservative management, incorporating neurodynamic and neurobiology education, nonneural tissue interventions, and neurodynamic techniques can be effective in addressing musculoskeletal presentations of altered neurodynamics. Patient education involves a discussion of the role of the nervous system in movement and pain related to mechanical loading. Interventions such as joint or soft tissue mobilization or motor control training to regain optimal function may reduce mechanical forces on sensitive neural tissues. For example, limitation in hip mobility may alter the mechanical load on the sciatic nerve over time, resulting in mechanosensitivity during an SLR. Direct treatment of the hip mobility deficits and reassessment of the SLR may result in diminished mechanosensitivity and improvement in the SLR. Treatment of nonneural impairments should be followed by reassessment of subjective complaints, nonneural impairments, and positive NDTs. Absence of improvement related to nonneural techniques indicates a need for neurodynamic mobilization procedures. In other words, after intervention for hip mobility deficits, reassess positive NDTs such as SLR. If the NDT does not improve, neurodynamic intervention is considered.

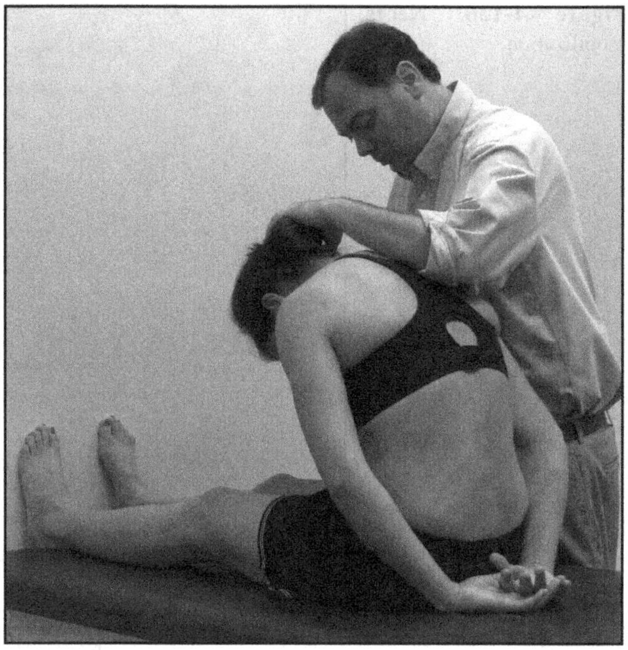

Figure 4-125. Slump stretching.

Neurodynamic mobilization procedures are passive or active movements centered on regaining the neural tissue's ability to move and withstand the stresses of normal daily activities. Nonprovocative gliding techniques are thought to result in a larger longitudinal excursion with a minimal increase in strain and to produce sliding movement between neural structures and adjacent nonneural tissue.[424] The cervical lateral glide (Figure 4-127) performed in the study by Allison et al[727] is an example of a sliding technique. These techniques are performed in an on-and-off or oscillatory manner and not performed as stretching techniques. Figure 4-128 illustrates a passive neurodynamic slider technique biasing the tibial branch of the sciatic tract with passive knee extension with ankle plantar flexion followed by passive knee flexion with passive ankle DF.[725] Tensile loading techniques, as performed in the Cleland et al[728] slump stretching study (see Figure 4-125), are more aggressive since tension is taken up from both ends of the nervous system at the same time and not indicated in patients with neurological signs of impaired conduction such as weakness, impaired sensation, and diminished DTRs.[725] Evidence supporting the effectiveness of neurodynamic techniques is limited. As discussed by Nee and Butler,[725] a conservative management approach using neurobiology education, nonneural tissue interventions, and neurodynamic techniques requires sound clinical reasoning using the concept of assess, treat, and reassess within and between sessions.

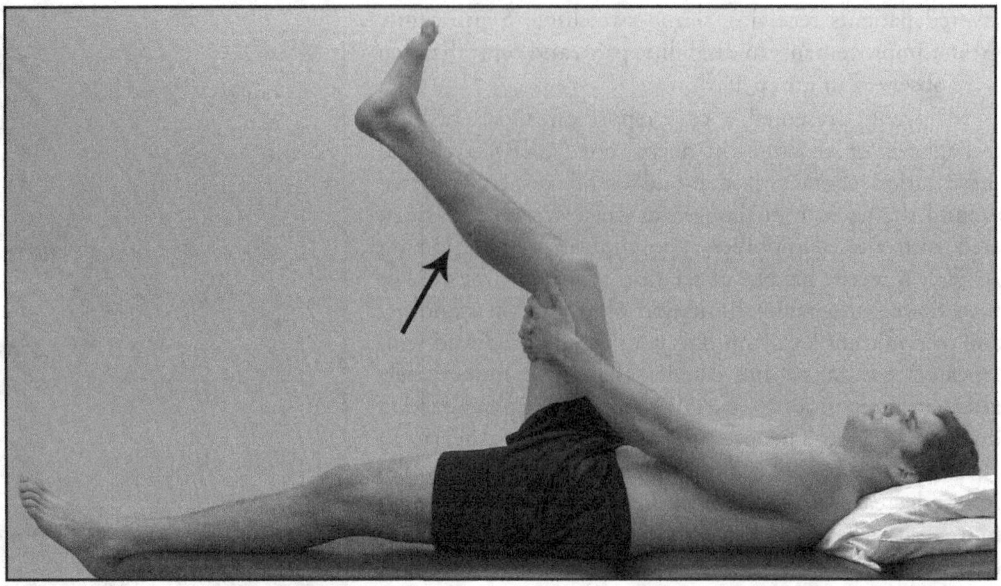

Figure 4-126. Neural mobilization.

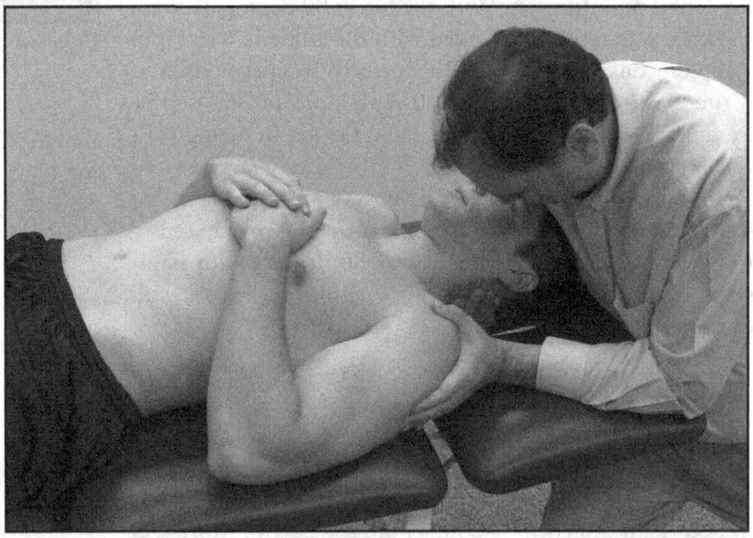

Figure 4-127. Cervical lateral glide technique. The head and cervical spine are translated in an oscillatory fashion away from the affected upper extremity that can be placed in a neurodynamic unloaded or loaded position at the therapist's discretion.

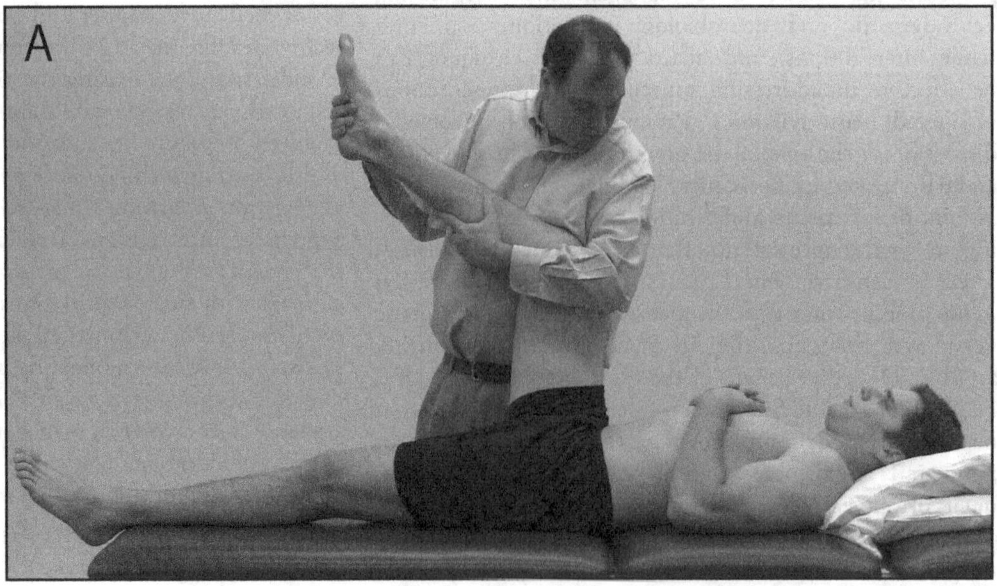

Figure 4-128. Neurodynamic slider technique: (A) passive knee extension is performed with the hip in 90 degrees of flexion and ankle plantarflexion. *(continued)*

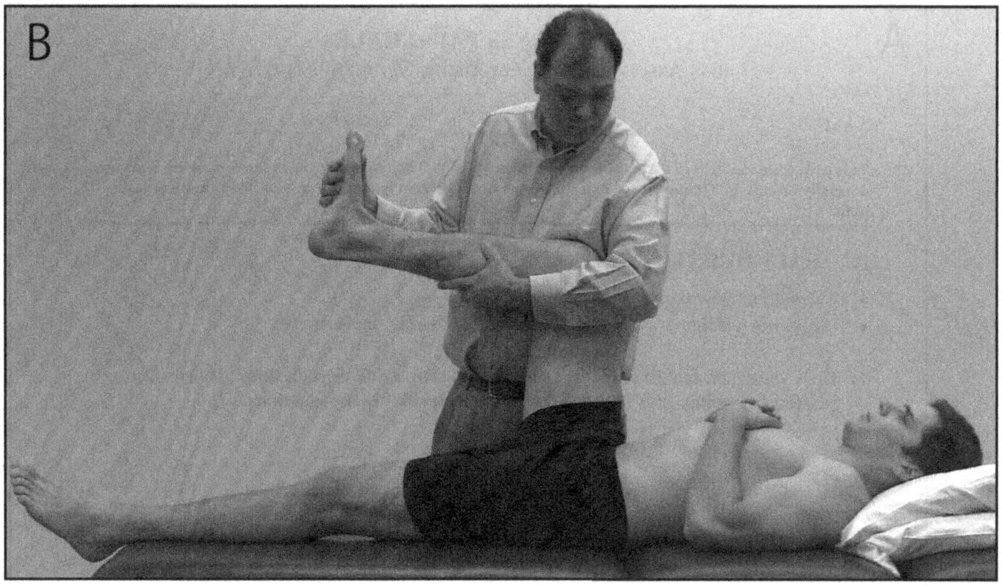

Figure 4-128 (continued). Neurodynamic slider technique: (B) passive knee flexion is performed with passive ankle DF.

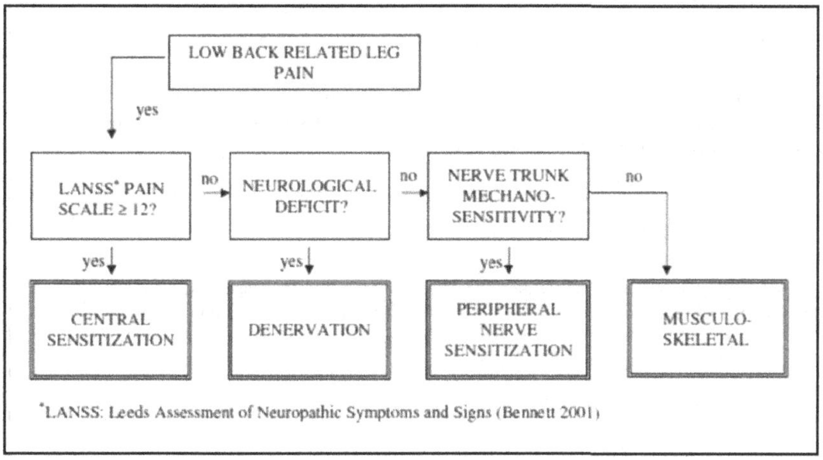

Figure 4-129. Classification algorithm of LBRLP. The classification is hierarchical and mutually exclusive. If criteria are met for the first category (neuropathic sensitization), then the classification is determined even if criteria are met for one of the other categories. LANNS = Leeds Assessment of Neuropathic Symptoms and Signs.[733] (Reprinted from *Man Ther*, 14, Schäfer A, Hall T, Briffa K, Classification of low back related leg pain—a proposed pathomechanism-based approach, 222-230, Copyright 2009, with permission from Elsevier.)

Mechanism-Based Classification of Low Back-Related Leg Pain

LBP with related leg pain can be a predictor of both severity and associated chronicity. Differentiating potential sources of radiating leg pain in patients with LBP facilitates a diagnosis and individualized treatment based on predominating pathomechanisms. Schäfer et al[732] have described a subclassification of persons with LBRLP based on distinct symptoms and signs associated with 4 predominating mechanisms (see Table 4-6): central sensitization, peripheral nerve sensitization, denervation, and musculoskeletal referred pain. To assist with clinical decision making, a classification algorithm[732] is also proposed (Figure 4-129).

The Leeds Assessment of Neuropathic Symptoms and Signs (LANSS; Figure 4-130), a reliable and valid tool for identifying patients with dominant neuropathic pain mechanisms, is a component of the examination protocol.[733] The LANSS scale is valid for discrimination between neuropathic and nociceptive pain regardless of disease-based diagnostic methods. If a patient scores 12 or more out of 24 on this scale, there is a strong likelihood that neuropathic pain is present to some degree. If the score is less than 12, neuropathic mechanisms are unlikely to be contributing to the patient's pain. A self-report LANSS score that does not require a clinical examination component has also been found reliable and valid.[734] The Self-Administered LANSS (S-LANSS; Figure 4-131) consists of 7 "yes" and "no" questions, a body chart, and an 11-point NPRS in response to, "How bad has your pain been in the last week?" The S-LANSS can be administered by self-report or through clinician interview. The S-LANSS score correctly identified 75% of pain types when self-reported and 80% when interviewed. Optimum cutoff score for self-report is 12 or more and 10 or more for interview completion.[734]

LBRLP arising from neural structures is classified as neuropathic pain, and LBRLP arising from musculoskeletal structures is classified as nociceptive pain. The neuropathic leg pain classification is further divided into

Figure 4-130. LANSS. *(continued)*

A

THE LANSS PAIN SCALE

Leeds Assessment of Neuropathic Symptoms and Signs

NAME____________________ **DATE**________________

This pain scale can help to determine whether the nerves that are carrying your pain signals are working normally or not. It is important to find this out in case different treatments are needed to control your pain.

A. PAIN QUESTIONNAIRE

- Think about how your pain has felt over the last week.
- Please say whether any of the descriptions match your pain exactly.

1) Does your pain feel like strange, unpleasant sensations in your skin? Words like pricking, tingling, pins and needles might describe these sensations.

a) NO - My pain doesn't really feel like this.............................. (0)

b) YES - I get these sensations quite a lot.................................. (5)

2) Does your pain make the skin in the painful area look different from normal? Words like mottled or looking more red or pink might describe the appearance.

a) NO - My pain doesn't affect the colour of my skin.................... (0)

b) YES - I've noticed that the pain does make my skin look different from normal .... (5)

3) Does your pain make the affected skin abnormally sensitive to touch? Getting unpleasant sensations when lightly stroking the skin, or getting pain when wearing tight clothes might describe the abnormal sensitivity.

a) NO - My pain doesn't make my skin abnormally sensitive in that area......... (0)

b) YES - My skin seems abnormally sensitive to touch in that area.................... (3)

4) Does your pain come on suddenly and in bursts for no apparent reason when you're still. Words like electric shocks, jumping and bursting describe these sensations.

a) NO - My pain doesn't really feel like this .... (0)

b) YES - I get these sensations quite a lot .... (2)

5) Does your pain feel as if the skin temperature in the painful area has changed abnormally? Words like hot and burning describe these sensations

a) NO - I don't really get these sensations... (0)

b) YES - I get these sensations quite a lot .... (1)

3 subgroups: central sensitization, denervation, and peripheral nerve sensitization. The 4 categories of LBRLP[732,735] (see Table 4-6) are as follows:

1. Neuropathic central sensitization (NCS) comprising major features of neuropathic pain with sensory sensitization such as allodynia, hyperalgesia, and paroxysmal pain
2. Neuropathic denervation arising from significant axonal compromise with clear sensory and motor deficits
3. Neuropathic peripheral nerve sensitization (NPNS) arising from nerve trunk inflammation with distinct nerve mechanosensitivity
4. Nociceptive musculoskeletal (NM) with pain referred from nonneural structures such as the disc or facet joints

Patients with LBRLP may have an overlap of more than one mechanism, so the subgrouping is determined in a hierarchical fashion, with priority given to NCS followed by denervation, NPNS, and finally NM. With regard to disability and psychosocial factors, Walsh and Hall[736] observed that the NPNS subgroup had significantly greater disability compared to all other subgroups and significantly greater fear-avoidance beliefs about physical activity compared to the NCS and denervation subgroups.

Interrater reliability of the classification system is good ($\kappa = 0.72$).[735] Predictive validity has been tested by

B

B. SENSORY TESTING

Skin sensitivity can be examined by comparing the painful area with a contralateral or adjacent non-painful area for the presence of allodynia and an altered pin-prick threshold (PPT).

1) ALLODYNIA

Examine the response to lightly stroking cotton wool across the non-painful area and then the painful area. If normal sensations are experienced in the non-painful site, but pain or unpleasant sensations (tingling, nausea) are experienced in the painful area when stroking, allodynia is present.

a) NO, normal sensation in both areas .... (0)

b) YES, allodynia in painful area only .... (5)

2) ALTERED PIN-PRICK THRESHOLD

Determine the pin-prick threshold by comparing the response to a 23 gauge (blue) needle mounted inside a 2 ml syringe barrel placed gently on to the skin in a non-painful and then painful areas.

If a sharp pin prick is felt in the non-painful area, but a different sensation is experienced in the painful area e.g. none / blunt only (raised PPT) or a very painful sensation (lowered PPT), an altered PPT is present.

If a pinprick is not felt in either area, mount the syringe onto the needle to increase the weight and repeat.

a) NO, equal sensation in both areas .... (0)

b) YES, altered PPT in painful area .... (3)

SCORING:

Add values in parentheses for sensory description and examination findings to obtain overall score.

TOTAL SCORE (maximum 24) ....

If score < 12, neuropathic mechanisms are **unlikely** to be contribution to the patient's pain

If score ≥ 12, neuropathic mechanisms are **likely** to be contributing to the patient's pain

Figure 4-130 (continued). LANSS. (Bennett MI. The LANSS Pain Scale: the Leeds assessment of neuropathic symptoms and signs. *Pain.* 2001;91:147-157. This appendix has been reprinted with permission of the International Association for the Study of Pain (IASP). The appendix may not be reproduced for any other purpose without permission.)

investigating differences in somatosensory profiles of subjects classified using quantitative sensory testing. Significant differences in sensory thresholds were found in groups supporting the mechanism-based classification system.[737]

Specific guidelines are not yet available for treatment based on this classification system, but a recent case report[738] provides an example of MT intervention of 7 sessions over 6 weeks provided to a patient with LBRLP due to overlapping mechanisms of NPNS and NM. MT intervention to the lumbar spine (ie, CPA PAIVM, PPIVM, and therapeutic exercise) began with addressing the musculoskeletal impairments for the first 2 sessions. The manual techniques included CPA PAIVM to L4, sustained grade IV (see Figure 4-89A), and lumbar PPIVM sustained in flexion and left LF. With minimal improvement, impairments associated with NPNS were first addressed through seated slump in knee extension, adding ankle DF as a home exercise program and progressing to adding cervical flexion (see Figure 4-40E). At the 4th session, prone PAIVM and side-lying PPIVM (Figure 4-132) in combination with lower extremity SLR neurodynamic mobilization were initiated with full resolution of symptoms by the sixth session.[738]

To determine whether pain and disability outcomes differ for subclassification of LBRLP, 74 patients with LBRLP greater than 6 weeks were classified into 1 of the 4 categories following a standardized examination protocol.[739] All patients received 7 neural mobilization sessions 2 times per week that included the following (Figure 4-133):

Figure 4-131. S-LANSS. *(continued)*

A

APPENDIX

THE S-LANSS PAIN SCORE

Leeds Assessment of Neuropathic Symptoms and Signs (self-complete)

NAME______________________ **DATE**______________

- This questionnaire can tell us about the type of pain that you may be experiencing. This can help in deciding how best to treat it.
- Please draw on the diagram below where you feel your pain. If you have pain in more than one area, **only shade in the one main area where your worst pain is.**

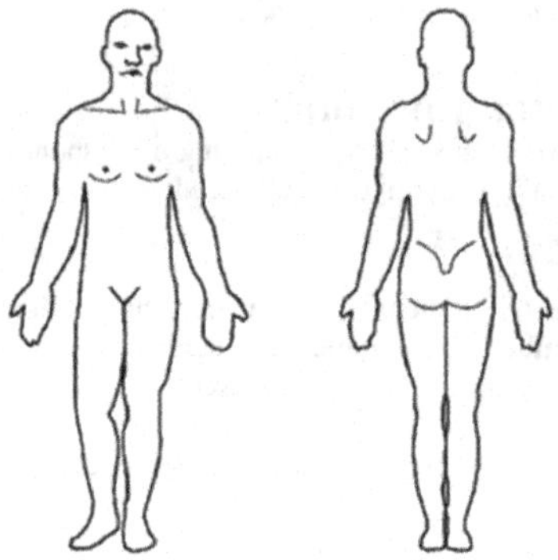

- On the scale below, please indicate how bad your pain (that you have shown on the above diagram) has been in the last week where: '0' means no pain and '10' means pain as severe as it could be.

NONE 0 1 2 3 4 5 6 7 8 9 10 **SEVERE PAIN**

- On the other side of the page are 7 questions about your pain (the one in the diagram).
- Think about how your pain that you showed in the diagram has felt **over the last week.** Please circle the descriptions that best match your pain. These descriptions may, or may not, match your pain no matter how severe it feels.
- Only circle the responses that describe your pain. **Please turn over.**

- Lumbar LF in side-lying away from the painful side at the affected level for 60 seconds at a frequency of 1 Hz to increase the size of the intervertebral foramen
- Side-lying hip and knee flexion followed by hip and knee extension for 30 seconds at a frequency of 0.5 Hz for nerve gliding proposed to decrease venous congestion and endoneurial pressure

Both procedures were repeated 5 times in a pain-free manner, and a home exercise program (which was not described) was included. This approach is theorized to desensitize an overly sensitized peripheral nervous system. Outcomes were NPRS (2.5 points), RMDQ (30% improvement), and a 7-point global perceived change scale from 1 (completely recovered) to 7 (worse than ever). A report of 1 (completely recovered) or 2 (much improved) was a successful outcome. The proportion of responders was significantly greater in the NPNS group (56%) compared to the other 3 groups (NCS 11%, neurodynamics 15%, and NM 11%) with no differences between these 3 groups. After adjusting for baseline differences, mean improvement of outcome measures was significantly greater in the NPNS group.[739] This single-arm study provides preliminary support for continued study of the LBRLP classification system. Preliminary findings suggest that, among patients receiving a specific neural mobilization treatment, the LBRLP classification system identified a subgroup of patients—NPNS—with a more favorable prognosis.[739] The ability to differentiate between neuropathic and nociceptive pain mechanisms may lead to improved pain

B

S-LANSS

1. **In the area where you have pain, do you also have 'pins and needles', tingling or prickling sensations?**

a)	NO – I don't get these sensations	(0)
b)	YES – I get these sensations often	(5)

2. **Does the painful area change colour (perhaps looks mottled or more red) when the pain is particularly bad?**

a)	NO – The pain does not affect the colour of my skin	(0)
b)	YES – I have noticed that the pain does make my skin look different from normal	(5)

3. **Does your pain make the affected skin abnormally sensitive to touch? Getting unpleasant sensations or pain when lightly stroking the skin might describe this.**

a)	NO – The pain does not make my skin in that area abnormally sensitive to touch	(0)
b)	YES – My skin in that area is particularly sensitive to touch	(3)

4. **Does your pain come on suddenly and in bursts for no apparent reason when you are completely still? Words like 'electric shocks', jumping and bursting might describe this.**

a)	NO – My pain doesn't really feel like this	(0)
b)	YES – I get these sensations often	(2)

5. **In the area where you have pain, does your skin feel unusually hot like a burning pain?**

a)	NO – I don't have burning pain	(0)
b)	YES – I get burning pain often	(1)

6. **Gently <u>rub</u> the painful area with your index finger and then rub a non-painful area (for example, an area of skin further away or on the opposite side from the painful area). How does this rubbing feel in the painful area?**

a)	The painful area feels no different from the non-painful area	(0)
b)	I feel discomfort, like pins and needles, tingling or burning in the painful area that is different from the non-painful area	(5)

7. **Gently <u>press</u> on the painful area with your finger tip then gently press in the same way onto a non-painful area (the same non-painful area that you chose in the last question). How does this feel in the painful area?**

a)	The painful area does not feel different from the non-painful area	(0)
b)	I feel numbness or tenderness in the painful area that is different from the non-painful area	(3)

Scoring: a score of 12 or more suggests pain of predominantly neuropathic origin

Figure 4-131 (continued). S-LANSS. (Reprinted from *J Pain,* 6(3), Bennett MI, Smith BH, Torrance N, Potter J. The S-LANSS score for identifying pain of predominantly neuropathic origin: validation for use in clinical and postal research, 149-158, Copyright 2005, with permission from Elsevier.)

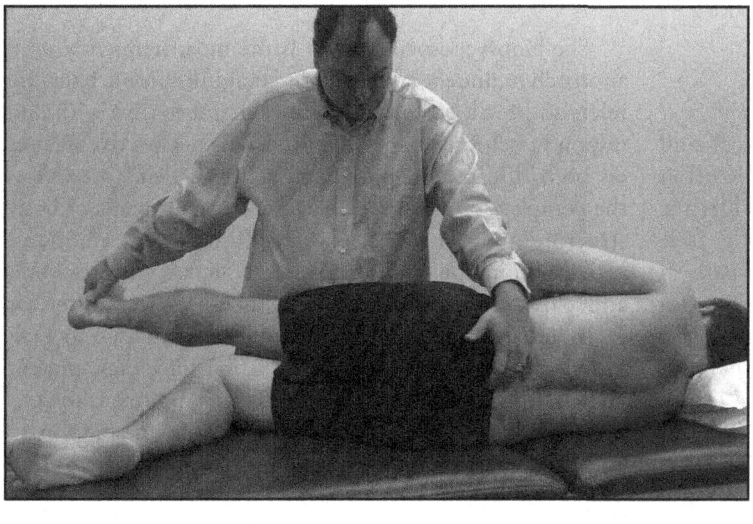

Figure 4-132. Side-lying PPIVM in combination with lower extremity (SLR) neurodynamic mobilization.

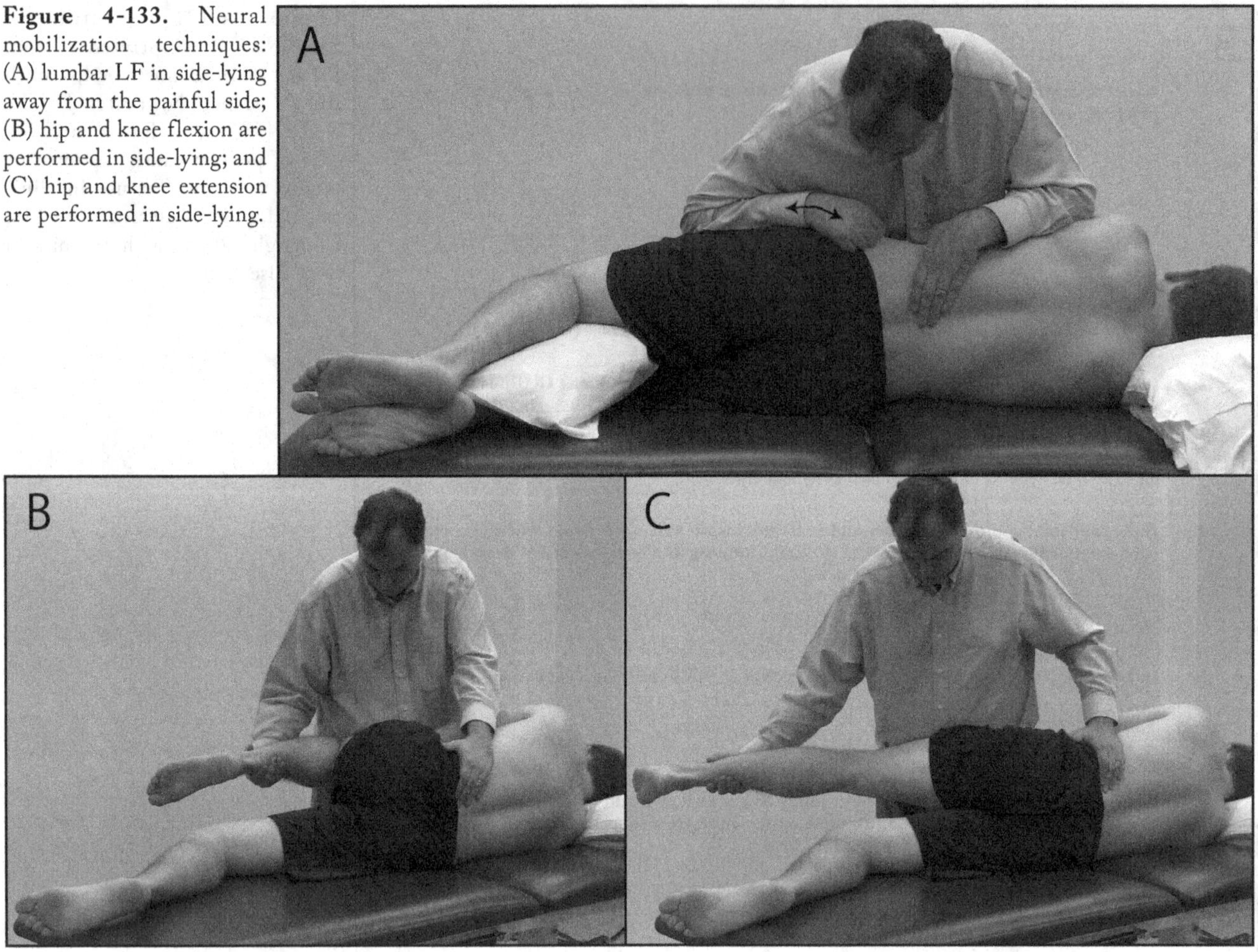

Figure 4-133. Neural mobilization techniques: (A) lumbar LF in side-lying away from the painful side; (B) hip and knee flexion are performed in side-lying; and (C) hip and knee extension are performed in side-lying.

control, comparison of treatment for patients with similar pain generating mechanisms, and the development of treatments tailored to specific pain mechanisms.[739] The next section considers the classification of CLBP.

Chronic Low Back Pain Classification

Chronic Low Back Pain

Chronic pain is a prevalent and costly physical and mental health problem in the United States. Von Korff et al[740] estimated a 19% annual prevalence and 29% lifetime prevalence for chronic spinal pain. Approximately 57% of adult Americans reported recurrent or chronic pain in the past year, while 62% of those reported being in pain for more than 1 year, with 40% in constant pain. Pain accounts for more than 80% of all physician visits with $70 billion annually related to lost productivity and health care costs. Persons 50 years of age or older are twice as likely to have chronic pain.[741,742] Though definitions vary considerably, chronic pain is often defined as a persistent pain for at least 3 months, or recurrent pain over months to years mixed together with pain-free periods. CLBP is a complex problem, different for each person, and resistant to intervention requiring a multidimensional management approach.[443,743]

Biopsychosocial Model

The biopsychosocial model is the most frequently used approach to understanding and managing chronic pain and refers to how a person and family members live with and respond to chronic pain disability. This perspective focuses on both disease and illness, with illness being viewed as the complex interaction of biological impairments of body structure and functions, psychological beliefs, emotions, activity limitation, and social factors such as culture, work, and participation restrictions.[744] These factors differ for each patient, making the pain experience unique to each individual, but their relative contributions may present yellow flags for the clinician. The clinician's role is to consider all factors in the patient presenting with spinal pain and to understand the underlying mechanisms causing the patient's problem within a biopsychosocial context. Specific best evidence treatments are then directed to the underlying mechanism to affect an optimal outcome.

Understanding and Addressing Pain From a Biopsychosocial Model

Patient beliefs and expectations are potential influences on adherence and behavioral change and are also mediators of outcome.[745] Each patient has a different expectation or goal for seeking care: a cure, symptom relief, or reassurance. A clinician's failure to understand each patient's expectations often leads to confusion and distress for the patient.[745] When assessing a patient with chronic pain, adhere to the basics of eye contact and listening, avoid interruption, summarize and clarify, use clear language, avoid unnecessary diagnostic detail, and encourage self-disclosure of relevant psychosocial concerns. Recognition of central pain mechanisms is important to integrate the role of cognitive and emotional influences into patient education. A therapeutic climate facilitates self-disclosure of psychosocial concerns and supports successful identification of patients' beliefs and expectations.[745]

Main et al[745] offered key points for addressing patient beliefs and expectations. For example, a simple question, "What in your body do you think is causing your pain?" allows the patient to explain his or her understanding. Knowledge that a patient's focus on a structural label such as degenerative disc disease may heighten attention on pain, enhance the vulnerability of the body to damage, and increase the patients' health care consumption gives the clinician an opportunity to educate with appropriate language and to assist the patient to reconceptualize the perceived threat.[746,747] Early recognition of specific concerns and clarification of mistaken beliefs facilitate an improved outcome and development of a mutual plan of care.[748] The clinician should provide a credible but simple explanation of the difference between acute and chronic pain, the importance of central pain mechanisms, and the development of disability. The use of terminology that is easily understood helps to frame the patient's beliefs and expectations in a positive manner and optimizes pain coping strategies.[745]

Developing a cognitive behavioral component to the treatment plan includes additional key characteristics.[749] The clinician should do the following:

- Assess patient complaints in terms of contributing biological, psychological, and social or environmental factors.
- Encourage the patient to play an active rather than a passive role in the plan.
- Identify specific behavioral and functional goals the patient wants to achieve.
- Develop a plan to achieve these goals and to deal with identified barriers to progress.
- Monitor and reinforce with recognition and performance of planned tasks and establish a plan for dealing with relapse.[749]

Establishing a plan for relapse should be individualized for each patient and include maintenance of a regular exercise plan, remaining active, and self-management and evaluation strategies.[749]

Neuroscience of Pain

Traditionally, pain is thought of as a signal of injury, potential injury, or symptom due to pathology with the amount of pain being directly related to the amount of pathology. When the pathology resolves, the pain goes away. In some patients, however, pain is present even if the pathology resolves or no pathology can be found.

Pain is modulated by many influences that result in a multidimensional experience. These influences are variable and depend on the meaning of pain to the individual. When tissue is perceived to be under threat, CNS outputs occur. However, it is the individual's perception of the degree of threat that determines the outputs, not the state of tissues or the actual threat to tissues.[750] The neuromatrix theory of pain proposes that pain is produced by output of a widely distributed neural network in the brain rather than purely by sensory input evoked by trauma, inflammation, or other pathology.[751,752] The neuromatrix is a combination of cortical mechanisms that produce pain when activated but requires no actual sensory input such as noxious stimulus, tissue injury, or inflammation to produce pain experiences. Pain is produced by the brain when it perceives that body tissue is in danger and that action is required.[750-752]

In the presence of injury and chronic stress, the body-self neuromatrix or the brain's neural network integrates cognitive, sensory, and motivational inputs and proposes that output patterns engage perceptions, behaviors, homeostatic controls, and autonomic system responses that produce a multidimensional pain experience. Cognitive inputs such as past experience and beliefs combine with cutaneous or visual sensory inputs and motivational inputs such as emotions, altered homeostasis, immune mechanisms, and stress that produce a complex neural pattern that results in pain.[751-753] A synthesis of nerve impulses associated with cognition, emotion, coping strategies, and social interaction, along with cortisol and stress regulation via immune, endocrine, and autonomic systems result in an altered neuromatrix output, often associated with altered movement performance and chronic pain.[752]

Two interdependent mechanisms can contribute to chronicity: nociceptive or peripheral mechanisms including immune-related dysfunction that stimulates nociceptive structures, and non-nociceptive or central mechanisms including cognitive-evaluative mechanisms. These mechanisms persuade the CNS that body tissue is in danger,

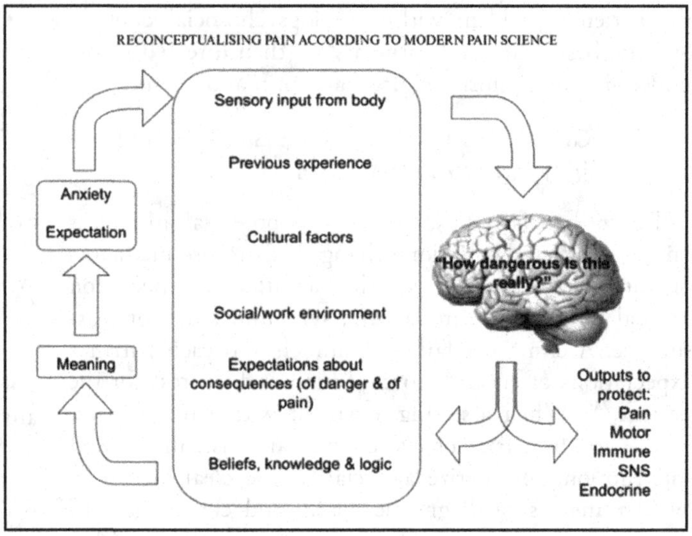

Figure 4-134. Reconceptualizing pain. (Reprinted with permission from Moseley GL. Reconceptualising pain according to modern pain science. *Phys Ther Rev.* 2007;12:169-178. The online version is available at http://www.maney.co.uk/journals/ptr and http://www.Ingentaconnect.com/content/maney/ptr.)

neuromatrix activity increases, and less input is needed for activation (ie, sensitization occurs). When pain persists, sensitivity to noxious and non-noxious stimuli increases and the integrity of motor output is altered, providing the patient and clinician with the following challenges:

- An unclear relationship between pain and tissue input
- Unpredictable flare-ups
- Poor tolerance of normal therapeutic approaches
- Problems with physical and functional improvement
- Difficulty transferring gains to other activities[746]

To assist in understanding the complexity of the pain experience, Moseley[750] proposed 4 key points based on modern pain science:

1. Pain does not reflect the state of tissues.
2. Pain is modulated by many factors from across somatic, psychological and social domains.
3. The relationship between pain and the state of the tissues becomes less predictable as pain persists.
4. Pain can be thought of as a conscious correlate of the perception that tissue is in danger and, therefore, is a conscious driver of behavior to protect those tissues.

The individual's perception of threat determines the CNS outputs of pain, fear, anxiety, or anger, not the state of the tissues or the actual threat of danger to the tissues[750] (Figure 4-134).

When tissue is under threat, the body part is reflexively withdrawn, inflammatory mediators are released, and rapid changes in blood flow and in the excitability of peripheral nociceptors or peripheral sensitization occur.[754] The nociceptive system transforms this threat into electrical activity in the peripheral nervous system. If this message reaches the CNS, immune mediators are released into the blood stream,[755] voluntary and postural muscle activity are altered,[756] and conscious knowledge of the threat emerges as pain. Within this theory, pain will not result until the nociceptive input to the brain has been evaluated. Pain is dependent on the perceived degree of threat and is merely one output of the CNS. The theory does not describe how the threat is evaluated, but the complex interactions of biological changes, psychological status, and sociocultural context must be considered. Basic neuroscience processes of pain are reviewed next, but a detailed discussion is beyond the scope of this reference.

Gatchel et al[744] provided a summary of neuroscience research related to chronic pain. Genetic factors may play a role in the initiation and maintenance of chronic pain. An excess or reduced amount of neurotransmitters may increase the sensitivity of neurons. Neurons in the somatosensory system are connected in certain patterns but are dynamic and easily modified by incoming signals from various connections. Chronic pain depends on the psychosocial status of the patient and may change within hours, days, or weeks, possibly related to hormone concentrations. Noninvasive technology such as CT, functional MRI, or positron emission tomography aids in understanding the dynamic activation of the brain in response to certain stimuli and how the brain changes in people with CLBP.[757]

Cortical changes in people with CLBP, when compared with healthy controls, are described as neurochemical, structural, or functional. Wand et al[757] detailed cortical changes, which are briefly discussed here. Neurochemical markers are altered by increasing or decreasing with the magnitude of change, increasing overall as the duration and intensity of pain increase.[758] Though not well understood, fewer brain cells or gray matter in certain regions are found in persons with CLBP compared to healthy controls. The primary somatosensory cortex (S1) of the back is different in persons with CLBP, specifically in those who are distressed, suggesting an emotional factor to CLBP.[759,760] The primary motor cortex representation (M1) is also different in CLBP. The primary motor cortical representation of TrA contraction is shifted and enlarged in recurrent LBP indicative of cortical reorganization. Both the location and size are associated with slower onset of the TrA during a rapid arm movement, suggesting that this reorganization is associated with deficits in postural control.[761] In CLBP, an expanded area of cortical activity was noted in preparation for arm movement and a decrease in cortical activity associated with TrA delay.[762]

Speculative clinical implications for altered brain activity in CLBP as described by Wand et al[757] are briefly discussed next. Most likely, neurochemical and functional changes result in sensitization of the neural networks promoting pain and nociception, creating the potential of widespread dysfunction of normal cortical mechanisms. Clinically, this might be observed as lower mechanical pain thresholds locally in the lumbar spine and at distant sites, widespread and more intense pain, and diffuse tenderness. CLBP patients have impairments in emotional decision making,[763] memory, language skills, and mental flexibility.[764,765] Cortical changes may be a contributor to psychological dysfunction. Altered cortical representation may possibly alter one's body perception. Persons with CLBP have impaired proprioception[766] and tactile acuity and find it difficult to draw an outline of their back when asked.[767]

Based on cortical changes in CLBP, Wand et al[768] propose that training the brain in persons with CLBP using tactile discrimination and graded motor imagery to activate movement related networks without eliciting pain[769] are potential strategies requiring additional research. A single case design[768] for 3 subjects with disabling nonspecific CLBP was used to describe the effects of a 10-week graded sensorimotor retraining program on pain intensity, pain interference with daily life, and self-reported disability. Retraining involved stimulus localization, graphesthesia training, laterality recognition, imagery, repositioning, and SSE. Improvement was noted in all 3 outcomes.

Preliminary research also shows that patients can gain voluntary control over activation of specific brain regions, possibly providing new avenues for treatment.[770] In response to a noxious thermal stimulus, increased activation of the brain resulted in an increased perception of pain, whereas decreased activation resulted in a decreased perception of pain. In subjects with CLBP, Tsao et al[771] observed a shift in cortical representation of the TrA associated with voluntary contraction training of the TrA. Reorganization of the motor cortex toward that of healthy controls is also associated with changes in motor coordination, but it is not found in subjects who performed only an unskilled walking exercise. These findings suggest that motor skill training may reverse cortical neuroplastic changes associated with pain. Motor cortex reorganization related to skilled motor training may be an underlying mechanism that drives recovery in this population. Emerging evidence supports that cortical neuroplastic changes in the sensorimotor system may be a key factor in the maintenance of persistent pain.

Emotional distress such as anxiety, depression, or anger may predispose people to experience pain, amplify or inhibit the severity of pain, or be a result of persistent pain. Persons with persistent pain are anxious and worried about pain increasing and future disability. Anxiety-related pain and fear may contribute to avoidance behavior, inactivity, and potentially greater disability.[772] Continual monitoring of pain and painful activities and belief that these activities are harmful lessens the pain threshold and may augment muscle tension and physiological arousal, resulting in a maintained pain experience.[744,773] Depression may be the cause or result of chronic pain. Jarvik et al[774] reported that patients with depression are 2.3 times more likely to report back pain compared to those who did not report depression. Two factors appear to mediate the relationship between depression and pain. Patients who believe they can continue to function with pain and maintain some control over their lives are less likely to become depressed.[775,776] Anger may be related to frustration with persistent symptoms, limited information about etiology, and unsuccessful treatment, and directed to themselves, employers, insurance agents, medical personnel, and family members. Okifuji et al[777] reported that anger is significantly correlated with pain intensity ($r = 0.30$ to 0.35), disability ($r = 0.26$), and depression ($r = 0.52$).

Cognitive factors are related to the appraisal and beliefs about pain or how the patient assigns meaning to pain; its significance as a threat or not; the ability to control it by adaptive or maladaptive coping mechanisms; assumptions about harm versus hurt; and understanding or misunderstanding of causes, prognosis, or treatment.[744] Appraisal and beliefs impact the affective and behavioral response to pain. If the perception of threat is believed to be harmful or associated with actual or potential tissue damage, the pain may be perceived as more intense and unpleasant and result in more escape or avoidance behavior.[744]

Maladaptive beliefs about pain are components of the fear-avoidance model of pain. Such maladaptive beliefs view pain as a warning of damage, see painful activities as those that should be avoided, or believe pain leads to a permanent, uncontrollable problem.[778] Following injury, a person's beliefs determine the extent to which pain is interpreted. A maladaptive belief can result in a catastrophic response of physiological arousal, avoidance behavior, and fears, which enhances the threat perception and creates a continued catastrophic appraisal.[779] Addressing maladaptive beliefs through advice to remain active and through graded exposure to alter fear-avoidance beliefs and behaviors is a component of management for CLBP. Graded exposure therapy involves engagement in a hierarchy of feared activities. Each step confronts or challenges the patient's beliefs until the harmful appraisals are reduced or eliminated while gradually progressing to the most fearful activities. Graded exposure may prove to be an effective treatment for diminishing maladaptive beliefs and reducing pain and disability in chronic pain patients with high levels of fear-avoidance.[780-782]

Individuals with high self-efficacy may be more motivated to engage in wellness behaviors and adhere to treatment recommendations because of personal expectations of success and persistence in the face of obstacles such as pain and activity limitations to recovery. In contrast to negative factors for chronic pain and disability, optimism is associated with better general health, adaptation to chronic disease, and recovery after surgery,[783] perhaps because optimism results in more flexible coping strategies.[744]

In the presence of multiple influences on chronic spinal pain, the neuromatrix theory allows clinicians to evaluate physical, psychological, and social factors and use them to guide treatment and educate patients.[750,751] Moseley[746] proposes the following guidelines:

- Reduce threatening input via education to decrease activity of the pain neuromatrix and thereby reduce its value.
- After assessing baseline function, target activation of specific components of the neuromatrix without activating the pain neuromatrix.
- Upgrade physical and functional tolerance by graded exposure to threatening inputs across sensory and nonsensory domains.

The main goal of education is to decrease the threat value associated with pain by increasing understanding of human physiology, assuming an appropriate cognitive and behavior and motor response follows. Compassionate and respectful teaching about pain science leads to altered beliefs and attitudes about pain[784] and increased pain thresholds during relevant tasks.[785] Integrating pain education into PT management in patients with chronic pain reduces pain and disability.[746,786] Patient management is directed by clinicians determining the effect of physical, psychological, and social factors on the patient's perception of threat. Identifying which factor or factors play a role in exaggerating the patient's perception of threat may be relevant to selecting interventions directed at reducing threat perception and, therefore, the pain experience.[750] Clinicians treating patients with acute or chronic pain must consider the patient's emotional and cognitive status as well as physical or somatic factors in order to maximize the probability of a successful outcome. A negative affect resulting in maladaptive cognitive and behavioral pain responses is likely to influence motivation and compliance with the plan of care.

In patients with chronic pain, assessment involves determining baseline movements or activities that target specific components of the neuromatrix without activating the pain. The goal is to use as much of the task or activity as possible without activating the pain threshold.[746] For example, if forward bending to lift a box is a threatening movement, the clinician must modify the task to make it nonthreatening. The task may be broken down into components and performed at a different speed, amplitude, or duration. The context may need to be changed to work, home, or recreation or may need to begin with the patient imagining lifting a box in a pain-free manner that activates the pain neuromatrix, but in a nonthreatening way.[746] A baseline is not the point where a patient would have a flare-up or exacerbation. Instead, a pain-free level is established by clear communication with the patient. The clinician asks the patient to start at a level of activity that the patient can definitely perform and uses that level as a baseline. Conservative or small and frequent goals are set to increase tolerance and avoid flare-ups and progressed to involve exposure to more threatening inputs. Overall focus is on reducing the sensitivity and pain by reducing the perceived threat.[746]

While evidence is limited, MT in a pain-free manner in addition to a graded exercise approach might have a place in the comprehensive management of a subgroup of patients with CLBP. Clinicians, aware of central sensitization (ie, markedly reduced sensory thresholds), should adapt hands-on techniques and exercise programs accordingly. In the presence of central sensitization, Nijs and Van Houdenhove[787] proposed that MT hands-on techniques more often than once every 3 seconds are likely to trigger pain amplification. Low- to moderate-intensity exercise programs and aerobic exercises using multiple recovery periods are recommended. Stress management and breathing techniques may be useful. Any intervention triggering more pain serves as a new peripheral source of nociceptive input and sustains the process of central sensitization. Soft tissue mobilization should be initiated superficially and then progressed to deep cross-fiber techniques, while ischaemic compression for trigger points is likely to amplify the pain experience. MT aimed at improving motor control in symptomatic regions and joints is likely to have its place in the prevention of chronicity. In cases of poor movement patterns due to deconditioning or joint tissue damage and altered proprioception, incongruence between motor activity and sensory feedback is likely to occur. The motor control system may alert the individual to the mismatch between motor activity and sensory feedback by generating warning signals such as pain or sensory changes. Fear of movement and catastrophizing are important to chronic pain patients and patients with inappropriate beliefs at the acute and subacute stages, and it may contribute to poor performance and adherence with exercise.[787]

In summary, the biopsychosocial model views pain as a result of the complex interaction among physiologic, psychological, and social factors that perpetuate or worsen the pain experience. Patients with chronic pain are at increased risk for emotional disorders, maladaptive cognition, physical deconditioning and activity limitation, and altered neuromatrix output. Interdisciplinary management based on a biopsychosocial model and embracing a cognitive behavioral treatment approach must address all of these factors in order to be effective.

Classification and Management of Chronic Low Back Pain

Considering the multidimensional nature of CLBP, it is not surprising that classification is challenging and complex. Most persons with CLBP present with a combination of factors. The clinician's role is to evaluate and identify the dominant influences and the underlying pain mechanism(s) driving the disorder. This information guides targeted intervention strategies. Many classification approaches focus on a single dimension (pathoanatomy, neurophysiology, psychosocial issues, signs and symptoms, biomechanical loading theory, and MCIs), but as a single dimension, all appear unsuccessful for managing CLBP.[23] Using the biopsychosocial model, O'Sullivan[443] proposed 3 main subgroups (see Figure 4-1) that present with chronic, disabling lumbopelvic pain related to MCIs and whether the patient has adapted to the disorder in a positive or negative manner. The following subgroup descriptions are based on the work of O'Sullivan.[443,788,789]

First Group: Adaptive or Protective Altered Motor Response to an Underlying Disorder[443]

Characteristics of this group are high pain levels, disability, and movement and/or control impairments that are secondary and adaptive to an underlying pathological process. Pathological processes include red flag conditions; symptomatic pathology such as disc, stenosis, radiculopathy, spondylolisthesis, inflammatory disorders, and neuropathic; and centrally or sympathetically mediated pain disorders. Though these patients present with altered movement patterns and motor control, attempts to normalize these impairments result in exacerbation or no improvement because these deficits are adaptive and driven by pathology. If the passage of time or targeted medical or surgical management resolves the pathological process, then the signs and symptoms should resolve. These conditions represent a small group severely disabled with CLBP. Some patients in this subgroup may benefit from PT management in conjunction with the primary medical and/or surgical intervention.[443]

Second Group: Altered Motor Response and Centrally Mediated Pain Secondary to Dominant Psychosocial Factors[443]

In the second small group, the pain disorder is driven by psychological and/or social nonorganic factors. While many persons with CLBP have some negative psychosocial influences, a small number have these psychosocial issues as the dominant coexisting, precipitating, or aggravating factor.[108] The result is high levels of disability, altered central pain processing, enhanced constant pain, and movement and MCIs. Common dominant psychosocial traits include pathological anxiety, fear, anger, depression, negative beliefs, emotional issues, poor coping strategies, and negative social influences.[108,790]

In this group, a pathological process cannot be found and consistent aggravating and easing factors such as the absence of peripheral nociceptor drivers are not present. Aggravating factors are inconsistent with abnormal out-of-proportion pain, emotion, and disability responses. Patients may be dependent on analgesic medication and more passive forms of health care. Consultation with clinical psychology or psychiatry is valuable to confirm the classification of this subgroup. A focused treatment of the movement and control impairments through exercise alone is unlikely to result in a successful outcome. Interdisciplinary care is indicated, which might include cognitive behavioral therapy (CBT), psychological intervention, and graded exposure to functional activity.[443]

Third Group: Maladaptive Motor Control Patterns That Drive the Pain Disorder[443]

This group is considered the largest, where maladaptive movement or MCIs (Figure 4-135) and poor coping strategies produce chronic abnormal tissue loading of excessive or reduced spinal stability, leading to ongoing pain, disability, and distress. Patients in this group are classified as having either MI presenting with pain avoidance behavior or MCIs presenting with pain provocation behavior as the driver of CLBP. Persons in this subgroup may have a specific pathoanatomical diagnosis or are classified as nonspecific CLBP, but they commonly have psychosocial and neurophysiological (ie, central sensitization) factors as contributors, not drivers, of the pain. The intervention is a cognitive behavioral approach, but specific management is different. This subgroup seems appropriate for primary PT intervention to address the movement and control deficits and added intervention for the secondary cognitive influences.[443]

Subgroup: Movement Impairment Classification of Pain Avoidance Behavior[443]

The MI subgroup presents with a painful loss or impairment of active and passive physiological movement in one or more directions associated with high levels of muscle guarding and cocontraction when moving in the impaired range. The MI results in excessive compressive loading and

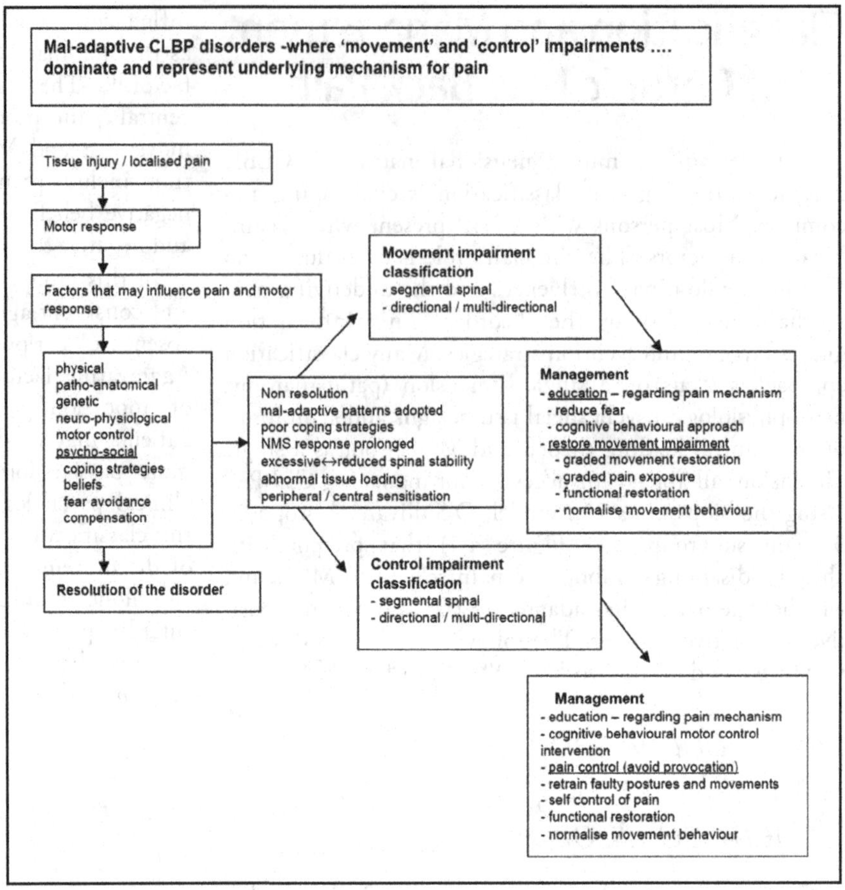

Figure 4-135. Maladaptive CLBP disorders. (Reprinted from *Man Ther,* 10, O'Sullivan P, Diagnosis and classification of chronic low back pain disorders: maladaptive movement and motor control impairments as underlying mechanisms, 242-255, Copyright 2005, with permission from Elsevier.)

movement restriction or rigidity (ie, excessive stability), providing a potential mechanism for tissue strain and continued peripheral nociceptor sensitization. These patients fear moving into the painful direction and perceive pain as damaging. The fear of movement has likely been reinforced by beliefs of harm, anxiety, and hypervigilance, reinforcing poor cognitive coping strategies and resulting in pain amplification and continued muscle guarding. The response is maladaptive since the compensation for the pain becomes the mechanism that drives the disorder. Patients can exhibit unidirectional MI in flexion, extension, rotation, LF, or multidirectional MI.[443]

Management involves both the dominant physical and secondary cognitive factors. The patient is educated that the pain is not harmful or damaging and that compensation strategies used to avoid movement are incorrect and now help to maintain the disorder. The goal is to restore normal movement through desensitizing the nervous system and reducing fear of movement and muscle guarding in the painful direction. Graded movement strategies into the painful range and cognitive strategies to alter fear beliefs are augmented by MT such as mobilization, manipulation, or soft tissue techniques to reduce the movement deficit. Active management to restore movement includes relaxation, breathing control, postural training, graded exposure exercise, cardiovascular exercise, and graded functional restoration to normalize motor control. A reduction in MI and fear result in less pain and disability. Intervention strategies that usually result in avoiding movement are generally contraindicated. Focus on pain and stabilization exercises tends to reinforce avoidance of movement behavior.[443]

Subgroup: Motor Control Impairment Classification of Pain Provocation Behavior[443]

According to O'Sullivan,[443] this subgroup is common in clinical practice. In contrast to the MI subgroup, the MCI group has no MI or painful loss of movement in the direction of pain. The MCI group is associated with a loss of functional control around the neutral zone of the motion segment due to specific motor control deficits, and muscle guarding in some patients of the spinal stabilizing muscles in the primary direction of pain. These patients demonstrate through range pain or painful arc and end-range pain during both static and dynamic tasks potentially stressing pain sensitive tissue. These patients appear to develop compensatory strategies to stabilize the motion segment toward an end-range position of flexion, extension, or lateral shift. MCI patients also adopt postures and movements that are provocative but have no awareness that they are assuming altered patterns, possibly due to poor proprioceptive awareness of the lumbopelvic region[766] or a gradual onset of pain and absence of a withdrawal reflex. MCI, like MI, is a maladaptive response providing a strong mechanism for disability and persistent pain both peripherally and centrally mediated. Patients have movement-related fear due to use of provocative movement strategies and failure to respond to general exercise programs. MCIs may present in a unidirectional manner of flexion or extension (either active or passive) and lateral shift or multidirectional combinations. Five clinically observed directional patterns of flexion, lateral shift, passive extension, active extension, and multidirectional are described in detail by O'Sullivan[788,789] and summarized next.*

Management of the MCI group is based on a cognitive behavioral training model that aims to change movement behavior through physical and cognitive learning processes. Once again, the goal is to desensitize the nervous system by educating the patient to control postures and movement patterns to avoid repetitive strain to painful tissues, reduce peripheral nociceptive drive, and improve function. Improved motor control should reduce stress on painful tissue, which then diminishes peripheral nociceptive input, allowing the patient to manage the disorder with reduced fear and increased levels of function. The role of MT is limited only to improving movement away from the direction of pain if impaired or preventing motor control in this direction with gains in motion followed by active control procedures in that direction. Motor learning interventions using SSEs have been discussed previously and are briefly discussed as intervention strategies in the management of the MCI group based on current reports in the literature.[649,766,788,789]

Flexion Pattern

O'Sullivan[789] described this as the most common pattern. Patients have a primary complaint of central LBP related to a single or repeated flexion/rotation injury. Aggravating factors involve control of flexed spinal postures and movements or sustained flexion or semiflexed postures. Easing factors include upright or lordotic postures. Examination findings[789] are detailed next.

Posture and Movement Analysis—Flexion Pattern[789]

- *Standing*: Flat lumbar lordosis
- *Sitting*: Loss of segmental lumbar lordosis worse in sitting or flexed postures with a tendency to position in a posterior pelvic tilt and associated with increased upper lumbar and lower thoracic ES muscle tone and thoracic spine lordosis
- *AROM flexion*: Increased segmental flexion at the symptomatic level and increased upper lumbar lordosis; a painful arc may be present with difficulty returning to upright without use of the hands
- *AROM extension*: Increased extension above the symptomatic segment; reduced extension at the symptomatic segment
- *Movement*: Inability to perform anterior pelvic tilt and extend lower lumbar spine independent of thorax in supine, sitting, and 4-point kneeling
- *Movement*: In sitting, an inability to reposition to neutral with a tendency to favor flexion at the symptomatic segment
- *Movement*: Squatting, sitting with knee extension, and hip flexion reveal inability to control segmental lordosis and an anterior pelvic tilt with a tendency to flex at the symptomatic segment and posteriorly tilt the pelvis
- *PPIVM*: Testing reveals excessive segmental flexion and rotation at the symptomatic site; extension may be stiff
- *PAIVM*: PA motion may be stiff at the symptomatic segment

Specific Muscle Performance Tests

- Inability to activate deep muscles without breath holding; bracing of superficial abdominal muscles, excessive thoracolumbar ES activation, and a tendency to flex the lumbar spine and posteriorly rotate the pelvis resulting in a compensatory stabilization strategy that appears to hold the symptomatic segment in end-range flexion rather than providing control within the neutral zone
- Apical breathing pattern may be present with poor ability to perform diaphragmatic breathing; the diaphragm may act as a stabilizing muscle compromising its respiratory function.
- Inability to assume a neutral lumbar lordosis in 4-point kneeling and sitting
- Other: Gluteus maximus weakness and long, short hip flexors

Motor Learning Intervention Strategies—Cognitive Stage[789]

- Education patient with video or mirrors to gain awareness of the relationship between pain and how each patient controls the spine.
- Achieve control of neutral lordosis independent of thorax and hips through individualized training for each pattern.

*Information on pp 265-269 is adapted with permission from O'Sullivan P. Clinical instability of the lumbar spine: its pathological basis, diagnosis, and conservative management. In: Boyling JD, Jull GA, eds. *Grieve's Modern Manual Therapy*. 3rd ed. Philadelphia, PA: Elsevier; 2004:311-331. Copyright 2004 Elsevier.

- Facilitate anterior pelvic tilt and low lumbar lordosis in supine, crook-lying, 4-point kneeling, and sitting.
- When neutral lordosis is achieved, cocontraction of LM and TrA often occurs automatically. If not, LM and TrA contraction must be trained.
- Focus is more on LM and psoas with coactivation of pelvic floor and TrA without dominant ES.
- In the presence of a high load stabilizing strategy such as breath holding, dominant global muscle activation, or fixation of the rib cage during LM, TrA, and pelvic floor training, lateral costal diaphragmatic breathing training with independent TrA and pelvic floor activation is used to inhibit the dominant global system and achieve low-level voluntary cocontraction. Daily concentrated practice of 10 to 15 minutes progressing up to 5-minute holds is recommended before integration into functional tasks and aerobic activities. In patients with chronic disabling pain, this process may take up to 4 to 5 weeks.
- When low-level cocontraction of deep muscles in neutral lordosis with good breathing control and without global muscle substitution in sitting and standing is attained, reduction in pain should occur in these postures.

Motor Learning Intervention Strategies—Associative Stage[789]

- Focus is on integrating cocontraction of the local muscles while maintaining a neutral spine into dynamic tasks or static holding postures with the intent to refine individualized poor movement patterns during activities such as sit-to-stand, walking, lifting, forward bending, backward bending, and reaching.
- Provocative movement patterns are broken down into simple steps. Each step is practiced in neutral spine posture with high repetitions up to 40 to 50. Individual steps are carried out at home on a daily basis with pain control. Awareness of optimal posture and movements throughout the day is reinforced.
- Regular exercise such as walking or swimming while maintaining a low-level stabilizing cocontraction for 30 minutes is recommended. This stage varies from weeks to months as patients gain the ability to carry out daily activities with minimal discomfort. Formal PT stops at this point.

Motor Learning Intervention Strategies—Autonomous Stage[789]

- Minimal attention is now required for correct task performance.
- Higher load activities and cardiovascular programs are initiated.
- This approach requires a high level of patient motivation, compliance, awareness or concentration on daily and quality performance with the goal of allowing each patient the opportunity to gain control of his or her pain.

Lateral Shift Pattern

O'Sullivan[789] suggested that a lateral shift is usually associated with a flexion/lateral shift pattern or, more rarely, an extension/lateral shift pattern. The mechanism of injury is a traumatic or repetitive flexion/rotation injury that usually presents with unilateral LBP. Aggravating factors include reaching or rotating in one direction while in a flexed posture with minimal movement. Easing factors include extended positions. Examination findings[789] are detailed next.

Posture and Movement Analysis—Lateral Shift Pattern[789]

- *Standing*: Decreased lordosis with or without segmental lateral shift; palpation of LM in standing reveals atrophy on the side contralateral to the shift
- *Single-limb stance*: Enhances the shift on the ipsilateral side and during gait
- *AROM flexion*: Increased flexion and lateral trunk deviation above the symptomatic segment; return to upright reveals thoracolumbar extension, but the symptomatic segment remains flexed
- *AROM extension*: Increased extension above the symptomatic segment with lateral deviation; reduced extension at the symptomatic segment
- *Movement*: Squatting, sitting, and sit-to-stand are similar to the flexion pattern with a tendency to shift
- *PPIVM*: Unidirectional segmental increase into flexion, rotation, and LF to the side of the shift

Specific Muscle Performance Tests[789]

- Dominant thoracolumbar ES and LM on the ipsilateral side of the shift and a loss of rotary and lateral trunk control in the direction of the shift contralateral LM deficit
- Inability to reposition the lumbar spine within the neutral zone with a tendency to overshoot into flexion and laterally deviate toward the shift
- Inability to cocontract the LM and deep abdominal muscles on the side opposite to the segmental lateral shift
- The compensatory strategy to stabilize the symptomatic segment involves lumbar ES, quadratus lumborum, and, in some cases, LM on the ipsilateral side of the shift; breath holding and abdominal bracing may occur. This strategy appears to hold the symptomatic

segment in flexion and LF rather than within the neutral zone.

- Other: Unilateral gluteus maximus weakness, iliopsoas weakness, and long or short hip flexors

Motor Learning Intervention Strategies—Cognitive Stage[789]

- Patient education with video or mirrors is the same as the flexion pattern.
- Achieve control of neutral lordosis independent of thorax and hips through individualized training for each pattern.
- Facilitate anterior pelvic tilt and low lumbar lordosis in supine, crook-lying, 4-point kneeling, and sitting; ensure central loading of the spine over the pelvis (ie, correct the shift), especially when training in sitting.
- When neutral lordosis is achieved, cocontraction of deep muscles often occurs automatically. If not, LM and TrA contraction must be trained.
- Focus is on activation of unilaterally inhibited LM and psoas in cocontraction of the TrA while maintaining neutral spine posture.
- In the presence of a high load stabilizing strategy, the guidelines are the same as in the flexion pattern.
- When low-level cocontraction of deep muscles in neutral lordosis with good breathing control and without global muscle substitution in sitting and standing is attained, reduction in pain should occur in these postures.

Motor Learning Intervention Strategies—Associative and Autonomous Stages[789]

Guidelines are the same as discussed under the flexion pattern.

Active Extension Pattern

O'Sullivan[789] reported that this group has central LBP that is worse with extension movements. In active extension, the lumbar spine is actively held in extension with high levels of muscle activity from the segmental back extensors and iliopsoas. The mechanism of injury is related to a single or repetitive extension/rotation injury often associated with sporting activities. Aggravating factors include standing; erect sitting; forward bending with the spine held in extension; overhead activities; and inability to walk fast, run, and swim. Easing factors include flexed postures. Examination findings[789] are detailed next.

Posture and Movement Analysis—Active Extension Pattern[789]

- *Standing*: Tendency to hold the lumbar spine in hyperlordosis at the symptomatic segment during upright postures and tasks; the pelvis is often in anterior pelvic tilt with the thorax relatively anterior to the pelvis
- *Sitting*: The hyperlordotic posture and anterior pelvic rotations with difficulty relaxing the lumbar spine and posteriorly tilting the pelvis
- *AROM flexion*: Increased hip flexion with a tendency to hold the lumbar spine in lordosis, especially at the symptomatic segment with or without mid-range loss of flexion and a painful arc; return to neutral reveals a tendency to increase lordosis at the symptomatic segment before the upright posture with pain on return and the need to assist with the hands
- *AROM extension*: Increased extension at the symptomatic segment with anterior pelvic rotation
- *Movement*: Squatting, sit-to-stand, and gait reveal increased lumbar spine lordosis
- *PPIVM*: Increased extension and rotation at the symptomatic segment; flexion may be stiff
- *PAIVM*: Painful increase in PA motion

Specific Muscle Performance Tests[789]

- Inability to cocontract the deep muscles in neutral spine with a tendency to hyperextend lower lumbar spine with dominant ES, breath holding, or apical breathing
- Inability to initiate posterior pelvic tilt independent of hip flexion
- Hip and knee extension in prone reveal a loss of cocontraction of the deep abdominals and a dominant ES pattern, resulting in excessive segmental lumbar spine extension at the symptomatic level.
- Inability to reposition the spine in the neutral zone with a tendency to overshoot into extension
- The compensatory strategy to stabilize the lumbar spine involves dominant lumbar spine ES, iliopsoas, and some superficial LM and abdominal bracing by the diaphragm and superficial abdominal muscles holding the symptomatic segment in extension rather than in the neutral zone.
- Other: Weak gluteus maximus, overactive psoas with a tendency to extend the lumbar spine, and short hip flexors

Motor Learning Intervention Strategies—Cognitive Stage[789]

- Patient education with video or mirrors is the same as the flexion pattern.
- Achieve control of neutral lordosis independent of thorax and hips through individualized training.

- Facilitate posterior pelvic tilt and flex the spine toward a more neutral lordosis in supine crook-lying; ensure disassociation of posterior pelvic tilt from the hip; inhibit dominant hip flexors and superficial LM.
- When neutral lordosis is achieved, cocontraction of LM and TrA often occurs automatically; if not, LM and TrA contraction must be trained.
- Focus is on deep muscle system to reduce lordosis without dominant ES.
- In the presence of a high load stabilizing strategy, the guidelines are the same as in the flexion pattern.
- When low-level cocontraction of deep muscles in neutral lordosis with good breathing control and without global muscle substitution in sitting and standing is attained, reduction in pain should occur in these postures.

Motor Learning Intervention Strategies—Associative and Autonomous Stages[789]

Guidelines are the same as discussed under the flexion pattern.

Passive Extension Pattern[789]

In contrast to the active extension pattern, these patients present with low tone of the LM, iliopsoas, and ES muscles and do have the ability to reverse their lumbar lordosis. The mechanism of injury is traumatic or repetitive injury in extension. Aggravating factors include extension activities and standing postures. Easing factors include flexion activities and postures. Examination findings[789] are detailed next.

Posture and Movement Analysis—Passive Extension Pattern[789]

- *Standing*: Swayback posture with the thorax posterior to the pelvis with hinging of the symptomatic segment into extension; muscle tone is reduced in the transverse abdominal wall, LM, ES, and gluteal muscles with tonic activation of the superficial abdominals; compression through the shoulders increases the segmental hinging and increases the symptoms
- *Sitting*: Slumped posture
- *AROM flexion*: Usually pain-free with a tendency to overshoot and hinge into extension
- *AROM extension*: Increased extension at the symptomatic segment; reduced extension above the symptomatic segment; excessive pelvic sway; a painful arc is possible with end-range symptoms
- *Movement*: In sitting and 4-point kneeling, inability to extend the thoracolumbar spine above the symptomatic segment with a tendency to hinge into extension at the symptomatic segment
- *Movement*: Inability to posteriorly rotate the pelvis without dominant superficial abdominals and flexion of the thorax
- *PPIVM*: Increased extension

Specific Muscle Performance Tests[789]

- Tendency to flex the thorax and upper lumbar spine with dominant upper abdominal wall, breath holding, or apical breathing with attempts to activate the TrA and pelvic floor
- Inability to activate LM at and above the symptomatic segment
- The compensations strategy involves dominant activation of the superficial abdominals with inhibition of the deep abdominals and psoas, resulting in hinging of the symptomatic segment.
- Other: Weak gluteus maximus bilaterally, weak iliopsoas, and long or short hip flexors

Motor Learning Intervention Strategies—Cognitive Stage[789]

- Patient education is the same as in the flexion pattern discussed previously.
- Achieve control of neutral lordosis independent of thorax and hips through individualized training for each pattern.
- In sitting with the thorax anterior to the pelvis, which inhibits superficial abdominals, facilitate a neutral lordosis above the symptomatic segment while maintaining a neutral lordosis below the symptomatic segment.
- When neutral lordosis is achieved, cocontraction of LM and TrA often occurs automatically; if not, LM and TrA contraction must be trained.
- Focus is on LM and psoas in cocontraction with the TrA while inhibiting the superficial abdominals while maintaining neutral spine posture.
- In the presence of a high load stabilizing strategy, guidelines are the same as in the flexion pattern.
- When low-level cocontraction of deep muscles in neutral lordosis with good breathing control and without global muscle substitution in sitting and standing is attained, reduction in pain should occur in these postures.

Motor Learning Intervention Strategies—Associative and Autonomous Stages[789]

Guidelines are the same as discussed under the flexion pattern.

Multidirectional Pattern

O'Sullivan[789] described this pattern as the most debilitating of the clinical presentations. Provocative movements are multidirectional in nature with high levels of pain and functional disability. The patient describes "locking" of the spine after sustained flexion and extension. All weightbearing postures are painful. Easing positions are difficult to find in weightbearing. Examination findings[789] are detailed next.

Posture and Movement Analysis—Multidirectional Pattern[789]

- Assumed postures are variable.
- Movements in all directions can be painful with segmental shifting, hinging patterns, and observable lumbar ES guarding.
- There is difficulty with assuming neutral lumbar lordosis.
- Neutral zone repositioning is impaired in variable directions.

Specific Muscle Performance Tests[789]

- Attempts to activate the deep muscle system result in a global system strategy, breath holding, and pain.
- In the presence of high irritability, all compressive loading positions are painful.
- The compensatory stabilization strategy is variable, with difficulty attaining and maintaining neutral positions.
- Variable compensatory strategies at end-range segmental positions are used to achieve stability.
- Other: Bilateral gluteus maximus weakness; iliopsoas may or may not be weak; and short hip flexors are long.
- Prognosis is poor for conservative management, but management would follow the previous concepts for enhancing motor control.*

Reliability and Validity of the Chronic Low Back Pain Classification System Using a Mechanism-Based Classification Method

The nature of CLBP is complex with a definite need to understand the biopsychosocial mechanisms underlying the pain disorder. In some patients, maladaptive MI and MCIs result in either excessive or impaired static and dynamic spinal stability that becomes the mechanism for ongoing pain. This classification identifies subgroups of patients for whom PT intervention is indicated or contraindicated, as well as provides guidance for specifically directed interventions to address the primary and secondary drivers of pain.

Several studies show acceptable reliability using a mechanism-based classification for CLBP.[790-792] Based upon a comprehensive clinical examination, Dankaerts et al[791] reported almost perfect agreement (κ = 0.96; 97% agreement) between 2 expert clinicians when classifying 35 patients with nonspecific CLBP into the 5 subgroups of MCI. Also in this study, 25 of the 35 patients were randomly selected and classified by 13 different raters. Agreement among the 13 raters was moderate to excellent (mean κ = 0.61; agreement 70%). Fersum et al[792] examined the intertester reliability of 4 trained clinicians to independently classify 26 patients with nonspecific LBP using the mechanism-based classification by O'Sullivan.[443] Reliability was determined at 6 levels of the diagnostic clinical reasoning process (see Figure 4-2). All patients were classified with nonspecific LBP (98% agreement—level 1). All patients had a peripheral pain source (98% agreement—level 2). One patient was classified with PGP (100% agreement) and the rest with LBP (99% agreement—level 3). Level 4 considered subgrouping as MCI (24 patients, 99% agreement), MI (1 patient, 75% agreement), or increased or decreased force closure for pelvic pain (1 patient, 100% agreement). At level 5, classification of the primary directional pattern of provocation demonstrated a mean κ of 0.82 (0.66 to 0.90) and mean agreement of 86% (73% to 92%). For detecting psychosocial influence (level 6), mean κ was 0.65 (0.57 to 0.74) and mean agreement was 87% (85% to 92%). Substantial clinician agreement supports the clinical usefulness and face validity of this classification system.

Dankaerts et al[386,444,793,794] provide evidence for the construct validity of this classification system. Usual and slump sitting postures of subjects with nonspecific CLBP classification (20 flexion pattern; 13 active extension) patterns were compared to asymptomatic subjects. Patients with an active extension pattern sat with a more lordotic posture at the symptomatic lower lumbar spine. Patients with a flexion pattern sat with a more kyphotic posture when compared with healthy controls. Both groups had decreased ability to change their lumbosacral posture. Differences in sitting posture in these subgroups support the proposed MCI classification.[793]

The results of Dankaerts et al[793] demonstrated that, compared to controls, the active extension group presents with high levels of cocontraction of the superficial LM, thoracolumbar ES, and internal oblique during usual sitting. The flexion pattern group had less activation of these muscles than the active extension group and trended lower when compared to controls. The flexion relaxation ratio of the back muscles was lower for all nonspecific CLBP. These findings clearly discriminate 2 subgroups of CLBP from the asymptomatic group but need to be confirmed in a larger study.

Dankaerts et al[795] developed a statistical classification model to discriminate 2 subgroups of nonspecific CLBP, flexion pattern and active extension, and a pain-free control group using trunk muscle activation and lumbosacral kinematics during aggravating postures such as standing, usual and slump sitting, and movements of AROM flexion and return and extension. The following variables correctly classified 96.4% of the cases: lower lumbar kinematics in sitting and forward bending and lack of flexion relaxation of the superficial LM in slump sitting and end-range flexion. This study demonstrated differences between the 3 groups (no LBP, flexion pattern, and active extension) in trunk muscle activation and lumbosacral kinematics that supports the classification system based on different underlying mechanisms of pain proposed by O'Sullivan et al.[649,766,788,789]

Using a case study, Dankaerts et al[795] illustrated a targeted motor learning intervention to describe a successful outcome of normalized motor control in a patient classified with a multidirectional MCI. The improvement in motor control was associated with reduced pain, disability, and fear related to movement at 3, 6, and 12 months. Objective laboratory tests, surface EMG, and spinal kinematics were performed on the subject and a pain-free control. Patient management included motor control learning based on a cognitive behavioral model progressed during 8 visits over 14 weeks. During the cognitive stage, a clinician provided patient education to the patient—a 37-year-old mother of 2 who worked as a nurse—regarding the mechanism of ongoing pain sensitization, mechanics of the spine, ongoing tissue sensitization due to habitual adoption of end-range postures, and the importance of the muscle system. The patient was made aware that the habitual postures and patterns of movement adopted had in fact resulted in maintaining the pain. She was made aware that she had no sense or control of neutral spine, nor an ability to preferentially activate the deep muscle system and gluteal muscles. The first exercise was to control the lumbopelvic region through the mid-range independent from the thorax in supine crook lying. Then, cocontraction of the deep muscles was performed in side-lying. In sitting, the patient was taught to maintain a posture of neutral lordosis and relaxation of the thoracolumbar region with cocontraction of the TrA/internal oblique and progressed to standing. When cocontraction in neutral was achieved in sitting and standing, instruction progressed to the associative stage, which included static holding and dynamic tasks such as single leg stance, sit-to-stand, squatting, and lifting. Additional recommendations for exercises during this stage included gentle aerobic activities such as walking or cycling with low-level cocontraction of the TrA and abdominal wall with neutral spine posture. At 10 weeks, hand weights were added to squats and sit-to-stand to increase global strength. The autonomous stage was reached when the patient could carry out functional movement tasks with a low degree of attention. At discharge, the patient was asked to remain aware of spinal posture and maintain cardiovascular fitness, alternating between walking and exercise biking.[795]

The authors hypothesized that the reduction in pain intensity and disability was primarily due to improvement in spinal control, which in turn reduced the peripheral nociceptive driver of pain. Cognitive factors such as patient awareness, better coping strategies, and improved function played a role in reducing central drivers of pain. This case provides low-level evidence to document successful outcomes from the use of this classification to direct specific intervention, but the case does not tell us whether pain caused the motor control changes or whether motor control changes resulted in pain.[795]

Luomajoki et al[796] performed a controlled case series study on 38 patients (21 females, 17 males) with a diagnosis of nonspecific CLBP subclassified as MCI to investigate the effects of a specific exercise approach intervention. MCI subclassification was not further classified into specific directional patterns. Treatment effects were evaluated using 6 movement control tests (MCT) that are reliable with face validity (Figure 4-136), patient-specific PSFS, and RMDQ. Average treatment sessions were 9 (SD 4.6). MCT improved 59% from 3.2 (max 6) to 1.3 ($d = 1.3$, $P < .001$), complaints (PSFS, max 10) decreased 41% from 5.9 points to 3.5 ($d = 1.3$, $P < .001$) and disability (RMDQ, max 24) decreased 43% from 8.9 points to 5.1 ($d = 1.0$, $P < .001$). Despite lack of a control group, this study provides preliminary evidence for continued study using this classification system.

Fersum et al[797] examined the efficacy of classification-based cognitive functional PT targeting maladaptive cognition, lifestyle, pain, and movement according to the O'Sullivan[443] system as compared to MT and exercise in patients with nonspecific CLBP of more than 52 weeks duration. The classification-based cognitive functional therapy was more effective than MT and exercise for localized nonspecific CLBP at 1-year follow-up, providing preliminary support for this approach. However, longitudinal studies are needed to document outcomes in the specific subgroups of nonspecific CLBP following a targeted intervention.

Current Evidence for Nonsurgical Management of Chronic Low Back Pain

Considering the wide variation of intervention strategies for CLBP, van Middelkoop et al[798] examined 83 RCTs up to December 2008 to determine the effectiveness of physical rehabilitation interventions for nonspecific CLBP. Selection criteria consist of adults 18 years and older with nonspecific CLBP persisting for at least 12 weeks. PPPP and postoperative studies were excluded. No statistically significant difference in reduction of pain and disability was found between exercise therapy (ET) and no

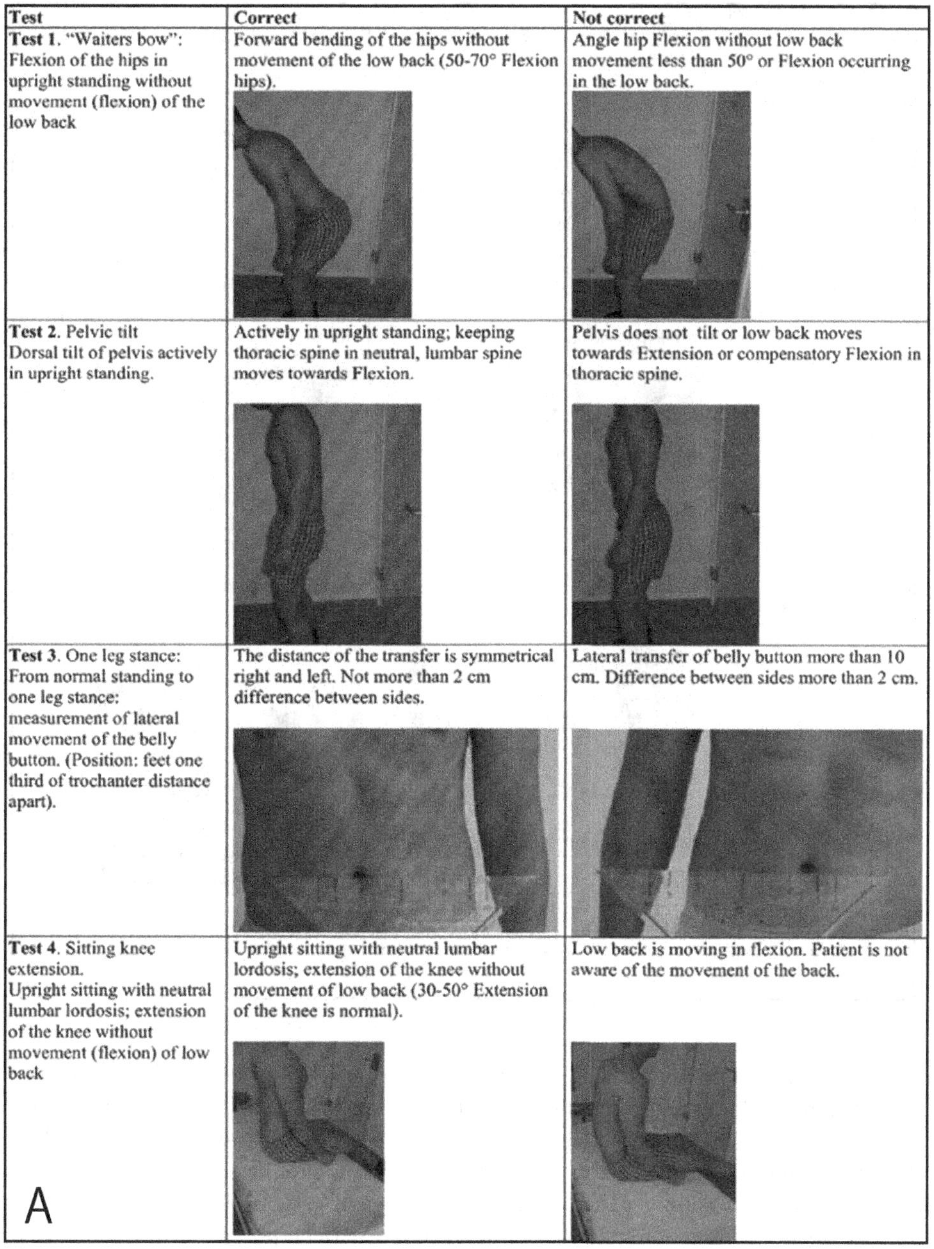

Test	Correct	Not correct
Test 1. "Waiters bow": Flexion of the hips in upright standing without movement (flexion) of the low back	Forward bending of the hips without movement of the low back (50-70° Flexion hips).	Angle hip Flexion without low back movement less than 50° or Flexion occurring in the low back.
Test 2. Pelvic tilt Dorsal tilt of pelvis actively in upright standing.	Actively in upright standing; keeping thoracic spine in neutral, lumbar spine moves towards Flexion.	Pelvis does not tilt or low back moves towards Extension or compensatory Flexion in thoracic spine.
Test 3. One leg stance: From normal standing to one leg stance: measurement of lateral movement of the belly button. (Position: feet one third of trochanter distance apart).	The distance of the transfer is symmetrical right and left. Not more than 2 cm difference between sides.	Lateral transfer of belly button more than 10 cm. Difference between sides more than 2 cm.
Test 4. Sitting knee extension. Upright sitting with neutral lumbar lordosis; extension of the knee without movement (flexion) of low back	Upright sitting with neutral lumbar lordosis; extension of the knee without movement of low back (30-50° Extension of the knee is normal).	Low back is moving in flexion. Patient is not aware of the movement of the back.

A

Figure 4-136. Description of 6 MCTs. *(continued)*

treatment/waiting list controls, between ET compared to back school education, and between exercise and behavioral therapy. Compared to usual care in the short term, pain intensity and disability were significantly reduced by ET and function improved in the long term. No consensus exists regarding the optimal exercise approach. No difference in effect was found between ET compared to TENS, laser, ultrasound, massage on pain, and disability at short-term follow-up. TENS is not supported compared to placebo in the management of CLBP. No difference was found between exercise compared to MT or manipulation at short- and long-term follow-up. No studies reported on the effectiveness of lumbar supports. This systematic review highlights the inability to draw firm conclusions and inform decision making from low-quality research on heterogeneous populations with CLBP, and it supports the need for continued research on specific subgroups of patients with CLBP using a biopsychosocial approach.

Van Middelkoop et al[798] underscored the use of biopsychosocial approaches such as interdisciplinary or behavioral as the most promising interventions for CLBP. In this review, behavioral therapy had an effect on pain intensity possibly related to the combined different strategies to modify behavior, cognition, and physical function. Because of the lack of or conflicting evidence on the effectiveness of different interventions, only interdisciplinary treatment, behavioral treatment, and ET should be provided as conservative treatment for CLBP. However, no consensus exists regarding the most effective program design. Further research based on subgroups and matching intervention is needed to provide optimal management of this population.[798]

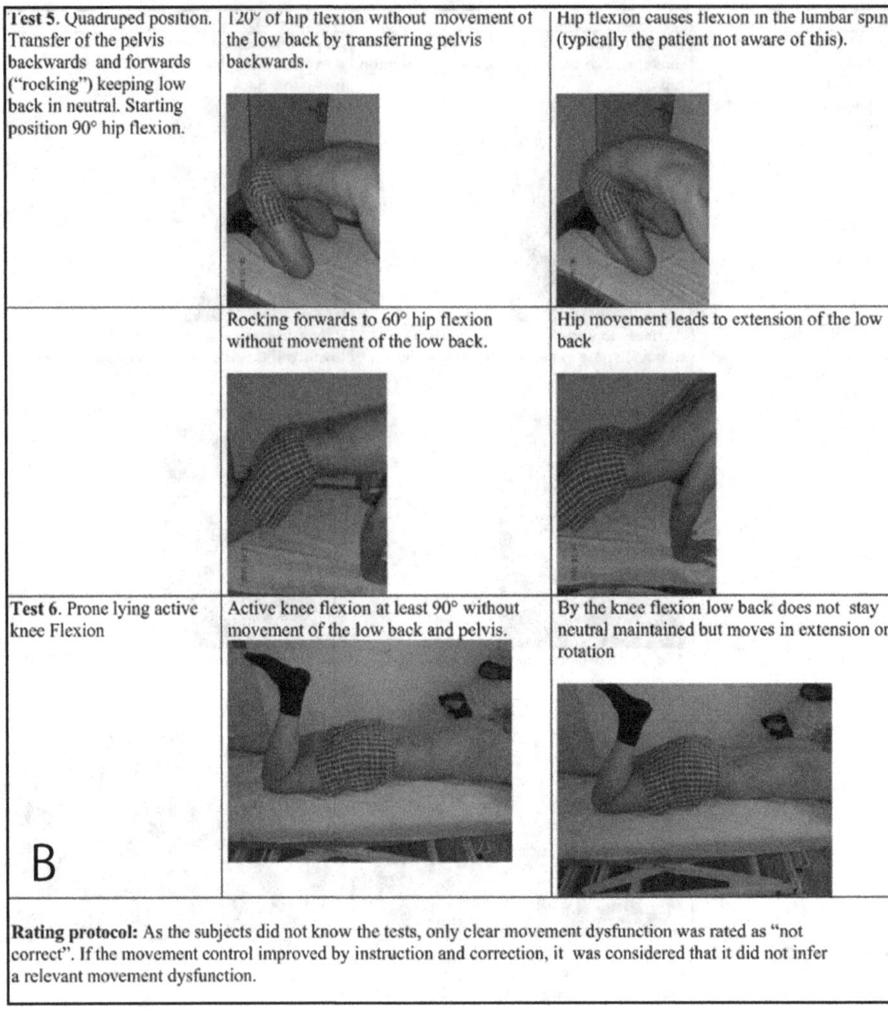
Test 5. Quadruped position. Transfer of the pelvis backwards and forwards ("rocking") keeping low back in neutral. Starting position 90° hip flexion.
120° of hip flexion without movement of the low back by transferring pelvis backwards.
Hip flexion causes flexion in the lumbar spine (typically the patient not aware of this).
Rocking forwards to 60° hip flexion without movement of the low back.
Hip movement leads to extension of the low back
Test 6. Prone lying active knee Flexion
Active knee flexion at least 90° without movement of the low back and pelvis.
By the knee flexion low back does not stay neutral maintained but moves in extension or rotation
B
Rating protocol: As the subjects did not know the tests, only clear movement dysfunction was rated as "not correct". If the movement control improved by instruction and correction, it was considered that it did not infer a relevant movement dysfunction.

Figure 4-136 (continued). Description of 6 MCTs. (Reprinted with permission from Luomajoki H, Kool J, de Bruin ED, Airaksinen O. Improvement in low back movement control, decreased pain and disability, resulting from specific exercise intervention. *Sports Med Arthrosc Rehabil Ther Technol.* 2010;2:11. Available at: http://www.smarttjournal.com/content/2/1/11. Accessed March 7, 2011. © 2008 Luomajoki et al; licensee BioMed Central Ltd. Available at http://www.biomedcentral.com/1471-2474/9/170. This is an Open Access article distributed under the terms of the Creative Commons Attribution License [http://creativecommons.org/licenses/by/2.0], which permits unrestricted use, distribution, and reproduction in any medium, provided that the original work is properly cited.)

MT intervention for CLBP is not included in the previous review, but it is the subject of several reviews. Bokarius and Bokarius[799] performed an evidence-based review of MT efficacy in the treatment of chronic musculoskeletal pain, with 11 trials related to CLBP meeting the inclusion criteria. The reviewers report conflicting evidence and conclude that strong evidence supports HVLA manipulation, MET, and spinal stabilization for treating CLBP. However, lower-level evidence does not support manipulation and mobilization for CLBP. No clear conclusions can be drawn regarding the best MT treatment for CLBP.

Rubinstein et al[800] also reported on the effectiveness of SMT for CLBP by examining 26 RCTs, 9 with low risk of bias. The authors reported high-quality evidence that SMT has a small, statistically significant, but not clinically relevant, short-term effect on pain relief and functional status compared to other interventions such as ET, standard medical care, or PT in general. Low- to high-quality evidence suggests that SMT, when added to another intervention, has a significant short-term effect on pain and functional status. Very low-quality evidence suggests that SMT alone is no more effective than passive intervention or sham SMT for short-term pain relief or function. No serious complications are recorded with SMT. Very little data are available related to recovery, return-to-work, quality of life, and costs of care. Clinicians should exercise caution when generalizing the findings of systematic reviews to clinical practice. Differences in patient populations are likely to be included in reviews, and distinguishing characteristics such as severity are not always available. Additionally, definitions of level of evidence vary. A wide variation of manipulation, mobilization, and PT approaches are applied with little to no written description of the specific interventions, which may affect outcomes. In the absence of robust data from systematic reviews and meta-analysis of classified subgroups of patients with CLBP, clinicians should review individual high-quality RCTs for applicability to particular patients.

Considering the importance of classification in clinical research and emerging evidence regarding the potential benefits of MT and exercise over exercise alone in some patients, Fersum et al[801] reviewed the literature on RCTs evaluating MT treatment and ET for patients with nonspecific CLBP. Additionally, the focus of this review examines the integration of subclassification in these RCTs as well as the treatment effects of the studies with subclassification and matched treatments. A total of 767 RCTs were identified. Only 68 focused on MT or ET. Only 5 studies had some form of subclassification beyond general inclusion and exclusion criteria. While the data should be interpreted with caution due to low numbers of studies, meta-analysis of these 5 studies indicates a statistically significant effect favoring matched intervention where subclassification is used. Significant effects were for the short term for pain and disability and the long term of 36 to 52 weeks follow-up for pain intensity, but not disability. Studies involving subgroups are extremely limited. The authors support the need for future research using subgroup classification consistent with the biopsychosocial model and interventions targeting the underlying mechanisms.

Despite a large number of randomized controlled clinical trials evaluating the effectiveness of treatment for non-specific CLBP, a lack of evidence for successful outcomes is apparent for generic, single-focus interventions. The majority of RCTs include heterogeneous study groups that may hinder finding a treatment effect. Any positive effects for a particular subgroup are diluted because of an absent effect in other subgroups. Interdisciplinary approaches that target maladaptive cognitive, neurophysiological, and social influences and relevant physical impairments that often underlie and drive nonspecific CLBP may be the key to better outcomes.

Evidence for a Cognitive Behavioral Approach for Chronic Low Back Pain

Cognitive behavioral therapies are psychological interventions for CLBP designed to enhance a patient's control over pain and increase function. Most approaches are part of interdisciplinary treatment including medical and PT, usually over 8 to 12 individual or group sessions. Many techniques use quotas or goals for gradual return to activities, family involvement, reframing of affective and cognitive responses, and introduction of positive coping and relaxation skills. Patients must incorporate these skills into their lifestyle through practice, self-evaluation and monitoring, and social reinforcement. The basis of this therapy centers on the role that a person's beliefs, attitudes, and behaviors play in determining the overall experience of pain.

A Cochrane review[802] examined 30 studies to evaluate 3 behavioral approaches for CLBP:

1. *Operant*: Acknowledges that external factors such as compensation, family attention, and diagnostic labels reinforce pain behavior
2. *Cognitive*: Deals with thoughts, feelings, beliefs, or a combination of the 3 that can trigger pain
3. *Respondent*: Deals with interrupting muscle tension with progressive relaxation techniques or biofeedback of muscle activity

For pain relief, there was moderate quality evidence that operant therapy was more effective than waiting list controls in the short term; there was little or no difference between operant therapy, cognitive therapy, or a combination of behavioral therapies in the short or intermediate term; and behavioral treatment was more effective than usual care of PT, back school, and/or medical treatments in the short term, but there was no difference in the intermediate to long term or functional status. Over a longer term, little or no difference exists between behavioral treatment and group exercise for pain relief or reduced depressive symptoms. The addition of behavioral therapy to inpatient rehabilitation did not appear to increase the effect of inpatient rehabilitation alone.

Operant conditioning, concerned with movement behavior, is suggested as the best approach for use by physical therapists[803] because its key concepts are active participation based on graded functional goals and quota-based activity agreed upon by the patient and clinician. The clinician uses positive reinforcement of appropriate pain behaviors ensuring that pain does not interfere with activity progression. Additional benefits are possible if modification of negative pain behavior interrupts the fear-avoidance cycle.[185] In acute or subacute LBP, the goal is to prevent progression to a chronic pain state. In CLBP, the goal is to reduce disability.[804]

Bunzli et al[805] reviewed current literature on whether physical therapist-led operant conditioning (POC) is more effective than comparison interventions in reducing LBP disability. Eight of 15 trials subgrouped as acute, subacute, and chronic reported a clinically significant difference. All active interventions and control interventions (ie, placebo or waiting list) were effective in reducing disability reflecting a likely placebo effect and the natural progression of LBP. The use of one active treatment such as exercise, usual care (ie, clinical practice guidelines or patient decides), or biomedical-based PT (ie, therapist discretion) over another is not supported by strong evidence. POC intervention was not inferior to any of the comparison interventions in reducing disability in any subgroup. Moderate evidence found that POC is more effective than other behavioral interventions in reducing long-term disability in CLBP. Moderate evidence showed POC may be more effective than other treatments in reducing posttreatment fear-avoidance beliefs in a subacute population, but less effective in reducing short-term fear-avoidance beliefs in a population with mixed LBP. POC was not found to have a clinically significant effect on disability in a mixed LBP population. Moderate evidence showed POC is more effective than a placebo intervention in reducing short-term pain in subacute LBP. Once again, heterogeneity of studies or variations in treatment techniques of the same name, dosage, and duration as wells as failure to subgroup CLBP patients appropriately were limitations in drawing firm conclusions. The authors concluded that POC may be considered efficacious in the treatment of acute, subacute, and CLBP with the added effect of reducing long-term disability in CLBP.[805]

Most CBT approaches for chronic pain incorporate several strategies such as education, graded exposure, graded exercise, and confrontation of negative beliefs and appraisals that are likely to be effective at reducing threat and fear-avoidance beliefs. Early reports have shown that a CBT approach can lead to reduced fear-avoidance beliefs and treatment success.[806,807] The CBT approach is not standardized but may include self-instruction such as imagery and motivational self-talk, relaxation or biofeedback, expansion of coping strategies such as assertiveness and reduction of negative cognition, changing maladaptive beliefs, and personal goal setting. The cost-effectiveness of comprehensive pain management programs is emerging in the evidence-based literature.[808]

Graded Exercise and Graded Exposure in Chronic Low Back Pain

Graded exercise and graded exposure utilize positive behavioral and cognitive influences to confront, prescribe, and dose functional activity without a goal of pain resolution. In graded exposure, the clinician and patient establish a set of most feared to least feared activities or situations. Exposure begins with the least feared activity addressing the feared consequences of exposure, incorrect appraisals, and beliefs, which leads to decreased anxiety about the activity and increased participation. Graded exercise and activity, as previously discussed, use operant conditioning to improve exercise and activity tolerance and reinforce healthy functional behaviors. More research in this area is needed, but preliminary results are promising

A systematic review by Macedo et al[809] evaluated the effectiveness of graded exercise and activity or graded exposure related to pain, disability, GPE, or work status outcomes for persistent or recurrent LBP of more than 6 weeks' duration. Graded exercise and activity are effective, but no form of exercise is superior to another. Graded exercise and activity are slightly more effective than a minimal intervention for pain and disability in the short and intermediate terms, but not more effective than other forms of exercise for pain, disability, and GPE in the short and intermediate terms. Graded exposure is no more effective than a minimal intervention or graded exercise and activity, but a small number of studies limit the strength of this conclusion.

Within an interdisciplinary rehabilitation program for CLBP, George et al[810] investigated whether pain and disability outcomes differed between PT supplemented with either graded exercise or graded exposure principles. Findings should be interpreted with caution since the study lacked a control and randomized treatment. The authors concluded that either graded exposure or graded exercise resulted in equivalent clinical outcomes for pain intensity and disability with modest treatment effects. Only 50% of patients met the minimally acceptable change for pain and 30% for disability. Reductions in pain and disability were associated with decreases in depression and catastrophizing, respectively, but not associated with the specific behavioral intervention. A clinical commentary and review of 2 patient cases using graded exposure in PT is available for further review.[811]

Further research supports the use of graded exercise in PT. Rasmussen-Barr et al[812] compared the effects of an 8-week supervised, graded exercise intervention of SSEs with a daily walking program for patients with recurrent nonspecific LBP who were still employed (n = 71; ages 18 to 60). The main outcomes were Oswestry LBP Questionnaire, pain on 100-mm VAS, a self-efficacy scale, modified FABQ, and SF-36 Health Survey. The stabilization program was individually progressed and based on daily low load endurance exercises.[492,493] The walking program consisted of unsupervised, 30-minute daily walks as fast as possible in a pain-free manner and general home exercises. The walking group met with a physical therapist during the first week and eighth week of the program. The stabilization group met weekly for a 45-minute session. The main results suggest that a graded exercise intervention focused on specific stability exercise improves perceived disability at 12 months and long term at 36 months and pain only in the short term. Long-term physical health ratings and self-efficacy beliefs improved in the graded exercise groups, but no effects were observed for fear-avoidance beliefs. The authors suggested that the exercises might change self-efficacy beliefs, resulting in reduced perceived disability and reduced need for recurrent treatment in the long term.[812]

As part of a cognitive behavioral approach of graded exercise, activity and exposure integrated with PT have potential as interventions for CLBP. Based on limited research, no form of exercise is superior to another and both strategies produce similar outcomes. A comprehensive approach to CBT should also include patient education and confrontation of negative beliefs in order to be effective at reducing threat and fear-avoidance beliefs.

The Role of Neurophysiology Education in Chronic Low Back Pain

MT, specific exercise, and education seem to promote successful outcomes by targeting specific mechanisms related to CLBP, but may not directly target psychosocial aspects of pain.[786] Generally, patient education alone or in combination with MT and/or exercise includes aspects of tissue healing, ergonomics, pathoanatomy, or biomechanics. In dealing with cognitive and behavioral aspects of CLBP, Mosely[786] suggested the use of pain education as a way to address psychosocial factors, reduce threatening input, and decrease activity of the pain neuromatrix, thereby reducing its value. The main goal of education is to decrease the threat value associated with pain by increasing patient understanding. Compassionate and respectful teaching about pain science leads to altered beliefs and attitudes about pain[784] and increased pain thresholds.[785]

Moseley[786] examined the efficacy of a 4-week, 2 times per week, PT treatment including MT, exercise, and pain education in patients with chronic disabling back pain. Fifty-seven patients were randomly assigned to receive therapist-directed mobilization or manipulation, soft tissue or neural mobilization, and SSE with no modalities. Each patient received 4 one-on-one sessions with a physical therapist specifically trained in neurophysiology of pain education. The control group was managed by a general practitioner. Both groups improved on pain and disability, the physiotherapy and pain education group significantly more than the medical care group. The therapy program reduced pain and disability by a mean of 1.5/10 points on an NPRS (95% CI: 0.7 to 2.3) and 3.9 points on the 18-point RMQ (95% CI: 2 to 5.8), respectively. The number needed to treat in order to gain a clinically meaningful change was 3 (95% CI: 3 to 8) for pain and 2 (95% CI: 2 to 5) for disability. A treatment effect was maintained at 1-year follow-up with patients in the treatment group seeking fewer health care visits.

Considering that the main goal of education is to decrease the threat value associated with pain by increasing a patient's understanding, Moseley[784] investigated the relationship between a change in pain cognition (ie, decreased neuromatrix input) and physical performance as measured by SLR and forward bending tests in patients with CLBP. A main assumption is that cognitive factors may cause persistent changes in movement patterns. Patients with CLBP (n = 121) participated in a single one-on-one, 3-hour education intervention. Patients were educated on either pain physiology or lumbar spine physiology during which they had no opportunity to move or be active. Subjects in the pain physiology group tended to shift toward a decrease in the threat value of back pain while the lumbar spine physiology group shifted toward an increase in the threat value of back pain. The direction of shift was matched by an effect on the physical tasks (ie, SLR and forward bending). The results suggest that providing information has an immediate impact on pain-related beliefs and attitudes. The author concluded that pain education has an immediate impact on pain thresholds during a physical task, implying that motor performance may be limited by pain beliefs, and that pain education should be included in the management of patients with CLBP.[784]

To further understand the effects of neurophysiology education, Moseley[785] investigated the effects on cognition, disability, and physical performance in patients with CLBP. Patients were randomly assigned to receive individual education of 2 types: pain biology or back school information such as lumbar spine anatomy and biomechanics. Both groups were given a workbook to review every day for 2 weeks. Patients in the pain biology group were less catastrophic about their pain, less likely to relate pain to tissue damage, and more likely to think that pain may be controllable without medications. Patients who received back school information were more likely to relate pain to tissue damage. The change in perceived disability was not clinically significant. The authors concluded that explaining pain biology does change how people think about pain, but does not impact perceived disability. Therefore, explaining pain is not enough on its own. Explaining pain changes conscious pain-related beliefs and should be included in interdisciplinary treatment approaches since it is likely to improve treatment effects.[785]

To further support the concept that motor performance may be limited by pain beliefs in CLBP, a case report[813] of a patient with disabling CLBP describes the changes in brain activity during a nonpainful task (ie, the abdominal drawing in maneuver) as observed on functional MRI. Brain activity was measured during the task and after 1 week of practice and before and after 2.5 hours of pain education. Before education, widespread brain activity was observed during performance of the task, including activity in cortical regions involved in pain. After education, widespread activity was absent with no evident brain activation outside of the primary somatosensory cortex. The results suggest that pain education markedly altered brain activity during performance of the task, offering a possible mechanism for difficulty in trunk muscle training in people with pain. The change in activity associated with education may reflect reduced threat related to the task, resulting in improved physical performance.[813]

The content of neurophysiology of pain education and associated clinical reasoning are described in detail using a case report. Louw et al[814] described the use of neuroscience education in combination with ROM, stretching, cardiovascular exercise, and aquatic therapy in the treatment of a patient with a 3-year history of CLBP. The treatment consisted of 8 sessions over 4 weeks. All outcome measures, NPRS, FABQW, FABQPA, Zung Depression Scale, and most notably the FABQ, were improved immediately after the initial evaluation and neuroscience education session and at 7-month follow-up.[814]

Research continues to support the use of pain physiology education aimed at decreasing the fear associated with movement. An improved understanding of how pain works allows the patient to reframe his or her problem, resulting in increased confidence and activity levels and reduced fear, depression, and disability. Specific education about pain and a graded exercise and activity approach should be used when indicated in the management of patients with CLBP.

Modalities for Chronic Low Back Pain

Therapeutic ultrasound does not demonstrate a level of evidence sufficient to warrant recommendation for the treatment of acute or chronic lumbopelvic pain.[815] In addition to the review by van Middelkoop et al[798] reported previously, studies comparing TENS with placebo for CLBP demonstrate conflicting evidence for reducing back pain intensity. Consistent evidence demonstrates that TENS did not improve disability, the use of medical services, or work status. The use of TENS is not supported in the routine care of acute or CLBP.[816]

Insufficient evidence exists to evaluate the effects of cold for LBP, and conflicting evidence exists for any differences between heat and cold for LBP. Moderate evidence demonstrated that heat wrap therapy provides a small short-term reduction in pain and disability in a mixed population with acute and subacute LBP and that the addition of exercise further reduces pain and improves function. In contrast, moderate evidence demonstrates that there is no difference in a heat wrap compared to an educational booklet or McKenzie exercise at 1 week.[817] The internal validity of some of the heat wrap trials is suspect due to funding by an affiliation of the research team with the manufacturer.[818] Application of heat via heating pads is a self-care option for short-term relief of acute LBP with insufficient evidence to recommend a cold pack. Evidence is conflicting regarding whether back supports are effective supplements to other interventions and unclear whether lumbar supports are more effective than no or other interventions for treating LBP.[819]

Clinicians should thoroughly investigate the treatment effects associated with modalities as compared to MT, exercise, pain education, and graded exercise interventions to determine the current best strategy (ie, most efficient and effective to achieve optimal outcomes) for each patient. Patients seek PT for skilled services that are better than the outcomes of self-care, usual medical care, and the passage of time. Current evidence does not support the routine, broad, first-line use of modalities in the management of LBP.

Conservative Management of Lumbar Radiculopathy in Chronic Low Back Pain

LBP with related leg pain can be a predictor of both severity and associated chronicity. Differentiating potential sources (ie, somatic referred or neurogenic) of radiating leg pain in patients with LBP facilitates a diagnosis and individualized treatment based on predominating pain mechanisms. As discussed earlier in this chapter, Schäfer et al[732] described a subclassification of persons with LBRLP based on distinct symptoms and signs associated with 4 predominating mechanisms (see Table 4-6): central sensitization, peripheral nerve sensitization, denervation, and musculoskeletal referred pain. To assist with clinical decision making, a classification algorithm[732] is also proposed (see Figure 4-129).

Other potential classifications for LBP related leg pain include the following:

- DSE classification also depicted as LBP with lower extremity referred pain (see Table 4-3)
- Traction classification for LBP with lower extremity radiating or related pain (see Table 4-4)
- An impairment-based classification for symptomatic LSS (see Table 4-5)
- An impairment-based classification for LBP with altered neurodynamics

The clinical characteristics and evidence supporting these classifications and matched conservative interventions are discussed earlier in this chapter and recommended for review. Evidence for invasive strategies for lumbar radiculopathy is provided later in this chapter.

Cardiovascular Exercise for Chronic Low Back Pain

Patients with acute or subacute LBP are advised to remain active rather than rest in bed. Recommendations for persons with CLBP often include some form of ET. Walking is often recommended for persons with acute, subacute, or CLBP and for postsurgical rehabilitation. However, there is little research related to specific activities or aerobic exercise such as walking for the management of LBP. For healthy adults under age 65, the ACSM[820] recommended moderately intense cardio 30 minutes a day or 10 000 steps[821] 5 days a week, or vigorously intense cardio 20 minutes a day 3 days a week and 8 to 10 strength-training exercises for 8 to 12 repetitions of each exercise twice a week to maintain health and reduce the risk of chronic disease. Healthy but sedentary persons who begin a regular walking program have improved risk factors associated with CVD.[822] Some persons with LBP are less physically active and have altered patterns of physical activity compared to active controls.[823] When compared to healthy controls, persons with CLBP took significantly less steps and failed to reach the recommended 10 000 steps.[823,824]

To determine the strength of evidence for walking as an intervention in the management of LBP, Hendrick et al[825] examined 4 studies with poor methodological quality and heterogeneity of design. The authors' report that findings are inconclusive with little evidence to support walking as having a positive effect on LBP. Additional studies are needed to either refute or support walking programs. Research also suggests that participation in recreational activities is inversely associated with LBP, related disability, and psychological distress.[826] Walking is a no-cost, easily implemented recreational activity and has the potential to be an effective component in the management of LBP. The challenge is to design effective walking programs and then motivate for adherence. An RCT[827] currently in progress may provide some additional evidence. The purpose of this trial is to investigate the difference in clinical effectiveness and costs of an individualized walking program and a supervised general exercise program compared to usual physiotherapy in people with CLBP. Follow-ups will occur at 3, 6, and 12 months.[827]

Cardiovascular exercise has been reported to improve outcomes in patients with chronic pain and central sensitization such as fibromyalgia.[828-833] These studies, while not specifically related to patients with LBP, provide some support for cardiovascular exercise in patients with CLBP who also have a component of central sensitization. Using ACSM[834] guidelines, Busch et al[831] analyzed the effects of aerobic exercise only in persons with fibromyalgia compared to a control group. In aerobics-only interventions, clinically significant improvements were found sporadically in 6 variables: depression, tender points, global well-being, physical function, self-efficacy, and symptoms. While this systematic review is not related to persons with CLBP, it does demonstrate the potential benefits of aerobic exercise for persons with chronic pain.

Summary of Evidence for Chronic Low Back Pain

Current evidence for nonspecific CLBP supports an interdisciplinary approach based on the biopsychosocial model including pain education, cognitive behavioral training such as graded exercise and graded exposure, SMT, and ET, although one intervention or form of exercise is not superior to another. The absence of strong recommendations or the presence of small treatment effects demonstrated in many of systematic reviews emphasizes the need for continued research and careful examination of individual RCTs rather than simply focusing on the summary statements.

All of the systematic reviews support future research based on subgrouping, identification of primary and secondary drivers to guide intervention, and dissolution of concepts related to treatment with a single-dimensional focus. Preliminary evidence supports patient subgrouping, pain education, matching to appropriate intervention, and adoption of the biopsychosocial model as important for managing the multifactorial nature of CLBP. Biopsychosocial factors differ for each patient, making the pain experience unique to each individual. These influences present barriers to recovery and contribute to maintenance of pain and the persistence of pain behavior and movement patterns, which in turn promote chronicity, but they also provide pathways to successful intervention. Each clinician is challenged to identify and understand the effects of physical, psychological, and social factors and to address each factor as it relates to the patient's expectations and goals.

Interventional Therapies, Interdisciplinary Rehabilitation, Pharmacology, and Surgery

Clinical Practice Guidelines for Interventional Therapies and Surgery[835]

Interventional treatment and surgery are widely available for nonspecific CLBP with increasing use, despite the inaccuracy of identifying specific anatomic causes of LBP and evidence that questions their clinical usefulness.[835] The American Pain Society clinical practice guidelines[835] for nonradicular LBP, radiculopathy with herniated disc, and symptomatic spinal stenosis are summarized next, along with a recommendation for shared decision making between the clinician and patient to weigh the potential benefits, harms, cost, and burdens of these treatments. In general, noninvasive therapies supported by evidence are recommended before consideration of interventional procedures or surgery. Guidelines are not applicable to all patients and clinical settings; therefore, review of the entire evidence-based guidelines and RCTs applicable to individual patients is advised.[835] The guidelines[835] recommend the following:

- Against the use of provocative discography for patients with chronic nonradicular LBP; insufficient evidence exists to evaluate validity or utility of diagnostic selective nerve root block, intraarticular facet joint block, medial branch block, or SIJ block as diagnostic procedures for LBP with or without radiculopathy
- Consideration of intensive interdisciplinary rehabilitation with a cognitive behavioral emphasis for nonradicular CLBP who do not respond to usual non-interdisciplinary care
- Against facet joint corticosteroid injection, prolotherapy, and intradiscal corticosteroid injections for patients with persistent nonradicular LBP; insufficient evidence exists to evaluate benefits of local injections, botulinum toxin injection, ESI, intradiscal electrothermal therapy (IDET), therapeutic medial branch block, radiofrequency (RF) denervation, SIJ steroid injection, or intrathecal therapy with opioids or other medications for nonradicular LBP

- In cases of nonradicular LBP, common degenerative changes and persistent disability, a discussion of risks and benefits of surgery with reference to rehabilitation as a similarly effective option for patients; the small to moderate average benefit from surgery versus non-interdisciplinary, nonsurgical therapy and the fact that the majority of such patients who have surgery do not experience an optimal outcome defined as minimum or no pain, discontinuation of or occasional pain medication use, and return of high level function
- Against vertebral disc replacement in patients with nonradicular LBP, common degenerative spinal changes, and persistent and disabling symptoms due to insufficient evidence
- Discussion of the risks and benefits of ESIs including review of evidence that shows moderate short-term benefits and lack of long-term benefit for patients with persistent radiculopathy due to herniated lumbar disc; insufficient evidence is available to evaluate benefits and harms of ESI for spinal stenosis
- Discussion of the risks and benefits of surgery that references moderate benefits that decrease over time (1 to 2 years) for patients with persistent and disabling radiculopathy due to herniated lumbar disc or persistent and disabling leg pain
- Discussion of risks and benefits of spinal cord stimulation including reference to the high rate of complications following stimulator placement for patients with persistent and disabling radicular pain following surgery for herniated disc and no evidence of a persistently compressed nerve root

Interdisciplinary Rehabilitation

For CLBP, interdisciplinary rehabilitation is moderately superior to non-interdisciplinary rehabilitation or usual care for improving short- and long-term functional status[836-838] and similar to the effectiveness of spinal fusion surgery for nonradicular LBP.[839-841] The most effective programs involve cognitive behavioral and supervised exercise components with at least 100 hours of treatment.[837] Interdisciplinary rehabilitation programs are expensive, not available in some areas, and have limited insurance coverage, but may reduce lost wages or time off from work.[842-844]

Pharmacology

Several medications have short-term benefits for patients with LBP. Acetaminophen is a safe, low-cost, first-line option for treatment of acute or CLBP.[845,846] Statistically significant effects were found for NSAIDs compared to placebo, but at the cost of significantly more side effects. NSAIDs are associated with a broad range of side effects including renal toxicity, exacerbation of hypertension, fluid retention, gastrointestinal complications, and cardiovascular events such as myocardial infarction. NSAIDs are not more effective than paracetamol (acetaminophen) for acute LBP, but paracetamol has less side effects. NSAIDs are not more effective than other drugs for acute LBP. Various types of NSAIDs, including cyclooxygenase-2 NSAIDs, are equally effective for acute LBP. Most studies have found that COX-2 selective inhibitors are associated with a lower risk of ulcers and ulcer complications than nonselective NSAIDs. In some studies, the difference is not significant.[847] All NSAIDs are associated with varying degrees of gastrointestinal and cardiovascular risks.[847] The increased risk of cardiovascular adverse events appears to be dependent on duration of exposure.[847] Insufficient evidence exists to recommend for or against the use of aspirin.[848] Gabapentin for radiculopathy has small, short-term benefits.[849] Benzodiazepines are similarly effective to skeletal muscle relaxants for short-term pain relief for acute or CLBP but have increased risk of abuse and addiction.[850] Systemic corticosteroids are not more effective than placebo and not recommended for treatment of LBP with or without sciatica.[851,852]

Another review examined the effectiveness of pharmacological interventions for nonspecific CLBP.[853] Seventeen randomized trials were included related to NSAIDs, antidepressants, and opioids. No trials were located for muscle relaxants. The overall quality of evidence was low, reporting only short-term effects of less than 3 months. NSAIDs and opioids seem to provide a higher relief in pain in the short term when compared to placebo. Opioids have a small effect in improving function but result in an exacerbation of symptoms after stopping medication. Both NSAIDs and opioids provide more adverse effects than placebo with no difference observed between antidepressants for pain relief and placebo in patients with nonspecific CLBP. Due to limited evidence in the long-term, Chou et al[311] recommended extended use of medications for patients who continually benefit without major adverse events.

Surgery

Back surgery rates are on the rise in the United States.[854] For lumbar radiculopathy due to herniated disc and spinal stenosis, surgery is generally indicated for serious or progressive neurological deficits.[855] In the absence of neurological deficit and persistent nonradicular LBP, the indications are less clear.

For nonradicular LBP with common degenerative changes, fair evidence suggests that fusion is no more effective than intensive cognitive behavioral rehabilitation, but slightly to moderately more effective than standard, nonintensive, nonsurgical therapy for improved pain and function.[855] Standard open and microdiscectomy procedures for chronic disabling radiculopathy with herniated disc are associated with moderate short-term benefits over 6 to 12 weeks when compared to conservative therapy, but outcomes diminish or are no longer present after 1 to 2 years in some studies.[855-860] Surgical discectomy for carefully selected patients with sciatica due to a prolapsed lumbar disc appears to provide faster relief from the acute onset than nonsurgical management.[860] Surgical success rates for lumbar discectomy range between 60% and 90%, while poor outcomes of continued pain and loss of movement and function range from 10% to 40%. Three to 12% of patients who have disc surgery are likely to develop another prolapsed disc and require reoperation.[861] Decompressive laminectomy for persistent disabling leg pain due to spinal stenosis is associated with moderate benefits compared to nonsurgery, but once again, benefits tend to diminish through 2 years.[862-865]

The effectiveness of surgery versus conservative treatment on pain, disability, and quality of life for LSS was analyzed by Kovacs et al.[866] Conservative treatments included orthosis, PT, exercise, modalities, analgesics, NSAIDs, and epidural steroids. Surgery showed better results for pain, disability, and quality of life, although not for walking ability. Results are similar among patients with and without spondylolisthesis and slightly better among those with neurogenic claudication than among those without it. Benefits of surgery are noticeable at 3 to 6 months and remain for up to 2 to 4 years, but differences tend to be smaller at the end of that period. The authors concluded that the implantation of a specific device and decompressive surgery with or without fusion are more effective than continued conservative treatment when that treatment has failed for 3 to 6 months.[866] Patients with dominant leg pain and degenerative spondylolisthesis and spinal stenosis appear to have better outcomes at 1 and 2 years compared to patients with dominant LBP.[867]

Evidence for Rehabilitation After Lumbar Disc Surgery

Two systematic reviews[868,869] have reached different conclusions related to the effectiveness of rehabilitation programs after first-time lumbar discectomy. Ostelo et al[868] report that exercise programs starting 4 to 6 weeks postsurgery for persons age 18 to 65 years seem to lead to a faster decrease in pain and disability than no treatment. High-intensity exercise programs as opposed to low-intensity programs also lead to a faster decrease in pain and disability. Supervised and home exercise programs provide similar benefits for pain relief, disability, or GPE. The authors conclude that it is not harmful to return to activity after lumbar disc surgery, but the study did not provide guidance on how to appropriately return to activity or if specific limitations are warranted. An increased reoperation rate due to postsurgery active exercise programs is not supported.[868]

Rushton et al[869] examined RCTs through December 2009 and concluded that, although evidence from 2 trials suggests that rehabilitation intervention might reduce short-term disability of less than 3 months and more intensive exercise may be more beneficial than less intensive exercise, the pooled effects for intervention versus control and for more versus less intensive exercise did not demonstrate statistically significant effects. Evidence does not support that rehabilitation improves flexion ROM or overall impairment short term, or disability or back pain longer than 12 months. Intensity of the exercise intervention does not appear to affect back pain in the short or longer term, ROM short term, or patient's satisfaction with outcome longer term. All interventions occurred in outpatient clinics ranging from 1 day to 2.8 years postsurgery. Duration of rehabilitation ranged from 1 day to 6 weeks. Interventions included group and individualized treatment; behavioral and multimodal approaches excluding MT but including posture, trunk, and extremity strengthening; aerobic exercise; stretching; hip and spine mobility; aquatics; dynamic lumbar stabilization; and neural mobilization, with many of the descriptions and dosage parameters not included in the discussion. Evidence for the effectiveness of outpatient physiotherapy post-first lumbar discectomy provides little information to inform clinical decision making. Best practice remains unclear based on this review, with substantial heterogeneity of 16 RCTs from 11 countries. Once again, the key to absence of a treatment effect is possibly due to lack of homogeneous subgroups for comparison.

An RCT[870] published after Rushton et al[869] reviewed the effectiveness and cost-effectiveness of a rehabilitation program and an education booklet for the postoperative management of patients undergoing discectomy for lateral nerve root decompression each compared with usual care. Four subgroups are included: rehabilitation only, booklet only, rehabilitation plus booklet, and usual care only. All patients were assessed for functional ability using the ODI, pain VAS, and satisfaction preoperatively and then at 6 weeks; 3, 6, and 9 months; and 1 year postoperatively. All patients received the booklet[871] entitled, *Your Back Operation* upon discharge. Rehabilitation started 6 to 8 weeks after surgery. The program was 12 standardized, 1-hour classes run twice weekly by an experienced therapist and included general aerobic fitness; stretching; stability exercises; strengthening and endurance training for the back, abdominal, and leg muscles; ergonomic training; advice on lifting and setting targets; and self-motivation along with an open group discussion at the end of each class. Usual care was based on the surgeon's practice. Only the rehabilitation group had a significant reduction in average leg pain and the difference between leg and back pain at 1 year. Disability at 12 months was not significantly better in patients receiving education or those receiving rehabilitation. However, all 4 groups improved significantly from baseline. Rapid improvement in symptoms occurred

Figure 4-137. Trunk strength and endurance assessment at varying angles against gravity. Backstrong apparatus. Levels of difficulty of the Backstrong Spinal Rehabilitation Apparatus (Backstrong LLC), from easiest (level 1) to most difficult (level 6). (Reprinted from Selkowitz DM, Kulig K, Poppert EM, et al; and the Physical Therapy Clinical Research Network. The immediate and long-term effects of exercise and patient education on physical, functional, and quality-of-life outcome measures after single-level lumbar microdiscectomy: a randomized controlled trial protocol. *BMC Musculoskelet Disord.* 2006;7:70. Available at: http://www.biomedcentral.com/1471-2474/7/70. © 2006 Selkowitz et al; licensee BioMed Central Ltd. This is an Open Access article distributed under the terms of the Creative Commons Attribution License [http://creativecommons.org/licenses/by/2.0], which permits unrestricted use, distribution, and reproduction in any medium, provided that the original work is properly cited.)

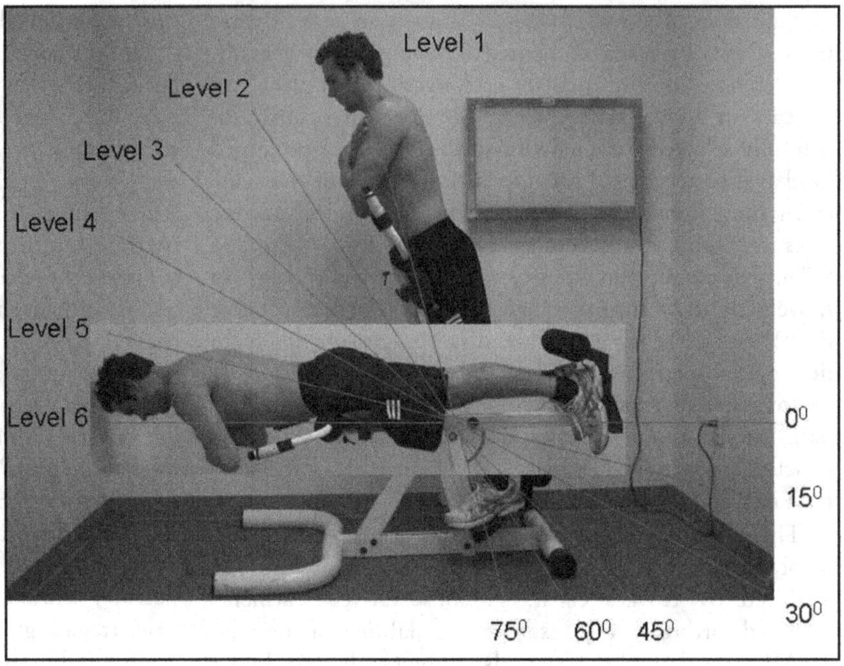

in the initial 3 months after surgery across all groups, possibly due to a natural course of recovery.[870]

Many questions remain regarding who needs postsurgical rehabilitation, when should it be initiated, and what duration and interventions should be included, perhaps explaining the current variability in practice of postsurgical rehabilitation.[872] While some individual RCTs suggest that postsurgical rehabilitation can be safe and effective, more research is needed to provide evidence-based guidelines with the ability to target the approach to each patient's activity limitations based on the history and physical examination. Preliminary evidence for rehabilitation after lumbar disc surgery is presented next, with emphasis on the clinical reasoning process and the results of 1 RCT and 1 case report.

Selkowitz et al[873] published an RCT training protocol to assess intermediate- and long-term outcomes of an exercise program targeting the trunk and lower extremities after single-level, first-time microdiscectomy. Subjects from 18 to 60 years of age were randomized to 2 groups: one session of back care education and a back care education session followed by the 12-week University of Southern California Spine Exercise Program (USCSEP). Education was a 1-hour one-on-one education session guided by an education booklet 4 to 6 weeks after surgery and included anatomy of the spine, anatomy of disc herniation, strategies to protect the back, and commonly asked questions, followed by a 10-question quiz. The USCSEP consists of back extensor strength and endurance and mat and upright therapeutic exercises 3 times per week for 12 weeks. Primary outcomes were ODQ, RMDQ, SF-36 quality of life assessment, Subjective Quality of Life Scale, 50-ft walk, repeated sit-to-stand, pain VAS, and a modified Sorensen test assessed before and after the 12-week program and every 6 months to 1 year after surgery and ending 5 years after surgery.[873]

The trunk and endurance protocol is prescribed in a graded manner determined by a pretest of strength and endurance of the trunk at varying angles against gravity using Backstrong Spinal Rehabilitation Apparatus (Backstrong LLC; Figure 4-137). The goal is for subjects to hold the Sorensen test position,[874] prone horizontal body position with spine and lower extremity joints in neutral position with arms crossed at the chest, lower extremities and pelvis supported with the upper trunk unsupported against gravity for 180 seconds. Training is performed 3 days per week with repetitions, sets, and rest periods designed to provide a safe progression of resistance. The mat and upright exercise program is an individualized progression to develop strength, endurance, and control of movement by the trunk and lower extremity musculature in supine, quadruped, and standing positions (Figure 4-138). Test performance is based upon individual symptoms, technique, and rate of perceived exertion. Details of the mat and upright exercise program are described in Table 4-24.

Using the protocol described by Selkowitz et al,[873] Kulig et al[875] randomized subjects to 2 groups: education only and exercise and education. Some subjects who did not adhere to group allocation attended PT at a clinic of their choosing, creating a third group called the usual PT group with unknown interventions. The exercise and education group showed a significantly greater reduction in ODI scores following the 12-week intervention at 4.5 months postsurgery. The ODI scores were reduced in both groups but only reached significance in the exercise

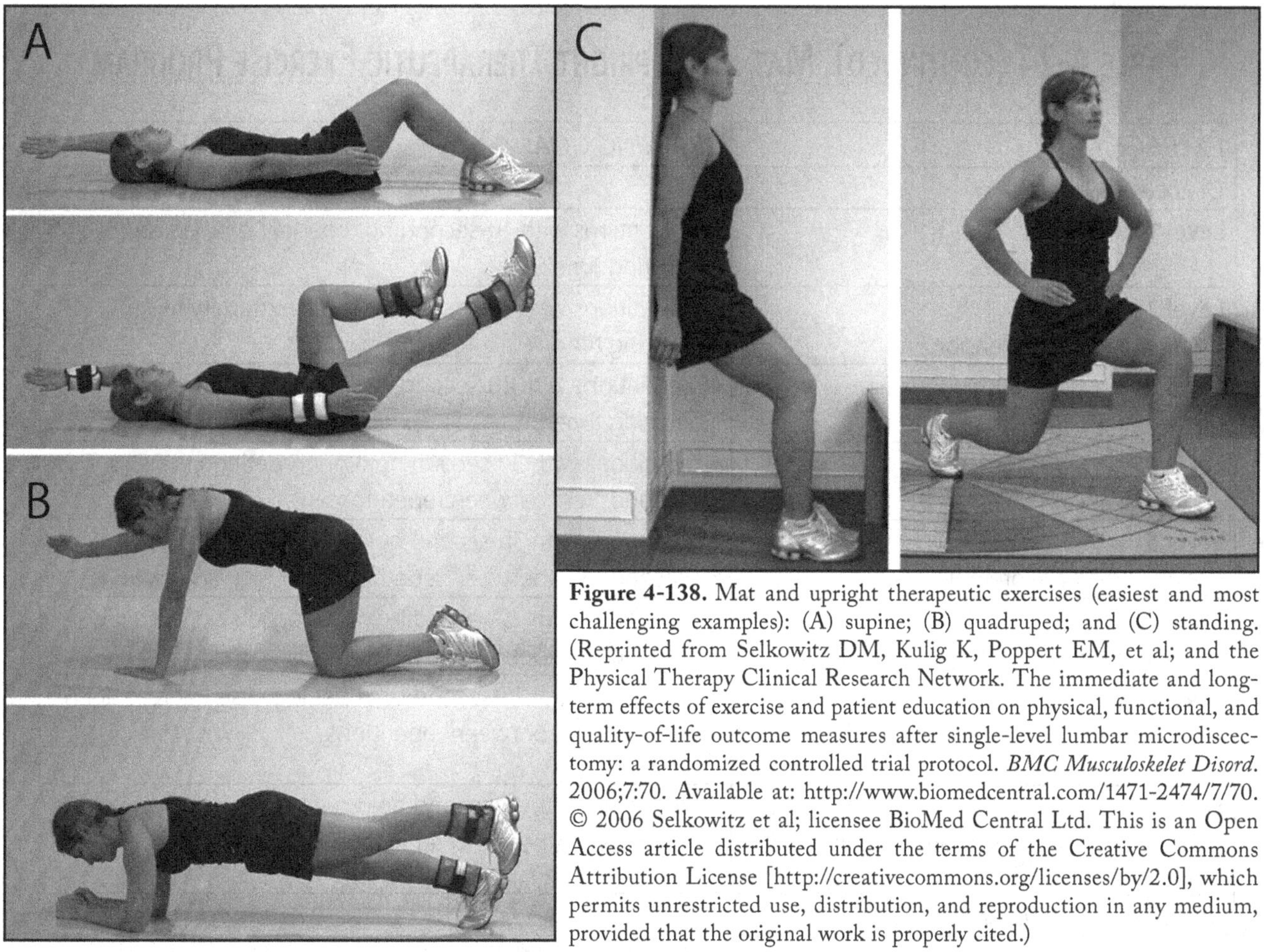

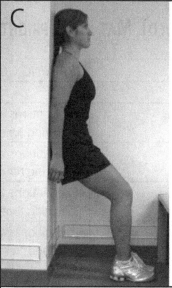

Figure 4-138. Mat and upright therapeutic exercises (easiest and most challenging examples): (A) supine; (B) quadruped; and (C) standing. (Reprinted from Selkowitz DM, Kulig K, Poppert EM, et al; and the Physical Therapy Clinical Research Network. The immediate and long-term effects of exercise and patient education on physical, functional, and quality-of-life outcome measures after single-level lumbar microdiscectomy: a randomized controlled trial protocol. *BMC Musculoskelet Disord.* 2006;7:70. Available at: http://www.biomedcentral.com/1471-2474/7/70. © 2006 Selkowitz et al; licensee BioMed Central Ltd. This is an Open Access article distributed under the terms of the Creative Commons Attribution License [http://creativecommons.org/licenses/by/2.0], which permits unrestricted use, distribution, and reproduction in any medium, provided that the original work is properly cited.)

TABLE 4-24. MAT AND UPRIGHT THERAPEUTIC EXERCISE PROGRAM

EXERCISE	*TRAINING GOAL*
ABDOMINAL PROGRESSION	
Level 1 Supine alternating upper extremity flexion	3 sets of 1 minute continuous motion 1 minute rest between sets
Level 2 Supine alternating lower extremity extension	3 sets of 1 minute continuous motion 1 minute rest between sets
Level 3 Supine alternating upper extremity flexion and lower extremity extension	3 sets of 1 minute continuous motion 1 minute rest between sets
Level 4 Supine leg extension unsupported	3 sets of 2 minutes continuous motion 2 minutes rest between sets
Level 5 Supine leg extension unsupported with alternating arms	3 sets of 2 minutes continuous motion 2 minutes rest between sets
Level 6 With 1- and 3-lb weights	3 sets of 2 minutes continuous motion 2 minutes rest between sets
Level 7 With 2- and 5-lb weights	3 sets of 2 minutes continuous motion 2 minutes rest between sets

(continued)

TABLE 4-24 (CONTINUED). MAT AND UPRIGHT THERAPEUTIC EXERCISE PROGRAM

EXERCISE	TRAINING GOAL
QUADRUPED PROGRESSION	
Level 1 Alternating arm raises	10 repetitions with 10-second hold per extremity raise No resting time
Level 2 Alternating leg extension	10 repetitions with 10-second hold per extremity raise No resting time
Level 3 Alternating arm and leg raises	10 repetitions with 10-second hold per extremity raise No resting time
Level 4 Prone plank on knees	6 repetitions with 30-second hold per repetition 30 seconds rest between repetitions
Level 5 Prone plank on forefoot	6 repetitions with 30-second hold per repetition 30 seconds rest between repetitions
Level 6 Prone plank with alternating leg lift	6 repetitions with 15-second hold per leg raise per repetition 30 seconds rest between repetitions
Level 7 Prone plank with alternating leg lift with 3-lb weight	6 repetitions with 15-second hold per leg raise per repetition 30 seconds rest between repetitions
Level 8 Prone plank with alternating leg lift with 5-lb weight	6 repetitions with 15-second hold per leg raise per repetition 30 seconds rest between repetitions
SQUAT/LUNGE PROGRESSION	
Level 1 Wall squat to 45 degrees knee flexion	3 sets of 20 repetitions 5-second hold per repetition; 2 minutes rest between sets
Level 2 Free standing squats to 90 degrees hip flexion	3 sets of 20 repetitions 2 minutes rest between sets
Level 3 Forward lunges	3 sets of 20 repetitions 2 minutes rest between sets
Level 4 Lunge series	3 sets of 2 cycles 2 minutes rest between sets
Level 5 Lunge series	3 sets of 2 cycles 2 minutes rest between sets

and education group. Improvement in ODI scores, 5-minute walk distance, and 50-ft walk time was significantly greater in the exercise and education group compared with either the education-only group or the usual PT group. Even with limitations of nonadherence to group allocation, unequal clinician contact time, and multiple use of univariate analyses that increases the risk of type I error, the USCSEP provides patients with the option to choose between education and exercise or education alone after lumbar microdiscectomy, and it provides clinicians with a standardized approach that may reduce disability.

Another postoperative program for a patient following a left L5-S1 lumbar microdiscectomy that began 10 days after surgery is described by Herbert et al.[876] Postoperative rehabilitation over 8 weeks was supervised 1 day per week by a physical therapist who emphasized motor control exercises and daily home exercise to restore trunk muscle function. The treatment approach included education and training about neutral spine strategies during daily activities, ROM, aerobic, and stabilization exercises. Initial motor control exercises addressed voluntary isometric activation of the TrA and LM in quadruped, and progressed to supine, seated, and standing positions. After 3 postoperative weeks, endurance of TrA, LM, and other trunk muscles was initiated using quadruped arm and/or leg lifting and horizontal side support with the knees flexed or extended. Initial dosage was a 5-second contraction for 30 repetitions per day and progressed at the clinician's discretion. A favorable clinical response in pain (NPRS) and disability (ODI) was observed at 1, 10, and 24 weeks. Using a rehabilitation ultrasound imaging procedure, a percent thickness change was estimated by assessing changes in thickness of the LM and TrA from rest to contraction during the abdominal drawing-in maneuver, ASLR, and a prone arm lift. The TrA and LM at the L4-L5 level demonstrated substantial improvement in muscle activation with the LM at L5-S1, showing a higher proportion of intramuscular fat and minimal improvement in activation. The significance of minimal improvement in muscle activation at the operated level of L5-S1 is unknown and should be the subject of further research.[876]

Trunk endurance and strength training are common in rehabilitation programs after lumbar spine surgery, with limited evidence to support their efficacy. As part of an unpublished doctoral thesis, Hebert[877] reported on the efficacy of 2 exercise approaches—motor control and general trunk strengthening—following lumbar disc surgery and the relationship between the change in muscle function and clinical outcome. Exercise begins 2 weeks after surgery. No between group differences were noted, but there was a relationship between improved LM function on the side of surgery and global improvement, suggesting the importance of maximizing LM function following lumbar disc surgery.[877]

As with all postsurgical rehabilitation, communication with the surgeon is important to know the surgical procedure, precautions and guidelines for progression, follow-up surgical appointments, expected outcomes from the surgeon's perspective, and plan for an appropriate evaluation for the patient. The outpatient evaluation process is the same as discussed earlier in this chapter, keeping in mind the stage of tissue healing, severity, irritability, nature, stage, and stability of the patient's presentation and the patient's response to examination. An appropriate rationale for the plan of care, clinical reasoning process, and PT evaluation should be individualized to each patient's needs.

Postoperative referrals for rehabilitation vary considerably from no rehabilitation to immediate postoperative rehabilitation, are delayed for 4 to 6 weeks, or occur on an as-needed basis. Standardized guidelines do not assist for postoperative lumbar spine rehabilitation and wide variation exists in outpatient rehabilitation evaluation and management strategies with no guidelines known to be superior to another. In the absence of research describing optimal criteria for postsurgical rehabilitation, the clinician relies on the clinical reasoning process, tissue healing, surgical procedure, surgeon prescription, applied sciences, and patient to guide clinical decision making.

Evidence for Rehabilitation After Lumbar Fusion Surgery

Spinal fusion for CLBP due to fractures, persistent infections, progressive deformity, or radiographic instability with spondylolisthesis has been shown to be beneficial. Seventy to 90% of patients with isthmic spondylolisthesis who received fusion benefits included return to full occupational function, minimal impairment, and discontinuation of all narcotic medication,[878,879] but research is limited related to the need for and/or the effectiveness of postoperative rehabilitation after lumbar spinal fusion.

Abbott et al[880] investigated the effectiveness of 2 rehabilitation programs, a psychomotor program compared with ET applied during the first 3 months after lumbar fusion. Subjects ages 18 to 65 with back pain and/or sciatica longer than 12 months who failed conservative treatment and were diagnosed with spinal stenosis, spondylosis, degenerative or isthmic spondylolisthesis, or degenerative disc disease were included. During the inpatient phase and after surgery, all patients were instructed in respiratory and circulatory exercises, training of transfers, walking, and other activities of daily living relevant for the patient. Before discharge from the hospital, patients in the ET group received a 20-minute instruction of a home exercise program. Exercises included 3 sets of 10 repetitions of supine bridging, quadruped contralateral arm and leg lifts, prone push-ups, standing semi-squats, forward lunges, and step-ups. Stretching included 30-second holds, 2 times bilaterally of hamstrings, hip abductor/external rotators, and quadriceps/iliopsoas muscle groups. Cardiovascular exercise was walking or stationary cycling for 20 to 30 minutes. Patients were restricted from activities such as contact sports, running, heavy lifting, and outer-range lumbar spine movements during the first 6 months after the operation.

The psychomotor therapy group received the same 20-minute instruction of a home program for lumbopelvic stabilization and three 90-minute outpatient sessions focusing on modifying maladaptive pain cognitions, behaviors, and motor control at 3, 6, and 9 weeks after surgery. A self-report diary was used to evaluate compliance with exercise and instructions in both groups. The psychomotor lumbopelvic stabilization training progressed as follows[880]:

- Home program 1 (0 to 3 weeks)[880]
  - o TrA and LM cocontraction with neutral spine in supine, sitting, standing for 10-second holds, 3 sets × 10 reps daily
- Outpatient session 1 (third postsurgical week)[880]
  - o Education on healing processes, physiological and psychological pain processes, relaxation techniques, and cognitive coping strategies for pain management
  - o Begin work and recreational time-contingent functional goals using patient priorities
  - o Diary review of self-monitoring of activity and home training based on quota, cognitions, and emotions and goal progress
  - o Introduction of home program 2
- Home program 2 (3 to 6 weeks)[880]
  - o Integrate lumbopelvic stabilization and closed kinetic chain functional exercise: seated overhead elastic band raises, wall-supported semi-squats and side lunges, forward lunges, and step-ups of 3 sets × 10 reps daily
- Outpatient session 2 (sixth postsurgical week)[880]
  - o Motivational discussion and positive reinforcement of goal progress
  - o Resource and hinder analysis for goal attainment
  - o Formulate action plan to manage barriers, setbacks and flare-ups, continued diary self-monitoring
  - o Introduction of home program 3
- Home program 3 (6 to 9 weeks)[880]
  - o Integration of stabilization exercise and more advanced closed kinetic chain functional exercises: semi-squats on uneven surfaces, semi-squats with elevated arms, wall-supported semi-squats with overhead hand weights, forward lunges with overhead hand weights, and step-ups with elevated arms (3 sets × 10 reps daily)
- Outpatient session 3 (ninth postoperative week)[880]
  - o Motivational discussion and positive reinforcement of goal progress and action plans for management of barriers, setbacks, and relapses
  - o Continued diary self-monitoring
  - o Introduction of home program 4
- Home program 4 (9 to 12 weeks)[880]
  - o Integration of stabilization and open kinetic chain function exercises: supine hip flexion, supine leg slide progressed to unsupported leg cycling, hip ABD in side-lying, hip flexion in a seated position, hip flexion in standing with wall support, 4-point kneeling shoulder flexion, 4-point kneeling hip flexion, and contralateral hip extension and shoulder flexion in a 4-point kneeling position for 3 sets × 10 reps daily

Both groups significantly improved in all outcome measures from baseline to 2 to 3 years after surgery with generally very large effect sizes for psychomotor therapy and medium-large effect sizes for ET. Psychomotor therapy (ie, stabilization exercise and a cognitive behavioral approach) significantly improved functional disability, self-efficacy, outcome expectancy, and fear of movement and reinjury more than ET. Both groups improved over time and generally regressed toward each other so that differences between the groups were less pronounced at long-term follow-up of 2 to 3 years. Patients in the psychomotor therapy group had more employment, less long-term sickness leave, and reduced health care use compared with the ET group. A higher reoperation rate was noted in the psychomotor group but within accepted ranges, suggesting no adverse effect of early training.[880]

Abbott et al[880] supported the results of an earlier trial[881] showing the importance of a biopsychosocial approach and initiating rehabilitation immediately after surgery. Christensen et al[881] analyzed the effect of 3 different rehabilitation programs after lumbar spinal fusion. Three months after surgery, 90 subjects were randomized to a video group of exercises for training with one-time instruction; a second group given the same video program supplemented with a meeting with other fusion patients 3 times over an 8-week period; or a third group receiving PT training 2 times per week for 8 weeks.

The exercises for the video group were designed to provide gradual dynamic muscular training to enhance endurance of the back, abdominal, and leg muscle groups. The training was aimed within normal ROM and included stretching of large muscle groups to be performed as a home exercise program. Subjects were not allowed to do contact sports, training on machines at a fitness center, jogging, or running. A videotape and written account of the exercises were given to patients.[880]

In addition to the video exercise program, the second group met 3 times with a physical therapist and other spinal fusion patients for reassurance and psychological support for 1.5 hours. The PT group received supervised training 2 times per week for 1.5 hours. The training included a 15-minute warm-up, aerobic condition of cycling and hop sequences, dynamic muscular endurance training at 7 to 10 reps, and stretching exercises of large muscle groups. A detailed description of the exercises was not reported. Functional outcomes were evaluated at 6, 12, and 24 months after surgery by use of the Low Back Pain Rating Scale and a questionnaire covering daily function, work status, and a patient's contact with primary care. At 24-week follow-up, the 2 video groups had less pain compared with the PT group. The second group was significantly better at performing daily functions such as carrying bags of groceries, getting up from a chair, and ascending stairs compared with the 2 other groups. In the second group, more subjects returned to work compared with the 2 other groups. The video group had significantly more contacts with health care providers compared with the second group and the PT group. The addition of a cognitive behavioral component to video exercises is favored to improve functional outcomes over video or exercise alone.[881]

The combined framework of a motor control and cognitive-behavioral approach for early rehabilitation emphasizes the importance of both physical and psychological interventions. Cognitive-behavioral intervention may be necessary in some patients to improve self-efficacy, anxiety, depression, and fear of movement and reinjury before motor control improvements can occur. Similarly, improvements in motor control reinforce improvements in self-efficacy, anxiety, depression, and fear of pain and reinjury. The evidence for rehabilitation after lumbar fusion surgery is scarce, with no consensus on the optimal guidelines for rehabilitation after lumbar spine fusion or if particular subgroups should receive rehabilitation. A spinal fusion requires sufficient time for the bone graft and bone to heal as well for bone to assimilate into any instrumentation. The healing rate may vary by procedure, age, or other patient characteristics. Therefore, communication with each surgeon is important to determine when movement and strengthening in the spinal area of fusion are initiated and progressed. The time to begin outpatient rehabilitation and progression is generally at the discretion of the surgeon.

Lumbar Spine Total Disc Replacement and Rehabilitation

Lumbar arthroplasty or total disc replacement (TDR) is a relatively new alternative procedure to lumbar spinal fusion for patients with symptomatic lumbar disc degeneration. Van den Eerenbeemt et al[882] examined the effectiveness and safety of the 2 procedures. Using the ProDisc device (DePuy Synthes), the results of TDR are contradictory when compared with anterior lumbar circumferential fusion. No clinically relevant differences were found on the primary outcomes between the Charité Artificial Disc (DePuy Spine) and the Bagby and Kuslick cage fusion at 2- and 5-year follow-up. High-quality prospective, controlled, long-term follow-up studies including economic evaluation are lacking. Existing evidence regarding long-term effectiveness and/or safety is insufficient to justify the widespread use of TDR over fusion for single-level degenerative disc. The overall success rate in treatment groups is small. Complications related to the surgical approach ranged from 2.1% to 18.7%, prosthesis-related from 2.0% to 39.3%, treatment-related from 1.9% to 62.0%, and general complications from 1.0% to 14.0%. No clinically relevant differences between TDR and fusion were found.[882]

No evidence-based guidelines for rehabilitation after total lumbar disc replacement are available. A synthesis of postoperative management discloses wide variation and a broad description of rehabilitation guidelines.[883] Guidelines[883] include the following. Hospitalization stay averages 3.4 days and return to work averages 6 weeks. PT begins during the immediate postoperative period with walking, an undefined abdominal flexion, and active and passive hip and knee flexion. After 4 weeks, PT is directed toward maintaining mobility, general conditioning, and strengthening. Lumbar spine rotation, side-bending, and abdominal strengthening begin at 6 weeks. A lumbar support is used by some surgeons up to 3 months. Patients should avoid lumbar hyperextension, heavy lifting, impact loading, twisting, and mechanical vibration or shock for about 3 months. Jumping, running, or contact sports are not recommended for 3 months. Swimming may be allowed at around 4 weeks.[883] Close communication with the surgeon is advised in planning postsurgical rehabilitation.

Continuing the review of postoperative rehabilitation for lumbar surgical procedures, a case report[884] describes the PT rehabilitation of a patient after an L5-S1 lumbosacral percutaneous nucleoplasty. A nucleoplasty procedure involves replacement of the nucleus pulposus and is recommended for early to moderate degenerative disc disease; this procedure requires an intact annulus to contain the prosthetic nucleus device.[885,886] No postsurgical rehabilitation was prescribed in the acute postoperative phase. At 7 weeks, per the surgeon's discretion and patient request, PT evaluation was initiated due to continuing LBP of an average 3/10 and functional deficits related to mobility, ODI 56%. Initial evaluation revealed decreased lumbar AROM in standing; PAIVM (PA) hypomobility and pain at L3-4, L4-5, and L5-S1; and decreased motor control to include poor TrA and LM prone using pressure-biofeedback. Based on the examination, the therapist planned a 3-phase program, 2 times per week for 8 weeks, which was progressed by continual reassessment.[884] The 3 phases are summarized next as described by Puentedura et al.[884]

Phase 1 (0 to 2 Weeks Through 7 to 9 Weeks Postsurgery)[884]

- Education at each session emphasized pain science, anatomy, biomechanics, stabilization, surgical procedure, safety issues, and appropriate and inappropriate activities.
- Gentle AROM exercises for the lumbar spine included pelvic tilts, bridging, and single knee to chest as graded movement to facilitate appropriate somatosensory input.
- SSE: Activation of TrA and LM (10 reps/10-second hold) first in quadruped, then prone over a pillow, side-lying, and supine
- Home program: Above exercises (10 to 15 reps/10-second hold), gradual increase in sitting, standing, and walking

Phase 2 (3 to 5 Weeks)[884]

- Main focus was to regain ROM and progressive stabilization exercises in weightbearing and closed kinetic chain activities.
- Lumbar rotation in supine hook-lying lumbar rotation was added to the ROM exercises carried over from phase 1.
- Prone extension was added. MT: PAIVM and CPA were added at L3-4, L4-5, and L5-S1 as grade III mobilization to improve extension.
- Deep muscle activation was emphasized during upper body ergometry and recumbent bicycling as reeducation for segmental control during perturbations caused by limb motions.
- Lat pull-downs and seated rowing were added with focus on slow, controlled movement and deep muscle activation.
- Balance and proprioceptive work were added on a wobble board and mini-trampoline for segmental control; these activities require segmental control while using superficial system to control lumbopelvic orientation.
- Work specific activities such as walking up and down a ladder with wrist cuff weights.

Phase 3 (6 to 8 Weeks)[884]

- Stabilization exercises were progressed to weightbearing, closed-chain activities related to ADL, work, and hobbies such as lifting.
- Squat lifts and weight work were added.

Outcomes at the end of phase 2 were as follows: ODI was 4% and pain was 0. By 6 weeks, the patient had returned fully to work and resumed recreational activities. ODI scores decreased from a preoperative 64% to 2% at 12 months. The pain scores decreased from a preoperative value of 7 to 0 at 12 months. In the absence of strong evidence-based guidelines to inform postoperative PT management for lumbar nucleoplasty, this case report emphasizes current best PT practice using a phased approach based on time that combines pain science education, graded movement, motor learning strategies, joint mobilization, home exercise, patient expectations, clinical reasoning, and continual reassessment for appropriate progression. The evidence-based framework appears to facilitate a functional recovery in the patient.[884]

Patient Expectations and Patient Satisfaction

Management of LBP has been discussed relative to clinical examination and current best evidence. The third component of the evidence-based practice includes patient expectations, values, and, ultimately, satisfaction with the care provided. As discussed earlier, psychosocial influences are likely to influence overall clinical outcomes related to PT management.[887,888] Patient expectations provide another set of multidimensional mechanisms not easily measured that mediate clinical outcomes,[889,890] influence behavior,[891,892] and modify satisfaction.[893,894]

Health care expectations are generally defined as a positive or negative belief that a clinical outcome will occur.[895,896] Predicted expectations are what the patient believes or thinks will occur[593,897,898]; ideal expectations are what the patient wants to occur[895,896,899]; normative expectations are what one believes should occur; and uninformed expectations are those that one is unable, unaware, or unwilling to express.[900]

Predicted expectations associated with clinical outcomes are the most frequently investigated and should be included as a prognostic indicator; however, a standardized measure of patient expectations does not exist.[901] Bialosky et al[901] suggested simply asking the patient. For example, "At the end of 4 weeks, what do you think the pain associated with your low back will be?" or "What do you believe your ability to return to work will be?" The response is then attached to a numeric rating scale from 0, meaning no better or no worse, to 10, meaning completely better or completely worse. Similar questions could be asked about intervention options. A link exists between predicted expectations and outcomes related to musculoskeletal pain, regardless of how expectations are measured.[901]

In a clinical perspective manuscript, Bialosky et al[901] suggested that current literature supports a prognostic value for patient expectation in the treatment of musculoskeletal pain that may exceed the treatment provided. Clinical outcomes may not depend entirely on the intervention, but they are shaped by patient expectations regarding the intervention. The physiological response, increased motivation, change in understanding a condition, conditioning to focus on specific aspects of the problem, and mediation of anxiety to decrease pain alter the musculoskeletal pain experience and suggest that clinician attention to enhance patient expectations may maximize treatment effects.[901]

Patient satisfaction is usually assessed as a component of quality of care because satisfied patients are more likely to adhere to recommendations, benefit from care, and lead a higher quality of life.[902,903] Patient characteristics, aspects of treatment, therapist qualities, the process and organization of care, treatment outcomes, and expectations are associated with patient satisfaction. Hush et al[904] report that patients are highly satisfied with musculoskeletal PT delivered across outpatient settings in Northern American, Europe, the United Kingdom, and Ireland. The interpersonal attributes of the therapist and the process of care are identified as key determinants of patient satisfaction. Treatment outcome was infrequently and inconsistently associated with patient satisfaction.[904]

Determinants of patient satisfaction are consistently described. For acute care conditions, the main determinant is the therapist, whereas for chronic conditions, organization of care was the best predictor.[905] Patients are more satisfied when treated by the same practitioner over the course of treatment.[906] The most consistent determinant of patient satisfaction is the therapist's attributes: professionalism; competence; friendliness; caring; ability to show empathy and respect; and the skill to communicate about the patient's condition, prognosis, and self-management.[907-910] High patient satisfaction with process of care is associated with timely and efficient treatment, adequate frequency, and follow-up.[910] Organization of care related to good access to services, convenient clinic hours, location, parking,[907,911] and available approachable support staff[911] add to patient satisfaction. In addition to pursuit of the best clinical outcomes, patient-therapist interactions and the process of care are keys to gaining patient rapport and inspiring loyalty.[904]

Pelvic Girdle Pain

The contribution of PGP (meaning SIJ and/or PS pain) to the occurrence of LBP is frequently a topic of substantial debate, as are the methods used for examination and intervention.[912] European guidelines[913] for the diagnosis and treatment of PGP provide a starting point for consensus, classification, and further discussion and research. Basic studies related to these guidelines are available at http://www.backpaineurope.org/web/files/WG4_Guidelines.pdf. The main summary findings[913] are presented as follows.

Epidemiology and Risk Factors[913]*

- PGP, as a form of LBP, occurs separately or in conjunction with LBP, but excludes gynecological or urological disorders. PGP is multifactorial and related to pregnancy (48% to 71% prevalence), trauma, arthritis, and OA (10% to 30% prevalence).[913]
- Although specific focus on PGP is possible, functionally, the pelvis cannot be studied in isolation from the thoracolumbar spine, hip, and lower extremity.[913]
- PGP is linked to nonoptimal stability of the lumbopelvic hip complex.[913]
- Anatomy of the SIJ, characterized by rough cartilage, a wedge-shaped sacrum, and a propeller-like shape of the joint surface, leads to the highest coefficient of friction of diarthrodial human joints, which can be altered by various loadings in order to stabilize the pelvic girdle.[913]
- Flexion or nutation of the sacrum relative to the ilia is generally the end result of load bearing to stabilize the pelvic girdle.[913]
- More research is needed to verify whether anterior rotation of the ilia relative to the sacrum in load-bearing situations denotes nonoptimal stability.[913]
- Point prevalence of pregnant women with PGP is about 20%. Risk factors for developing PGP during pregnancy are a history of previous LBP and/or previous pelvic trauma. Conflicting evidence does not favor pluripara and high workload as risk factors. Non-risk factors include contraceptive pills, time since last pregnancy, height, weight, smoking, and possibly younger age. The risk factors for non-pregnant women to suffer from PGP are unknown.[913]

Diagnosis and Imaging[913]*

- Diagnosis occurs after exclusion of a symptomatic lumbar spine.[913]
- Pain or functional disturbance related to PGP must be reproduced by the following clinical tests:
  - *SIJ pain*: P4 test, Patrick's or FABER's test, palpation of the LDL, and Gaenslen's test[913]
  - *PS pain*: Palpation of the symphysis and modified Trendelenburg's test of the pelvic girdle—while standing on one leg with the contralateral hip and knee flexed to 90 degrees, pain at the PS is a positive test[913]
  - *Functional test*: ASLR test[913]

*With kind permission from Springer Science+Business Media: *Eur Spine J*, European guidelines for the diagnosis and treatment of pelvic girdle pain, 17(6), 2008, 794-819, Vleeming A, Albert HB, Östgaard HC, Sturesson B, Stuge B.

- A history related to specific provocation of pain during prolonged standing and/or sitting is recommended. A precise location of the area of pain may be important and should be noted by the patient and clinician on a pain diagram.[913]
- Due to poor sensitivity in detecting early stages of SIJ degeneration and arthritis of the SIJ, indications for conventional radiography are limited.[913]
- In most cases of non-AS PGP, imaging has little value. Computer tomography and conventional radiography are not recommended as a diagnostic alternative when MRI is available because of radiation exposure and the fact that no further information is gained. MRI is best to discriminate changes in and around the SIJ; early AS and tumors can be easily detected. Bone scintigraphy for PGP is not recommended. To establish the diagnosis of PGP, imaging techniques are generally only needed in AS, for patients with red flags, and when surgical intervention procedures are considered.[913]
- Local SIJ injections are not recommended to aid diagnosis for PGP. A combination of manual diagnostic tests with high sensitivity and specificity should be used to analyze a wide range of PGP complaints.[913]

Treatment Recommendations[913]*

- Individualized exercises in pregnancy with a focus on stabilization for control and stability as part of multifactorial treatment postpartum.[913]
- Intraarticular SIJ injection under imaging guidance for AS.[913]
- Medication as necessary for pain relief, excluding pregnant women, with first choice paracetamol and second choice NSAIDs.[913]
- Adequate information and reassurance as part of a multifactorial intervention.[913]

Basic Science Research Related to the Pelvic Girdle

The exact cause of nonspecific PGP is unknown, but plausible hypotheses include effects of the hormone relaxin, neurophysiological factors, and biomechanical factors such as failed load transfer from the legs to the trunk. Biomechanically, the optimal position for load transfer occurs with a self-locking mechanism of the SIJ described as sacral nutation and relative posterior tilt or rotation of the ilium with optimal stability based on the principles of form and force closure.[914] Relative to joint mobility and stability, form closure describes the role of joint structure or the osteoligamentous system, and force closure describes the role of the neuromuscular system. Theoretically, optimizing force and/or form closure is thought to enhance pelvic girdle stability with deficits in either one potentially leading to poor loading strategies and nonoptimal stability.[914] For example, facilitating a posteriorly tilted ilium or sacral nutation is most likely to be a more stable position than an anteriorly tilted ilium, whereas anterior rotation of the ilium or relative sacral counternutation at the SIJ and PS are nonoptimal positions for stability and may result in a pain experience. Theoretically, Vleeming et al[915] proposed that it is possible for the SIJ to move and assume a new position of displacement that cannot be detected by radiography. The biomechanical factors of form and force closure theory, along with motor control and cognitive behavioral influences, are components of a proposed classification for PGP[916] and used to explain the transfer of loads through the lumbopelvic hip complex.

The SIJ is inherently stable and designed to safely transfer load.[914,915,917] In weightbearing, the SIJs have a small amount of motion (ie, 0.4 to 4.3 degrees rotation coupled with < 0.7 mm translation)[918] and may have more motion in nonweightbearing.[919] SIJ motion varies among individuals, but within an individual, motion appears to be symmetrical between right and left sides.[920] Asymmetrical laxity of the SIJs as measured with Doppler imaging correlates with symptoms in subjects with peripartum PGP.[921] Compared to healthy subjects, pelvic girdle joint motion is 32% to 68% larger in patients with PGP or LBP during the last months of pregnancy and the first 3 weeks after delivery, supporting the idea that increased motion is one factor that may cause PGP and gives rationale for treatment to reduce this motion.[922]

Movement of the SIJ cannot be reliably assessed by motion palpation tests.[921-926] Intraarticular displacement or positional faults of the SIJ have not been identified using a valid instrument.[927] Asymmetry of the pelvis perceived clinically is likely to occur secondary to changes in pelvic and trunk muscle activity or mechanical loads resulting in positional strain, not positional changes within the SIJs themselves,[927,928] and asymmetry does not always mean pathology or altered function. Pelvic manipulation does not appear to alter the position of the pelvic joints.[927] As previously discussed, the mechanism of pain relief due to manipulation is most likely a neurophysiological response. When clinical signs of reduced force closure such as a positive ASLR have been identified, the increased movement is observed at the symphysis pubis, not the SIJ.[929]

Altered motor control strategies and respiratory function have been found in subjects with PGP.[930] Compared to healthy controls during a positive ASLR, subjects with PGP had increased minute ventilation, decreased diaphragmatic excursion, and increased pelvic floor descent. Manual compression through the ilia theorized to augment

*With kind permission from Springer Science+Business Media: *Eur Spine J*, European guidelines for the diagnosis and treatment of pelvic girdle pain, 17(6), 2008, 794-819, Vleeming A, Albert HB, Östgaard HC, Sturesson B, Stuge B.

pelvic stability reversed these differences.[930] Altered motor responses are proposed as an attempt by the neuromuscular system to compensate for a lack of ability to transfer load through the lumbopelvic region due to a deficit in form and/or force closure.[930] During an ipsilateral ASLR, pain-free subjects show greater abdominal and chest wall activation on the same side as the ASLR, with minimal change in intra-abdominal pressure (IAP), respiration, and pelvic floor position. In contrast, subjects with chronic PGP show increased muscle activation bilaterally through the anterior abdominal wall and the ipsilateral chest wall, increased IAP, pelvic floor descent, and a decrease in diaphragmatic motion thought to be a splinting action in conjunction with increased IAP.[931,932] The strategy observed in subjects with PGP is a bracing strategy usually observed in high-load tasks and reflects an altered motor control pattern.[932]

Many muscles act to provide stability through force closure by increasing compression of joint surfaces and creating stiffness to allow for effective load transfer through the lumbopelvic hip complex during a variety of functional tasks.[914,915,917,920,930,933-942] Excessive muscle activation, as well as insufficient activation (ie, poor motor control), of the deep and superficial lumbopelvic and hip musculature[916,930,936,941,942] can be associated with PGP.

Superficial Muscle System

The theoretical role of this system is to control lumbopelvic movement, orientation in space, and balance.[943] When compared to healthy controls, women with postpartum PGP walk slower[944] and have decreased hip muscle strength[944-948] and trunk muscle endurance.[944,948]

Four groups of superficial muscle slings are theorized to provide pelvic girdle stability.[914,934] The anterior oblique sling provides links between the external oblique, the anterior abdominal fascia, the contralateral internal oblique, and the thigh adductors. The posterior oblique sling contains links between the latissimus dorsi and the gluteus maximus through the thoracolumbar fascia. The lateral sling includes stabilizers of the hip joint, gluteus medius, gluteus maximus, and TFL. The longitudinal sling connects peronei, the biceps femoris, the sacrotuberous ligament, the deep lamina of the thoracolumbar fascia, and the ES. Hungerford et al[941] reported delayed onset of the LM, internal oblique, and gluteus maximus in patients with SIJ pain. Through Doppler imaging, SIJ stiffness was increased by contraction of the ES, latissimus dorsi, biceps femoris, and gluteus maximus.[937]

Deep Muscle System

Contraction of the TrA is thought to provide some stiffness to the SIJ[923] due to its attachment to the thoracolumbar fascia.[949] The TrA,[950] deep LM,[951] and diaphragm are activated in a feed-forward manner prior to initiation of rapid arm movement in anticipation of lumbopelvic stabilization. The PFM are located inside the pelvis and form the floor of the abdominal cavity. The PFM together with other muscles surrounding the abdominal cavity generate and maintain IAP, controlling bladder and bowel continence and evacuation, and providing stability in the lumbopelvic region.[942,952,953] The PFM can be contracted voluntarily, resulting in an inward, upward lift and tightening around the urethra, vagina, and anus[954] and are vital for urinary and fecal continence during daily activities.[955,956] A biomechanical analysis of the upright standing posture has shown that cocontraction of the TrA and PFM could decrease vertical SIJ shear forces and increase pelvic stability.[952] Theoretically, coordination between the superficial and deep systems ensures stability and motion control.

Pregnancy and vaginal delivery can lead to deficits in PFM contractions and problems. PFM dysfunction can cause urinary and fecal incontinence, pelvic organ prolapse, pain, and sexual disorders.[955] Neuromuscular disturbance of the PFM has been observed in women with pregnancy-related lumbopelvic pain.[930,942] For example, the PFM showed a significant increase in EMG activity during prolonged contractions and pushing in women with pregnancy-related lumbopelvic pain compared with healthy controls.[936] An increase in PFM activity might be an attempt to compensate for functional pelvic instability.[954]

In addition, a relationship between urinary incontinence (UI) and LBP has been observed. Eliasson et al[957] described the occurrence of UI in women ages 17 to 45 with LBP to a reference group of comparable age, language, culture, and parity (ie, number of deliveries). Seventy-eight percent of the women with LBP reported UI. The prevalence of UI and altered PFM activation were significantly increased in the LBP group. The authors concluded that the condition of LBP and PFM dysfunction described as the inability to stop urine flow are risk factors for UI regardless of parity.[957] During the first 3 months postpartum, pooled prevalence of any postpartum UI was 33% (95% CI: 32% to 36%) in all women. The mean prevalence of weekly and daily incontinence was 12% (95% CI: 11% to 13%) and 3% (95% CI: 3% to 4%), respectively, and doubled after vaginal delivery (31%, 95% CI: 30% to 33%) compared to the cesarean section (15%, 95% CI: 11% to 18%). Prevalence within the first year postpartum showed only small changes.[958] Increased risk of long-term UI is associated with prepartum stress UI.[959] About 52% of women with pregnancy-related LBP and PGP had PF dysfunction characterized by UI, sexual dysfunction, and/or constipation,[942] having social and psychological implications. Clinicians treating patients with nonspecific PGP or pregnancy-related LBP and PGP should inquire about the presence of bladder, bowel, and/or sexual dysfunction and include assessment and treatment of the PFM in addition to the other deep and superficial muscles of the lumbopelvic hip region.

Classification for Pelvic Girdle Pain

PGP is a specific form of LBP occurring on its own or in conjunction with LBP.[913] Though presented here as a separate classification, clinically and functionally, the pelvis is not isolated from the thoracolumbar spine, hip, lower extremity, or, in some instances, the cervicothoracic spine and upper extremities. Though subject to debate, diagnosis can be reached after exclusion of medical disease or red flag conditions and after exclusion of a symptomatic lumbar spine as the lumbar spine refers to the pelvic girdle/SIJ region and/or hip. At a minimum, nonspecific PGP is likely a combination of factors related to nonoptimal stability of the lumbopelvic hip region. As with all musculoskeletal problems, the clinician must use current best evidence, clinical examination, clinical expertise, and the patient to clinically reason why the patient is presenting with PGP.

Emerging research supports a subgroup classification[916] of nonspecific CLBP patients presenting with PGP and is based on a diagnostic clinical reasoning model to identify the underlying mechanisms that drive the pain and guide patient management. This process has been discussed previously related to CLBP within a biopsychosocial framework and a neurophysiological perspective, indicating that ongoing pain can be mediated centrally and peripherally. Intertester reliability of the PGP classification was examined in the previously described study[792] for nonspecific CLBP (see Figures 4-1 and 4-2) with MCIs. In this classification, PGP is a subclassification of CLBP. One patient out of 26 was identified with PGP with 100% agreement between 4 trained examiners. The proposed classification for PGP (see Figure 4-3) is not presented as all-inclusive and complete but instead as a framework to guide clinical decision making.[916]

Chronic PGP disorders are subgrouped as specific pelvic pain disorders and nonspecific pelvic pain disorders[916] (see Figure 4-3). The specific subgroup includes PGP associated with pathology such as fracture or infection that requires medical management. The nonspecific subgroup includes pelvic pain disorders that are centrally mediated or peripherally mediated with a small group presenting with inflammatory pain. The centrally mediated subgroup may have dominant or nondominant psychosocial factors as the drivers of pain. The peripherally mediated subgroup has physical factors such as reduced or excessive force closure with or without cognitive psychosocial factors as drivers of the pain experience and guide intervention.[916] The subgroups are summarized in the next section.

Specific Pelvic Girdle Pain Disorders

The lumbar spine and hip should be thoroughly evaluated to assess for dominant, coexisting, or contributing influences. The timing, manner, and extent of the examination are at the clinician's discretion. However, as previously discussed in the lumbar spine examination, the use of a test item cluster[501,502] of distraction, compression, thigh thrust, Gaenslen's, and sacral thrust and no centralization or peripheralization is advocated to identify a symptomatic SIJ. If 3 or more tests are positive, sensitivity was 0.91 (95% CI: 0.62 to 0.98), specificity was 0.87 (95% CI: 0.68 to 0.96), +LR was 6.97 (95% CI: 2.70 to 20.27), and –LR was 0.11 (95% CI: 0.02 to 0.44). Using only 4 tests (distraction, thigh thrust, sacral thrust, and compression) and no centralization or peripheralization, only 2 of the 4 tests need to be positive for a diagnosis of SIJ-related pain: Sn 0.88 (0.64, 0.97), Sp 0.78 (0.61, 0.89), +LR 4.0 (2.13, 8.08), and –LR (0.04, 0.47). If all 6 tests do not produce familiar pain, the SIJ can be ruled out.[501,502]

When a symptomatic SIJ or PS is identified, the clinician must first decide whether the PGP is specific or nonspecific in nature (see Figure 4-3). SIJ pain due to a specific systemic or pathological process must be ruled out or ruled in through appropriate referral for medical diagnosis and management. Specific SIJ diagnoses include inflammatory disorders such as AS, Reiter syndrome, psoriatic arthritis, or rheumatoid arthritis and may be associated with inflammatory bowel disorders. Infectious disorders include osteomyelitis or tuberculosis. Disorders of spondylogenic origin include fracture, osteoporosis, or Paget's disease. Systemic diseases that can refer pain to the sacrum include endocarditis, gynecological disorders, and gastrointestinal disorders. Primary tumors are rare, but metastasis from prostate cancer, colorectal cancer, or multiple myeloma is possible with a history of cancer. Any organ disease or systemic condition of the pelvic or abdominal cavity can cause primary pelvic pain or referred musculoskeletal pain in the lumbopelvic hip region. Conversely, the hip, SIJ, pelvis, or lumbar spine can be the source of referred pelvic pain.[33]

While these pathological processes can be associated with altered motor control, the patterns are adaptive or protective in nature. Treatment with MT and exercise is not appropriate and the outcomes will not be successful. However, PT may be indicated to address the effects of certain disorders such as AS or in postfracture management.[916]

Nonspecific Pelvic Girdle Pain Disorders

O'Sullivan and Beales[916] subclassify nonspecific PGP disorders into 3 groups (see Figure 4-3): nonspecific inflammatory pain disorders, peripherally mediated nonspecific PGP with or without cognitive or psychosocial factors that amplify central pain, and centrally mediated PGP. In a small case series, these authors present 3 case studies to describe the clinical usefulness of this classification system.[960] The characteristics of these groups as described by O'Sullivan and Beales[960] are presented next.

Nonspecific Inflammatory Pelvic Girdle Pain Disorder[916]

A small group of PGP presents as inflammatory, distinguished by constant, unremitting pain; increased with weightbearing, compression, and pain provocation tests; and relieved by NSAIDs or local steroid injection, but does not have a specific inflammatory disorder or known etiology. These cases are unresponsive to PT intervention and referral for medical management is appropriate.[916]

Peripherally Mediated Pelvic Girdle Pain Disorder (see Figure 4-4)[916]

Characteristics of this classification include a well-defined localized SIJ pain and associated connective tissue or myofascial structures with or without complaints of PS pain. The pain is usually unilateral, intermittent, aggravated, and eased by specific postures or movements, often related to vertical loading or directional loading in weightbearing. Pain is not usually provoked or associated with spinal movement. Mechanism or timing of onset is clear, perhaps due to repeated activity or direct trauma such as a fall onto a buttock or landing hard onto one leg to the pelvis or peripartum. Consistent local motor control changes that inhibit the deep system or overactivate the superficial system are present, which negatively impacts force closure during various functional tasks. Suboptimal strategies for load transfer may repetitively strain sensitive tissues and serve as a cause of recurrent or chronic PGP or LBP. Cognitive and psychosocial influences may amplify pain and disability to varying levels in nonspecific PGP, even though the dominant driver is peripherally mediated. Strategies to promote positive beliefs and active coping strategies are needed in addition to addressing the physical impairments. O'Sullivan and Beales[960] proposed 2 subgroups: reduced force closure or excessive force closure, with details described next. For additional study, Lee and Lee[351] provided advanced concepts integrating research and clinical reasoning related to the lumbar spine, pelvic girdle, and hip regions.

1. *Reduced force closure or insufficient compressive force*: In this group, the peripheral driver is most likely excessive strain to the sensitized SIJs/PS and surrounding structures secondary to ligamentous laxity (ie, reduced form closure or passive stability)[921] and motor control deficits (ie, reduced force closure) across the pelvic girdle.[916,941,960] The motor control deficits, while initially secondary to pain, are now maladaptive or provocative in that reduced force closure leads to impaired load transfer through the pelvis, serving as an ongoing peripheral nociceptive mechanism for pain.
   - Reduced force closure is associated with postpartum PGP and a positive ASLR normalized with pelvic compressions.[930,961]
   - Motor control deficits are linked to reduced cocontraction of the deep muscles, iliopsoas, and gluteal muscles and compensation by overactivation of superficial muscles such as quadratus lumborum, thoracic ES, external oblique, RA, and internal oblique.
   - Functional impairments include walking, sitting, standing, or loaded rotational activities such as cycling and rowing.
   - Patients assume postures such as swayback in standing, slump sitting, habitual standing on one leg, or thoracic upright sitting[385,386,793,962,963] and are unable to disassociate pelvic and thoracic movement.
   - Lumbar spine-related pain or impairment and centralization or peripheralization are not present, although clinically, mixed presentations of nonspecific LBP and PGP do occur.
   - Pain may be eased with an SIJ belt[938,964] and by training optimal postural alignment and functional cocontraction strategies across the pelvis with relaxation of the overactivated superficial musculature.[916]
   - Based on clinical observation, mobilization, MET, soft tissue massage, and manipulation of the SIJs may provide short-term relief.[916]
   - Management focuses on retraining optimal loading strategies to enhance force closure of specific motor control deficits in order to control pain and restore functional capacity with evidence to support this approach[916,961]; regional interdependence influences should be addressed.
2. *Excessive force closure or excessive compressive force*[916]: This group has a peripheral nociceptive driver based on excessive, abnormal, and sustained loading of sensitized SIJ and PS structures from excessive activation of the motor system local to the pelvis or perhaps hypomobility (ie, increased form closure) due to stiffness in articular structures usually related to trauma or joint fusion.
   - Pain is usually localized to the SIJs/PS and associated tissues and pain provocation tests are positive. However, the ASLR is negative, while manual or belt compression and stabilization exercises are often provocative or do not reduce effort to lift the leg.
   - Habitual postures may show varied patterns of high levels of cocontraction, including both deep muscles and superficial muscles such as ES and gluteals.
   - Lee and Lee[351] described 3 muscles that, when overactive, can compress various parts of the SIJ:

ischiococcygeus, piriformis and superficial LM. The authors[351] described a bilateral "butt-gripping strategy," resulting in a large divot posterior to the greater trochanter, the pelvis in posterior tilt, lower lumbar spine in flexion, and the lower extremities externally rotated. If unilateral, the pelvis may be rotated in the transverse plane.

- Motor control strategies may be due to excessive cognitive muscle training or protective guarding and are provocative.
- Easing factors are cardiovascular exercise, relaxation, stretching, soft tissue mobilization, MET, manipulation, and discontinuation of stabilization exercises.
- Some clinicians believe that the pelvis is unstable or displaced with all PGP and that an intervention strategy of more muscle contraction is beneficial. In this subgroup, the driver is an overactivation or high-load motor control strategy, even when unnecessary. These individuals may be anxious, under high levels of stress, and highly active individuals. The initial intervention involves strategies to reduce the overactive muscles (ie, reduce force closure).
- Management for excessive activation of the motor control systems may involve reducing force closure across the pelvic girdle through relaxation strategies, diaphragmatic breathing, muscle inhibitory techniques, and cardiovascular exercise. Management due to hypomobility from stiff articular structures involves mobilization or manipulation and specific retraining of optimal loading strategies. Influences from the lumbar spine, hip, and lower extremity should be addressed.

Centrally Mediated Pelvic Girdle Pain[916]

This group is similar to the nonspecific CLBP with centrally mediated pain and presents with widespread, severe, and constant nonmechanical pain. A peripheral driver or pathology is not identified. Widespread allodynia, generalized hyperalgesia, physical impairment, and inconsistent motor control deficits are secondary to central sensitization, which is often associated with dominant cognitive and psychosocial influences such as fear, anxiety, depression, and catastrophizing. These PGP disorders are very disabling and unresponsive to PT management. An interdisciplinary approach targeting functional rehabilitation, graded exposure, pain neurophysiology education with medical management for CNS modulation, and psychological management with coping strategies is required.[916]

Pregnancy-Related Pelvic Girdle Pain

During the first 3 months postdelivery, the prevalence of women with PGP falls substantially, reaching about 25%.[965] Eight to 10% of the women with PGP continue to have pain for 1 to 2 years.[965-967] About one-fifth of those with PGP postpartum are assumed to have serious problems and diminished quality of life.[968] About 50% of all women suffer from lumbopelvic pain as a complication of pregnancy, with 20% reporting PGP.[965] Pregnancy-related PGP is usually located between the posterior iliac crest and the gluteal fold, most often near the SIJ, and can be referred to the posterior thigh with or without pain in the PS or may be only experienced in the PS. The classification for chronic PGP described by O'Sullivan and Beales[916] is applicable to pregnancy-related PGP and will assist in developing appropriate management strategies. However, since women with pregnancy-related lumbopelvic pain have varying clinical presentations,[936,969,970] subgroup classification is being investigated on pregnant and peripartum women to further assist in defining optimal management strategies. Investigations are ongoing to describe the varying clinical presentations in women with pregnancy-related lumbopelvic pain.

In a cohort of 215 postpartum women of whom 86/262 had lumbopelvic pain, a standardized classification system identified 3 subgroups: PGP (45/262), lumbar pain (27/262), and combined PGP and lumbar pain (14/262).[944] In another study using this classification system,[971] women with combined PGP and lumbar pain recovered to a lower degree (17 of 51) than those with PGP (56 of 85) or lumbar pain (21 of 29). Predictors for persistent PGP or combined pain after delivery include low back flexor endurance, older age, combined pain during 12 to 18 weeks gestation, and work dissatisfaction explaining 30% of the variance.[971] Subsequently, the reliability of this classification system was measured for lumbopelvic pain to determine its ability to differentiate between lumbar pain and PGP in pregnancy.[972] Thirty-one pregnant women with nonspecific lumbopelvic pain were evaluated by 2 physical therapists using a standardized history and examination protocol. The protocol included ROM of the back and hip, repeated movements of the lumbar spine, a neurological examination, ASLR, and 5 pelvic pain provocations tests (ie, distraction, P4 [thigh thrust], Gaenslen's test, compression, and sacral thrust).[972]

Based on the examination, subjects were classified as either a PGP group, a lumbar pain group, or a combined group. Criteria for being assigned to the PGP group[972] were as follows:

- Pain experienced distal to L5 between the posterior iliac crest and the gluteal fold with or without radiation in the posterior thigh and calf and with or without pain in the PS
- Pain reproduced by at least 2 out of 5 provocation tests
- No centralization or peripheralization phenomenon and no change in lumbar pain or the ROM during repeated movements
- PGP onset was related to pregnancy[972]

Criteria for being assigned to the lumbar pain group[972] were as follows:

- Pain experienced in the lumbar region with or without radiation to the leg
- Reproducible pain and/or a change in the ROM from repeated movements or different positions of the lumbar spine or centralization and/or peripheralization during examination
- Less than 2 positive provocation tests[972]

Criteria for being assigned to the combined pain group[972] were as follows:

- Lumbar region pain as well as between the posterior iliac crest and gluteal fold with or without radiation in the posterior thigh and calf and with or without pain in the symphysis
- 2 or more positive provocation tests
- Pain and/or a change in ROM from repeated movements or different positions of the lumbar spine or centralization and/or peripheralization[972]

Agreement for the 3 groups (ie, LBP, PGP, combined pain) in pregnant women with nonspecific lumbopelvic pain was 87% (27/31) with a κ coefficient of 0.79 (95% CI: 0.60 to 0.98). This classification system, in contrast to the O'Sullivan and Beales' classification system,[916] includes only biomedical factors and does not include psychosocial factors. Use of this classification system may assist in differentiating nonspecific LBP from nonspecific PGP. Further subgrouping of the lumbopelvic classification[972] in peripartum women is needed to develop matched interventions, and psychosocial factors as well as muscle performance should be considered in subgroup analysis.

Components of the Subjective Examination for Persons With Pelvic Girdle Pain

The importance of a thorough subjective examination has been discussed in Chapter 2. Patients complaining of pregnancy-related PGP or PGP due to other causes may also have LBP or a combination of the two. Despite its poor diagnostic utility, the subjective examination attempts to distinguish among these different disorders that seem to have overlapping or similar complaints.

The patient's description of pain provides important information related to diagnosis and classification of PGP. Pain related to the SIJ is located primarily over the joint, inferior to the PSIS, and may refer distally to the buttock, groin, or posterior thigh but does not refer to the low back. Several studies describe SIJ pain referral features:

- A unilateral area 3-cm wide by 10-cm long just inferior to the PSIS[973,974]
- Groin pain only present in SIJ patients[975]
- Only non-SIJ patients had pain above L5[976]
- Decreased likelihood of SIJ pain radiating below the knee in older patients[977]
- Absence of lumbar pain and pain when rising from sitting
- 3 or more positive P4 tests[978]

In patients suspected of SIJ pain undergoing SIJ block with lumbar causes excluded, Fukui and Nosaka[979] reported all had pain over the SIJ, 68.7% in the medial buttock, 37.5% at the greater trochanter and lateral thigh region, 31.2% in the posterior thigh, and 9.3% in the groin area. Anecdotally, symptoms may present on the contralateral side from the initial dysfunction.

Potential mechanisms of injury for PGP are similar to those for nonspecific LBP. Slipman et al[980] reported various mechanisms of injury: falls or lifting with torsional stresses; trauma; sudden heavy lifting; prolonged lifting and bending; rising from a stooped position; MVA with same side on the brake; and repeated torsional stresses such as golf, bowling, skating. In 194 subjects with SIJ pain confirmed by diagnostic block, Chou et al[981] reported the following inciting events: 44% traumatic including MVA, fall onto buttock, immediately postpartum, football, and one pelvic fracture; 21% nontraumatic cumulative injury including lifting, running, a lower extremity injury, training injury, and forceful hip extension; and 35% spontaneous or idiopathic SIJ pain.

Aggravating factors for LBP such as sitting, standing, and walking are commonly considered by clinicians as aggravating factors for patients with PGP. Schwarzer et al[975] reported that these items do not discriminate between patients with or without PGP. Dreyfuss et al[976] reported that no aggravating or easing factors had value in differentiating patients with or without PGP. For aggravating factors, the results are as follows: cough/sneeze (Sn 0.45, Sp 0.47, +LR 0.9), bowel movements (Sn 0.38, Sp 0.63, +LR 1.3), wearing heels/boots (Sn 0.26, Sp 0.56, +LR 0.8), and job activities (Sn 0.20, Sp 0.74, +LR 1.5). Easing factors revealed the following: standing (Sn 0.07, Sp 0.98, +LR 3.0), walking (Sn 0.13, Sp 0.77, +LR 1.3), sitting (Sn 0.07, Sp 0.80, +LR 1.2), lying down (Sn 0.53, Sp 0.49, +LR 1.1), and lying down with painful side up (Sn 0.75, Sp 0.23, +LR 1.0).[976] Though aggravating and easing factors may not help with diagnosis, they are useful to set goals and can be analyzed for nonoptimal movement patterns and MCIs that become targets for intervention.

As discussed in Chapter 4, related to CLBP, PGP can present with peripherally or centrally mediated pain drivers. The following subjective information should be considered to assist with differentiation[916]:

- Pain area whether localized or widespread
- Levels of disability and impairment
- History related to specific and surrounding events as contributors to the development of symptoms
- Family history of PGP
- Presence of active or passive coping strategies
- The patient's pain beliefs and the presence of psychosocial and fear-avoidance behaviors
- Pacing patterns
- Presence of incontinence and/or sexual dysfunction[916]

Overall, the history appears to provide little to no statistically significant diagnostic value for PGP. However, the patient's story is still valuable from a clinical reasoning perspective to understand the patient's problem, generate hypotheses, and to assist in planning the objective examination. The PSFS may be useful as well as listening to the patient's story and asking targeted questions related to activity limitations for purposes of developing outcome measures. Clinicians should also rely on relevant outcomes such as pain intensity, functional status, quality of life, perception of improvement, impact on employment, and measurements from the physical examination.[913]

Components of the Physical Examination for Persons With Pelvic Girdle Pain

The examination process to determine whether the pelvic girdle, meaning the SIJ, PS, or both, is the source of a patient's pain is a subject of much debate and varies considerably in clinical practice. While subject to much scientific inquiry, little useful information has resulted for examination and diagnosis. The European Guidelines[913] for diagnosis of PGP state SIJ pain disorders can be diagnosed using a clinical examination[501,502,978,982] and includes pain primarily located to the inferior sulcus of the SIJs, positive SIJ pain provocation tests, and an absence of painful lumbar spine impairment. These general evidence-based guidelines are recommended to determine the pelvic girdle as a source of pain, but they provide no guidance related to intervention.

Functional Tests, Active Range of Motion, and Repeated Movements

Relevant functional tests should be analyzed for quality of movement, from a biomechanical viewpoint, from a motor control perspective, and for provocation. During biomechanical analysis, nonoptimal strategies may provide clues to deficits in form and force closure. As described for LBP, standard cardinal plane AROM tests or tests of combined movements are not useful to discriminate between patients with or without SIJ pain[983] but may be useful as a functional baseline of provocative movement and a measure of dynamic motor control when altered or asymmetrical movement occurs between the left and/or right sides of the pelvis. As previously discussed, strong evidence supports that the response to repeated movements seeks to establish the presence or absence of centralization or peripheralization and assists in ruling in or out a lumbar spine component.

Passive Range of Motion and Passive Accessory Motion Tests

Asymmetry or side-to-side differences in laxity or stiffness correlates with SIJ pain in peripartum patients.[932] Passive physiological motion tests, anterior and posterior tilt of the ilium commonly performed in side-lying (Figure 4-139) are reported in the clinical literature, but the reliability and diagnostic accuracy are unknown. Passive accessory movements (Figure 4-140) take many forms and generally compare one side to another, but no studies have assessed their diagnostic utility. Anterior-to-posterior movement (see Figure 4-140) is assessed in supine through the ASIS; PA movement is assessed in prone through the PSIS; and CPA movement is also assessed directly on the sacrum to the coccyx (see Figure 4-139C). Using a pisiform contact, superior-to-inferior glide at the PS is performed in supine (Figure 4-141).

Hip Examination

As with LBP, a hip problem may contribute to or present as PGP. Tests and measures for the hip are discussed under components of the physical examination for the lumbar spine (see Figures 4-46 to 4-70). Two useful test item clusters for the hip[984] may be important to identify or rule out a symptomatic hip OA as a component or contributor to LBP or PGP. The first test item cluster is hip pain, hip IR ROM less than 15 degrees, and hip flexion ROM less than or equal to 115 degrees. If hip IR ROM is greater than or equal to 15 degrees, the following test item cluster is recommended: age greater than 50 years, morning hip stiffness less than or equal to 60 minutes, and hip pain with IR. Diagnostic accuracy for both test item clusters is a +LR of 3.4 if all components are present and a –LR of 0.19 if all 3 are absent.[985] Finally, a relationship between asymmetrical hip rotation of ER greater than IR and LBP has been reported in patients with a variety of diagnoses of LBP as compared to persons without LBP.[985,986]

One hip test adds to the diagnosis of SIJ pain. The resisted hip ABD test has acceptable diagnostic accuracy

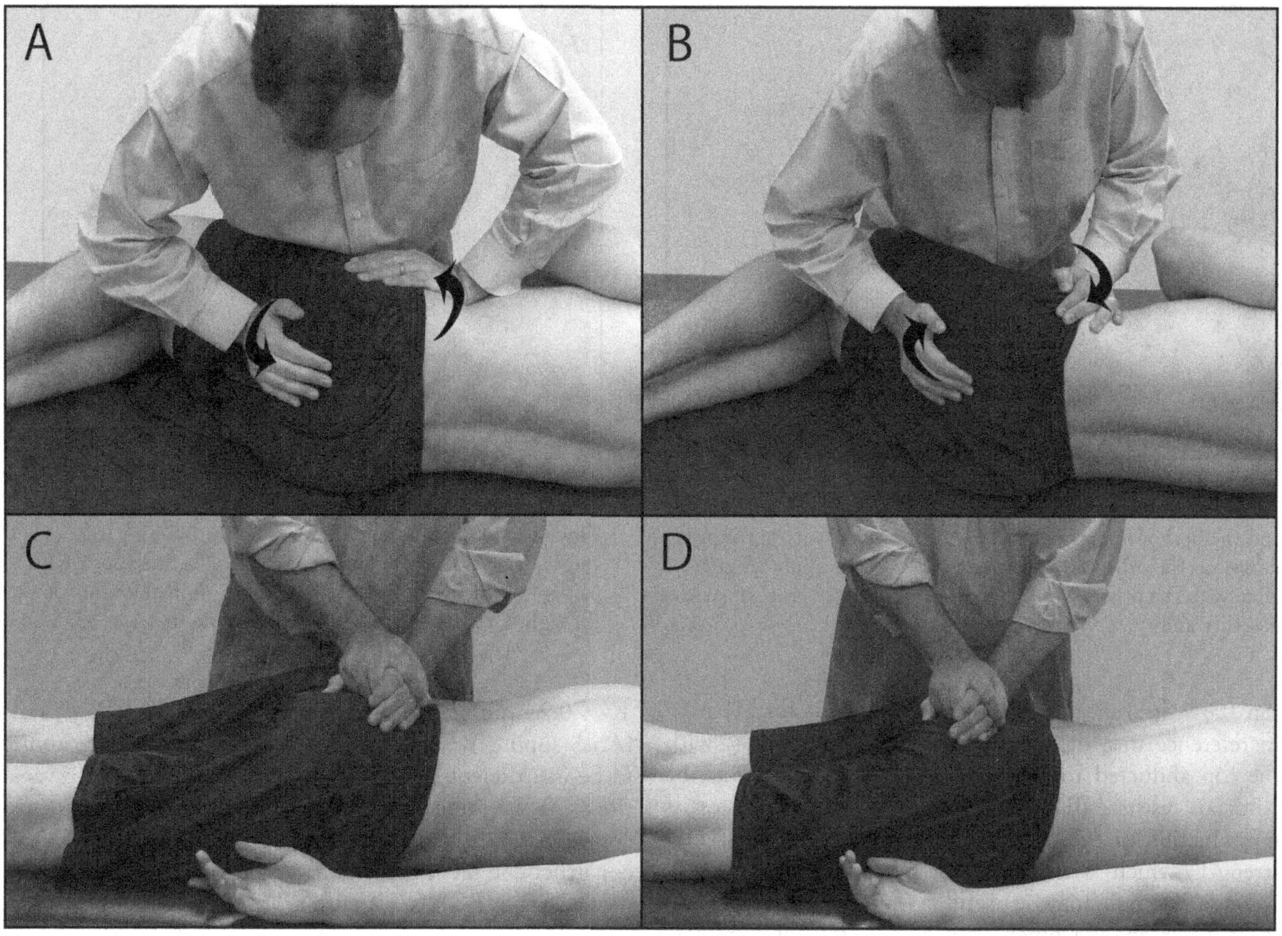

Figure 4-139. Passive physiological ROM, anterior and posterior tilt of the ilium and sacral nutation and counternutation: (A) anterior tilt; (B) posterior tilt of the ilium; in side-lying while supporting the uppermost knee in the clinicians abdomen or resting on top of the other leg table supported on a pillow, the SIJ is taken through full ROM into anterior tilt and posterior tilt by gently grasping the ilium in both hands; (C) sacral nutation (relative posterior tilt of the ilium); apply a PA force to the base of the sacrum centrally; assess mobility and pain response; and (D) sacral counternutation (relative anterior tilt of the ilium); apply a PA force to the apex of the sacrum.

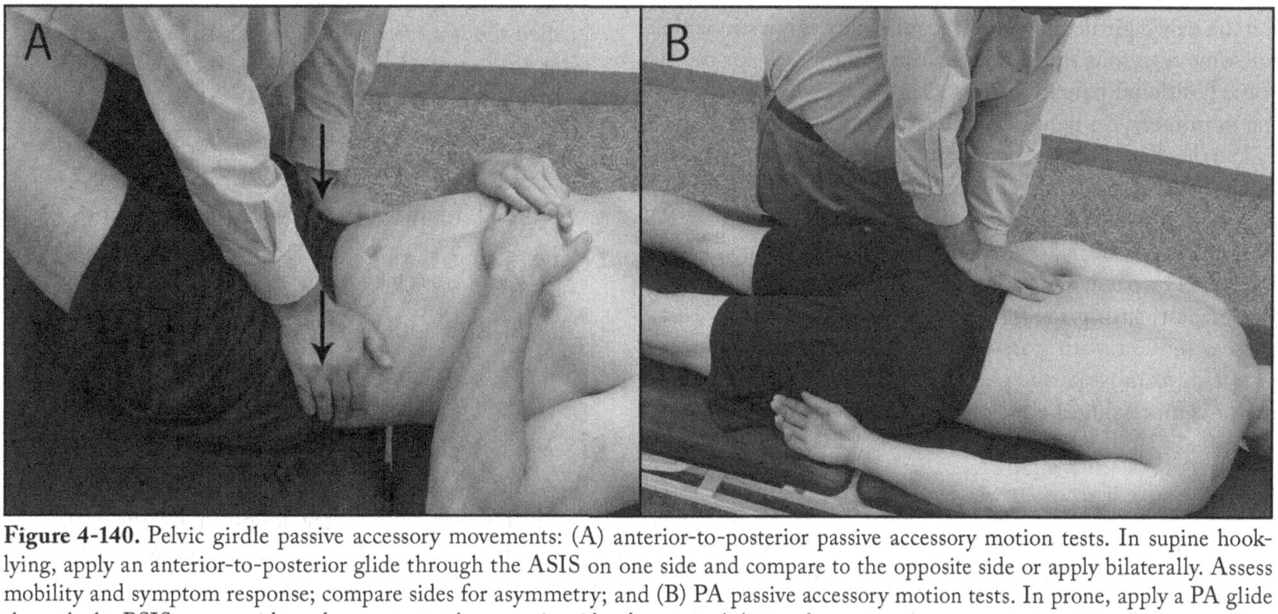

Figure 4-140. Pelvic girdle passive accessory movements: (A) anterior-to-posterior passive accessory motion tests. In supine hook-lying, apply an anterior-to-posterior glide through the ASIS on one side and compare to the opposite side or apply bilaterally. Assess mobility and symptom response; compare sides for asymmetry; and (B) PA passive accessory motion tests. In prone, apply a PA glide through the PSIS on one side and compare to the opposite side. Assess mobility and symptom response.

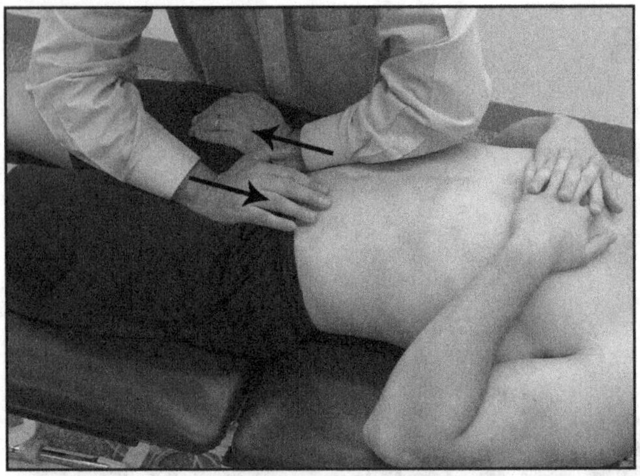

Figure 4-141. Superior-inferior glide at the PS. Use the heel of one hand on the superior aspect of the pubic ramus on one side and the heel of the other hand on the inferior aspect of the pubic ramus on the other side. Stabilize one side and apply an inferior glide with the other; switch hands and repeat the process. Assess mobility and symptom response.

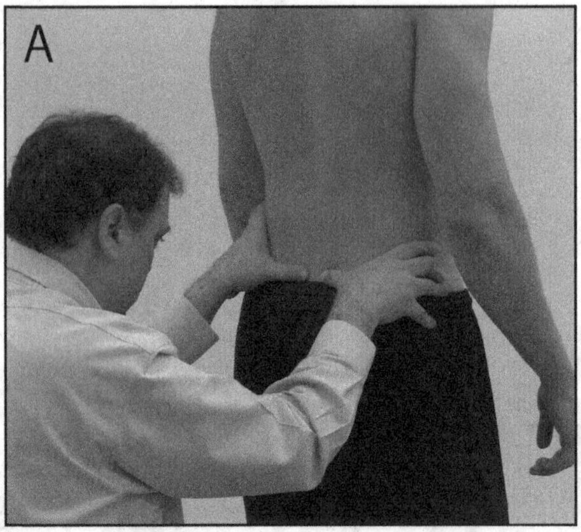

Figure 4-142. Standing hip flexion test, Gillet test, or stork test on the nonweightbearing side. (A) Start position; palpate S2 SP with the left thumb; the right thumb is on the right PSIS and hand on ilium. *(continued)*

(Sn 0.87, Sp 1.0; –LR.13, +LR NA) to test for SIJ pain in reference to a diagnostic SIJ block.[987] In supine with the hip abducted to 30 degrees and knee extended, the clinician resists ABD (see Figure 4-56). A positive test is reproduction of the patient's SIJ pain. Loss of hip ADD strength, which is tested in side-lying (see Figure 4-57), secondary to pain may be useful in implicating postpartum PGP.[947] Pregnant women with gluteus medius weakness are 6 to 8 times more likely to have LBP than those without weakness.[988]

Special Tests

Three categories of tests are traditionally used to examine the pelvic girdle; however, the reliability is questionable for some tests and the validity is unsubstantiated for most tests. Positional palpation tests aim to diagnose by detecting asymmetry in pelvic bony landmarks of the ASIS and PSIS, the iliac crests, the greater trochanters, the sacral sulcus, and the inferolateral angle of the sacrum. Motion palpation tests are designed to diagnose PGP by the detection of motion of relative abnormal pelvic landmarks during active or passive motion tests, such as the standing hip flexion test, sitting flexion test, or abnormal resistance to passive motion with passive accessory tests. Provocation tests aim to provoke the patient's specific pain by stretching or compressing the SIJ or PS and associated structures.

Positional Palpation Tests

Postural assessment was introduced earlier. In general, the absence or presence of bony pelvic asymmetry demonstrates poor to moderate interrater reliability (PSIS standing, $\kappa = 0.13$; PSIS sitting, $\kappa = 0.23$; iliac crest, $\kappa = 0.23$; pubic tubercle in supine, $\kappa = -0.04$),[140] and (ASIS supine $\kappa = 0.15$),[989] which is considered by some to be insufficient reliability to guide manual PT interventions. At the same time, positional palpation tests are not considered a valid measure of SIJ position. The theoretical construct connecting positional asymmetry to hypomobility or LBP or PGP is not currently supported.[989-998]

Motion Palpation Tests

General consensus related to the following tests is that they are not considered sufficiently reliable or valid indicators to PT intervention. Motion palpation tests include the following:

- The standing hip flexion test[999] (Figure 4-142), also called the *stork test*, performed on the nonweightbearing side, and Gillet test ($\kappa = 0.23$)[140]; +LR 1.31, –LR 0.83[976]
- The standing flexion test ($\kappa = 0.08$)[140]; +LR 0.81, –LR 1.05[993,999] (Figure 4-143)[999-1001]
- Modified Trendelenburg test[915] (Figure 4-144)
- The sitting flexion test ($\kappa = 0.08$)[140]; +LR 1.29, –LR 0.98[140,993,1000] (Figure 4-145)
- The PKB ($\kappa = 0.21$)[140,999] (Figure 4-146)
- Supine-to-sit test ($\kappa = 0.08$)[140]; +LR 1.22, –LR 0.88[993] (Figure 4-147)[991,996,999,1001-1003]
- Sacral springing ($\kappa = -0.06$)[1004]; +LR 1.14, –LR 0.81[976]

Clinically, positional and motion palpation tests seek to establish pelvic asymmetry followed by interventions to restore asymmetry. However, identifying reliable and accurate tests to quantify asymmetry remains a substantial challenge.

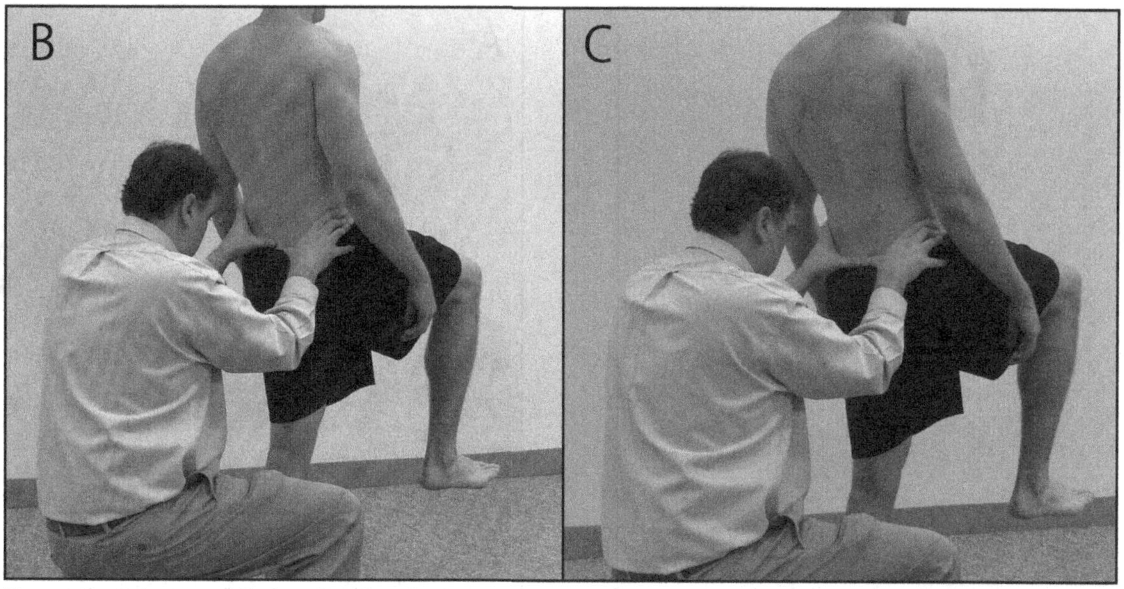

Figure 4-142 (continued). Standing hip flexion test, Gillet test, or stork test on the nonweightbearing side. (B) In standing, the patient is asked to raise the right knee toward the ceiling (ie, flex the right hip). The clinician maintains palpation of the S2 SP with the left thumb; the right thumb on the right PSIS and hand on ilium and monitors movement of the right PSIS and ilium. The right ilium should move into posterior tilt relative to the sacrum. Results are compared between left and right sides. (C) Theoretically, the PSIS that does not move posteriorly and inferior relative to S2 is considered a positive test.[136]

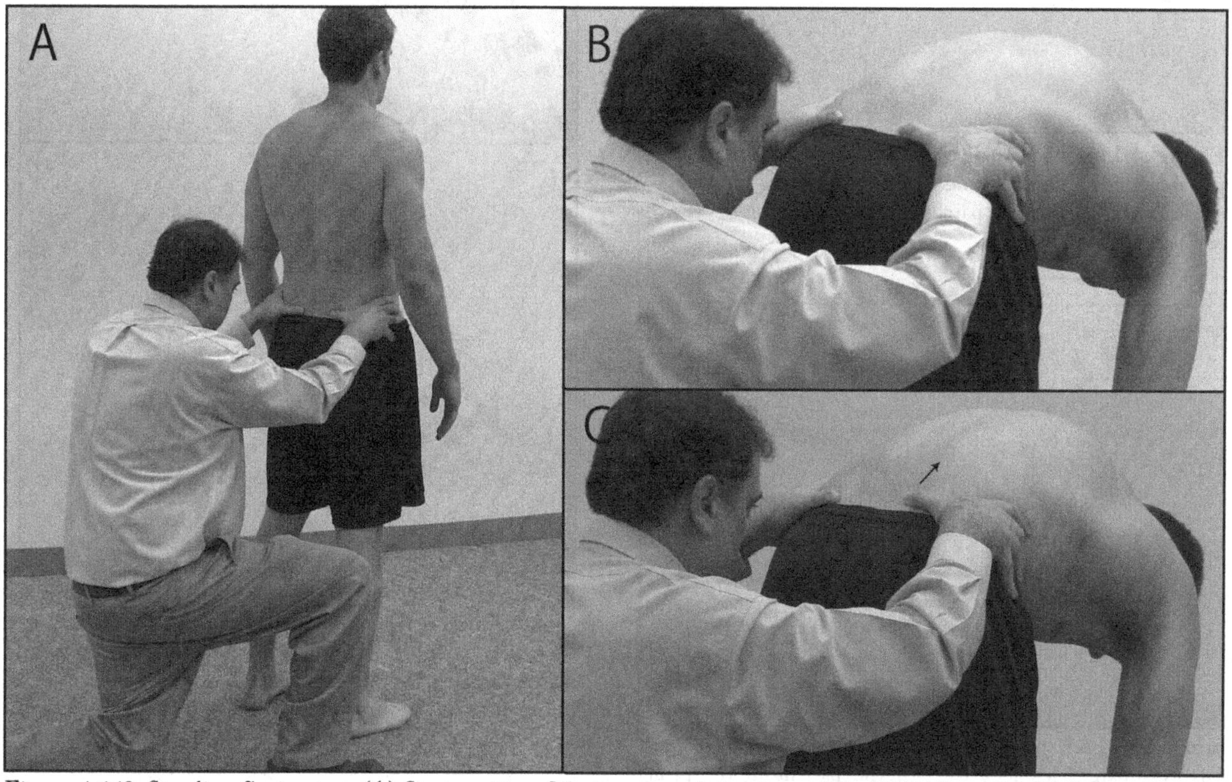

Figure 4-143. Standing flexion test. (A) Start position. Monitor the inferior slope of the PSIS bilaterally. (B) In standing, the patient is asked to bend forward. The clinician maintains palpation with the inferior slope of the PSIS/ilium bilaterally and monitors movement of the PSISs and ilia during forward bending. The normal response is symmetrical anterior tilt of both ilium over the femoral heads without deviation from the sagittal plane. (C) The side that moves further cranially is suggested as the dysfunctional side with an observable minimal difference between sides estimated at 2.54 cm or at least 1 inch.[1012]

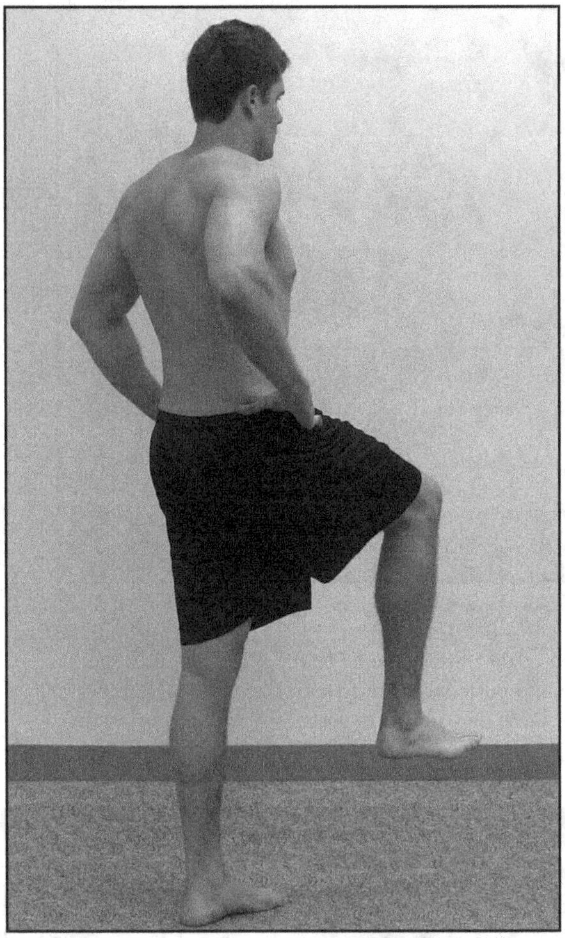

Figure 4-144. Modified Trendelenburg test.[925] The patient stands on one leg and flexes the opposite hip with the knee at 90 degrees. If pain is experienced in the PS, the test is considered positive.

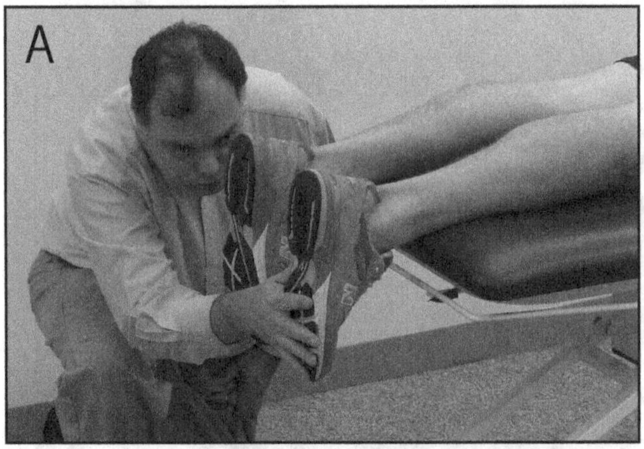

Figure 4-146. PKB or prone knee flexion test. (A) This test compares apparent leg lengths with the patient in the prone when both knees are extended to when both knees are flexed to 90 degrees by visually examining the left and right soles of the heel with shoes on. When the patient is lying prone with both knees fully extended, a finding of a shorter leg compared to the opposite side suggests, but does not confirm, a posteriorly rotated innominate. *(continued)*

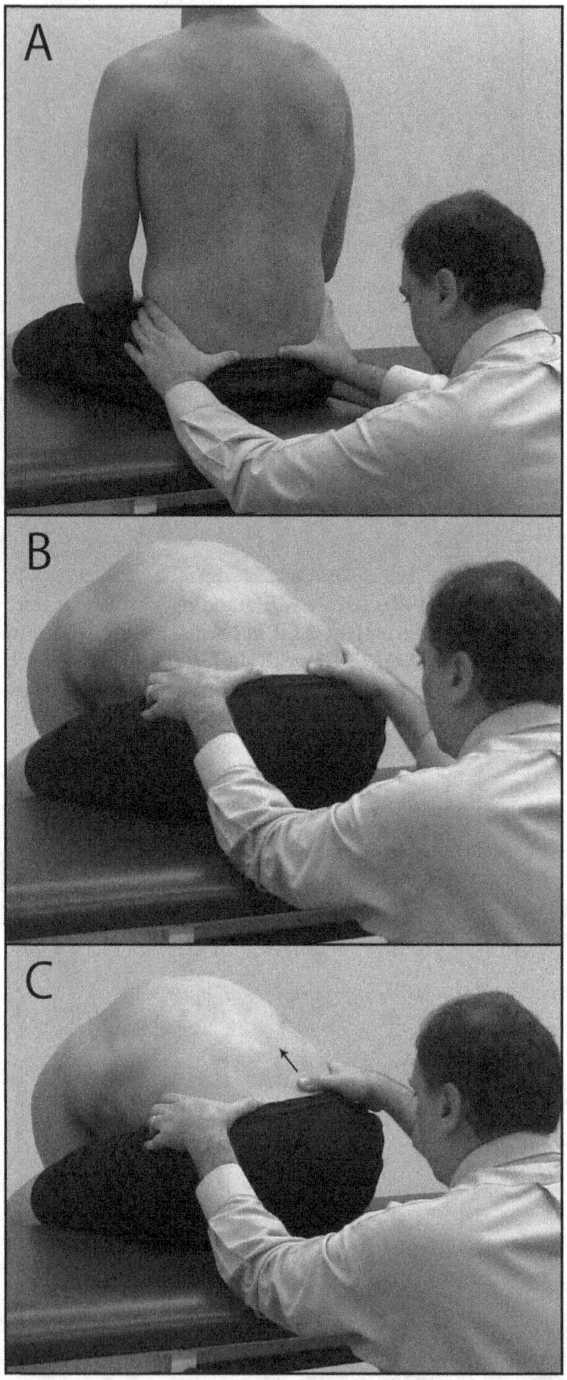

Figure 4-145. Sitting flexion test. (A) Start position. Monitor the inferior slope of PSIS bilaterally. (B) In sitting, the patient is asked to bend forward. The clinician maintains palpation with the inferior slope of the PSIS and ilium bilaterally and monitors movement of the PSISs and ilia during forward bending. The normal response is symmetrical anterior tilt of both ilium over the femoral heads without deviation from the sagittal plane. (C) The side that moves further cranially is suggested as the dysfunctional side and may indicate failure of load transfer. In the fully flexed position, a change in the relationship of one PSIS relative to the other indicates a positive test.[136]

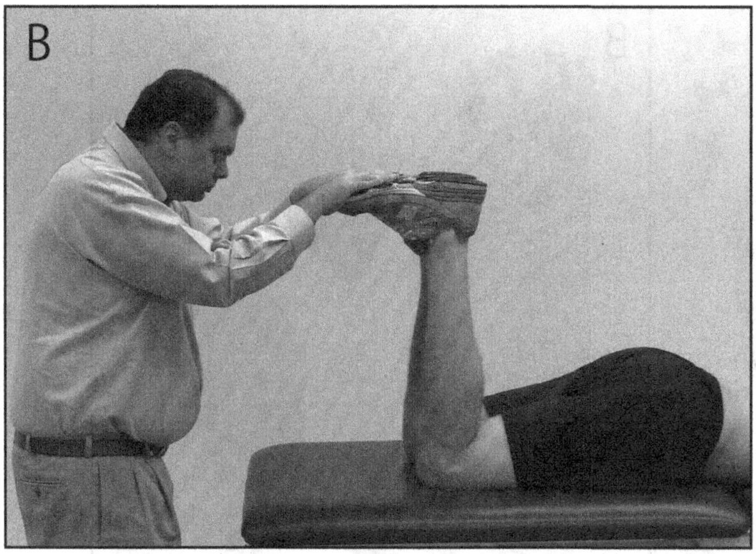

Figure 4-146 (continued). PKB or prone knee flexion test. (B) While both heels of the patient's shoes are held, the patient's knees are passively flexed to 90 degrees. An observable minimum difference estimated visually at 2.54 cm between the prone knee flexed and prone knee extended position is a positive test.[1012] Theoretically, an observed difference indicates a posteriorly rotated innominate.[1012]

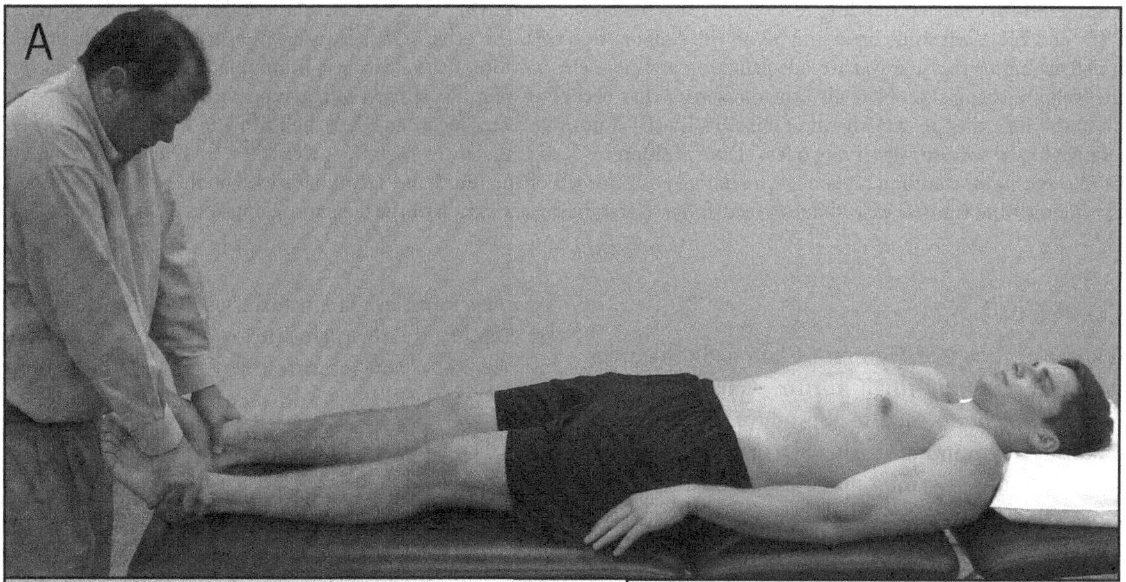

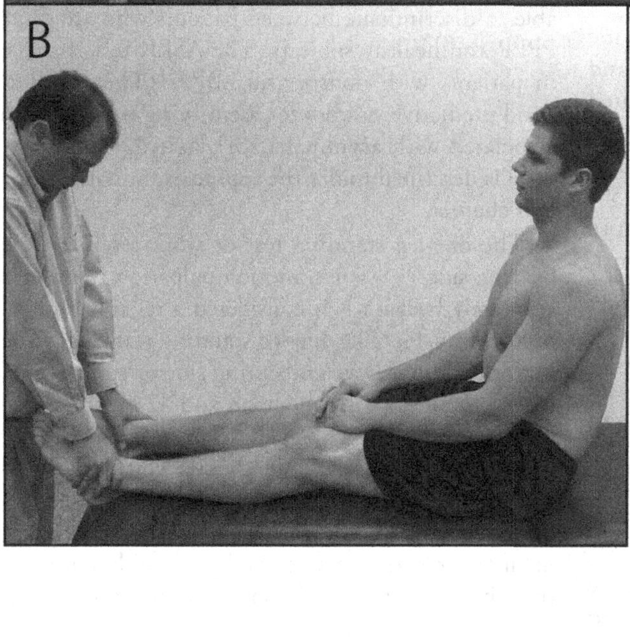

Figure 4-147. Supine-to-sit test or long-sitting test. The supine-to-sit test compares apparent leg lengths in the supine and long-sitting positions. In the supine position, the lengths of the inferior aspects of both medial malleoli are compared. The finding of a shorter leg when compared to the opposite side suggests a posteriorly rotated innominate. Theoretically, a posterior innominate rotates the acetabulum superior carrying the leg with it, giving the appearance of a short leg while supine. (A) Start position; holding the inferior medial borders of the medial malleoli with the thumbs and (B) the patient comes to a long-sitting position. An apparent lengthening of the short leg, an observable minimum difference between the supine and long-sitting position estimated visually at 2.54 cm is a positive test. The reverse would occur with an anteriorly rotated innominate.[1012]

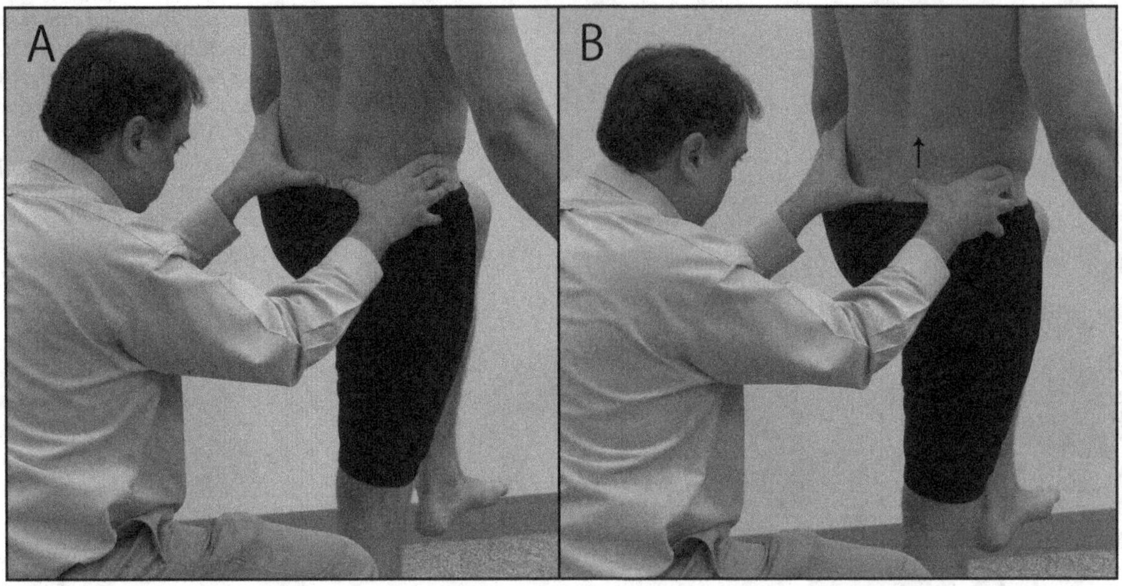

Figure 4-148. One-leg standing test or stork test on the weightbearing side. (A) On the weightbearing side, palpate PSIS and ilium with one hand and S2 on the support side with the other hand. Instruct the patient to flex the contralateral hip or the side you are not palpating and note the motion of the PSIS and ilium relative to the sacrum on the weightbearing side. Note also the movement that occurs as weight is shifted to the supporting leg; the PSIS and ilium should either posteriorly tilt or remain still. (B) A positive test is recorded when the PSIS and ilium tilt anteriorly relative to the sacrum, signifying a less stable position for load transfer through the pelvis.[451,1018] During movement from standing to standing on one leg, a relative posterior tilt of the ilium and sacral nutation should result in optimal SIJ stability and transfer of load due to feed-forward stabilizing activation of the deep muscle system prior to the move.

Provocation Tests

This cluster of tests (see Figures 4-81 to 4-85) includes distraction, compression, thigh thrust, Gaenslen's, and sacral thrust[502,503] performed to reproduce or increase a patient's familiar symptoms in the SIJ in an attempt to implicate or rule out a symptomatic SIJ. The tests have good to excellent interrater reliability (K): distraction (0.69), compression (0.73), thigh thrust (0. 88), Gaenslen's (0.76), and sacral thrust (0.56).[503] Laslett et al[502,503] reported the following statistics to suggest a symptomatic SIJ in patients having positive SIJ diagnostic injections and no centralization or peripheralization based on a repeated movement examination. If 3 or more of the previously mentioned tests are positive, Sn is 0.91 (95% CI: 0.62 to 0.98), Sp is 0.87 (95% CI: 0.68 to 0.96), +LR is 6.97 (95% CI: 2.70 to 20.27), and –LR is 0.11 (95% CI: 0.02 to 0.44). Using only 4 tests of distraction, thigh thrust, sacral thrust, and compression, only 2 of the 4 tests need to be positive for a diagnosis of SIJ-related pain: Sn 0.88 (0.64, 0.97), Sp 0.78 (0.61, 0.89), +LR 4.0 (2.13, 8.08), and –LR (0.04, 0.47). If all 6 tests do not produce familiar pain, the SIJ can be ruled out. Each test position is held 7 to 10 seconds and performed as follow.[502,503]

Transfer of Load Tests and Muscle Performance Tests

The ASLR (see Figure 4-43) assesses the ability of the lumbopelvic region to transfer loads between the trunk and lower extremities. The transfer of load requires both articular stability (ie, form closure) and adequate neuromuscular control (ie, force closure).[442] Patients with nonspecific LBP,[443-447] PPPP,[448] and sacroiliac disorders[442,443] show changes in movement patterns and force closure during the ASLR. Test-retest reliability of the ASLR in women with PPPP is ICC 0.83. The best balance between specificity (0.94) and sensitivity (0.87) occurs when scores 1 to 10 are designated as positive and 0 as negative.[450] The ASLR is able to discriminate between patients who are disabled by PPPP and healthy subjects. The ASLR test is also reliable in patients with nonspecific LBP.[451] The ASLR test has good predictive validity for identifying patients with PPPP associated with asymmetric SIJ laxity.[452] The test procedure is described under the supine examination for LBP in this chapter.

The one-leg standing test or stork test on the weightbearing side[941,1005] is a motion palpation test and covered separately because it is considered a reliable and valid test of load transfer. The one-leg standing test (Figure 4-148) is performed on the weightbearing side or stance side by palpating the PSIS with one hand and S2 on the support side with the other hand. The clinician instructs the patient to flex the contralateral hip (ie, the side you are not palpating) and notes the motion of the ilium (PSIS) relative to the sacrum on the weightbearing side. Also noted is the movement that occurs as weight is shifted to the supporting leg; the ilium and thus PSIS should either posteriorly tilt or

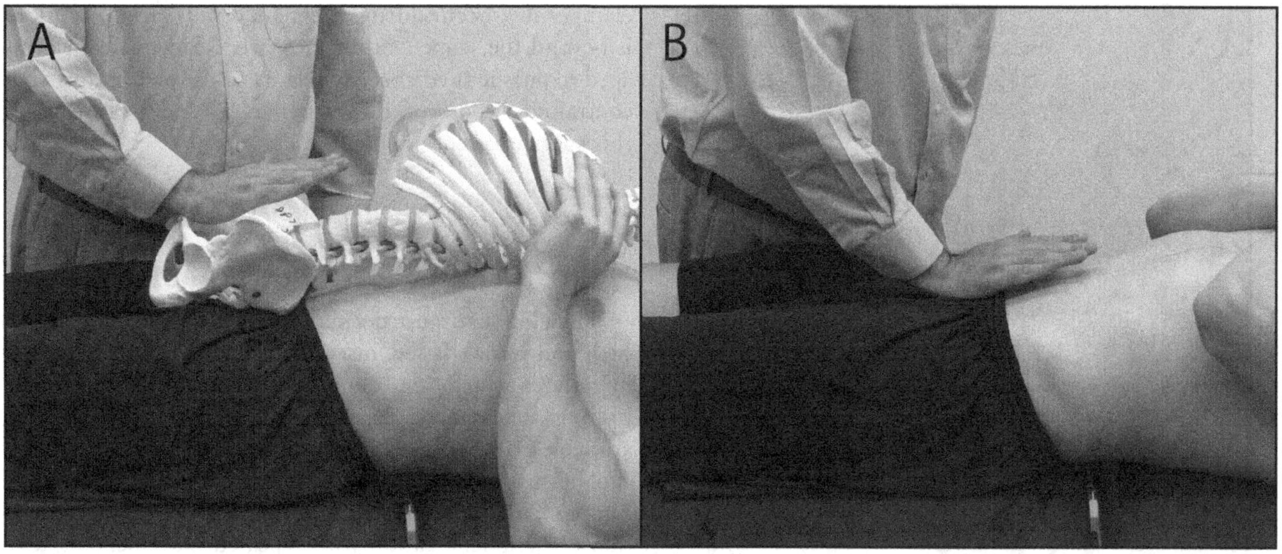

Figure 4-149. PS and pubic tubercle palpation: (A) the clinician should demonstrate to the patient on a skeleton where you will be placing your hands; (B) the clinician uses the heel of the hand to locate the PS or asks the patient to locate it first. *(continued)*

remain still. A positive test is recorded when the ilium or PSIS anteriorly tilts relative to the sacrum, implying a less stable position for load transfer through the pelvis.[941,1005] During movement from standing to standing on one leg, a relative posterior tilt of the ilium or sacral nutation should result in optimal stability and load transfer due to feed-forward activation of the deep muscle system prior to movement.[941,1005]

Hungerford et al[1006] investigated this hypothesis in 14 male subjects with PGP in the SIJ region aggravated by weightbearing on the symptomatic side compared to healthy controls. All subjects with SIJ pain had a positive active ASLR, positive stork test, and passive joint glide tests on the side of pain. In healthy subjects, the internal oblique and LM onset on the side of weightbearing occurred prior to movement to that leg. Onset of biceps femoris, adductor longus, gluteus maximus, gluteus medius, and tensor fascia lata occurred after initiation of movement. The ilium on the weightbearing side posteriorly tilted relative to the sacrum. In subjects with PGP, onset of the internal oblique, LM, and gluteus maximus were significantly delayed on the symptomatic side, suggesting an altered motor control strategy and ineffective stabilization. Onset of the biceps femoris occurred significantly earlier on the weightbearing side, theoretically a compensation strategy to augment force closure. The ilium anteriorly tilted relative to the sacrum on the symptomatic side, indicating failure of load transfer or the self-bracing mechanism. When a 2-point scale of either positive or negative was used, inter-therapist agreement on the pattern of intrapelvic motion during load transfer showed good reliability (left $\kappa = 0.67$, right $\kappa = 0.77$), and the percentage of agreement was high (left = 91.9%, right = 89.9%). A 3-point scale measuring the superior, inferior, or remaining neutral position of the PSIS resulted in moderate reliability for both the left and the right sides (left $\kappa = 0.59$, right $\kappa = 0.59$), and percentage of agreement decreased to left = 82.8%, right = 79.8%.[1006]

Palpation

Palpation of the PS and LDL are common tests useful for diagnostic purposes. Location and palpation of the PS and pubic tubercles are demonstrated in Figure 4-149. Albert et al[995,1007] described the clinical usefulness of PS palpation in symphysiolysis: reliability (0.89) and Sn 0.81, Sp 0.99; +LR 4.68. The clinician gently palpates the entire front side of the PS. If the palpation pain lasts more than 5 seconds after removal of the clinician's hand, pain is recorded. If the pain does not last >5 seconds, tenderness is recorded. Vleeming et al[1008] reported that palpation of the LDL may be useful in diagnosis. In prone, the LDL is palpated just inferior to the PSIS. The pain is scored on a 4-point scale: no pain (0); mild (1); moderate (2); and unbearable (3). The scores on both sides are added for a range from 0 to 6 with ≥2 as the cutoff. Vleeming et al[1009] reported that sensitivity was 76% in a group of 133 women with peripartum PGP. In women who scored positive on both the ASLR and P4 tests, sensitivity for LDL palpation was 86%.

Precautions During Examination and Treatment

Diastasis recti abdominis (DRA) is characterized as a midline separation of the RA muscle along the linea alba. Assessment procedures and grading criteria vary. The separation, visible as a midline bulge, is assessed 1 inch above or below the umbilicus, palpated during a head lift

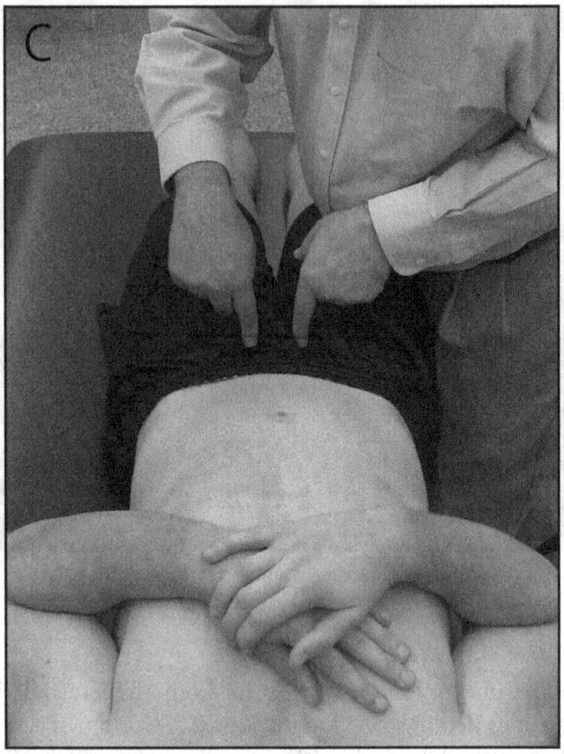

Figure 4-149 (continued). PS and pubic tubercle palpation: (C) the clinician gently palpates the front side of the PS, noting location of symptoms and symmetry of the pubic tubercles.

maneuver or partial sit-up with scapulae off the table and arms extended reaching forward.[1010] In supine with the hips and knees flexed and feet flat on the table, DRA is graded by the number of finger widths at approximately 1.5 cm per finger width between the medial edges of the RA muscle.[1010] According to Noble,[1010] a DRA of 3 or more finger widths requires corrective exercise, crossing the hands over the abdomen and pulling the bands of muscle toward the midline during a partial sit-up until the separation is decreased to 2 cm or less. Training of the TrA is also recommended.[1011,1012] DRA may be related to a variety of PFM dysfunctions such as UI, fecal incontinence, and pelvic organ prolapse.[1013] A higher degree of abdominal or pelvic region pain is associated with DRA.[1014]

After the first trimester, the enlarging uterus may compress the vena cava, abdominal aorta, and iliac arteries when lying in a supine position.[1015] This compression may result in decreased cardiac output and orthostatic hypotension, causing supine hypotensive syndrome. The patient may experience dizziness, nausea, paleness or flushing, and a sense of claustrophobia when lying on the back. The compression is usually relieved by shifting to the left lateral decubitus position. The American College of Obstetricians and Gynecologists[1016] recommended that pregnant women avoid supine positions during exercise as much as possible. A description of the anatomical and physiological changes that occur during pregnancy and warrant caution is beyond the scope of this reference. Readers are encouraged to pursue further study related to the precautions and contraindications for PT examination and treatment of this special patient population.

Pelvic Girdle Pain Examination Summary

The clinician must decide on the best examination for each individual based on the history, location of pain, hypothesis generation, clinical experience, relevant exam findings, movement deficits, and understanding of the available evidence. An initial diagnosis of nonspecific PGP can be made from a detailed history and exclusion of a symptomatic lumbar spine and hip, absence of centralization or peripheralization with repeated movements, a test item cluster of positive pain provocation tests, palpation of PS and long dorsal ligament, assessment of the deep and superficial muscle performance of lumbopelvic hip complex, a neurological examination, resisted hip ABD and ADD, and special tests of load transfer such as the ASLR and stork test on the weightbearing side. Little evidence supports the use of positional, motion palpation, and passive mobility tests for patients with PGP.

A diagnosis of nonspecific PGP is possible as outlined above, but a specific diagnosis or subgroup classification is more challenging. O'Sullivan and Beales[916] proposed a mechanism-based classification system for PGP within a biopsychosocial framework (see Figures 4-3 and 4-4) developed from a synthesis of current evidence and clinical expertise. A subclassification of PGP includes both specific and nonspecific musculoskeletal PGP disorders that are both complex and multifactorial in nature with the potential for both peripheral and central pain drivers. Within dominant peripherally mediated PGP disorders, a further classification is proposed, dividing patients into either reduced or excessive force closure of the lumbopelvic hip region resulting in abnormal stress on pain sensitive pelvic structures. Identification of either reduced or excessive force closure through examination of muscle performance helps to guide appropriate management. Further research is required to establish the validity of this classification system. RCTs related to clinical outcomes using this system have not been conducted. A classification of pregnancy-related LBP that includes LBP, PGP, or a combination of both[972] was presented, but the validity and ability to guide interventions has not been investigated. Patients who do not fit these classifications or present with disorders of urinary or fecal incontinence, pelvic pain with sexual intercourse, or complicated or high-risk pregnancy and delivery may require consultation with or referral to a physical therapist with specialized training in women's health.

Lee and Lee[351] described an integrated model of function related to the lumbopelvic hip complex with a focus on how the pelvis transfers loads during functional tasks. The authors reported that the model provides a framework that addresses why the pelvis is painful through identification of deficits in form closure, force closure, motor control, and emotions, and suggested a method to subgroup patients with failed load transfer according to the primary deficit. The examination process and details of integrated management of this complex region are beyond the scope of this chapter. Interested readers are encouraged to review this excellent reference.[351] Additional reading related to research of the lumbopelvic hip complex is also found in this text.[1017]

Evidence of Conservative Management of Pelvic Girdle Pain

While some progress has been made related to a framework of classification within the biopsychosocial model, very little evidence is available to guide intervention in nonspecific PGP. Therefore, a treatment prescription for PGP must be developed based on relevant impairments or deficits hypothesized to explain nonoptimal stabilization strategies for the lumbopelvic hip complex, continual use of assessment and reassessment, clinical reasoning, and the highest external evidence. At the end of the physical examination and excluding specific red-flag PGP disorders, the patient may be classified as nonspecific PGP or peripherally mediated, centrally mediated, or a combination of both, with emphasis on the establishment of a primary driver. Consideration of the guidelines for intervention from O'Sullivan and Beales[916,960] is appropriate. As previously discussed, peripherally mediated PGP may be further classified as excessive force closure (too much compressive force) or reduced force closure (insufficient compressive force). Specific examination findings on motor control strategies (ie, excessive or reduced force closure and timing), mobility deficits (ie, excessive or reduced form closure), impairment of muscle performance (ie, strength, endurance), and cognitive behavioral issues (ie, fear, anxiety, depression, stress) are identified, prioritized, and targeted for intervention.

Several risk factors have been identified for continued pregnancy-related PGP beyond 3 months postdelivery. Prolonged duration of labor, age greater than 29 years, VAS pain intensity of more than 6/10, early gestation pain onset, combined LBP and PGP in pregnancy and pain in more than one of the pelvic joints, a high number of positive provocation diagnostic tests, a low index of mobility, unskilled work history, and multiparity may be associated with poor prognosis.[1018] Expectations of a positive outcome and a positive ASLR test of less than 4 support a favorable prognosis.[1019]

Systematic Reviews

Strong comparative evidence for various treatments of pregnancy-related PGP across multiple medical disciplines is lacking. To manage prenatal-related LBP and PGP, a variety of procedures may be useful in addition to usual care. For women with LBP, strengthening exercises, sitting pelvic tilt exercises, and water gymnastics reduced pain intensity and back pain-related sick leave better than usual prenatal care alone.[1020] For PGP, stabilizing exercises and acupuncture was more effective than usual prenatal care. For women with both LBP and PGP pain, acupuncture was more effective than physiotherapy in reducing pain intensity. Stretching exercises reduced total pain (60%) more than usual care (11%). Usual prenatal care alone resulted in more use of analgesics, physical modalities, and sacroiliac belts.[1020] While the effects are small, the authors concluded that the addition of pregnancy-specific exercises, physiotherapy, or acupuncture to usual prenatal care is better at reducing back or PGP than usual prenatal care alone.[1020]

Evidence to support the use of acupuncture in pregnant women with PGP is mixed. Acupuncture in pregnancy is considered safe, but certain points must be avoided.[1021] Sixty percent of those receiving acupuncture reported less intense pain compared to 14% receiving usual prenatal care.[1020] In contrast to older studies, acupuncture for women with PGP showed no significant effect on pain or on sick leave compared to nonpenetrating sham acupuncture, although some daily activities improved as measured by the disability rating index. No significant differences in quality of life, discomfort of PGP, and recovery were found between groups.[1022] The role of acupuncture in reducing pain during pregnancy is unclear.[916]

Another review[1021] of treatment options for PGP and LBP in pregnancy reports benefits for some individuals from patient education on ergonomics and posture, the use of pelvic stabilization belts, acupuncture, and tailored postpartum aquatic exercises. Pregnant women with a previous history of LBP may benefit from education and exercise.[1023] Patient education is useful and may include energy conservation and lifting strategies, avoiding fatigue, maintenance of good postures, and rolling in bed with knees flexed and squeezed together.[913,1024,1025] The use of an abdominal support pillow in the lateral recumbent position and pillows to support other parts of the body appears to aid in decreasing pain and insomnia during late pregnancy.[1025,1026] No evidence supports a recommendation of massage, rest, or electrotherapy as stand-alone treatments for PGP.[913] Pelvic belts decrease SIJ mobility and work best when applied below the ASIS rather than at the level of the PS,[938] but no support exists for use of a pelvic belt alone for treatment[913] with recommended use limited to brief periods for symptomatic relief. Use of a pelvic belt during hip ABD in side-lying resulted in a significant decrease in

EMG activity of the quadratus lumborum and a significant increase in EMG activity of the gluteus medius and LM in healthy subjects.[1027]

Based on these systematic reviews, high-quality comparative evidence to guide clinical decisions with regard to treatment options for persons with nonspecific PGP is scarce. Exercises postpartum are generally recommended as effective for PGP and pregnancy-related LBP.[913,1028] Joint mobilization or manipulation may be used to assess for symptomatic relief, but only for a few treatments.[925] The recommended postpartum model is an individualized, supervised treatment program based on examination findings and focused on SSE as part of a multimodal plan for PGP. For all subgroups of PGP, examination findings related to motor control strategies (ie, excessive or reduced force closure and timing), mobility deficits (ie, excessive or reduced form closure), impairment of muscle performance (ie, strength, endurance), and cognitive behavioral factors (ie, fear, anxiety, depression, stress) are identified, prioritized, and targeted for intervention.

Manual Therapy and Exercise Intervention in Pregnancy-Related Low Back Pain

Little evidence supports or does not support the use of MT in pregnancy-related LBP. Vleeming et al[913] reported no evidence to support manipulation or mobilization for PGP, but suggested MT be used to assess for pain relief applied only for a few treatments because of increasing ligamentous laxity. Khorsan et al[1029] found that evidence to support effectiveness or lack of effectiveness for SMT including manipulation, mobilization, manual traction, and massage during pregnancy is lacking. The authors concluded that clinicians may want to consider SMT as a treatment option for patients who have a preference for this approach if no contraindications are present.[1029] Proposed contraindications to spinal manipulation may include vaginal bleeding, cramping, sudden onset of pelvic pain, premature labor, ruptured amniotic membranes, placenta abruption, ectopic pregnancy, and moderate to severe toxemia.[1030]

In antenatal and postpartum periods, adverse events associated with SMT (ie, HVLA thrust) to any region of the spine may be related to ligamentous laxity and hypercoagulable disorders (ie, venous stasis, vessel wall changes, and changes in blood composition).[1030] A review of the safety of SMT reported the following adverse events:

- *For cervical spine manipulation*: Stroke, epidural hematoma, and fracture
- *For lumbar manipulation*: Mild and transient reports of increased pain that resolved within a few days.[1031]

In this review, the authors suggested that the etiology of the adverse events is unknown and recommended informing patients of the risks associated with SMT, and making them aware of the signs and symptoms of possible neurovascular complications.[1031]

Another study[1032] in subjects between the 28th and 30th weeks of pregnancy compared usual obstetrical care (UOBC) and osteopathic manipulative treatment (OMT) (UOBC + OMT), UOBC and sham ultrasound treatment (SUT) (UOBC + SUT), and UOBC only. Outcomes included average pain levels and the RMDQ to assess back-specific functioning. Subjects with high-risk pregnancy were excluded. OMT was provided by an osteopathic physician over 7 weekly visits lasting 30 minutes. OMT included soft tissue, myofascial release, muscle energy, and ROM mobilization based upon the physician's identification of specific somatic dysfunctions in the cervical, thoracic, and lumbar spine; thoracic outlet and clavicles; rib cage and diaphragm; and pelvis and sacrum. A cranial compression technique of the fourth ventricle was not allowed due to risk of inducing premature labor. HVLA techniques were not allowed because of the potential risk related to increasing ligamentous laxity in late pregnancy.[1032] Intention-to-treat analyses of 144 subjects showed RMDQ scores worsened during pregnancy; however, back-specific functioning declined less in the UOBC + OMT group (effect size 0.72; 95% CI: 0.31 to 1.14; P = .001 versus UOBC only; and effect size 0.35; 95% CI: –0.06 to 0.76; P = .09 versus UOBC + SUT). Although between-group differences were not significant, during pregnancy, back pain decreased in the UOBC + OMT group, remained unchanged in the UOBC + SUT group, and increased in the UOBC only group. The authors concluded that OMT may slow or halt the deterioration of back-specific functioning during the third trimester of pregnancy.[1032]

A study by Murphy et al[1033] described the successful outcomes of a prospective cohort of consecutive pregnant women with pregnancy-related lumbopelvic pain, subgrouped as LBP, PGP, or a combination of both, who were examined and treated according to a diagnosis-based CDR[1034] (Figures 4-150 and 4-151). The decision rule[1034] allows the clinician to develop a working diagnosis upon which treatment decisions are made. Baseline data on 115 patients at the beginning of treatment and 78 patients at the end of treatment were collected. Disability was measured using the Bournemouth Disability Questionnaire (BDQ); pain intensity was measured using the NRS. Patients were also asked to self-rate their improvement. Care was provided by a chiropractic physician/physical therapist team. Exclusion criteria were systemic illness, red flags for complications to the pregnancy such as bleeding, spotting, unusual discharge, bouts of diarrhea, or feeling "as if the baby is going to fall out." Contraindications to treatments were spinal fracture, spinal infection, blood dyscrasias, CES, inflammatory arthropathy, inability to communicate well in English, worker's compensation or personal injury cases, and pain prior to the pregnancy.

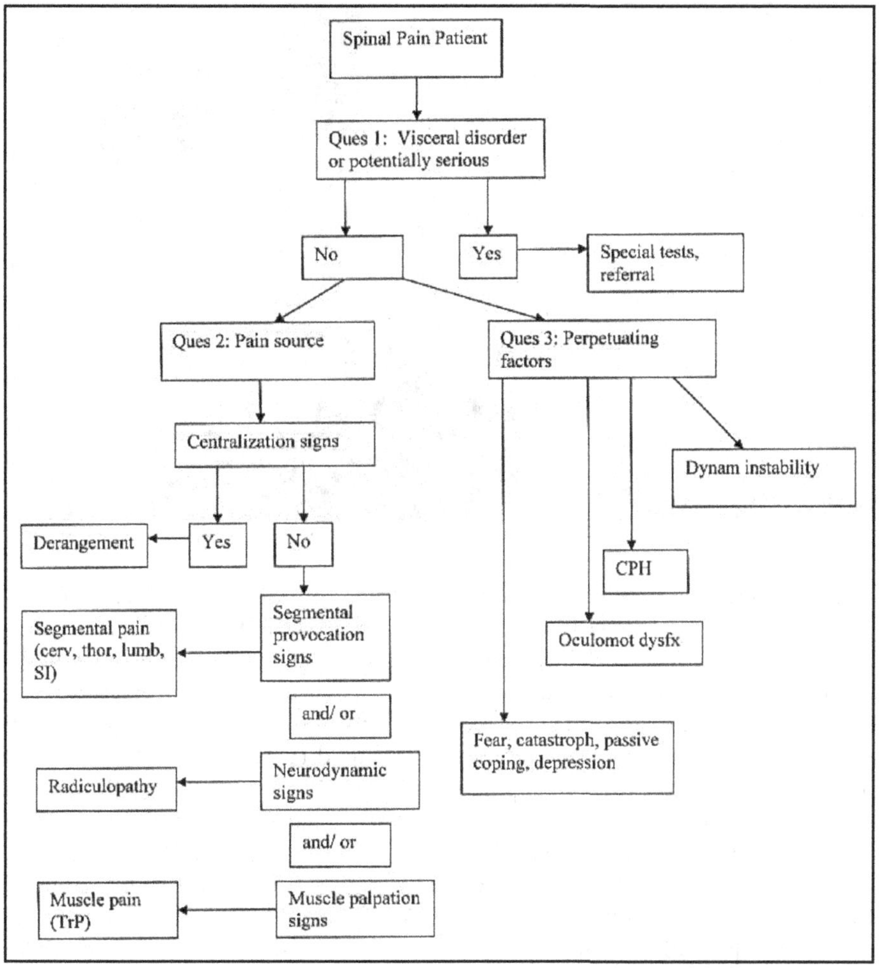

Figure 4-150. Diagnosis-based clinical decision rule for pregnancy-related lumbopelvic pain. Abbreviations: cerv, cervical; thor, thoracic; lumb, lumbar; SI, sacroiliac; TrP, trigger point; CPH, central pain hypersensitivity; dysfx, dysfunction; catastroph, catastrophizing. (Reprinted from Murphy DR, Hurwitz EL. A theoretical model for the development of a diagnosis-based clinical decision rule for the management of patients with spinal pain. *BMC Musculoskelet Disord*. 2007;8:75. © 2007 Murphy and Hurwitz; licensee BioMed Central Ltd. This is an Open Access article distributed under the terms of the Creative Commons Attribution License [http://creativecommons.org/licenses/by/2.0], which permits unrestricted use, distribution, and reproduction in any medium, provided that the original work is properly cited.)

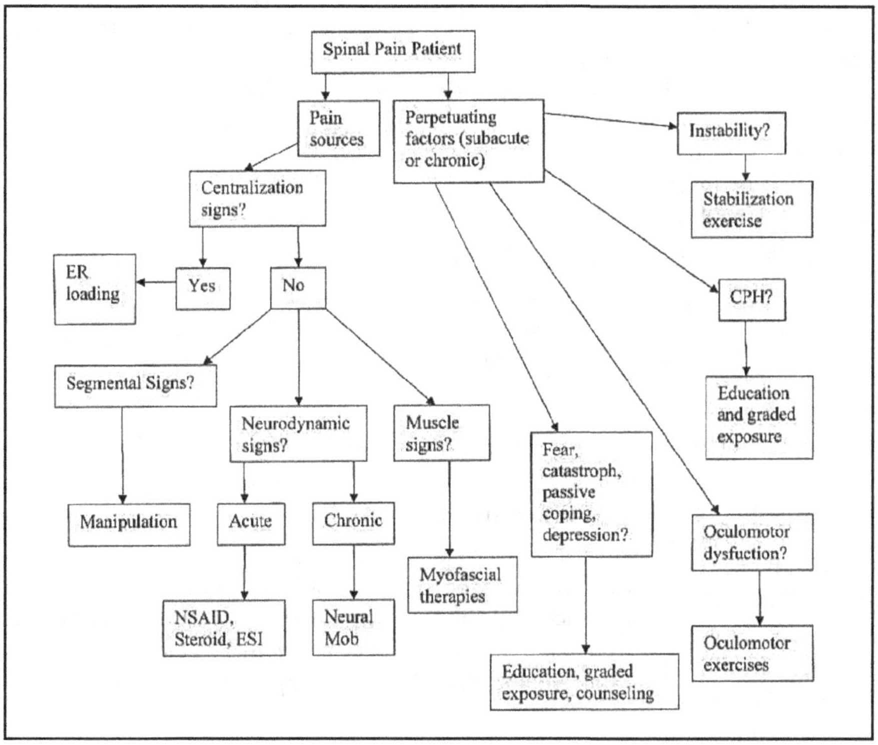

Figure 4-151. Management algorithm for the diagnosis-based clinical decision rule. Abbreviations: ER, end range; mob, mobilization; CPH, central pain hypersensitivity. (Reprinted from Murphy DR, Hurwitz EL. A theoretical model for the development of a diagnosis-based clinical decision rule for the management of patients with spinal pain. *BMC Musculoskelet Disord*. 2007;8:75. © 2007 Murphy and Hurwitz; licensee BioMed Central Ltd. This is an Open Access article distributed under the terms of the Creative Commons Attribution License [http://creativecommons.org/licenses/by/2.0], which permits unrestricted use, distribution, and reproduction in any medium, provided that the original work is properly cited.)

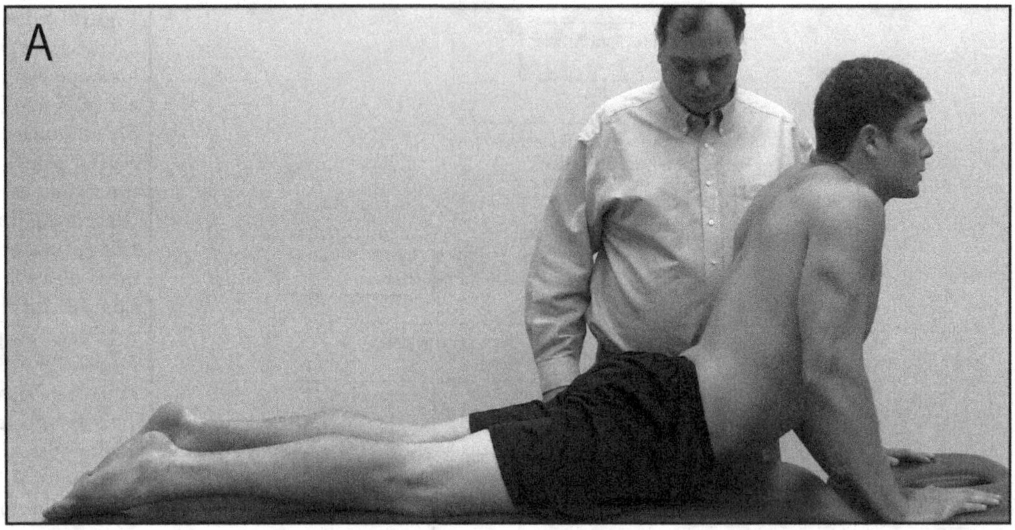

Figure 4-152. Hand heel rock ROM exercise. In quadruped, rest some of the weight on the hands and arms with the hands slightly in front of the shoulders: (A) a forward rock is done by transferring weight more to the hands, keeping the elbows straight while looking up and allowing the abdomen to sag. A brief pause at the end of range occurs before moving back toward neutral. *(continued)*

Patients were seen an average 6.8 visits. The treatment each patient received was based on the diagnosis. All but 10 patients received some form of MT in the form of lumbar or SIJ mobilization or manipulation with oscillatory mobilization in the prone position and wedges under the pelvis to attempt to counterrotate the ilia or manipulation in side-lying. Other interventions included end-range repeated movements, lumbopelvic stabilization exercise, neural mobilization, myofascial therapy, education, and graded exposure.[1033]

Fifty-seven patients (73%) reported either excellent or good improvement, with a mean improvement in pain of 2.9/10 points. Fifty-one percent of the patients experienced clinically significant improvement in disability; 67% had clinically significant improvement in pain. Upon 11-month follow-up, 85.5% of patients rated improvement as either excellent or good with a mean improvement in pain of 3.5 points. Seventy-three percent of the patients had clinically significant improvement in disability and 82% had clinically significant improvement in pain. Patients with combined pain in both areas were significantly less likely to experience a meaningful outcome in disability compared to the other 2 groups with the difference decreasing at long-term follow-up. Improvement in pain followed a similar pattern but was not significantly different. The authors conclude that this management strategy is a safe option that results in favorable outcomes.[1033] Lack of randomization and a control group limit interpretation of clinical effectiveness.

Similar to LBP, a CPR may assist with determining if a patient with PGP is likely to respond to manipulation. Al-Sayegh et al[1035] determined preliminary CPRs to identify postpartum women with LBP or PGP who are likely to respond to a lumbopelvic thrust manipulation technique (see Figure 4-100) followed by 10 repetitions of a hand-heel rock ROM exercise in quadruped (Figure 4-152). Sixty-nine women aged 18 to 45, within 1 year of giving birth, with LBP and pelvic pain, with or without referral to the lower extremities, and baseline ODQ scores of at least 30% were included in the study. Subjects with radiculopathy, a history of spinal surgery, a new pregnancy, or fracture were excluded. The study protocol over 3 sessions is similar to previous protocols[140,141] used to develop a CPR using the same manipulation technique in subjects with LBP.

Fifty-five subjects (80%) had success defined as 50% improvement in 48 to 72 hours after one intervention session with the supine HVLA thrust; 14 subjects (20%) were scored as a failure. No subjects in the failure group had more disability or pain after the intervention. The mean functional disability score (ODQ) at baseline was 42.26 ± 9.21. After the first intervention, it was 13.54 ± 11.47. Mean percentage improvement in the ODQ was 69 ± 25.25% (range, 10.5% to 100%). A CPR for success with 4 criteria[1035] was identified:

1. Pain not extending below the knee
2. Symmetrical PSIS test in the seated position
3. A positive seated flexion test
4. A positive PKB test[1035]

The presence of 2 of 4 criteria (+LR = 3.05) increased the probability of success from 80% to 92%. A CPR for treatment failure with 3 criteria was identified[1035]:

1. Age > 35
2. VAS of higher than 3/10 rated as the best level in the past 24 hours
3. A negative PKB test

The presence of 2 of 3 criteria (+LR = 11.79) increased the probability of treatment failure from 20% to 75%; the presence of 3 variables increased the probability of failure from 20% to 87%. These preliminary findings must be validated and should include long-term follow-up.[1035]

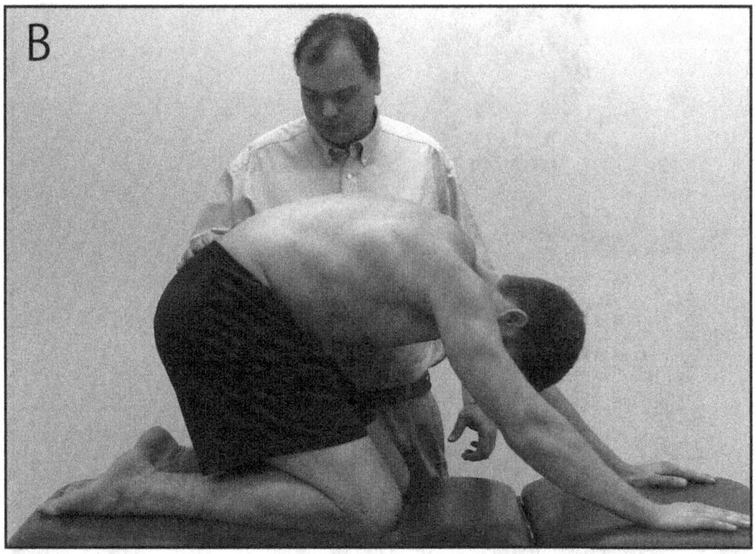

Figure 4-152 (continued). Hand heel rock ROM exercise. In quadruped, rest some of the weight on the hands and arms with the hands slightly in front of the shoulders: A brief pause at the end of range occurs before moving back toward neutral and (B) the backward rock is done while slowly moving toward sitting on the heels, allowing the back to round out.

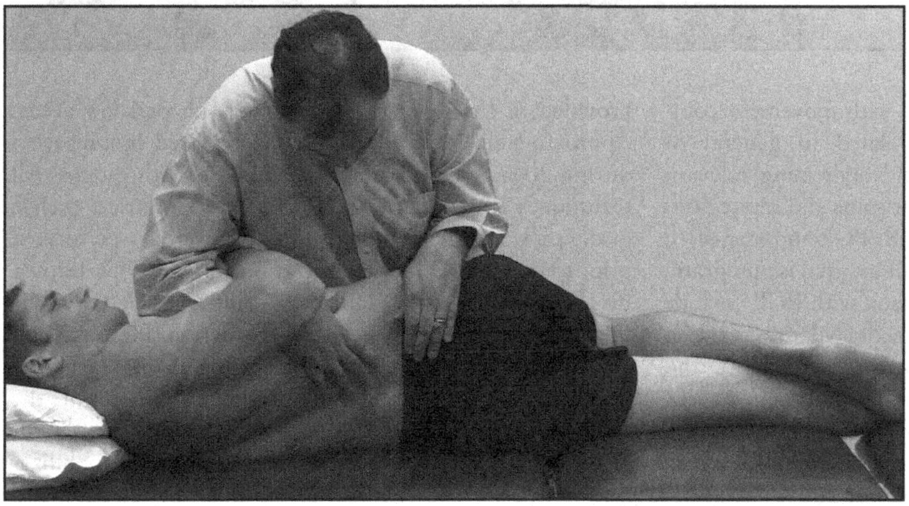

Figure 4-153. SIJ posterior distraction HVLA technique. In left sidelying with the lower leg extended and upper hip and knee flexed, the trunk is rotated to the right until L5-S1 is fully rotated to the right. With L5-S1 stabilized, the innominate is rotated internally about a horizontal axis, resulting in a distraction of the posterior aspect of the SIJ. The thrust technique can be focused through the stiffest segment of the sacrum (S1, S2, S3). Reassessment of the SIJ mobility and neuromuscular systems is mandatory to determine the response to the intervention.[358]

Manual Therapy and Exercise in Nonspecific Pelvic Girdle Pain

Other than the classification-based recommendations of O'Sullivan and Beales[916] that include pregnancy-related PGP, evidence is lacking to inform clinicians of optimal guidelines for PT management of non–pregnancy-related PGP. Using the models of form and force closure and/or a targeted impairment-based strategy based on examination findings, the ultimate goal is to promote and develop optimal movement strategies for load transfer through the SIJ. Mobility deficits from reduced form or excessive force closure are most likely targeted with joint mobilization and manipulation and soft tissue techniques and/or addressing motor control deficits, respectively.

When asymmetric motion of the SIJs is identified, joint mobilization, manipulation, or MET may be necessary to optimize form closure. Improving mobility and decreasing pain may improve motor recruitment and activation patterns or at least provide a foundation for developing motor control. Since the need for specificity of technique remains controversial, an SIJ HVLA distraction technique[351] (Figure 4-153) is presented as a treatment option for patients with examination findings of reduced SIJ mobility and with no contraindications or precautions. Reassessment after manual intervention is mandatory to determine the patient's response, effectiveness, and prescription for exercise to augment the manual technique. Current best practice for manual or exercise interventions for reduced SIJ mobility is at the discretion of the clinician, and one MT technique or approach is not known to be more effective than another for PGP. Excessive or reduced force closure and timing strategies are most likely targeted through motor control exercise, although optimal exercise procedures have not been identified for PGP. Cognitive behavioral issues are generally addressed through graded exposure, graded exercises, or psychological referral as needed throughout rehabilitation.

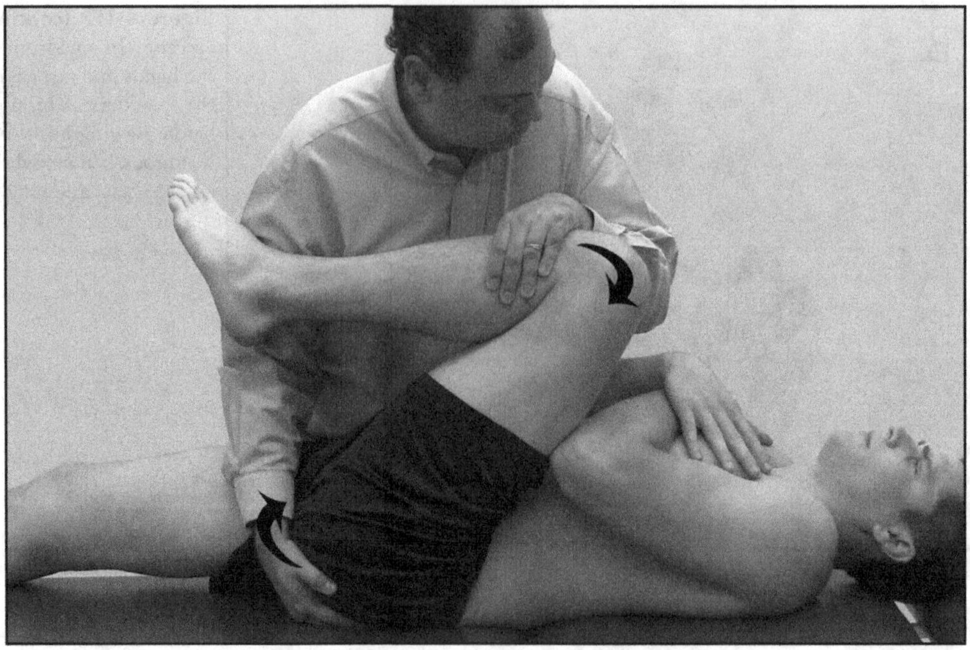

Figure 4-154. Direct mobilization. The knee is flexed and brought to the axilla with one hand placed under the ischial tuberosity and the other on the top of the patient's knee. The pelvis is rotated posteriorly by pushing down on the shaft of the femur and lifting up firmly, with the thenar eminence hand on the ischial tuberosity.[330]

Under the classification for LBP with movement coordination impairments, exercises related to general or specific stabilization approaches and addressing relevant contributors from the thoracolumbar spine and hip regions should be considered for patients with PGP and identified impairments. General components of an exercise program, although not indicated for every person with PGP, include addressing optimal muscle recruitment; balance between the superficial and deep systems of the lumbopelvic and hip regions; training during activities relevant to the patient; and muscle length issues, strength, or endurance. Little research is available to guide exercise prescription in persons with PGP, but the concepts are similar to those discussed for nonspecific LBP with an emphasis on SSE and a motor learning approach.[671,961]

A study designed to test the concepts of form and force closure in women with PGP evaluated the effectiveness of SSE.[671] Subjects with PGP located distal and/or lateral to the L5-S1 area in the buttocks and/or in the PS, pain onset during pregnancy or within 3 weeks after delivery, most recent delivery within 6 to 16 weeks, and willingness to participate with informed consent were included. Diagnostic criteria included the P4 test (ie, thigh thrust), ASLR test, pain provocation of LDL, PS palpation, and modified Trendelenburg test. Persons with LBP, radiculopathy, serious pathology or disease, or neurological compromise were excluded. Eighty-one women with PGP were assigned randomly to 2 treatment groups for 20 weeks. One group received PT with SSE. The control group received individualized PT without SSE. Treatment was based on individual exam findings in both groups.[671]

Information, coping strategies, ergonomic advice, continuation of normal activities, mobilization and self-mobilization treatments, massage, relaxation, and stretching were provided in both groups specific to each person's needs. Approximately 70% of the women received mobilization during 20% of the treatment sessions in both groups. All techniques were pain-free. When asymmetrical pelvic girdle motion was identified, mobilization was performed prior to exercise. Direct mobilization was either performed by the therapist with oscillatory techniques between the ilium and sacrum (Figure 4-154) or traction (Figures 4-155 and 4-156) or by self-mobilization using an MET (Figure 4-157) toward posterior rotation to theoretically restore the self-bracing mechanism or optimize form closure.[1036] For all subjects with asymmetrical SIJ motion, joint mobilization was performed to influence optimal force closure and possibly enhance the ability to perform exercise without pain. However, the main focus in the SSE group was on exercise and training

With a multimodal intervention strategy similar for both groups except for the exercise prescription, the main question of the study was to determine if an SSE approach was more effective than a nonspecific exercise approach. The SSE program was based on specific training of the transversely oriented abdominal muscles with coactivation of the LM at the lumbosacral region, training of the gluteus maximus, latissimus dorsi, external oblique, internal oblique, ES, quadratus lumborum, hip adductors, and abductors. Initially, the focus was on specific contraction of the deep muscles. After approximately 4 weeks, loading was progressively increased. Subjects exercised for 30 to 60 minutes 3 days a week for 18 to 20 weeks with supervision by the physical therapist once a week or every second week. Exercises were performed in a pain-free manner with cocontraction of the deep muscles encouraged during daily activities. Subjects kept individual records of resistance, number of repetitions, and compliance. Specialized sling

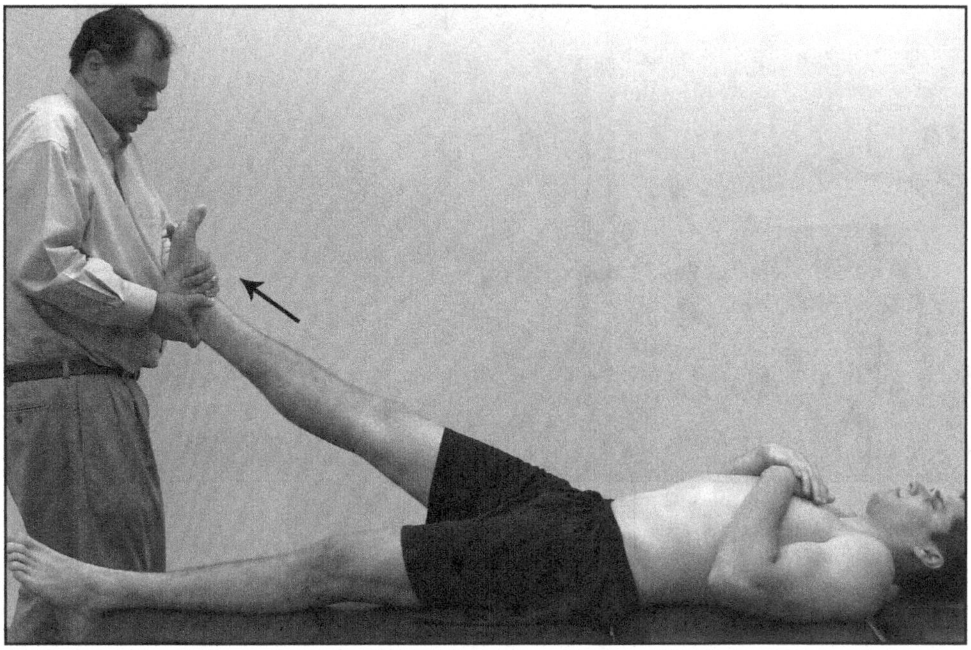

Figure 4-155. Traction. The ankle is grasped at about 45 degrees of passive SLR, providing a strong pull on the leg in the long axis for about 5 seconds. During distraction, the patient tightens the abdominal muscles to facilitate posterior pelvic rotation. Traction is done on each leg one at a time for 4 to 5 repetitions. Reassess frequently.[330]

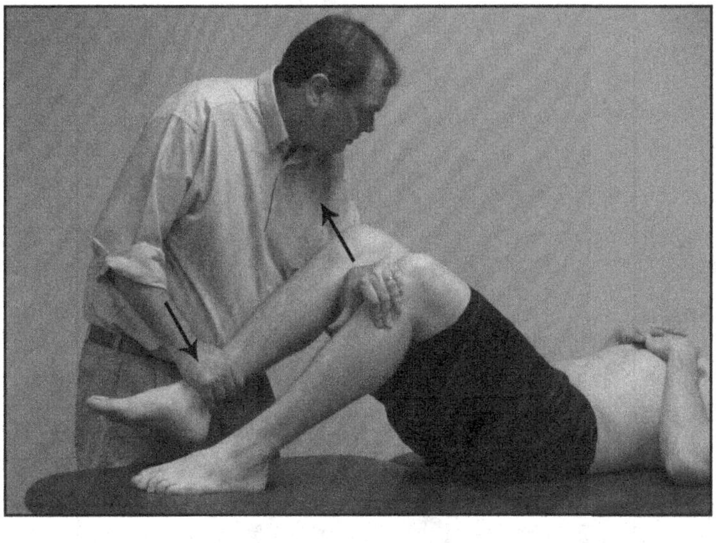

Figure 4-156. Traction. This technique is used to traction the leg if unable to traction through the ankle. For the right side, place the left forearm under the right knee and the left hand over the front of the left knee. Stabilize the right ankle with the right hand holding the knee in flexion. The clinician tractions the leg through the left forearm using the left hand to lever the traction, which lifts the buttock on that side. Reassess frequently.[330]

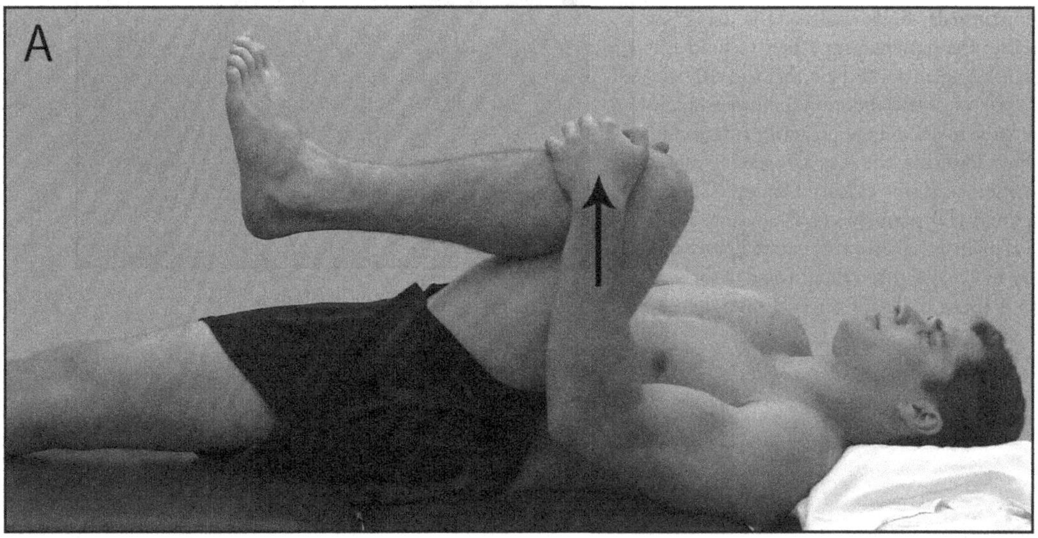

Figure 4-157. Self-mobilization using an MET: (A) in supine, the patient grasps the knee with both arms, holds firmly, and pushes hard against the arms for 5 to 10 seconds. *(continued)*

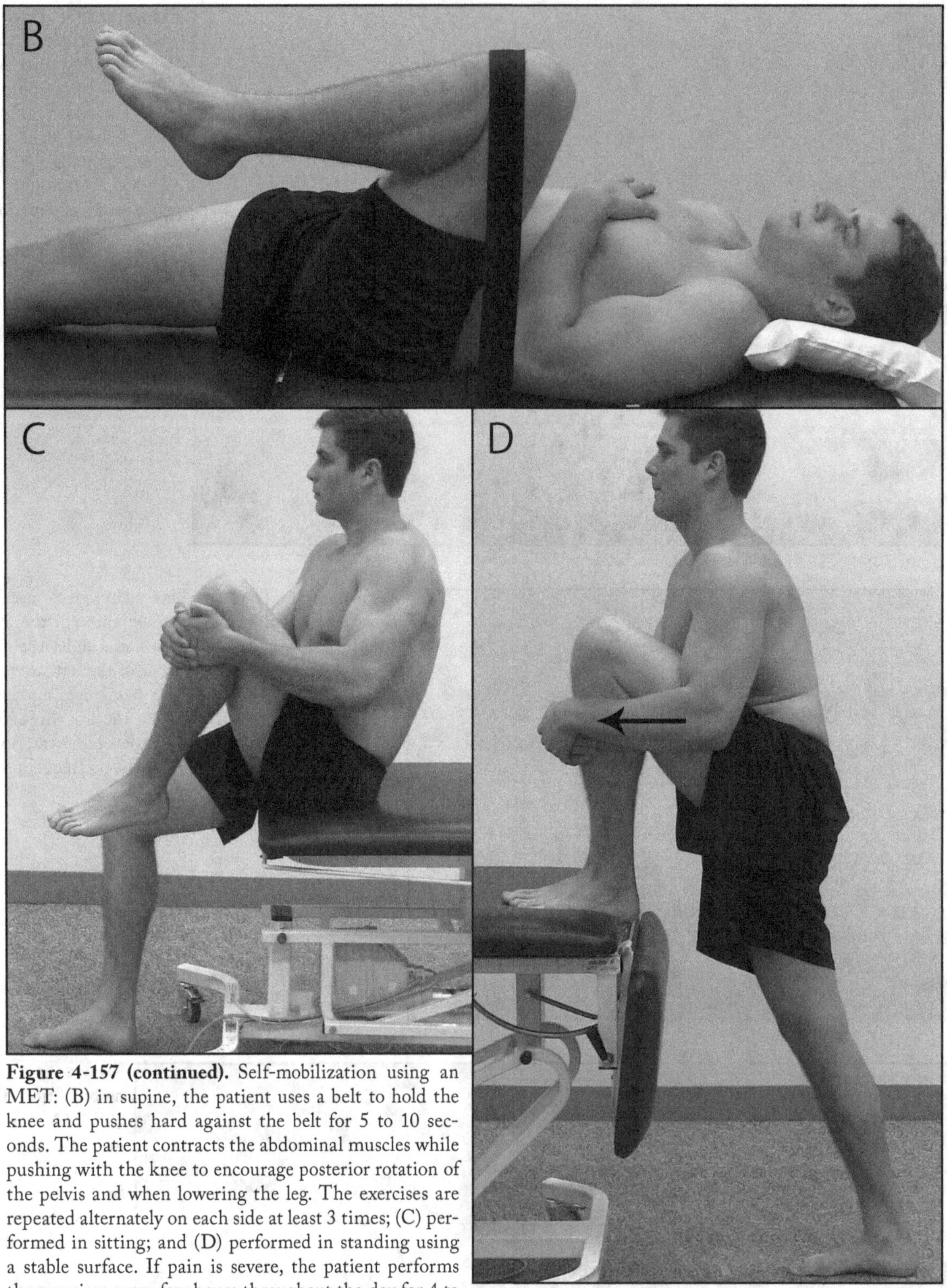

Figure 4-157 (continued). Self-mobilization using an MET: (B) in supine, the patient uses a belt to hold the knee and pushes hard against the belt for 5 to 10 seconds. The patient contracts the abdominal muscles while pushing with the knee to encourage posterior rotation of the pelvis and when lowering the leg. The exercises are repeated alternately on each side at least 3 times; (C) performed in sitting; and (D) performed in standing using a stable surface. If pain is severe, the patient performs the exercises every few hours throughout the day for 4 to 5 days, then 3 to 4 times daily for a week, and then as needed.[330]

exercise equipment was installed at each subject's home during the intervention period. The control group received the same instructions and a variety of PT intervention based on the examination similar to the SSE group. Mobilization and strengthening exercises and promotion of activities in an ergonomically safe manner were included. However, no SSE was given to the control group. Subjects were treated about every second week individually, supervised over 20 weeks. The average number of treatments was 11 for both groups.[671,961]

Immediately after intervention and 1-year postpartum, the SSE group showed statistically and clinically significant lower pain intensity, lower disability, and higher quality of life compared with the control group. The group difference in median values for evening pain was 30 mm on VAS. Disability was reduced by more than 50% for the exercise group, with minimal changes in the control group. All objective test measures showed significant differences in favor of the SSE group. Due to high-quality study design, control of cointerventions, blinded assessor, no dropouts, and high compliance with treatment in both groups, the authors concluded that the results provide strong evidence for the effectiveness of an individualized, multimodal treatment program focusing on SSE for persons with PGP.[671] A 2-year follow-up was published by the same authors.[961] Significant differences between groups in functional status, pain, and physical health were maintained. In the SSE group, 85% reported minimal disability compared to 47% in the control group. The control group showed significant improvement in functional status from year 1 to 2. In the SSE group, 68% reported minimal evening pain compared to 23% in the control group. Subjects with the highest levels of disability and greatest potential for improvement recovered the most, regardless of group. This study provides strong evidence for an individualized, multimodal approach including MT with a focus on SSE.

In the presence of limited evidence, the prescription for stabilizing exercise in PGP should be based on individual impairments related to activity limitations. Certain subgroups may benefit from stabilization exercises and others may not. The clinician's challenge is to identify the key characteristics of patients who are likely to respond favorably and those who are not.

In a broad review of interdisciplinary treatment for all classifications of PGP, Vanelderen et al[1037] maintain that treatment of pelvic girdle (SIJ) pain is necessary and may include pharmacological, CBT, manual medicine, exercise, and, as needed, psychiatric evaluation and interventional pain management. In persons with chronic, nonspecific PGP who do not respond to conservative treatment, an SIJ intraarticular injection with a local anesthetic and corticosteroids is recommended. If this procedure fails or produces only short-term effects, cooled RF treatment to the lateral branches of S1 to S4 is recommended. If this procedure is not available, pulsed RF targeting the L5 posterior ramus and lateral branches of S1-S3 should be considered.[1037] Complications of these procedures are low but include infection, neural damage, hematoma, gas and vascular embolism, weakness due to extra-articular extravasation, and complications related to drug administration.[1037] Fusion of the pelvis is considered an end-stage option in the presence of persistent disabling symptoms.[913]

Pelvic Floor Muscle Training

Some patients with LBP and/or PGP may have incontinence or PFM dysfunction, while other patients may not. In addition to contributing to continence the PFM function is part of the trunk stabilizing mechanism due to its integrated function with the abdominal muscles.[1038] Sapsford[1038] recommended initiating PFM training using a staged rehabilitation program as a part of a comprehensive approach to PFM dysfunction, which is appropriate for most common problems. The 5 stages are as follows:

1. Diaphragmatic breathing in sitting and supine (see Chapter 5)
2. Tonic activation of the TrA and PFM
3. Strengthening of the TrA, PFM, and internal oblique
4. Functional expiratory patterns such as sneezing and coughing
5. Progressions to impact activities such as running and jumping[1038]

In patients with overactive superficial abdominals, retraining of diaphragmatic breathing in lying and sitting is the first step, with a focus to minimize upper rib cage elevation. Next, PFM training is begun with retraining of a tonic PFM action as gentle, prolonged holds or contractions. Strong PFM contractions are not encouraged. Using selective activation of the TrA helps to ensure a low-level PFM contraction. In subjects without LBP, PFM training is begun in standing. TrA and PFM activation are slowly incorporated into standing and walking. The progression to impact activities is described in Figure 4-158.[1038]

Hung and colleagues[1039] performed an RCT to investigate the effectiveness of Sapsford's program[1038] in 70 women with stress UI or mixed UI. Seventy women were randomized into 2 groups. The training group received 8 individual sessions and followed Sapford's staged exercise program[1038] (see Figure 4-158). The control group performed a home program of self-monitored PFM exercises. After 4 months, 96.7% of subjects in the training group reported that they were cured or improved versus 66.6% in the control group. Furthermore, the amount and number of leaks were significantly lower in the training group compared to the control group, and quality of life improved significantly more in the training group. Maximal vaginal squeeze pressure, however, decreased slightly in both groups. The authors concluded that coordinated retraining

Stage and Exercise Regimen

I. Diaphragmatic breathing (wk1~4)

- Position: lying, sitting, standing: Home exercise: 30 repetitions x 3 sets/day

II-1. Tonic TrA and PFM activation (wk2~5): Prerequisite: correct diaphragmatic breathing

- Position: standing; Instruction: Try to lift up your lower abdomen cranially with normal diaphragmatic breathing. The spinal and pelvic motion was prohibited.
- Feedback: in front of a mirror to see the lower abdominal movement; tactile input medial to ASIS by both therapist and participant; participant's subjective feeling of tensioning response around periurethral, perivaginal, & perianal regions.
- Home exercise: 5 repetitions x 5 sets/day, holding the contraction as long as possible, and gradually increase the holding time to 40 s up.

II-2.Tonic activation with ADL, walking (wk4~7): Prerequisite: the participant can hold the tonic TrA/PFM co-contraction into daily activities in standing and walking

- Position: upright position
- Instruction: incorporate the co-contraction into daily activities in standing and walking
- Feedback: participant's subjective feeling of tensioning response around periurethral, perivaginal, and perianal region.
- Home exercise: 6 tasks x 2 sets/day, target holding contraction with walking for more than 15 s

III. Muscle strengthening (wk6~16): Prerequisite: tonic TrA/PFM co-contraction can be maintained easily during walking for more than 15 s

- Position: standing
- Instruction: start with the gentle lower abdominal activation used in the previous stage, then keep pulling the lower abdomen in towards the spine and pulling up the periurethral PFM as far as possible. Spinal movement was avoided to minimize activity of rectus abdominal muscle.

IV. Functional expiratory patterns (wk8~16): (Nose blowing) (wk8~9)

- Position: begin sitting upright without support, progress to standing, slumped supported sitting
- Instruction: begin with diaphragmatic breathing for 3-5x, make sure the anterior-posterior diameter of the abdomen increased during inspiration. After the last full inspiration, incorporate a strong cognitive abdominal pulling in contraction as the nose blowing takes place.
- Feedback: in front of a mirror to see the chest and abdomen motion: hand palpation at lower abdomen; the abdominal wall should be pulled in and the lower rib cage should be widened laterally; participant's subjective feeling of tensioning response around peripurethral, perivaginal, and perianal regions.
- Home exercise: 5 repetitions x 2 sets/day
- (Coughing) (wk10~16); Note: requires stronger/faster abdominal muscle contraction
- (Laughing) (wk10~16); Note: requires the ability to repeat and sustain the contraction of the abdominal muscles and PFM
- (Sneezing) (wk12~16); Note: require the greatest muscle power and correct timing

V. Impact activities (wk10~16):

- Prequisite: tonic TrA/PFM co-contraction can be maintained easily during walking for more than 15 s
- Instruction: incorporate the tonic TrA/PFM contraction into impact activities, such as running, jumping, dancing
- Home exercise: according to participant's activity schedule

Figure 4-158. PFM training. (Reprinted from *Man Ther,* 15, Hung H-C, Hsiao S-M, Chih S-Y, Lin H-H, Tsauo J-Y, An alternative intervention for urinary incontinence: retraining diaphragmatic, deep abdominal and pelvic floor muscle coordinated function, 273-279, Copyright 2010, with permission from Elsevier.)

of diaphragmatic muscles, deep abdominal, and PFM function could improve symptoms and quality of life.[1039]

Many aspects of PFM training associated with PGP are beyond the scope of this reference, except to reiterate the importance of identifying patients with LBP or PGP who also have stress, urge, or mixed UI and referring appropriately to a medical or PT specialist. Cochrane review[1040] recommends that PFM training be included as a first-line intervention for women with stress, urge, or mixed UI. PFM training seems to be effective in women with stress UI alone who participate in a supervised PFM training program for at least 3 months. Women who received PFM training were more likely to report a cure or improvement, better continence, better quality of life, and fewer incontinence episodes per day than women who did not receive PFM training. The authors concluded that PFM training is better than no treatment, placebo drug, or inactive control treatments for women with stress, urge, or mixed UI.[1040] PFM training should be considered for treatment of certain types of incontinence and/or as a component of PGP intervention.

Despite a paucity of evidence-related treatment for PGP, use of the highest levels of available evidence applicable to the individual patient is recommended. Considering the complexity and lack of consensus in the examination and management of PGP or SIJ pain, an impairment-based strategy is supported with emphasis on a multimodal biopsychosocial consideration and integration of MT and exercise where indicated.

Summary

The examination and treatment of persons with LBP and PGP should be informed with the most current evidence. Clinicians must keep in mind the interplay of research, clinical expertise, patient expectations, and clinical reasoning to guide decision making related to initial and continued intervention. Patients who present with LBP are complex and may fit neatly into one classification, may have key findings of more than one classification, or may not fit neatly in one of these classifications. Additional complexity occurs with changes throughout the course of treatment that require reassessment and can result in a different focus of intervention. Continual assessment and reassessment is mandatory throughout the plan of care in order to monitor the multiple influences that either facilitate or hinder recovery.

The subjective examination seeks to identify and understand key detailed information within a multidimensional context of physical and psychological factors specific to the individual patient. A careful and thorough history provides the basis to form initial diagnostic hypotheses or classifications that then guide the focus and comprehensiveness of the physical examination. Accurate, relevant data from the patient history aid in diagnostic triage, planning the tests and measures, and implementing an effective management strategy.

The physical examination is not simply the routine application of tests, but instead a planned collection of additional data to test the working diagnostic hypotheses. The reliability and diagnostic usefulness of tests and measures must be considered before they are selected. Appropriate selection of examination procedures should result in the data to support or negate working hypotheses by altering the pretest probability beyond the treatment threshold. Key history and exam findings are used to place the patient into a diagnostic classification or impairment-based category of LBP that initially guides PT intervention.

With little evidence to support classification based on a pathoanatomical source, current evidence favors the use of a classification system that identifies subgroups of patients who are most likely to respond to specific interventions with the potential to maximize outcomes. Many LBP classifications exist with no classification system known to be superior to another.

Key history and exam findings are used to define homogeneous subgroups and place a patient into a diagnostic classification or impairment-based category of LBP that initially guides PT intervention. For patients with LBP, subgroup classifications are described through integration of clinical practice guidelines, clinical reasoning, and evidence-based clinical characteristics, along with evidence to support matched interventions. The subgroups include the following:

- Manipulation and mobilization plus exercise LBP subgroup also depicted as LBP mobility deficits
- Stabilization exercise LBP subgroup also depicted as LBP with movement coordination impairments
- DSE classification also depicted as LBP with lower extremity referred pain
- Traction classification for LBP with lower extremity radiating or related pain
- An impairment-based classification for symptomatic LSS
- An impairment-based classification for LBP with altered neurodynamics
- LBRLP based on predominating pain mechanisms (ie, central sensitization, peripheral nerve sensitization, denervation, and musculoskeletal referred pain)
- CLBP or chronic, disabling lumbopelvic pain classification related to MCIs based on a biopsychosocial approach
- PGP classification based on a biopsychosocial and neurophysiological pain mechanisms classification
- Pregnancy-related PGP classification

In a best-evidence approach, an LBP diagnostic classification assists the clinician with matching the patient's clinical presentation to the most suitable initial treatment in order to optimize outcomes. In an impairment-based LBP category, the clinician identifies relevant physical impairments such as limited ROM, joint or muscle stiffness or hypermobility, and/or muscle coordination deficits. Evidence-based interventions are selected to target the prioritized impairments to address activity limitations or functional deficits important to the patient. Current evidence supports the use of diagnostic classification to guide PT intervention and to achieve improved outcomes over no classification.

Considering the complex nature of LBP or PGP, patients often present with criteria from more than one subgroup. In this situation, clinicians utilize clinical reasoning to prioritize criteria and classification in deciding on the best initial treatment or pursue an impairment-based approach to management. Continued assessment and reassessment of the patient's response to treatment provide additional criteria for reclassification and progression of treatment. The majority of persons with LBP or PGP require multimodal treatment. The ultimate goal is to facilitate the earliest, most effective management to enhance recovery and prevent progression to a chronic, persistent stage.

The appendix section provides case studies for each region (Appendices C, D, and E—2 LBP and 1 PGP) to illustrate the clinical reasoning framework. Each case study allows for practice taking a history and planning a physical examination. The data from the history and physical examination are then synthesized using current best evidence to determine appropriate diagnostic classification, prognosis, and initial management strategies. The case study process provides an opportunity to practice using clinical reasoning and an evidence-based framework.

References

1. Deyo RA, Mirza SK, Martin BI. Back pain prevalence and visit rates. Estimates from US national surveys, 2002. *Spine.* 2006;31:2724-2727.
2. Martin BI, Deyo RA, Mirza SK, et al. Expenditures and health status among adults with back and neck problems. *JAMA.* 2008;299:656-664.
3. Martin BI, Turner JA, Kirza SK, et al. Trends in health care expenditures, utilization, and health status among US adults with spine problems, 1997-2006. *Spine.* 2009;34:2077-2084.
4. Katz JN. Lumbar disc disorders and low back pain: socioeconomic factors and consequences. *J Bone Joint Surg Am.* 2006;88(suppl 2):21-24.
5. Gellhorn AC, Chan L, Martin B, Friedly J. Management patterns in acute low back pain. The role of physical therapy. *Spine (Phila Pa 1976).* 2012;37:775-782.
6. Fritz JM, Cleland JA, Speckman M, et al. Physical therapy for acute low back pain: associations with subsequent healthcare costs. *Spine.* 2008;33:1800-1805.
7. Wand BM, Bird C, McAuley JH, et al. Early intervention for the management of acute low back pain: a single-blind randomized controlled trial of biopsychosocial education, manual therapy, and exercise. *Spine.* 2004;29:2350-2356.
8. Fritz JM, Childs JD, Wainner RS, Flynn TW. Primary care referral of patients with low back pain to physical therapy: impact on future healthcare utilization and costs. *Spine (Phila Pa 1976).* 2012;37(25):2114-2121.
9. van Tulder MW, Assendelft WJ, Koes BW, Bouter LM. Spinal radiographic findings and nonspecific low back pain. A systematic review of observational studies. *Spine.* 1997;22:427-434.
10. Deyo RA. Practice variations, treatment fads, rising disability. Do we need a new clinical research paradigm? *Spine.* 1993;18:2153-2162.
11. Chou R, Qaseem A, Snow V, et al. Diagnosis and treatment of low back pain: a joint clinical practice guideline from the American College of Physicians and the American Pain Society. *Ann Intern Med.* 2007;147:478-491.
12. Jarvik JG, Deyo RA. Diagnostic evaluation of low back pain with emphasis on imaging. *Ann Intern Med.* 2002;137:586-597.
13. Deyo RA, Rainville J, Kent DL. What can the history and physical examination tell us about low back pain? *JAMA.* 1992;268:760-765.
14. Delitto A, George SA, Van Dillen L, et al. Low back pain. Clinical practice guidelines linked to the International Classification of Functioning, Disability, and Health from the orthopaedic section of the American Physical Therapy Association. *J Orthop Sports Phys Ther.* 2012;42(4):A1-A57.
15. Delitto A. Research in low back pain: time to stop seeking the elusive "magic bullet". *Phys Ther.* 2005;85:206-208.
16. Kent P, Keating J. Do primary care clinicians think that nonspecific low back pain is one condition? *Spine.* 2004;29:1022-1031.
17. Li LC, Bombardier C. Physical therapy management of low back pain: an exploratory survey of therapist approaches. *Phys Ther.* 2001;81:1018-1028.
18. Mikhail C, Korner Bitensky N, Rossignol M, Dumas JP. Physical therapists' use of interventions with high evidence of effectiveness in the management of a hypothetical typical patient with acute low back pain. *Phys Ther.* 2005;85:1151-1167.
19. Fritz J, Delitto A, Erhard RE. Comparison of classification-based physical therapy with therapy based on clinical practice guidelines for patients with acute low back pain: a randomized clinical trial. *Spine.* 2003;28:1363-1371.
20. Brennan GP, Fritz JM, Hunter SJ, Thackeray A, Delitto A, Erhard RE. Identifying subgroups of patients with acute/subacute "nonspecific low back pain. Results of a randomized clinical trial. *Spine.* 2006;31:623-631.
21. Hall H, McIntosh G, Boyle C. Effectiveness of a low back pain classification system. *Spine J.* 2009;9:648-657.
22. Riddle DL. Classification and low back pain: a review of the literature and critical analysis of selected systems. *Phys Ther.* 1998;78:708-737.
23. McCarthy CH, Arnall FA, Strimpakos N, Freemont A, Oldham J. The biopsychosocial classification of non-specific low back pain: a systematic review. *Phys Ther Rev.* 2004;9:17-30.
24. Karayannis NV, Jull GA, Hodges PW. Physiotherapy movement based classification approaches to low back pain: a comparison of subgroups through review and developer/expert survey. *BMC Musculoskelet Disord.* 2012;13:24.

25. Kovacs FM, Abraira V, Zamora J, Fernández C; Spanish Back Pain Research Network. The transition from acute to subacute and chronic low back pain: a study based on determinants of quality of life and prediction of chronic disability. *Spine (Phila Pa 1976)*. 2005;30(15):1786-1792.
26. Negrini SA, Giovannoni S, Minozzi S. Diagnostic therapeutic flow-charts for low back pain patients: the Italian clinical guidelines. *Eura Medicophys*. 2006;42;151-170.
27. Balague F, Mannion AF, Pellise F. Clinical update: low back pain. *Lancet*. 2007;369:726-728.
28. Hestbaek L, Leboeuf-Yde C, Manniche C. Low back pain: what is the long-term course? A review of studies of general patient populations. *Eur Spine J*. 2003;12:149-165.
29. Stanton TR, Latimer J, Maher CG, Hancock MJ. How do we define the condition "recurrent low back pain"? A systematic review. *Eur Spine J*. 2010;19:533-539.
30. Dunn KM, Jordan K, Croft PR. Characterizing the course of low back pain: a latent class analysis. *Am J Epidemiol*. 2006;163:754-761.
31. Croft PR, Macfarlane GH, Papageorgiou AC, Thomas E, Silman JS. Outcome of low back pain in general practice: a prospective study. *BMJ*. 1998;316:1356-1359.
32. Sackett DL, Rennie D. The science of the art of the clinical examination. *JAMA*. 1992;267:2650-2652.
33. Goodman CC, Snyder TE. *Differential Diagnosis for Physical Therapists: Screening for Referral*. Philadelphia, PA: Saunders; 2007.
34. Henschke N, Maher CG, Refshauge KM. Screening for malignancy in low back pain patients: a systematic review. *Eur Spine J*. 2007;16(10):1673-1679.
35. Deyo RA, Diehl AK. Cancer as a cause of back pain: frequency, clinical presentation, and diagnostic strategies. *J Gen Intern Med*. 1988;3:230-238.
36. Suarez-Almazor ME, Belseck E, Russell AS, Mackel JV. Use of lumbar radiographs for the early diagnosis of low back pain. Proposed guidelines would increase utilization. *JAMA*. 1997;277:1782-1786.
37. Atlas SJ, Deyo RA. Evaluating and managing acute low back pain in the primary care setting. *J Gen Intern Med*. 2001;16(2):120-131.
38. Refshauge KM, Maher CG. Low back pain investigations and prognosis: a review. *Br J Sports Med*. 2006;40:494-498.
39. Guillodo Y, Botton E, Saraux A, et al. Contralateral spondylolysis and fracture of the lumbar pedicle in an elite female gymnast: a case report. *Spine*. 2000;25:2541-2543.
40. Millson HB, Gray J, Stretch RA, et al. Dissociation between back pain and bone stress reaction as measured by CT scan in young cricket fast bowlers. *Br J Sports Med*. 2004;38:586-591.
41. Van den Bosch M, Hollingworth W, Kinmonth AL, Dixon AK. Evidence against the use of lumbar spine radiography for low back pain. *Clin Radiol*. 2004;59:69-76.
42. Raisz L. Screening for osteoporosis. *N Engl J Med*. 2005;353:164-171.
43. National Osteoporosis Foundation. NOF releases new data detailing the prevalence of osteoporosis. http:/www.nof.org/news/1009. Published April 18, 2013. Accessed September 20, 2013.
44. Henschke N, Maher CG, Refshauge KM. A systematic review identifies "red flags" to screen for vertebral fracture in patients with low back pain. *J Clin Epidemiol*. 2008;61:110-118.
45. Waldvogel F, Vasey H. Osteomyelitis: the past decade. *N Engl J Med*. 1980;303:360-370.
46. Lurie JD. What diagnostic tests are useful for low back pain? *Best Pract Res Clin Rheumatol*. 2005;19:557-575.
47. Sapico FL, Montgomerie JZ. Pyogenic vertebral osteomyelitis: repot of nine cases and review of the literature. *Rev Infect Dis*. 1979;1:754-776.
48. Baker AS, Ojemann RG, Swartz MN, et al. Spinal epidural abscess. *N Engl J Med*. 1975;293:463-468.
49. Johnston KW, Rutherford RB, Tilson D, Shah DM, Hollier L, Stanley JC. Suggested standards for reporting on arterial aneurysms. Subcommittee on reporting standards for arterial aneurysms, ad hoc committee on reporting standards, society for vascular surgery and North American chapter, international society for cardiovascular surgery. *J Vasc Surg*. 1991;13:452-458.
50. Lederle FA, Johnson GR, Wilson Se, et al. Rupture rate of large abdominal aortic aneurysms in patients refusing or unfit for elective repair. *JAMA*. 2002;287:2968-2972.
51. Gillum RF. Epidemiology of aortic aneurysm in the United States. *J Clin Epidemiol*. 1995;48:1289-1298.
52. Lindholt JS, Henneberg EW, Fasting H, Juul S. Mass or high-risk screening for abdominal aortic aneurysm. *Br J Surg*. 1997;84:40-42.
53. Scott RA, Bridgewater SG, Ashton HA. Randomized clinical trial of screening for abdominal aortic aneurysm in women. *Br J Surg*. 2002;89:283-285.
54. Edwards JZ, Weinder SD. Chronic back pain caused by an abdominal aortic aneurysm: case report and review of the literature. *Orthopedics*. 2003;26:191-192.
55. Mechelli F, Preboski Z, Boissonnault W. Differential diagnosis of a patient referred to physical therapy with low back pain: abdominal aortic aneurysm. *J Orthop Sports Phys Ther*. 2008;38:551-557.
56. Fleming C, Whitlock EP, Beil TL, Lederle FA. Screening for abdominal aortic aneurysm: a best-evidence review for the US Preventive Services Task Force. *Ann Intern Med*. 2005;142:203-211.
57. Fleming C, Whitlock EP, Beil T, Lederle F. *Primary Care Screening for Abdominal Aortic Aneurysm*. Evidence Synthesis, No. 35. Rockville, MD: Agency for Healthcare Research and Quality; 2005. http://www.ncbi.nlm.nih.gov/books/NBK42895/. Accessed September 20, 2013
58. Fink HA, Lederle FA, Roth CS, Bowles CA, Nelson DB, Haas MA. The accuracy of physical examination to detect abdominal aortic aneurysm. *Arch Intern Med*. 2000;160:833-836.
59. Federle FA, Walker FM, Reinke DB. Selective screening for abdominal aortic aneurysms with physical examination and ultrasound. *Arch Intern Med*. 1988;148:1753-1756.
60. Ahn UM, Ahn NU, Buchowski JM, Garrett ES, Sieber AN, Kostuik JP. Cauda equina syndrome secondary to lumbar disc herniation: a meta-analysis of surgical outcomes. *Spine*. 2000;25:1515-1522.
61. Busse JW, Bhandari M, Schnittker JB, Reddy K, Dunlop RB. Delayed presentation of cauda equine syndrome secondary to lumbar disc herniation: functional outcomes and health-related quality of life. *CJEM*. 2001;3:285-291.
62. Shapiro S. Cauda equine syndrome secondary to lumbar disc herniation. *Neurosurgery*. 1993;32:743-746.
63. Shapiro S. Medical realities of cauda equina syndrome secondary to lumbar disc herniation. *Spine*. 2000;25:348-351.
64. Crowell MS, Gill NW. Medical screening and evacuation: cauda equina syndrome in a combat zone. *J Orthop Sports Phys Ther*. 2009;39:541-549.
65. O'Laoire SA, Crockard HA, Thomas DG. Prognosis for sphincter recovery after operation for cauda equine compression owing to lumbar disc prolapsed. *BMJ*. 1981;282:1852-1854.

66. Tay Eck, Chacha PB. Midline prolapsed of a lumbar intervertebral disc with compression of the cauda equina. *J Bone Joint Surg Br.* 1979;61:43-46.
67. Haswell K, Gilmour J, Moore B. Clinical decision rules for identification of low back pain patients with neurologic involvement in primary care. *Spine.* 2008;33:68-73.
68. Kostuik JP, Harrington I, Alexander D, Rand W, Evans D. Cauda equina syndrome and lumbar disc herniation. *J Bone Joint Surg Am.* 1986;68:386-391.
69. Sliwa J, Wiesner S, Novick A, Charuk G. Concurrent musculoskeletal pain in a patient with symptomatic lower extremity arterial insufficiency. *Arch Phys Med Rehabil.* 1989;70:848-850.
70. Goodman CC, Snyder TEK. *Differential Diagnosis for Physical Therapists. Screening for Referral.* St Louis, MO: Saunders; 2007.
71. Lyden S, Joseph D. The clinical presentation of peripheral arterial disease and guidance for early recognition. *Cleve Clin J Med.* 2006;73(suppl 4):S15-S21.
72. Hooi JD, Stoffers HE, Kester AD, et al. Risk factors and cardiovascular diseases associated with asymptomatic peripheral arterial occlusive disease: the Limburg PAOD Study. *Scand J Prim Health Care.* 1998;16:177-182.
73. Khan MA. Update on spondyloarthropathies. *Ann Intern Med.* 2002;136:896-907.
74. Braun J, Sieper J. Ankylosing spondylitis. *Lancet.* 2007;369:1379-1390.
75. Jois RN, Macgregor AJ, Gaffney K. Recognition of inflammatory back pain and ankylosing spondylitis in primary care. *Rheumatology.* 2008;47:1364-1366.
76. Calin A, Porta J, Fries JF, Scheurmann DJ. Clinical history as a screening test for ankylosing spondylitis. *J Am Med Assoc.* 1997;237:2613-2614.
77. Gran JT. An epidemiological survey of the signs and symptoms of ankylosing spondylitis. *Clin Rheumatol.* 1985;4:161-169.
78. Van der Linden SM, Fahrer H. Occurrence of spinal pain syndromes in a group of apparently healthy and physically fit sportsmen (orienteers). *Scand J Rheumatol.* 1988;17:475-481.
79. Van der Linden S, Valkenburg HA, Cats A. Evaluation of diagnostic criteria for ankylosing spondylitis: a proposal for modification of the New York criteria. *Arthritis Rheum.* 1984;27:361-368.
80. Rudwaleit M, Metter A, Listing J, Sieper J, Braun J. Inflammatory back pain in ankylosing spondylitis: a reassessment of clinical history for application as classification and diagnostic criteria. *Arthritis Rheum.* 2006;54:569-578.
81. Reynolds PMG. Measurement of spinal mobility: a comparison of three methods. *Rheumatol Rehabil.* 1975;14:180-185.
82. Rae PS, Waddell G, Venner RM. A simple technique for measuring lumbar spinal flexion. *J R Coll Surg Edinb.* 1984;29:281-284.
83. Moll JMH, Wright V. An objective clinical study of chest expansion. *Ann Rheum Dis.* 1972;31:1-8.
84. Potter NA, Rothstein JM. Intertester reliability for selected clinical tests of the sacroiliac joint. *Phys Ther.* 1985;65:1671-1675.
85. Russell AS, Maksymowych W, LeClercq S. Clinical examination of sacroiliac joints: a prospective study. *Arthritis Rheum.* 1981;24:1575-1577.
86. Blower PW, Griffin AJ. Clinical sacroiliac tests in ankylosing spondylitis and other causes of low back pain. *Ann Rheum Dis.* 1984;43:192-195.
87. Wolff MW, Levine LA. Cervical radiculopathies: conservative approaches to management. *Phys Med Rehabil Clin North Am.* 2002;13:589-608.
88. Heliovaara M, Impivaara O, Sievers K, et al. Lumbar disc syndrome in Finland. *Epidemiol Community Health.* 1987;41:251-258.
89. Manninen P, Riihimaki H, Heliovaara M. Incidence and risk factors of low-back pain in middle-aged farmers. *Occup Med.* 1995;45:141-146.
90. Health Council of the Netherlands. *Management of the Lumbosacral Radicular Syndrome (Sciatica).* The Hague: Health Council of the Netherlands; 1999; publication no. 1999/18.
91. Kelsey JL. Epidemiology of radiculopathies. *Adv Neurol.* 1978;19:385-398.
92. Katz JN. Lumbar disc disorders and low-back pain: socioeconomic factors and consequences. *J Bone Joint Surg Am.* 2006;88(suppl 2):21-24.
93. Vroomen PCAJ, de Krom MCTFM, Wilmink JT, et al. Diagnostic value of history and physical examination in patients suspected of lumbosacral nerve root compression. *J Neurol Neurosurg Psychiatry.* 2002;72:630-634.
94. Lauder TD, Dillingham TR, Andary M, et al. Effect of history and exam in predicting electrodiagnostic outcome among patients with suspected lumbosacral radiculopathy. *Am J Phys Med Rehabil.* 2000;79:60-68.
95. Spangfort V. Lumbar disc herniation: a computer aided analysis of 2504 operations. *Acta Orthop Scand.* 1972;(suppl 142):1-93.
96. Alpers BJ. The neurological aspects of sciatica. *Med Clin North Am.* 1953;37:503-510.
97. Murphy DR, Hurwitz, EL, Gerrard JK, Clary R. Pain patterns and descriptions in patients with radicular pain: does the pain necessarily follow a specific dermatome. *Chiropr Osteopat.* 2009;17:9.
98. Deville WLJM, Windt DAWM, van der Dzaferagic A, Bezemer PD, Bouter LM. The test of Lasegue: systematic review of the accuracy in diagnosing herniated discs. *Spine.* 2000;25:1140-1147.
99. de Graaf I, Prak A, Bierma-Zeinstra S, Thomas S, Peul W, Koes B. Diagnosis of lumbar spinal stenosis. A systematic review of the accuracy of diagnostic tests. *Spine.* 31:1168-1176.
100. Konno S, Kikuchi S, Tanaka Y, et al. A diagnostic support tool for lumbar spinal stenosis: a self-administered, self-reported history questionnaire. *BMC Musculoskeletal Disorders.* 2007;8:102.
101. Katz JN, Dalgas M, Stucki G, et al. Degenerative lumbar spinal stenosis. Diagnostic value of the history and physical examination. *Arthritis Rheum.* 1995;38:1236-1241.
102. Fritz JM, Erhard RE, Delitto A, et al. Preliminary results of the use of a two-stage treadmill test as a clinical diagnostic tool in the differential diagnosis of lumbar spinal stenosis. *J Spinal Disord.* 1997;10:410-416.
103. Kendall NAS. Psychosocial approaches to the prevention of chronic pain: the low back paradigm. *Baillieres Best Pract Res Clin Rheumatol.* 1999;13:545-554.
104. Fritz JM, George SZ, Delitto A. The role of fear-avoidance beliefs in acute low back pain: relationships with current and future disability and work status. *Pain.* 2001;94:7-15.
105. Fritz JM, George SZ. Identifying psychosocial variables in patients with acute work-related low back pain: the importance of fear-avoidance beliefs. *Phys Ther.* 2002;82:973-983.
106. Picavet HS, Vlaeyen JW, Schouten JS. Pain catastrophizing and kinesiophobia: predictors of chronic low back pain. *Am J Epidemiol.* 2002;156:1028-1034.
107. Sieben JM, Vlaeyen JWS, Tuerlinckx S, et al. Pain-related fear in acute low back pain: the first two weeks of a new episode. *Eur J Pain.* 2002;6:229-237.

108. Kopec JA, Sayre EC, Esdaile JM. Predictors of back pain in a general population cohort. *Spine (Phila Pa 1976).* 2004;29(1):70-77.
109. Swinkels-Meewisse IE, Roelofs J, Verbeek AL, et al. Fear of movement/(re)injury, disability and participation in acute low back pain. *Pain.* 2003;105:371-379.
110. Linton SJ. A review of psychological risk factors in back and neck pain. *Spine.* 2000;25:1148-1156.
111. Pengel LH, Herbert RD, Maher CG, Refshauge KM. Acute low back pain: systematic review of its prognosis. *BMJ.* 2003;327:323.
112. Pincus T, Burton AK, Vogel S, Field AP. A systematic review of psychological factors as predictors of chronicity/disability in prospective cohorts of low back pain. *Spine.* 2002;27:E109-E120.
113. Gurcay E, Bal A, Eksioglu E, Tasturk AE, Gurcay A, Cakci A. Acute low back pain: clinical course and prognostic factors. *Disabil Rehabil.* 2009;31:840-845.
114. Heneweer H, Aufdemkampe G, van Tulder MW, Kiers H, Stappaerts KH, Vanhess L. Psychosocial variables in patients with (sub)acute low back pain: an inception cohort in primary care physical therapy in The Netherlands. *Spine.* 2007;32:586-592.
115. Eccleston C, Crombez G. Pain demands attention: a cognitive-affective model of the interruptivefunction of pain. *Psychol Bull.* 1999;125:356-366.
116. Crombez G, Vlaeyen JW, Heuts PH, Lysens R. Pain related fear is more disabling than pain itself: evidence on the role of pain-related fear in chronic back pain disability. *Pain.* 1999;80:329-339.
117. Slade PD, Troup JDG, Lethem J, Bentley G. The fear-avoidance model of exaggerated pain perception: II. *Behav Res Ther.* 1983;21:409-416.
118. Lethem J, Slade PD, Troup JDG, Bentley G. Outline of a fear avoidance model of exaggerated pain perception: I. *Behav Res Ther.* 1983;21:401-408.
119. Leeuw M, Goossens ME, Linton SJ, Crombez G, Boersma K, Vlaeyen JW. The fear-avoidance model of musculoskeletal pain: current state of scientific evidence. *J Behav Med.* 2007;30:77-94.
120. Myers SS, Phillips RS, Davis RB, et al. Patient expectations as predictors of outcome in patients with acute low back pain. *J Gen Intern Med.* 2008;23(2):148-153.
121. Verbeek J, Sengers MJ, Riemens L, Haafkens J. Patient expectations of treatment for back pain: a systematic review of qualitative and quantitative studies. *Spine (Phila Pa 1976).* 2004;29(20):2309-2318.
122. Shaw WS, Saia A, Pransky G, Winters T, Patterson WB. Perceptions of provider communication and patient satisfaction for treatment of acute low back pain. *J Occup Environ Med.* 2005;47:1036-1043.
123. Iles RA, Davidson M, Taylor NF. Psychosocial predictors of failure to return to work in non-chronic non-specific low back pain: a systematic review. *Occup Environ Med.* 2008;65:507-517.
124. Gatchel RJ. Psychosocial factors that can influence the self-assessment of function. *J Occup Rehabil.* 2004;14:197-206.
125. Swinkels-Meewisse IE, Roelofs J, Oostendorp RA, et al. Acute low back pain: pain-related fear and pain catastrophizing influence physical performance and perceived disability. *Pain.* 2006;120:36-43.
126. Swinkels-Meewisse IE, Roelofs J, Verbeek AL, et al. Fear-avoidance beliefs, disability, and participation in workers and non-workers with acute low back pain. *Clin J Pain.* 2006;22:45-54.
127. Gheldof EL, Vinck J, Vlaeyen JW, et al. The differential role of pain, work characteristics and pain-related fear in explaining back pain and sick leave in occupational settings. *Pain.* 2005;113:71-81.
128. Waddell G, Newton M, Henderson I, et al. A Fear-Avoidance Beliefs Questionnaire (FABQ) and the role of fear-avoidance beliefs in chronic low back pain and disability. *Pain.* 1993;52:157-168.
129. Pincus T, Vlaeyen WS, Kendall N, Von Korff MR, Kalauakalani DA, Reis S. Cognitive-behavioral therapy and psychosocial factors in low back pain. Directions for the future. *Spine.* 2002;27(5):E133-E138.
130. Jarvik JG, Hollingworth W, Heagerty PJ, et al. Three-year incidence of low back pain in an initially asymptomatic cohort: clinical and imaging risk factors. *Spine.* 2005;30:1541-1548.
131. Carroll LJ, Cassidy JD, Cote P. Depression as a risk factor for onset of an episode of troublesome neck and low back pain. *Pain.* 2004;107:134-139.
132. Currie SR, Wang JL. Chronic back pain and major depression in the general Canadian population. *Pain.* 2004;107:54-60.
133. Sullivan MJ, Adams H, Thibault P, et al. Initial depression severity and the trajectory of recovery following cognitive-behavioral intervention for work disability. *J Occup Rehabil.* 2006;16:63-74.
134. Paykel ES. Depression: major problem for public health. *Epidemiol Psychiatr Soc.* 2006;15:4-10.
135. Dewa CS, Goering P, Lin E, et al. Depression-related short-term disability in an employed population. *J Occup Environ Med.* 2002;44:628-633.
136. Goldberg RJ, Steury S. Depression in the workplace: costs and barriers to treatment. *Psychiatr Serv.* 2001;52:1639-1643.
137. Jette DU, Halbert J, Iverson C, Miceli E, Shah P. Use of standardized outcome measures in physical therapist practice: perceptions and applications. *Phys Ther.* 2009;89(2):125-135.
138. George SZ, Fritz JM, Childs JD. Investigation of elevated fear-avoidance beliefs for patients with low back pain: a secondary analysis involving patients enrolled in physical therapy clinical trials. *J Orthop Sports Phys Ther.* 2008;38(2):50-58.
139. Lansky D, Butler JBV, Waller FT. Using health status measures in the hospital setting: from acute care to outcomes management. *Med Care.* 1992;30:MS57-MS73.
140. Flynn T, Fritz J, Whitman J, et al. A clinical prediction rule for classifying patients with low back pain who demonstrate short-term improvement with spinal manipulation. *Spine.* 2002;27:2835-2843.
141. Childs JD, Fritz JM, Flynn TW, et al. A clinical prediction rule to identify patients with low back pain most likely to benefit from spinal manipulation: a validation study. *Ann Intern Med.* 2004;141:920-928.
142. Portney LG, Watkins MP. *Foundations of Clinical Research: Application to Practice.* 2nd ed. Upper Saddles River, NJ: Prentice Hall Health; 2000.
143. Binkley JM, Stratford PW, Lott SA, et al. The Lower Extremity Functional Scale (LEFS): scale development, measurement properties, and clinical application. North American Orthopaedic Rehabilitation Research Network. *Phys Ther.* 1999;79:371-383.
144. Resnik L, Dobrzykowski E. Guide to outcomes measurement for patients with low back pain syndromes. *J Orthop Sports Phys Ther.* 2003;33:307-316.
145. Jaeschke R, Singer J, Guyatt GH. Measurement of health status. Ascertaining the minimal clinically important difference. *Control Clin Trials.* 1989;10(4):407-415.

146. Ostelo RW, de Vet HC. Clinically important outcomes in low back pain. *Best Pract Res Clin Rheumatol.* 2005;19:593-607.
147. Longo UG, Loppini M, Denaro L, Maffulli N, Denaro V. Rating scales for low back pain. *Br Med Bull.* 2010;94:81-144.
148. Roland MO, Morris RW. A study of the natural history of back pain. Part 1: development of a reliable and sensitive measure of disability in low back pain. *Spine.* 1983;8:141-144.
149. Roland M, Fairbank J. The Roland-Morris Disability Questionnaire and the Oswestry Disability Questionnaire. *Spine.* 2000;25:3115-3124.
150. Bombardier C. Outcome assessments in the evaluation of treatment of spinal disorders: summary and general recommendations. *Spine.* 2000;25:3100-3103.
151. Stratford PW, Binkley JM, Riddle DL. Development and initial validation of the back pain functional scale. *Spine.* 2000;25:2095-2102.
152. Davies CC, Nitz AJ. Psychometric properties of the Roland-Morris Disability Questionnaire compared to the Oswestry Disability Index: a systematic review. *Phys Ther Rev.* 2009;14:399-408.
153. Stratford PW, Binkley JM, Riddle DL, Guyatt GH. Sensitivity to change of the Roland-Morris Back Pain Questionnaire: part 1 [see comments]. *Phys Ther.* 1998;78:1186-1196.
154. Ostelo RWJG, Deyo RA, Stratford P, et al. Interpreting change scores for pain and functional status in low back pain. Toward international consensus regarding minimal important change. *Spine.* 2008;33:90-94.
155. Beurskens AJ, de Vet HC, Koke AJ. Responsiveness of functional status in low back pain: a comparison of different instruments. *Pain.* 1996;65:71-76.
156. Fairbank JC, Couper J, Davies JB, O'Brien JP. The Oswestry low back pain disability questionnaire. *Physiotherapy.* 1980;66:271-273.
157. Fritz JM, Irrgang JJ. A comparison of a modified Oswestry Low Back Pain Disability Questionnaire and the Quebec Back Pain Disability Scale. *Phys Ther.* 2001;81:776-788.
158. Leclaire R, Blier F, Fortin L, Proulx R. A cross-sectional study comparing the Oswestry and Roland-Morris Functional Disability scales in two populations of patients with low back pain of different levels of severity. *Spine.* 1997;22:68-71.
159. Fritz JM, Hebert J, Koppenhaver S, Parent E. Beyond minimally important change. Defining a successful outcomes of physical therapy for patients with low back pain. *Spine.* 2009;34:2803-2809.
160. Hicks GE, Manal T. Psychometric properties of commonly used low back disability questionnaires: are they useful for older adults with low back pain? *Pain Med.* 2009;10:85-94.
161. Lauridsen HH, Hartvigsen J, Manniche C, Korsholm L, Grunnet-Nilsson N. Responsiveness and minimal clinically important difference for pain and disability instruments in low back pain patients. *BMC Musculoskelet Disord.* 2006;7:82.
162. Stratford PW, Gill C, Westaway M, Binkley JM. Assessing disability and change on individual patients: a report of a patient-specific measure. *Physiother Can.* 1995;47:258-263.
163. Pengel LH, Refshauge KM, Maher CG. Responsiveness of pain, disability, and physical impairment outcomes in patients with low back pain. *Spine.* 2004;29:879-883.
164. Kamper SJ, Maher CG, Mackay G. Global rating of change scales: a review of strengths and weaknesses and considerations for design. *J Man Manip Ther.* 2009;17(3):163-170.
165. Jaeschke R, Singer J, Guyatt GH. Measurement of health status. Ascertaining the minimal clinically important difference. *Control Clin Trials.* 1989;10:407-415.
166. Costa LOP, Maher CG, Latimer J, et al. Clinimetric testing of three self-report outcome measures for low back pain patients in Brazil: which one is the best? *Spine.* 2008;33:2459-2463.
167. Fischer D, Stewart AL, Bloch DA, Lorig K, Laurent D, Holman H. Capturing the patient's view of change as a clinical outcomes measure. *JAMA.* 1999;282:1157-1162.
168. Deyo RA, Centor RM. Assessing the responsiveness of functional scales to clinical change: an analogy to diagnostic test performance. *J Chronic Dis.* 1986;39:897-906.
169. Stratford PW, Binkley JM, Solomon P, Gill C, Finch E. Assessing change over time in patients with low back pain. *Phys Ther.* 1994;74:528-533.
170. Childs JD, Piva S, Fritz JM. Responsiveness of the numeric pain rating scale in patients with low back pain. *Spine.* 2005;30:1331-1334.
171. Lauridsen HH, Hartvigsen J, Korsholm I, Grunnet Nilsson N, Manniche C. Choice of external criteria in back pain research: does it matter? Recommendations based on analysis of responsiveness. *Pain.* 2007;131:112-120.
172. Ferreira ML, Ferreira PH, Herbert RD, Latimer J. People with low back pain typically need to feel "much better" to consider intervention worthwhile: an observational study. *Aust J Physiother.* 2009;55(2):123-127.
173. Leeuw M, Goossens ME, Linton SJ, Crombez G, Boersma K, Vlaeyen JW. The fear-aoidance model of musculoskeletal pain: current state of scientific evidence. *J Behav Med.* 2007;30:77-94.
174. Buer N, Linton SJ. Fear-avoidance beliefs and catastrophizing: occurrence and risk factor in back pain and ADL in the general population. *Pain.* 2002;99:485-491.
175. Gheldof ELM, Vinck J, Van den Bussche E, Vlaeyen JWS, Hidding A, Crombez G. Pain and pain-related fear are associated with functional and social disability in an occupational setting: evidence of mediation by pain-related fear. *Eur J Pain.* 2006;10:513-525.
176. Gheldof EL, Vinck J, Vlaeyen JWS, Hidding A, Crombez G. The differential role of pain, work characteristics and pain-related fear in explaining back pain and sick leave in occupational settings. *Pain.* 2005;113:71-81.
177. George SZ, Bialosky JE, Donald DA. The centralization phenomenon and fear-avoidance beliefs as prognostic factors for acute low back pain: a preliminary investigation involving patients classified for specific exercise. *J Orthop Sports Phys Ther.* 2005;35:580-588.
178. Boersma K, Linton SJ. Screening to identify patients at risk: profiles of psychological risk factors for early intervention. *Clin J Pain.* 2005;21:38-43.
179. Storheim K, Brox JI, Holm I, Bo K. Predictors of return to work in patients sick listed for sub-acute low back pain: a 12-month follow-up study. *J Rehab Med.* 2005;37:365-371.
180. Al-Obaidi SM, Nelson RM, Al-Awadhi S, Al-Shuwaie N. The role of anticipation and fear of pain in the persistence of avoidance behavior in patients with chronic low back pain. *Spine.* 2000;25:1126-1131.
181. Goubert L, Crombez G, Lysens R. Effects of varied-stimulus exposure on over predictions of pain and behavioural performance in low back pain patients. *Behav Res Ther.* 2005;43:1347-1361.
182. Pincus T, Vogel S, Burton AK, Santos R, Field AP. Fear avoidance and prognosis in back pain. A systematic review and synthesis of current evidence. *Arthitis Rheum.* 2006;54:3999-4010.
183. Jacob T, Baras M, Zeev A, Epstein L. Low back pain: reliability of a set of pain measurement tools. *Arch Phys Med Rehabil.* 2001;82:735-742.
184. Swinkels-Meewisse EJ, Swinkels RA, Verbeek AL, Vlaeyen JW, Oostendorp RA. Psychometric properties of the Tampa Scale for kinesiophobia and the fear-avoidance beliefs questionnairein acute low back pain. *Man Ther.* 2003;8:29-36.

185. George SZ, Fritz JM, McNeil DW. Fear-avoidance beliefs as measured by the fear-avoidance beliefs questionnaire: change in fear-avoidance beliefs questionnaire is predictive of change in self-report of disability and pain intensity for patients with acute low back pain. *Clin J Pain.* 2006;22:197-203.
186. Mannion AF, Junge A, Taimela S, Muntener M, Lorenzo K, Dvorak J. Active therapy for chronic low back pain: part 3. Factors influencing self-rated disability and its change following therapy. *Spine.* 2001;26:920-929.
187. Carragee EJ, Alamin TF, Miller JL, Carragee JM. Discographic, MRI and psychosocial determinants of low back pain disability and remission: a prospective study in subjects with benign persistent back pain. *Spine J.* 2005;5:24-35.
188. Jellema P, van der Horst HE, Vlaeyen JW, Stalman WA, Bouter LM, van der Windt DA. Predictors of outcome in patients with (sub)acute low back pain differ across treatment groups. *Spine.* 2006;31:1699-1705.
189. Klenerman L, Slade PD, Stanley IM, et al. The prediction of chronicity in patients with an acute attack of low back pain in a general practice setting. *Spine.* 1995;20:478-484.
190. Al-Obaidi SM, Beattie P, Al-Zoabi B, Al-Wekeel S. The relationship of anticipated pain and fear avoidance beliefs to outcome in patients with chronic low back pain who are not receiving workers' compensation. *Spine.* 2005;30:1051-1057.
191. George SZ, Fritz JM, Bialosky JE, Donald DA. The effect of a fear-avoidance-based physical therapy intervention for patients with acute low back pain: results of a randomized clinical trial. *Spine.* 2003;28:2551-2560.
192. Grotle M, Brox JI, Vøllestad NK. Reliability, validity and responsiveness of the fear-avoidance beliefs questionnaire: methodological aspects of the Norwegian version. *J Rehabil Med.* 2006;38:346-353.
193. Burton AK, Waddell G, Tillotson KM, Summerton N. Information and advice to patients with back pain can have a positive effect. A randomized controlled trial of a novel educational booklet in primary care. *Spine.* 1999;24:2484-2491.
194. Cleland JA, Fritz FM, Brennan GP. Predictive validity of initial fear avoidance beliefs in patients with low back pain receiving physical therapy: is the FABQ a useful screening tool for identifying patients at risk for a poor recovery? *Eur Spine J.* 2008;17(1):70-79.
195. Klaber Moffett JA, Carr J, Howarth E. High fear-avoiders of physical activity benefit from an exercise program for patients with back pain. *Spine.* 2004;29:1167-1172.
196. Werneke MW, Hart DL, George SZ, Stratford PW, Matheson JW, Reyes A. Clinical outcomes for patients classified by fear-avoidance beliefs and centralization phenomenon. *Arch Phys Med Rehabil.* 2009;90:768-777.
197. Hicks GE, Fritz JM, Delitto A, McGill SM. Preliminary development of a clinical prediction rule for determining which patients with low back pain will respond to a stabilization exercise program. *Arch Phys Med Rehabil.* 2005;86:1753-1762.
198. George SZ, Valencia C, Beneciuk JM. A psychometric investigation of fear-avoidance model measures in patients with chronic low back pain. *J Orthop Sports Phys Ther.* 2010;40(4):197-205.
199. Osman A, Breitenstein JL, Barrios FX, Gutierrez PM, Kopper BA. The Fear of Pain Questionnaire-III: further reliability and validity with nonclinical samples. *J Behav Med.* 2002;25:155-173.
200. Albaret MC, Munoz Sastre MT, Cottencin A, Mullet E. The Fear of Pain questionnaire: factor structure in samples of young, middle-aged and elderly European people. *Eur J Pain.* 2004;8:273-281.
201. Woby SR, Roach NK, Urmston M, Watson PJ. Psychometric properties of the TSK-11: a shortened version of the Tampa Scale for Kinesiophobia. *Pain.* 2005;117:137-144.
202. Roelofs J, Goubert L, Peters ML, Vlaeyen JW, Crombez G. The Tampa Scale for Kinesiophobia: further examination of psychometric properties in patients with chronic low back pain and fibromyalgia. *Eur J Pain.* 2004;8:495-502.
203. Sullivan M, Bishop SR, Pivik J. The pain catastrophizing scale: development and validation. *Psychol Assess.* 1995;7:524-532.
204. D'Eon JL, Harris CA, Ellis JA. Testing factorial validity and gender invariance of the Pain Catastrophizing Scale. *J Behav Med.* 2004;27:361-372.
205. Hill JJ, Keating JL. A systematic review of the incidence and prevalence of low back pain in children. *Phys Ther Rev.* 2009;14:272-284.
206. Tanner JM, Whitehouse RH, Marubii E, Resele LF. The adolescent growth spurt of boys and girls of the Harpenden Growth Study. *Ann Hum Biol.* 1976;3(2):109-126.
207. Salminem JJ, Erkintalo M, Laine M, et al. Low back pain in the young. A prospective three year follow-up study of subjects with and without low back pain. *Spine.* 1995;20:2101-2107.
208. Kovacs FM, Abraira V, Zamora J, Fernández C; Spanish Back Pain Research Network. The transition from acute to subacute and chronic low back pain: a study based on determinants of quality of life and prediction of chronic disability. *Spine (Phila Pa 1976).* 2005;30(15):1786-1792.
209. Hestbaek L, Leboeuf-Yde C, Kyvik KO, et al. The course of low back pain from adolescence to adulthood. *Spine.* 2006;31:468-472.
210. Lawrence RC, Helmick CG, Arnett FC, et al. Estimates of the prevalence of arthritis and selected musculoskeletal disorders in the United States. *Arthritis Rheum.* 1998;41:778-799.
211. Hurwitz EL, Morgenstern H. Correlates of back problems and back related disability in the United States. *J Clin Epidemiol.* 1997;50:669-681.
212. Waxman R, Tennant A, Helliwill P. A prospective follow-up study of low back pain in the community. *Spine.* 2000;25:2085-2090.
213. Kopec JA, Sayre EC, Esdaile JM. Predictors of back pain in a general population cohort. *Spine (Phila Pa 1976).* 2004;29(1):70-77.
214. Loney PL, Stratford PW. The prevalence of low back pain in adults: a methodological review of the literature. *Phys Ther.* 1999;79:384-396.
215. George SZ, Fritz JM, Childs JD, Brennan GP. Sex differences in predictors of outcomes in seleted physical therapy interventions for acute low back pain. *J Orthop Sports Phys Ther.* 2006;36:354-363.
216. Smith BH, Elliott AM, Hannaford PC, et al. Factors related to the onset and persistence of chronic back pain in the ommunity. Results from a general population follow-up study. *Spine.* 2004;29:1032-1040.
217. Thomas E, Silman AJ, Croft PR, et al. Predicting who develops chronic low back pain in primary care: a prospective study. *BMJ.* 1999;318:1662-1667.
218. Linton SJ, Hellsing AL, Hallden K. A population-based study of spinal pain among 35-45-year-old individuals. *Spine.* 1998;23:1457-1463.
219. Bressler HB, Keys WJ, Rochon PA, Badley E. The prevalence of low back pain in the elderly. A systematic review of the literature. *Spine.* 1999;24:1813-1819.
220. Hicks GE, Morone N, Weiner DK. Degenerative lumbar disc and facet disease in older adults: prevalence and clinical correlates. *Spine.* 2009;34:1301-1306.

221. Hartvigsen J, Christensen K, Frederiksen H. Back pain remains a common symptom in old age. A population-based study of 4486 Danish twins aged 70-102. *Eur Spine J.* 2003;12:528-534.
222. Cecchi F, Debolini P, Lova RM, et al. Epidemiology of back pain in a representative cohort of Italian persons 65 years of age and older. *Spine.* 2006;31:1149-1155.
223. Hicks GE, Simonsick EM, Harris TB, et al. Cross sectional associations between trunk muscle composition, back pain, and physical function in the health, aging and body composition study. *J Gerontol A Biol Sci Med Sci.* 2005;60:882-887.
224. Rubin DI. Epidemiology and risk factors for spine pain. *Neurol Clin.* 2007;25:353-371.
225. Waddell G, Burton AK. Occupational health guidelines for the management of low back pain at work: evidence review. *Occup Med.* 2001;51(2):124-135.
226. Thorbjornsson CB, Alfredsson L, Fredriksson K, et al. Physical and psychosocial factors related to low back pain during a 24-year period: a nested case-control analysis. *Spine.* 2000;25:369-375.
227. Hoogendoorn WE, van Poppel MN, Bongers PM, et al. Physical load during work and leisure time as risk factors for back pain. *Scand J Work Environ Health.* 1999;25:387-403.
228. Andersson GB. Epidemiology of low back pain. *Acta Orthop Scand.* 1998;281:28-31.
229. Hurwitz EL, Morgenstern H. Correlates of back problems and back related disability in the United States. *J Clin Epidemiol.* 1997;50:669-681.
230. Punnett L, Pruss-Ustun A, Nelson DI, et al. Estimating the global burden of low back pain attributable to combined occupational exposures. *Am J Ind Med.* 2005;48:459-469.
231. Macfarlane GJ, Thomas E, Papageorgiou AC, et al. Employment and physical work activities as predictors of future low back pain. *Spine.* 1997;22:1143-1149.
232. Lis AM, Black K, Korn H, Nordin M. Association between sitting and occupational LBP. *Eur Spine J.* 2007;16:283-298.
233. Burton AK, Erg E. Back injury and work loss: biomechanical and psychosocial influences. *Spine.* 1997;22:2575-2580.
234. Papageorgiou AC, Macfarlane GH, Thomas E, Croft PR, Jayson MIV, Silman AJ. Psychosocial factors in the workplace—do they predict new episodes of low back pain? Evidence from the South Manchester Back Pain Study. *Spine.* 1997;22:1137-1142.
235. Bakker EWP, Verhagen AP, van Trijffel E, Lucas C, Koes BW. Spinal mechanical load as a risk factor for low back pain. A systematic review of prospective cohort studies. *Spine.* 2009;34:E281-E293.
236. Watson KD, Papageorgiou AC, Jones GT, et al. Low back pain in schoolchildren: the role of mechanical and psychosocial factors. *Arch Dis Child.* 2003;88:12-17.
237. Rossignol AM, Morse EP, Summers VM, Pagnotto LD. Video display terminal use and reported health symptoms among Massachusetts clerical workers. *J Occup Med.* 1987;29:112-118.
238. Gunzburg R, Balagué F, Nordin M, et al. Low back pain in a population of school children. *Eur Spine J.* 1999;8:439-443.
239. Hakala PT, Rimpela AH, Saarni LA, Salminen JJ. Frequent computer-related activities increase the risk of neck-shoulder and low back pain in adolescents. *Eur J Pub Health.* 2006;16:536-541.
240. Campello M, Nordin M, Weiser S. Physical exercise and low back pain. *Scand J Med Sci Sports.* 1996;6:63-72.
241. Heneweer H, Vanhees L, Picavet H. Physical activity and low back pain: a U-shaped relation? *Pain.* 2009;143(1):21-25.
242. Jacob T, Baras M, Zeev A, Epstein L. Physical activities and low back pain: a community-based study. *Med Sci Sports Exerc.* 2004;36:9-15.
243. Dionne CE, Von Korff M, Deyo RA, et al. Formal education and back pain: a review. *J Epidemiol Community Health.* 2001;55:455-468.
244. Goubert L, Crombez G, Bourdeaudhuij ID. Low back pain, disability and back pain myths in a community sample: prevalence and interrelationships. *Eur J Pain.* 2004;8:385-394.
245. Feinstein B, Langton JNK, Jameson RM, Schiller F. Experiments on pain referred from deep somatic tissues. *J Bone Joint Surg Am.* 1954;36:981-997.
246. Fukui S, Kiyoshige O, Masahiro S, Ohno K, Karasawa H, Naganuma Y. Distribution of referred pain from the lumbar zygapophyseal joints and dorsal rami. *Clin J Pain.* 1997;13:303-307.
247. Hockaday JM, Whitty CWM. Patterns of referred pain in the normal subject. *Brain.* 1967;90:481-496.
248. Inman VT, Saunders JB. Referred pain from skeletal structures. *J Nerv Ment Dis.* 1944;99:481-496.
249. Kellgren JH. Observations on referred pain arising from muscle. *Clin Sci.* 1938;3:175-190.
250. Kellgren JH. On the distribution of pain arising from deep somatic structures with charts of segmental pain areas. *Clin Sci.* 1939;4:35-46.
251. Marks R. Distribution of pain provoked form lumbar facet joints and related structures during diagnostic spinal infiltration. *Pain.* 1989;39:37-40.
252. McCall IW, Park WM, O'Brien JP. Induced pain referral from posterior lumbar elements in normal subjects. *Spine.* 1979;4:441-446.
253. McCulloch JA, Waddell G. Variation of the lumbosacral myotomes with bony segmental anomalies. *J Bone Joint Surg.* 1980;62B:475-480.
254. Milette PC, Fontaine S, Lepanto I, Breton G. Radiating pain to the lower extremities caused by lumbar disk rupture without spinal nerve root involvement. *Am J Neuroradiol.* 1995;16:1605-1613.
255. Mooney V, Robertson J. The facet syndrome. *Clin Orthop.* 1976;115:149-156.
256. Ohnmeiss DD, Vanharanta H, Ekholm J. Degree of disc disruption and lower extremity pain. *Spine.* 1997;22:1600-1605.
257. Ohnmeiss DD, Vanharanta H, Ekholm J. Relation between pain location and disc pathology: study of pain drawings and CT/discography. *Clin J Pain.* 1999;15:210-217.
258. Smyth MJ, Wright V. Sciatica and the intervertebral disc. An experimental study. *J Bone Joint Surg.* 1959;40A:1401-1418.
259. Travell J, Rinzler SH. The myofascial genesis of pain. *Postgrad Med.* 1952;11:425-434.
260. Falconer MA, McGeorge M, Begg AC. Observations on the cause and mechanism of symptom-production in sciatica and low-back pain. *J Neurol Neurosurg Psychiatry.* 1948;11:13-26.
261. Kuslich SS, Ulstrom CL, Michael CJ. The tissue origin of low back pain and sciatica: a report of pain response to tissue stimulation during operations on the lumbar spine using local anesthesia. *Orthop Clin North Am.* 1991;22:181-187.
262. Wiberg G. Back pain in relation to the nerve supply of the intervertebal disc. *Acta Orthop Scand.* 1947;19:211-221.
263. Waddell G. A new clinical model of the treatment of low back pain. *Spine.* 1987;12(7):632-644.
264. Bogduk N. Lumbar dorsal ramus syndrome. *Med J Aust.* 1980;2:537-541.
265. Robinson JR. Lower extremity pain of lumbar spine origin: differentiating somatic referred and radicular pain. *J Man Manip Ther.* 2003;11:223-234.

266. Bogduk N. On the definitions and physiology of back pain, referred pain, and radicular pain. *Pain.* 2009;147:17-19.
267. Boden SD, Wiesel SW, Laws ER, Rothman R. *The Aging Spine: Essentials of Pathophysiology, Diagnosis, and Treatment.* Philadelphia, PA: WB Saunders Co; 1991.
268. Grieve GP. Referred pain and other clinical features. In: Boyling JD, Palastanga N, eds. *Grieve's Modern Manual Therapy: The Vertebral Column.* 2nd ed. New York, NY: Churchill Livingstone; 1994:277-279.
269. Maitland G, Hengeveld E, Banks K, English K. *Maitland's Vertebral Manipulation.* 6th ed. Boston, MA: Butterworth-Heinemann; 2001.
270. McCulloch JA, Waddell G. Variation of the lumbosacral myotomes with bony segmental anomalies. *J Bone Joint Surg.* 1980;62B:475-480.
271. Norlen G. On the value of the neurological symptoms in sciatica for the localization of a lumbar disc herniation. *Acta Chir Scand Supp.* 1944;95:1-96.
272. Smyth MJ, Wright V. Sciatica and the intervertebral disc. An experimental study. *J Bone Joint Surg.* 1959;40A:1401-1418.
273. Waddell G. *The Back Pain Revolution.* Edinburgh, Scotland: Churchill Livingstone; 2001.
274. Fritz JM, Cleland JA, Childs JD. Subgrouping patients with low back pain: evolution of a classification approach to physical therapy. *J Orthop Sports Phys Ther.* 2007;37:290-302.
275. Hall H. A simple approach to back pain management. *Patient Care.* 1992;15;77-91.
276. Krismer M, van Tulder M; Low Back Pain Group of the Bone and Joint Health Strategies for Europe Project. Strategies for prevention and management of musculoskeletal conditions. Low back pain (non-specific). *Best Pract Res Clin Rheumatol.* 2007;21(1):77-91.
277. Sieben JM, Portegijs PJ, Vlaeyen JW, Knottnerus JA. Pain-related fear at the start of a new low back pain episode. *Eur J Pain.* 2005;9:635-641.
278. Sieben JM, Vlaeyen JW, Portegijs PJ, et al. A longitudinal study on the predictive validity of the fear-avoidance model in low back pain. *Pain.* 2005;117:162-170.
279. Good M, Stiller C, Zauszniewski JA, Anderson GC, Stanton-Hicks M, Grass JA. Sensation and distress of pain scales: reliability, validity, and sensitivity. *J Nurs Meas.* 2001;9:219-238.
280. Finch E, Brooks D, Stratford PW, Mayo N. *Physical Rehabilitation Outcome Measures—A Guide to Enhanced Clinical Decision Making.* 2nd ed. Baltimore, MD: Lippincott Williams & Wilkins; 2002.
281. Jensen MP, Turner JA, Romano JM. What is the maximum number of levels needed in pain intensity measurement? *Pain.* 1992;57:387-392.
282. Jensen MP, Turner JA, Romano JM, et al. Comparative reliability and validity of chronic pain intensity measures. *Pain.* 1999;83:157-162.
283. von Korff M, Jensen MP, Karoly P. Assessing global pain severity by self-report in clinical and health services research. *Spine.* 2000;25:3140-3151.
284. Farrar JT, Young JP Jr, La Moreaux L, et al. Clinical importance of changes in chronic pain intensity measured on an 11-point numerical pain rating scale. *Pain.* 2001;94:149-158.
285. van der Roer N, Ostelo RS, Bekkering GE, et al. Minimal clinically important change I for pain intensity, functional status, and general health status in patients with nonspecific low back pain. *Spine.* 2006;31:578-582.
286. Carlsson AM. Assessment of chronic pain. I. Aspects of reliability and validity of the visual analogue scale. *Pain.* 1983;16:87-101.
287. Flaherty SA. Pain measurement tools for clinical practice and research. *AANA J.* 1996;64:133-140.
288. Collins S, Moore RA, McQuay HJ. The visual analogue pain intensity sale: what is moderate pain in millimeters? *Pain.* 1997;72(1-2):95-97.
289. Enebo BA. Outcome measures for low back pain: pain inventories and functional disability questionnaires. *J Chiropr Tech.* 1998;10:27-33.
290. Kelly AM. The minimum clinically significant difference in visual analogue scale pain score does not differ with severity of pain. *Emerg Med J.* 2001;18:205-207.
291. Hagg O, Fritzell P, Nordwall A. The clinical importance of changes in outcomes scores after treatment for chronic low back pain. *Eur Spine J.* 2003;12:12-20.
292. Grotle M, Vollestad NK, Veierod MB, Brox JI. Fear-avoidance beliefs and distress in relation to disability in acute and chronic low back pain. *Pain.* 2004;112:343-352.
293. Bolton JE, Wilkinson R. Responsiveness of pain scales: a comparison of three pain intensity measures in chiropractic patients. *J Manipulative Physiol Ther.* 1998;12:1-7.
294. Kahl C, Cleland JA. Visual analogue scale, numeric pain rating scale and the McGill Pain Questionnaire: an overview of psychometric properties. *Phys Ther Rev.* 2005;10:123-128.
295. Maitland G, Hengeveld E, Banks K, English K. *Maitland's Vertebral Manipulation.* 6th ed. Boston, MA: Butterworth-Heinemann; 2001.
296. Goodman CC, Fuller KS. *Pathology. Implications for the Physical Therapist.* 3rd ed. St Louis, MO: Saunders; 2009.
297. Boissonnault WG. Patient health history including identification of health risk factors. In: Boissonnault WG, ed. *Primary Care for the Physical Therapist. Examination and Triage.* Philadelphia, PA: Saunders; 2005:70.
298. Goodman CC, Fuller KS. *Pathology. Implications for the Physical Therapist.* 3rd ed. St Louis, MO: Saunders; 2009.
299. Idler EL, Benyamini Y. Self-rated health and mortality: a review of twenty-seven community studies. *J Health Soc Behav.* 1997;38:21-37.
300. Idler EL, Russell LB, Davis D. Survival, functional limitations, and self-rated health in the NHANES I Epidemiologic Follow-up Study 1992; first National Health and Nutrition Examination Survey. *Am J Epidemiol.* 2000;9:874-883.
301. Hagen KB, Tambs K, Bjerkedal T. A prospective cohort study of risk factors for disability retirement because of back pain in the general working population. *Spine.* 2002;27:1790-1796.
302. Shiri R, Karppinen J, Leino-Arjas P, Solovieva S, Viikari-Juntura E. The association between smoking and low back pain: a meta-analysis. *Am J Med.* 2010;123:87.e7-87.e35.
303. Mikkonen P, Leino-Arjas P, Remes J, Zitting P, Taimela S, Karppinen J. Is smoking a risk factor for low back pain in adolescents? A prospective cohort study. *Spine.* 2008;33:527-532.
304. Webb R, Brammah T, Lunt M, et al. Prevalence and predictors of intense, chronic, and disabling neck and back pain in the UK general population. *Spine.* 2003;28:1195-1202.
305. Croft PR, Papageorgiou AC, Thomas E, et al. Short term physical risk factors for new episodes of low back pain: prospective evidence from the South Manchester Back Pain Study. *Spine.* 1999;24:1556-1561.
306. Shiri R, Karppinen J, Leino-Arjas P, Solovieva S, Viikari-Juntura E. The association between obesity and low back pain: a meta-analysis. *Am J Epidemiol.* 2010;171:135-154.
307. Vismara L, Menegoni F, Zaina F, Galli M, Negrini S, Capodaglio P. Effect of obesity and low back pain on spinal mobility: a cross sectional study in women. *J Neuroeng Rehabil.* 2010;7:3.
308. Billek-Sawhney B, Sawhney R. Cardiovascular considerations in outpatient orthopedic physical therapy [abstract]. *J Orthop Sports Phys Ther.* 1998:27:57.

309. Scherer SA, Noteboom JT, Flynn TW. Cardiovascular assessment in the orthopaedic practice setting. *J Orthop Sports Phys Ther.* 2005;35:730-737.
310. Thompson WR, Gordon NG, Pescatello LS, eds. *ACSM's Guidelines for Exercise Testing and Prescription.* 8th ed. Philadelphia, PA: Wolters Kluwer Lippincott Williams & Wilkins; 2010.
311. Chou R, Huffman LH. Medications for acute and chronic low back pain: a review of the evidence for an American Pain Society/American College of Physicians Clinical Practice Guideline. *Ann Intern Med.* 2007;147:505-514.
312. Luo X, Pietrobon R, Curtis LH, Hey LA. Prescription of nonsteroidal anti-inflammatory drugs and muscle relaxants for back pain in the United States. *Spine.* 2004;29:E531-E537.
313. Luo X, Pietrobon R, Hey L. Patterns and trends in opioid use among individuals with back pain in the United States. *Spine.* 2004;29:884-890; discussion 891.
314. Bernstein E, Carey TS, Garrett JM. The use of muscle relaxant medications in acute low back pain. *Spine.* 2004;29:1346-1351.
315. Deyo RA, Weinstein JN. Low back pain. *N Engl J Med.* 2001;344:363-370.
316. Verbeek J, Sengers MJ, Riemens L, Haafkens J. Patient expectations of treatment for back pain: a systematic review of qualitative and quantitative studies. *Spine (Phila Pa 1976).* 2004;29(20):2309-2318.
317. Wilson IB, Dukes K, Greenfield S, Kaplan S, Hillman B. Patients' role in the use of radiology testing for common office practice complaints. *Arch Intern Med.* 2001;16:256-263.
318. Ash LM, Modic MT, Obushowski NA, Ross JS, Brant-Zawadzki MN, Grooff PN. Effects of diagnostic information, per se, on patient outcomes in acute radiculopathy and low back pain. *Am J Neuroradiol.* 2008;29:1098-1103.
319. Hart L, Deyo R, Cherkin D. Physician office visits for low back pain: frequency, clinical evaluation, and treatment patterns from a US national survey. *Spine.* 1995;20:11-19.
320. Reinus WR, Strome G, Zwemer FL. Use of lumbosacral spine radiographs in a level 11 emergency department. *Am J Roentgenol.* 1998;170:443-448.
321. Gilbert FJ, Grant AM, Gillan MG, et al. Low back pain: influence of early MR imaging or CT on treatment and outcomes—multicenter randomized trial. *Radiology.* 2004;231:343-351.
322. Kendrick D, Fielding K, Bentley E, Kerslake R, Miller P, Pringle M. Radiography of the lumbar spine in primary are patients with low back pain: randomized controlled trial. *BMJ.* 2001;322:400-405.
323. Kerry S, Hilton S, Dundas D, Rink E, Oakeshott P. Radiography for low back pain: a randomized controlled trial and observational study in primary care. *Br J Gen Pract.* 2002;52:469-474.
324. Lurie JD, Birkmeyer NJ, Weinstein JN. Rates of advanced spinal imaging and spine surgery. *Spine.* 2003;28:616-620.
325. Jarvik JG, Hollingworth W, Martin B, et al. Rapid magnetic resonance imaging versus radiographs for patients with low back pain: randomized controlled trial. *JAMA.* 2003;289:2810-2818.
326. van Tulder MW, Assendelft WJ, Koes BW, Bouter LM. Spinal radiographic findings and nonspecific low back pain. A systematic review of observational studies. *Spine.* 1997;22:427-434.
327. Jonsson B, Stromqvist B, Egund N. Anomalous lumbosacral articulations and low-back pain: evaluation and treatment. *Spine.* 1989;14:831-834.
328. Brault J, Smith J, Currier B. Partial lumbosacral transitional vertebra resection for contralateral facetogenic pain. *Spine.* 2001;26:226-229.
329. Liang M, Komaroff AL. Roentgenograms in primary care patients with acute low back pain: a cost-effectiveness analysis. *Arch Intern Med.* 1982;142:1108-1112.
330. Jensen MC, Brant-Zawadzki MN, Obuchowski N, et al. Magnetic resonance imaging of the lumbar spine in people without back pain. *N Engl J Med.* 1994;331:69-73.
331. Boden SD, Davis DO, Dina TS, et al. Abnormal magnetic-resonance scans of the lumbar spine in asymptomatic subjects: a prospective investigation. *J Bone Joint Surg Am.* 1990; 72:403-408.
332. Beattie PF, Meyers SP, Stratford P, Millard RS, Hollenberg GM. Associations between patient report of symptoms and anatomic impairment visible on lumbar magnetic resonance imaging. *Spine.* 2000;25:819-828.
333. Videman T, Battie MC, Gibbons LE, Maravoilla K, Manninen H, Kaprio J. Associations between back pain history and lumbar MRI findings. *Spine.* 2003;28:582-588.
334. Deyo RA, Diehl AK. Lumbar spine films in primary care: current use and effects of selective ordering criteria. *J Gen Intern Med.* 1986;1:20-25.
335. Chou R, Rongwei Fu, Carrino JA, Deyo RA. Imaging strategies for low back pain: systematic review and meta-analyisis. *Lancet.* 2009;373:463-472.
336. Kleinstück F, Dvorak J, Mannion AF. Are "structural abnormalities" on magnetic resonance imaging a contraindication fot he successful conservative treatment of chronic nonspecific low back pain? *Spine.* 2006;31:2250-2257.
337. Frymoyer JW. Back pain and sciatica. *N Engl J Med.* 1988;318:291-300.
338. Deyo RA, Bigos SJ, Maravilla KR. Diagnostic imaging procedures for the lumbar spine. *Ann Intern Med.* 1989;111:865-867.
339. Refshauge KM, Maher CG. Low back pain investigations and prognosis: a review. *Br J Sports Med.* 2006;40:494-498.
340. Mondloch MV, Cole DC, Frank JW. Does how you do depend on how you think you'll do? A systematic review of the evidence for a relation between patients' recovery expectations and health outcomes. *Can Med Assoc J.* 2001;165:174-179.
341. Myers SS, Phillips RS, Davis RB, et al. Patient expectations as predictors of outcome in patients with acute low back pain. *J Gen Intern Med.* 2008;23(2):148-153.
342. Bialosky JE, Bishop MD, Cleland JA. Individual expectation: an overlooked, but pertinent factor in the treatment of individuals experiencing musculoskeletal pain. *Phys Ther.* 2010;90:1345-1355.
343. American Academy of Orthopaedic Manual Physical Therapists. *Orthopaedic Manual Physical Therapy. Description of Advanced Clinical Practice.* Tallahassee, FL: Author; 2009.
344. Rubinstein SM, van Tulder M. A best-evidence review of diagnostic procedures for neck and low back pain. *Best Prac Res Clin Rheum.* 2008;22:471-482.
345. Bombardier C. Outcomes assessment in the evaluation of treatment of spinal disorders: summary and general recommendations. *Spine.* 2000;225:3100-3103.
346. Zuberbier OA, Kozlowski AJ, Hunt DG, et al. Analysis of convergent and discriminant validity of published lumbar flexion, extension, and lateral flexion scores. *Spine.* 2001;26:472-478.
347. Dionne CE, Von Kkorff M, Koepsell TD, et al. A comparison of pain, functional limitation, and work status indices as outcome measures in back pain research. *Spine.* 1999;24:2339-2345.
348. Waddell G, Somerville D, Henderson I, Newton M. Objective clinical evaluation of physical impairment in chronic low back pain. *Spine.* 1992;17:617-628.
349. Fritz JM, Piva SR. Physical impairment index: reliability, validity, and responsiveness in patients with acute low back pain. *Spine.* 2003;28:1189-1194.

350. Tubach F, Leclerc A, Landre M, Pietri-Taleb F. Risk factors for sick leave due to low back pain: a prospective study. *J Occup Environ Med.* 2002;44:451-458.
351. Lee D, Lee LF. *The Pelvic Girdle. An Integration of Clinical Expertise and Research.* 4th ed. Philadelphia, PA: Churchill Livingstone; 2011.
352. Keefe FJ, Hill RW. An objective approach to quantifying pain behavior and gait patterns in low back pain patients. *Pain.* 1985;21:153-161.
353. Simmonds MJ, Claveau Y. Measures of pain and physical function in patients with low back pain. *Physiother Theory Pract.* 1997;13:53-65.
354. Simmonds MJ, Olson SL, Jones S, et al. Psychometric characteristics and clinical usefulness of physical performance tests in patients with low back pain. *Spine.* 1998;23:2412-2421.
355. Hussein TM, Simmonds MJ, Olson SL, et al. Kinematics of gait in normal and low back pain subjects. *J Orthop Sports Phys Ther.* 1998;27:84.
356. Vogt L, Pfeifer K, Portscher M, et al. Influences of nonspecific low back pain on 3-dimensional lumbar spine kinematics in locomotion. *Spine.* 2001;26:1910-1919.
357. Simmonds MJ. Physical function and physical performance in patients with low back pain: what are the measures and what do they mean? Paper presented at: 9th World Congress on Pain; August 22-27, 1999; Vienna, Austria.
358. Winter DA. Kinematic and kinetic patterns in human gait: variability and compensating effects. *Hum Mov Sci.* 1984;3:51-76.
359. Lee CE, Simmonds M, Etnyre BR, Morris GS. Influence of pain distribution on gait characteristics in patient with low back pain. Part 1: vertical ground reaction force. *Spine.* 2007;32:1329-1336.
360. Nilsson J, Thorstensson A. Ground reaction forces at different speeds of human walking and running. *Acta Physiol Scand.* 1989;136:217-227.
361. Wosk J, Voloshin AS. Low back pain: conservative treatment with artificial shock absorbers. *Arch Phys Med Rehabil.* 1985;66:145-148.
362. Joffe D, Watkins M, Steiner L, et al. Treadmill ambulation with partial body weight support for the treatment of low back and leg pain. *J Orthop Sports Phys Ther.* 2002;32:202-213.
363. Al-Obaidi SM, Al-Zoabi B, Al-Shuwaie N, et al. The influence of pain and pain-related fear and disability beliefs on walking velocity in chronic low back pain. *Int J Rehabil Res.* 2003;26:101-108.
364. Lamoth CJC, Meijer OG, Wuisman PIJM, van Dieen JH, Levin MF, Beek PJ. Pelvis-thorax coordination in the transverse plane during walking in persons with nonspecific low back pain. *Spine.* 2002;27(4):E92-E99.
365. Lamoth CJ, Meijer OG, Daffertshofer A, Wuisman PI, Beek PJ. Effects of chronic low back pain on trunk coordination and back muscle activity during walking: changes in motor control. *Eur Spine J.* 2006;15:23-40.
366. Arendt-Nielsen L, Graven-Nielsen T, Svarrer H, et al. The influence of low back pain on muscle activity and coordination during gait: a clinical experimental study. *Pain.* 1995;64:231-240.
367. Marras WS, Wongsam P. Flexibility and velocity of the normal and impaired lumbar spine. *Arch Phys Med Rehabil.* 1986;67:213-217.
368. van der Hulst M, Vollenbroek-Hutten MM, Rietman JS, Hermens HJ. Lumbar and abdominal muscle activity during walking I subjects with chronic low back pain: support of the "guarding" hypothesis? *J Electromyogr Kinesiol.* 2010;20:31-38.
369. Saunders SWM, Coppeiters M, Magarey M, Hodges PW. Low back pain and associated changes in abdominal muscle activation during human locomotion. Paper presented at: Australia Conference of Science and Medicine in Sport: Hot Topics From the Red Centre; October 6-9, 2004; Alice Springs, Northern Territory, Australia.
370. McGregor AH, Hukins DW. Lower limb involvement in spinal function and low back pain. *J Back Musculoskelet Rehabil.* 2009;22(3):219-222.
371. Byl NN, Sinnot PL. Variations in balance and body sway. *Spine.* 1991;16:325-330.
372. Louto S, Aalto H, Taimela S, et al. One-footed and externally disturbed two-footed postural control in chronic low back pain patients: a controlled follow-up study. *Spine.* 1996;21:2621-2627.
373. Mok NW, Brauer S, Hodges PW. Hip strategy for balance control in quiet standing is reduced in people with low back pain. *Spine.* 2004;29:E107-E112.
374. Takala E, Viikari-Juntura E. Do functional tests predict low back pain? *Spine.* 2000;25:2126-2132.
375. Stovall BA, Kumar S. Anatomical landmark asymmetry assessment in the lumbar spine and pelvis: a review of reliability [abstract]. *PM R.* 2010;2:48-56.
376. Sabharwal S, Kumar A. Methods for assessing leg length discrepancy. *Clin Orthop Relat Res.* 2008;466:2910-2922.
377. Brady RJ, Dean JB, Skinner TM, Gross MT. Limb length inequality: clinical implications for assessment and intervention. *J Orthop Sports Phys Ther.* 2003;33:221-234.
378. Saulicz E, Bacik B, Saulicz M, Gnat R. [Pelvic asymmetry and symptoms of dysfunction of the sacroiliac joints. A study in people without ailments of the low lumbar.] *Manuelle Medizin.* 2001;39:312-319.
379. Gnat R, Saulicz E, Bialy M, Klaptocz P. Does pelvic asymmetry always mean pathology? Analysis of mechanical factors leading to the asymmetry. *J Hum Kinet.* 2009;21:23-35.
380. May S, Littlewood C, Bishop A. Reliability of procedures used in the physical examination of non-specific low back pain: a systematic review. *Aust J Phsiother.* 2006;52(2):91-102.
381. Leard JS, Crane BA, Ball KA. Intrarater and interrater reliability of 22 clinical measures associated with lower quarter malalignment. *J Manipulative Physiol Ther.* 2009;32:270-276.
382. Fedorak C, Ashworth N, Marshall J, Paull H. Reliability of visual assessment of cervical and lumbar lordosis: how good are we? *Spine.* 2003;28(16):1857-1859.
383. Adams MA, Dolan P, Marx C, Hutton WC. An electronic inclinometer technique for measuring lumbar curvature. *Clin Biomech (Bristol, Avon).* 1986;1:130-134.
384. Hicks GE, George SZ, Nevitt MA, Cauley JA, Vogt MT. Measurement of lumbar lordosis: interrater reliability, minimum detectable change and longitudinal variation. *J Spinal Disord Tech.* 2006;19:501-506.
385. O'Sullivan P, Mitchell T, Bulich P, Waller R, Holte J. The relationship between posture and back muscle endurance in industrial workers with flexion-related low back pain. *Man Ther.* 2006;11:264-271.
386. Dankaerts W, O'Sullivan P, Burnett A, Straker L. Differences in sitting postures are associated with nonspecific chronic low back pain disorders when patients are subclassified. *Spine.* 2006;31:698-704.
387. Tuzun C, Yorulmaz I, Cindas A, Vatan S. Low back pain and posture. *Clin Rheumatol.* 1999;18:308-312.
388. Widhe T. Spine: posture, mobility and pain. A longitudinal study from childhood to adolescence. *Eur Spine J.* 2001;10:118-123.

389. Scannell JP, McGill JM. Lumbar posture—should it, and can it, be modified? A study of passive tissue stiffness and lumbar position during activities of daily living. *Phys Ther.* 2003;83:907-917.
390. McKenzie RA. *The Lumbar Spine. Mechanical Diagnosis and Therapy.* Raumatic Beach, New Zealand: Spinal Publications; 1981.
391. Donahue MS, Riddle D, Sullivam MS. Intertester reliability of a modified version of McKenzie's lateral shift assessments obtained on patients with low back pain. *Phys Ther.* 1996;76:706-726.
392. Kilpikoski S, Airaksinen O, Kankaanpaa M, Leminen P, Videman T, Alen M. Interexaminer reliability of low back pain assessment using the McKenzie method. *Spine.* 2002;27:E207-E214.
393. Clare HA, Adams R, Maher CG. Reliability of detection of lumbar lateral shift. *J Manipulative Physiol Ther.* 2005;26:476-480.
394. Childs JD, Piva SR, Erhard RE, Hicks G. Side-to-side weight-bearing asymmetry in subjects with low back pain. *Man Ther.* 2003;8(3):166-169.
395. McKenzie RA. Manual correction of sciatic scoliosis. *N Z Med J.* 1972;484:194-199.
396. Porter RW, Miller CG. Back pain and trunk list. *Spine.* 1986;11:596-600.
397. Matsui H, Ohmori K, Kanamori M, Ishihara H, Tsuji H. Significance of sciatic scoliotic list in operated patients with lumbar disc herniation. *Spine.* 1998;23:338-342.
398. Suk KS, Lee HM, Moon SH, Kim NH. Lumbosacral scoliotic list by lumbar disc herniation. *Spine.* 2001;26:667-671.
399. Laslett M. Manual correction of an acute lumbar lateral shift: maintenance of correction and rehabilitation: a case report with video. *J Man Manip Ther.* 2009;17(2):78-85.
400. Grieve GP. Treating backache: a topical comment. *Physiotherapy.* 1983;69:316.
401. McKenzie R, May S. *The Lumbar Spine Mechanical Diagnosis and Therapy. Vol 2.* Raumatic Beach, New Zealand: Spinal Publications; 2003.
402. McKenzie R, May S. *The Lumbar Spine Mechanical Diagnosis and Therapy. Vol 1.* Raumatic Beach, New Zealand: Spinal Publications; 2003.
403. Robinson AJ, Russell S, Rimmer S. The value of ultrasonic examination of the lumbar spine in infants with specific reference to cutaneous markers of occult spinal dysraphism. *Clin Radiol.* 2005;60:72-77.
404. Hsu CH, Change YW, Chou WY, Chiou CP, Change WN, Wong CY. Measurement of spinal range of motion in healthy individuals using an electromagnetic tracing device. *J Neurosurg Spine.* 2008;8(2):125-142.
405. Hicks GE, Fritz JM, Delitto A, McGill SM. Preliminary development of a clinical prediction rule for determining which patients with low back pain will respond to a stabilization exercise program. *Arch Phys Med Rehabil.* 2005;86:1753-1762.
406. Breum J, Wiberg J, Bolton J. Reliability and concurrent validity of the BROM II for measuring lumbar mobility. *J Manipulative Physiol Ther.* 1995;18:497-502.
407. Saur P, Ensink F, Frese K, Seegar D, Hildebrandt J. Lumbar range of motion: reliability and validity of the inclinometer technique in the clinical measurement of trunk flexibility. *Spine.* 1996;21:1332-1338.
408. Fritz JM, Piva S, Childs JD. Accuracy of the clinical examination to predict radiographic instability of the lumbar spine. *Eur Spine J.* 2005;14:743-750.
409. Hunt D, Zuberbier O, Kozlowski A, et al. Reliability of lumbar flexion, lumbar extension, and passive straight leg raise test in normal populations embedded within a complete physical examination. *Spine.* 2001;26:2714-2718.
410. Delitto A, Erhardt R, Bowling R. A treatment-based classification approach to low back syndrome: identifying and staging patients for conservative treatment. *Phys Ther.* 1995;75:470-485.
411. Long A, Donelson R, Fung T. Does it matter which exercise? A randomized control trial of exercise for low back pain. *Spine.* 2004;29:2593-2602.
412. Werneke M, Hart DL, Cook D. A descriptive study of the centralization phenomenon. *Spine.* 1999;24:676-683.
413. Fritz JM, Delitto A, Vignovic M, Busse RG. Interrater reliability of judgments of the centralization phenomenon and status change during movement testing in patients with low back pain. *Arch Phys Med Rehabil.* 2000;81:57-61.
414. Kilpikoski S, Airaksinen O, Kankaanpaa M, Leminen P, Videman T, Alen M. Interexaminer reliability of low back pain assessment using the McKenzie method. *Spine.* 2002;27:E207-E214.
415. Werneke M, Hart DL. Discriminant validity and relative precision for classifying patients with non-specific neck and low back pain by anatomic pain patterns. *Spine.* 2003;28:161-166.
416. Laslett M, Öberg B, Aprill CN, McDonald B. Centralization as a predictor of provocation discopgraphy results in chronic low back pain, and the influence of disability and distress on diagnostic power. *Spine J.* 2005;5:370-380.
417. Werneke M, Hart DL. Centralization phenomenon as a prognostic factor for chronic low back pain and disability. *Spine.* 2001;26:758-765.
418. Edwards BC. Combined movements of the lumbar spine: examination and clinical significance. *Aust J Physiother.* 1979;25:147-152.
419. Barrett CJ, Singer R, Day R. Assessment of combined movements of the lumbar spine in asymptomatic and low back pain subjects using a three-dimensional electromagnetic tracking system. *Man Ther.* 1999;4:94-99.
420. Haswell K, Williams M, Hing W. Interexaminer reliability of symptom-provoking active sidebend, rotation and combined movement assessments of patients with low back apin. *J Man Manip Ther.* 2004;12:11-20.
421. McCarthy C. *Combined Movement Theory. Rational Mobilization and Manipulation of the Vertebral Column.* New York, NY: Churchill Livingstone; 2010.
422. Lyle MA, Manes S, McGuinness M, Ziaei S, Iversen MD. Relationship of physical examination findings and self-reported symptoms severity and physical function in patients with degenerative lumbar conditions. *Phys Ther.* 2005;85:120-133.
423. Cook CE. *Orthopedic Manual Therapy. An Evidence-Based Approach.* Upper Saddle River, NJ: Pearson Prentice Hall; 2007.
424. Butler DS. *The Sensitive Nervous System.* Adelaide, Australia: NOI Publications. 2000.
425. Butler DS. *Mobilisation of the Nervous System.* New York, NY: Churchill Livingstone; 1992.
426. Breig A, Marions O. Biomechanics of the lumbosacral nerve roots. *Acta Radiol.* 1962;1:1141-1160.
427. Troup JDG. Biomechanics of the lumbar spinal canal. *Clin Biomech.* 1986;1:31-43.
428. Philip K, Lew P, Matyas TA. The inter-therapist reliability of the slump test. *Aust J Physiother.* 1989;35:89-94.
429. Coppieters MW, Kurz K, Motensen TE, et al. The impact of neurodynamic testing on the perception of experimentally induced muscle pain. *Man Ther.* 2005;10:52-60.

430. Majlesi J, Togay H, Unalan H, Toprak S. The sensitivity and specificity of the slump and the straight leg raising tests in patients with lumbar disc herniation. *J Clin Rheumatol.* 2008;14:87-91.
431. Smith SA, Massie JB, Chesnut R, et al. Straight leg raising. Anatomical effects on the spinal nerve root without and with fusion. *Spine.* 1993;18:992-999.
432. Goddard MD, Reid JD. Movements induced by straight leg raising in the lumbo-sacral roots, nerves and plexus, and in the intrapelvic section of the sciatic nerve. *J Neurol Neurosurg Psychiatry.* 1965;28:12-18.
433. Strender LE, Sjoblom A, Sundell K, Ludwig R, Taube A. Interexaminer reliability in physical examination of patients with low back pain. *Spine.* 1997;22:814-820.
434. Vroomen PCAJ, de Krom M, Knottnerus JA. Consistency of history taking and physical examination in patients with suspected lumbar nerve root involvement. *Spine.* 2000;25:91-97.
435. Deville WL, van der Windt DA, Dzaferagic A, et al. The test of Lasegue: systematic review of the accuracy in diagnosing herniated discs. *Spine.* 2000;25:1140-1147.
436. Hicks GE, Fritz JM, Delitto A, Mishock J. Interrater reliability of clinical examination measures for identification of lumbar segmental instability. *Arch Phys Med Rehabil.* 2003;84:1858-1864.
437. Coppieters MW, Kurz K, Mortensen TE, et al. The impact of neurodynamic testing on the perception of experimentally induced muscle pain. *Man Ther.* 2005;10:52-60.
438. Shacklock M. Improving application of neurodynamic (neural tension) testing and treatments: a message to researchers and clinicians. *Man Ther.* 2005;10:175-179.
439. Walsh J, Hall T. Agreement and correlation between the straight leg raise and slump tests I subjects with leg pain. *J Manipulative Physiol Ther.* 2009;32:184-192.
440. Sweetman BJ, Anderson JA, Dalton ER. The relationships between little finger mobility, lumbar mobility, straight leg raising and low back pain. *Rheum Rehabil.* 1974;13:161-166.
441. Slater H. The effect of foot position on the SLR responses. In: Jones H, Jones MA, Milde MR, eds. *Proceedings of the Sixth Biennial Conference.* Adelaide, Australia: Manipulative Therapists Association of Australia; 1989:183-190.
442. Hungerford B, Gilleard W, Lee D. Altered patterns of pelvic bone motion determined in subjects with posterior pelvic pain using skin markers. *Clin Biomech.* 2004;19:456-464.
443. O'Sullivan P. Diagnosis and classification of chronic low back pain disorders: maladaptive movement and motor control impairments as underlying mechanisms. *Man Ther.* 2005;10:242-255.
444. Dankaerts W, O'Sullivan PB, Burnett A, Straker L, Skouen J. Towards a clinical validation of a classification method for non specific chronic low back pain patients with motor control impairment. *Man Ther.* 2006;11:28-39.
445. Silfies SP, Squillante D, Maurer P, Westcott S, Karduna A. Trunk muscle recruitment patterns in specific chronic low back pain populations. *Clin Biomech.* 2005;20:465-473.
446. Richardson CA, Snijders CJ, Hides JA, Damen L, Pas MS, Storm J. The relation between the transversus abdominis muscles, sacroiliac joint mechanics, and low back pain. *Spine.* 2002;27:399-405.
447. Shum GLK, Crosbie J, Lee RYW. Effect of low back pain on the kinematics and joint coordination of the lumbar spine and hip during sit-to-stand and stand-to-sit. *Spine.* 2005;30:1998-2004.
448. Mens JM, Vleeming A, Snijders CJ, Stam HJ, Ginai AZ. The active straight leg raising test and mobility of the pelvic joints. *Eur Spine J.* 1999;8:468-473.
449. O'Sullivan PB, Beales DJ, Beetham JA, et al. Altered motor control strategies in subjects with sacroiliac joint pain during the active straight-leg-raise test. *Spine.* 2002;27:E1-E8.
450. Mens JM, Vleeming A, Snijders CJ, Koes BW, Stam HJ. Reliability and validity of the active straight leg raise test in posterior pelvic pain since pregnancy. *Spine.* 2001;26:1167-1171.
451. Roussel NA, Nijs J, Truijen S, Smeuninx L, Stassijns G. Low back pain: clinimetric properties of the Trendelenburg test, active straight leg raise test, and breathing pattern during active straight leg raising. *J Manipiulative Physiol Ther.* 2007;30:270-278.
452. Damen L, Buyruk HM, Gueler-Ysal F, Lotgering FK, Snijders CJ, Stam HJ. The prognostic value of asymmetric laxity of the sacroiliac joints in pregnancy-related pelvic pain. *Spine.* 2002;27:2820-2824.
453. Lee D. *The Pelvic Girdle.* 3rd ed. Philadelphia, PA: Churchill Livingstone Elsevier; 2004.
454. de Groot M, Pool-Goudzwaard AL, Spoor CW, Snijders CJ. The active straight leg raising test (ASLR) in pregnant women: differences in muscle activity and force between patients and healthy subjects. *Man Ther.* 2008;13:68-74.
455. Teyhen DS, Williamson JN, Carlson NH, et al. Ultrasound characteristics of the deep abdominal muscles during the active straight leg raise test. *Arch Phys Med Rehabil.* 2009;90:761-767.
456. Boissonault WG. *Primary Care for the Physical Therapist. Examination and Triage.* 2nd ed. St Louis, MO: Elsevier Saunders; 2011.
457. Whitman JM, Flynn TW, Childs JD, et al. A comparison between two physical therapy treatment programs for patients with lumbar spinal stenosis: a randomized clinical trial. *Spine.* 2006;31:2541-2549.
458. Ellison JB, Rose SJ, Sahrmann SA. Patterns of hip rotation range of motion: a comparison between healthy subjects and patients with low back pain. *Phys Ther.* 1990;70:537-541.
459. Chesworth BM, Padfeld BJ, Helewa A, Stitt LW. A comparison of hip mobility in patients with low back pain and matched healthy subjects. *Physiother Can.* 1994;46:267-274.
460. Cibulka MT, Sinacore DR, Cromer GS, Delitto A. Unilateral hip rotation range of motion asymmetry in patients with sacroiliac joint regional pain. *Spine.* 1998;23:1009-1015.
461. Vad VB, Bhat AL, Basrai D, Gebeh A, Aspergren DD, Andrews JR. Low back pain in professional golfers: the role of associated hip and low back range-of-motion deficits. *Am J Sports Med.* 2004;32:494-497.
462. Nadler SF, Malanga GA, Feinberg JH, Prybicien M, Stitik TP, DePrince MS. Relationship between hip muscle imbalance and occurrence of low back pain in collegiate athletes: a prospective study. *Am J Phys Med Rehabil.* 2001;80:572-577.
463. Nourbakhsh MR, Ara AM. Relationship between mechanical factors and incidence of low back pain. *J Orthop Sports Phys Ther.* 2002;32:447-460.
464. Nadler SF, Malanga GA, DePrince M, Stitik TP, Feinberg JH. The relationship between lower extremity injury, low back pain, and hip muscle strength in male and female collegiate athletes. *Clin J Sport Med.* 2000;10(2):89-97.
465. Nadler SF, Malanga GA, Bartoli LA, Feinberg JH, Prybicien M, Deprince M. Hip muscle imbalance and low back pain in athletes: influence of core strengthening. *Med Sci Sports Exerc.* 2002;34:9-16.
466. Cibulka MT, White DM, Woehrle J, et al. Hip pain and mobility deficits—hip osteoarthritis: Clinical practice guidelines linked to the International Classification of Functioning, Disability, and Health from the orthopaedic section of the American Physical Therapy Association. *J Orthop Sports Phys Ther.* 2009;39(4):A1-A25.

467. Sutlive TG, Lopez HP, Schnitzer DE, et al. Development of a clinical prediction rule for diagnosing hip osteoarthritis in individuals with unilateral hip pain. *J Orthop Sports Phys Ther.* 2008;38:542-550.
468. Altman R, Alarcón G, Appelrouth D, et al. The American College of Rheumatology criteria for the classification and reporting of osteoarthritis of the hip. *Arthritis Rheum.* 1991;34:505-514.
469. Pua YH, Wrigley TV, Cowan SM, Bennell KL. Intrarater test-retest reliability of hip range of motion and hip muscle strength measurements in persons with hip osteoarthritis. *Arch Phys Med Rehabil.* 2008;89:1146-1154.
470. Perry J, Weiss WB, Burnfield JM, Gronley JK. The supine hip extensor manual muscle test: a reliability and validity study. *Arch Phys Med Rehabil.* 2004;85:1345-1350.
471. Pollard H, Lakay B, Tucker F, Watson B, Bablis P. Interexaminer reliability of the deltoid and psoas muscle test. *J Manipulative Physiol Ther.* 2005;28:52-56.
472. Cleland JA, Koppenhaver S. *Netter's Orthopaedic Clinical Examination. An Evidence-Based Approach.* 2nd ed. Philadelphia, PA: Saunders; 2011.
473. Oh JS, Cynn HS, Won JH, et al. Effects of performing an abdominal drawing-in maneuver during prone hip extension exercises on hip and back extensor muscle activity and amount of anterior pelvic tilt. *J Orthop Sports Phys Ther.* 2007;37:320-324.
474. Martin RL, Sekiya JK. The interrater reliability of 4 clinical tests used to assess individuals with musculoskeletal hip pain. *J Orthop Sports Phys Ther.* 2008;38:71-77.
475. Martin RL, Irrgang JJ, Sekiya JK. The diagnostic accuracy of a clinical examination in determining intra-articular hip pain for potential hip arthroscopy candidates. *Arthroscopy.* 2008;24:1013-1018.
476. Cliborne AV, Wainner RS, Rhon DI, et al. Clinical hip tests and a functional squat test in patients with knee osteoarthritis: reliability, prevalence of positive test findings, and short-term response to hip mobilization. *J Orthop Sports Phys Ther.* 2004;34:575-685.
477. Dreyfuss P, Michaelsen M, Pauza K, McLarty J, Bogduk N. The value of medical history and physical examination in diagnosing sacroiliac joint pain. *Spine.* 1996;21:2594-2602.
478. Ozgocmen S, Bozgeyik Z, Kalcik M, Yildirim A. The value of sacroiliac pain provocation tests in early active sacroilitis. *Clin Rheumatol.* 2008;10:1275-1282.
479. Page P, Frank C, Lardner R. *Assessment and Treatment of Muscle Imbalance. The Janda Approach.* Champaign, IL: Human Kinetics; 2010.
480. Piva SR, Fitzgerald K, Irrgang JJ, et al. Reliability of measures of impairments associated with patellofemoral pain syndrome. *BMC Musculoskelet Disord.* 2006;7:33.
481. Bandy WD, Irion JM. THe effect of time on static stretch on the flexibility of the hamstring muscles. *Phys Ther.* 1994;74:54-61.
482. Gajdoski RL, RIeck MA, Sullivan DK, et al. Comparison of four clinical tests for assessing hamstring muscle length. *J Orthop Sports Phys Ther.* 1993;18:614-618.
483. Cleland JA, Childs JD, Fritz JM, Whitman JM. Interrater reliability of the history and physical examination in patients with mechanical neck pain. *Arch Phys Med Rehabil.* 2006;87:1388-1395.
484. Borstad JD, Briggs MS. Reproducibility of a measurement for latissimus dorsi muscle length. *Physiother Theor Pract.* 2010;26(3):195-203.
485. Clapis PA, Davis SM, Davis RO. Reliability of inclinometer and goniometric measurements of hip extension flexibility using the modified Thomas test. *Physiother Theor Pract.* 2008;24:135-141.
486. Harvey D. Assessment of the lexibility of elite athletes using the modified Thomas test. *Br J Sports Med.* 1998;32:68-70.
487. Costa L, Costa L, Cancado R, Oliveira W, Ferreira P. Short report: intra-tester reliability of two clinical tests of transversus abdominis muscle recruitment. *Physiother Res Int.* 2006;11:48-50.
488. de Paula Lima PO, de Oliveira RR, Costa LO, Laurentinao GE. Measurement properties of the pressure biofeedback unit in the evaluation of transversus abdominis muscle activity: a systematic review. *Physiotherapy.* 2010;97(2):100-106.
489. Hodges P, Richardson C, Jull G. Evaluation of the relationship between laboratory and clinical tests of transversus abdominis function. *Physiother Res Int.* 1996;1:30-40.
490. Ghamkhar L, Emami M, Moseni-Bandpei MA, Behtash H. Application of rehabilitative ultrasound in the assessment of low back pain: a literature review. *J Bodyw Mov Ther.* 2011;15(4):465-477.
491. Koppenhaver SL, Hebert JJ, Fritz JM, Parent EC, Teyhen DS, Magel JS. Reliability of rehabilitative ultrasound imaging of the transversus abdominis and lumbar multifidus muscles. *Arch Phys Med Rehabil.* 2009;90:87-94.
492. Richardson C, Jull G, Hodges P, Hides J. *Therapeutic Exercise for Spinal Segmental Stabilization in Low Back Pain: Scientific Basis and Clinical Approach.* London, England: Churchill Livingstone; 1999.
493. Richardson C, Hodges P, Hides J. *Therapeutic Exercise for Lumbopelvic Stabilization: A Motor Control Approach for the Treatment and Prevention of Low Back Pain.* 2nd ed. London, UK: Churchill Livingstone; 2004.
494. Hides JA, Richardson CA, Jull GA. Multifidus muscle recovery is not automatic following resolution of acute first episode low back pain. *Spine.* 1996;21:2763-2769.
495. Kiesel KB, Uhl TL, Underwood FB, Rodd DW, Nitz AJ. Measurement of lumbar multifus muscle contraction with rehabilitative ultrasound imaging. *Man Ther.* 2007;12(2):161-166.
496. Hides J, Wilson S, Stanton W, et al. An MRI investigation into the function of the transversus abdominis muscle during "drawing-in" of the abdominal wall. *Spine.* 2006;31(6):175-178.
497. Teyhen DS, Gill NW, Whittaker JL, Henry SM, Hides JA, Hodges P. Rehabilitative ultrasound imaging of the abdominal muscles. *J Orthop Sports Phys Ther.* 2007;38:450-466.
498. Hodges PW, Pengel LH, Herbert RD, Gandevia SC. Measurement of muscle contraction with ultrasound imaging. *Muscle Nerve.* 2003;27:682-692.
499. McGill S. *Low Back Disorders. Evidence-Based Prevention and Rehabilitation.* 2nd ed. Champaign, IL: Human Kinetics; 2007.
500. Grenier SG, McGill SM. Quantification of lumbar stability by using 2 different abdominal activation strategies. *Arch Phys Med Rehabil.* 2007;88:54-62.
501. Laslett M, Young SB, Aprill CN, McDonald B. Diagnosing painful sacroiliac joints: a validity study of a McKenzie evaluation and sacroiliac joint provocation tests. *Aust J Physiother.* 2003;49:89-97.
502. Laslett M, Aprill C, McDonald B, Young S. Diagnosis of sacroiliac joint pain: validity of individual provocation tests and composites of tests. *Man Ther.* 2005;10:207-218.
503. Laslett M, Williams M. The reliability of selected pain provocation tests for sacroiliac joint pathology. *Spine.* 1994;19:1243-1249.
504. Kobayashi S, Suzuki Y, Asai T, Yoshizawa H. Changes in nerve root motion and intraradicular blood flow during intraoperative femoral nerve stretch test. Report of four cases. *J Neurosurg.* 2003;99(suppl):298-305.

505. McCarthy CJ, Gittins M, Roberts C, Oldham JA. The reliability of the clinical tests and questions recommended in international guidelines for low back pain. *Spine.* 2007;32:921-926.
506. Trainor K, Pinnington MA. Reliability and diagnostic validity of the slump knee bend neurodynamic test for upper/mid lumbar nerve root compression: a pilot study. *Physiotherapy.* 2011;97:59-64.
507. Billis EV, Foster NE, Wright CC. Reproducibility and repeatability: errors of three groups of physiotherapists in locating spinal levels by palpation. *Man Ther.* 2003;8:223-232.
508. Fritz JM, Whitman JM, Childs JD. Lumbar spine segmental mobility assessment: an examination of validity for determining intervention strategies with low back pain. *Arch Phys Med Rehabil.* 2005;86:1745-1752.
509. Kasai Y, Morishita K, Kawakita E, Kondao T, Uchida A. A new evaluation method for lumbar spinal instability: passive lumar extension test. *Phys Ther.* 2006;86:1661-1667.
510. Reese ND, Bandy WD. Use of inclinometer to measure flexibility of the iliotibial band using the Ober test and the modified Ober test: differences in magnitude and reliability of measurements. *J Orthop Sports Phys Ther.* 2003;33:326-330.
511. Olson KA. *Manual Physical Therapy of the Spine.* St Louis, MO: Saunders Elsevier; 2009.
512. Harding VR, Williams AC, Richardson PH, et al. The development of a battery of measures for assessing physical functioning of chronic pain patients. *Pain.* 1994;58:367-375.
513. Mayer TG, Barnes D, Kishino ND, et al. Progressive isoinertial lifting evaluation. I. A standardized protocol and normative database. *Spine.* 1988;13:993-997.
514. Lee CE, Simmonds MJ, Novy DM, Jones S. Self reports and clinician-measured physical function among patients with low back pain: a comparison. *Arch Phys Med Rehabil.* 2001;82:227-231.
515. Smeets RJ, Hijdra HJ, Kester AD, Hitters MW, Knottnerus JA. The usability of six performance tasks in a rehabilitation population with chronic low back pain. *Clin Rehabil.* 2006;20:989-998.
516. Smeets RJ, Van Geel AC, Kester AD, et al. Physical capacity tasks in chronic low back pain: what is the contributing role of cardiovascular capacity, pain and psychological factors? *Disabil Rehabil.* 2007;29:577-586.
517. Mayer TG, Barnes D, Nicholas G, et al. Progressive isoinertial lifting evaluation. II. A comparison with isokinetic lifting in a disabled chronic low-back pain industrial population. *Spine.* 1988;13:998-1002.
518. Mayer TG, Gatchel RJ, Barnes D, et al. Progressive isoinertial lifting evaluation. Erratum notice. *Spine.* 1990;15:5.
519. Andersson EI, Lin CC, Smeets RJ. Performance tests in people with chronic low back. Responsiveness and minimal clinically important change. *Spine.* 2010;35:E1559-E1563.
520. Shumway-Cook A, Brauer S, Woollacott M. Predicting the probabillity for falls in community-dwelling older adults using the time up and go test. *Phys Ther.* 2000;80:896-903.
521. Kristensen MT, Foss NM, Kehlet H. Timed "Up and Go" Tests as a predictor of falls within 6 months after hip fracture surgery. *Phys Ther.* 2007;87:24-30.
522. Bohannon RW. Reference values for the Timed Up and Go Test: a descriptive meta-analysis. *J Geriatr Phys Ther.* 2006;29(2):64-68.
523. Troosters T, Gosselink R, Decramer M. Six minute walking distance in healthy elderly subjects. *Eur Respir J.* 1999;14:270-274.
524. Harada ND, Chiu V, Stewart AL. Mobility-related function in older adults: assessment with a 6-minute walk test. *Arch Phys Med Rehabil.* 1999;80:837-841.
525. Focht B, Rejeski WJ, Ambrosius W, Katula J, Messier S. Exercise, self-efficacy, and mobility performance in overweight and obese older adults with knee osteoarthritis. *Arthritis Rheum.* 2005;53:659-665.
526. American Thoracic Society. ATS statement: guidelines for the six-minute walk test. *Am J Respir Crit Care Med.* 2001;166:111-117.
527. Lusardi MM, Pellecchia GL, Schulman PT. Functional performance in community living older adults. *J Geriatr Phys Ther.* 2003;26(3):14-22.
528. Salzman SH. The 6-min walk test: clinical and research role, technique, coding, and reimbursement. *Chest.* 2009;135:1345-1352.
529. Smith DR. Use of the 6-min walk test: a pro and con review. *American College of Chest Physicians.* http://69.36.35.38/accp/pccsu/use-6-min-walk-test-pro-and-con-review?page=0,3. Published June 15, 2009. Accessed September 20, 2013.
530. McGill SM, Grenier S, Bluhm M, Preuss R, Brown S, Russell C. Previous history of LBP with work loss is related to lingering effects in biomechanical, physiological, personal, and psychological characteristics. *Ergonomics.* 2003;46:731-746.
531. Jorgensen K, Nicholaisen T. Trunk extensor endurance: determination and relation to low back trouble. *Ergonomics.* 1987;30:259-267.
532. Roy SH, Deluca CJ, Casavant DA. Lumbar muscle fatigue and chronic low back pain. *Spine.* 1989;14:992-1001.
533. Ashmen KJ, Swanik CB, Lephart SM. Strength and flexibility characteristics of athletes with chronic low back pain. *J Sport Rehabil.* 1996;5:275-286.
534. O'Sullivan PB, Mitchell T, Bulich P, Waller R, Holte J. The relationship between posture and back muscle endurance in industrial workers with flexion-related low back pain. *Man Ther.* 2006;11:264-271.
535. Ito T, Shirado O, Suzuki H, Takahashi M. Lumbar trunk muscle endurance testing: an inexpensive alternative to a machine for evaluation. *Arch Phys Med Rehabil.* 1996;77:75-79.
536. Moffroid MT. Endurance of trunk muscles in persons with chronic low back pain: assessment, performance, training. *J Rehabil Res Dev.* 1997;34:440-447.
537. Malliou P, Gioftsidou A, Beneka A, Godolias G. Measurements and evaluations in low back pain patients. *Scand J Med Sci Sports.* 2006;16:219-230.
538. Corin G, Strutton PH, McGregor AH. Establishment of a protocol to test fatigue of the trunk muscles. *Br J Sports Med.* 2005;39:731-735.
539. McGill SM, Childs A, Liebenson C. Endurance times for low back stabilization exercises: clinical targets for testing and training from a normal database. *Arch Phys Med Rehabil.* 1999;80:941-944.
540. Alaranta H, Hurri H, Heliovaara M, Sonkka A, Harju R. Nondynamometric trunk performance tests: reliability and normative data. *Scand J Rehabil Med.* 1994;26:211-215.
541. McIntosh G, Wilson L, Affleck M, Hall H. Tunk and lower extremity muscle endurance: normative data for adults. *J Rehabil Outcomes Meas.* 1998;2(4):20-39.
542. American College of Radiology. ACR appropriateness criteria. http://www.acr.org/~/media/ACR/Documents/AppCriteria/Diagnostic/LowBackPain.pdf. Accessed September 20, 2013.
543. Masci L, Pike J, Malara F, Phillips B, Bennell K, Brukner P. Use of the one-legged hyperextension test and magnetic resonance imaging in the diagnosis of active spondylolysis. *Br J Sports Med.* 2006;40:940-946; discussion 946.
544. Jarvik JG. Imaging of adults with low back pain in the primary care setting. *Neuroimaging Clin N Am.* 2003;13:293-305.

545. Post MJ, Sze G, Quencer RM, Eismont FJ, Green BA, Gahbauer H. Gadolinium-enhanced MR in spinal infection. *J Comput Assist Tomogr.* 1990;14:721-729.
546. Modic MT, Obuchowski NA, Ross JS, et al. Acute low back pain and radiculopathy: MR imaging findings and their prognostic role and effect on outcome. *Radiology.* 2005;237:597-604.
547. Wiesel SW, Tsourmas N, Feffer HL, Citrin CM, Patronas N. A study of computer-assisted tomography. I. The incidence of positive CAT scans in an asymptomatic group of patients. *Spine.* 1984;9:549-551.
548. Billis EV, McCarthy CJ, Oldham JA. Subclassification of low back pain: a cross-country comparison. *Eur Spine J.* 2007;16:865-879.
549. Browder DA, Childs JD, Cleland JA, Fritz JM. Effectiveness of an extension-oriented treatment approach in a subgroup of subjects with low back pain: a randomized clinical trial. *Phys Ther.* 2007;87:1608-1618.
550. Fritz JM, George S. The use of a classification approach to identify subgroups of patients with acute low back pain. Interrater reliability and short-term treatment outcomes. *Spine.* 2000;25:106-114.
551. Fritz JM, Brennan GP, Clifford SN, Hunter SJ, Thackeray A. An examination of the reliability of a classification algorithm for subgrouping patients with low back pain. *Spine.* 2006;31:77-82.
552. Kiesel KB, Underwood FB, Mattacola CG, Nitz AJ, Malone TR. A comparison of select trunk muscle thickness change between subjects with low back pain classified in the treatment-based classification system and asymptomatic controls. *J Orthop Sports Phys Ther.* 2007;37:596-607.
553. Apeldoorn AT, Ostelo RW, van Helvoirt H, et al. A randomized controlled trial on the effectiveness of a classification-based system for sub-acute and chronic low back pain. *Spine (Phila Pa 1976).* 2012;37(16):1347-1356.
554. American Physical Therapy Association. Guide to Physical Therapist Practice, second edition. American Physical Therapy Association. *Phys Ther.* 2001;81:9-746.
555. Powers CM, Kulig K, Harrison J, Bergman G. Segmental mobility of the lumbar spine during a posterior to anterior mobilization: assessment using dynamic MRI. *Clin Biomech (Bristol, Avon).* 2003;18:80-83.
556. Kulig K, Landel R, Powers CM. Assessment of lumbar spine kinematics using dynamic MRI: a proposed mechanism of sagittal plane motion induced by manual posterior-to-anterior mobilization. *J Orthop Sports Phys Ther.* 2004;34(2):57-64.
557. Lee RY, McGregor AH, Bull AM, Wragg P. Dynamic response of the cervical spine to posteroanterior mobilisation. *Clin Biomech (Bristol, Avon).* 2005;20:228-231.
558. Ross JK, Bereznick DE, McGill SM. Determining cavitation location during lumbar and thoracic spinal manipulation: is spinal manipulation accurate and specific? *Spine.* 2004;29:1452-1457.
559. Beffa R, Mathews R. Does the adjustment cavitate the targeted joint? An investigation into the location of cavitation sounds. *J Manipulative Physiol Ther.* 2004;27:e2.
560. Flynn TW, Fritz JM, Wainner RS, Whitman JM. The audible pop is not necessary for successful spinal high-velocity thrust manipulation in individuals with low back pain. *Arch Phys Med Rehabil.* 2003;84:1057-1060.
561. Haas M, Groupp E, Panzer D, Partna L, Lumsden S, Aickin M. Efficacy of cervical endplay assessment as an indicator for spinal manipulation. *Spine.* 2003;28:1091-1096; discussion 1096.
562. Chiradejnant A, Maher CG, Latimer J, et al. Efficacy of "therapist-selected" versus "randomly selected" mobilization techniques for the treatment of low back pain: a randomized controlled trial. *Aust J Physiother.* 2003;491:223-241.
563. Grieve GP. *Common Vertebral Joint Problems.* 2nd ed. New York, NY: Churchill Livingstone; 1988.
564. Cook CE. *Orthopedic Manual Therapy: An Evidence-Based Approach.* Upper Saddle River, NJ: Pearson Prentice Hall; 2007.
565. Haldeman S, Rubenstein SM. Cauda equina syndrome in patients undergoing manipulation of the lumbar spine. *Spine.* 1992;17:1469-1473.
566. Assendelft WJ, Bouter LM, Knipschild PG. Complications of spinal manipulation: a comprehensive review of the literature. *J Fam Pract.* 1996;42:475-480.
567. Senstad O, Leboeuf-Yde C, Borchgrevink C. Frequency and characteristics of side iffects of spinal manipulative therapy. *Spine.* 1997;22:435-441.
568. Hurwitz EL, Morgenstern H, Vassilaki M, Chiang L. Frequency and clinical predictors of adverse reactions to chiropractic care in the UCLA neck pain study. *Spine.* 2005;30:1477-1484.
569. Caigne B, Vinck E, Beernaert A, Cambier D. How common are side effects of spinal manipulation and can these side effects be predicted? *Man Ther.* 2004;9(3):151-156.
570. Kerry R, Taylor AJ. Cervical arterial dysfunction assessment and manual therapy. *Man Ther.* 2006;11:243-253.
571. Childs JD, Flynn TW, Fritz JM, et al. Screening or vertebrobasilar insufficiency in patients with neck pain: manual therapy decision-making in the presence of uncertainty. *J Orthop Sports Phys Ther.* 2005;35:300-306.
572. Kerry R, Taylor AJ, Mitchell J, McCarthy C, Brew J. Manual therapy and cervical arterial dysfunction, directions for the future: a clinical perspective. *J Man Manip Ther.* 2008;16:39-48.
573. Cassidy JD, Boyle E, Cote P, et al. Risk of vertebrobasilar stroke and chiropractic care. *Spine.* 2008;33:S176-S183.
574. Rivett DA, Milburn P. A prospective study of complications of cervical spine manipulation. *J Manual Manipulative Ther.* 1996;4:166-170.
575. Di Fabio RP. Manipulation of the cervical spine: risks and benefits. *Phys Ther.* 1999;79:50-65.
576. Haldeman S, Kohlbeck FJ, McGregor M. Unpredictability of cerebrovascular ischemia associated with cervical spine manipulation therapy: a review of sixty-four cases after cervical spine manipulation. *Spine.* 2002;27:49-55.
577. Carnes D, Mars TS, Mullinger B, Froud R, Underwood M. Adverse events and manual therapy: a systematic review. *Man Ther.* 2010;15:355-363.
578. Dabbs V, Lauretti WJ. A risk assessment of cervical manipulation vs NSAIDs for the treatment of neck pain. *J Manip Physiol Ther.* 1995;18:530-536.
579. Oliphant D. Safety of spinal manipulation in the treatment of lumbar disk herniations: a systematic review and risk assessment. *J Manip Physiol Ther.* 2004;27(3):197-210.
580. Cleland JA, Childs JD, Fritz JM, Whitman JM, Eberhart SL. Development of a clinical prediction rule for guiding treatment of a subgroup of patients with neck pain: use of thoracic spine manipulation, exercise, and patient education. *Phys Ther.* 2010;90:1239-1250.
581. Cleland JA, Fritz JM, Kulig K, et al. Comparison of the effectiveness of three manual physical therapy techniques in a subgroup of patients with low back pain who satisfy a clinical prediction rule. *Spine.* 2009;34:2720-2729.

582. Bialosky JE, Bishop MD, Robinson ME, Barabas JA, George SZ. The influence of expectation on spinal manipulation induced hypoalgesia: an experimental study in normal subjects. *BMC Musculoskelet Disord.* 2008;9:19.
583. Bialosky JE, Bishop JE, George S, Robinson ME. Placebo response to manual therapy: something out of nothing? *J Man Manip Ther.* 2011;19:11-19.
584. Bialosky JE, Bishop MD, Price DD, Robinson ME, George SZ. The mechanisms of manual therapy in the treatment of musculoskeletal pain: a comprehensive model. *Man Ther.* 2009;4:531-538.
585. Degenhardt BJ, Darmani NA, Johnson JC, et al. Role of osteopathic manipulative treatment in altering pain biomarkers: a pilot study. *J Am Osteopath Assoc.* 2007;107:387-400.
586. McPartland JM, Guiffrida A, King J, Skinner E, Scotter J, Musty RE. Cannabimimetic effects of osteopathic manipulative treatment. *J Am Osteopath Assoc.* 2005;105:283-291.
587. Field T, Diego M, Cullen C, Hernandez-Reif M, Sunshine W, Douglas S. Fibromyalgia pain and substance P decrease and sleep improves after massage therapy. *J Clin Rheumatol.* 2002;8:72-76.
588. Smith LL, Keating MN, Holbert D, et al. The effects of athletic massage on delayed onset muscle soreness, creatine kinase, and neutrophil count: a preliminary report. *J Orthop Sports Phys Ther.* 1994;19:93-99.
589. Pickar JG, Wheeler JD. Response of muscle proprioceptors to spinal manipulative-like loads in the anesthetized cat. *J Manipulative Physiol Ther.* 2001;24:2-11.
590. Vicenzino B, Paungmali A, Buratowski S, Wright A. Specific manipulation therapy treatment for chronic lateral, epicondylalgia produces uniquely characteristic hypoalgesia. *Man Ther.* 2001;6:205-212.
591. Boal RW, Gillette RG. Central neuronal plasticity, low back pain and spinal manipulative therapy. *J Manipulative Physiol Ther.* 2004;27:314-326.
592. George SZ, Bishop MD, Bialosky JE, Zeppieri G, Robinson ME. Immediate effects of spinal manipulation on thermal pain sensitivity: an experimental study. *BMC Musculoskelet Disord.* 2006;7:68.
593. Kalauokalani D, Cherkin DC, Sherman KJ, Koepsell TD, Deyo RA. Lessons from a trial of acupuncture and massage for low back pain: patient expectations and treatment effects. *Spine.* 2001;26:1418-1424.
594. William NH, Hendry M, Lewis R, Russell I, Westmoreland A, Wilkinson C. Psychological response in spinal manipulation (PRISM): a systematic review of psychological outcomes in randomized controlled trials. *Complement Ther Med.* 2007;15:271-283.
595. Olson KA. *Manual Physical Therapy of the Spine.* St Louis, MO: Saunders Elsevier; 2009.
596. Fernandez-de-las-Penas C, Alonso-Blanco C, Cleland JA, Rodriguez-Blanco C, Alburquerque-Sendin F. Changes in pressure pain thresholds over C5-C6 zygapophyseal joint after a cervicothoracic junction manipulation in healthy subjects. *J Manipulative Physiol Ther.* 2008;31:332-337.
597. Krouwel O, Hebron C, Willett E. A investigation into the potential hypoalgesic effects of different amplitudes of PA mobilizations on lumbar spine as measured by pressure pain thresholds (PPT). *Man Ther.* 2010;15:7-12.
598. Chiradejnant A, Latimer J, Maher CG, Stepkovitch N. Does the choice of spinal level treated during posteroanterior (PA) mobilization affect treatment outcome? *Physiother Therory Pract.* 2002;18:165-174.
599. Schmidt A, Brunner F, Wright A, Bachmann LM. Paradigm shift in manual therapy? Evidence for a central nervous system component in the response to passive cervical joint mobilization. *Man Ther.* 2008;13:387-396.
600. Winkelstein BA. Mechanisms of central sensitization, neuroimmunology, and injury biomechanics in persistent pain: implications for musculoskeletal disorders. *J Electromyogr Kinesiol.* 2004;14:87-93.
601. Rygh LJ, Svendsen F, Fiska A, et al. Long term potentiation in spinal nociceptive systems: how acute pain may become chronic. *Psychoneuroendocrinology.* 2005;30:959-964.
602. Suter E, McMorland G, Herzog W, Bray R. Decrease in quadriceps inhibition after sacroiliac joint manipulation in patients with anterior knee pain. *J Manipulative Physiol Ther.* 1999;22:149-153.
603. Cleland J, Selleck B, Stowell T, et al. Short-term effects of thoracic manipulation on lower trapezius muscle strength. *J Manip Man Ther.* 2004;12(2):82-90.
604. Liebler EJ, Tufano-Coors L, Douris P, et al. The effect of thoracic sine mobilization on lower trapezius strength testing. *J Man Manip Ther.* 1986;9:207-212.
605. Cassidy JD, Lopes AA, Yong-Hing K. The immediate effect of manipulation versus mobilization on pain and range of motion in cervical spine: a randomized clinical trial. *J Manipulative Physiol Ther.* 1992;15:570-575.
606. Sterling M, Jull G, Wright A. Cervical mobilization: concurrent effects on pain, sympathetic nervous system activity and motor activity. *Man Ther.* 2001;6:72-81.
607. Shambaugh P. Changes in electrical activity in muscles resulting from chiropractic adjustment: a pilot study. *J Manipulative Physiol Ther.* 1987;10:300-304.
608. Gill NW, Teyhen DS, Lee IE. Improved contraction of the transversus abdominis immediately following spinal manipulation: a case study using real-time ultrasound imaging. *Man Ther.* 2007;12:280-285.
609. Raney NH, Teyhen DS, Childs JD. Observed changes in lateral abdominal muscle thickness after spinal manipulation: a case series using rehabilitative ultrasound imaging. *J Orthop Sports Phys Ther.* 2007;37:472-479.
610. Puentedura EJ, Landers MR, Hurt K, Meissner M, Mills J, Young D. Immediate effects of lumbar spine manipulation on the resting and contraction thickness of transversus abdominis in asymptomatic individuals. *J Orthop Sports Phys Ther.* 2011;41:13-21.
611. Fritz FM, Koppenhaver SL, Kawchuk GN, Teyhen DS, Hebert JJ, Childs JD. Preliminary investigation of the mechanisms underlying the effects of manipulation: exploration of a multi-variate model including spinal stiffness, multifidus recruitment, and clinical findings. *Spine (Phila Pa 1976).* 2011;36(21):1772-1781.
612. Koppenhaver SL, Fritz JM, Hebert JJ, et al. Association between changes in abdominal and lumbar multifidus muscle thickness and clinical improvement after spinal manipulation. *J Orthop Sports Phys Ther.* 2011;41(6):389-399.
613. Marshall P, Murphy B. The effect of sacroiliac joint manipulation on feed-forward activation times of the deep abdominal musculature. *J Manipulative Physiol Ther.* 2006;29:196-202.
614. Bialosky JE, George SZ, Bishop MD. How spinal manipulative therapy works: why ask why? *J Orthop Sports Phys Ther.* 2008;38:293-295.
615. Bronfort G, Haas M, Evans RL, Bouter LM. Efficacy of spinal manipulation and mobilization for low back pain and neck pain: a systematic review and best evidence synthesis. *Spine J.* 2004;4:335-356.

616. Rajadurai V, Murugan K. Spinal manipulative therapy for low back pain: a systematic review. *Phys Ther Rev.* 2009;14:260-271.
617. Dagenais S, Tricco AC, Haldeman S. Synthesis of recommendations for the assessment and management of low back pain from recent clinical practice guidelines. *Spine J.* 2010;10:514-529.
618. Fritz JM, Cleland JA, Brennan GP. Does adherence to the guideline recommendation for active treatments improve the quality of care for patients with acute low back pain delivered by physical therapists? *Med Care.* 2007;45:973-980.
619. Dagenais S, Gay RE, Tricco AC, Freeman MD, Mayer JM. NASS contemporary concepts in spine care: spinal manipulation therapy for acute low back pain. *Spine J.* 2010;10:918-940.
620. Fritz JM, Whitman JM, Flynn TW, et al. Factors related to the inability of individuals with low back pain to improve with a spinal manipulation. *Phys Ther.* 2004;4:173-190.
621. Hancock M, Maher CG, Latimer J, Herbert RD, McAuley JH. Independent evaluation of a clinical prediction rule for spinal manipulative therapy: a randomized controlled trial. *Eur Spine J.* 2008;17:936-943.
622. Hancock MJ, Maher CG, Latimer J. Spinal manipulative therapy for acute low back pain: a clinical perspective. *J Man Manip Ther.* 2009;16(4):198-203.
623. Powers CM, Beneck GJ, Kulig K, Landel RF, Fredericson M. Effects of a single session of posterior-to-anterior spinal mobilization and press-up exercise on pain response and lumbar spine extensions in people with nonspecific low back pain. *Phys Ther.* 2008;88:485-493.
624. Fryer G. Muscle energy technique: an evidence-informed approach. *Int J Osteopath Med.* 2011;14:3-9.
625. Greenman PE. *Principles of Manual Therapy.* 3rd ed. Philadelphia, PA: Lippincott Williams & Wilkins; 2003.
626. Schenk RJ, Adelman K, Rousselle J. The effects of MET technique on cervical range of motion. *J Man Manipulative Ther.* 1994;2:149-155.
627. Fryer G, Ruszkowski W. The influence of contraction duration in MET technique applied to the atlanto-axial joint. *J Osteopath Med.* 2004;7:79-84.
628. Lenehan KL, Fryer G, McLaughlin P. The effect of MET technique on gross trunk range of motion. *J Osteopath Med.* 2003;6:13-18.
629. Schenk RJ, MacDiarmid, Rousselle J. The effects of MET technique on lumbar range of motion. *J Man Manipulative Ther.* 1997;5:179-183.
630. Wilson E, Payton O, Donegan-Shoaf L, Dec K. MET technique in patients with acute low back pain: a pilot clinical trial. *J Orthop Sports Phys Ther.* 2003;33:502-512.
631. Licciardone JC, Stoll ST, Fulda KG, et al. Osteopathic manipulative treatment for chronic low back pain: a randomized controlled trial. *Spine.* 2003;28:1355-1362.
632. Niemistö L, Lahtinen-Suopanki T, Rissanen P, Lindgren K, Sarna S, Hurri H. A randomized trial of combined manipulation, stabilizing exercises, and physician consultation compared to physician consultation alone for chronic low back pain. *Spine.* 2003;28:2185-2191.
633. Fryer G, Alivizatos J, Lamaro J. The effect of osteopathic treatment on people with chronic and sub-chronic neck pain: a pilot study. *Int J Osteopath Med.* 2005;8:41-48.
634. Chown M, Whittamore L, Rush M, Allan S, Stott D, Archer M. A prospective study of patients with chronic back pain randomised to group exercise, physiotherapy or osteopathy. *Physiotherapy.* 2008;94:21-28.
635. Leone A, Guglielmi G, Cassar-Pullicino VN, Bonomo L. Lumbar intervertebral instability: a review. *Radiology.* 2007;245:62-77.
636. Cook C, Brismée JM, Sizer PS. Subjective and objective descriptors of clinical lumbar spine instability: a Dephi study. *Man Ther.* 2006;11:11-21.
637. Hodges P. Transversus abdominis: a different view of the elephant. *Br J Sports Med.* 2008;42:941-944.
638. Hodges P, Vanden Hoorn W, Dawson A, Cholewicki J. Changes in the mechanical properties of the trunk in low back pain may be associated with recurrence. *J Biomech.* 2009;24:61-65.
639. Cholewicki J, McGill SM. Mechanical stability of the in vivo lumbar spine: implications for injury and chronic low back pain. *Clin Biomech.* 1996;11:1-15.
640. McGill S. *Low Back Disorders: Evidence-Based Prevention and Rehabilitation.* 2nd ed. Champaign, IL: Human Kinetics; 2007.
641. Grenier SG, McGill SM. Quantification of lumbar stability by using 2 different abdominal activation strategies. *Arch Phys Med Rehabil.* 2007;88:54-62.
642. Danneels LA, Vanderstraeten GG, Cambier DC, et al. Effects of three different training modalities on the cross sectional area of the lumbar multifidus muscle in patients with chronic low back pain. *Br J Sports Med.* 2001;35(3):186-191.
643. Koumantakis GA, Watson PJ, Oldham JA. Trunk muscle stabilization training plus general exercise versus general exercise only: randomized controlled trial of patients with recurrent low back pain. *Phys Ther.* 2005;85:209-225.
644. Cairns MC, Foster NE, Wright C. Randomized controlled trial of specific spinal stabilization exercises and conventional physiotherapy for recurrent low back pain. *Spine.* 2006;31:E670-E681.
645. Tsao H, Hodges PW. Persistence of improvements in postural strategies following motor control training in people with recurrent low back pain. *J Electromyogr Kinesiol.* 2008;18:559-567.
646. Tsao H, Hodges PW. Immediate changes in feedforward postural adjustments following voluntary motor training. *Exp Brain Res.* 2007;181:537-546.
647. Rissanen A, Kalimo H, Alaranta H. Effect of intensive training on the isokinetic strength and structure of lumbar muscles in patients with chronic low back pain. *Spine.* 1995;20:333-340.
648. Hides JA, Richardson CA, Jull GA. Multifidus muscle recovery is not automatic after resolution of acute, first-episode low back pain. *Spine.* 1996;21:2763-2769.
649. O'Sullivan PB, Phyty GD, Twomey LT, et al. Evaluation of specific stabilizing exercise in the treatment of chronic low back pain with radiologic diagnosis of spondylolysis or spondylolisthesis. *Spine.* 1997;22:2959-2967.
650. Hides JA, Jull GA, Richardson CA. Long-term effects of specific stabilizing exercises for first episode low back pain. *Spine.* 2001;26:E243-E248.
651. Koumantakis GA, Watson PJ, Oldham JA. Supplementation of general endurance exercise with stabilisation training versus general exercise only. Physiological and functional outcomes of a randomised controlled trial of patients with recurrent low back pain. *Clin Biomech (Bristol, Avon).* 2005;20:474-482.
652. Rasmussen-Barr E, Nilsson-Wikmar L, Arvidsson I. Stabilizing training compared with manual treatment in sub-acute and chronic low-back pain. *Man Ther.* 2003;8:233-241.
653. Goldby LJ, Moore AP, Doust J, et al. A randomized controlled trial investigating the efficiency of musculoskeletal physiotherapy on chronic low back disorder. *Spine.* 2006;31:1083-1093.
654. Ferreira PH, Ferreira ML, Maher CG, et al. Specific stabilisation exercise for spinal and pelvic pain: a systematic review. *Aust J Physiother.* 2006;52:79-88.

655. Tsao H, Druitt TR, Schollum TM, Hodges PW. Motor training of the lumbar paraspinal muscles induces immediate changes in motor coordination in patients with recurrent low back pain. *J Pain*. 2010;11:1120-1128.
656. Hauggaard A, Persson AL. Specific spinal stabilisation exercises in patients with low back pain—a systematic review. *Phys Ther Rev*. 2007;12:233-248.
657. May S, Johnson R. Stabilisation exercises for low back pain: a systematic review. *Physiotherapy*. 2008;94:179-189.
658. Macedo LG, Maher CG, Latiner J, McAuley JH. Motor control for persistent, nonspecific low back pain: a systematic review. *Phys Ther*. 2009;89:9-25.
659. Kriese M, Clijsen R, Taeymans J, Cabri J. Segmental stabilization in low back pain: a systematic review [abstract]. *Sportverletz Sportschaden*. 2010;24:17-25.
660. McGill SM. Estimation of force and extensor moment contributions of the disc and ligaments at L4-L5. *Spine*. 1988;13:1395-1402.
661. Richardson CA, Jull GA. Muscle control-pain control: what exercises would you prescribe? *Man Ther*. 1995;1:2-10.
662. McGill S, Juker D, Kropf P. Quantitative intramuscular myoelectric activity of quadratus lumborum during a wide variety of lift tasks. *Clin Biomech (Bristol, Avon)*. 1996;11:170-172.
663. Hodges PW, Richardson CA. Contraction of the abdominal muscles associated with movement of the lower limb. *Phys Ther*. 1997;77(2):132-142.
664. McGill SM. Low back exercises: evidence for improving exercise regimens. *Phys Ther*. 1998;78:754-764.
665. Lee JH, Hoshino Y, Nakamura K, Kariya Y, Saita K, Ito K. Trunk muscle weakness as a risk factor for low back pain a 5-year prospective study. *Spine*. 1999;24:54-57.
666. McGill SM. Low back stability: from formal description to issues for performance and rehabilitation. *Exerc Sports Sci Rev*. 2001;29:26-31.
667. Hebert JJ, Koppenhaver SL, Magel JS, Fritz JM. The relationship of transversus abdominis and lumbar multifidus activation and prognostic factors for clinical success with a stabilization exercise program: a cross-sectional study. *Arch Phys Med Rehabil*. 2010;91:78-85.
668. Alqarni AM, Schneiders AG, Hendrick PA. Clinical tests to diagnose lumbar segmental instability: a systematic review. *J Orthop Sports Phys Ther*. 2011;41(3):130-140.
669. Abbott JH, McCane B, Herbison P, Moginie G, Chapple C, Hogarty T. Lumbar segmental instability: a criterion-related validity study of manual therapy assessment. *BMC Musculoskelet Disord*. 2005;6:56-64.
670. Kasai Y, Morishita K, Kawakita E, Kkondo T, Uchilda A. A new evaluation method for lumbar spinal instability: passive lumbar extension test. *Phys Ther*. 2006;86:1661-1667.
671. Stuge B, Laerum E, Kirkesola G, Vøllestad N. The efficacy of a treatment program focusing on specific stabilizing exercises for pelvic girdle pain after pregnancy. A randomized controlled trial. *Spine*. 2004;29:351-359.
672. Ostgaard HC, Zetherstrom G, Roos-Hansson E. The posterior pelvic pain provocation test in pregnant women. *Eur Spine J*. 1994;3:258-260.
673. Vleeming A, Vries HJ, Mens JM, et al. Possible role of the long dorsal sacroiliac ligament in women with peripartum pelvic pain. *Acta Obstet Gynecol Scand*. 2002;81:430-436.
674. Albert H, Godskesen M, Westergaard J. Evaluation of clinical tests used in classification procedures in pregnancy-related pelvic joint pain. *Eur Spine J*. 2000;9:161-166.
675. Hodges PW, Ferreira PH, Ferreira N. Lumbar spine: treatment of instability and sisorders of movement control. In: Magee DJ, Zachazewski JE, Quillen WS, eds. *Pathology and Intervention in Musculoskeletal Rehabilitation*. St Louis, MO: Saunders Elsevier; 2009:389-425.
676. Fitts PM, Posner MI. *Learning and Skilled Performance in Human Performance*. Belmont, CA: Brooks-Cole; 1967.
677. Richardson C, Hodges P, Hides J. *Therapeutic Exercise for Lumbopelvic Stabilization*. 2nd ed. Philadelphia, PA: Churchill Livingstone; 2004.
678. Kavcic N, Grenier S, McGill SM. Determining the stabilizing role of individual torso muscles during rehabilitation exercises. *Spine*. 2004;29:1254-1265.
679. Kavcic N, Grenier S, McGill SM. Quantifying tissue loads and spine stability while performing commonly prescribed low back stabilization exercises. *Spine*. 2004;29:2319-2329.
680. Machado LA, Maher CG, Herbert RD, Clare H, McAuley JH. The effectiveness of the McKenzie method in addition to first-line care for acute low back pain: a randomized controlled trial. *BMC Med*. 2010;8:10.
681. Machado LA, de Souza MS, Ferreira PH, et al. The McKenzie method for low back pain: a systematic review of the literature with a meta-analysis approach. *Spine*. 2006;31(9):E254-E262.
682. Cook C, Ramey K, Hegedus E. Physical therapy exercise intervention based on classification using the patient response method: a systematic review of the literature. *J Man Manip Ther*. 2005;13(3):152-162.
683. Erhard R, Delitto A, Cibulka M. Relative effectiveness of an extension program and a combined program of manipulation and flexion and extension exercises in patients with acute low back syndrome. *Phys Ther*. 1994;74:1093-1100.
684. Miller ER, Schenk RJ, Karnes JL, et al. A comparison of the McKenzie approach to a specific spine stabilization program for chronic LBP. *J Man Manip Ther*. 2005;13(2):103-112.
685. Peterson T, Kryger P, Ekdahl C, Olsen S, Jacobsen S. The effect of McKenzie therapy as compared with that of intensive strengthening training for the treatment of patients with subacute or chronic low back pain: a randomized controlled trial. *Spine*. 2002;27:1702-1709.
686. Long A, May S, Fung T. The comparative prognostic value of directional preference and centralization: a useful tool for front-line clinicians? *J Man Manip Ther*. 2008;16:248-254.
687. Gillan MG, Ross JC, McLean IP, Porter RW. The natural history of trunk list, its associated disability and the influence of McKenzie management. *Eur Spine J*. 1998;7:480-483.
688. Harrison DE, Cailliet R, Betz JW, et al. A non-randomized clinical control trial of Harrison mirror image methods for correcting trunk list (lateral translations of the thoracic cage) in patients with chronic low back pain. *Eur Spine J*. 2005;14:155-162.
689. Johnsson KE, Rosen I, Uden A. The natural course of lumbar spinal stenosis. *Clin Orthop*. 1992;279:82-86.
690. Simotas AC, Dorey FJ, Hansraj KK, Cammisa F Jr. Nonoperative treatment for lumbar spinal stenosis. Clinical and outcome results and a 3-year survivorship analysis. *Spine*. 2000;25(2):197-203.
691. Watters WC, Baisden J, Gilbert TJ, et al. Degenerative lumbar spinal stenosis: an evidence-based clinical guideline for the diagnosis and treatment of degenerative lumbar spinal stenosis. *Spine J*. 2008;8:305-310.
692. Reindl R, Steffen T, Cohen L, Aebi M. Elective lumbar spinal decompression in the elderly: is it a high risk operation? *Can J Surg*. 2003;46:43-46.
693. Weinstein JN, Lurie JD, Tosteson TD, et al. Surgical versus nonsurgical treatment for lumbar degenerative spondylolisthesis. *N Engl J Med*. 2007;356:2257-2270.
694. Weinstein JN, Tosteson TD, Lurie JD, et al. Surgical versus nonsurgical therapy for lumbar spinal stenosis. *N Engl J Med*. 2008;358:794-810.

695. Weinstein JN, Tosteson, Lurie JD, et al. Surgical versus nonoperative treatment for lumbar spinal stenosis four-year results of the spine patient outcomes research trial. *Spine.* 2010;35:1329-1338.
696. Malmivaara A, Slätis P, Heliövaara M, et al. Surgical or non-operative treatment for lumbar spinal stenosis? A randomized controlled trial. *Spine.* 2007;32:1-8.
697. Slätis P, Malmivaara A, Heliövaara M, et al. Long-term results of surgery for lumbar spinal stenosis: a randomized controlled trial. *Eur Spine J.* 2011;20(7):1174-1181.
698. Steurer J, Nydegger A, Held U, et al. The LumbSten: the lumbar spinal stenosis outcome study. *BMC Musculoskelet Disord.* 2010;11:254.
699. Koc Z, Ozcakir S, Sivrioglu K, Gurbet A, Kucukoglu S. Effectiveness of physical therapy and epidural steroid injections in lumbar spinal stenosis. *Spine.* 2009;34:985-989.
700. Whitman JM, Flynn TW, Fritz JM. Nonsurgical management of patients with lumbar spinal stenosis: a literature review and a case series of three patients managed with physical therapy. *Phys Med Rehabil Clin N Am.* 2003;14:77-101.
701. Pua Y, Cai C, Lim K. Treadmill walking with body weight support is no more effective than cycling when added to an exercise program for lumbar spinal stenosis: a randomized controlled trial. *Aust J Physiother.* 2007;53:83-89.
702. Reiman MP, Harris JY, Cleland JA. Manual therapy interventions for patients with lumbar spinal stenosis: a systematic review. *N Z J Physiother.* 2009;37:17-28.
703. Backstrom KM, Whitman JM, Flynn TW. Lumbar spinal stenosis—diagnosis and management of the aging spine. *Man Ther.* 2011;16:308-317.
704. Rademeyer I. Manual therapy for lumbar spinal stenosis: a comprehensive physical therapy approach. *Phys Med Rehabil Clin N Am.* 2003;14:103-110.
705. Harte AA, Gracey JH, Baxter GD. Current use of lumbar traction in the management of low back pain: results of a survey of physiotherapists in the United Kingdom. *Arch Phys Med Rehabil.* 2005;86:1164-1169.
706. Harte AA, Baxter GD, Gracey JH. The efficacy of traction for back pain: a systematic review of randomized controlled trials. *Arch Phys Med Rehabil.* 2003;84:1542-1553.
707. Clarke JA, van Tulder MW, Blomberg SE, et al. Traction for low-back pain with or without sciatica. *Cochrane Database Syst Rev.* 2007;(2):CD003010.
708. Chou R, Huffman LH. Nonpharmacologic therapies for acute and chronic low back pain: a review of the evidence for an American Pain Society/American College of Physicians clinical practice guideline. *Ann Intern Med.* 2007;147:492-504.
709. Saunders HD. Lumbar traction. *J Orthop Sports Phys Ther.* 1979;1:36-45.
710. Saunders HD, Saunders R. *Evaluation, Treatment, and Prevention of Musculoskeletal Disorders: Vol 1. Spine.* Bloomington, MN: Educational Opportunities; 1993.
711. Krause M, Refshauge KM, Dessen M, Boland R. Lumbar spine traction: evaluation of effects and recommended application for treatment. *Man Ther.* 2000;5(2):72-81.
712. Fritz JM, Lindsay W, Matheson JW, et al. Is there a subgroup of patients with low back pain likely to benefit from mechanical traction? Results of a randomized clinical trial and subgrouping analysis. *Spine.* 2007;32:E793-E800.
713. Fritz JM, Thackeray A, Childs JD, Brennan GP. A randomized clinical trial of the effectiveness of mechanical traction for sub-groups of patients with low back pain: study methods and rationale. *BMC Musculoskelet Disord.* 2010;11:81.
714. Harte AA, Baxter GD, Gracey JH. The effectiveness of motorised lumbar traction in the management of LBP with lumbosacral nerve root involvement: a feasibility study. *BMC Musculoskelet Disord.* 2007;8:118.
715. Maitland GD. *Vertebral Manipulation.* 8th ed. Edinburgh, Scotland: Churchill and Livingstone; 2001.
716. Cyriax J. *Textbook of Orthopaedic Medicine.* Vol 1, 8th ed. London, England: Bailliere Tindall; 1982.
717. Gagne AR, Hasson SM. Lumbar extension exercises in conjunction with mechanical traction for the management of a patient with a lumbar herniated disc. *Physiother Theor Pract.* 2010;26:256-266.
718. Murphy DR, Hurwitz EL, McGovern EE. A nonsurgical approach to the management of patients with lumbar radiculopathy secondary to herniated disk: a prospective observational cohort study with follow-up. *J Manipulative Physiol Ther.* 2009;32:723-733.
719. Gudavalli M, Cambron J, McGregor M, et al. A randomized clinical trial and subgroup analysis to compare flexion-distraction with active exercise for chronic low back pain. *Eur Spine J.* 2005;15:1070-1082.
720. Stern PJ, Cote P, Cassidy JD. A series of consecutive cases of low back pain with radiating leg pain treated by chiropractors. *J Manipulative Physiol Ther.* 1995;18:335-342.
721. Chaitow L, Liebenson C. *Muscle Energy Techniques.* 2nd ed. Edinburgh, Scotland: Churchill Livingstone; 2001.
722. Lavelle W, Smith HS. Myofaxcial trigger points. *Anesthesiology Clin.* 2007;25:841-852.
723. Stanton TR, Fritz JM, Hancock MJ, et al. Evaluation of a treatment based classification algorithm for low back pain: a cross-sectional study. *Phys Ther.* 2011;91:496-509.
724. Shacklock M. Neurodynamics. *Physiotherapy.* 1995;81:9-16.
725. Nee RJ, Butler D. Management of peripheral neuropathic pain: integrating neurobiology neurodynamics, and clinical evidence. *Phys Ther Sport.* 2006;7:36-49.
726. Ellis RF, Hing WA. Neural mobilization: a systematic review of randomized controlled trials with and analysis of therapeutic efficacy. *J Man Manip Ther.* 2008;16:8-22.
727. Allison GT, Nagy BM, Hall T. A randomized clinical trial of manual therapy for cervico-brachial pain syndrome: a pilot study. *Man Ther.* 2002;7(2):95-102.
728. Cleland JA, Childs JD, Palmer JA, Eberhart S. Slump stretching in the management of non-radicular low back pain: a pilot clinical trial. *Man Ther.* 2007;11:279-286.
729. Scrimshaw S, Maher C. Randomized controlled trial of neural mobilization after spinal surgery. *Spine.* 2001;26:2647-2652.
730. George SZ. Characteristics of patients with lower extremity symptoms treated with slump stretching: a case series. *J Orthop Sports Phys Ther.* 2002;32:391-398.
731. Melbye M. An adherent nerve root—classification and exercise therapy in a patient diagnosised with lumbar disc prolapsed. *Man Ther.* 2010;15:126-129.
732. Schäfer A, Hall T, Briffa K. Classification of low back related leg pain—a proposed patho-mechanism-based approach. *Man Ther.* 2009;14:222-230.
733. Bennett MI. The LANSS Pain Scale: the Leeds assessment of neuropathic symptoms and signs. *Pain.* 2001;91:147-157.
734. Bennett MI, Smith BH, Torrance N, Potter J. The S-LANSS score for identifying pain of predominantly neuropathic origin: validation for use in clinical and postal research. *J Pain.* 2005;6(3):149-158.
735. Schäfer A, Hall T, Lüdtke K, Mallwitz J, Briffa K. Interrater reliability of a new classification system for patients with low back related leg pain. *J Man Manip Ther.* 2009;17:109-117.

736. Walsh J, Hall T. Classification of low back-related leg pain: do subgroups differ in disability and psychosocial factors? *J Man Manip Ther.* 2009;17(2):118-123.
737. Hall T, Schäfer A, Rolke R, et al. QST profiles of subgroups of patients with sciatica: do they differ? Paper presented at: 12th World Congress on Pain; August 17-22, 2008; Glasgow, Scotland.
738. Petersen SM, Scott DR. Application of a classification system and description of a combined manual therapy intervention: a case with low back related leg pain. *J Man Manip Ther.* 2010;18(2):89-96.
739. Schäfer A, Hall T, Müller G, Briffa K. Outcomes differ between subgroups of patients with low back and leg pain following neural manual therapy: a prospective cohort study. *Eur Spine J.* 2011;20:482-490.
740. Von Korff M, Crane P, Lane M, et al. Chronic spinal pain and physical-mental comorbidity in the United States: results from the National Comorbidity Survey Replication. *Pain.* 2005;113:331-339.
741. Gatchel RJ. Award for distinguished professional contributions to applied research. *Am Psychol.* 2004;59:794-805.
742. Gatchel RJ. Comorbidity of chronic pain and mental health: the biopsychosocial perspective. *Am Psychol.* 2004;59:792-794.
743. McCarthy CH, Arnall FA, Strimpakos N, Freemont A, Oldham J. The biopsychosocial classification of non-specific low back pain: a systematic review. *Phys Ther Rev.* 2004;9:17-30.
744. Gatchel RJ, Peng YB, Peters ML, Fuchs PN, Turk DC. The biopsychosocial approach to chronic pain: scientific advances and future directions. *Psychol Bull.* 2007;133:581-624.
745. Main CG, Buchbinder R, Porcheret M, Foster N. Addressing patient beliefs and expectations in the consultation. *Best Pract Res Clin Rheumatol.* 2010;24:219-225.
746. Moseley GL. Joining forces—combining cognition-targeted motor control training with group or individual pain physiology education: a successful treatment for chronic low back pain. *J Man Manip Ther.* 2003;11:88-94.
747. Nachemson AL. Newest knowledge of low back pain. A critical look. *Clin Orthop.* 1992;279:8-20.
748. Gask L, Usherwood T. ABC of psychological medicine: the consultation. *BMJ.* 2002;324:1567-1569.
749. Hush JM, Nicholas MK. Cognitive behavioral treatment for low back pain. *J Clin Outcomes Manag.* 2011;18(2):85-95.
750. Moseley GL. Reconceptualising pain according to modern pain science. *Phys Ther Rev.* 2007;12:169-178.
751. Melzack R. Pain and the neuromatrix in the brain. *J Dent Educ.* 2001;65:1378-1382.
752. Melzack R. Evolution of the neuromatrix theory of pain. The Prithvi Raj lecture: presented at the third world congress of world institute of pain, Barcelona 2004. *Pain Pract.* 2005;5(2):85-94.
753. Melzack R, Casey KL. Sensory motivational and central control determinants of pain: a new conceptual model. In: Kenshalo D, ed. *The Skin Senses.* Springfield, IL: Thomas; 1968:423-443.
754. Bevan S. Nociceptive peripheral neurons: cellular properties. In: Wall P, Melzack R, eds. *The Textbook of Pain.* 4th ed. Edinburgh, Scotland: Churchill Livingstone; 1999:85-103.
755. Watkins L, Maier S. The pain of being sick: implications of immune-to-brain communication for understanding pain. *Annu Rev Psychol.* 2000;51:29-57.
756. Hodges PW, Moseley GL. Pain and motor control of the lumbopelvic region: effect and possible mechanisms. *J Electromyogr Kinesiol.* 2003;13:361-370.
757. Wand BM, Parkitny L, O'Connell NE, et al. Cortical changes in chronic low back pain: current state of the art implications for clinical practice. *Man Ther.* 2011;16:15-20.
758. Grachev ID, Fredrickson BE, Apkarian AV. Dissociating anxiety from pain: mapping the neuronal marker N-acetyl aspartate to perception distinguishes closely interrelated characteristics of chronic pain. *Mol Psychiatry.* 2001;6:256-258.
759. Flor H, Braun C, Elbert T, Birbaumer N. Extensive reorganization of primary somatosensory cortex in chronic back pain patients. *Neurosci Lett.* 1997;224:5-8.
760. Lloyd D, Findlay G, Roberts N, Nurmikko T. Differences in low back pain behavior are reflected in the cerebral response to tactile stimulation of the lower back. *Spine.* 2008;33:1372-1377.
761. Tsao H, Galea MP, Hodges PW. Reorganization of the motor cortex is associated with postural control deficits in recurrent low back pain. *Brain.* 2008;131:2161-2171.
762. Jacobs JV, Henry SM, Nagle KJ. Low back pain associates with altered activity of the cerebral cortex prior to arm movements that require postural adjustment. *Clin Neurophysiol.* 2010;121:431-440.
763. Apkarian AV, Sosa Y, Krauss BR, et al. Chronic pain patients are impaired on an emotional decision-making task. *Pain.* 2004;108:129.
764. Weiner DK, Rudy TE, Morrow L, Slaboda J, Lieber S. The relationship between pain neuropsychological performance, and physical function in community-dwelling older adults with chronic low back pain. *Pain Med.* 2006;7:60-70.
765. Lourenco JL, Gerard C, Revel M. Evidence of memory dysfunction and maladaptive coping in chronic low back pain and rheumatoid arthritis patients: challenges for rehabilitation. *Eur J Phys Rehabil Med.* 2009;45:469-477.
766. O'Sullivan PB, Burnett A, Floyd AN, et al. Lumbar repositioning deficit in a specfic low back pain population. *Spine.* 2003;28:1074-1079.
767. Moseley GL. I can't find it! Distorted body image and tactile dysfunction in patients with chronic back pain. *Pain.* 2008;149:239-243.
768. Wand BM, O'Connell NE, Di Pietro F, Bulsara M. Managing chronic nonspecific low back pain with a sensorimotor retraining approach: an exploratory multiple-baseline study of 3 participants. *Phys Ther.* 2011;91:535-546.
769. Moseley GL. Graded motor imagery for pathologic pain: a randomized controlled trial. *Neurology.* 2006;67:2129-2134.
770. deCharms RC, Maeda F, Glover GH, et al. Control over brain activation and pain learned by using real-time functional MRI. *Neuroscience.* 2005;102:18626-18631.
771. Tsao H, Galea MP, Hodges PW. Driving plasticity in the motor cortex in recurrent low back pain. *Eur J Pain.* 2010;14:832-839.
772. Boersma K, Linton SJ. Psychological processes underlying the development of a chronic pain problem: a prospective study of the relationship between profiles of psychological variables in the fear avoidance model in disability. *Clin J Pain.* 2006;22:160-166.
773. Robinson ME, Riley JL. The role of emotion in pain. In: Gatchel RJ, Turk DC, eds. *Psychosocial Factors in Pain: Critical Perspectives.* New York, NY: Guilford; 1999:74-78.
774. Jarvik JG, Hollingworth W, Heagerty PJ, Haynor DR, Boyco EJ, Deyo RA. Three-year incidence of low back pain in an initially asymptomatic cohort. Clinical and imaging risk factors. *Spine.* 2005;30:1541-1548.
775. Turk DC, Okifuji A, Scharff L. Chronic pain and depression: role of perceived impact and perceived control in different age cohorts. *Pain.* 1995;61:93-101.

776. Rudy TE, Kerns RD, Turk DC. Chronic pain and depression: toward a cognitive behavioral mediational model. *Pain.* 1988;35:129-140.
777. Okifuji A, Turk DC, Curran SL. Anger in chronic pain: investigations of anger targets and intensity. *J Psychosom Res.* 1999;61:771-780.
778. Turner JA, Jensen MP, Romano JM. Do beliefs, coping, and catastrophizing independently predict functioning in patients with chronic pain? *Pain.* 2000;85:115-125.
779. Asmundson GJ, Norton PJ, Vlaeyen JWS. Fear avoidance models of chronic pain: an overview. In: Asmundson GJ, Vlaeyen WS, Crombez G, eds. *Understanding and Treating Fear of Pain.* Oxford, England: Oxford University Press; 2004:3-24.
780. Boersma K, Linton S, Overmeer T, Jansson M, Vlaeyen J, de Jong J. Lowering fear-avoidance and enhancing function through exposure in vivo: a multiple baseline study across six patients with back pain. *Pain.* 2004;108:8-16.
781. de Jong JR, Vlaeyen JWS, Onghena P, Goossens ME, Geilen M, Mulder H. Fear of movement/(re)injury in chronic low back pain: education or exposure in vivo as mediator to fear reduction? *Clin J Pain.* 2005;21:9-17.
782. Vlaeyen JW, de Jong JR, Onghena P, Kerckhoffs-Hanssen M, Kole-Snijders AM. Can pain-related fear be reduced? The application of cognitive-behavioural exposure in vivo. *Pain Res Manag.* 2002;7:144-153.
783. Scheier MF, Carver CS. Effects of optimism on psychological and physical well-being: theoretical overview and empirical update. *Cognit Ther Res.* 1992;16:201-228.
784. Moseley GL, Nicholas MK, Hodges PW. A randomized controlled trial of intensive neurophysiology education in chronic low back pain. *Clin J Pain.* 2004;20:324-330.
785. Moseley GL. Evidence for a direct relationship between cognitive and physical change during an education intervention in people with chronic low back pain. *Eur J Pain.* 2004;8:39-45.
786. Moseley GL. Combined physiotherapy and education is effective for chronic low back pain. A randomised controlled trial. *Aus J Physiother.* 2002;48:297-302.
787. Nijs J, Van Houdenhove B. From acute musculoskeletal pian to chronic widespread pain and fibromyalgia: application of pain neurophysiology in manual therapy practice. *Man Ther.* 2009;14:3-12.
788. O'Sullivan P. Lumbar segmental instability: clinical presentation and specific exercise management. *Man Ther.* 2000;5:2-12.
789. O'Sullivan P. Clinical instability of the lumbar spine: its pathological basis, diagnosis, and conservative management. In: Boyling JD, Jull GA, eds. *Grieve's Modern Manual Therapy.* 3rd ed. Philadelphia, PA: Elsevier; 2004:311-331.
790. Bergstrom G, Bodin L, Jensen I, Linton S, Nygren A. Long term, nonspecific spinal pain: reliable and valid sub-groups of patients. *Behav Res Ther.* 2001;39:75-78.
791. Dankaerts W, O'Sullivan PB, Straker LM, Burnett AF, Skouen JS. The inter-examiner reliability of a classification method for non-specific chronic low back pain patients with motor control impairment. *Man Ther.* 2006;11:28-39.
792. Fersum KV, O'Sullivan PB, Kvåle A, Skouen JS. Inter-examiner reliability of a classification system for patients with non-specific low back pain. *Man Ther.* 2009;14:555-561.
793. Dankaerts W, O'Sullivan PM, Straker LM. Altered patterns of superficial trunk muscle activation during sitting in non-specific chronic low back pain patients: importance of subclassification. *Spine.* 2006;31:2017-2023.
794. Dankaerts W, O'Sullivan PM, Straker LM, Davey P, Gupta R. Discriminating healthy controls and two clinical subgroups of nonspecific chronic low back pain patients using trunk muscle activation and lumbosacral kinematics of postures and movement: a statistical classification model. *Spine.* 2009;34:1610-1618.
795. Dankaerts W, O'Sullivan PB, Burnett AF, Straker LM. The use of a mechanism-based classification system to evaluate and direct management of a patient with non-specific chronic low back pain and motor control impairment—a case report. *Man Ther.* 2007;12:181-191.
796. Luomajoki H, Kool J, de Bruin ED, Airaksinen O. Improvement in low back movement control, decreased pain and disability, resulting from specific exercise intervention. *Sports Med Arthrosc Rehabil Ther Technol.* 2010;2:11. http://www.smarttjournal.com/content/2/1/11. Accessed March 7, 2011.
797. Fersum KV, O'Sullivan P, Kvale A, et al. Classification based cognitive functional therapy for the management of non-specific low back pain (NSLBP)—a randomized control trial. Paper presented at: Melbourne International Forum XI, Primary Care Research on Low Back Pain; March 15-18, 2011; Melbourne, Australia.
798. van Middelkoop M, Rubinstein SM, Kuijpers T, et al. A systematic review on the effectiveness of physical rehabilitation interventions for chronic non-specific low back pain. *Eur Spine J.* 2011;20:19-39.
799. Bokarius AV, Bokarius V. Evidence-based review of manual therapy efficacy in treatment of chronic musculoskeletal pain. *Pain Pract.* 2010;10:451-458.
800. Rubinstein SM, van Middelkoop M, Assendelft WJ, DeBoer MR, van Tulder MW. Spinal manipulative therapy for chronic low back pain. *Cochrane Database Syst Rev.* 2011;(2):CD008112.
801. Fersum KV, Dankaerts W, O'Sullivan PB, et al. Integration of subclassification strategies in randomized controlled clinical trials evaluating manual therapy treatment and exercise therapy for non-specific chronic low back pain: a systematic review. *Br J Sports Med.* 2010;44:1054-1062.
802. Henschke N, Ostelo RWJG, van Tulder MW, et al. Behavioural treatment for chronic low-back pain. *Cochrane Database Syst Rev.* 2010;(7):CD002014.
803. Bekkering G, Hendriks H, Koes B, et al. Dutch physiotherapy guidelines for low back pain. *Physiotherapy.* 2003;89(2):82-95.
804. Hlobil H, Staal JB, Twisk J, et al. The effects of a graded activity intervention for low back pain in occupational health on sick leave, functional status and pain: 12 month results of a randomized controlled trial. *J Occup Rehabil.* 2005;15:569-580.
805. Bunzli S, Gillham D, Esterman A. Physiotherapy-provided operant conditioning in the management of low back pain disability: a systematic review. *Physiother Res Int.* 2011;16:4-19.
806. Jensen MP, Turner JA, Romano JM. Changes in beliefs, catastrophizing, and coping are associated with improvement in multidisciplinary pain treatment. *J Consult Clin Psychol.* 2001;69:655-662.
807. McCracken LM, Gross RT, Eccleston C. Multimethod assessment of treatment process in chronic low back pain: comparison of reported pain-related anxiety with directly measured physical capacity. *Behav Res Ther.* 2002;40:585-594.
808. Gatchel RJ, Okifuji A. Evidence-based scientific data documenting the treatment- and cost-effectiveness of comprehensive pain programs for chronic pain management. *J Pain.* 2006;7:779-793.

809. Macedo LG, Smeets RJEM, Maher CG, Latimer J, McAuley JH. Graded activity and graded exposure for persistent nonspecific low back pain: a systematic review. *Phys Ther.* 2010;90:860-879.
810. George SZ, Wittmer VT, Fillingim RB, Robinson ME. Comparison of graded exercise and graded exposure clinical outsomes for patients with chronic low back pain. *J Orthop Sports Phys Ther.* 2010;40:694-704.
811. George SZ, Zeppieri G. Physical therapy utilization of graded exposure for patients with low back pain. *J Orthop Sports Phys Ther.* 2009;39:496-505.
812. Rasmussen-Barr E, Ang B, Arvidsson I, Nilsson-Wikmar L. Graded exercise for recurrent low-back pain. A randomized, controlled trial with 6-, 12-, and 36 month follow-ups. *Spine.* 2009;34:221-228.
813. Moseley GL. Widespread brain activity during an abdominal task markedly reduced after pain physiology education: fMRI evaluation of a single patient with chronic low back pain. *Aust J Physiother.* 2004;51:49-52.
814. Louw A, Puentedura EL, Mintken P. Use of an abbreviated neuroscience education approach in the treatment of chronic low back pain: a case report. *Physiother Theory Pract.* 2012;28(1):50-62.
815. Philadelphia Panel. Philadelphia Panel evidence-based clinical practice guidelines on selected rehabilitation interventions for low back pain. *Phys Ther.* 2001;81:1641-1672.
816. Khadilkar A, Odebiyi DO, Brosseau L, Wells GA. Transcutaneous electrical nerve stimulation (TENS) versus placebo for chronic low-back pain. *Cochrane Database Syst Rev.* 2008;(4):CD003008.
817. French SD, Cameron M, Walker BF, Reggars JW, Esterman AJ. Superficial heat or cold for low back pain. *Cochrane Database Syst Rev.* 2006;(1):CD004750.
818. Cook C, Learman K. *Low Back Pain and the Evidence of Effectiveness of Physical Therapy Interventions. Independent Study Course 18.1.6.* La Crosse, WI: Orthopaedic Section, American Physical Therapy Association; 2008.
819. van Duijvenbode I, Jellema P, van Poppel M, van Tulder MW. Lumbar supports for prevention and treatment of low back pain. *Cochrane Database Syst Rev.* 2008;(2):CD001823.
820. American College of Sports Medicine. http://www.acsm.org. Accessed September 20, 2013.
821. Tudor-Locke C, Hatano Y, Pangrazi RP, Kang M. Revisiting "how many steps are enough?" *Med Sci Sports Exerc.* 2008;40(7 suppl):s537-s543.
822. Murphy MH, Nevill AM, Murtagh EM, Holder RL. The effect of walking on fitness, fatness and resting blood pressure: a meta-analysis of randomised, controlled trials. *Prev Med.* 2007;44:377-385.
823. Ryan CG, Grant PM, Dall PM, Gray H, Newton M, Granat M. Individuals with chronic low back pain have a lower level, and an altered pattern of physical activity compared with matched controls: an observational study. *Aust J Physiother.* 2009;55:53-58.
824. Hurley DA, Brady L, O'Brien E, McDonough S, Baxter GD, Neneghan C. Subjective and objective evaluation of the physical activity profiles of people with low back pain and age-matched controls over 7 consecutive days. *J Bone Joint Surg Br.* 2010;92B(suppl):234.
825. Hendrick P, Te Wake AM, Tikkisetty AS, Wulff L, Yap C, Milosavljevic S. The effectiveness of walking as an intervention for low back pain: a systematic review. *Eur Spine J.* 2010;19:1613-1620.
826. Hurwitz EL, Morgenstern H, Chiao C. Effects of recreational physical activity and back exercises on low back pain and psychological distress: findings from the UCLA Low Back Pain Study. *Am J Public Health.* 2005;95:1817-1824.
827. Hurley DA, O'Donoghue G, Tully MA, et al. A walking programme and a supervised exercise class versus usual physiotherapy for chronic low back pain: a single-blinded randomized controlled trial (The Supervised Walking in comparison to Fitness Training for Back Pain (SWIFT) Trial). *BMC Musculoskelet Disord.* 2009;10:79.
828. Bonifazi M, Suman AL, Cambiaggi C, et al. Changes in salivary cortisol and corticosteroid receptor-alpha mRNA expression following a 3-week multidisciplinary treatment program in patients with fibromyalgia. *Psychoneuroendocrinology.* 2006;31:1076-1086.
829. Brosseau L, Wells GA, Tugwell P, et al. Ottawa Panel evidence-based clinical practice guidelines for aerobic fitness exercises in the management of fibromyalgia. Part 1. *Phys Ther.* 2008;88:857-871.
830. Brosseau L, Wells GA, Tugwell P, et al. Ottawa Panel evidence-based clinical practice guidelines for strengthening exercises in the management of fibromyalgia. Part 2. *Phys Ther.* 2008;88:873-886.
831. Busch AJ, Barber KA, Overend TJ, Peloso PM, Schachter CL. Exercise for treating fibromyalgia syndrome. *Cochrane Database Syst Rev.* 2008;(4):CD003786.
832. Carville SF, Arendt-Nielsen S, Bliddal H, et al. EULAR evidence-based recommendations for the management of fibromyalgia syndrome. *Ann Rheum Dis.* 2008;67:536-541.
833. Rooks DS, Gautam S, Romeling M, et al. Group exercise, education, and combination self-management in women with fibromyalgia: a randomized trial. *Arch Int Med.* 2007;167:2192-2200.
834. American College of Sports Medicine. *ACSM's Guidelines for Exercise Testing and Prescription.* 7th ed. Baltimore, MD: Lippincott Williams & Wilkins; 2006.
835. Chou R, Loeser JD, Owens DK, et al, and the American Pain Society Low Back Pain Guideline Panel. Interventional therapies, surgery, and interdisciplinary rehabilitation for low back pain: an evidence-based clinical practice guideline from the American Pain Society. *Spine.* 2009;34:1066-1077.
836. Guzman J, Esmail R, Karjalainen K, et al. Multidisciplinary rehabilitation for chronic low back pain: systematic review. *BMJ.* 2001;322:1511-1516.
837. Guzman J, Esmail R, Karjalainen K, et al. Multidisciplinary bio-psychosocial rehabilitation for chronic low-back pain. *Cochrane Database Syst Rev.* 2002;(1):CD000963.
838. van Geen J, Edelaar MJ, Janssen ME, et al. The long-term effect of multidisciplinary back training. *Spine.* 2007;32:249-255.
839. Fairbank J, Frost H, Wilson-MacDonald J, et al. Randomised controlled trial to compare surgical stabilisation of the lumbar spine with an intensive rehabilitation programme for patients with chronic low back pain: the MRC Spine Stabilisation Trial. *BMJ.* 2005;330:1233.
840. Brox J, Reikeras O, Nygaard O, et al. Lumbar instrumented fusion compared with cognitive intervention and exercises in patients with chronic back pain after previous surgery for disc herniation: a prospective randomized controlled study. *Pain.* 2006;122:145-155.
841. Brox JI, Sorensen R, Friis A, et al. Randomized clinical trial of lumbar instrumented fusion and cognitive intervention and exercises in patients with chronic low back pain and disc degeneration. *Spine.* 2003;28:1913-1921.

842. Skoen JS, Grasdal AL, Haldorsen EMH, et al. Relative cost-effectiveness of extensive and light multidisciplinary treatment programs versus treatment as usual for patients with chronic low back pain on long-term sick leave. *Spine.* 2002;27:901-910.
843. Loisel P, Lemaire J, Poitras S, et al. Cost-benefit and cost-effectiveness analysis of a disability prevention model for back pain management: a six year follow up study. *Occup Environ Med.* 2002;59:807-815.
844. Gatchel RJ, Polatin PB, Noe C, et al. Treatment- and cost-effectiveness of early intervention for acute low-back pain patients: a one-year prospective study. *J Occup Rehabil.* 2003;13:1-9.
845. Zhang W, Jones A, Doherty M. Does paracetamol (acetaminophen) reduce the pain of osteoarthritis? A meta-analysis of randomized controlled trials. *Ann Rheum Dis.* 2004;63:901-907.
846. Rahme E, Pettitt D, LeLorier J. Determinants and sequelae associated with utilization of acetaminophen versus traditional nonsteroidal anti-inflammatory drugs in an elderly population. *Arthritis Rheum.* 2002;46:3046-3054.
847. Conaghan PG. A turbulent decade for NSAIDs: update on current concepts of classification, epidemiology, comparative efficacy, and toxicity. *Rheumatol Int.* 2012;32:1491-1502.
848. Derry S, Loke YK. Risk of gastrointestinal haemorrhage with long term use of aspirin: meta-analysis. *BMJ.* 2000;321:1183-1187.
849. Yildirim K, Sisecioglu M, Karatay S, et al. The effectiveness of gabapentin in patients with chronic radiculopathy. *The Pain Clinic.* 2003;15:213-218.
850. van Tulder M, Touray T, Furlan A, Solway S, Bouter L; the Cochrane Back Review Group. Muscle relaxants for nonspecific low back pain: a systematic review within the framework of the Cochrane Collaboration. *Spine.* 2003;28:1978-1992.
851. Finckh A, Zufferey P, Schurch MA, Balagué F, Waldburger M, So AK. Short-term efficacy of intravenous pulse glucocorticoids in acute discogenic sciatica. A randomized controlled trial. *Spine.* 2006;31:377-381.
852. Friedman BW, Holden L, Esses D, et al. Parenteral corticosteroids for Emergency Department patients with non-radicular low back pain. *J Emerg Med.* 2006;31:365-370.
853. Kuijpers T, van Middelkoop M, Rubinstein SM, et al. A systematic review on the effectiveness of pharmacological interventions for chronic non-specific low-back pain. *Eur Spine J.* 2011;20:40-50.
854. Deyo RA, Gray DT, Kreuter W, et al. United States trends in lumbar fusion surgery for degenerative conditions. *Spine.* 2005;30:1441-1445.
855. Chou R, Baisden J, Carragee EJ, Resnick DK, Shaffer WO, Loeser JD. Surgery for low back pain. A review of the evidence for an American Pain Society clinical practice guideline. *Spine.* 2009;34:1094-1109.
856. Osterman H, Seitsalo S, Karppinen J, et al. Effectiveness of microdiscectomy for lumbar disc herniation: a randomized controlled trial with 2 years of follow-up. *Spine.* 2006;31:2409-2414.
857. Peul WC, van Houwelingen HC, van den Hout WB, et al. Surgery versus prolonged conservative treatment for sciatica. *N Engl J Med.* 2007;356:2245-2256.
858. Peul W, van den Hout W, Brand R, et al. Prolonged conservative care versus early surgery in patients with sciatica caused by lumbar disc herniation: two year results of a randomised controlled trial. *BMJ.* 2008;336:1355-1358.
859. Weinstein JN, Tosteson TD, Lurie JD, et al. Surgical vs nonoperative treatment for lumbar disk herniation: the Spine Patient Outcomes Research Trial (SPORT): a randomized trial. *JAMA.* 2006;296:2441-2450.
860. Gibson JA, Waddell G. Surgical interventions for lumbar disc prolapse. *Cochrane Database Syst Rev.* 2007;(2):CD001350.
861. Ostelo RWJG, Costa LOP, Maher CG, de Vet HCW, van Tulder MW. Rehabilitation after lumbar disc surgery. *Cochrane Database Syst Rev.* 2008;(4):CD003007.
862. Amundsen T, Weber H, Nordal H, et al. Lumbar spinal stenosis: conservative or surgical management? A prospective 10-year study. *Spine.* 2000;25:1424-1436.
863. Malmivaara A, Slatis P, Heliovaara M, et al. Surgical or non-operative treatment for lumbar spinal stenosis? A randomized controlled trial. *Spine.* 2007;32:1-8.
864. Weinstein JN, Lurie JD, Tosteson TD, et al. Surgical versus nonsurgical treatment for lumbar degenerative spondylolisthesis. *N Engl J Med.* 2007;356:2257-2270.
865. Weinstein J, Tosteson T, Lurie J, et al. Surgical versus non-surgical therapy for lumbar spinal stenosis. *N Engl J Med.* 2008;358:794-810.
866. Kovacs FM, Urrótia G, Alarcón JD. Surgery versus conservative treatment for symptomatic lumbar spinal stenosis: a systematic review of randomized controlled trials. *Spine (Phila Pa 1976).* 2011;36(20):E1335-E1351.
867. Bruggeman AJ, Decker RC. Surgical treatment and outcomes of lumbar radiculopathy. *Phys Med Rehabil Clinics N Am.* 2011;22:161-177.
868. Ostelo RWJG, Costa LOP, Maher CG, de Vet HCW, van Tulder MW. Rehabilitation after lumbar disc surgery. An update Cochrane review. *Spine.* 2009;34:1839-1848.
869. Rushton A, Wright C, Goodwin P, Calvert M, Freemantle N. Physiotherapy rehabilitation post-first lumbar discectomy: a systematic review and meta-analysis of randomized controlled trials. *Spine.* 2011;36(14):E961-E972.
870. McGregor AH, Doré C, Morris TP, Morris S, Jamrozik K. ISSLS prize winner: Function After Spinal Treatment, Exercise, and Rehabilitation (FASTER): a factorial randomized trial to determine whether the functional outcome of spinal surgery can be improved. *Spine (Phila Pa 1976).* 2011;36(21):1711-1720.
871. Waddell G, Sell P, McGregor AH, et al. *Your Back Operation.* London, England: The Stationery Office; 2005.
872. Williamson E, White L, Rushton A. A survey first time post-operative management for patients following first time lumbar discectomy. *Eur Spine J.* 2007;16:795-802.
873. Selkowitz DM, Kulig K, Poppert EM, et al; the Physical Therapy Clinical Research Network. The immediate and long-term effects of exercise and patient education on physical, functional, and quality-of-life outcome measures after single-level lumbar microdiscectomy: a randomized controlled trial protocol. *BMC Musculoskelet Disord.* 2006;7:70.
874. Biering-Sorensen F. Physical measurements as risk indicators for low-back trouble over a one-year period. *Spine.* 1984;9:106-119.
875. Kulig K, Beneck GJ, Selkowitz DM, et al; the Physical Therapy Clinical Research Network. An intensive, progressive exercise program reduces disability and improves functional performance in patients after single-level lumbar microdiskectomy. *Phys Ther.* 2009;89:1145-1157.
876. Hebert JJ, Marcus RL, Koppenhaver SL, Fritz JM. Postoperative rehabilitation following lumbar discectomy with quantification of trunk muscle morphology and function: a case report and review of the literature. *J Orthop Sports Phys Ther.* 2010;40:402-412.

877. Hebert JJ. Stabilization exercise and disorders of the lumbar spine: neuromuscular implications and clinical efficacy in nonoperative and postoperative populations. http://gradworks.umi.com/34/12/3412866.html. Accessed March 12, 2011.
878. Moller H, Hedlund R. Surgery versus conservative management in adult isthmic spondylolisthesisda prospective randomized study: part 1. *Spine.* 2000;25:1716-1721.
879. Swan J, Hurwitz E, Malek F, et al. Surgical treatment for unstable low-grade isthmic spondylolisthesis in adults: a prospective controlled study of posterior instrumented fusion compared with combined anterior-posterior fusion. *Spine J.* 2006;6:606-614.
880. Abbott AD, Tyni-Lenné R, Hedlund R. Early rehabilitation targeting cognition, behavior, and motor function after lumbar fusion. *Spine.* 2010;35:848-857.
881. Christensen FB, Laurberg I, Bünger CE. Importance of the back-café concept to rehabilitation after lumbar spinal fusion: a randomised clinical study with a 2-year follow-up. *Spine.* 2003;28:2561-2569.
882. van den Eerenbeemt KD, Ostelo RW, van Royen BJ, Peul WC, van Tulder MW. Total disc replacement surgery for symptomatic degenerative lumbar disc disease: a systematic review of the literature. *Eur Spine J.* 2010;19:1262-1280.
883. Villavicencio AT, Burneikiene S, Johnson JP. Spinal artificial disc replacement: lumbar arthroplasty. Part II. *Contemp Neurosurg.* 2005;27(19):1-5.
884. Puentedura EJ, Brooksby CL, Wallman HW, Landers MR. Rehabilitation following lumbosacral percutaneous nucleoplasty: a case report. *J Orthop Sports Phys Ther.* 2010;40:214-224.
885. Sagi HC, Bao QB, Yuan HA. Nuclear replacement strategies. *Orthop Clin North Am.* 2003;34:263-267.
886. Di Martino A, Vaccaro A, Lee JY, Denaro V, Lim MR. Nucleus pulposus replacement: basic science and indications for clinical use. *Spine.* 2005;30:S16-S22.
887. George SZ, Hirsh AT. Distinguishing patient satisfaction with treatment delivery from treatment effect: a preliminary investigation of patient satisfaction with symptoms after physical therapy treatment of low back pain. *Arch Phys Med Rehabil.* 2005;86:1338-1344.
888. Breen A, Breen R. Back pain and satisfaction with chiropractic treatment: what role does the physical outcome play? *Clin J Pain.* 2003;19:263-268.
889. O'Malley KJ, Roddey TS, Gartsman GM, Cook KF. Outcome expectancies, functional outcomes, and expectancy fulfillment for patients with shoulder problems. *Care.* 2004;42:139-146.
890. Iles RA, Davidson M, Taylor NF. Psychosocial predictors of failure to return to work in non-chronic non-specific lowback pain: a systematic review. *Occup Environ Med.* 2008;65:507-517.
891. Lin CC, Ward SE. Perceived self-efficacy and outcome expectancies in coping with chronic low back pain. *Res Nurs Health.* 1996;19:299-310.
892. Booth-Kewley S, Larson GE, Highfill-McRoy RM. Psychosocial predictors of return to duty among Marine recruits with musculoskeletal injuries. *Mil Med.* 2009;174:139-152.
893. Bell RA, Kravitz RL, Thom D, et al. Unmet expectations for care and the patient physician relationship. *J Gen Intern Med.* 2002;17:817-824.
894. Eisler T, Svensson O, Tengstrom A, Elmstedt E. Patient expectation and satisfaction in revision total hip arthroplasty. *J Arthroplasty.* 2002;17:457-462.
895. Uhlmann RF, Inui TS, Carter WB. Patient requests and expectations: definitions and clinical applications. *Med Care.* 1984;22: 681-685.
896. Wiles R, Cott C, Gibson BE. Hope, expectations and recovery from illness: a narrative synthesis of qualitative research. *J Adv Nurs.* 2008;64:564-573.
897. Hill JC, Lewis M, Sim J, et al. Predictors of poor outcome in patients with neck pain treated by physical therapy. *Clin J Pain.* 2007;23:683-690.
898. Myers SS, Phillips RS, Davis RB, et al. Patient expectations as predictors of outcome in patients with acute low back pain. *J Gen Intern Med.* 2008;23(2):148-153.
899. Leung KK, Silvius JL, Pimlott N, et al. Why health expectations and hopes are different: the development of a conceptual model. *Health Expect.* 2009;12:347-360.
900. Thompson AG, Sunol R. Expectations as determinants of patient satisfaction: concepts, theory and evidence. *Int J Qual Health Care.* 1995;7:127-141.
901. Bialosky JE, Bishop MD, Cleland JA. Individual expectation: an overlooked, but pertinent, factor in the treatment of individuals experiencing musculoskeletal pain. *Phys Ther.* 2010;90:1345-1355.
902. Safran DG, Taira DA, Rogers WH, et al. Linking primary care performance to outcomes of care. *J Fam Pract.* 1998;47:213-220.
903. Guldvog B. Can patient satisfaction improve health among patients with angina pectoris? *Int J Qual Health Care.* 1999;11:233-240.
904. Hush JM, Cameron K, Mackey M. Patient satisfaction with musculoskeletal physical therapy care: a systematic review. *Phys Ther.* 2011;91:25-36.
905. Hills R, Kitchen S. Satisfaction with outpatient physiotherapy: a survey comparing the views of patients with acute and chronic musculoskeletal conditions. *Physiother Theory Pract.* 2007;23:21-36.
906. Beattie PF, Dowda M, Turner C, et al. Longitudinal continuity of care is associated with high patient satisfaction with physical therapy. *Phys Ther.* 2005;85:1046-1052.
907. May SJ. Patient satisfaction with management of back pain. *Physiotherapy.* 2001;87:4-20.
908. MacDonald CA, Cox PD, Bartlett DJ. Productivity and client satisfaction: a comparison between physical therapists and student-therapist pairs. *Physiother Can.* 2002;54:92-101.
909. Cooper KS, Blair H, Hancock E. Patient-centredness in physiotherapy from the perspective of the low back pain patient. *Physiotherapy.* 2008;94:244-252.
910. Hills R, Kitchen S. Satisfaction with outpatient physiotherapy: focus groups to explore of patients with acute and chronic musculoskeletal conditions. *Physiother Theory Pract.* 2007;2:1-20.
911. Casserley-Feeney SN, Phelan M, Duffy F, et al. Patient satisfaction with private physiotherapy for musculoskeletal pain. *BMC Musculoskelet Disord.* 2008;9:50.
912. Hazle CR, Nitz Arthur J. Evidence-based assessment and diagnosis of pelvic girdle disorders: a proposal for an alternate diagnostic category. *Phys Ther Rev.* 2008;13:25-36.
913. Vleeming A, Albert HB, Östgaard HC, Sturesson B, Stuge B. European guidelines for the diagnosis and treatment of pelvic girdle pain. *Eur Spine J.* 2008;17:794-819.
914. Snijders C, Vleeming A, Stoeckart R. Transfer of lumbosacral load to iliac bones and legs. Part 1: biomechanics of self-bracing of the sacroiliac joints and its significance for treatment and exercise. *Clin Biomech.* 1993;8:285-294.
915. Vleeming A, Stoeckart R, Volkers C, Snijders C. Relation between form and function in the sacroiliac joint. Part 1: clinical anatomic aspects. *Spine.* 1990;15:130-132.

916. O'Sullivan PB, Beales DJ. Diagnosis and classification of pelvic girdle pain disorders—part 1: a mechanism based approach within a biopsychosocial framewori. *Man Ther.* 2007;12:86-97.
917. Vleeming A, Volkers AC, Snijders CJ, Stoeckart R. Relation between form and function in the sacroiliac joint. Part II: biomechanical aspects. *Spine.* 1990;15(2):133-136.
918. Jacob HA, Kissling RO. The mobility of the sacroiliac joints in healthy volunteers between 20 and 50 years of age. *Clin Biomech.* 1995;10:352-361.
919. Lund PJ, Krupinsi EA, Brooks WJ. Ultrasound evaluation of sacroiliac motion in normal volunteers. *Acad Radiol.* 1996;3:192-196.
920. Damen L, Stijnen T, Roebroeck ME, Snijders CJ, Stam HJ. Reliability of sacroiliac joint laxity measurement with Doppler imaging of vibrations. *Ultrasound Med Biol.* 2002;28:407-414.
921. Damen L, Buyruk HM, Guler-Uysal F, Lotgering FK, Snijders CJ, Stam HJ. Pelvic pain during pregnancy is associated with asymmetric laxity of the sacroiliac joints. *Acta Obstet Gynecol Scand.* 2001;80:1019-1024.
922. Mens JM, Pool-Goudzwaard A, Stam JH. Mobility of the pelvic joints in pregnancy-related lumbopelvic pain: a systematic review. *Obstet Gyecol Surv.* 2009;64:200-208.
923. Sturesson B, Uden A, Vleeming A. A radiostereometric analysis of movements of the sacroiliac joints during the standing hip flexion test. *Spine.* 2000;25:364-368.
924. van der Wurff P, Hagmeijer RH, Meyne W. Clinical tests of the sacroiliac joint. A systemic methodological review. Part 1: reliability. *Man Ther.* 2000;5(1):30-36.
925. van der Wurff P, Meyne W, Hagmeijer RH. Clinical tests of the sacroiliac joint. A systematic methodological review. Part 2: validity. *Man Ther.* 2000;5(2):89-96.
926. Robinson HS, Brox JI, Robinson R, Bjelland E, Solem S, Telje T. The reliability of selected motion and pain provocation tests for the sacroiliac joint. *Man Ther.* 2007;12:72-79.
927. Tullberg T, Blomberg S, Branth B, Johnsson R. Manipulation does not alter the position of the sacroiliac joint. A roentgen stereophotogrammetric analysis. *Spine.* 1998;23:1124-1128; discussion 1129.
928. Gnat R, Saulicz E, Gialy M, Klaptocz P. Does pelvic asymmetry always mean pathology? Analysis of mechanical factors leading to the asymmetry. *J Hum Kinet.* 2009;21:23-25.
929. Mens JM, Vleeming A, Snijders CJ, Stam HJ, Ginai AZ. The active straight leg raising test and mobility of the pelvic joints. *Eur Spine J.* 1999;8:468-474.
930. O'Sullivan PB, Beales DJ, Beetham JA, et al. Altered motor control strategies in subjects with sacroiliac joint pain during the active straight-leg-raise test. *Spine.* 2002;27:E1-E8.
931. De Groot M, Bool-Goudzwaaard AL, Spoor CW, Snijders CJ. The active straight leg raising test (ASLR) in pregnant women: differences in muscle activity and force between patients and health subjects. *Man Ther.* 2008;13:68-74.
932. Beales DJ, O'Sullivan PB, Briffa NK. Motor control patterns during an active straight leg raise in chronic pelvic girdle pain subjects. *Spine.* 2009;34:861-870.
933. Snijders CJ, Ribbers MT, de Bakker HV, Stoeckart R, Stam HJ. EMG recordings of abdominal and back muscles in various standing postures: validation of a biomechanical model on sacroiliac joint stability. *J Electromyogr Kines.* 1998;8:205-214.
934. Vleeming A, Pool-Goudzwaard AL, Stoeckart R, van Wingerden JP, Snijders CJ. The posterior layer of the thoracolumbar fascia. Its function in load transfer from spine to legs. *Spine (Phila Pa 1976).* 1995;20:753-758.
935. Richardson CA, Snijders CJ, Hides JA, Damen L, Pas MS, Storm J. The relation between the transversus abdominis muscles, sacroiliac joint mechanics, and low back pain. *Spine.* 2002;27:399-405.
936. Pool-Goudzwaard A, Hoek Van Dijke G, Van Gurp M, Mulder P, Snijders C, Stoeckart R. Contribution of pelvic floor muscles to stiffness of the pelvic ring. *Clin Biomech.* 2004;19:564-571.
937. van Wingerden JP, Vleeming A, Buyruk HM, Raissadat K. Stabilization of the sacroiliac joint in vivo: verification of muscular contribution to force closure of the pelvis. *Eur Spine J.* 2004;13:199-205.
938. Mens JM, Damen L, Snijders CJ, Stam HJ. The mechanical effect of a pelvic belt in patients with pregnancy-related pelvic pain. *Clin Biomech.* 2006;21(2):122-127.
939. Snijders CJ, Hermans PF, Kleinrensink GJ. Functional aspects of cross-legged sitting with special attention to piriformis muscles and sacroiliac joints. *Clin Biomech.* 2006;21(2):116-121.
940. Pel JJM, Spoor CW, Pool-Goudzwaard AL, Hoek van Dijke GA, Snijders CJ. Biomechanical analysis of reduction sacroiliac joint shear load by optimization of pelvic muscle and ligament forces. *Ann Biomed Eng.* 2008;6:415-424.
941. Hungerford B, Gilleard W, Hodges P. Evidence of altered lumbopelvic muscle recruitment in the presence of sacroiliac joint pain. *Spine.* 2003;28:1593-1600.
942. Pool-Goudzwaard AL, Slieker Ten Hove MC, Vierhout ME, et al. Relations between pregnancy related low back pain, pelvic floor activity and pelvic floor dysfunction. *Int Urogynecol J Pelvic Floor Dysfunct.* 2005;16:468-474.
943. Bergmark A. Stability of the lumbar spine. A study in mechanical engineering. *Acta Orthop Scand Suppl.* 1989;230:1-54.
944. Gutke A, Ostgaard HC, Oberg B. Association between muscle function and low back pain in relation to pregnancy. *J Rehabil Med.* 2008;40:304-311.
945. Mens JM, Vleeming A, Snijders CJ, Koes BW, Stam HJ. Validity of the active straight leg raise test for measuring disease severity in patients with posterior pelvic pain after pregnancy. *Spine (Phila Pa 1976).* 2002;27(2):196-200.
946. Mens JM, Vleeming A, Snijders CJ, Koes BW, Stam HJ. Reliability and validity of the active straight leg raise test in posterior pelvic pain since pregnancy. *Spine (Phila Pa 1976).* 2001;26:1167-1171.
947. Mens JM, Vleeming A, Snijders CJ, Ronchetti I, Stam HJ. Reliability and validity of hip adduction strength to measure disease severity in posterior pelvic pain since pregnancy. *Spine (Phila Pa 1976).* 2002;27:1674-1679.
948. Noren L, Ostgaard S, Johansson G, Ostgaard HC. Lumbar back and posterior pelvic pain during pregnancy: a 3-year follow-up. *Eur Spine J.* 2002;11(3):267-271.
949. Barker PJ, Briggs CA. Attachments of the posterior layer of lumbar fascia. *Spine (Phila Pa 1976).* 1999;24:1757-1764.
950. Hodges PW, Richardson CA. Inefficient muscular stabilization of the lumbar spine associated with low back pain. A motor control evaluation of transversus abdominis. *Spine (Phila Pa 1976).* 1996;21:2640-2650.
951. Moseley GL, Hodges PW, Gandevia SC. Deep and superficial fibers of the lumbar multifidus muscle are differentially active during voluntary arm movements. *Spine (Phila Pa 1976).* 2002;27(2):E29-E36.
952. Ashton-Miller JA, Howard D, Delancey JO. The functional anatomy of the female pelvic floor and stress continence control system. *Scand J Urol Nephrol.* 2001;(207):1-7; discussion 106-125.

953. Sapsford R, Hodges P. Contraction of the pelvic floor muscles during abdominal manoeuvres. *Arch Phys Med Rehabil.* 2001;82:1081-1088.
954. Bo K, Sherburn M. Evaluation of female pelvic-floor muscle function and strength. *Phys Ther.* 2005;85:269-282.
955. Ashton-Miller JA, Delancey JO. On the biomechanics of vaginal birth and common sequelae. *Annu Rev Biomed Eng.* 2009;11:163-176.
956. Stoker J. Anorectal and pelvic floor anatomy. *Best Prac Res Clin Gastroenterol.* 2009;23:463-475.
957. Eliasson K, Elfving B, Nordgren B, Mattsson E. Urinary incontinence in women with low back pain. *Man Ther.* 2008;13:206-212.
958. Thom DH, Rortveit G. Prevalence of postpartum urinary incontinence: a systematic review. *Acta Obstet Gynecol Scand.* 2010;89:1511-1522.
959. Viktrup L, Rortveit G, Lose G. Risk of stress urinary incontinence twelve years after the first pregnancy and delivery. *Obstet Gynecol.* 2006;108:248-254.
960. O'Sullivan PB, Beales DJ. Diagnosis and classification of pelvic girdle pain disorders. Part 2: illustration of the utility of a classification system via case studies. *Man Ther.* 2007;12:e1-e12.
961. Stuge B, Veierod MB, Laerum E, Vollestad N. The efficacy of a treatment program focusing on specific stabilizing exercises for pelvic girdle pain after pregnancy: a two-year follow-up of a randomized clinical trial. *Spine.* 2004;29(10):E197-E203.
962. O'Sullivan PB, Grahamslaw KM, Kendell M, Lapenskie SC, Moller NE, Richards KV. The effect of different standing and sitting postures on trunk muscle activity in a pain-free population. *Spine.* 2002;27:1238-1244.
963. Sapsford RR, Richardson CA, Stanton WR. Sitting posture affects pelvic floor muscle activity in parous women: an observational study. *Aust J Physiother.* 2006;52:219-222.
964. Ostgaard HC, Zetherstrom G, Roos-Hansson E, Svanberg B. Reduction of back and posterior pelvic pain in pregnancy. *Spine.* 1994;19:894-900.
965. Wu WH, Meijer OG, Uegaki K, et al. Pregnancy-related pelvic girdle pain (PPP), I: terminology, clinical presentation, and prevalence. *Eur Spine J.* 2004;13:575-589.
966. Ostgaard HC, Andersson GBJ. Previous back pain and risk of developing back pain in a future pregnancy. *Spine.* 1991;16:432-436.
967. Rost CC, Jacqueline J, Kaiser A, Verhagen AP, Koes BW. Prognosis of women with pelvic pain during pregnancy: a long-term follow-up study. *Acta Obstet Gynecol Scand.* 2006;85:771-777.
968. Robinson HS, Mengshoel AM, Veierød MB, Vøllestad N. Pelvic girdle pain: potential risk factors in pregnancy in relations to disability and pain intensity three months postpartum. *Man Ther.* 2010;15:522-528.
969. Sturesson B, Uden G, Uden A. Pain pattern in pregnancy and "catching" of the leg in pregnant women with posterior pelvic pain. *Spine.* 1997;22:1880-1883; discussion 1884.
970. Ostgaard HC, Zetherstrom G, Roos-Hansson E, Svanberg B. Reduction of back and posterior pelvic pain in pregnancy. *Spine.* 1994;19:894-900.
971. Gutke A, Ostgaard HC, Oberg B. Predicting persistent pregnancy-related low back pain. *Spine* (Phila Pa 1976). 2008;33:E386-E393.
972. Gutke A, Kjellby-Wendt G, Öberg B. The inter-rater reliability of a standardized classification system for pregnancy-related lumbopelvic pain. *Man Ther.* 2010;15:13-18.
973. Fortin JD, Aprill CN, Ponthieux B, Pier J. Sacroiliac joint: pain referral maps upon applying a new injection/arthrography technique. Part II: clinical evaluation. *Spine.* 1994;19:1483-1489.
974. Fortin JD, Dwyer AP, West S, Pier J. Sacroiliac joint: pain referral maps upon applying a new injection/arthrography technique. Part I: asymptomatic volunteers. *Spine.* 1994;19:1475-1482.
975. Schwarzer AC, Aprill CN, Bogduk N. The sacroiliac joint in chronic low back pain. *Spine.* 1995;20:31-7.
976. Dreyfuss P, Michaelsen M, Pauza K, McLarty J, Bogduk N. The value of medical history and physical examination in diagnosing sacroiliac joint pain. *Spine.* 1996;21:2594-2602.
977. Slipman CW, Jackson HB, Lipetz JS, Chan KT, Lenrow D, Vresilovic EJ. Sacroiliac joint pain referral zones. *Arch Phys Med Rehabil.* 2000;81:334-338.
978. Young S, Aprill C, Laslett M. Correlation of clinical examination characteristics with three sources of chronic low back pain. *Spine J.* 2003;3:460-465.
979. Fukui S, Nosaka S. Pain patterns originating from the sacroiliac joints. *J Anesth.* 2002;16:245-247.
980. Slipman CW, Patel RK, Whyte WS, et al. Diagnosing and managing sacroiliac pain. *J Musculoskel Med.* 2001;18:325-332.
981. Chou LH, Slipman CW, Bhagia SM, et al. Inciting events initiating injection-proven sacroiliac joint syndrome. *Pain Med.* 2004;5:26-32.
982. Laslett M, McDonald B, Tropp H, Aprill CN, Oberg B. Agreement between diagnoses reached by clinical examination and available reference standards: a prospective study of 216 patients with lumbopelvic pain. *BMC Musculoskelet Disord.* 2005;6:28.
983. Levangie PK. The association between static pelvic asymmetry and low back pain. *Spine.* 1999;24:1234-1242.
984. Altman R, Alarcon G, Appelrouth D, et al. The American College of Rheumatology criteria for the classification and reporting of osteoarthritis of the hip. *Arthritis Rheum.* 1991;34:505-514.
985. Mellin G. Correlations of hip mobility with degree of back pain and lumbar spinal mobility in chronic low-back pain patients. *Spine.* 1988;13:668-670.
986. Ellison JB, Rose SJ, Sahrmann SA. Patterns of hip rotation range of motion: comparison between healthy subjects and patients with low back pain. *Phys Ther.* 1990;70:537-541.
987. Broadhurst NA, Bond MJ. Pain provocation tests for the assessment of sacroiliac joint dysfunction. *J Spinal Disord.* 1998;11:341-345.
988. Bewyer KJ, Bewyer DC, Messenger D, Kennedy CM. Pilot data: association between gluteus medius weakness and low back pain during pregnancy. *Iowa Orthop J.* 2009;29:97-99.
989. Tong HC, Heyman OG, Lado DA, Isser MM. Interexaminer reliability of three methods of combining test results to determine side of sacral restriction, sacral base position, and innominate bone position. *J Am Osteopath Assoc.* 2006;106:464-468.
990. Mann M, Glasheen-Wray M, Nyberg R. Therapist agreement for palpation and observation of iliac crest heights. *Phys Ther.* 1984;64:334-338.
991. Potter NA, Rothstein JM. Intertester reliability for selected tests of the sacroiliac joint. *Phys Ther.* 1985;65:1671-1675.
992. Tullberg T, Blomberg S, Branth B, Johnsson R. Manipulation does not alter the position of the sacroiliac joint: a Roentgen stereophotogrammetric analysis. *Spine.* 1998;23:1124-1128.
993. Levangie PK. The association between static pelvic asymmetry and low back pain. *Spine.* 1999;24:1234-1242.

994. O'Haire C, Gibbons P. Inter-examiner and intra-examiner agreement for assessing sacroiliac anatomical landmarks using palpation and observation. *Man Ther.* 2000;5:13-20.
995. Albert H, Godskesen M, Westergaard J. Evaluation of clinical tests used in classification procedures in pregnancy-related pelvic joint pain. *Eur Spine J.* 2000;9:161-166.
996. Riddle DL, Freburger JK, and the North American Orthopaedic Rehabilitation Research Network. Evaluation of the presence of sacroiliac region dysfunction using a combination of tests: a multicenter intertester reliability study. *Phys Ther.* 2002;82:772-781.
997. Krawiec CJ, Denegar CR, Hertel J, Salvaterra GF, Buckley WE. Static innominate asymmetry and leg length discrepancy in asymptomatic collegiate athletes. *Man Ther.* 2003;8:207-213.
998. Stovall BA, Kumar S. Anatomical landmark asymmetry assessment in the lumbar spine and pelvis: a review of reliability. *PM R.* 2010;2:48-56.
999. Cibulka MT, Koldehoff R. Clinical usefulness of a cluster of sacroiliac joint tests in patients with and without low back pain. *J Orthop Sports Phys Ther.* 1999;29(2):83-92.
1000. Wiles MR. Reproducibility and interexaminer correlation of motion plapation findings of the sacroiliac joints. *J Can Chiropr Assoc.* 1980;24:59-69.
1001. Carmichael JP. Inter- and intra-examiner reliability of palpation for sacroiliac joint dysfunction. *J Manipulative Physiol Ther.* 1987;10:164-171.
1002. Bowman C, Gribble R. The value of the forward flexion tests and three tests of leg length changes in the clinical assessment of movement of the sacroiliac joint. *J Orthop Med.* 1995;17:66-67.
1003. Vincent-Smith B, Gibbons P. Inter-examiner and intra-examiner reliability of the standing flexion test. *Man Ther.* 1999;4:87-93.
1004. Robinson HS, Brox JI, Robinson R, Bjelland E, Solem S, Telje T. The reliability of selected motion and pain provocation tests for the sacroiliac joint. *Man Ther.* 2007;12:72-79.
1005. Hungerford B, Gilleard W, Lee D. Altered patterns of pelvic bone motion determined in subjects with posterior pelvic pain using skin markers. *Clin Biomech.* 2004;19:456-464.
1006. Hungerford B, Gilleard W, Moran M, Emmerson C. Evaluation of the ability of Physical Therapists to palpate intrapelvic motion with the stork test on the support side. *Phys Ther.* 2007;87:879-887.
1007. Albert H, Godskesen M, Westergaard J. Prognosis in four syndromes of pregnancy-related pelvic pain. *Acta Obstet Gynecol Scand.* 2001;80:505-511.
1008. Vleeming A, Pool-Goudzwaard AL, Hammudoghlu D, Stoeckart R, Snijders CJ, Mens JM. The function of the long dorsal sacroiliac ligament: its implication for understanding low back pain. *Spine.* 1996;21:556-562.
1009. Vleeming A, de Bries JH, Mens JMA, van Wingerden JP. Possible role of the long dorsal sacroiliac ligament in women with peripartum pelvic pain. *Acta Obstet Gynecol Scand.* 2002;81:430-436.
1010. Noble E. *Essential Exercises for the Childbearing Year.* 2nd ed. Boston, MA: Houghton Mifflin Co; 1982.
1011. Lo T, Candido G, Janssen P. Diastasis of the recti abdominis in pregnancy: risk factors and treatment. *Physiother Can.* 1999;51:32-37.
1012. Sheppard S. The role of transversus abdominis in post partum correction of gross divarication recti. *Man Ther.* 1996;1:214-216.
1013. Spitznagle TM, Leong FC, Va Dillen LR. Prevalence of diastasis recti abdominis in a urogynecological patient population. *Int Urogynecol J.* 2007;18:321-328.
1014. Parker MA, Millar AL, Dugan SA. Diastasis rectus abdominis and lumbo-pelvic pain and dysfunction—are they related? *J Womens Health Phys Ther.* 2009;33(2):15-22.
1015. Bieniarz J, Yoshida T, Romero-Salinas G, Curuchet E, Caldeyro-Barcia R, Crottogini JJ. Aortocaval compression by the uterus in late human pregnancy. IV. Circulatory homeostasis by preferential perfusion of the placenta. *Am J Obstet Gynecol.* 1969;103:19-31.
1016. ACOG Committee Opinion No. 267. Exercise during pregnancy and the postpartum period. *Obstet Gynecol.* 2002;99:171-173. http://mail.ny.acog.org/website/SMIPodcast/Exercise.pdf. Accessed April 5, 2011.
1017. Vleeming A, Mooney V, Stoeckart R. *Movement, Stability and Lumbopelvic Pain.* 2nd ed. Philadelphia, PA: Churchll Livingstone; 2007.
1018. Kanakaris N, Roberts CS, Giannoudis PV. Pregnancy-related pelvic girdle pain and update. *BMC Med.* 2011;9:15.
1019. Vøllestad NK, Stuge B. Prognostic factors for recovery from postpartum pelvic girdle pain. *Eur Spine J.* 2009;18:718-726.
1020. Pennick VE, Young G. Interventions for preventing and treating pelvic and back pain in pregnancy. *Cochrane Database Syst Rev.* 2007;(2):CD001139.
1021. Vermani E, Mittal R, Weeks A. Pelvic girdle pain and low back pain in pregnancy: a review. *Pain Pract.* 2010;10:60-71.
1022. Elden H, Fagevik-Olsen M, Ostgaard HC, Stener-Victorin E, Hagberg H. Acupuncture as an adjunct to standard treatment for pelvic girdle pain in pregnant women: randomized double-blinded controlled trial comparing acupuncture with non-penetrating sham acupuncture. *BJOG.* 2008;115:1655-1668.
1023. Ostgaard HC, Zetherstrom G, Roos-Hansson E. Back pain in relation to pregnancy: a 6-year follow-up. *Spine.* 1997;22:2945-2950.
1024. Association of Chartered Physiotherapists in Women's Health. Pregnancy-related pelvic girdle pain (PGP)—for health professionals. *ACPWH Web site.* http://acpwh.csp.org.uk/publications/pregnancy-related-pelvic-girdle-pain-pgp-health-professionals. Accessed September 20, 2013.
1025. Lile J, Perkins J, Hammer RL, Loubert PV. Diagnostic and management strategies for pregnant women with back pain. *JAAPA.* 2003;16:31-44.
1026. Thomas IL, Nicklin J, Pollock H, Faulkner K. Evaluation of a maternity cushion (Ozzlo pillow) for backache and insomnia in late pregnancy. *Aust N Z J Obstet Gynaecol.* 1989;29:133-138.
1027. Park KM, Kim SY, Oh DW. Effects of the pelvic compression belt on gluteus medius, quadratus lumborum, and lumbar multifidus activities during side-lying hip abduction. *J Electromyogr Kinesiol.* 2010;20:1141-1145.
1028. Kanakaris NK, Roberts CS, Giannoudis PV. Pregnancy-related pelvic girdle pain: an update. *BMC Med.* 2011;9:15.
1029. Khorsan R, Hawk C, Lisi A, Kizhakkeveettil A. Manipulative therapy for pregnancy and related conditions: a systematic review. *Obstet Gynecol Surv.* 2009;64:416-427.
1030. Borggren CL. Pregnancy and chiropractic: a narrative review of the literature. *J Chiropr Med.* 2007;6:70-74.
1031. Stuber KJ, Wynd S, Weis CA. Adverse events from spinal manipulation in the pregnant and postpartum. *Chiropr Man Ther.* 2012;20:8.

1032. Licciardone JC, Buchanan S, Hensel KL, King HH, Fulda KG, Stoll ST. Osteopathic manipulative treatment of back painand related symptoms during pregnancy: a randomized controlled trial. *Am J Obstet Gynecol.* 2010;202:43.e1-43.e8.
1033. Murphy DR, Hurwitz EL, McGovern EE. Outcome of pregnancy-related lumbopelvic pain treated according to a diagnosis-based decision rule: a prospective observational cohort study. *J Manipulative Physiol Ther.* 2009;32:616-624.
1034. Murphy DR, Hurwitz EL. A theoretical model for the development of a diagnosis-based clinical decision rule for the management of patients with spinal pain. *BMC Musculoskelet Disord.* 2007;8:75.
1035. Al-Sayegh NA, George SE, Boninger ML, Rogers JC, Whitney SL, Delitto A. Spinal mobilization of postpartum low back and pelvic girdle pain: an evidence-based clinical rule for predicting responders and nonresponders. *PM R.* 2010;2:995-1005.
1036. DonTigny RL. Mechanics and treatment of the sacroiliac joint. In: Vleeming A, Mooney V, Dorman T, Snijders C, Stoeckart, eds. *Movement, Stability & Low Back Pain. The Essential Role of the Pelvis.* London, England: Churchill Livingstone; 1997:461-476.
1037. Vanelderen P, Szadek K, Cohen SP, et al. Evidence-based interventional pain medicine according to clinical diagnoses. Sacroiliac joint pain. *Pain Pract.* 2010;10:470-478.
1038. Sapsford R. Rehabilitation of pelvic floor muscles utilizing trunk stabilization. *Man Ther.* 2004;9:3-12.
1039. Hung H-C, Hsiao S-M, Chih S-Y, Lin H-H, Tsauo J-Y. An alternative intervention for urinary incontinence: retraining diaphragmatic, deep abdominal and pelvic floor muscle coordinated function. *Man Ther.* 2010;15:273-279.
1040. Dumoulin C, Hay-Smith J. Pelvic floor muscle training versus no treatment, or inactive control treatments, for urinary incontinence in women. *Cochrane Database Syst Rev.* 2010;(1):CD005654.

Please visit www.routledge.com/9781556429323 to access additional material.

Chapter 5

Evidence-Based Physical Therapy Practice for Thoracic Spinal Pain

In comparison to low back pain (LBP) and cervical pain, research related to thoracic back pain is scarce. Thoracic spinal pain (TSP) or thoracic spine-related pain may be located on the anterior, lateral, or posterior thorax between the 1st and 12th thoracic vertebrae. In this region, numerous sources of musculoskeletal or nonmusculoskeletal pain or other symptoms challenge the clinician. The thorax can be a significant source of local pain and symptoms as well as referred pain from visceral structures, the cervical spine, thoracic spine, and rib cage. In addition to protection of vital organs (ie, heart and lungs), the thorax serves as a transitional zone for transfer of load or forces to and from the upper and lower halves of the body.

The thorax is biomechanically and functionally related to the lumbar spine, pelvic girdle, hip, cervical, and shoulder girdle regions. Many muscles that control the cervicobrachial regions and lumbopelvic regions have attachments in the thorax. The cervical spine is often a source of referred pain to the upper and mid-thoracic spine. Reduced or excessive mobility or poor motor control of the thoracic spine may cause or contribute to pain and dysfunction in the cervical spine, lumbar spine, or shoulder girdle. For example, during functional activity, stiffness of the thorax places more movement demands on the cervical spine and shoulder regions. As discussed in the previous chapter, pain in the lumbar spine alters activation patterns of the superficial trunk muscles that span the thoracolumbar regions and may produce secondary pain and limited motion in the thorax. Since these regions are interdependent, the thoracic spine must be examined in persons presenting with LBP, neck pain, and shoulder complaints as well as in those presenting with a primary complaint of thoracic pain.

Prevalence, Incidence, and Risk Factors

Prevalence data are highly variable, based on age, gender, and definitions of thoracic pain. In general, thoracic pain is less prevalent than LBP or cervical pain in adults,[1] but studies report a higher prevalence during childhood and adolescence, specifically in females.[2] Prevalence for any thoracic pain ranged from 0.5% to 23.0% (7 days), 15.8% to 34.8% (1 month), 15.0% to 27.5% (1 year), and 12.0% to 31.2% (lifetime). A trend for prevalence to increase in middle adult years of 40 to 50 with a decrease into the later adult years of greater than 70 is observed.[1] Incidences were at 1 month (0% to 0.9%), 6 months (10.3%),[1] 1 year (3.8% to 35.3%), and 25 years (9.8%).[2] Thoracic pain was significantly associated with concurrent musculoskeletal pain; differences in growth, physical activity, lifestyle, social activity, and backpack usage; and postural, psychological, and environmental factors. In adolescents, risk factors included being older and having poorer mental health. During adolescence, performing less than 10 minutes of high physical activity a day substantially increased the odds (odds ratio [OR] = 7.2) of developing thoracic back pain over the next 3 years in 9- and 12-year-olds.[3] Boys and girls with pain at age 13 are 6.3 and 2.8 times more likely to report thoracic pain at age 17.[4]

Stetts DM, Carpenter JG. *Physical Therapy Management of Patients With Spinal Pain: An Evidence-Based Approach (pp 343-446).*

Risk factors for the development of thoracic back pain in adults, other than thoracic pain in adolescence, are unknown. The economic burden of thoracic back pain has not been established. However, some studies suggest that thoracic back pain results in reduced physical activity, increased care-seeking,[5] and difficulties with activities of daily living (ADL),[4] and it is a predictor of failure to return to work in individuals with LBP who present to primary care.[6] Considering the prevalence and impact on function, future studies are needed to investigate the economic impact of thoracic back pain.

Classification of Thoracic Spinal Pain

The medical diagnostic model, based on a pathoanatomical source, is the most common classification for persons with symptoms related to the thorax or TSP. Neuromusculoskeletal sources of pain include, but are not limited to, degenerative disc disease, disc herniation, spinal stenosis, fracture or dislocation of the vertebra or ribs, muscle strain, rib syndromes, costochondritis, osteoarthritis, intercostals neuralgia, thoracic outlet syndrome (TOS), trigger points, and scoliosis. Similar to LBP, a precise anatomical tissue cannot be reliably identified as the cause or pain generator for mechanical TSP. In a magnetic resonance imaging (MRI) thoracic spine study of asymptomatic subjects, Wood et al[7] found high prevalence of anatomic irregularities such as disc herniation (37%), deformation of the spinal cord (29%), and Scheuermann end plate irregularities or kyphosis (38%). Scheuermann's disease generally presents at ages 8 to 16 years with multilevel Schmorl's nodes, vertebral wedging, and endplate degenerative changes of the mid-lower thoracic and upper lumbar spine resulting in a rigid thoracic kyphosis, which may or may not be painful.[7]

Twenty subjects with 48 asymptomatic thoracic disc herniations were followed for a mean period of 26 months.[8] The disc herniations were generally unchanged, and large herniations tended to decrease in size. All subjects remained asymptomatic during follow-up. Differentiation between symptomatic and asymptomatic thoracic disc herniation is not easily determined by MRI.[8] In another MRI study,[9] degenerative changes in the thoracic spine were observed in 47% of subjects at 1 or more intervertebral levels. Positive MRI findings included decreased signal intensity in intervertebral discs (37.2%), posterior disc protrusion (30.9%), anterior dural sac compression (29.8%), and disc space narrowing (4.3%). MRI findings increased with age.[9] Classification of TSP using pathoanatomical diagnoses has not been validated. However, some anatomic diagnoses such as compressions fractures and thoracic myelopathy are important to rule in or rule out.

After excluding medical disease and neurological compromise such as radiculopathy or myelopathy, limitations of the medical model for TSP lead to a diagnostic category of mechanical or nonspecific thoracic pain. A reliable and valid classification of persons with nonspecific thoracic pain into subgroups with key diagnostic criteria does not exist. However, characteristics of the LBP subgroup classifications discussed in Chapter 4 provide a plausible framework to aid in the diagnosis and management of TSP.

Most clinicians would agree that patients with mechanical thoracic pain with or without pain related to the rib cage do not have a homogeneous condition. Other than pathoanatomy, classification approaches can be based on various factors such as length of symptoms (acute, subacute, chronic); a biomechanical model of form/force closure, motor control, and emotions[10]; movement impairments; response to repeated movements[11,12]; and/or biopsychosocial factors, but clinical trials have not been completed to investigate any of these systems for TSP.

The concepts from several classification systems are used to develop the proposed classification of TSP in this reference. The response to repeated movements generates a diagnostic classification similar to LBP.[11] After exclusion of nonmechanical causes of TSP, medical disease, and neurological disorders, Olson[13] described an impairment-based classification for nonspecific mechanical TSP. This diagnostic classification (Table 5-1) is supported by key examination findings and proposed interventions, but reliability and validity are unknown. Lee and Lee[14] propose an integrated model that provides the basis for assessment and treatment of TSP with the goal of regaining optimum function. These authors define optimum function of the thorax as a balance of stability and mobility specific to the load, predictability, and threat of the immediate task while maintaining a normal breathing pattern and intra-abdominal pressure.[14] Nonoptimal function results in failure of load transfer between the upper and lower body requiring assessment of form closure, force closure, motor control strategies, and emotions to determine why load failure has occurred.[14]

A TSP classification system with strong current evidence to support its use and ability to improve patient outcomes is not available, but it is likely that persons with nonspecific TSP can be classified into subgroups based on patterns of signs and symptoms. To assist the clinician with matching a patient's clinical presentation to an appropriate intervention, a proposed impairment-based classification system for TSP is presented, integrating current best research, concepts used in the classification of LBP, and a clinical reasoning process to guide decision making toward best treatment strategies of TSP.

TABLE 5-1. IMPAIRMENT-BASED CLASSIFICATION FOR THORACIC SPINE PAIN DISORDERS

CLASSIFICATION	EXAMINATION FINDINGS	PROPOSED INTERVENTIONS
Thoracic hypomobility	• Restricted active range of motion (AROM) • Restricted PPIVM and/or PAIVM • No upper extremity radicular symptoms • Muscle imbalances • Postural deviations	• Mobility exercises • Thoracic spine and rib mobilization/manipulation • ULNDT exercise • Postural exercise
Thoracic hypomobility with upper extremity referred pain	• Restricted AROM • Restricted PPIVM and/or PAIVM of the upper thoracic spine and ribs • Upper extremity symptoms • Positive upper limb neurodynamic tests (ULNDT) • Muscle imbalances • Postural deviations	• Mobility exercise • Thoracic spine and rib mobilization/manipulation • ULNDT mobilization/exercise • Self-mobilization techniques • Postural exercise
Thoracic hypomobility with neck pain	• Symptoms <30 days • No symptoms distal to the shoulder • No aggravation of symptoms with looking up • Fear-Avoidance Beliefs Questionnaire with physical activity scale <12 • Diminished upper thoracic spine kyphosis (visual observation) • Cervical extension ROM <30 degrees by inclinometer	• Thoracic and rib mobilization/manipulation • Mobility exercises • Treatment of cervical impairments
Thoracic hypomobility with shoulder impairments	• Stiff thoracic spine with shoulder AROM • Restricted PPIVM or PAIVM in the upper thoracic spine and ribs • Shoulder impingement/rotator cuff signs • Muscle imbalances • Postural deviations	• Mobility exercises • Thoracic and rib mobilization/manipulation • Self-mobilization techniques • Postural exercises
Thoracic hypomobility with LBP	• Stiff thoracic spine with thoracolumbar AROM • Restricted PPIVM or PAIVM • Lumbar impairments • Muscle imbalances • Postural deviations	• Mobility exercises • Thoracic and rib mobilization/manipulation • Lumbar rehabilitation • Self-mobilization techniques • Postural exercises
Thoracic clinical instability	• History of trauma or thoracic surgery • Provocation of symptoms with sustained weight-bearing posture • Relief of symptoms with nonweightbearing postures • PPIVM or PAIVM hypermobility (loose end feel) • Poor strength (2/5 of thoracic multifidus, erector spinae, and parascapular muscles) • Shaking/poorly controlled (aberrant) motion with thoracic AROM	• Postural education • Thoracic stabilization exercise program • Parascapular exercises • Mobilization/manipulation above and below hypermobilities • Ergonomic correction

PPIVM indicates passive physiological intervertebral movement; PAIVM, passive accessory intervertebral movement
Adapted from *Manual Physical Therapy of the Spine*, Olson KA, Copyright 2009, with permission from Elsevier.

History

Chapter 2 reviews the components of the subjective examination (see Table 2-3). Specifically, the section on medical screening assists in identifying systemic disease or illness that can mimic neuromusculoskeletal symptoms or conditions. While there is little to no evidence of the reliability and validity of data obtained from the history related to TSP, the importance of a detailed history should not be underestimated.

Diagnostic Triage

Diagnostic triage occurs in the same manner as for LBP. A focused history and physical examination are used to classify patients into 1 of 3 categories: nonspecific TSP, TSP with potential radiculopathy or myelopathy, or TSP potentially due to serious spinal pathology. The process of classifying persons with TSP begins with ruling out serious underlying disease or nonspinal pathology and determines if the patient is appropriate for physical therapy (PT) services or if a medical referral is needed. The disease or systems capable of referring pain or other symptoms to the thoracic spine are infection, cardiovascular, oncology, pulmonary, renal, and gastrointestinal (GI).[15] Among 24 620 primary care encounters, Verdon et al[16] reported on 672 consecutive patients presenting with thoracic pain. At 3-month follow-up, the main diagnoses were: thoracic wall pain 51%, chest wall syndrome (CWS) 44.6%, traumatic 4%, divers 2.4%, cardiovascular diseases (CVD) 16%, coronary artery diseases (CAD) 12.5%, non-CAD 3.4%, psychogenic pain 11%, respiratory diseases 10%, GI disorders 8%, and no diagnosis 4%. CWS of 300 cases represented 1.2% of all consultations and was more common than CAD of 84 cases or 0.34%. For CWS, 155 were women and 145 were men, with the overall mean age of 50.3 ± 18.2 years and included teenagers and patients more than 75. In CWS, 62% of cases were new, 35% were old or recurrent, and 3% undetermined. In half of the patients, a thoracic pain complaint was the principal one. Comorbidity was noted for 250 patients or 83% as follows: 50% or 149 psychiatry disorders, 33.3% or 100 patients with CVD, 20.7% or 62 patients with rheumatologic disease, and 2 cases of spondylarthritis, but no rheumatoid diseases. Six patients had neoplastic disease that included 2 lung cancers.[16]

Serious pathology in the thorax is associated with key clinical findings. Differential diagnosis includes a detailed history, identification of risk factors, examination findings, and continual reassessment to determine the response to treatment. Figure 2-3 in Chapter 2 depicts common visceral referral patterns. Goodman and Snyder[15] provide an excellent reference for additional study related to the clinical presentation of medical disease in patients presenting with musculoskeletal complaints.

Screening for Red Flags of Serious Thoracic Spine Pathology

Screening for Infection as a Cause of Thoracic Spinal Pain

Spinal infection related to LBP was discussed in Chapter 4, and the screening concepts are applicable to the thorax. Vertebral osteomyelitis commonly targets the thoracic spine and may occur after surgery, open fractures, skin breakdown and ulcers, and systemic infections.[17] Susceptible individuals are diabetics, intravenous drug users, alcoholics, persons on corticosteroid drugs, the elderly, or any individual who is immunocompromised.[16,18] In general, vertebral osteomyelitis presents with constant pain that is more severe at night; all movements are painful with localized tenderness and muscle guarding; ESR is likely to be elevated; and fever and sweating are common but not always present.[17] Discitis or disc space infection is another form of osteomyelitis commonly affecting the lower thoracic and lumbar spines. Discitis can occur after discectomy, urinary tract infection, upper respiratory infection, or gastroenteritis.[17]

Screening for Cardiovascular Causes of Thoracic Spinal Pain

The most common CVD causes of TSP are associated with angina, myocardial infarction, and aneurysm.[17] Screening for an abdominal aortic aneurysm was discussed in Chapter 4. Patients with CVD risk factors should be examined closely for pain referral patterns; symptom descriptors such as constant, deep, boring pain; or throbbing and pulsating symptoms. The absence of aggravating factors related to movement and with increasing pain with activity that requires increased cardiac output such as climbing stairs is often present and eased when the activity stops.[17] Location of the aneurysm determines the symptoms. Typical complaints of pain with aortic dissection of the ascending aorta or just distal to left subclavian artery are severe, acute, anterior chest pain that radiates to the upper back region. Radial pulses may be unequal.[19]

Pain from angina or myocardial infarction can present as isolated mid-thoracic back pain in men or postmenopausal women with or without varying patterns of the jaw, neck, shoulder, arm, or chest symptoms such as substernal pressure, tightness, or squeezing complaints. Classically, the presentation of pain is in the left chest and left upper extremity (UE), but for women and the elderly, epigastric; mid-thoracic; or right shoulder, neck, jaw, and teeth pain are more likely. Since the heart is innervated by C3 through T4 spinal nerves, pain may be experienced in any part of the body innervated by these levels.[17] Additional symptoms such as diaphoresis, nausea, vomiting, and shortness of breath are often present, but up to 25% of myocardial infarctions are silent or go unrecognized.[17,19]

Screening for risk factors of CVD and assessment of vital signs must be performed.

Screening for Cancer as a Cause of Thoracic Spinal Pain

Cancer as a cause of LBP was discussed in Chapter 4 (see Table 4-2). In 1975, 316 patients (16%) presenting to primary care with spinal pain had thoracic spine pain.[20] Two of these patients, or 0.63%, had cancer-related thoracic pain while a similar percentage (0.66%) had cancer-related LBP. Deyo and Diehl[20] reported 4 clinical findings with the highest positive likelihood ratios (+LR) for detecting the presence of metastatic cancer in spinal pain: (1) previous history of non-skin cancer (+LR 14.7), (2) failure of conservative management in past month (+LR 3.0), (3) age >50 years (+LR 2.7), and (4) unexplained weight loss of more than 4.5 kg in 6 months (+LR 2.7). The absence of all 4 of these clinical findings essentially rules out cancer (Sn 1.0, Sp 0.6). Of these 4 red flags, the most useful is a previous history of cancer with a pooled +LR of 23.7, while the other 3 had +LRs of 3.[21] Laboratory test results had the following significant LRs[20]:

- Erythrocyte sedimentation rate (ESR) >50 mm/h (+LR 18.0, –LR 0.46)
- Presence of anemia (+LR 3.9, –LR 0.53)
- Hematocrit 30% (+LR 18.2)
- White blood cell count >12000 (+LR 4.1)

Since the spine is a common site for metastasis (Figure 5-1), a previous history of cancer is a red flag for a patient presenting with thoracic pain. Brihaye et al[22] reviewed 1477 cases of spinal metastases with epidural compromise and found that 16.5% were from primary breast tumor, 15.6% from the lung, 9.25% from the prostate, and 6.5% from the kidney. In addition to persistent thoracic back pain and movement impairment, painful or painless neurological deficit associated with cord compression often occurs.[23]

The most common primary cancer of the spine is multiple myeloma, a cancer of plasma cells often resulting in osteoporosis and compression fractures.[17] In the earliest stages, cancer can present as mechanical TSP, making the differential diagnosis difficult. When suspicion is high for cancer-related spinal pain, the clinician must complete a detailed history: ask for symptoms anywhere else in the body, the presence of night pain, the presence of constitutional symptoms such as fever and unexplained weight loss, and the presence of a previous history of cancer. Local pain with percussion of the involved spinous process (SP), movement impairment, and muscle guarding are present.[17] Because a thoracic radiculopathy or myelopathy may be present, a neurological examination is required. A progressive worsening of symptoms overtime is likely along with failure of conservative management within the past month.[23]

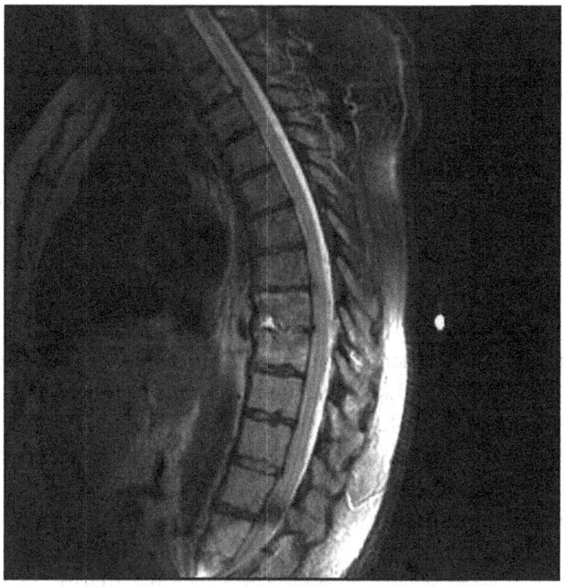

Figure 5-1. MRI of metastases to the thoracic spine.

Screening for Pulmonary Causes of Thoracic Spinal Pain

Common disorders that refer pain to the thorax are pleuritis, pneumonia, pneumothorax, pulmonary embolus, cor pulmonale, and pleurisy. When taking a history of a patient presenting with upper quarter pain or symptoms, a recent history of any pulmonary disorder is a red flag.[17] Pleuritis or inflammation of the membranes that line the chest cavity is a common cause of chest pain, usually described as sharp; well localized; and made worse with breathing, sneezing, or coughing.[24] Pleuritis may occur with pneumonia; pulmonary embolism; lung cancer; or lower respiratory infections such as bronchitis, influenza, and pneumonia due to overuse of the chest wall muscles during coughing. Associated symptoms of lung disease include persistent cough, sputum, hemoptysis, shortness of breath, rapid heartbeat, anxiety, faintness, cyanosis, general malaise, or other constitutional symptoms.[17] Pulmonary embolism presents with acute onset of dyspnea; pleuritic chest pain; severe hypoxia; and risk factors that might include recent surgery, a bed ridden or sedentary state, neoplasm, and trauma or fractures of the extremities. The most common cause of pulmonary embolus is deep vein thrombosis of the lower extremity.[17,19]

Chest or back pain may vary with the respiratory cycle such as inspiration or coughing, but this does not rule in a pulmonary cause of TSP nor does it rule out a musculoskeletal cause.[17] Autosplinting, or lying on the involved side to ease symptoms, may be present. This position reduces respiratory movements and pain. Vital sign assessment and chest auscultation should be performed.[17]

Screening for Renal Causes of Thoracic Spinal Pain

The upper urinary tract most commonly refers to the posterior subcostal thoracic spine, costovertebral area, or ipsilateral shoulder if the diaphragm is irritated, and less often across the low back with referral around the flank to the lower abdomen and groin. The lower urinary tract usually refers to the lumbopelvic and sacral regions. A history of trauma to the area, a recent urinary tract infection, urinary frequency or urgency, dysuria, hematuria, and testicular pain increase the suspicion for a renal source of symptoms.[17] Disorders such as perinephric abscess or pyelonephritis (ie, kidney infection) may present as a dull, constant pain and associated symptoms of fever, chills, frequent urination, or blood in the urine. Percussion to the costovertebral angle may reproduce back or flank pain; percussion to this area should produce no pain or discomfort. Lower thoracic or upper lumbar pain radiating to the flank or iliac crest may be due to kidney stones. As the kidney stone passes, intermittent severe pain is produced radiating down the ureter into the groin and often associated with nausea, vomiting, sweating, tachycardia, and bloody urine.[17]

Screening for Gastrointestinal Causes of Thoracic Spinal Pain

Thoracic pain is commonly due to upper GI problems such as esophageal or stomach ulcers that present with sternal, epigastric, shoulder, scapular, or mid-back symptoms.[17,19] Associated symptoms include dysphagia, painful swallowing, early satiety, and weight loss. Long-term use of NSAIDs, alendronate, or other medications increases the risk of GI disturbances.[19] TSP made better or worse by eating is a red flag. Immediate change to within 30 minutes of eating suggests the upper GI tract is involved whereas a change 2 to 4 hours after eating suggests the lower GI tract, which is more likely associated with LBP. Pain linked to a duodenal ulcer occurs when the stomach is empty, may occur in waves, and is eased by antacids and relieved temporarily. Ulcers may hemorrhage, perforate, or cause obstruction and lead to additional symptoms. Nausea, vomiting, and weight loss may occur. Bleeding may occur as bright red vomit, coffee ground vomit, or melena or dark tarry stool.[17] The liver, gallbladder, and pancreas are also potential causes of referred pain to the thorax. Disorders of these organs are all related to the eating cycle. Pancreatitis or pancreatic carcinoma may refer pain to the upper back and midscapular areas. Acute pancreatitis results in a constant, boring epigastric pain and alcoholism, cholelithiasis, and hypertriglyceridemia should raise the index of suspicion.[19] Additional symptoms for the liver and gallbladder include fever, chills, nausea, indigestion, or jaundice. Specific questions should be pursued related to the function of these systems to assist in ruling in or ruling out a disease process.[17]

Screening for Fracture as a Cause of Thoracic Spinal Pain

Screening for fracture as a cause of LBP was discussed in Chapter 4 and is applicable to the thoracic spine. Because vertebral fractures in the absence of major trauma present similarly to acute nonspecific LBP, only 30% are identified in clinical practice.[21] Therefore, accurate diagnosis for the clinician is vital to appropriate management. In a review of 12 studies and 9 categories of clinical features, Henschke et al[25] identified 5 features based on methodological quality that could raise or lower the probability of vertebral fracture:

1. Age > 50 years (+LR 2.2, –LR 0.34)
2. Female gender (+LR 2.3, –LR 0.67)
3. Major trauma (+LR 12.8, –LR 0.37)
4. Pain and tenderness (+LR 6.7, –LR 0.44)
5. A distracting painful injury (+LR1.7, –LR 0.78)

Trauma with neurological signs and structural deformity or neurological deficit were also significant features (+LR 14.4 and +LR 46.4), while corticosteroid use and altered consciousness did not significantly alter the probability of fracture.[25] Deyo et al[26] reported from unpublished data that LBP and long-term corticosteroid therapy has a specificity of 0.995. A compression fracture is considered likely until proven otherwise.

Fractures of the thoracic spine and/or ribs associated with major trauma are most commonly due to motor vehicle accidents, violence, sporting activities, or falls. Approximately half of the injuries occur in the thoracic, lumbar, and sacral regions. The other half occur in the cervical spine and may result in spinal cord damage.[27] Pathologic fractures are related to osteomalacia, osteoporosis, Paget's disease, metastatic bone disease, inflammation, or infection.[17] Approximately 25% of postmenopausal women are affected by vertebral compression fractures (VCFs)[28] with increasing prevalence reaching 40% in women 80 years of age.[29] Compression fractures occur in older men, although they are less common.[30] In cases of moderate to severe osteoporosis a minor trauma such as a sneeze, lifting a light object, or attempting to lift a heavy object may result in fracture. Pain, physical limitation, and increased risk of subsequent fractures lead to diminished quality of life, psychosocial issues, further disability, and a higher mortality rate compared to those who do not experience compression fractures.

Details of the mechanism of injury are important to understand the forces involved in the injury. However, some fractures occur without any history of increased force on the spine. Onset can be insidious with only moderate pain early in the course of progressive disease.[31] Multiple fractures result in loss of height and kyphosis reducing thoracic and abdominal space with the potential for reduced pulmonary function, early satiety, and weight loss.[32] Pain may continue after the fracture has healed. In addition to pain, symptoms suggesting neurological compromise such as numbness, tingling, or weakness should be specified. Easing factors include lying supine, while walking and standing are aggravating.[31] Pain and tenderness are located over the area of acute fracture, increased kyphosis may be noted, and a neurological examination should be performed. When the index of suspicion is high, a referral for radiographic imaging is required.[23,31]

Clinical Signs and Symptoms of Thoracic Spinal Pain Associated With Neurological Involvement

Screening for Thoracic Spinal Pain With Radiculopathy or Myelopathy

Thoracic disc herniations are much less common than those found in the cervical and lumbar regions. However, asymptomatic thoracic disc herniations are relatively common. Wood et al[7] found a high prevalence (37%) of thoracic anatomic irregularities such as disc herniation. Even with a relatively high frequency of asymptomatic disc herniations, symptomatic herniations are uncommon, ranging from 1 in 1000 to 1 in 1 million persons. Neurological findings associated with thoracic disc herniations occur about 1 in 1 million annually.[33] Most herniated thoracic discs are central or centrolateral and below the level of T7.[34] If symptomatic, central protrusions may cause spinal cord compression. Centrolateral protrusions may present as a Brown-Séquard syndrome, and lateral protrusion may cause nerve root compression or radiculopathy.

Thoracic discogenic pain is difficult to diagnose, partially due to its rarity. The clinical presentation is often insidious with a dull thoracic pain as the initial symptom, but trauma such as twisting, lifting, and repetitive movements may also be the mechanism of injury. The exam findings are generally mechanical in nature but nonspecific to a precise anatomical tissue in the thoracic spine. The cervical and lumbopelvic regions must be examined as a source or contributor of symptoms. Depending on the location and extent of the herniation, patients may present with signs and/or symptoms of radiculopathy or more commonly myelopathy. Lower thoracic herniations may manifest as LBP and upper disc lesions as cervical pain.[33] Most patients are managed conservatively with surgical intervention reserved for neurological involvement.[33]

In addition to thoracic disc herniations, fracture, thoracic spine degenerative changes, and diabetes mellitus are common etiologies of thoracic pain with or without myelopathy or radiculopathy.[33,35] In general, clinical presentations related to neurological compromise include spinal cord compression (myelopathy) or nerve root compression (radiculopathy). Thoracic myelopathic symptoms may include bilateral leg weakness and paresthesia, increased lower extremity muscle tone, hyperreflexia, gait ataxia, widespread sensory impairment below the level of compression, and urinary and bowel dysfunction, with urgency most common.[34,36] Contralateral pain; temperature loss with ipsilateral spastic paresis below the level of the lesion; and ipsilateral loss of tactile discrimination, vibration, and position sense below the level of the lesion are suggestive of Brown-Séquard syndrome or hemisection of the spinal cord. Hyperactive patellar or Achilles reflexes, or clonus and Babinski's sign are usually present on exam.

Thoracic radiculopathy may present with axial pain and intermittent or constant electric, burning, or shooting pains in a band-like distribution (see thoracic dermatomes Figures 2-4 and 2-5) referred to the anterior thorax, chest, or abdomen.[33,35] Numbness or paresthesias typically in a unilateral dermatomal distribution is often reported. On physical exam, sensation to light touch and pinprick may be impaired in a dermatomal pattern. T4 at the nipple line, T7 at the xiphoid process, and T10 at the umbilicus are commonly used landmarks. When absent bilaterally, the superficial abdominal reflex indicates an upper motor neuron problem, and when absent unilaterally, it indicates a lower motor neuron problem from T7 to T12 segmental levels. The superficial abdominal reflex (see Figure 3-22) is tested using the end of a reflex hammer or tongue blade to stroke each quadrant of the abdomen in supine in a triangular fashion around the umbilicus and then graded as present or absent. The stimulus is out and away from the umbilicus. A normal response is abdominal contraction with movement of the umbilicus toward the quadrant of the stimulus. T8 to T10 are tested above the umbilicus and T10 to T12 below the umbilicus. In normal young adults, superficial abdominal reflex testing responses show wide variability such as asymmetry and absence in some or all quadrants.[37] Abdominal muscle strength tests can be evaluated through the use of standardized positions or observation of the umbilicus during a partial sit-up. The umbilicus normally does not change position. In the presence of lower abdominal weakness or paralysis, the upper rectus abdominis fibers are dominant and pull the umbilicus upward, indicating a positive Beevor's sign.[38]

Differentiation between thoracic radiculopathy and intercostal neuralgia is challenging because the description of symptoms is similar. However, intercostal neuralgia is less likely to be aggravated with trunk movements in comparison to thoracic radiculopathy. The intercostal nerves are peripheral nerves that generally run with the vascular bundle on the inferior surface of each rib and may become irritated post-thoracotomy or after other forms of trauma, resulting in intercostal neuralgia. The symptoms of intercostal neuralgia are quite similar to thoracic radiculopathy and may mimic the pain of herpes zoster or shingles but without rash. Clinicians and patients should carefully monitor the skin associated with any intercostal symptoms over at least 3 to 5 days for the appearance of a rash, suggesting a diagnosis of herpes zoster. Early referral and intervention help to reduce or prevent postherpetic neuralgia.[39]

Shingles is a syndrome that presents with a painful, vesicular rash on the chest wall, usually in a unilateral dermatomal distribution. The varicella zoster virus spreads down the spinal nerve toward the skin. When the virus reaches the skin, it causes the typical blistering rash of shingles. Pain and/or itching typically precede the appearance of rash by several days. The rash typically lasts for about 2 weeks. Precipitating factors are stress, trauma, infection, and immune suppression. Shingles usually has a benign course, but some patients develop systemic complications or progress to a chronic phase of postherpetic neuralgia. Postherpetic neuralgia, a frequent complication increasing with age, can result in severe and incapacitating chronic pain. Pharmacological treatment for acute shingles includes analgesics and antivirals to decrease pain, inhibit viral replication, promote tissue healing, and prevent or reduce the severity of postherpetic neuralgia. Intravenous antivirals are recommended with dissemination of acute herpes zoster in the immunocompromised patient.[39]

Screening for Yellow Flags

In addition to medical red flag screening, the clinician also assesses for the presence of yellow flags or psychological risk factors. Yellow flags raise the index of suspicion for the potential to develop a chronic problem that may require appropriate cognitive and behavioral management strategies. Depression, pain-related fear-avoidance beliefs and behaviors, and patient expectations must be identified to determine risk factors that may interfere with the normal recovery process and when needed to prescribe appropriate treatment.

Standardized Self-Report Outcome Measures

Standardized instruments measure various factors related to current level of pain, function, activities, participation, quality of life, or health status. No self-report measures are available specifically for thoracic spine or associated rib cage symptoms. The following instruments are used for patients presenting with thoracic pain, but the reliability, responsiveness, or validity has not been determined for use with this population. The Oswestry Low Back Pain Disability Index (ODI) and Neck Disability Index (NDI) are commonly used for symptoms below T4 and above T4, respectively. The Patient-Specific Functional Scale (PSFS) and Global Rate of Change (GROC) scale are also used for this patient population.

The Functional Rating Index (FRI), available at http://www.chiroevidence.com, is a 10-item, region-specific measure designed to reflect the patient's perception of function and pain related to the cervical, thoracic, or lumbar spine musculoskeletal system.[40] Items from the NDI and ODI are combined and fall within 4 constructs: pain, sleep, work, and daily activity. Each of the 10 items is scored from 0 to 4 with a maximum score of 40, taking about 1 minute to complete and 20 seconds to score. Higher scores indicate a higher level of disability. To score, the items are summed and multiplied by 2.5 and reported as a percentage.[41] Feise and Menke[41] reviewed 10 studies that provided psychometric data and concluded that the FRI demonstrates reasonable reliability, validity, and responsiveness. Effect size scores varied from 0.14 to 2.92 with 50% of scores >0.80. Feise and Menke[40] reported population effect sizes as 1.24 ($n=36$) for cervical pain; 1.61 ($n=5$) for thoracic pain; and 1.24 ($n=14$) for lumbar pain. In subjects with LBP, the minimal clinically important difference for the FRI is about 9 points, having comparable responsiveness and validity to the ODI but less reliability.[42]

Stewart et al[43] evaluated the responsiveness of several pain and disability measures in a cohort of patients with chronic whiplash. The PSFS (effect size: 0.84% confidence interval (CI): 1.22 [1.06, 1.37]) was more responsive than the FRI (effect size: 84% CI: 0.65 [0.54, 0.76]), but no differences were found among the NDI (effect size: 84% CI: 0.77 [0.66, 0.87]), FRI, and Copenhagen scale (effect size: 84% CI: 0.65 [0.54, 0.76]), meaning that any of these measures could be used for patients with whiplash. The Numeric Rating Scale (NRS) of pain bothersomeness (effect size: 84% CI: 1.17 [1.01, 1.31]) was the most responsive pain measure when compared with the NRS of pain intensity (effect size: 84% CI: 0.75 [0.61, 0.89]) and the 36-Item Short Form Health Survey (SF36) bodily pain score (effect size: 84% CI: 0.49 [0.36, 0.61]).[43]

Components of the History (Subjective Examination)

Clinical and occupational research related to thoracic pain is scarce, resulting in little to no studies on diagnostic accuracy of the historical information obtained for patients with TSP. Similar to LBP, a patient's experience of TSP is likely to be multifactorial, consisting of individual, occupational, and psychosocial factors with variable contributions as they relate to the development and persistence of symptoms. However, the goals (Table 5-2) for obtaining relevant history during the patient interview are consistent. During the interview, the clinician reflects on the patient responses and the context in which the patient presents as potential key factors to developing a preliminary PT diagnosis, prognosis, and plan for the physical examination. The information obtained through the interview guides decision making throughout the episode of care. Patients vary in their ability to accurately recall events and understand and answer questions. Patience, care, and good technique in the patient-therapist relationship are important to obtain accurate information.

TABLE 5-2. GOALS OF THE SUBJECTIVE EXAMINATION

- Obtain a patient demographic profile.
- Make a preliminary decision regarding whether the patient is appropriate for PT intervention.
- Obtain a detailed description of all of the patient's symptoms and determine whether a link exists between the presenting symptoms.
- Determine the aggravating factors, easing factors, and 24-hour behavior of each of the symptoms.
- Determine contraindications or precautions to examination and treatment.
- Obtain a sequential history (present and past) of the patient's problem.
- Determine patient expectations.
- Develop a diagnostic hypothesis, classification, or pretest probability of the disorder.
- Evaluate the data from the patient history.
- Establish a baseline level of symptoms, activity limitations, and participation restrictions from which progress is measured.
- Establish a basis for planning the physical examination and selecting appropriate diagnostic tests—determine what should be examined and in what detail.

Demographic Profile Considerations for Patients With Thoracic Spinal Pain

Age, Gender, Race, and Ethnicity Considerations

Studies report a higher prevalence during childhood and adolescence, specifically in females.[44] Up to 10% of adolescents had TSP that interrupted school or leisure activities. A trend for prevalence to increase in middle adult years (40 to 50) with a decrease in the later adult years (>70) was observed.[1] Epidemiological characteristics are lacking.

Occupational, Leisure and Sport and Socioeconomic Considerations

TSP can be disabling and contribute to the economical burdens of the individual and community. The patient's occupation and leisure activities involve various risks. Static postures and work-related activities produce variable biomechanical loads that may predispose to TSP. Some of these risks, such as work demands or pain-related fear, may be potential barriers to a successful outcome.

The prevalence of TSP varies according to occupation. Although not age adjusted, populations reporting the highest prevalence of TSP are health professionals (77% lifetime), manufacturers (47% 3 months, 38% 1 week), manual laborers (38% 1 month), and performing artists (44% point prevalence).[44] Individual factors significantly associated with TSP are concurrent musculoskeletal symptoms, exercising, premenstrual tension, and female gender. Other significant factors include high work load and intensity, perception of economic issues in the workplace, work in specialized areas such as PT private practice, internal medicine, electronics, assembly line tasks, tedious work, employment duration, certain year levels of study, driving specialized vehicles, and a large number of flying hours. Physical work-related factors include manual PT procedures, climbing stairs, and high physical stress. Psychosocial risk factors include perceived risk of injury and high mental pressure. The impact of these factors (ie, individual, general work, physical work, and psychosocial) on worker function, disability, and absenteeism is unknown, but the data support a biopsychosocial framework for the development and study of theories related to etiology, modifiable risk factors, and prognosis.[44] The relationship between low educational level, socioeconomic status, and TSP is unknown but is likely to be similar to that of LBP.[44]

Roelen et al[45] investigated whether perceived physical and mental workload and job demands are associated with self-reported health complaints. Physical workload was related to musculoskeletal symptoms. Standing work predicted leg pain, thoracic pain, and LBP, while sedentary work predicted LBP. Repetitive movements predicted arm pain, thoracic pain, and LBP. Mental workload was related to fatigue and chest pain. Working behind schedule and under pressure is not related to self-reported health complaints.

Clinicians should know and understand the individual's occupation and associated postural stresses as well as whether the patient is off work at present or remaining at work. In light of the limited evidence, knowledge and consideration of individual risk factors related to all daily physical activities and potential spinal loads, not just work, are important with respect to prevention and management. Returning to work and recreational activities are often a primary rehabilitation outcome.

Thoracic pain was significantly associated with concurrent musculoskeletal pain and differences in growth; physical activity; lifestyle; social activity; backpack usage; and postural, psychological, and environmental factors in adolescents. Risk factors included postural changes associated with backpack wear, participation in sports, chair height at school, difficulty with homework, and having poorer mental health. During adolescence, performing less than 10 minutes of high physical activity a day increased the odds (OR = 7.2) of developing thoracic back pain over the next 3 years in 9 and 12 year olds.[3] Boys and girls with pain at age 13 are 6.3 and 2.8 times more likely, respectively, to report thoracic pain at age 17.[4]

Thoracic and chest wall pain in athletes may be linked to musculoskeletal, GI, respiratory, and cardiac causes. Musculoskeletal causes are either a result of macrotrauma or repetitive microtrauma. Rib stress fractures, costochondritis, muscle strain, myofascial trigger points, gastroesophageal reflux, and exercise-induced asthma are common causes. Psychogenic causes can be common in children and adolescents.[46]

Chief Complaint

Eliciting the chief complaint usually begins with an open-ended question such as, "In your own words, please tell me what your main problem is?" giving the patient a chance to express immediate concerns and reasons for seeking treatment. The primary problem usually includes a report of pain, but some patients have no pain and instead report symptoms of weakness, stiffness, balance, dizziness, or numbness and tingling sensations. Documentation of the chief complaint using a body diagram includes recording the exact location and pattern of symptoms as well as the quality; depth (ie, superficial or deep); variability such as constant and varying, constant and nonvarying, or intermittent; worst area; intensity; and any relationship among or between symptoms. Obtaining a detailed description of patient symptoms is discussed in Chapter 2.

Description and Assessment of Symptoms for Patients With Thoracic Spinal Pain

Completion of the body chart and patient's description of symptoms provide information to initiate and/or continue the process of diagnostic triage, hypothesis generation, and classification. The patient should be adequately undressed so that the clinician is able to precisely note the area and extent of symptoms, usually pain and/or paresthesia. When the patient points to the area of pain, the clinician confirms the location by placing a hand on the patient and tracing the distribution. In persons presenting with primary thoracic pain, the clinician should clear areas that the patient has not reported as symptomatic. Certain areas should be routinely questioned: (a) the chest wall, abdomen, cervical spine, and UE regions, circumferentially; (b) lumbosacral spine (unilaterally and centrally), bilateral buttocks, both lower extremities, circumferentially; and (c) if not offered by the patient, specifically ask for numbness and tingling or other sensations that do not feel normal.

Pain patterns may be classified as nonmusculoskeletal or musculoskeletal, or have components of both disorders. Widespread allodynia and generalized hyperalgesia may suggest a component of centrally mediated pain or central sensitization, whereas a more localized, intermittent pain pattern suggests a peripherally mediated nociceptive driver. The patient's description and pattern of pain or other symptoms often inform the initial impression or working diagnosis, which in turn focuses the rest of the history and identifies areas for further questioning and clarification.

Nonmusculoskeletal or Visceral Referred Pain

Visceral referred thoracic pain or chest wall pain is most likely the result of infection, cardiovascular, oncology, pulmonary, renal, or GI disease.[15] Figure 2-3 in Chapter 2 depicts the common visceral referral patterns.[15] If the pain pattern generates an initial hypothesis for a nonmusculoskeletal disorder, clinicians should question for clusters of symptoms and signs that may suggest a particular system is involved.

Musculoskeletal Somatic Referred Pain and Radicular Pain

Listen to everything the patient tells you. Accurate documentation helps to understand the patient's experience and establish a baseline of symptoms for use as an outcome measure, prognosis, or classification. A description of thoracic radicular symptoms discussed previously is associated with damage or injury to or inflammation of the spinal nerve, nerve roots, or dorsal root ganglion. Keep in mind that variability and overlap of dermatomes is considerable, making the levels of radicular numbness and pain difficult to distinguish from one another. Pain or numbness and tingling may be distributed anywhere along the dermatome or in specific locations within the dermatome, not always a continuous line traveling along the dermatome.

Thoracic zygapophyseal joints (z-joints) cause both local and referred pain. In asymptomatic subjects, Dreyfuss et al[47] examined T3-4 through T10-11 z-joints through intra-articular injection (Figure 5-2). In 8 subjects, 72.5% of joints injected produced a mild pain of mean 3 out of 10, most often described as a deep, dull ache sensation that was different from the sensation of needle advancement through the soft tissues. The most intense area of pain occurred 1 segment inferior and slightly lateral to the injected joint. No subject reported pain as sharp, electric, burning, tingling, or localized to a specific point. Referral areas did not cross midline. No joint referred pain more

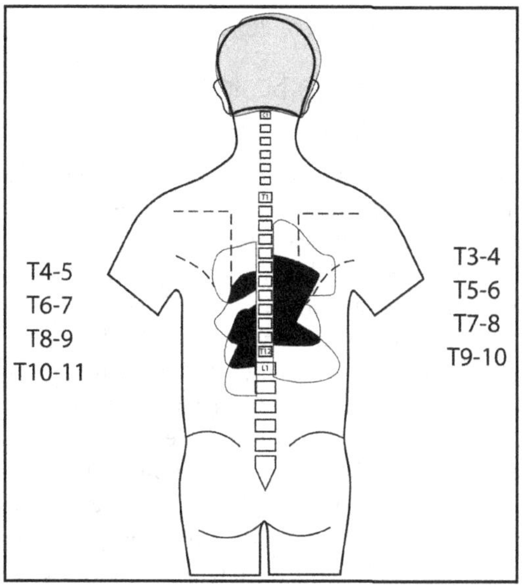

Figure 5-2. A composite map of referral patterns from the T3/T4 to T10/T11 thoracic zygapophyseal joints. (Reprinted with permission from Dreyfuss P, Tibiletti C, Dreyer SJ. Thoracic zygapophyseal joint pain patterns: a study in normal volunteers. *Spine*. 1994;19(7):807-811.)

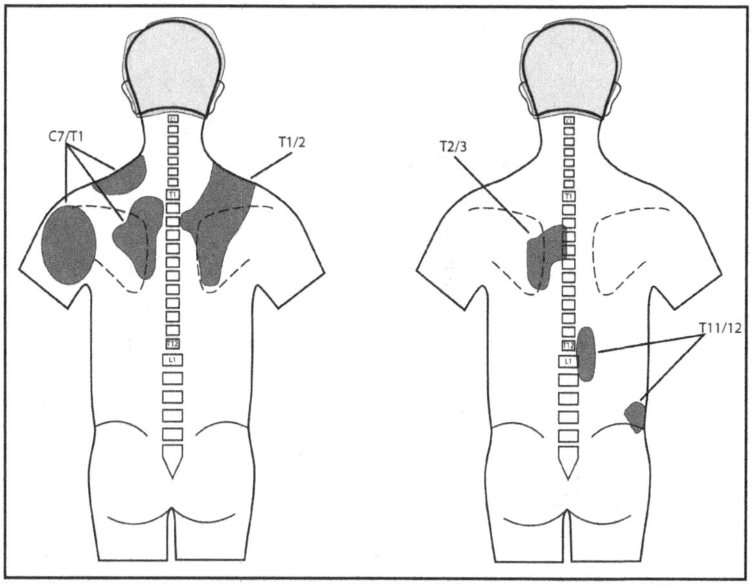

Figure 5-3. Composite pain referral map as described by Fukui et al[48] for the thoracic zygapophyseal joints from C7/T1 to T2/T3 and for the T11/T12 joint. (Reprinted from *Reg Anesth*, Vol 22, Fukui S, Ohseto K, Shiotani M, Patterns of pain induced by distending the thoracic zygapophyseal joints, pp 332-336, Copyright 1997, with permission from Elsevier.)

superior than one-half the vertical height of that vertebral segment. Distal referral was up to 2.5 segments below the injected level. When T3/T4 and T4/T5 were injected, 2 subjects had anterior chest wall and sternal pain. Evoked referral patterns were consistent in all subjects with significant overlap in the referral patterns with most thoracic regions sharing 3 to 5 different joint referral zones. No referral areas could be localized to 1 thoracic zygapophyseal joint.[47]

Fukui et al[48] injected C7/T1 through T2/T3, and T11/T12 z-joints in 15 patients with complaints of TSP. A total of 21 joints were studied. Composite pain distribution maps for the thoracic z-joints from C7/T1 to T2/T3 and for the T11/T12 joint revealed the following: suprascapular region pain was referred from C7/T1 and T1/T2; superior angle of the scapula pain from C7/T1 and T1/T2; mid-scapular region pain from C7/T1, T1/T2, and T2/T3; and pain local to the site of injection and the area over the iliac crest from T11/T12. Significant overlap occurred for C7/T1 to T2/T3 z-joints (Figure 5-3).[48]

In 8 asymptomatic male volunteers Young et al[49] studied the pain referral patterns of T2 to T7 costotransverse joints (Figure 5-4). Average verbal pain was 3.3 out of 10 and described as an ipsilateral deep, dull ache and pressure sensation. Only 1 subject reported a sharp burning pressure on the left at T5; another subject described a sharp pressure at the same level. Generally, pain sensations were local to the injected joint. Only the right T2 segment referred approximately 2 vertebral segments superior and inferior from the target joint. Chest wall, UE, or pseudovisceral symptoms were not reported.[49]

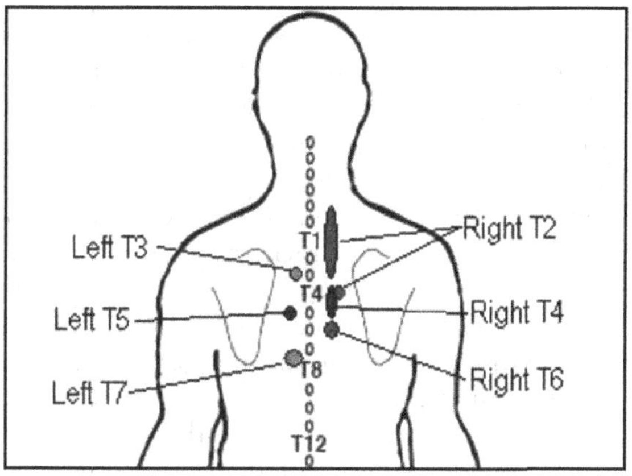

Figure 5-4. Costotransverse joint pain referral patterns. (Reprinted from Young B, Gill H, Wainner R, Flynn T. Thoracic costotransverse joint pain patterns: a study in normal volunteers. *BMC Musculoskelet Disord*. 2008;9:140. http://www.biomedcentral.com/1471-2474/9/140. © 2008 Young et al; licensee BioMed Central Ltd.)

Since the cervical spine is capable of referring pain into the upper and middle thoracic spine, UE, chest, and face,[50-53] examination of the cervical spine is mandatory in patients presenting with symptoms in these regions. In 5 asymptomatic subjects, Dwyer et al[50] examined cervical spine z-joint pain patterns for C2/C3 through C6/C7 (Figure 5-5) through intra-articular injection with blocking of the medial branches of the dorsal primary rami. Pain was described as a deep ache with a mean of 2 on a 10-cm Visual Analog Scale (VAS). Each joint produced a clinically characteristic pattern of pain that may assist in determining the segmental location of a painful cervical zygapophyseal joint.[50]

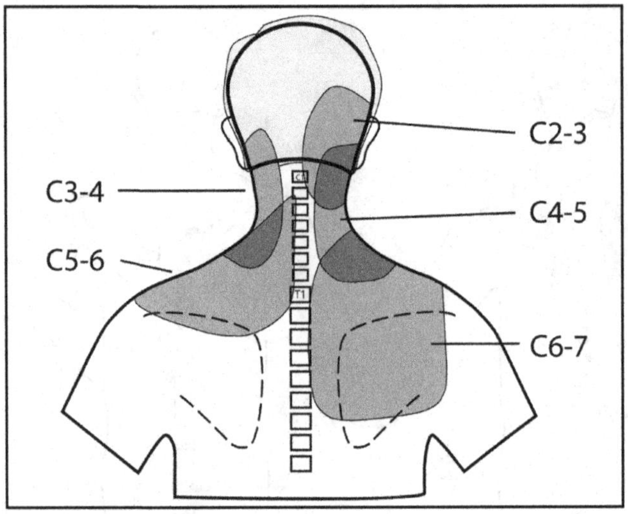

Figure 5-5. A composite of referral patterns from cervical zygapophyseal joints C2-C3 to C6-C7. (Reprinted with permission from Dwyer A, Aprill C, Bogduk N. Cervical zygapophyseal joint pain patterns. I: a study in normal volunteers. *Spine.* 1990;15(6):453-457.)

In subjects undergoing cervical discography, 101 symptom provocation maps were recorded.[52] The C2/C3 disc referred pain to the neck, suboccipital, and face; C3/C4 disc to the neck, suboccipital, trapezius, anterior neck, face, shoulder, interscapular area, and limb; C4/C5 disc to the neck, shoulder, interscapular area, trapezius, extremity, face, chest, and suboccipital; C5/C6 disc to the neck, trapezius, interscapular, suboccipital, anterior neck, chest, and face; C6/C7 disc to the neck, interscapular, trapezius, shoulder, extremity, and suboccipital; and C7/T1 to the neck and interscapular regions. Predominantly unilateral symptoms were provoked just as often as bilateral symptoms. In general, the results of Slipman et al[52] were similar to Schellhas et al.[53] Exceptions were that the Slipman et al[52] study did not produce anterior chest wall symptoms at the C6/C7 disc and the Schellhas et al[53] study did not produce facial symptoms at C5/C6. Both studies produced anterior chest wall symptoms at C4/C5 and C5/C6 and head and facial symptoms at C3/C4 and C4/C5. The sternoclavicular joint produces local pain over the joint and referred pain to the ipsilateral anterior trapezial fold along the lateral clavicle to the anterior shoulder, neck, and jaw.[54]

Both thoracic z-joints, costotransverse joints, cervical spine, and associated musculotendinous structures are potential pain generators for the upper quadrant that may relate to observed clinical pain syndromes, but due to significant overlap, pain referral patterns alone are not enough to determine an exact source of pain in patients presenting with a primary complaint of TSP or chest wall pain. Careful and unbiased attention to patients' descriptions of symptoms quickly reveals that spinal musculoskeletal pain presents in a highly variable form but provides valuable information to assist with diagnostic triage, classification, and intervention.

Pain Intensity Outcomes

Numeric Pain Rating Scale or Visual Analog Scale

Either the NPRS or VAS may be used to assess the patient's pain intensity even though these measures have not been studied in patients presenting with only TSP or chest wall pain. The reliability and responsiveness of these measures for LBP are discussed in Chapter 4 and recommended for use in patients with TSP. Ostelo and de Vet[55] suggested that the minimally clinically important change (MCIC) for acute LBP and chronic LBP should be 3.5 and 2.5, respectively. Empirical values for the minimally important change (MIC) on the 10-point NPRS are 1.0 to 4.5 points, representing a 30% improvement from baseline.[56] An absolute cutoff of the MIC proposed by consensus is 2 on the NPRS.[56] Ostelo and deVet[55] suggested that the MCIC should not be a fixed value. For the VAS and patients with acute LBP, subacute LBP, and chronic LBP, the MCIC should be at least 35, 20, and 20 mm, respectively. Empirical values for the VAS MCIC pain score (0 to 100 mm) were reported as 2 to 29 with an absolute cutoff of 15 proposed by consensus.[56]

History of the Current Episode

Details of the current episode should establish the manner in which the symptoms began, the progression of those symptoms, and the stage and stability of the problem.[57] The clinician should elicit chronological details about the mode of onset (ie, macro- or microtraumatic versus nontraumatic), the date of onset, the progression of symptoms, all treatments to date and their effects, and the overall progression of the problem. Details of the current episode help to define the nature (ie, musculoskeletal or nonmusculoskeletal), stage (ie, acute, subacute, or chronic), and stability (ie, getting better, worse, or staying the same) of the problem. When the most recent episode of symptoms is not the first episode, the quickest way to obtain relevant data is to start with the present episode.

Mode and Date of Onset

Careful inquiry by the clinician often reveals the cause of the patient's problem. Asking "How/when did the problem begin?" allows the clinician to explore the exact mechanism of injury or nature of the onset. If the onset is sudden or related to a specific event such as a fall, the clinician should determine the activity, position, direction, and magnitude of forces related to the injury. Injury related to lifting or a motor vehicle accident may provide information related to the potential or extent of injured structures, severity of onset, and intervention. If the onset is gradual or insidious, the clinician must ask for predisposing factors such as unusual or repetitive activity, change in work, training, recent illness, or stress. Gradual may mean over one day or over weeks to months. Spinal loads with cumulative or repetitive stress and biomechanical creep loading may subject some tissues to fatigue damage. A truly insidious onset merits concern about the underlying cause of the condition and raises the suspicion of a nonmusculoskeletal problem.

Progression of Symptoms

Using a completed body chart, the clinician asks for the progression of each symptom since onset. Changes in area and severity of symptoms provide clues regarding the relationship and stability of the problem. For example, if a patient reports the onset of right-sided, mid-TSP 3 days ago and now has right shoulder pain radiating to the right elbow and numbness and tingling in the ulnar border of the right hand, the clinician may infer the condition is worsening. A condition may worsen if the pain or symptom distribution becomes more widespread and distal (ie, peripheralizes). Likewise, a patient whose UE symptoms have resolved over the past week and now has only right-sided TSP describes a condition that is likely improving with time. A condition in which the symptom distribution becomes more localized and moves proximally toward the midline of the thoracic spine normally indicates improvement or centralization.

Treatments and Effects

To determine the effects of current or previous treatment, the clinician asks, "Have you had any treatment? Did it help?" If yes, "In what way?" Specific details of the exact treatment and patient response (ie, if better or worse) helps with treatment planning. Treatment that has worked in the past may again be appropriate; however, treatment that was unsuccessful is unlikely to be recommended. Symptoms unchanged, worsened, or improved and then worse again despite appropriate PT intervention are considered a red flag. An inconsistent response to PT intervention suggests a nonmusculoskeletal problem, a musculoskeletal problem that is not amenable to PT at this time, or perhaps a centrally mediated pain disorder.

Stability

Determining the stability of the problem is established by asking, "Compared to when this first started, is it getting better, worse, or staying the same?" If better or worse, the clinician should then ask, "In what way?" Changes in the intensity, severity, duration, and location of symptoms reveal the stability of the problem and assist with prognosis and the rate and level of recovery. When a patient reports worsening symptoms, clinicians should look for red flags, lifestyle risk factors such as mechanical factors, or yellow flags that may be delaying recovery. When symptoms are improving, contributing risk factors are addressed to prevent recurrence.

History of the Previous Episode(s) of a Similar Problem

The history of previous episodes begins with the question, "Have you had this problem before?" If the patient is not sure, "Is it similar to what you are feeling now?" With a long history of recurrence, the clinician chronologically determines the initial manner of onset, severity, previous treatment and effects, frequency of recurrences, time to recover, level of recovery, and status between episodes. The initial onset and mechanism of injury should be described in detail. Frequency and duration of episodes and level of recovery from the last episode or between episodes may affect the potential for recovery. Is there a pattern to the manner of onset? For example, if each episode of TSP is associated with prolonged use of the UEs, an important aspect of intervention and recurrence involves addressing this functional activity. Previous treatment and effects and level of recovery put the present injury in perspective, help to establish reasonable goals and likelihood of recurrence, and provide data on the stability of the problem over time.[57] If the symptoms are easier to provoke and last longer with each episode, and full recovery does not occur between episodes, then the clinician infers the problem is getting worse over time and the possibility of a favorable prognosis may be less likely.

As discussed in Chapter 4, chronic pain is the result of the complex interaction among physiologic, psychological, and social factors that perpetuate or worsen the pain experience. Patients with chronic pain are at increased risk for emotional disorders such as anxiety, depression, and anger; maladaptive cognitions of fear, catastrophizing, and poor coping skills; physical deconditioning and activity limitation due to decreased physical activity and fear of reinjury; and altered neuromatrix output. Early identification and interdisciplinary management based on a biopsychosocial model and a cognitive behavioral treatment approach are needed to address all contributing dimensions.

Symptom Behavior: Aggravating Factors, Easing Factors, and 24-Hour Behavior

The purpose of determining symptom behavior is to understand how the symptoms respond to activity, postures, movement, and the time of day. Some musculoskeletal problems get better with certain positions or movements while others get worse. In-depth questioning about which postures or movements result in a change in the location, intensity, or quality of a patient's symptoms helps to determine the mechanical nature of the problem and the severity or impact on function and irritability or ease of symptom provocation. A consistent pattern of aggravating and easing factors guides the classification, prognosis, and intervention. An inconsistent pattern of aggravating and easing factors may suggest a centrally mediated disorder. Symptoms that do not alter with posture and movement may suggest a nonmusculoskeletal disorder. Chapter 2 details the process for obtaining specific symptom behavior.

Aggravating Factors

The structure of the thoracic spine lends itself to 3 subregions: upper, middle, and lower. The upper thoracic spine consists of the first through the fourth (T1 through T4) thoracic vertebrae and ribs biomechanically and functionally linked with the cervicobrachial region. The middle region includes T4 through T9 or T10 and functionally may be involved with either the upper or lower half of the body. The lower region consists of T10 through T12 segments more closely related to function of the lumbopelvic region. The thoracic spine and chest wall serve as the transitional zone between the cervicobrachial and lumbopelvic regions. Considering the range of motion (ROM) and stability inherent in the thoracic spine, a wide variety of movements, activities, and postures may result in or present as aggravating factors.

Questions of movement and posture are asked to assist with ruling in and ruling out a spinal region, peripheral joint, or viscera as either a source or contributor to the patient's complaints. For symptoms related to the lower thoracic region, patients often report activities that also involve the lumbopelvic region or lower extremities such as bending; twisting; repetitive lifting; walking; running; recreational or sports-related movements; and daily care activities of dressing, bathing, or laundry. Although not exclusive of the lower thoracic spine, symptoms of the mid- and upper thoracic regions are commonly produced by activities that require the use of UEs such as arm elevation, reaching for a seat belt, twisting, pushing or pulling activities, coughing or sneezing, deep breathing, or involving movement of the cervical spine. Questions related to movement of the cervical spine (ie, looking up, turning the head, or postures) are routine for patients presenting with a primary complaint of thoracic pain. Sustained postures such as standing, sitting, or bending may affect any or all of the subregions of the thoracic spine.

Aggravating factors that might support a hypothesis of visceral referred pain include questions about symptoms with or after eating or drinking, pain with exertion such as climbing stairs, or determination of pain unrelated to position or movement. Aggravating and easing factors may also reveal patterns of centralization, peripheralization, or a directional preference.

A patient identifies the exact movement or posture and amount of time, distance, or repetitions it takes to produce or increase each symptom and how long it takes for the provoked symptom or symptoms to ease. Additional aggravating factors may be obtained from self-report measures such as the PSFS, ODI, or NDI. These activities should be analyzed to determine the general requirements for motion and stability of the thoracic spine and associated regions. Daily activity limitations and participation restrictions associated with a person's complaint are documented at baseline. The baseline aggravating factors are then used to set functional goals and reassessed to evaluate intervention effectiveness over the episode of care. Analysis of the aggravating movements or posture and the patient's response provides guidance for the selection of specific tests and measures or interventions.

Easing Factors

Easing factors such as movement, positions, medication, or other treatments should be sought for all symptoms and may serve as a factor in the initial intervention or the overall management of the patient's problem. Similar to the analysis of aggravating factors, the thoracic spine and associated cervicobrachial and lumbopelvic regions should be considered for requirements of movement or postural control that result in a decrease or elimination of the patient's symptoms. For example, a patient who reports walking as an easing factor for thoracic pain requires specific analysis of gait and possibly a specific dosage of walking as exercise intervention. A clinician should also ask patients if they have good days and bad days to determine what movements or positions create good days, providing data that are equally as important as determining the aggravators on bad days. The patient with a chronic problem and a central sensitization component may require a multidisciplinary approach with a graded focus on resolving relevant activity limitations rather than resolution of pain.

24-Hour Behavior

Clinicians must inquire about the behavior of symptoms over a 24-hour period with specific emphasis on a patient's ability to sleep through the night. The quality of sleep is important for restoration of body function. With a disruptive sleep pattern, the body and mind are not capable of optimal function. In addition to pain, medication side effects, increased urination, and night sweats are a few factors related to sleep deprivation that can interfere with the rehabilitation process.[58]

Night

Pain at night is often deemed a symptom of cancer, but further clarification is needed when a patient answers "yes" to the question, "Does it wake you at night?" The clinician might then ask, "What is it that wakes you?" Pain at night is typical of mechanical problems when the patient reports an inability to lie on the involved side or reports waking with symptoms that are simply relieved by a change of position and return to sleep. If the pain is the most intense at night and the patient is unsure of what wakes him or her, reports he or she must get up and walk around, and has difficulty returning to sleep, the clinician should consider the possibility of an active inflammatory component or more serious pathology such as neoplasm.[59] If night pain is a primary mechanical complaint, the clinician should determine the frequency, provocative position, and symptoms produced. This information is helpful to reassess at subsequent visits as one aspect of treatment effectiveness.

Morning

Most musculoskeletal problems are better in the morning and eased by rest. Some degenerative joint disorders are better or less painful in the morning, but patients often report pain and/or stiffness that are eased with movement within 30 to 60 minutes. Systemic inflammatory disorders such as ankylosing spondylitis (AS) or rheumatoid arthritis are usually better with rest but present with the most stiffness first thing in the morning, usually lasting longer than 60 minutes.[58] Symptoms that are worse in the morning may be due to poor sleeping posture. Symptoms that are unchanged in the morning may be nonmechanical or minor mechanical problems.

Evening

Clinicians should ask patients how symptoms change throughout the day or vary with workdays versus nonworkdays. Symptoms that are improved in the morning and remain better with movement throughout the day are likely mechanical in nature and a good prognostic indicator. Symptoms that are improved in the morning but worsen with activities of the day are mechanical, may have a limited prognosis, and should be identified for assessment and as potential barriers to recovery. Symptoms that do not vary with daily activities are minor mechanical problems or suggestive of a more serious pathology.

Review of the Medical Screening Questionnaire and General Medical History

Review of the medical screening questionnaire is a limited discussion of general health; a systems review; and an evaluation of past medical, surgical, medication, and diagnostic test histories. This review screens for systemic disease that may mimic musculoskeletal conditions and requires referral to another medical provider or may identify precautions or contraindications related to PT intervention. Synthesis of this information helps the clinician formulate a diagnosis, prognosis, plan of care, and select direct interventions.

The clinician must be alert for the presence of red or yellow flags during the history and physical examination. Screening for red flags (ie, cancer; infection; thoracic abdominal aortic aneurysm; fracture; renal disorder; and CVD, pulmonary, GI, and neurological involvement) was discussed earlier. Please see Chapter 2 (Tables 2-7 and 2-8) to review fear-avoidance beliefs and behaviors and the characteristics of systemic disease. The following discussion is a brief review of general health factors that may influence the examination or management of patients referred to PT.

General Health Status Considerations Related to Thoracic Spinal Pain

Clinicians frequently ask, "In general, how would you rate your health?" Most patients respond with excellent, very good, good, fair, or poor. Self-assessment of general health is a complex process related to patient experience with and knowledge of diseases. Health status rated as poor is predictive of future mortality,[60] functional limitations,[61] and the development of chronic conditions.[62] The patient's response to the general health question is a potential warning signal, but as with all risk factors or red flags, it should be considered in the context of the whole person and the clinical presentation. Exploring general health status gives insight into the patient's clinical presentation and the prognosis for rehabilitation.

Persons with a perception of poor health status are more likely to have back pain.[63,64] These same individuals have a variety of health problems including headaches; respiratory, cardiac, or GI diseases; and other joint diseases such that the presence of back pain is only one factor related to a perception of poor health rather than the cause of perceived poor health.[65] Persons with poor general health due to comorbidities are likely to progress slowly with rehab and are at risk for delay in the normal healing process.

Smoking, Obesity, and Cardiovascular Considerations

According to the United States Department of Health and Human Services,[66,67] the harms to smokers and nonsmokers are well known. Cancers related to cigarette smoking include lung, esophagus, larynx, mouth, throat, kidney, bladder, pancreas, stomach, cervix, and acute myeloid leukemia. Smokers are at risk for developing respiratory infections, pneumonia, heart disease, stroke, aortic aneurysm, chronic obstructive pulmonary disease (COPD), emphysema, asthma, hip fractures, and cataracts. The risk of disease is substantially reduced by quitting.[66,67]

Obesity, recognized as a major public health problem associated with musculoskeletal problems, is only a weak risk factor for back pain. In a study[68] of healthy obese persons (n = 23) with and without chronic LBP, obesity was characterized by a generally reduced ROM of the spine, specifically reduced pelvic and thoracic levels with a static postural adaptation of an increased anterior pelvic tilt or lumbar lordosis and reduced lateral bending when compared to obese persons without LBP and healthy nonobese women. Specifically, thoracic ROM was significantly lower in obese women without LBP. In this group, forward flexion was performed mainly by the lumbar spine. The authors concluded that thoracic stiffness with normal lumbar ROM appears to be a feature of obesity. Hypothetically, reduced thoracic ROM may pose additional demands for mobility on both the cervical and lumbar spine. However, additional studies are needed to determine a cause and effect relationship.[68]

Screening for CVD was discussed previously as part of diagnostic triage. Billek-Sawhney and Sawhney[69] report that 62% of patients examined in an orthopedic PT practice have CVD. To minimize the risk of an adverse cardiac event related to physical activity or exercise, baseline screening should determine if CVD exists or if CVD risk factors are present.[70] Screening is generally accomplished during the interview process. CVD screening is recommended to identify individuals with medical precautions or contraindications to physical activity and exercise.

Medication Usage

Any person who seeks medical care for musculoskeletal thoracic pain is likely to receive pharmacological therapy. Clinicians should inquire about all types of medication, the purpose and duration of use, dosage, tolerance, adherence, and effectiveness. Because these medications may hide symptoms, documentation of any medication and its effectiveness prior to the visit is important.

Since studies are not available relative to the TSP, most common medications are those used for cervical and musculoskeletal LBP. As presented in Chapter 4, Chou and Huffman[71] summarized the benefits and risks of the most common medications used to treat acute and chronic LBP. These medications include acetaminophen, nonsteroidal anti-inflammatory drugs (NSAIDs), antidepressants, benzodiazepines, antiepileptic drugs, skeletal muscle relaxants, opioid analgesics, tramadol, and systemic corticosteroids for acute or chronic LBP with or without leg pain. Of these medications, the most commonly prescribed are NSAIDs, skeletal muscle relaxants, and opioid analgesics.[72-74] Recommendations for first-line medications for LBP are acetaminophen or NSAIDs.[71] Common side effects are as follows[15,71]:

- *NSAIDs*: Back and/or shoulder pain due to retroperitoneal bleeding, GI symptoms, kidney and liver problems, or myocardial infarction
- *Corticosteroids*: Avascular necrosis of the femoral head, osteoporosis, immunosuppression, and steroid-induced myopathy
- *Antidepressants*: Movement disorders
- *Skeletal muscle relaxants*: Sedation
- *Statins*: Related musculoskeletal pain
- *Opioids*: Nausea, constipation, dry mouth, dizziness, and addiction

Imaging and Other Diagnostic Test Results

The traditional role of imaging has been to provide accurate, diagnostic anatomic information that guides the treatment decision-making process. However, even with extensive testing, a pathological cause for TSP cannot be reliably identified since many structural abnormalities are common in persons with and without LBP.[7-9] Diagnostic imaging is often a common procedure for most patients with thoracic and/or chest wall pain presenting in a primary care setting. In the absence of a clear indication, radiography is often done to reassure patients, to meet patient expectations, or for financial reimbursement purposes.[75,76] However, imaging is associated with a potential negative effect of labeling a patient with a diagnosis based on irrelevant imaging findings.[77] Imaging may not affect treatment, may increase direct costs,[78-80] and may lead to increased use of expensive, unnecessary invasive procedures.[81]

Diagnostic imaging practice guidelines[82] for spinal disorders including musculoskeletal thoracic or chest wall pain suggest that radiographs are not usually indicated for nonspecific acute, subacute, or persistent back and neck pain in the absence of red flags. Conventional radiography is considered after blunt trauma or acute injuries such as falls, motor vehicle accidents according to decision rules, no improvement with 4 to 6 weeks of conservative care, or the presence of increasing disability. Conventional radiography and specialized imaging (ie, MRI, computed tomography (CT), or nuclear medicine) should be considered for radicular syndrome and the presence of red flags. Severe or progressive neurologic deficit, sphincter or gait disturbance, saddle anesthesia, and suspicion of systemic illness such as cancer or infection or vascular causes such as aortic aneurysm or cervical artery dissection present urgent indications for specialized imaging of neck pain, thoracic pain, and LBP.[82] Osteoporosis risk in postmenopausal women should be assessed by history, physical examination, and diagnostic testing.[83] The medical history and physical examination should solicit clinical risk factors for osteoporosis and fracture and also evaluate for secondary causes of osteoporosis and fracture. This includes the World Health Organization's Fracture Risk Assessment Tool,[84] risk factors such as personal history of fracture after age 40, history of hip fracture in a parent, cigarette smoking, excess alcohol consumption, glucocorticoid use, rheumatoid arthritis, or other secondary causes of osteoporosis. This tool, available online at http://www.shef.ac.uk/FRAX and used with guidelines for treatment thresholds, is very helpful in identifying candidates for pharmacotherapy. Osteoporosis can be diagnosed by bone density testing in postmenopausal women and men over age 50. The results of a bone density exam (ie, dual-energy x-ray absorptiometry [DEXA] scan) are reported in 2 ways. A t-score compares a patient's bone density to the optimal peak bone density for gender reported as number of standard deviations (SDs) below the average. A t-score of >–1 is considered normal; –1 to –2.5 is considered osteopenia or a risk for developing osteoporosis; and <–2.5 is diagnostic of osteoporosis. A z-score compares a patient's results to others of the same age, weight, ethnicity, and gender and is useful to determine unusual contributors to bone loss. A z-score of <–1.5 raises concern of factors such as use of glucocorticoid medication, tobacco, high alcohol intake, malnutrition, or metabolic disorders, other than aging as contributing to osteoporosis.

Routine laboratory tests such as ESR, urinalysis, or complete blood count are not needed for persons with thoracic pain unless the history or examination suggests serious pathology as a cause. ESR may be helpful to screen for cancer or infection since this test is more sensitive and less specific than plain radiographs.[85] In suspected cases of bladder or kidney infection, a urinalysis is a useful test.[86]

Clinicians should carefully consider the role and relative impact of imaging on the overall management of individual patients with TSP. Serious visceral or spinal pathology can present as thoracic or chest wall pain and clinicians should perform adequate screening to recognize these presentations with re-evaluation on a frequent basis. For individuals who do not respond quickly within 4 to 6 weeks of onset, selective investigations or referral may be warranted.[87]

Patient Expectations or Goals

Clinicians generally ask patients to describe their functional goals or expectations from PT treatment. Previous research has documented an association between positive patient expectations and improved health outcomes.[88] In a secondary analysis, Myers et al[89] investigated the association between patients' general expectations for recovery from acute LBP and their functional outcomes. Patients were asked to rate on a 0 to 10 scale (0 = no improvement, 10 = complete recovery) the amount of improvement they expected in 6 weeks. The mean expectation for recovery was 8.8 (SD 1.7). The patient's response appears to have some predictive value. Based on their findings, patients with higher expectations for a speedy recovery are likely to show more improvement. Establishing patient goals provides an opportunity to listen to patient concerns and assists with tailoring interventions to achieve a specific functional recovery.

Interview Summary

At the end of the formal interview, the clinician should ask, "Are there any other problems or concerns that you would like to tell me about or that we have not discussed?" The clinician should then present a brief summary of the key findings from the interview and discuss the plan for the physical examination.

Clinical Reasoning Guide to Plan the Physical Examination

At the end of the formal interview, clinicians should briefly review the subjective data and begin planning the physical examination. For the novice clinician, this reflection provides an opportunity to identify anatomical and biomechanical relationships, movement impairments, pain patterns, activity limitations, and risk and prognostic factors that direct the search for further information and might influence the rehabilitation process. This deliberate approach allows for a systematic review of the important points of the history, provides a database that initially dictates the focus and comprehensiveness of the physical examination, and provides a baseline that can be used in the reassessment of the patient's progress. As a clinician gains experience and more easily recognizes patterns emerging from the history, this process occurs with less deliberation; however, this reflective process is always a useful exercise with any patient, the complex patient, or a patient that is not responding as expected.

The process of planning the examination was discussed in Chapter 2. A form for planning the examination (see Table 2-9) was presented to assist the clinician with analyzing the information gained from the history, plan the appropriate tests and measures, and increase the probability of performing an efficient and appropriate examination. To plan the extent and vigor of the physical examination, the clinician considers the severity, irritability, nature, stage, and stability of the patient's symptoms or problem.[90] The clinician also considers risk factors associated with the development of persistent TSP or other factors contributing to the condition such as posture, ergonomics, conditioning, depression, job requirements, body awareness and sensorimotor integrity, trauma, previous episodes, and other medical problems. The end result of this process is to generate a working diagnostic classification or working hypothesis(es) of the patient's thoracic or chest wall symptoms and a plan to test the working hypothesis(es) through the physical examination and continued reassessment. The clinician should establish a clear plan of what needs to be examined at the first session and over the next 1 to 2 sessions. Sample case studies in Appendices F and G include a form for planning the examination.

Summary of Diagnostic Triage and Subjective Examination

In comparison to LBP and cervical pain, research related to thoracic back pain is scarce. Musculoskeletal or nonmusculoskeletal thoracic pain with or without chest wall complaints often presents a challenge to the clinician. Functionally, the thorax is related to the lumbopelvic and cervicobrachial regions responsible for load transfer

TABLE 5-3. COMPONENTS OF THE PHYSICAL EXAMINATION

- Observation (anthropometric: height, weight, body fat composition, girth)
- Gait
- Posture
- Functional tests
- Active range of motion
- Passive range of motion (physiological, accessory, segmental motion testing)
- Resisted tests
- Neurological screening examination
- Muscle length/flexibility tests
- Muscle performance (strength/power/endurance)
- Screen region/joints above and below
- Special tests
- Palpation

between the upper and lower halves of the body. Since these regions are interdependent, the thoracic spine must be examined in persons presenting with LBP and neck and shoulder complaints as well as in those presenting with a primary complaint of thoracic pain.

Considering the prevalence of thoracic pain with or without chest wall symptoms and the potential impact on function, the importance of the data gained from the subjective examination cannot be underestimated. The subjective examination seeks to identify key information from all patients with the context and details specific to the patient's presenting problems. This early information provides the basis to develop initial diagnostic hypotheses or classifications, which then guide the focus and comprehensiveness of the physical examination. Obtaining accurate, relevant data from the patient history aids in diagnostic triage, planning the physical examination, and implementing an effective management strategy.

Components of the Physical Examination

This section details and sequences the thoracic spine examination. The physical examination continues the process of diagnostic triage and diagnostic classification seeking to confirm (ie, rule in) or refute (ie, rule out) a serious underlying pathological condition, any condition resulting in neurological compromise, or other competing medical disease.[91] Basic components and general procedures of the physical examination are discussed in Chapter 3. Table 5-3 is a list of the basic components for the physical examination of persons with TSP including chest wall symptoms. Table 5-4 describes a list of commonly used tests and measures sequenced by patient position (ie, standing, sitting, supine, prone, and side-lying) to assist with organizing the physical examination. The sequence is varied by patient and condition, and not all tests and measures should be performed on every patient. The reliability and diagnostic accuracy of tests and measures must be considered before they are selected. In the thoracic spine, data supporting the reliability and validity of physical examination procedures are limited. Initially, the history guides prioritization of the tests and measures that will be conducted at the initial session.

In addition to pain and disability in patients with thoracic pain, physical impairments of body structure and function are routinely used by physical therapists to assess progress and treatment effectiveness. However, not all measurements used in the clinic are equally useful in the diagnosis and management of mechanical thoracic pain. In general, impairment measurements have uncertain convergent validity with patient satisfaction, pain, or disability measures and have poor ability to distinguish between symptomatic and asymptomatic individuals.[92,93] Due to the lower responsiveness of physical impairments (ie, ROM, strength), the use of self-report pain and functional activity measures such as the PSFS, FRI, and ODI should be emphasized to determine if meaningful change has occurred.

The physical examination is a continuation of the history designed to test hypotheses generated by subjective information. To establish a diagnostic classification, the clinician uses key findings from the history and physical examination to place a patient with thoracic pain into a specific subgroup or subgroups intended initially to guide appropriate intervention.

Goals of the Physical Examination

The goals of the physical examination are to (1) reproduce the patient's symptoms in patterns consistent with the information obtained in the patient interview; (2) determine the impact of posture, movement, work, or recreational psychosocial factors as causes of, contributors to, or perpetuator's of the patient's problem; (3) establish the treatment threshold for a diagnostic classification for the

TABLE 5-4. EXAMINATION OUTLINE FOR THE THORACIC REGION

STANDING

- General observation and baseline vital signs
- Functional activity, gait, balance
- Neurological exam: Manual muscle test toe/heel walk L4/5; S1/S2
- Posture
- Screen lumbar spine if indicated: active range of motion (AROM), overpressure (OP): flexion, extension, lateral flexion, with OP
  - Repeated lumbar movements: repeated extension in standing, repeated flexion in standing
- Screen shoulder as indicated by history

SITTING

- Observation/posture/correct deformity if present/chest expansion as needed
- Resting symptoms
- For upper T-spine (C7 through T5), test cervical spine
  - AROM, OP; repeated movements—retraction/retraction-extension
- For T5 through T12: test thoracic movements in sitting
  - AROM: flexion, extension, lateral flexion, rotation; AROM with OP
  - Repeated flexion, extension, rotation right/left
  - As needed combined movements: flexion/left rotation, flexion/right rotation, extension/left rotation, extension/right rotation
- Neurological screen
- Passive segmental mobility testing
  - T1 through T4 via palpation of the transverse processes
  - Passive physiological intervertebral movement (T5 through T12): sitting flexion, extension, lateral flexion, rotation via palpation of spinous process
- Special test: sitting arm lift
- Slump test and/or sympathetic slump test
- Cervical rotation lateral flexion test

SUPINE

- Cervical/thoracic/chest wall/rib anterior palpation
  - Breathing assessment, palpation of rib cage during respiration
- Anterior rib cage mobility assessment: rib anterior-to-posterior along the sternum
- First rib mobility assessment
- Active straight leg raise
- Muscle performance: motor control, length, strength, endurance
- Other as indicated: upper limb neurodynamic test, screen cervicobrachial or lumbopelvic regions

PRONE

- Repeated movements:
  - Sustained thoracic extension in lying (prone on elbows)
  - Repeated extension in standing with or without clinician OP
- Palpation soft tissue, bony landmarks, rib angle
- Thoracic passive accessory intervertebral movement: central and unilateral, cervicothoracic/CV and rib angles, first rib (inferior glide)
- Prone arm lift

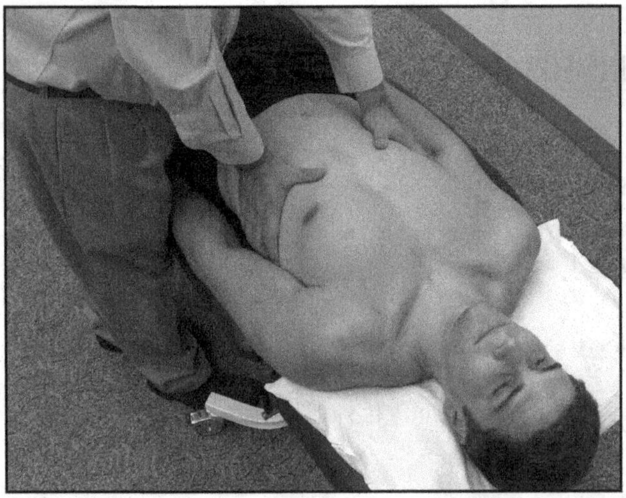

Figure 5-6. Palpation of rib cage during respiration.

person presenting with TSP; and (4) establish an accurate, data baseline or outcome measures from which to evaluate and progress treatment. Appropriate selection of examination procedures should result in the data to support or negate working hypotheses by altering the pretest probability beyond the treatment threshold or the point where the examination ends and treatment begins.

Physical Examination of the Thoracic Region

Examination Procedures in Standing

- General observation, baseline vital signs, respiration
- Functional activity
- Gait screen
- Balance
- Neurological exam
- Posture
- Lumbar spine screen
- Shoulder screen

General Observation and Baseline Vital Signs

Observation begins when first meeting the patient and continues throughout the examination. Initial observations include facial expression, postural characteristics, general fitness and well-being, quality of movement, rising from the waiting room chair, transitions of supine to sitting, sitting, walking, and willingness to move. The patient's unwillingness to move is related to poor outcomes[94,95] and may be a behavior related to fear of pain or reinjury that should be addressed. Prior to the interview or formal observations and during the physical examination, baseline data such as height, weight, pulse, respirations, or blood pressure are collected. At the start of the physical examination, baseline symptoms should be documented and then monitored as the examination continues. Establishing resting symptoms prior to each test and during each test or measure enables the clinician to ensure the symptoms are not getting worse and to document an accurate response to posture, movement, and activity. Observation requires adequate exposure of the thoracic region or areas of interest.

Respiration

Altered breathing patterns such as breath holding or upper chest breathing have been observed in patients with back pain.[96,97] Patterns such as rapid shallow breathing produce a decrease in CO_2 blood levels (ie, increase in pH or respiratory alkalosis) causing smooth muscle constriction, electrolyte balance, decreased tissue oxygenation, increased excitability of the corticospinal system, heightened pain, and hyperirritability of motor and sensory axons.[98] Capnography measures CO_2 levels at the end of exhalation known as *end tidal* CO_2. Normal values are 35 to 45 mm Hg, which closely reflects arterial CO_2 in subjects with healthy cardiopulmonary function. Capnography is considered an accurate and time-sensitive arterial CO_2 measure.[99]

During normal quiet inspiration, the descent of the diaphragm results in abdominal expansion and a lateral, posterior, and anterior expansion of the lower rib cage. Lee[10] described the assessment of respiration as follows. Respiration should be observed over several respiratory cycles looking for movement in the upper chest (ie, apical breathing), lower lateral rib cage (ie, lateral costal expansion), and upper and lower abdomen, noting where most of the movement occurs. Next, palpation of the lateral lower rib cage is used to monitor the side-to-side symmetry and amount of movement during breathing (Figure 5-6). Most movement should occur in the lower lateral rib cage (ie, lateral costal expansion). Further inspiration involves the vertebrosternal rib cage and an increase in the anteroposterior dimension of the thorax. Expiration occurs passively as the diaphragm relaxes.[10] To assess for excessive trunk muscle activity, rib cage rigidity, or restriction of movement, the clinician applies a gentle lateral translation force to the right and left (Figure 5-7) on the lateral aspect of the rib cage. Lateral movements to the right and left should be symmetrical with minimal resistance to movement.[100]

In standing, sitting, and supine or during functional activity, observation of breathing and its affect on spinal position or the effect of spinal position on breathing is important. Nonoptimal patterns of breathing, bilateral or unilateral, have been described by several authors.[10,100] A lower rib cage may be limited by stiffness in the thorax or by excessive activity of the superficial muscles, external or internal oblique, or erector spinae (ES). Absent or reduced lateral or posterolateral rib cage expansion on inspiration may result in abdominal breathing making it difficult to maintain contraction of the deep muscle system, or upper chest breathing and excessive use of accessory respiratory muscles.[10] Apical breathing is often associated with excessive thoracolumbar extension from T11 to L1. Other common observations are overactive external and/or internal oblique or ES muscles, resulting in abdominal bracing and continued restriction of the thorax. If a normal breathing pattern is not observed and/or not maintained, retraining and integration of the normal breathing into postural control is important to facilitate optimal coordination of the deep and superficial stabilization systems, reduce trunk rigidity or bracing strategies, and maintain mobility gained from manual intervention for thoracic hypomobility.[10]

Contraction of the diaphragm maintains ventilation and results in increased intra-abdominal pressure and trunk stiffness without excessive activity of abdominal or back muscles.[101,102] In healthy subjects, normal breathing is sustained while the diaphragm performs all of these tasks simultaneously, even when trunk stability is challenged.[103] Using visual inspection, palpation, and a pressure feedback unit, Roussel et al[97] compared breathing patterns at rest, with deep breathing, and during motor control tests in healthy subjects and subjects with chronic LBP. Diaphragmatic breathing was defined as a normal pattern. A paradoxical breathing pattern, upper chest breathing, a mixed pattern, and breath holding were considered altered or asynchronous motions[104] since these breathing patterns are likely to prevent effective alveolar ventilation.[105] Breathing patterns were similar in both groups in supine during quiet breathing, but significantly more altered breathing patterns were observed in the subjects with chronic LBP during deep breathing in standing and motor control tests. Changes in breathing patterns were not related to pain severity but were related to motor control dysfunction when trunk stability was challenged using the bent knee fall out and active straight leg raise (ASLR).[97] In a subgroup of patients with back pain, breath holding and increased diaphragmatic activity may be a compensatory strategy to increase trunk stability.[106,107] If the deep stabilizing system fails to provide optimal load transfer, the diaphragm may be used to enhance spinal stability through breath holding or decreased diaphragmatic excursion, thereby reducing respiratory activity. Other patients with back pain may use the global muscles or pelvic floor to compensate. As a potential compensation strategy for poor trunk control, breathing patterns should be assessed in supine, while standing, and during motor control tests.

Functional Activity

During all tests and measures, the clinician should observe the quality and quantity of motion involved and ask the patient what the effect was in order to determine the symptom response. If appropriate, the clinician asks the patient to perform a functional activity or patient-reported movement from the history that reproduces or increases the patient's symptoms. The therapist may select a specific movement from the history for further analysis or allow the patient to select one. Functional activities should be important to the patient and may include motions of the thoracic spine such as bending or twisting, elevation of one or both arms as in reaching or dressing, deep breathing, pushing, pulling, or lifting. If the lower thoracic spine is symptomatic, tasks that reproduce symptoms are similar to the lumbopelvic region such as bending, sitting, sit to stand, or walking. If the upper thoracic spine is symptomatic, activities such as looking up or down or turning the head to the right or left may be reported by the patient as provocative.

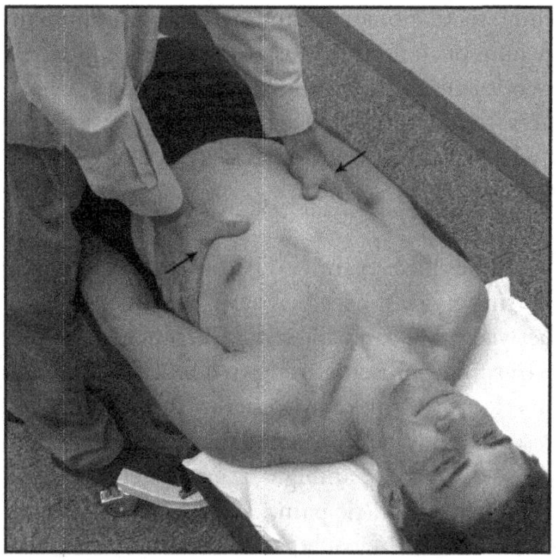

Figure 5-7. Lateral rib cage translation.

Analysis of painful movement or postures should reveal poor alignment, such as areas of hypomobility or hypermobility and/or poor muscle activation patterns (ie, excessive or insufficient), that either perpetuate or contribute to continued nociceptive input. In addition to qualitative analysis of the motion and postural control, these functional movements are often baseline provocative measures and indicators of nonoptimal motor control strategies, and they are useful for reassessment within or between sessions.

Analysis of functional movement requires development of observational and palpation skills. An observational framework for qualitative assessment of optimal movement strategies[10] includes the following:

- Optimal lumbopelvic function
- The ability to attain neutral thoracic posture relative to the cervical and lumbopelvic regions
- The ability to maintain and control neutral thoracic posture during increased loading from the upper or lower extremities
- The ability to move in and out of neutral thoracic spine posture with segmental control
- The ability to maintain optimal load transfer during daily functional tasks, work, and sport-specific activities[10]

Failure to demonstrate any of these components suggests a nonoptimal, altered motor control strategy.[10] This framework can be used to qualitatively assess all tests and measures that require movement to generate hypotheses about why the motor control strategy is altered.

Gait Screen

Few studies have examined trunk muscle activation patterns during gait. No studies have examined the relationship between TSP and altered gait. Since the abdominal and paraspinal musculature provide both stability and mobility for the trunk, hypothetically, information from LBP research may be considered when walking is provocative or observed to be antalgic or asymmetrical in patients presenting with thoracic pain. The control of trunk muscle activity is affected by back pain and often visualized clinically as trunk rigidity. In subjects with chronic LBP van der Hulst and colleagues[108] demonstrated increased superficial muscle activity of the ES and rectus abdominis (RA) but not of the external oblique abdominals. These differences were present irrespective of gait velocity. Increased coactivation of the ES and RA may serve to control spinal movement and support the hypothesis of guarding or trunk rigidity. Saunders et al[109,110] demonstrated a loss of tonic, transverse abdominis electromyography (EMG) activity during walking in subjects with LBP. Patients with thoracic pain who have difficulty walking should be assessed for altered motor control of the trunk in the context of regional interdependence. Walking may need to be broken down into the kinematics of specific components (ie, heel strike, toe off) and analyzed to determine why walking has become provocative. Studies that may be relevant to thoracic pain but related to trunk muscle activation in LBP were presented in Chapters 3 and 4.

Balance

Postural control is a requirement for all ADL. An optimal balance strategy should result in bilateral or unilateral maintenance of the normal standing posture with minimal effort and normal breathing patterns. Qualitatively, spinal curves, pelvis, and lower extremities should remain stable in all planes. Deformity or loss of control in any plane or region indicates the need for further examination of the neuromuscular system.

The relationship of osteoporosis, vertebral fracture, kyphosis, and balance impairment is complex. Many factors are likely to influence balance in persons with osteoporotic vertebral fractures and increased kyphosis such as pain,[111,112] poor muscle control,[113] fear of falling,[114] and the effects of postural changes.[115,116] A relationship between impaired balance and increased thoracic kyphosis has been reported.[117,118]

Sinaki et al[113] examined the influence of osteoporosis-related kyphosis on balance and falls in 12 community-dwelling women age 76 ± 5.1 years with a 50- to 65-degree kyphosis angle and 13 healthy women controls age 71 ± 4.6 years. Gait was assessed during level walking and during stepping over obstacles. Balance was assessed with computerized dynamic posturography consisting of the sensory organization test. Back extensor strength, grip strength, and all lower extremity muscle groups were significantly weaker in the kyphosis group, except for right ankle plantar flexors. Significant differences for all velocity measures were found for the kyphosis group during all walking tasks. The osteoporosis-related kyphosis subjects had significantly greater balance abnormalities on computerized dynamic posturography. The authors concluded that hyperkyphosis on a background of reduced muscle strength is an important factor in increased body sway, gait unsteadiness, and risk of falls in osteoporosis.[113]

Greig et al[119] investigated the independent effects of osteoporotic vertebral fracture and thoracic kyphosis on balance. In 22 subjects with osteoporosis with (n = 10) and without (n = 12) radiologically diagnosed fractures, a comparison of balance measures suggest that vertebral fracture, but not thoracic kyphosis, is associated with impaired balance or poorer sway strategy scores and greater reliance on hip strategies for balance compared with the control group. The relationship between vertebral fracture and thoracic kyphosis is not clear, but a stronger positive relationship develops with greater severity of kyphosis and numbers of vertebral fractures.[115,116] Standing and single limb balance tests should be examined at some point throughout the examination process but may not be appropriate or safe if weightbearing is painful. Baseline balance measures may be useful if viewed as important functional activities for the individual patient or for individuals who have increased kyphosis, have osteoporosis-related vertebral fracture, or are at risk for falls.

Excessive kyphosis of the thoracic spine common in older adults may result in impairments of mobility, slower gait speed, difficulty climbing stairs, poor ability to make a 360-degree turn, and poor balance.[113,120-123] Katzman and colleagues[124] used longitudinal data from the Fracture Intervention Trial to determine the relationship between increasing kyphosis angle and worsening mobility as measured by the timed up and go test (TUG) after controlling for other established risk factors, age, baseline kyphosis, health status, body mas index, grip strength, change in hip bone mineral density (BMD), and new vertebral fractures. The primary predictor was a change in kyphosis angle over a mean of 4.4 years. Kyphosis angle was measured using a Debrunner kyphometer (Proteck AG, Bern, Switzerland), a protractor-like instrument that measures Cobb's angle of kyphosis by placing the arms of the device over the SP of C7 and T12.[116] Interrater reliability of the kyphometer measurement of kyphosis angle assessed using intraclass correlation coefficients (ICCs) ranged from 0.98 to 0.99.[125] Greater kyphosis angle predicted longer mobility performance times ($P < .001$). For every 5 degrees increase in kyphosis angle, TUG performance times increased by 0.02 seconds (95% CI: 0.01 to 0.03) more than the increase in mobility time of 0.01 seconds (95% CI: 0.005 to 0.03) over 1 year observed in this cohort. Increasing kyphosis angle is independently related to worsening disability.[124] Therefore, kyphosis angle measured as a baseline and over time is likely an important clinical measure. Interventions to prevent or reduce increasing kyphosis are needed in addition to studies that demonstrate a meaningful change in mobility. Kyphotic posture, balance, and gait seem to be closely related.

Neurological Exam

Toe and heel walk are quick functional tests for the L4/L5 and S1/S2 myotomes. S1/2 may also be tested and graded in the manual muscle test position for the gastrocsoleus complex in standing as discussed in Chapter 3 (see Figure 3-17I).

Posture

Formal examination usually begins with observation of the patient's posture in standing, but clinicians should specifically analyze any posture that aggravates the patient's symptoms. The clinician initially observes global posture anteriorly, posteriorly, and laterally from both sides, gradually focusing on the thoracic spine. Observation of posture was discussed in Chapters 3 and 4. Specific details related to the thoracic spine are covered here.

Ideally, a primary thoracic kyphosis should be maintained with no visible lordosis. The thorax using the manubriosternal junction as a landmark should be in line with the pubic symphysis and the anterior superior iliac spine as viewed laterally. Anteriorly, the manubrium and sternum should be vertical and the clavicles horizontal or with a slight inclination laterally. Posteriorly, the scapulae rest on the chest wall with the medial border parallel to the spine or in 2 to 3 degrees upward rotation, slight anterior tilt, and about 30 degrees of internal rotation. The T2/T3 SP is at the level of the spine of the scapula and T7 to T9 SPs at the level of the inferior angle of the scapula. Muscular symmetry, tone, hypertrophy, or atrophy is also observed along with the position of the head and neck on the thorax in all 3 planes. Visible asymmetry or deviation of the thorax in all 3 planes is common but not always associated with or relevant to the patient's complaint.

Muscular Analysis

Muscular dysfunction is associated with injury, repetitive overuse, or sustained postural habits resulting in patterns of muscle imbalance and altered motor patterns. Muscle imbalance can lead to postural asymmetry and postural asymmetry to muscle imbalance. Clinicians should observe and palpate resting muscle tone, shape, and size for signs of atrophy or weakness and hypertrophy, overactivity, or trigger points as contributors to altered movement patterns.

The thoracolumbar spinal extensors may exhibit hypertrophy bilaterally or unilaterally to compensate for poor deep stabilizers, weak hip extensors, or stiff hip flexors. A protruding abdominal wall suggests generalized abdominal weakness and poor trunk stabilization. Stiffness of the RA, internal obliques, and external obliques may be observed as anterior rib cage depression, an increased infrasternal angle, and a decreased infrasternal angle, respectively. Stiffness of the pectoral muscles is associated with a rounded and protracted shoulder position often found in the upper-crossed syndrome (UCS; see Figure 3-3). Medial rotation of the arms with greater than one-third of the humeral head anterior to the acromion process suggests dominance of the shoulder girdle internal rotators. Common to UCS is the forward head posture linked to weak deep neck flexors and stiffness of the suboccipitals, scalenes, and sternocleidomastoid process.[126] Visual observation related to a hypothesis of muscle length must be confirmed with additional mobility testing.

Upper-Crossed Syndrome[127]

Postural changes associated with UCS include forward head, increased cervical lordosis and thoracic kyphosis, elevated and protracted shoulders, and abduction or winging of the scapulae. Possible joint dysfunction related to this pattern involves the atlantooccipital joint, C4/C5 segment, cervicothoracic joint, T4/T5 segment, and reduced glenohumeral motion. The pectoral muscles are stiff anteriorly and the upper trapezius and levator scapulae are stiff posteriorly. Weakness is noted in the deep neck flexors and middle and lower trapezius.[127] Additional tests are needed to confirm altered muscle length or motor control related to UCS.

Kyphosis

Excessive thoracic kyphosis and reduced kyphosis occur in all age groups and both genders. A reduction or reversal of the normal thoracic kyphosis appears flat or extended and may occur at a single segment or include multiple segments of the upper, middle, or lower thoracic spine. In a flat upper thoracic spine, the medial borders of the scapula appear to wing but are most likely in the optimum position with the spine being in extension rather than flexion. A reduced thoracic kyphosis in the upper or mid-thoracic spine may result in loss of flexion mobility, placing increased demands on the cervical spine. Likewise, an excessive kyphosis in the lower thoracic spine may result in loss of extension mobility and is likely to place more demands for extension on the lumbar spine. Palpation of the individual spinal segments assists in confirming visible observation of the thoracic spine curvature.

Excessive kyphosis has many causes such as postural slouching, degenerative changes associated with age, osteoporosis, fracture, Scheuermann's disease, neuromuscular disease such as cerebral palsy, posttrauma or postsurgery, vitamin D deficiency, and tuberculosis of the spine. As

TABLE 5-5. DEGREE OF KYPHOSIS IN MALES AND FEMALES BY AGE

AGE	MALE KYPHOSIS (DEGREES) MEAN ± SD	FEMALE KYPHOSIS (DEGREES) MEAN ± SD
2 to 9	20.88 ± 7.85	23.87 ± 6.67
10 to 19	25.11 ± 8.16	26.00 ± 7.43
20 to 29	26.27 ± 8.12	26.83 ± 7.98
30 to 39	29.04 ± 7.93	28.42 ± 8.63
40 to 49	29.75 ± 6.93	32.66 ± 6.72
50 to 59	33.00 ± 6.46	40.71 ± 9.88
60 to 69	34.67 ± 5.12	44.86 ± 7.80
70 to 79	40.67 ± 7.57	41.67 ± 9.00

Data extracted from Fon GT, Pitt MJ, Thies AC. Thoracic kyphosis: range in normal subjects. *AJR Am J Roentgenol.* 1980;134:979-983.

discussed previously, excessive kyphosis is associated with impairments of mobility, slower gait speed, difficulty climbing stairs, poor ability to make a 360-degree turn, and poor balance. Additionally, thoracic spine associations with impaired respiratory function,[128,129] cervical pain,[130,131] headaches, and shoulder problems[132,133] have been reported.

Griegel-Morris et al[134] identified postural deviations using a plumb line visual assessment of the thoracic, cervical, and shoulder regions in healthy subjects ages 20 to 50. Interrater and intrarater reliability for postural assessment were K = 0.611 and K = 0.825, respectively. Sixty-six percent had forward head, 38% kyphosis, and 78% round shoulders. No relationship was found between the severity of postural abnormality and the severity or frequency of pain. A significant increase in the incidence of pain was noted in subjects with more severe postural deviations: kyphosis and rounded shoulders increased the incidence of interscapular pain, and forward-head posture increased the incidence of cervical, interscapular, and headache pain. The authors suggest a relationship between the presence of more severe postural deviations and the incidence of pain.[134] Posture-related pain may be due to emotional, neural, articular, or muscular factors, or insidious onset. Individual differences are usually normal variations with ideal posture being uncommon. Additional examination procedures are needed to determine relevance of postural deviations to individual patients.

A standardized definition of normal, excessive, or reduced thoracic kyphosis does not exist. Fon et al[135] measured thoracic kyphosis in 316 normal subjects ages 2 to 77 using a modified Cobb technique.[136] Using a lateral chest radiograph, lines are drawn extending anteriorly along the superior border of the upper vertebra and along the superior border of the lower vertebra. Perpendicular lines are drawn from these 2 lines with the angle measured at the intersection.[135] This study shows that the normal range of kyphosis is related to both patient age and gender with the degree of kyphosis increasing with age. The rate of increase is higher in females than males, becoming more obvious after age 40. The degree of kyphosis in females and males by age is presented in Table 5-5.[135] The authors suggested that their results serve as a useful guideline for predicting normal thoracic kyphosis.[135]

Bartynski et al[137] measured the thoracic kyphotic angle (TKA) in older subjects without vertebral body abnormalities compared to a younger population. A lateral thoracic spine digital radiograph was used to measure the Cobb angle in 90 subjects older than 65 years, 60 subjects between 51 and 65 years, 67 subjects between 36 and 50 years, and 63 subjects between 18 and 35 years of age. In patients older than 65, average TKA was 41.9 degrees, but the distribution was bimodal or nonnormal) with a low mode of 28.3 degrees and an upper mode of 51.5 degrees (P<.001). Elderly women and men independently demonstrate a bimodal TKA distribution with two-thirds of elderly women and half of elderly men having a TKA greater than 40 degrees (ie, upper mode). In younger patients, average TKA was 26.8 degrees. In middle-aged patients, TKA was intermediate with a normal distribution. This study identified a subpopulation of elderly subjects who develop excessive kyphosis in the absence of VCFs and a subgroup who remains near baseline of the younger thoracic curve. In the absence of VCFs, the authors attribute the development of extreme kyphosis to asymmetric disk degeneration, weakened muscular tone, intrinsic hypermobility, and endocrine-related collagen weakening, or some patients may simply have a stiffer spine that has retained its shape over time.[137] The TKA increases with age but not symmetrically. Significant differences exist between men and women. In men, the TKA distribution is normal in the young but shifts with age to become bimodal in the elderly. In women, the TKA distribution is bimodal in the young, becomes symmetric and greater than in men in late middle age, and becomes bimodal in the elderly. Considering the biomechanical effects of severe thoracic kyphosis, this distribution in the elderly suggests a population at risk for compression fracture. As previously discussed, excessive kyphosis and decreased extension occurring over time or as a result of compression fractures may alter mechanical stresses and increase demands for extension in regions above and below the kyphosis, warranting examination and appropriate intervention.

A variety of methods are available to measure thoracic curvature. Visual observation of the thoracic curvature is measured using a grading scale: normal (ie, no deviation), excessive kyphosis (ie, increased convexity), and diminished kyphosis (ie, flattening of the convexity of the thoracic spine). This scale may be used for grading the contour of the thoracic spine for the following subdivisions: C7 to T2 or cervicothoracic junction, T3 to T5, and T6 to T10. Moderate to substantial agreement has been demonstrated using this scale: C7 to T2 excessive kyphosis (k = 0.79 [0.51 to 1.0]); T3 to T5 excessive kyphosis (k = 0.69 [0.3 to 1.0]); T3 to T5 decreased kyphosis (k = 0.58 [0.22 to 0.95]); T6 to T10 excessive kyphosis (k = 0.9 [0.74 to 1.0]); and T6 to T10 decreased kyphosis (k = 0.9 [0.73 to 1.0]).[138]

Greendale et al[125] described the reliability of 3 clinical measures of kyphosis (ie, Debrunner kyphosis angle, flexicurve kyphosis index, and flexicurve kyphosis angle). The Cobb angle using T4 and T12 was measured in standing with a lateral thoracolumbar radiograph. To perform a flexicurve measurement, the flexicurve ruler is gently pressed onto the back from C7 to T12 to approximate the thoracic and/or lumbar curves to L5 to S1 interspace. A trace of the ruler's shape is made on paper and the kyphosis index or angle is calculated. Women with a kyphotic index greater than or equal to 13 have diminished cardiovascular fitness, muscle strength, and physical function.[139,140] Calculations were described by Greendale et al[141] and MacIntyre et al.[142] Each of the clinical measurements had similar reliability and validity. Characteristics of low cost, ease of use, and accommodation to variations in spine contour favor a flexicurve ruler in longitudinal assessments.

MacIntyre et al[142] compared the flexicurve ruler to digital inclinometer measurements of spinal curves to determine intertrial and interrater reliability in postmenopausal women with osteoporosis. The flexicurve ruler was used to calculate the kyphosis index as described previously. Landmarks from the traced curves were used to draw a vertical line to connect the C7 mark and the L5 to S1 interspace, and a perpendicular line drawn at the thoracolumbar junction. The kyphosis index is calculated as thoracic width × 100 divided by thoracic length. Thoracic width is the greatest width from the thoracic curve to the vertical line. Thoracic length is the distance from the C7 mark to the junction of the thoracic and lumbar curves. The digital inclinometers were placed at the C7/T1 interspace, T12/L1 interspace, and sacral midpoint from which the lumbosacral interspace was identified 3.0 cm superiorly. All measures of spine curvature and the kyphosis index in this study had acceptable reliability.[142]

Test-retest reliability of gravity-dependent inclinometer measurements of thoracic kyphosis was established on subjects with and without shoulder pain.[143] The base or feet of the inclinometer was placed over the SPs of T1 and T2 and over T12 and L1 as determined by palpation during relaxed standing. Two sets of 3 measurements were taken with 30 minutes of rest between sets. The thoracic kyphosis angle was the sum of the angle recorded over T1 and T2 and over T12 and L1. The thoracic angle measurement has excellent intrarater reliability for both subjects with and without symptoms. ICC (first measurement) for the subjects without symptoms was 0.95 (95% CI: 0.91 to 0.97). ICC (average) was 0.97 (95% CI: 0.95 to 0.99). The results for subjects with symptoms were ICC 0.93 (95% CI: 0.88 to 0.96) for ICC (first measurement) and for ICC (average) 0.97 (95% CI: 0.94 to 0.98). Standard error of the mean results for subjects without and with symptoms were 1.0 and 1.7 degrees, respectively. While this method appears to be very reliable, the validity is unknown.[143]

Since postural asymmetry and varying degrees of kyphosis are common, the clinician must link the postural findings to the patient's symptoms on an individual basis. For example, 2 studies[132,133] have demonstrated effects of thoracic posture on shoulder pain. In some patients, postural correction in the thoracic spine is related to increasing shoulder motion and decreasing pain. As indicated by the history, posture can be observed in both static and dynamic positions and its contribution individually determined by continued examination and noting the symptom response to altering the patient's observed posture or the demands of postural control.

Lumbar Spine Screen

A working hypothesis that involves a primary complaint of symptoms in the region of T10 and below is most likely best examined using a similar process as described in Chapter 4 for the lumbopelvic region, but it also includes examination procedures directed toward the rib cage as well as selected procedures discussed in this chapter.

Shoulder Screen

The amount of shoulder examination is dictated by the patient's history. No standard examination is available to screen the shoulder. However, bilateral or unilateral shoulder elevation in standing is often assessed because of the regional interdependence between the thoracic spine and UE.

Theodoridis and Ruston[144] investigated upper thoracic movement patterns in 25 asymptomatic women ages 45 to 64. In this study, the predominant pattern is upper thoracic extension coupled with ipsilateral lateral flexion and rotation during unilateral elevation of the arm in the sagittal and scapular planes. In 32 healthy women, Crosbie et al[145] found consistent patterns of thoracic extension during bilateral arm elevation with more extension in the lower thoracic spine than the upper in all 3 elevation planes. No bilateral arm elevation evoked any statistically or functionally significant trunk side flexion or axial rotation. Ipsilateral upper thoracic lateral flexion and axial rotation occur predominantly with unilateral elevation. Lumbar spine motion appears insignificant for all arm elevations. Mobility deficits of the thoracic spine are associated with functional limitation of arm elevation,[146-148] and mobility

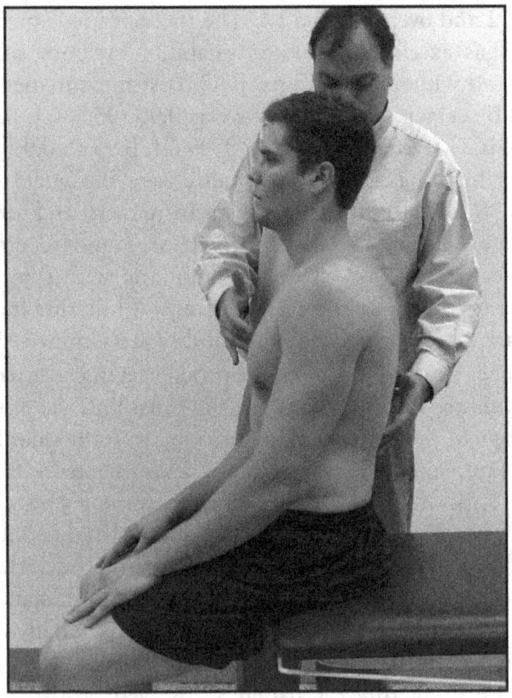

Figure 5-8. Sitting posture lateral view.

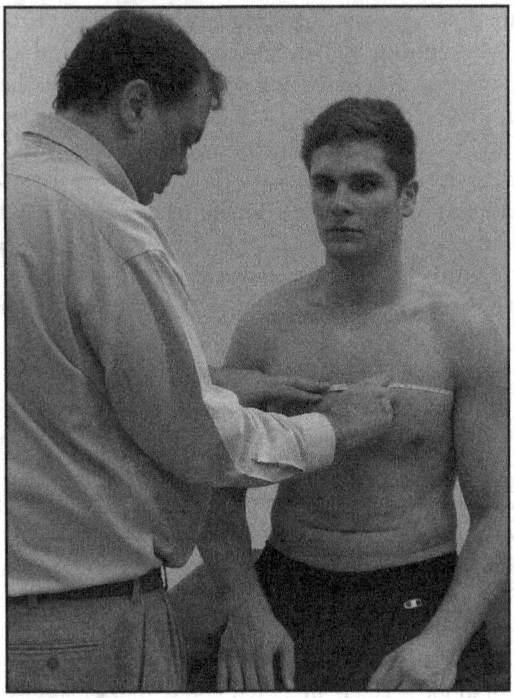

Figure 5-9. Chest expansion measurement.

deficits of the shoulder girdle are likely to create demands or compensatory movements in the thoracic and cervical spine. The interdependence of these 2 regions demands assessment of both regions for patients with mechanical thoracic or shoulder girdle symptoms.

Unilateral shoulder elevation in the sagittal or scapular planes may be used as a screen for limited upper thoracic mobility. Observations that suggest upper thoracic mobility deficits include limited shoulder elevation, limited or absent thoracic extension and ipsilateral lateral flexion and rotation, or compensatory contralateral lateral flexion and rotation. The diagnostic accuracy of unilateral shoulder elevation as a screen for upper thoracic mobility is unknown, but deviations from the expected pattern suggest the need for passive segmental motion of the thoracic spine as well as further examination of the shoulder girdle.

Examination Procedures in Sitting

- Observation, posture, resting symptoms, palpation posteriorly
- Chest expansion
- Thoracic spine active range of motion (AROM)
- Repeated movements
- Neurological screen
- Sitting arm lift (SAL)
- Passive physiological intervertebral movement (PPIVM) test
- Slump test and/or sympathetic slump test (SST)
- Cervical rotation lateral flexion (CRLF) test

Observation, Posture, Resting Symptoms, Palpation Posteriorly

The process of assessing sitting posture (Figure 5-8) and the analysis of lumbopelvic upright, thoracic upright, and slump sitting postures on muscle activation patterns is detailed in Chapter 3. The patient's feet should be supported with the hips at 80 degrees flexion. Resting symptoms and posture are noted. Posture is corrected as needed to assess the effect on symptoms. The patient's ability to find neutral or lumbopelvic upright sitting posture may also be assessed.

If asymmetry is noted in standing, reassessment in sitting may provide additional information since any contributions from the lower extremity are lessened in the seated position. Asymmetry in standing that is no longer present in sitting may be related to the lower extremity or clinician error. Asymmetry in standing that remains in sitting may be structural or related to impairments in the lumbopelvic hip complex or clinician error. Palpation of the posterior thoracic region may be done in sitting and is discussed in the section Examination Procedures in Prone on page 384.

Chest Expansion

Moll and Wright[149] measured chest expansion in 262 normal subjects 111 men and 151 women ages 15 to 75+ years with a tape measure (Figure 5-9). Chest expansion is defined as the difference between maximal inhalation and maximum exhalation. Measurements were made in standing with hands on head and arms flexed in the frontal plane at the level of the fourth intercostal space. The results revealed a wide scatter of normal values in all decades with a gradual but considerable 50% to 60% decrease with advancing age. Male expansion values exceeded female expansion by 13% to 22%. A previously recommended measure of <2.5 cm[150] as the baseline for abnormal expansion is not recommended.

Bockenhauer et al[151] assessed the reliability of using a cloth tape measure in standing to determine chest expansion in 9 healthy male subjects. Upper thoracic circumferential measurements were taken at the level of the fifth thoracic SP and third intercostal space at the midclavicular line. Lower thoracic circumferential measurements were taken at the xiphoid process and at the level of the fifth thoracic SP. Interrater reliability was excellent for upper and lower thoracic measurements with ICCs of 0.86 to 0.91 and 0.81 to 0.84, respectively. Bockenhauer et al[151] reported upper thoracic expansion measured at 2 different sessions ranging from 1 to 7 cm with a mean (SD) of 4.2 (0.8) cm and 1.7 to 6.6 cm with a mean (SD) of 3.6 (0.6) cm. Lower thoracic expansion ranged from 1.5 to 7.8 cm with a mean (SD) of 5.9 (0.5) cm and 1.7 to 7.3 cm with a mean (SD) of 4.9 (0.6) cm. Measuring chest expansion using a cloth tape measure is reliable and may be useful in measuring change associated with pulmonary problems such as asthma or COPD and AS.

Thoracic Spine Active Range of Motion

AROM varies widely among individuals. Therefore, the quality of movement and symptom response may be more important than the gross available range. While nonpainful AROM measures do not correlate highly with function or disability, a gain or loss from baseline in pain-limited AROM often indicates a positive or negative response to treatment. Pain-limited AROM is used to determine a baseline response and reveal impairments or a directional preference for movement. In the thoracic region, mean values in degrees + SDs of 26 + 9 for flexion, 17 + 10 for extension, 49 + 9 for left rotation, 42 + 9 for right rotation, 27 + 6 for left lateral flexion, and 26 + 4 for right lateral flexion were reported for healthy men mean age 31 years (range 24 to 36).[152] General AROM test procedures should be reviewed in Chapter 3. Standard procedures for testing AROM of the thoracic spine do not exist.

Since the upper thoracic spine (T1 to T4/T5) is closely related to the cervical spine and is a common site for referral from the cervical spine, AROM of this region is performed in the same manner as active motion assessment for the cervical spine. Initial cervical spine AROM assessment includes flexion, extension, lateral flexion, rotation, repeated movements of retraction, and retraction with extension and flexion. AROM for the cervical spine is discussed in Chapter 6.

Initial AROM of the mid-thoracic region (T4/T5 to T10) includes flexion, extension, lateral flexion, and rotation with or without overpressure (OP) observing the quality, quantity, and symptom response. Observations include ease of movement and recovery from movement, the presence of aberrant movements, deviation from the tested plane, gross range of movement, change in intensity or location of symptoms from baseline, and where in the range the symptoms occur. Segmental or intervertebral movement is observed and palpated for the presence or absence of a smooth curve or of a fulcrum or sharp angulation that suggests altered (ie, reduced or excessive) segmental mobility. A clearing examination for the cervical spine and/or lumbar spine may be necessary to differentiate symptoms referred from these regions to the thoracic spine.

Lee and Lee[153] noted that thoracic rotation, a primary movement of the thoracic spine and a key element of functional activity, is often limited during AROM testing. Rotational activities require motion control between the thorax and pelvis, thorax and neck, and thorax and shoulder girdle, and segmental control within the thorax.[154] In normal subjects, the contralateral longissimus thoracis should exhibit decreased activity during rotation. Patients with overactivity or cocontraction of the trunk muscles (ie, trunk rigidity) may have decreased rotation in one or both directions as a result of overactivity in the superficial muscles, a nonoptimal control strategy.[155]

Proposed biomechanics for segmental rotation of the thorax include a contralateral translation of the third through sixth thoracic rings.[153] A thoracic ring consists of 2 vertebrae, the intervertebral disc, associated right and left ribs, ligaments, and the anterior sternal attachments. The proposed biomechanics during rotation to the right include translation of the sixth ring to the left. The T5 vertebra rotates and laterally flexes to the right and translates to the left relative to T6. The right sixth rib posteriorly rotates and translates to the left anteromedially, and the left sixth rib anteriorly rotates and translates to the left posterolaterally (Figure 5-10A).[10] Nonoptimal or failed load transfer is defined as no contralateral translation, excessive contralateral translation, ipsilateral translation, or no translation to either side. This concept of failed load transfer can be applied to static positions or a variety of tasks requiring the transfer of forces through the thorax.[153] Using the same concepts in Chapter 4 related to lumbopelvic pain, failed load transfer in the thorax may be due to deficits of form closure, force closure, and/or motor control.[153]

Palpation posterolaterally along the rib cage, using the index fingers along the lateral borders and thumbs along the posterior rib borders at the thoracic ring of interest, is used to assess a dysfunctional pattern or failed load transfer at a specific level during trunk rotation (Figure 5-10B). If manual correction of the dysfunctional pattern can be corrected with a decrease in symptoms and increase in rotation motion, a motor control deficit is hypothesized. Inability to

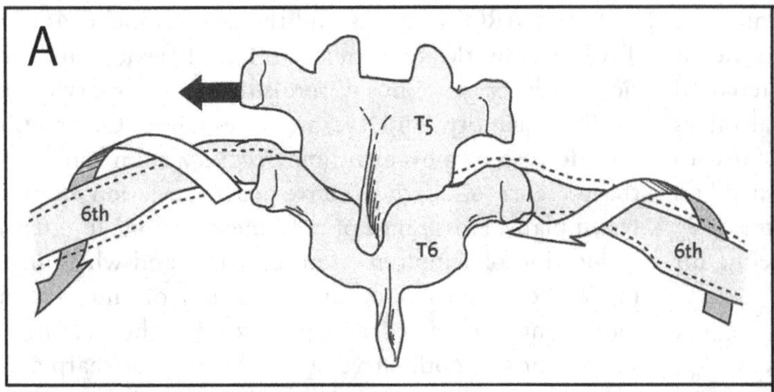

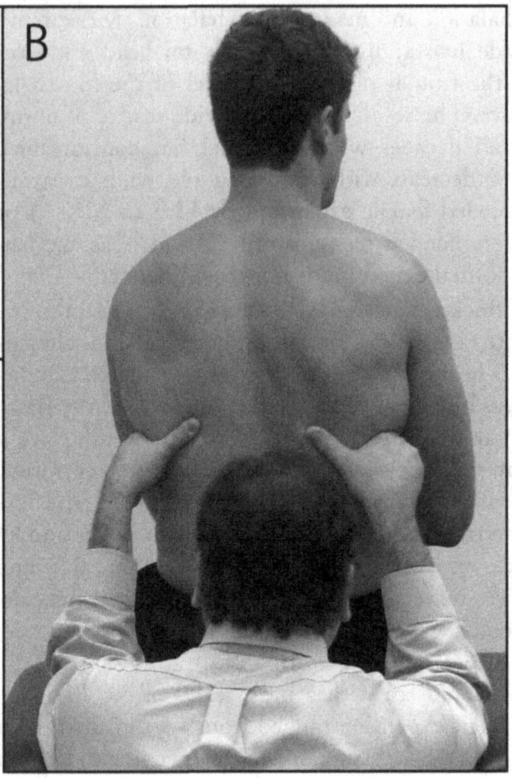

Figure 5-10. Thoracic right rotation. (A) The proposed biomechanics during right rotation are translation of the sixth ring to the left. The T5 vertebra rotates and laterally flexes to the right and translates to the left relative to T6. The right sixth rib posteriorly rotates and translates to the left anteromedially and the left sixth rib anteriorly rotates and translates to the left posterolaterally. (Reprinted with permission from Lee D. *The Thorax. An Integrated Approach.* 2nd ed. White Rock, British Columbia: Diane G. Lee Physiotherapist Corporation; 53.) (B) Palpation posterolaterally along the rib cage during right rotation.

manually correct the dysfunctional pattern suggests a pattern related to stiffness such as joint hypomobility or overactive superficial muscles.[153] Additional testing such as the SAL or prone arm lift (PAL; discussed later in this section) are required for confirmation. Lee and Lee[153] also advocate for palpation of thoracic ring biomechanics as described previously during neurodynamic tests such as slump and upper limb neurodynamic testing (ULNDT).

AROM of the thoracic spine in sitting is shown in Figures 5-11 and 5-12. With the patient's feet supported and arms across the chest or hands clasped behind neck, the patient is instructed to perform AROM. From behind and/or a lateral view, the clinician observes for symptom response (ie, change in location and intensity from baseline), gross and segmental mobility, and deviations from the tested plane. Depending on the location of symptoms, the clinician may want to allow cervical motion with all of the motions or attempt to maintain the cervical spine in neutral to assist in differentiation of the cervical and thoracic spine. If AROM fails to provoke the patient's symptoms, add OP.

Active Range of Motion Measurement—Inclinometry (Figure 5-13)

Normative values for thoracic spine motion are not established. In 31 subjects without thoracic pathology, Lee et al[156] reported moderate reliability for standing single inclinometry measurements of flexion (F), extension (E), and right and left lateral flexion (LF) of the thoracic spine (T1 to T12) on 2 different days (mean 4.2 days). The measurements allowed cervical motion. Intrarater ICCs (rater 1) were 0.84, 0.79, 0.84, and 0.86 for F, E, R LF, and L LF, respectively. Intrarater ICCs (rater 2) were 0.88, 0.48, 0.84, and 0.78 for F, E, R LF, and L LF, respectively. Interrater ICCs (day 1) were 0.81, 0.65, 0.45, and 0.88 for F, E, R LF, and L LF, respectively. Interrater ICCs (day 2) were 0.85, 0.86, 0.46, and 0.75 for F, E, R LF, and L LF, respectively. Validity for lateral flexion compared to a radiographic reference was poor to moderate (ICCs 0.43 to 0.66). The high values of the smallest detectable difference, range 8 to 15 degrees, are not sensitive enough to detect meaningful change in thoracic AROM using this method.[156] Reliability may be compromised by many factors such as palpation, instructions to the patient, pain, structural abnormalities such as adolescent or adult idiopathic scoliosis,[157] and the starting position of the patient. Thoracic rotation is measured using a standard goniometer or visual estimate. Further research is needed for the thoracic spine.

Differentiation of Cervical and Thoracic Spine

Since symptoms in the upper to mid-thoracic spine may be referred from the cervical spine and when both the cervical and thoracic spine are involved in the provocative movement, differentiating the source of thoracic spine symptoms is often difficult. Magarey[158] offered a differentiation process using the following examples. If combined cervical and thoracic rotation to the right is

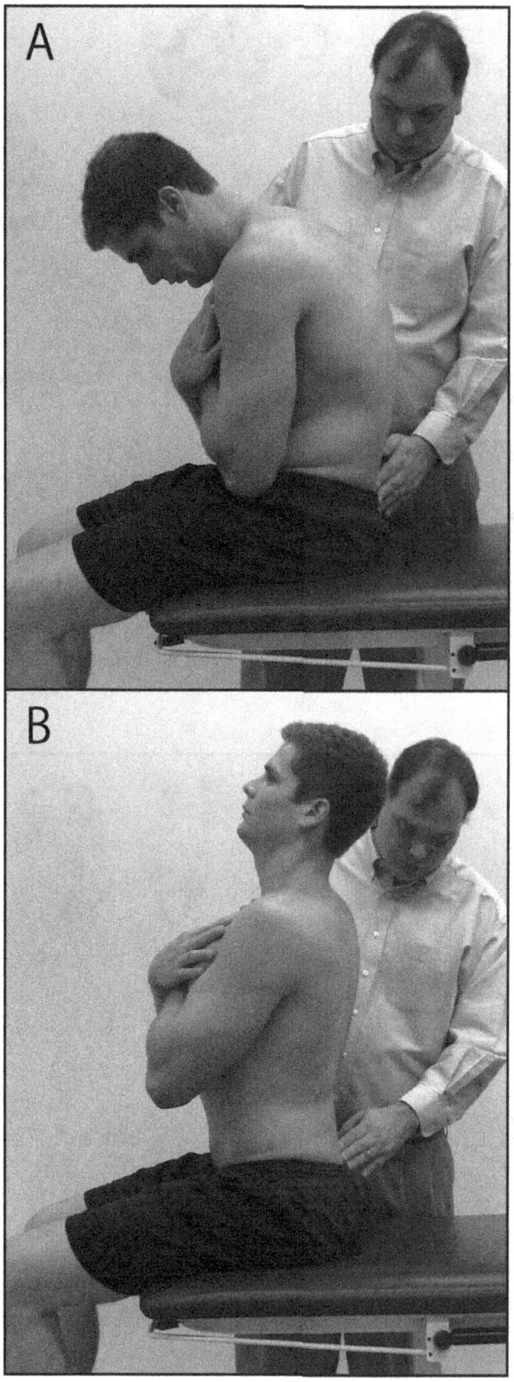

Figure 5-11. AROM. (A) Flexion. Instruct the patient to move by pulling the elbows in toward the groin. (B) Extension. Instruct the patient to raise the elbows upward or elevate the arms overhead.

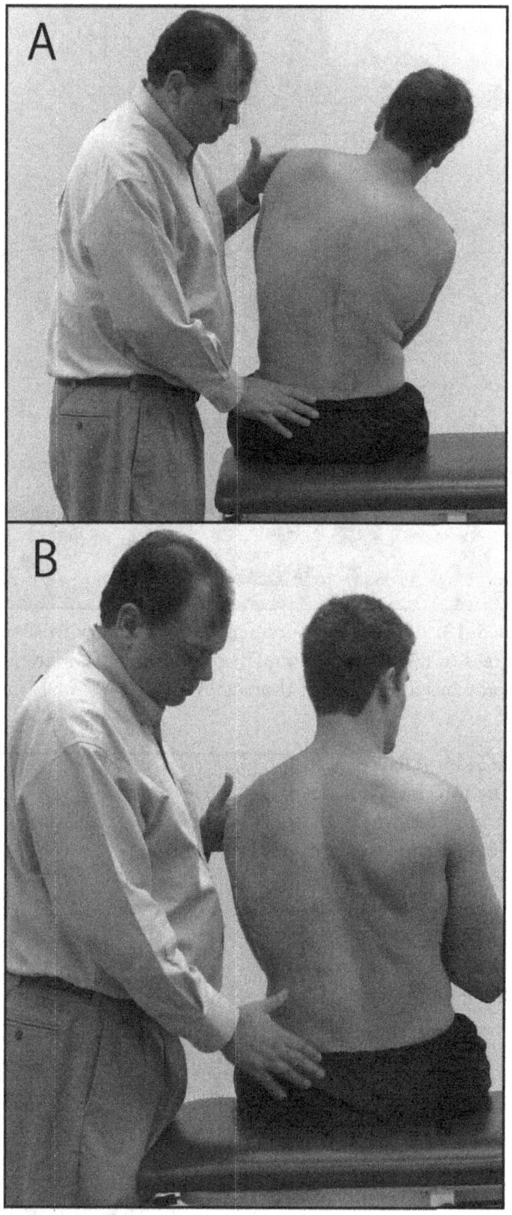

Figure 5-12. AROM. (A) Right lateral flexion. Instruct the patient to bend to the right. The pelvis should remain stable in the frontal plane with the ischial tuberosities firmly on the table. (B) Right rotation. Instruct the patient to twist to the right with ischial tuberosities firmly on the table. Left lateral flexion and left rotation are performed in a similar manner.

provocative, cervical rotation is maintained while thoracic rotation is further increased slightly to the right, resulting in increased stress in the thoracic spine but decreased stress in the cervical spine. If the symptoms are increased, the thoracic spine is implicated. If the symptoms decrease or remain the same, the cervical spine is implicated. This response is confirmed by slight thoracic rotation to the left while maintaining cervical rotation, which results in an increased stress on the cervical spine and decreased stress on the thoracic spine. If symptoms remain the same or increase, the cervical spine is implicated. If the symptoms decrease, the thoracic spine is implicated. Ultimately, a detailed examination of each region may be necessary, but attempts to differentiate which region is involved serve to guide the rest of the examination.

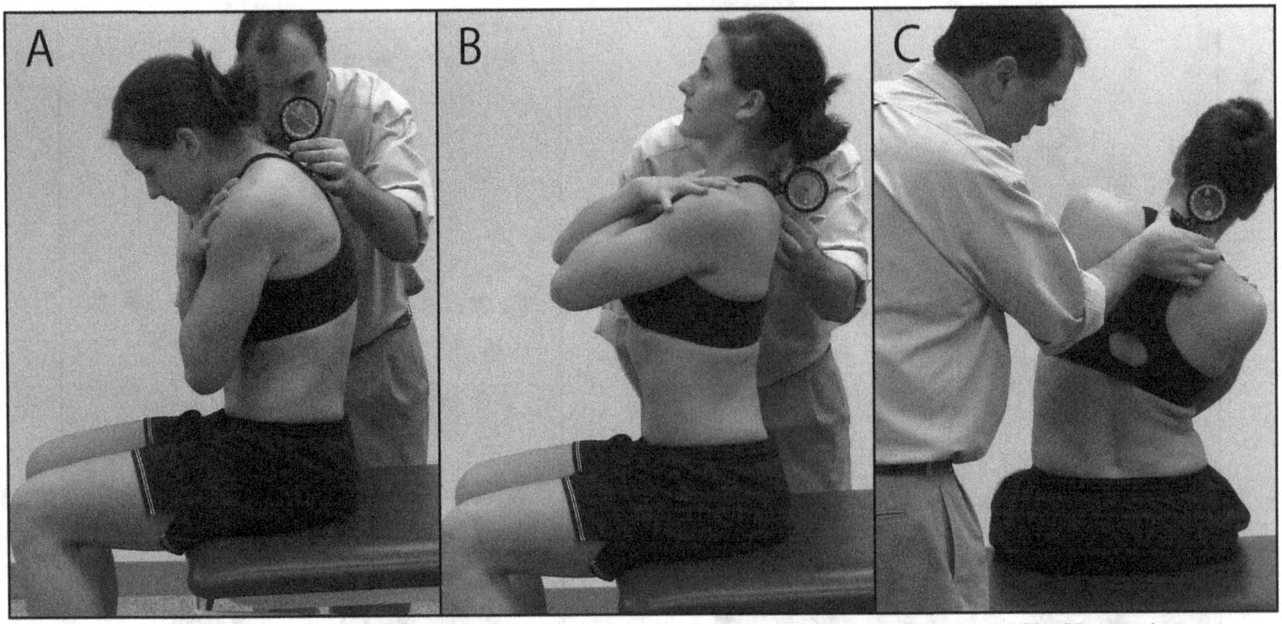

Figure 5-13. AROM measurement—inclinometry in sitting. One inclinometer placed and zeroed at the T1 SP provides a measure in degrees of (A) total flexion, (B) extension, or (C) lateral flexion. The process is repeated at the T12 SP. The difference (T1 minus T12) provides a measure of thoracic AROM.

Figure 5-14. AROM with OP. The inferior hand stabilizes at T12 while the mobilizing hand oscillates through the trunk as close as possible to T1: (A) flexion; (B) extension. *(continued)*

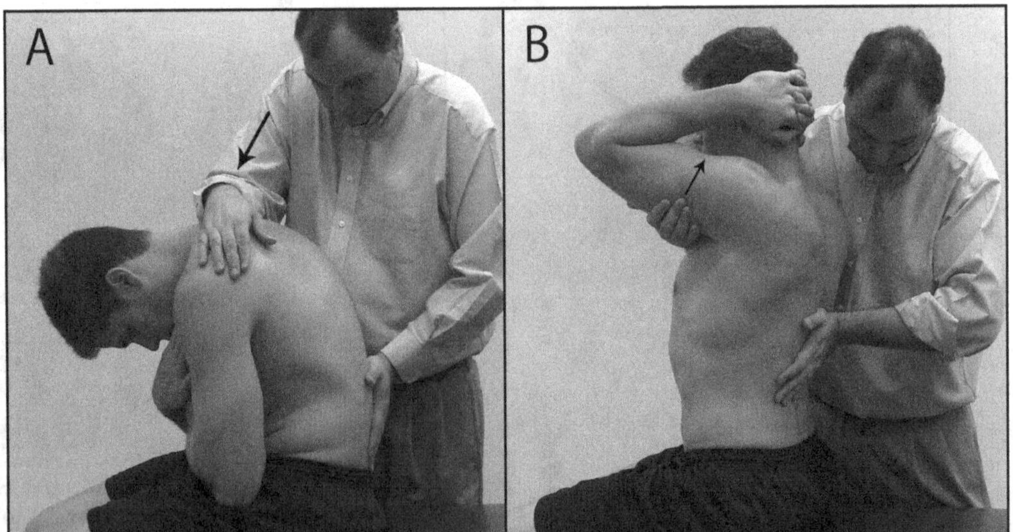

Active Range of Motion With Overpressure

If it is indicated and safe for the patient and AROM is full range and painless, passive OP performed in an oscillatory manner at the limit of the movement confirms the end-feel and effect on symptoms. If AROM with OP is normal (Figure 5-14), try repeated movements, sustained movements, or combined movements to reproduce the patient's symptoms.

Repeated Movements (Figure 5-15)

Assessment using repeated movements in the thoracic spine is the same as used in the lumbar spine. When a patient's symptoms centralize during repeated movements such as flexion, extension, or rotation, the direction that produces the centralization suggests a subgroup classification that is likely to respond to repeated movements in the direction that resulted in centralization.[159] For example, if centralization occurs with repeated thoracic extension, repeated extension is the recommended intervention.

Sagittal plane movements of repeated flexion or extension are tested first. As needed, rotation is tested toward the side of pain when the response to sagittal plane movements is nonresponsive or inconclusive or with unilateral or asymmetrical symptoms. Clear communication is necessary

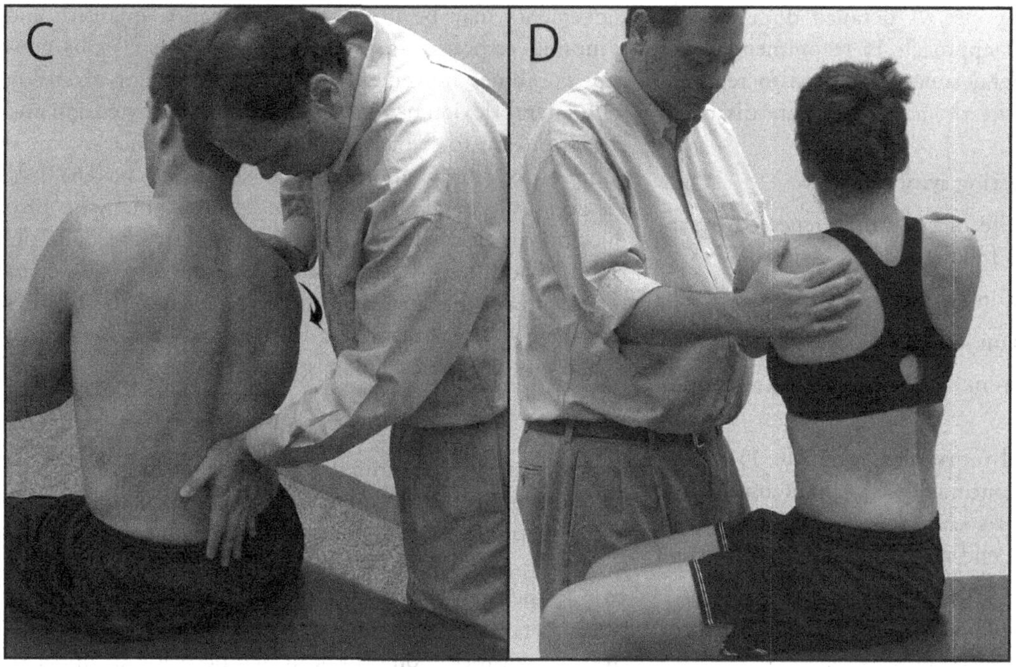

Figure 5-14 (continued). AROM with OP. The inferior hand stabilizes at T12 while the mobilizing hand oscillates through the trunk as close as possible to T1: (C) lateral flexion; and (D) rotation. OP may be localized to various levels by changing the position of the stabilization hand.

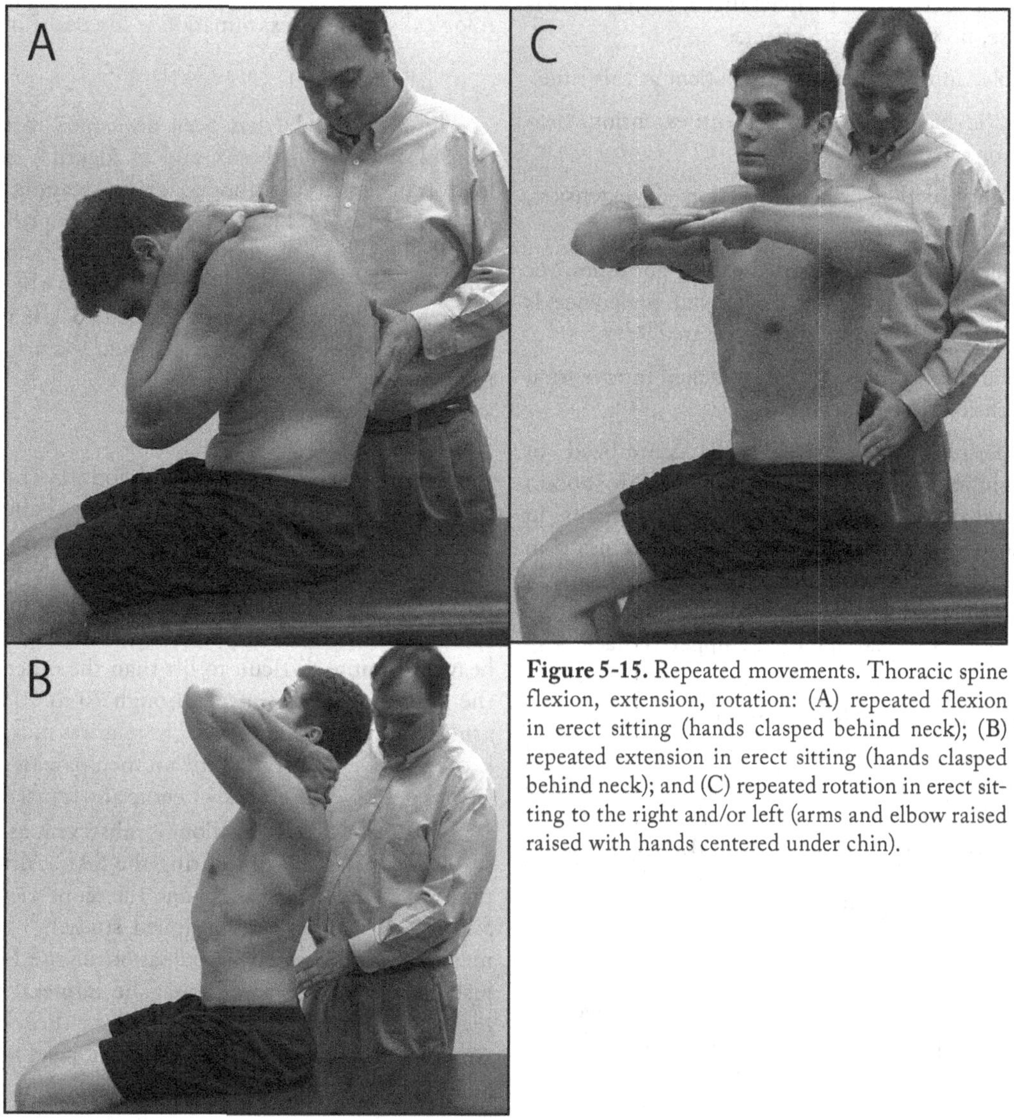

Figure 5-15. Repeated movements. Thoracic spine flexion, extension, rotation: (A) repeated flexion in erect sitting (hands clasped behind neck); (B) repeated extension in erect sitting (hands clasped behind neck); and (C) repeated rotation in erect sitting to the right and/or left (arms and elbow raised raised with hands centered under chin).

to correctly note the response. A detailed discussion of the repeated movements approach is recommended for further study.[159,160] General concepts related to repeated movement testing[159] in the thoracic region are discussed as follows:

- Establish baseline resting symptoms.
- Explain the procedure of end-range repeated movements and assess the following:
    - Repeated flexion in erect sitting
    - Repeated extension in erect sitting
    - Repeated rotation in erect sitting to the right and/or left
- During the repeated movements of 10 to 15 repetitions, the clinician continually asks about any change in symptom behavior such as location, intensity, during movement, or at end-range and notes any change in quantity of movement.
- Record the response about 1 to 2 minutes after the movements.
- Responses: centralized, peripheralized, better, no better, worse, no worse, or no effect.
- If possible, appropriately classify patient at this time.
    - Specific exercise or derangement: extension, flexion, or rotation
    - Mobility deficits or dysfunction of extension, flexion, or rotation
- If a repeated movement decreases, abolishes, or centralizes symptoms or a directional preference is obtained, further testing is unnecessary.[159,160]
    - If centralized, proceed with matched intervention (extension, flexion, rotation).
    - If peripheralized or partially centralized in weightbearing, the clinician attempts to obtain centralization through repeated movements in unloaded positions such as repeated extension in lying (REIL; prone for lower thoracic segments) or repeated extension supine as described in Chapter 6 for the cervical spine and upper thoracic segments.
    - If the response is limited motion and end-range pain only (ie, produced, increased, or no worse) and no centralization or peripheralization occurs, further examination such as passive accessory intervertebral movement (PAIVM) or PPIVM are indicated. The clinician considers a classification of TSP with mobility deficits.

Combined Movement Testing

If AROM and repeated movements are full range and do not provoke a patient's symptoms or are inconclusive, combined movements of any combination of thoracic movements may be used to assess quality, quantity and symptom response. Introduced by Edwards,[161] this concept combines movements of either flexion or extension with lateral flexion or rotation. For example, extension and lateral flexion to the left are thought to produce maximal compression forces to the spinal structures on the left. Flexion and lateral flexion to the left are thought to produce maximal tensile stresses to the spinal structures on the right. In addition to being used as a provocative test, combined movements may help to direct positioning during treatment.[161] Diagnostic utility of combined movement testing in the thoracic spine is unknown.

Neurological Screen

A neurological examination is required for all patients who exhibit cervicothoracic pain or thoracolumbar pain with symptoms extending into the extremities, weakness, numbness, paresthesia, anesthesia, radicular pain, referred pain to the chest wall or abdomen, a history of neurological deficit, or with symptoms of an unknown origin. Details from the history should indicate the need for an upper or lower motor neuron or cranial nerve examination. The neurological screening examination is discussed in Chapter 3.

Sitting Arm Lift (Figure 5-16)

The SAL[14,153,162] has been developed to test interring control within the thorax and to identify areas of failed load transfer in the thorax, spine, scapula, and glenohumeral joint.[153] The SAL is based on principles of the ASLR. The test is recommended for all patients with upper quadrant symptoms as a guide to focus the initial treatment for failed load transfer related to UE movement or another task relevant to the patient.[153] Diagnostic utility is unknown.

Test Procedure

The patient is seated with hands resting on thighs without postural correction to observe habitual pattern. The patient raises the uninvolved arm into flexion with the thumb up and then raises the involved arm in the same manner. In addition to the quality of movement and symptom response, the patient is then asked if one arm is heavier or more difficult to lift than the other, keying into the initiation of movement through 70 to 90 degrees. The arm that is reported as heavier or requires more effort to lift is the positive side. The clinician then palpates the thoracic ring as described previously to note any translation.[14,153,162]

The scapula rest position is observed as well as the scapulohumeral rhythm during the SAL. Altered scapular position or movement is beyond the scope of this reference and recommended for continued study.[163] The glenohumeral joint is assessed by palpation of the humeral head just inferior to the acromion. The humeral head should remain centered on the glenoid fossa through elevation. Anterior translation of the humeral head is considered failed load transfer of the glenohumeral joint.

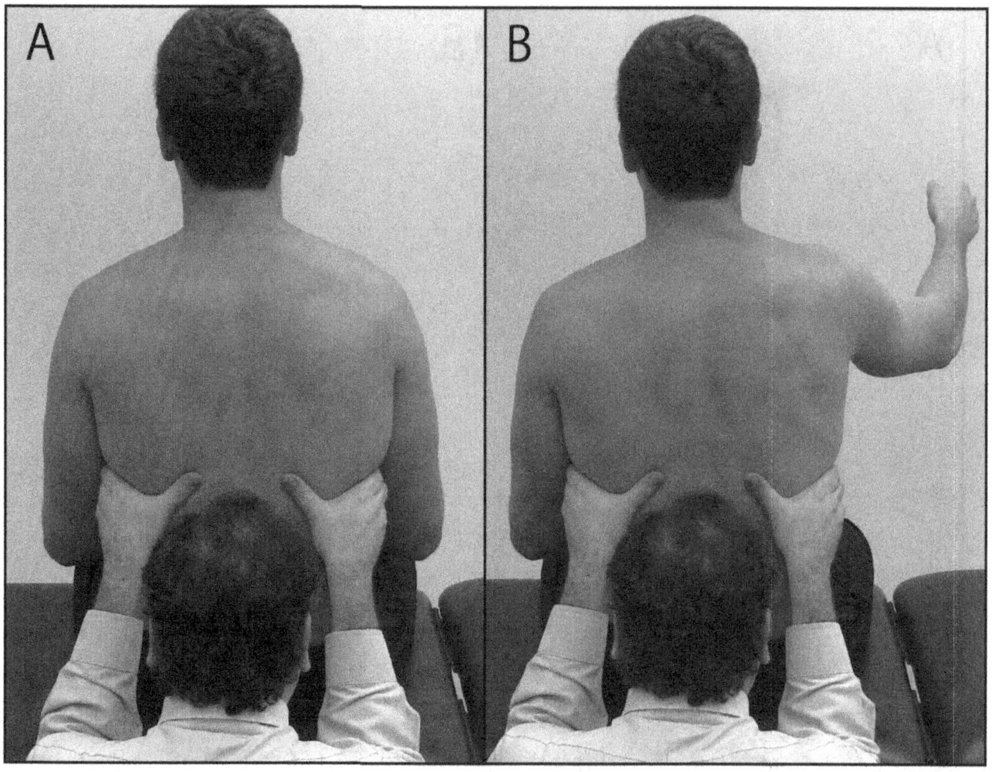

Figure 5-16. SAL: (A) starting position and (B) normal response.

During the SAL, the C2 to C7 motion segments are palpated bilaterally along the lateral aspect of the articular pillars. Failed load transfer is observed through anterior, posterior, or lateral translation of a superior vertebra relative to an inferior vertebra. Slight cervical extension, lateral flexion, and rotation to the same side occur through the cervical levels at the end of elevation. Excessive translation at one level (ie, often translation to the same side and rotation to the opposite side) is identified as poor segmental control.

Normal Response

At the beginning of raising the arm, the thorax provides a stable base with no shifts or translations in any direction within the thorax. As discussed in Chapter 4, the trunk is stabilized by central nervous system muscle feed forward activation in preparation for moving the UE. The spinal curve relationship of thorax to head and thorax to pelvis should be maintained. Near the end of arm elevation, the upper thoracic spine extends, rotates, and laterally flexes to the same side.[14,153,162]

Positive Test

A positive test for failed load transfer is palpated when one or more of the thoracic rings or its components translates along any axis or rotates in any plane. Loss of control is usually noted on initiation to mid-range of elevation with lateral translation occurring to the same side or opposite of the arm lift. Similar to the altered timing observed in the lumbopelvic region, the lateral translation is thought to occur by altered timing and recruitment between the long superficial thoracic longissimus muscles and the deep multifidus segmental muscles. Preliminary evidence supports this hypothesis during trunk perturbation requiring rotational control.[164] As discussed previously, failed load transfer may occur at the scapula, glenohumeral joint, or cervical spine.[14,153,162]

Correction of the Identified Areas of Failed Load Transfer

General postural correction is made and the SAL repeated. If the arm is easier to lift, then postural re-education is indicated. Any abnormal translation at rest or during movement is manually corrected by the clinician and the SAL is repeated, noting any difference in symptoms or effort. For the cervical and thoracic spine, a gentle traction force is applied along with the correction of the translation. In addition to identifying areas of failed load transfer, the response to the addition of manual correction of increased stability or compression during the SAL is used to guide intervention.[14,153,162]

If manual correction reduces symptoms or effort to lift the arm, intervention is directed toward improving motor control and stability through stabilization exercises, postural re-education, and activity and movement retraining in that area. If symptoms are worse or the effort to raise the arm is increased, the region most likely has sufficient or excessive compression. Intervention is directed toward improving mobility through joint mobilization or

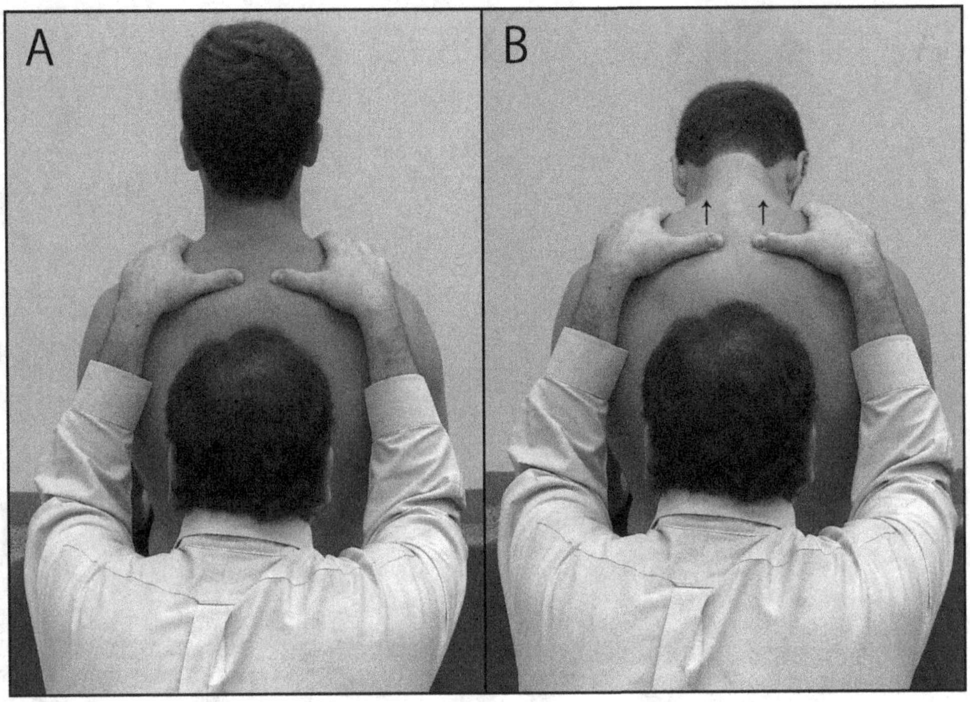

Figure 5-17. Segmental mobility testing for T1 to T4: (A) starting position; (B) symmetrical motion for flexion. *(continued)*

manipulation or reducing excessive muscle tone through breathing retraining, postural re-education, or soft tissue mobilization. Additional testing of PAIVM or PPIVM testing, palpation of multifidus, or other trunk muscles is required to determine specific interventions to improve mobility and stability.

Passive Physiological Intervertebral Movement Test

Several models[10,165,166] exist for assessment of thoracic spine segmental mobility with no system known to be superior to another. For T1 to T4 motion segments, the osteopathic model is used for segmental mobility testing by following the transverse processes (TPs) of one segment through an arc of motion.[166] For T4 to T10 motion segments, PPIVMs are performed primarily in sitting to assess flexion, extension, lateral flexion, and rotation to determine if movement at an appropriate spinal segment reproduces the patient's symptoms and whether the segmental motion is normal, hypomobile, or hypermobile for purposes of diagnostic classification and guiding intervention.[165] The PPIVM quality, quantity, and symptom response are not used in isolation, but instead combined with key subjective and objective examination findings to form a diagnostic classification. T10 to T12 PPIVMs are assessed in side-lying as described for the lumbar spine.

Interrater reliability studies involving PPIVM of the thoracic spine are limited. Brismée et al[167] demonstrated fair to substantial interrater reliability for PPIVM at T5 to T7 on healthy subjects. For the upper 8 segments of the thoracic spine during sitting motion palpation, prone motion palpation, and palpation for tenderness, Christensen et al[168] reported good intraobserver reliability but poor interobserver reliability for motion palpation only. Paraspinal tenderness showed good interobserver reliability. Haas et al[169] examined T3 to L1 rotation PPIVM to identify hypomobile segments resulting in fair reliability. Similar to the lumbar and cervical spine uncertainty exists regarding the reliability of these manual assessments. No studies have examined validity in the thoracic spine.

Segmental Motion Testing for T1 to T4 (Figure 5-17)

This method of segmental motion assessment is based upon the biomechanical model of motion in the thoracic spine.[166] Flexion occurs when both inferior facets of superior vertebrae glide upward on the superior facets of the inferior vertebra as the superior vertebral body rolls and glides anteriorly. The reverse occurs during thoracic extension.

With the patient seated in neutral, the clinician palpates the TPs of T1 with his or her thumbs and instructs the patient to bend his or her head and neck forward into flexion. Normal motion is perceived when the TPs move symmetrically in a superior and anterior direction. If one or both sides do not move in the anticipated direction, motion at that segment is considered abnormal, suggesting a flexion motion restriction on that side or on both sides at the T1/T2 motion segment. A unilateral flexion restriction may also include limitation in contralateral lateral flexion and rotation. Similarly, while palpating the TP of T1, the patient is instructed to extend the head and neck. Normal motion is perceived when the TPs move symmetrically in an inferior and posterior direction. If one or both sides

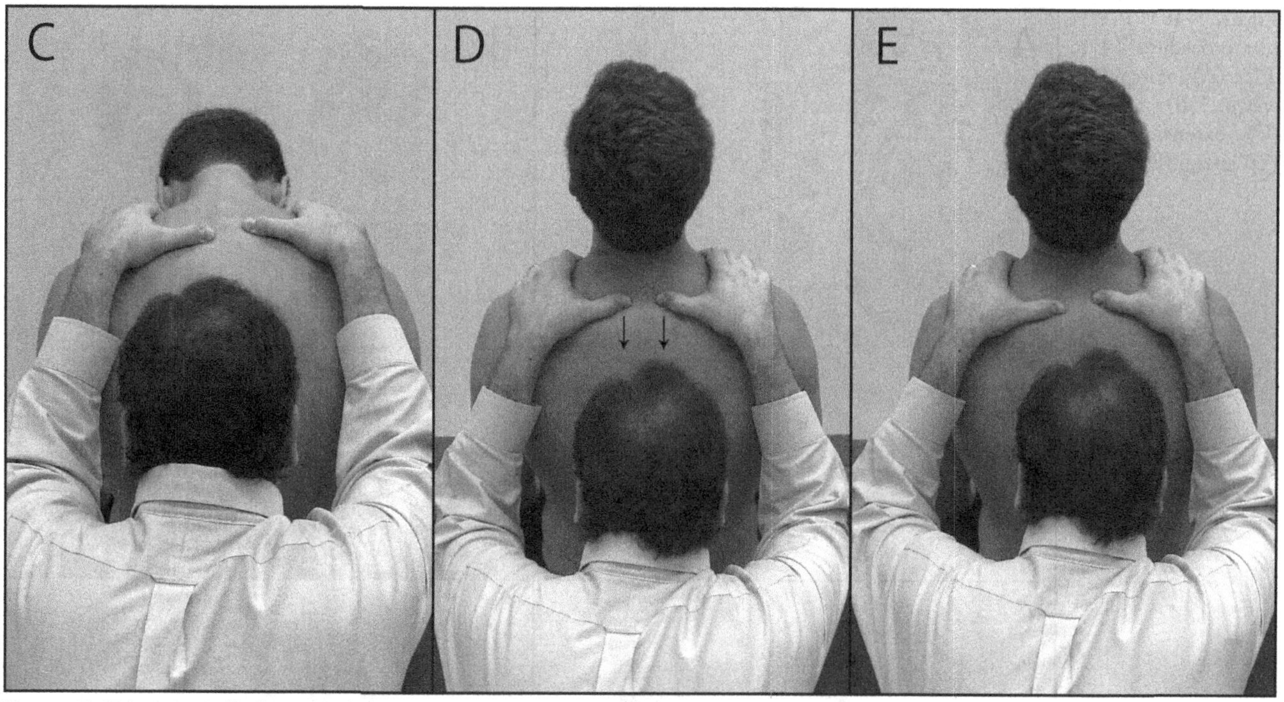

Figure 5-17 (continued). Segmental mobility testing for T1 to T4: (C) asymmetrical motion for flexion suggesting a flexion motion deficit on the left side; (D) symmetrical motion for extension; and (E) asymmetrical motion for extension suggesting an extension motion deficit on the right side.

do not move in the anticipated direction, motion at that segment is considered abnormal, suggesting an extension motion restriction on that side or both sides at the T1/T2 motion segment. A unilateral extension restriction may also include limitation in ipsilateral lateral flexion and rotation. Correlation or additional testing with active motion findings, PPIVM or PAIVM, and/or muscle length tests may be necessary for confirmation.

Passive Physiological Intervertebral Movement Flexion (Figures 5-18A and B)

The patient is seated with hands clasped behind his or her neck. The motion segment of T5/T6 is used as an example. The clinician stands to the side of the patient to support the trunk with one arm and palpate at the interspinous space (see Figure 5-18A) with the pad of the index or middle finger. A neutral position for each segment should be the starting position for assessment. The trunk is slowly flexed from the neutral position until motion is felt at the interspinous space. When T6 SP starts to move, the end of segmental flexion is reached. The clinician assesses the amount of opening at the interspinous space and returns to neutral. Each segment is graded as normal, hypomobile, or hypermobile.[165]

Passive Physiological Intervertebral Movement Extension (Figure 5-18C)

The motion segment of T5/T6 is used as an example. Extension is performed in a similar manner except that the trunk is slowly extended until motion is felt at the interspinous space. A neutral position for each segment should be the starting position for assessment. The clinician assesses the amount of closing at the interspinous space and returns to neutral. Each segment is graded as normal, hypomobile, or hypermobile.[165]

Passive Physiological Intervertebral Movement Lateral Flexion Left/Right (Figure 5-18D)

The motion segment of T5/T6 is used as an example. Lateral flexion is performed by slowly moving the trunk into left or right lateral flexion until motion is felt at the interspinous space. The clinician stands on the side of the direction of motion (ie, left side for left lateral flexion). A neutral position for each segment should be the starting position for assessment. A closing motion at the interspinous space is felt as the T5 SP moves toward T6 into the palpating finger for left lateral flexion. The clinician assesses the amount of closing and returns to neutral. Each segment is graded as normal, hypomobile, or hypermobile.[165]

Passive Physiological Intervertebral Movement Rotation Left/Right

The motion segment of T5/T6 is used as an example. Rotation is performed by slowly moving the trunk into left or right rotation until motion is felt at the interspinous space. The clinician stands on the side of the direction of

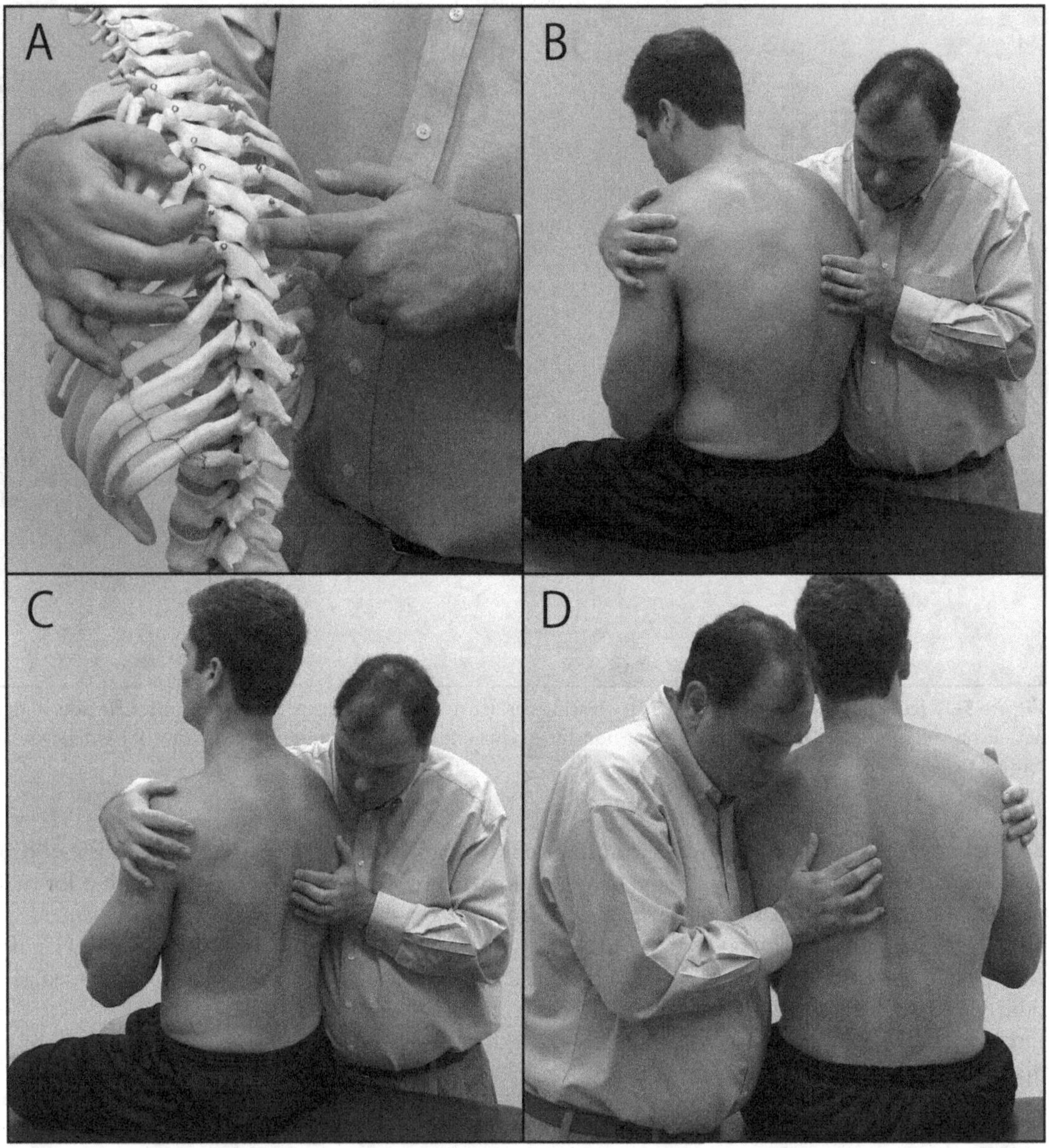

Figure 5-18. PPIVM test procedure T4 to T10: (A) interspinous space; (B) flexion; (C) extension; and (D) lateral flexion.

motion (ie, left side for left rotation). A neutral position for each segment should be the starting position for assessment. The palpating finger at the interspinous space of T5/T6 notes that the T5 SP move into the pad of the middle finger. When T6 starts to move, the end of segmental rotation is reached. The clinician assesses the amount of motion and returns to neutral. Each segment is graded as normal, hypomobile, or hypermobile.

Slump Test and/or Sympathetic Slump Test

The sympathetic nervous system (SNS) may be linked to conditions such as complex regional pain syndrome (CRPS), T4 syndrome, and TOS. CRPS presents with continuous pain, usually out of proportion to the severity of the injury or continuing beyond the time expected for healing. Regions affected include the extremities, hands, and feet with complaints of intense burning pain, sensitivity to touch, sweating, and edema as well as alteration in the color and temperature of skin. The cause is unknown, but in some individuals the SNS is thought to contribute to or sustain the pain.[170] Several studies indicate that it is possible to influence peripheral sympathetic function with increases in skin conductance and decreases in skin temperature in response to spinal mobilization.

Sympathetic preganglionic nerves leave the central nervous system between T1 and L2 to join the sympathetic ganglia, which form chains running anteriorly along the rib heads and costovertebral joints. Postganglionic nerves leave the ganglia to supply their target organ, skin, blood vessels, nerves, and skeletal muscle. Postganglionic nerves supply every part of the peripheral nervous system from the dorsal root ganglion to the peripheral pain receptors. The sympathetic neurons to the head and neck arise from T1 to T4, the UE from T1 to T9; to the thorax T3 to T6; to the abdomen T7 to T11; and the lower extremity from T12 to L2.[171] The role of the SNS is beyond the scope of this reference, but the SNS has the potential to exert widespread effects on its target tissues that potentially influence the rate and extent of pain and tissue repair after injury. Evaluation and treatment using the SST is largely based on basic science,[172-175] clinical speculation, and case reports.[176]

Clinically, impaired mobility of the thorax appears to be linked with local and referred pain to the trunk and extremities. Clinical reasoning leads to the possibility that deficits in thoracic spine mobility might be accompanied by altered sympathetic neurodynamics or other thoracic neurodynamics of the spinal nerve or nerve root. Mechanical compromise (ie, irritation, compression, or stretching) of the sympathetic neural tissues theoretically can occur with trauma, postsurgery, sustained or repetitive microtrauma, or altered postures or movement of the extremities, resulting in altered mechanosensitivity. Clinical observations suggest that spinal manipulation of the thoracic region can alter symptoms associated with a positive slump test or SST.

The SST, also known as the long sit slump test and a variation of the slump test, is theoretically designed to mechanically load the sympathetic trunk and sympathetic peripheral nervous system and assess its mobility and mechanosensitivity.[172] The SST is recommended when the sympathetic trunk is suspected of contributing to symptoms such as hyper or hypohidrosis, altered skin color, or temperature; the history suggests a slumped, provocative position (ie, reading in bed) or position of injury; a thoracic neurogenic disorder is suspected; or the slump test does not adequately reproduce the patient's symptoms.[172] Precautions and contraindications for the slump test are discussed in Chapter 3.

Reliability and validity of the SST are unknown. Slater et al[172] used a randomized, repeated measures, double-blind, placebo-controlled protocol (n = 22) to evaluate the effects of SST, placebo, and control conditions on skin conductance and skin temperature in the UEs. The SST produced a significantly greater increase in skin conductance than either placebo or control. A greater increase in skin conductance was observed in the right UE compared to the left UE. The technique used in this study consisted of a grade IV, posterior-to-anterior (PA) mobilization to the right T6 costovertebral joint thought to bias the right sympathetic trunk. Significant changes in skin temperature occurred for both SST and placebo compared to control, but there was no significant difference between SST and placebo. The authors concluded that the SST technique influences peripheral SNS function and has the capacity to differentially increase sympathetic activity in the ipsilateral UE.[172]

In asymptomatic subjects and subjects with frozen shoulder, the SST technique with T6 costovertebral mobilization produced significant increases in sudomotor activity and reduction in skin temperature at the hand with a trend toward decreases in skin conductance and temperature in the involved side. The authors interpreted the response as a sympathoexcitatory effect.[177]

Cleland et al[175] assessed sympathetically mediated peripheral sudomotor (ie, sweating) and vasomotor (ie, temperature) responses in the feet of healthy, asymptomatic individuals (n = 10) during the SST or long sitting slump. The SST was performed using a grade IV, PA mobilization to the right, 10th costovertebral joint for 30 seconds. The same position was used as the control with the hand placed at the right, 10th costovertebral joint, but no mobilization provided. The results of this study did not support a sympathoexcitatory response to SST, only a trend toward increased skin conductivity and decreased skin temperature in the ipsilateral lower extremity, perhaps due to the low number of subjects.[175] The neurophysiological effects of spinal manipulative therapy (SMT) were discussed in Chapter 4. Speculation about the effects mediated by the SNS through thoracic SMT are discussed later under intervention.

Test Procedure

Butler and Slater[173] proposed the sympathetic trunk is unilaterally lengthened in the long sit position by adding contralateral thoracic lateral flexion, contralateral thoracic rotation, and contralateral cervical lateral flexion. Care is required at each step to assess range of movement, quality of movement, and symptom response. A sequence of test procedures is provided as follows (Figure 5-19)[173,174]:

- Patient is in the long sit position with knees extended and thoracic and lumbar spine in neutral; therapist position is standing beside patient.
- *Step 1*: Establish resting symptoms, explain the procedure, and begin with the uninvolved side.
- *Step 2*: Ask patient to slump (ie, thoracic and lumbar flexion) but do not allow neck flexion; assess response.
- *Step 3*: Gently over press thoracic and lumbar spine position, add cervical flexion; assess response.
- *Step 4*: Gently over press and maintain Step 3 position; add contralateral lateral thoracic flexion; assess response; sensitize by releasing cervical flexion or adding knee flexion.
- *Step 5*: Gently over press and maintain Step 4 position; add contralateral lateral thoracic rotation; assess response; sensitize by releasing cervical flexion or adding knee flexion.
- *Step 6*: Gently over press and maintain Step 5; add cervical contralateral lateral flexion; assess response; sensitize by releasing cervical flexion or adding knee flexion.
- *Step 7*: Repeat steps on involved side.
- *Note*: If symptoms decrease or disappear with sensitization, slowly increase range of the limited component until symptoms reappear.

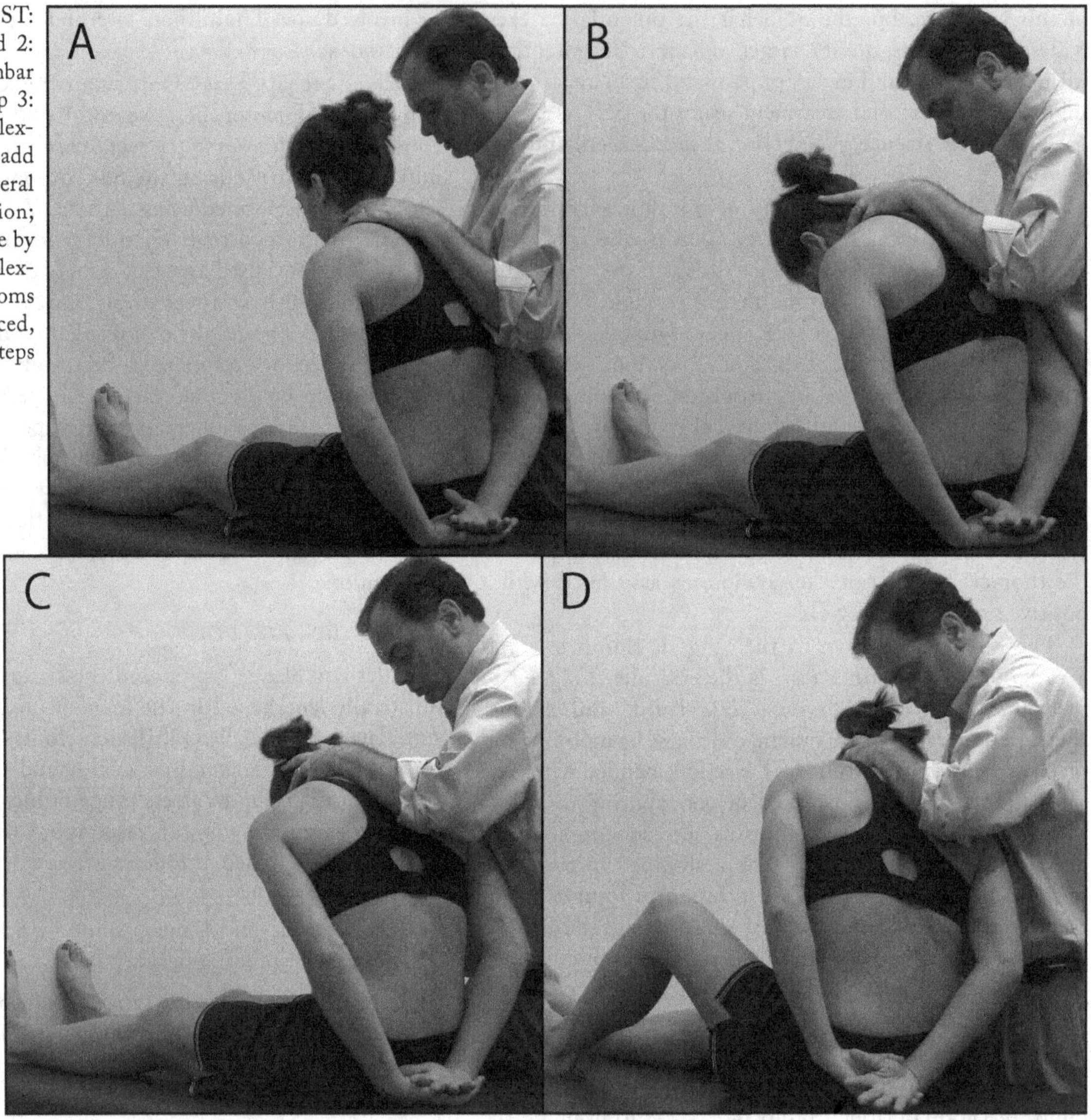

Figure 5-19. SST: (A) Steps 1 and 2: thoracic and lumbar flexion; (B) Step 3: add cervical flexion; (C) Step 4: add contralateral lateral thoracic flexion; and (D) sensitize by adding knee flexion. If symptoms are not produced, continue with steps 5, 6, and 7.

Positive Test

A positive test is defined as reproduction of some or all of the patient's symptoms, asymmetry from uninvolved to involved sides, and a positive sensitizing maneuver. A positive test suggests sensitivity of the sympathetic peripheral nervous system but does not indicate that the sympathetic system is the cause of the symptoms or the source of the symptoms. Normal responses to the SST in asymptomatic subjects have not been reported.

Cervical Rotation Lateral Flexion Test

The CRLF test (Figure 5-20) is purported to determine the presence of first rib hypomobility in patients with brachialgia and TOS.[178,179] With the patient in sitting, the clinician passively and maximally rotates the head and neck away from the side being tested. While maintaining this position, the cervical spine is flexed, bringing the ear toward the chest. If the lateral flexion is restricted compared to the opposite side, the test is considered positive for a hypomobile first rib.[178] Reliability is excellent ($\kappa = 1.0$) with good agreement ($\kappa = 0.84$) with cineradiographic findings of first rib hypomobility during inspiration and expiration.[178,180] A positive CRLF test is an indication to assess first rib hypomobility, which is done in supine, prone, or sitting using a similar procedure. The diagnostic utility of the CRLF test is unknown.

Examination Procedures in Supine

- Cervical and anterior thorax palpation and breathing assessment
- Anterior-to-posterior (AP) rib passive mobility assessment

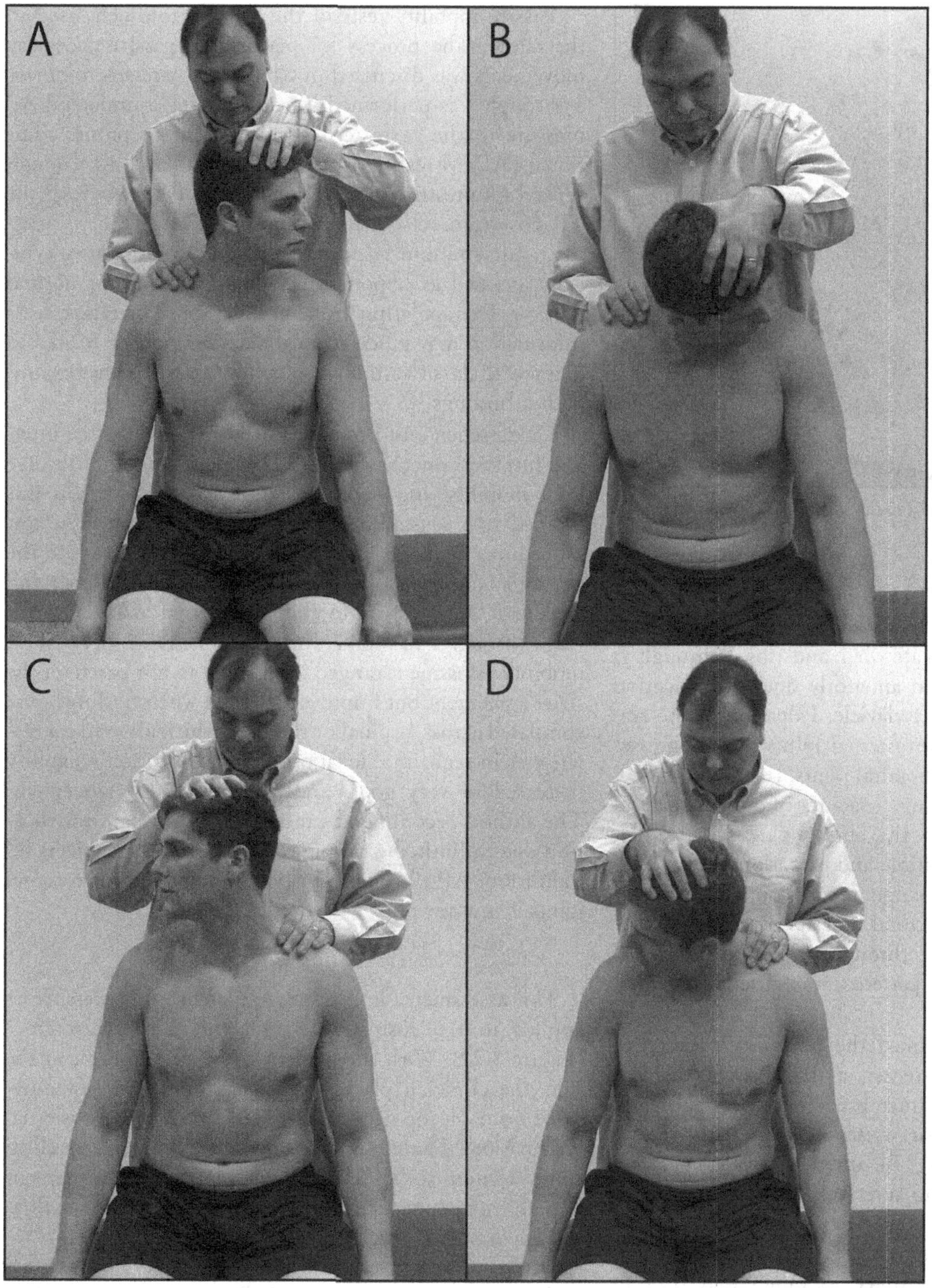

Figure 5-20. CRLF test: (A) cervical rotation to the left; (B) lateral flexion component assessing the right side; (C) cervical rotation to the right; and (D) lateral flexion component assessing the left side.

- First rib mobility assessment
- Muscle performance: motor control, length, strength, endurance
- ASLR
- Other as indicated: ULNDT, screen peripheral joints, sacroiliac joint provocation, screen hip if indicated: flexion, internal rotation, external rotation, flexion/adduction with OP as indicated

Cervical and Anterior Thorax Palpation and Breathing Assessment

Palpation

Palpation of the chest and abdominal regions in supine should include any area of the patient's symptoms beginning anteriorly and moving laterally, seeking changes in temperature, sweating, tissue texture, lymph nodes, and soft tissue. Bony landmarks such as the sternum, manubrium, xiphoid process, and sternoclavicular joints

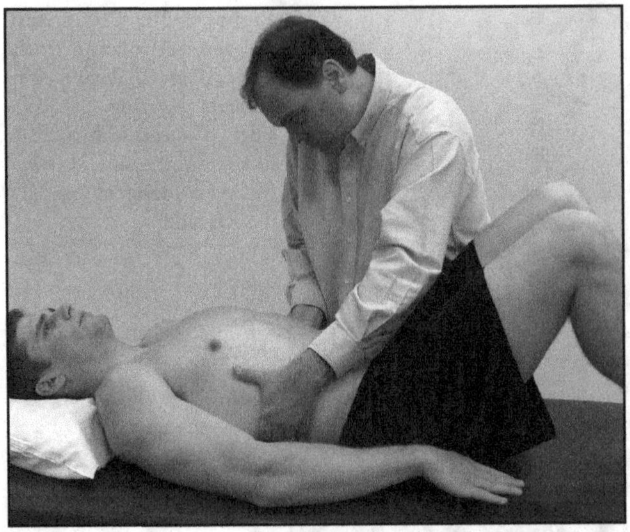

Figure 5-21. Palpation of rib cage during respiration in supine.

are palpated as needed. The second rib articulates at the junction between the sternum and manubrium. This landmark is utilized to locate rib 1 and ribs 3 through 7. Rib 1 may be hard to find anteriorly due to its location both behind and below the clavicle. Palpation of the ribs begins anteriorly at the costosternal joints and progresses laterally toward the costochondral joints. Intercostal spaces are palpated for thickening, spacing, prominence, and tenderness. Assessment of the abdominal area includes general inspection, observation, and palpation of breathing patterns (Figure 5-21); palpation; percussion; and auscultation as needed.[181] The pectoral and abdominal musculature are generally palpable through overlying soft tissue. Assessment of breathing patterns was discussed earlier under respiration.

Few studies have examined the reliability of anterior chest wall palpation. Christensen et al[182] assessed the day-to-day and hour-to-hour interobserver and intraobserver reliability of palpation for muscular tenderness in the anterior chest wall using 14 intercostal and pectoral predetermined areas of the anterior chest wall in sitting. Tenderness was rated as absent or present. Pooled data revealed generally poor agreement. Interrater κ values were 0.22 to 0.31 and intrarater κ values were 0.21 to 0.28 for the day-to-day reliability and 0.44 to 0.49 for the hour-to-hour reliability.

Anterior-to-Posterior Rib Passive Mobility Assessment

The thorax is subject to hypomobility or hypermobility impairments for many reasons, including altered posture, muscle stiffness, trauma, or joint dysfunction. These mobility impairments are associated with various pain syndromes of the upper and lower quarter and could be the cause of or contribute to the patient's problem.[131,183-186]

Passive mobility tests of the ribs are routinely used in the clinic. The process for performing passive accessory movements was discussed in Chapter 3. Assessment of ribs 1 through 7 is performed in supine using a unilateral AP pressure to the costosternal articulation. In prone, additional PAIVM testing is performed to T1 to T12 through central PA pressure to the SP, unilateral PA pressure to the TP, costotransverse articulation, and ribs. Quality, quantity, and symptom response are noted with quantity typically assessed as hypomobility, hypermobility, or normal motion. Extrapolating from lumbar spine literature, this information may guide clinical decision making related to diagnostic classification when combined with other examination findings.[187]

Heiderscheit and Boissonnault[188] investigated the inter- and intraexaminer reliability of thoracic spine and rib cage joint mobility and pain in 9 healthy subjects. Pain was defined as a sensation other than just pressure. The test procedures included PAIVM of central PA pressure to the SP, unilateral PA to the TP and rib angles in prone, and unilateral AP pressure to the costosternal articulation of ribs 1 through 7 in supine. Intraexaminer reliability of joint mobility assessment ranged from slight to fair based on the strict agreement but improved to good when findings were compared across 1 spinal or rib level, which allowed for differences in segmental location. Pain provocation reliability increased to very good under the expanded agreement. The authors recommend caution related to pain provocation due to limited pain prevalence in healthy subjects.[188] Validity of AP rib mobility assessment at the costosternal joints is unknown.

Test Procedure

For assessment in supine, unilateral AP pressure is applied to the costosternal joints of ribs 1 through 7 (Figure 5-22). With the patient in supine and arms at the side, the clinician places his or her thumb pads side-by-side or one on top of the other across the first costosternal articulation. The elbows are straight, allowing the clinician's sternum to be directly over the first rib. Assessment is performed superficial to deep in a progressive, oscillatory manner to assess symptom response and quality of movement through range and at end range. For comfort and appropriate technique, the AP movement is produced by the clinician's trunk and not the thumb flexors. The procedure is repeated for ribs 2 through 7. The AP mobility assessment, when needed, can be performed at the costochondral articulation or along the rib anteriorly. In addition, the angle of application can be varied superiorly, inferiorly, or medially and laterally.

First Rib Mobility Assessment

In supine, mobility of the first rib is assessed with an AP pressure at the sternocostal joint as discussed previously or posteriorly with an inferior glide at the first costotransverse

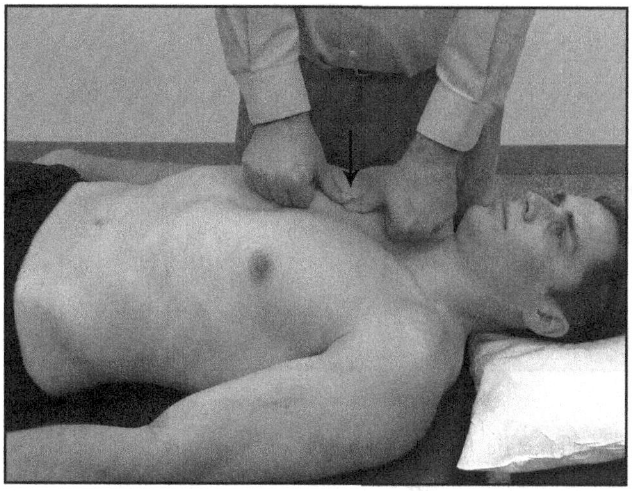

Figure 5-22. Anterior rib cage passive accessory motion assessment. Unilateral AP costosternal joints, ribs 2 through 7.

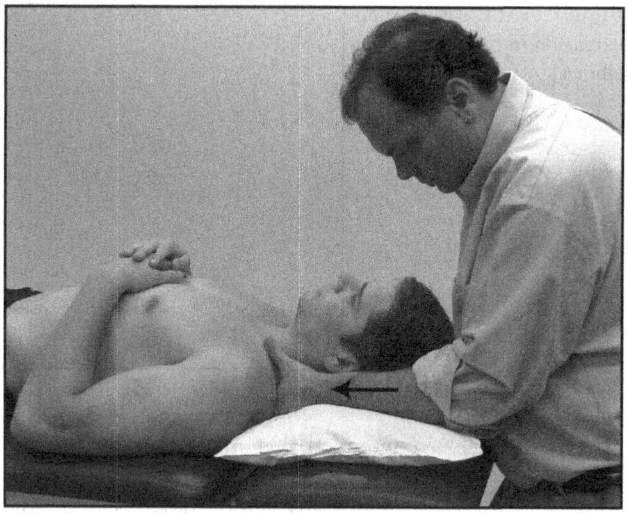

Figure 5-23. First rib mobility assessment—inferior glide supine.

joint (Figure 5-23). With the patient in supine, the cervical spine may be rotated and laterally flexed to the tested side to reduce tension from the scalene muscles. When testing the right side, the left hand stabilizes the left T1 TP with the index finger metacarpophalangeal (MCP) and locates the posterolateral aspect of the right first rib with the index finger MCP of the right hand. The examiner applies an inferior glide to the first rib. The angle of application may be varied slightly in an anterior or posterior direction. Quality, quantity, and symptom response are noted with comparison of uninvolved and involved sides. In subjects with various shoulder girdle complaints, Nomden et al[189] assessed first rib mobility (normal or restricted), pain (present or absent), and joint stiffness (present or absent). Interrater reliability was $\kappa = 0.26$ (66% agreement), $\kappa = 0.66$ (82% agreement), and $\kappa = 0.09$ (68% agreement), respectively. In subjects with cervical spine pain, interrater reliability was $\kappa = 0.35$ (70% agreement).[190] Hypomobility of the first rib could be associated with local thoracic pain and cervicobrachial pain.[180]

Muscle Performance: Motor Control, Length, Strength, Endurance

The thoracic spine and rib cage require complex neuromuscular control to meet functional demands of mobility on stability. In comparison to the lumbar spine musculature, few studies have investigated the control of the deep and superficial thoracic musculature.

During sagittal plane loading, preliminary investigations reveal that both deep multifidus and superficial thoracic longissimus are active prior to predictable loading, such as holding a bucket with elbow at 90 degrees flexion with no EMG differences in onset and no differences in pattern of EMG activity in different regions (T5, T8, T11).[191] These findings are in contrast to the lumbar paraspinals, where a predictable load induced preparatory deep multifidus EMG activity but not superficial multifidus activity.[192] The authors postulated that the greater potential for sagittal plane motion in the lumbar spine requires discrete control of the deep and superficial lumbar multifidus during predictable loading whereas reduced availability of sagittal plane motion in the thorax does not require this level of neuromuscular control.[191] The findings of similar deep and superficial activity at all thoracic levels is consistent with previous recruitment during anticipatory postural adjustments associated with fast bilateral arm flexion and extension, where rotation movement is minimal.[164] Where rotation requirements are increased, such as unilateral arm movements[164] and seated trunk rotation,[193] differential control between the deep and superficial thoracic muscles is used. The right multifidus is active with rotation to either side, suggesting control of intervertebral orientation, while the right longissimus is more active during ipsilateral trunk rotation, suggesting control of the center of mass.[193] However, the right longissimus was more active with left arm movements, and the right multifidus with right arm movements.[193] Observation and assessment of bilateral or unilateral arm movements, the SAL test, PAL test, trunk rotation, or trunk loading in the sagittal plane such as holding weight with elbows at 90 degrees flexion could be important tasks for identifying nonoptimal load transfer in the thorax.[193] These preliminary findings are from healthy subjects. Despite a lack of studies related to thoracic spine neuromuscular control, trunk stabilization exercises remain integral to achieving the patient's functional goals in postoperative outpatient rehabilitation such as spinal fusion in adolescent idiopathic scoliosis.[194] Additional studies are necessary on both healthy subjects and subjects with thoracic pain.

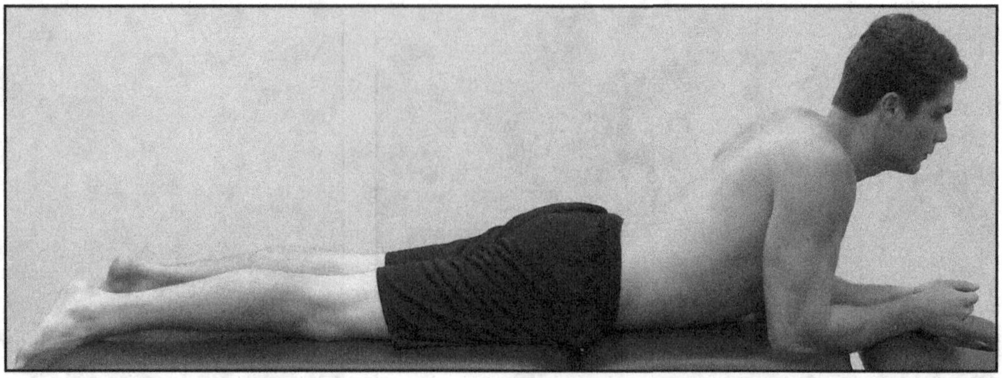

Figure 5-24. Sustained extension in lying (prone on elbows).

Lee and Lee[153] contended that many muscles become overactive, unilaterally or bilaterally, in patients with thoracic pain such as ES, latissimus dorsi, rhomboids, trapezius, rotator cuff, serratus anterior, scalenes, levator scapulae, pectoralis major and minor, quadratus lumborum, internal and external obliques, intercostals, rectus abdominis, and superficial lumbar multifidi. These authors recommend palpation for tone and muscle bulk at rest during respiration and during functional activity.[153] Similar to the lumbopelvic region, altered control in the thorax often presents with overactivity of the superficial system and inhibition of the deep muscle system, resulting in pain and thoracic rigidity. Identification of poor movement patterns serves as a guide to focus the training of optimal motor control strategies.[153]

Muscle Length

The examination of latissimus dorsi length was discussed in Chapter 4. Trapezius, scalenes, suboccipital muscles, and levator scapulae length tests are reviewed in Chapter 6. Muscle imbalance implies that a person has an inadequate balance of mobility and stability during specific functional movements. A postural and movement analysis may suggest a pattern of muscle imbalance that requires specific muscle length testing. A stiff muscle is most likely only one component of a nonoptimal movement pattern. For example, excessive kyphosis or limited upper thoracic extension may be related to stiff pectoral muscles, weak trunk extensors, limited thoracic spine or rib cage joint mobility, stiffness in the abdominal muscles, or poor lumbopelvic trunk control. All factors related to creating a balance of mobility and stability during thoracic extension must be examined. Page et al[126] provided a review of procedures for the assessment and treatment of muscle imbalance.

Active Straight Leg Raise

While the ASLR (see Figure 4-39) has not been investigated in subjects with thoracic pain, the test requires the clinician to observe for poor motor control strategies to stabilize the thorax, low back, and pelvis. A positive test suggests a lack of dynamic stabilization and impaired load transfer. The lack of stabilization is thought to occur in the lumbopelvic regions, resulting in poor control of the thorax, but it is possible that poor control is due to impairments in the thorax or the patient may have problems in both areas. Further examination of the thorax is indicated. If the ASLR is positive, Lee[162] recommended palpation of the thoracic ring that was positive during previous tests (ie, trunk rotation or SAL) during initiation of the leg lift on the side of the positive ASLR. If poor thoracic control contributes to reduced lumbopelvic control, manual correction of the thoracic ring translation should reduce the effort of lifting the leg, more so than pelvic compression. Assessment and treatment of the thorax may be necessary.[162] The ASLR is not indicated for all patients with thoracic pain, but in some, it may provide additional information if load transfer is not optimal through the thorax or if lumbopelvic control is a component of the patient's problem. Further examination of the lumbopelvic hip and lower extremity may be necessary in some patients. A cervical spine examination and ULNDT as described in Chapter 6 are often required in patients with thoracic complaints.

Examination Procedures in Prone

- Repeated movements
- Palpation
- Thoracic PAIVM
- PAL

Repeated Movements

Resting posture in prone is observed for provocative and easing postures. If peripheralization or partial centralization occurs during repeated extension in sitting for mid- and lower thoracic symptoms, continuation of the repeated movement examination occurs in prone in an attempt to obtain centralization. Sustained prone lying in extension (Figure 5-24) for a maximum of 3 minutes is attempted with the patient leaning on his or her elbows, allowing the spine to sag, which provides a passive OP to the thoracic spine.[159,160] Alternatively, REIL as performed in the lumbar spine may be tested. In prone with hands under the shoulders, the patient raises the upper half of the body by gradually straightening the arms. The pelvis and thigh remain relaxed and allow the abdomen to sag. Initially, the response to 10 to 15 repetitions is observed. As needed, clinician OP is applied using a cross-arm technique to place one hypothenar eminence of each hand over the thoracic TPs at the appropriate level (Figure 5-25).[159,160]

Test Procedure

The procedure is the same as that listed under repeated movements in sitting and the response is recorded. If centralization occurs, diagnostically classify as direction-specific exercise for extension or derangement and proceed to matched intervention. If the response is limited motion and end-range pain only (ie, produced, increased, or no worse) and no centralization or peripheralization occurs, further examination such as PAIVM or PPIVM is indicated. The clinician considers a classification of TSP with mobility deficits.

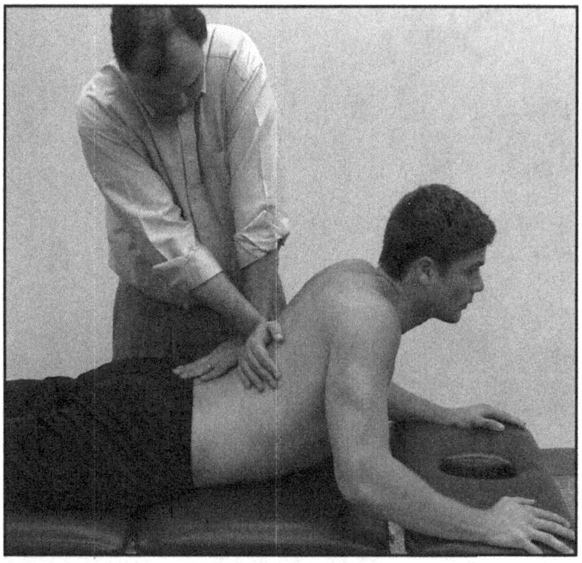

Figure 5-25. Extension in lying with clinician OP.

Palpation

Palpation in prone should include any area of the patient's symptoms. An approach to palpation of this area is discussed next, but not all areas are palpated on every patient. General guidelines are to begin with palpation for changes in temperature and sweating with progression in a layered manner to assess tone, texture, and mobility of skin and soft tissue structures and bony symmetry. The skin and muscles should be soft and easy to move. Areas of tenderness are noted in a side-to-side and above-to-below comparison. Final palpation involves segmental passive movement tests to assess PAIVM. Palpation procedures are not standardized in the literature.

The patient should be relaxed with arms resting at the side, soft tissue as relaxed as possible, and the cervical spine in neutral. During both soft tissue and joint motion assessment, clinicians attempt to identify painful tissues or segments and local changes in tissue texture for diagnosis and application of treatment techniques. The SPs are usually the first bony landmarks used to identify thoracic vertebral level and palpated with the pad of the index or middle fingers. Depending on the region to be examined, each SP is palpated, moving slowly to the interspinous space and the next SP. T1 may be identified by palpating what is believed to be the most posterior projecting SP, usually C7 and an adjacent SP. Ask the patient to gently flex and extend the neck. If the superior of the 2 SPs move away from your palpating finger during extension and the inferior remains stationary, then the upper SP is thought to be C6 and the lower one C7. If both SPs do not move, then most likely you are palpating C7 and T1 SPs. Using the method of flexion and extension and identifying the lowest freely moving SP as C6 and the stationary SP as C7 is more accurate than simply identifying the most prominent cervical SP as C7.[195] The SP may also be found by counting up from the lumbar spine. Holmaas et al[196] reported that only 26.7% of thoracic intervertebral spaces from T7 to T12 were accurately identified by anaesthesiologists in 92 patients. The success rate for identifying the thoracic interspaces was significantly higher when using the iliac crest or intercristal line (L4 to L5) as a starting point as opposed to the C7 reference point. Robinson et al[197] reported acceptable inter-therapist surface palpation agreement of 65% at C7 and 85% at L5 using these methods, but the procedures failed to identify the correct SP as determined by x-ray.

Palpation of thoracic TPs is used by some clinicians to assess spinal segmental motion via position testing as described previously or to perform unilateral PA PAIVM as described in the next section. The rule of 3s is the traditional method used to locate the level of the TP relative to the SP.[198] The rule of 3s identifies the TPs as follows: T1 through T3 TPs are in the same plane as the tip of the SP of the same vertebra; T4 through T6 TPs are one-half a level above the corresponding SP; T7 through T9 TPs are a full level above the corresponding SP; T10 TP is similar to T9; T11 TP is one-half a level above its SP; and T12 TP is at the same level of its SP. Geelhoed et al[199] proposed that the rule of 3s cannot be validated anatomically and suggested a more accurate model to palpate thoracic TPs.[200] Based on a dissection of 15 cadavers, the TPs can be found lateral to the most prominent aspect of the SP of the vertebra one level above.[199] Palpation of the ribs at the costotransverse joint, rib angles, and intercostal spaces may also be indicated.

Between the skin and zygapophyseal joints are layers of subcutaneous tissue and muscle. The trapezius lies immediately below the subcutaneous tissue. Under the lower half of the lower trapezius superficial to deep are the latissimus dorsi

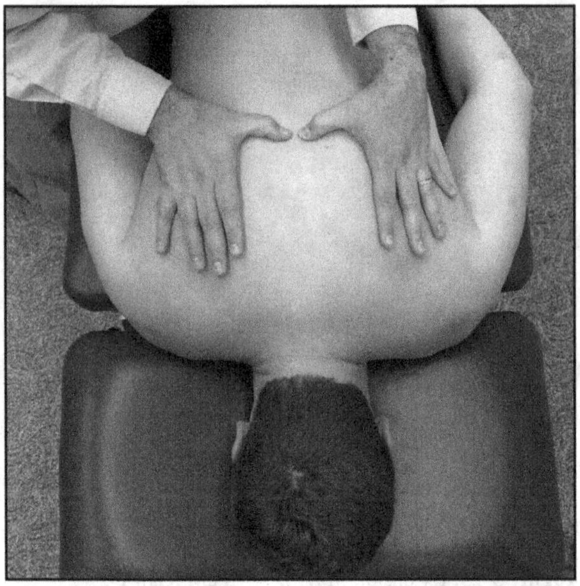

Figure 5-26. Palpation of deep thoracic paraspinal muscles.

or thoracolumbar fascia. Under the upper half of the trapezius are the rhomboids, serratus posterior superior, and splenius cervicis. Within the paravertebral gutter or the space between the SP and TP are the rotators, multifidus, semispinalis cervicis and thoracis, and spinalis thoracis at various levels. The longissimus thoracis overlies the costotransverse regions but is lateral to the semispinalis thoracis.[201]

The thoracic zygapophyseal joints cannot be palpated,[201] but the soft tissue in the paravertebral gutter and medial to the ES may provide information on the tension of the deep paraspinals (Figure 5-26). Changes in tone that are increased or decreased should be compared from side to side and to levels above and below. Clinically, atrophy of the multifidus and rotatores can be palpated as loss of stiffness or resistance to manual pressure, unilaterally or bilaterally close to the SP.[153] Lee and Lee[153] suggested that a decrease in muscle tone in the paravertebral gutter and decreased activation may be associated with failed load transfer during active rotation of the SAL or PAL. If there is excessive tone in the ES, reduced tone in the paravertebral gutter may not be palpable until tone in the superficial muscles is reduced. Conversely, increased tissue tension and/or tenderness are also thought to suggest local joint dysfunction. Tender areas with abnormal tissue texture demonstrate a lower pressure pain threshold than nontender tissues[202] and may be associated with increased EMG signal or increased resting motor activity of deep paraspinals.[203]

Thoracic Passive Accessory Intervertebral Movement Assessment

PAIVM are used to determine whether movement at an appropriate spinal segment reproduces the patient's symptoms and which segments are normal, hypomobile, or hypermobile for purposes of diagnostic classification and guiding intervention. Definitions of mobility are based on the clinician's perception of the mobility at each spinal segment relative to the segments above and below the tested segment and based on the clinician's experience and perception of normal mobility. Pain provocation is judged as painful or not painful relative to the patient's complaint.[165]

Intrarater and interrater reliability were fair for identifying mobility dysfunction using strict agreement of spinal levels, but they increased to good to moderate with expanded agreement to include one segment above or below.[188] Between each segment of the thoracic spine from T1 to T9, Cleland et al[138] reported weighted κ values for thoracic spine mobility from slight to moderate, while pain provocation during mobility testing in the thoracic spine ranged from no agreement to substantial agreement in subjects with neck pain. The 95% CI were large, suggesting continued uncertainty regarding the reliability of mobility testing in the thoracic spine. The weighted κ values for mobility were higher than previous reports.[204,205] Reliability of PA passive accessory tests for rib cage mobility was fair for strict agreement of spinal levels but improved to good with expanded agreement.[188] For rib cage mobility in healthy subjects with strict agreement, passive accessory tests for intrarater reliability of pain provocation ranged from no agreement to moderate and no agreement for interrater reliability, but they improved to complete agreement and good for intrarater and interrater reliability, respectively.[188] Despite the low reliability associated with PAIVM tests, clinician assessments of hypomobility or hypermobility may prove useful for clinical decision making when combined with other examination findings. The predictive validity of thoracic segmental motion tests is unknown. However, using the concepts from the research related to the lumbar spine, PAIVM in combination with other clinical findings may be useful for determining intervention and outcome. Findings of thoracic hypomobility may be an indication for mobilization or manipulation, while hypermobility may indicate the need for stabilization exercise.

Test Procedure

In prone with the neck in neutral rotation, thoracic PA PAIVM is performed between T1 to T12 centrally on the SP, unilaterally just lateral to the SP, or on the TP. Rib motion is assessed by PA over the rib angles in prone or AP at the costosternal joints in supine as previously discussed. If the patient has difficulty in this position, a pillow may be placed under the chest or abdomen for comfort.

Central Posterior-to-Anterior Passive Accessory Intervertebral Movement[57]

With the patient in prone arms at the side, the clinician places the thumb pads on the SP or hypothenar eminence just distal to the pisiform over the SP of the target thoracic

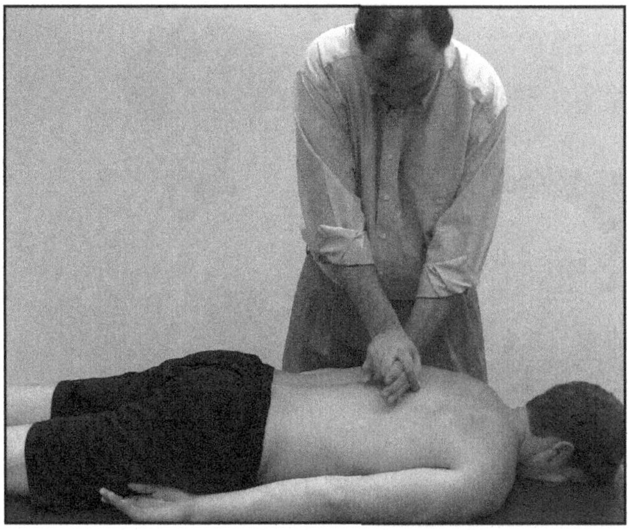

Figure 5-27. Central PA thoracic PAIVM (T1 to T12).

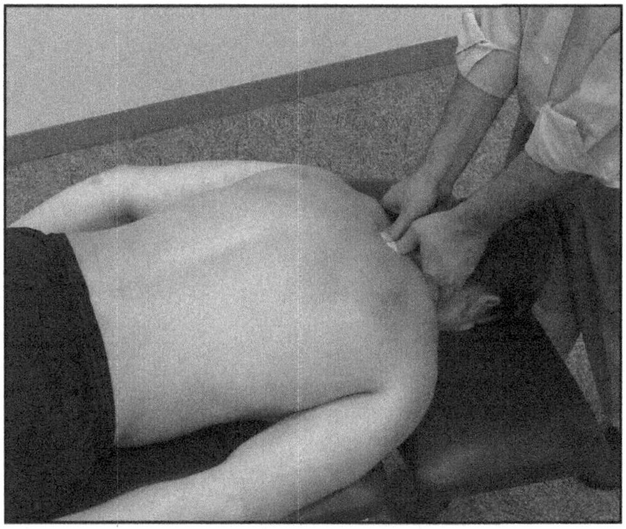

Figure 5-28. Central PA thoracic PAIVM (T1 to T5).

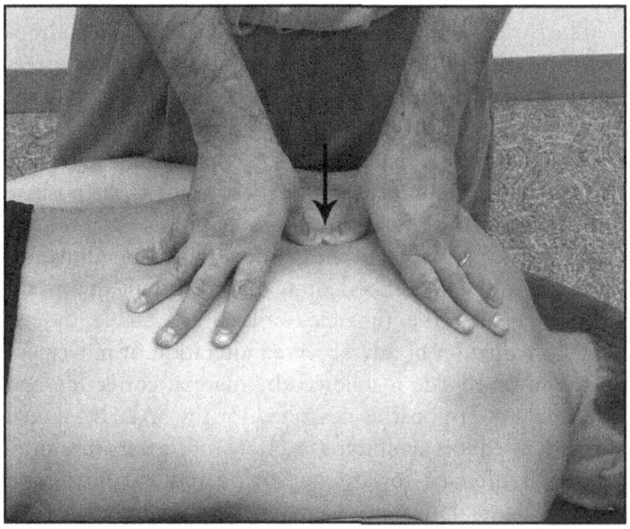

Figure 5-29. Unilateral PA thoracic PAIVM lateral to SP or on TP.

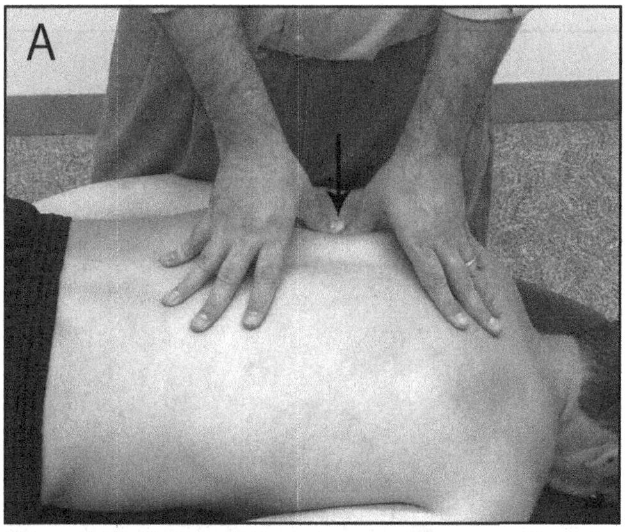

Figure 5-30. Unilateral PA passive accessory test at rib angles: (A) thumbs on rib angle. *(continued)*

vertebra (T1 to T12; Figure 5-27). The other hand is gently placed on top of this hand and assists in keeping the wrist extended. The elbows are straight, allowing the clinicians sternum to be directly over the SP. Assessment is performed superficial to deep in a progressive, oscillatory manner to assess symptom response and quality of movement through range and at end range. The clinician does not push on the spine, but instead leans forward, translating the weight of the trunk through the arms to the spine. Alternatively for T1 to T5 (Figure 5-28), the clinician may be at the head of the patient with his or her shoulders over the area to be assessed. The thumb pads are placed on the SP with the fingers spread gently along the neck or across the posterior chest wall.

Unilateral Posterior-to-Anterior Passive Accessory Intervertebral Movement[57]

In the same position as described for central PA PAIVM, the clinician uses both thumbs to produce the passive accessory movement. The thumbs are placed just lateral to the SP or on the TP beginning on the uninvolved side, making a side-to-side and segment above or below comparisons (Figure 5-29).

Unilateral Posterior-to-Anterior Rib Angles[57]

Passive accessory assessment is made with the thumbs placed along the rib angle so that maximum surface area contact is made between the thumbs and rib (Figure 5-30). The ulnar border of the hand may also be used for assessment.

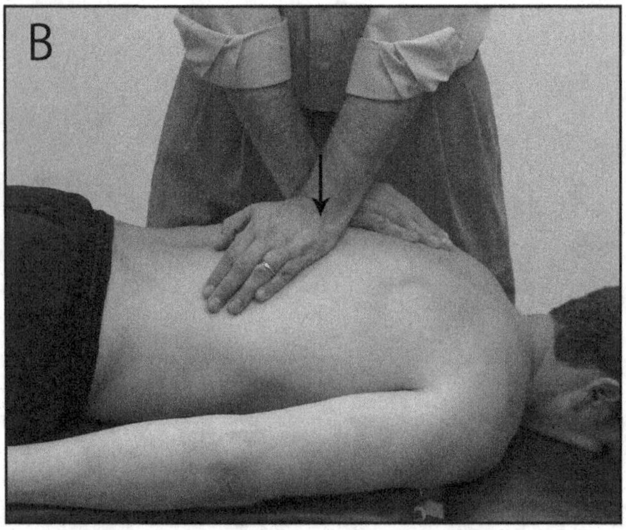

Figure 5-30 (continued). Unilateral PA passive accessory test at rib angles: (B) ulnar border of hand on rib angle.

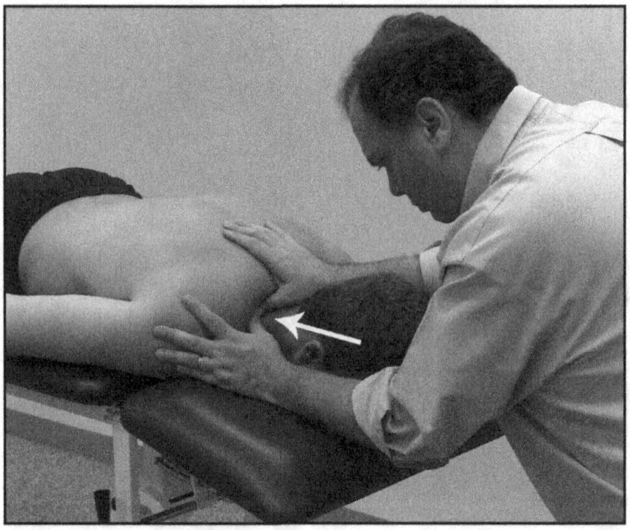

Figure 5-31. Inferior glide first rib prone.

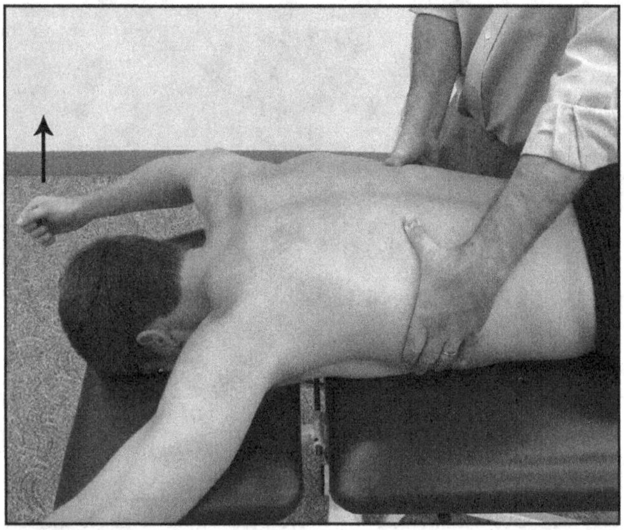

Figure 5-32. PAL on right.

First Rib Passive Accessory Movement Test—Inferior Glide

With the clinician at the head of the patient, the thumbs are placed just anterior to the trapezius on the superior and posterior aspect of the first rib. Mobility and symptom response are assessed in a superior-to-inferior direction (Figure 5-31).

Prone Arm Lift[14]

The PAL is similar to the SAL, but the PAL uses a position of higher load at 120 degrees shoulder flexion to assess the ability to lift the arm (Figure 5-32). Use of this test is important in patients whose functional activities, work, and recreation require this position or in patients who find this position provocative.

The patient is in prone at the head of the table in a drop-down position. With both arms overhead in 120 degrees shoulder flexion and supported on the treatment table, the patient is asked to lift one arm about 2 cm (1 inch) and then lower it. The test is repeated on the opposite side. The side that the patient reports as the heaviest to lift is the positive side for failed load transfer. Any production of symptoms is also noted. Observation of the quality of movement involves flexion at the glenohumeral joint, a stable scapula in upward rotation against the thoracic wall, and a stable thorax. Manual palpation of any observed alteration of movement on the involved side is followed by manual correction and assessment of response as described for the SAL. If manual correction reduces symptoms or effort to lift the arm, intervention is directed toward improving motor control and stability (ie, stabilization exercises, postural re-education, activity, and movement retraining) in that area. If symptoms are worse or the effort to raise the arm is increased, the region most likely has sufficient or excessive compression. Intervention is directed toward improving mobility through joint mobilization or manipulation or reducing excessive muscle tone (ie, breathing retraining, postural re-education, or soft tissue mobilization). Additional tests of PAIVM or PPIVM testing, multifidus or other trunk muscle palpation, etc are needed to determine interventions to improve mobility and stability.

Imaging Guidelines

At this point in the examination, the clinician may consider whether to recommend diagnostic imaging and/or refer to a medical colleague or subspecialist. The index of suspicion for recommending diagnostic imaging should be high enough that it is likely to change the intervention or alter the treatment threshold. Clinical decision making to use diagnostic imaging requires careful consideration of the history, physical examination, and if initiated, the response to intervention.

The American College of Radiology has established appropriateness criteria to assist providers in making the most appropriate imaging decisions.[206] For acute chest pain with low probability of CAD, the American College of Radiology recommends the following. Chest radiographs can diagnose pneumothorax, pneumomediastinum (ie, air in the mediastinum), fractured ribs, infection, and cancer. Initially, rib or thoracic spine radiographs are indicated when suspicion of skeletal pathology is high.

For suspected thoracolumbar spine trauma indications to image the thoracolumbar spine include back pain or midline tenderness, local signs of thoracolumbar injury, abnormal neurological signs, cervical spine fracture, Glasgow Coma Score < 15, major distracting injury, and alcohol or drug intoxication. Fractures identified in one level of the spine indicate an increased risk of spinal fractures elsewhere and suggest a need to image the rest of the spine. MRI is indicated in patients who have possible spinal cord injury or clinical suspicion for cord compression due to disk protrusion or hematoma and ligamentous instability. Review of the guidelines for acute LBP presented in Chapter 4 is suggested. In the absence of trauma, referral for imaging is indicated when historical data and examination findings suggest the presence of osteoporotic fracture, cancer, infection, neurological signs, or other serious spinal pathology.

Concluding the Physical Examination

At the conclusion of the physical examination, the clinician briefly reflects on whether the goals of the examination have been met. Did the physical examination do the following:

- Reproduce the patient's symptoms in patterns consistent with the information obtained in the patient interview?
- Result in a determination of the impact of posture, movement, work, recreational, and psychosocial factors as causes, contributors, or perpetuators of the patient's problem?
- Establish the treatment threshold for a diagnostic classification?
- Establish an accurate functional baseline or outcome measures from which to evaluate and progress treatment?

Review of examination findings should provide data that refine, support, or negate competing hypotheses to the point where the examination ends and treatment begins. Key history and exam findings are used to place the patient into a diagnostic classification or impairment-based category of mechanical thoracic spine or mechanical chest wall pain that initially guides PT intervention. A clinical decision-making algorithm process is in Figure 5-33.

Diagnostic Classification and Impairment-Based Management

At this point in the evaluation, the clinician designates a baseline diagnostic classification and proceeds with PT intervention. The medical diagnostic model, based on a pathoanatomical source, is the most common classification for persons with symptoms related to the thorax or thoracic spine. Neuromusculoskeletal sources of pain include but are not limited to degenerative disc disease, disc herniation, spinal stenosis, fracture or dislocation of the vertebra or ribs, muscle strain, rib syndromes, costochondritis, osteoarthritis, intercostal neuralgia, TOS, trigger points, and scoliosis. Similar to LBP, a precise anatomical tissue cannot be reliably identified as the cause or pain generator for mechanical TSP.

After excluding medical disease, serious spinal pathology, and neurological compromise such as radiculopathy or myelopathy, limitations of the medical model lead to a diagnostic classification of mechanical or nonspecific TSP. A reliable and valid classification of persons with nonspecific TSP does not exist. However, characteristics of the treatment-based classification for acute and chronic LBP provide a plausible framework that may aid in the classification and management of TSP.

Most clinicians would agree that patients with thoracic pain with or without pain related to the rib cage do not have a homogeneous condition. Other than pathoanatomy, classification approaches can be based on various factors such as length of symptoms (ie, acute, subacute, chronic); a biomechanical model of form/force closure, motor control, and emotions[10]; movement impairments; response to repeated movements[11,12]; and/or biopsychosocial factors, but clinical trials have not been completed to investigate any of these classification systems in this population.

A thoracic pain classification system with strong current evidence to support its use and ability to improve patient outcomes is not available, but it is likely that persons with nonspecific TSP can be classified into subgroups based on patterns of signs and symptoms. To assist the clinician with matching a patient's clinical presentation to an appropriate intervention, a proposed impairment-based classification system for subgroups of TSP is presented, integrating current best research, concepts used in the classification of LBP, and a clinical reasoning process to guide decision making toward best treatment strategies. In an impairment-based approach, the clinician identifies relevant physical impairments such as limited ROM, joint or muscle stiffness or hypermobility, and/or muscle coordination deficits. Evidence-based interventions are selected to target the prioritized impairments to address activity limitations or functional deficits important to the patient.

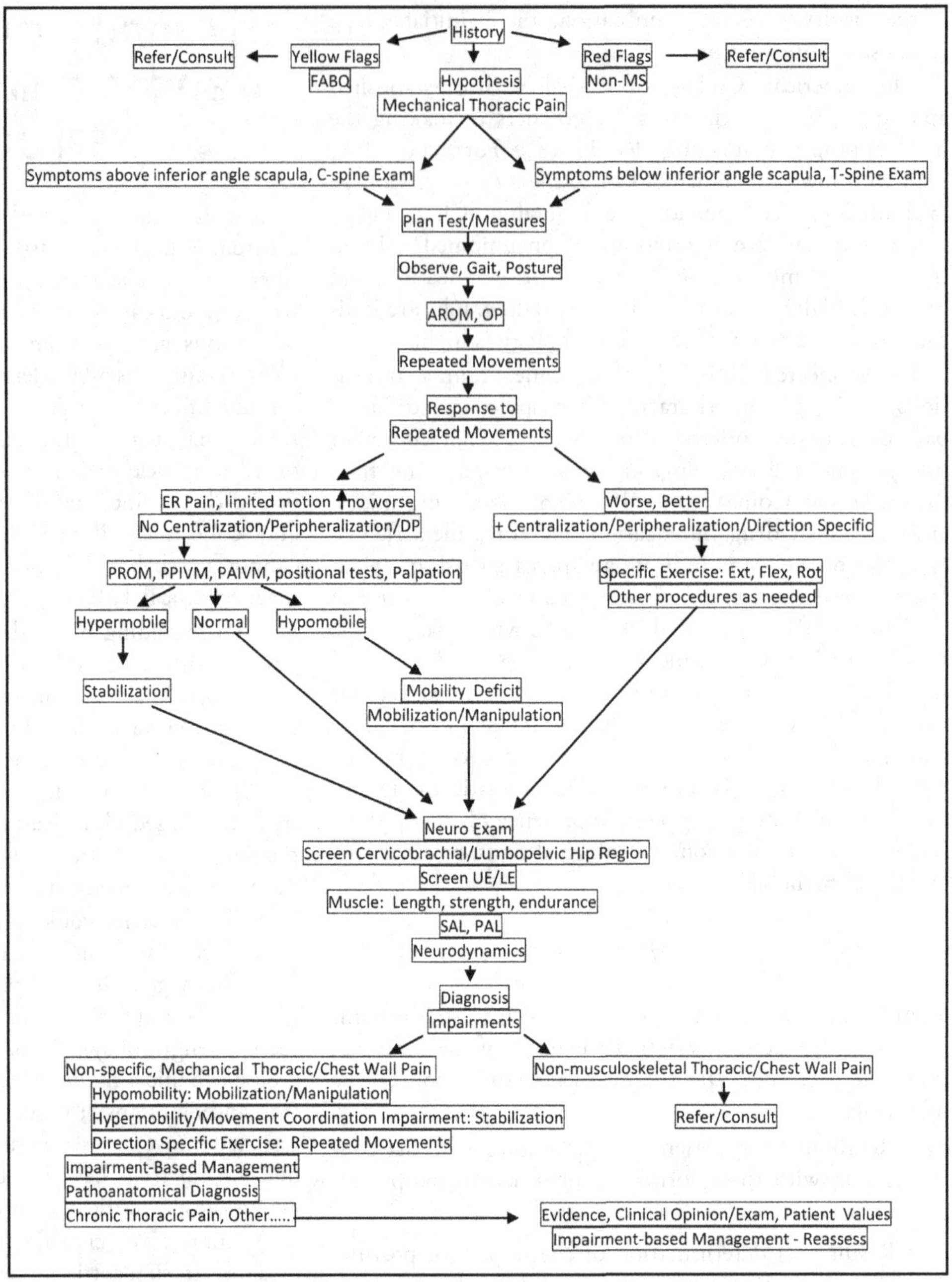

Figure 5-33. Clinical decision-making algorithm.

Proposed Direction-Specific Exercise Classification and Matched Intervention

Similar to LBP, a symptomatic response to repeated end-range movements is a reasonable method to classify patients who preferentially respond to exercises in a specific direction.[159,160] Three subgroups for thoracic pain may be identified using centralization as the primary examination finding: an extension subgroup, flexion subgroup, or a rotation subgroup.[159,160] Each subgroup is identified by the movement direction that results in centralization. If a repeated movement decreases, abolishes, or centralizes symptoms, further examination may not be required as a treatment threshold is reached. The matched intervention for a direction-specific exercise subgroup is the use of repeated or sustained end-range movements such as thoracic flexion, extension, or rotation in the direction that causes centralization during the examination. If peripheralization or partial centralization occurs in weightbearing, assessment continues in unloaded positions such as REIL in an attempt to obtain maximum centralization. Based on a centralization response to repeated movements in unloaded positions, matched intervention begins in an unloaded position. If no centralization or peripheralization occurs and the response is limited mobility with end-range pain that is no worse or no better, a classification of TSP

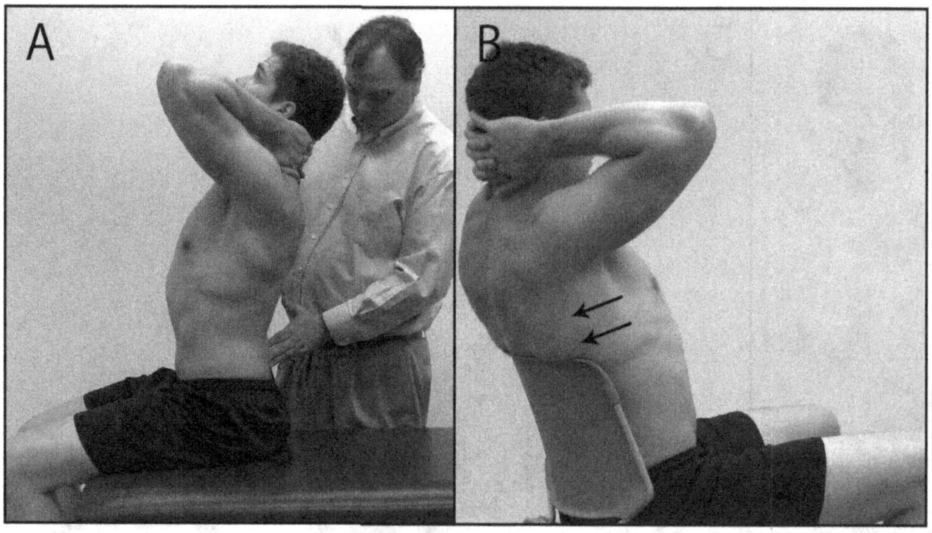

Figure 5-34. Repeated extension exercises. (A) Extension in sitting. With the hands interlaced behind the neck for support, the patient extends the thoracic spine and maintains the position briefly before returning to the start position. Repeat 10 times, increasing the range to maximum. (B) Extension in sitting with patient OP. With the hands interlaced behind the neck for support, the patient extends the thoracic spine using the back of the chair as a hinge and maintains the position briefly before returning to the start position. Repeat 10 times, increasing the range to maximum. *(continued)*

with mobility deficits is considered. With additional examination (ie, segmental mobility tests) to confirm mobility deficits, a matched intervention includes manual therapy and exercise to improve mobility in the direction of the motion limitation. A response of status quo to all repeated movements is a factor against a direction-specific exercise subgroup classification. Reliability, validity, and outcomes as a result of this proposed classification and treatment system for TSP are unknown.

Extension Subgroup and Matched Intervention

These guidelines represent a brief overview of the clinical picture and intervention strategies based on the response to repeated movements.[159,160] An extensive discussion related to the management of persons with TSP using repeated movements is available for review.[159,160]

The clinical presentation varies from acute to chronic thoracic pain with or without varying degrees of referred pain in bands around the trunk, in the front of the chest, or in isolated patches of pain over the trunk. The most distal symptoms are felt anteriorly or laterally. A summary[159,160] of the interview includes a flexion-related manner of onset: flexion activities such as sitting or bending produce or worsen symptoms, while extension activities such as standing or walking decrease or abolish symptoms. Exam findings include a slouched posture, excessive thoracic kyphosis, reduced lumbar lordosis, and a painful extension AROM deficit greater than flexion; repeated flexion produces, worsens or peripheralizes symptoms; and PAIVM are provocative. In the mid-thoracic region, repeated extension in sitting abolishes, reduces, or centralizes symptoms and increases extension ROM. Therefore, the specific exercise prescription is repeated extension. The home exercise program includes postural correction, temporary avoidance of flexion activities, and the appropriate level of extension exercise repeated 10 times every 2 to 3 hours.[159,160]

Commonly prescribed repeated extension exercises, patient and therapist assisted, are provided in Figure 5-34.[160] All patients do not progress through each level. The starting point is determined by the clinician, with progression determined by patient response. If the response to repeated extension is described as end-range pain that is increased but not worse and no centralization or peripheralization occurs, a mobility deficit is considered. However, further examination is warranted to assign a diagnostic classification. These same exercises are appropriate for thoracic extension mobility deficits. Extension in sitting is for the mid-thoracic region; extension in supine for the upper thoracic region is the same as for the cervical spine (see Chapter 6); and extension in prone is for the mid- and lower thoracic spine.

Flexion Subgroup and Matched Intervention

The clinical presentation is uncommon and not well defined.[159,160] Patients generally prefer flexion activities such as sitting to extension activities such as standing or walking. Flexion AROM may be limited with extension AROM full range. PAIVM may be provocative. Repeated extension produces, worsens, or peripheralizes symptoms; repeated flexion abolishes, reduces, or centralizes symptoms and may increase flexion ROM. Therefore, the specific exercise prescription is the appropriate level of repeated flexion performed 10 times every 2 to 3 hours.[159,160] Commonly prescribed flexion exercises are flexion and flexion in sitting (Figure 5-35). These same exercises are appropriate for thoracic flexion mobility deficits.[159,160] If the response to repeated flexion is described as end-range pain that is increased but not worse with no centralization or peripheralization, a mobility deficit is considered. However, further examination is warranted to assign a diagnostic classification.

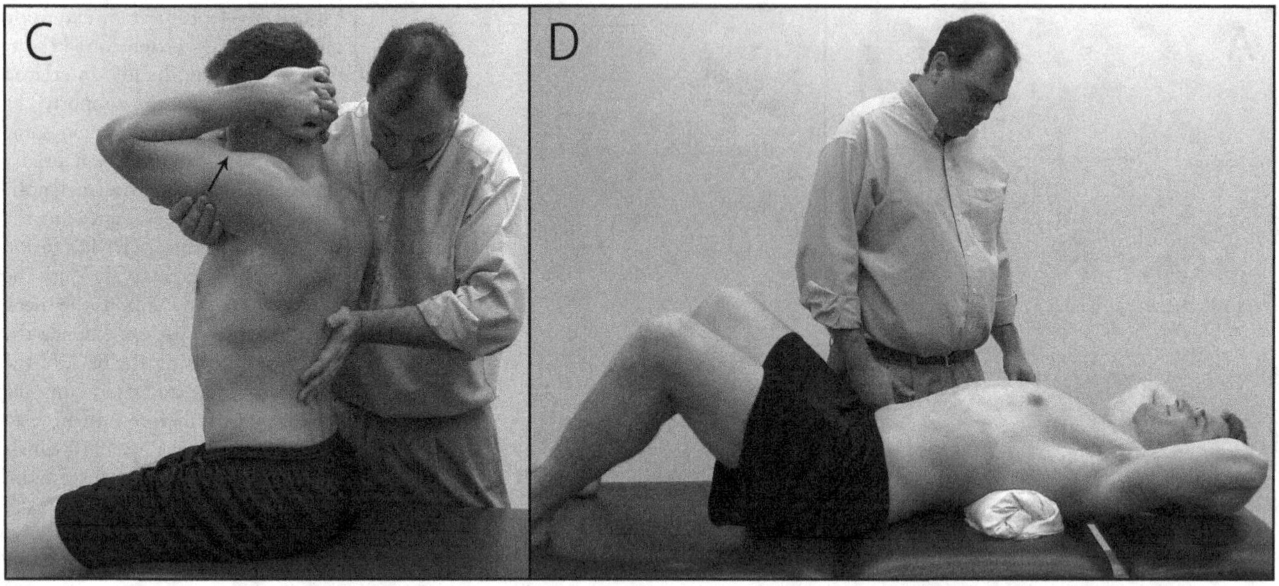

Figure 5-34 (continued). Repeated extension exercises. (C) Extension in sitting with clinician OP. With the hands interlaced behind the neck for support, the patient extends the thoracic spine and maintains the position briefly before returning to the start position. The clinician lifts up on the elbows, applying OP at the SP through the heel of his or her hand at the appropriate thoracic segment. Repeat 5 to 6 times, increasing the range to maximum. (D) Mid-thoracic sustained extension in supine. The patient lies supine with a towel rolled and positioned under the thoracic spine. Further extension is attained by placing the hands interlaced behind the neck.

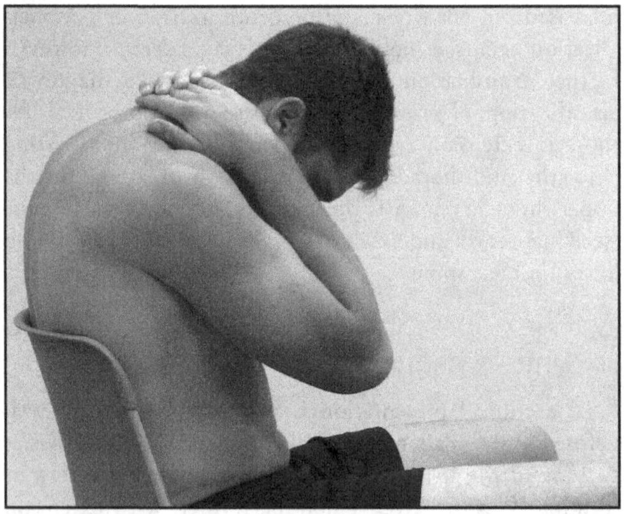

Figure 5-35. Repeated flexion exercises. (1) Flexion in sitting. With the hands interlocked behind the lower cervical and upper thoracic spine, the patient slouches into the fully flexed position, maintains for a few seconds, and returns to upright. Repeat about 10 times. (2) Flexion in sitting with patient OP. In the same position as for Figure 5-33A, the patient applies OP at the end of the movement by pulling through the upper thoracic spine, maintains for a few seconds, and returns to upright. Repeat about 10 times.

Rotation Subgroup and Matched Intervention

Patients with asymmetrical or unilateral symptoms that respond partially to extension movements may require rotation exercises toward the side of pain followed by extension for centralization to occur.[160] Common exercises prescribed for rotation directional preference are rotation in sitting (see Figure 5-15C), rotation in sitting with patient OP provided through increased speed and force of movement, and rotation in sitting with clinician OP (Figure 5-36).[159,160] These exercises may also be appropriate for thoracic rotation mobility deficits. If the response to repeated rotation is described as end-range pain that is increased but not worse with no centralization or peripheralization, a mobility deficit is considered. However, further examination is warranted to assign a diagnostic classification.

For all persons in the subgroups responding to direction-specific repeated movements, management focuses on self-treatment through knowledge of posture, activities, and movements that centralize symptoms. In the early stages, movements that cause peripheralization are avoided. Exercises should be discontinued only if peripheralization occurs. When the patient is asymptomatic for a period of several days, recovery of function begins.[159,160] The patient begins exercise in the direction that has been avoided or that initially produced peripheralization. For example, in the extension subgroup, flexion in sitting exercises are prescribed as 5 to 6 reps 5 to 6 times per day followed by repeated extension over 1 to 2 days. If no return of symptoms, flexion may progress slowly to sitting followed by repeated extension in sitting exercises.[159,160] Reassessment throughout the episode of care and further examination may identify additional areas for intervention.

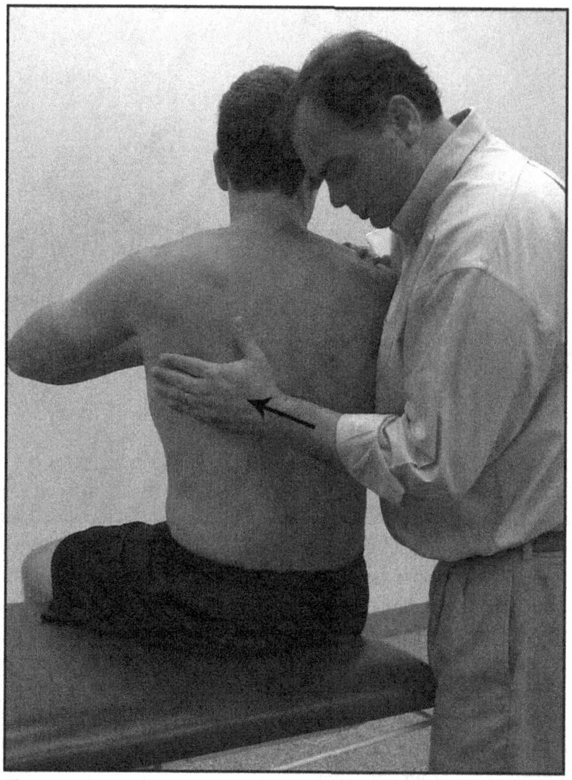

Figure 5-36. Repeated rotation exercises in sitting with clinician OP. With the patient at end-range rotation, the clinician applies OP with one hand anteriorly on the shoulder and the other hand posteriorly on the thorax to further increase rotation. Repeat 5 to 6 times.

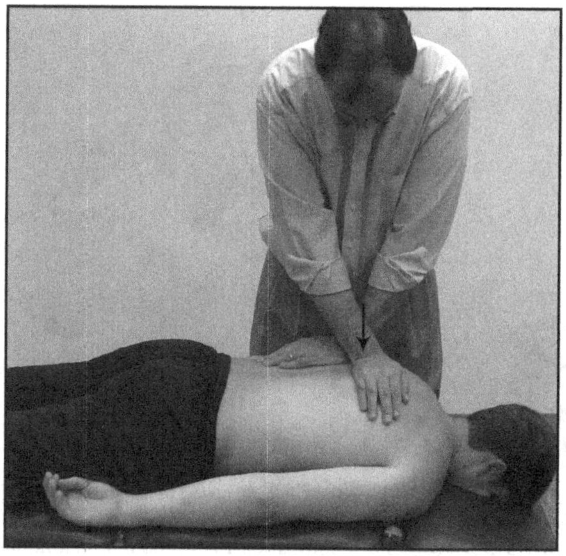

Figure 5-37. A cross-hand PA thrust manipulation on adjacent thoracic segments. The patient is prone with the head and neck in a comfortable neutral position. The clinician is at the patient's left side. At the T4 to T5 segment, place left hypothenar eminence on the left TP of T5, the hypothenar eminence of the right hand on the right TP of T4. Obtain a skin lock, lean your body weight over your hands, apply a PA force to achieve tension toward the end of available range, and apply a high-velocity low amplitude thrust using the minimum amount of force necessary. This procedure is also used as a mobilization.

Proposed Mobilization and Manipulation Classification for Thoracic Spinal Pain With Mobility Deficits

After exclusion of nonmechanical causes such as medical disease and neurological disorders, Olson[13] described an impairment-based classification (see Table 5-1) for nonspecific, mechanical TSP. The diagnostic classification is supported by key examination findings and proposed interventions, but reliability and validity are unknown. Clinical findings commonly associated with this proposed classification[13] are listed as follows and expanded as proposed subgroups within a mobilization and manipulation classification based on current research, clinical reasoning, and the concept of regional interdependence.

Thoracic Hypomobility[13]

Examination findings suggestive of mobility deficits with or without thoracic spinal and/or chest wall symptoms but no referral to the UE include limited AROM, limited passive ROM (PROM), no centralization or peripheralization with repeated movements, hypomobility, and/or pain provocation with PPIVM and/or PAIVM of the thoracic spinal segments and/or ribs. Postural deviations such as forward head posture and excessive or reduced kyphosis may be present along with associated muscle imbalances in the region. Muscle imbalances include weakness of the middle and lower trapezius and deep neck flexors and short pectoral muscles, latissimus dorsi, upper trapezius, scalenes, and/or levator scapulae. Mobility deficits of the thorax may exist unilaterally or bilaterally in extension, flexion, lateral flexion, or rotation or functional combinations of the cardinal plane motions.

Evidence for Thoracic Mobilization and Manipulation Classification in Patients With Thoracic Hypomobility

Research examining the effects of manual therapy on mechanical or nonspecific thoracic pain is limited. When compared to a no treatment control in a convenience sample of chiropractic students, Haas et al[207] concluded that spinal manipulation using a cross-hand technique on adjacent thoracic segments to produce rotation (Figure 5-37) in a specific direction resulted in a moderate short-term change from restricted to normal in rotary thoracic end-play restrictions. A comparison of 3 groups (control, mobility tests only, and mobility tests plus manipulation) for a single session demonstrated immediate changes in

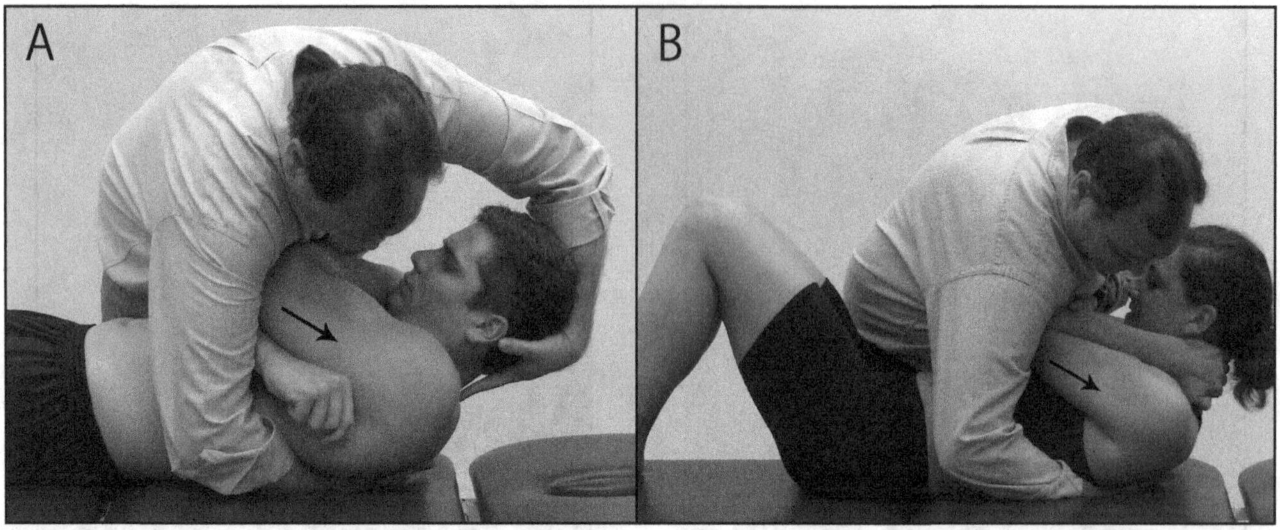

Figure 5-38. T3 to T8 mobilization/manipulation techniques. (A) Supine mid-thoracic AP thrust manipulation with a flexion bias toward the T4/T5 motion segment. With the patient in supine, arms hugging the upper body and/or a towel, and the away arm on top forming a "V," the clinician stands on the patient's right side and reaches the lower hand across to locate and stabilize the inferior segment at the TP of T5. A variety of hand positions (see Figure 5-39) are available to localize forces to the thoracic spine or rib cage. Keeping the right hand in place, the clinician rolls the patient back into supine and uses his or her left hand and forearm to support the patient's head, neck, and upper thoracic spine. The clinician flexes the patient's head, neck, and upper thoracic spine until tension is felt at the T4/T5 segment. The clinician then rests his or her sternum or upper abdomen on the patient's elbows and applies an AP thrust through the patient's arms and chest toward T4 to T5. Note the direction of the arrow in the photo. (B) Alternative patient position: the patient may interlock his or her hands behind the neck, keeping the elbows together.

Figure 5-39. Various hand positions to stabilize the inferior segment (ie, TPs) and localize forces: (A) pistol grip. *(continued)*

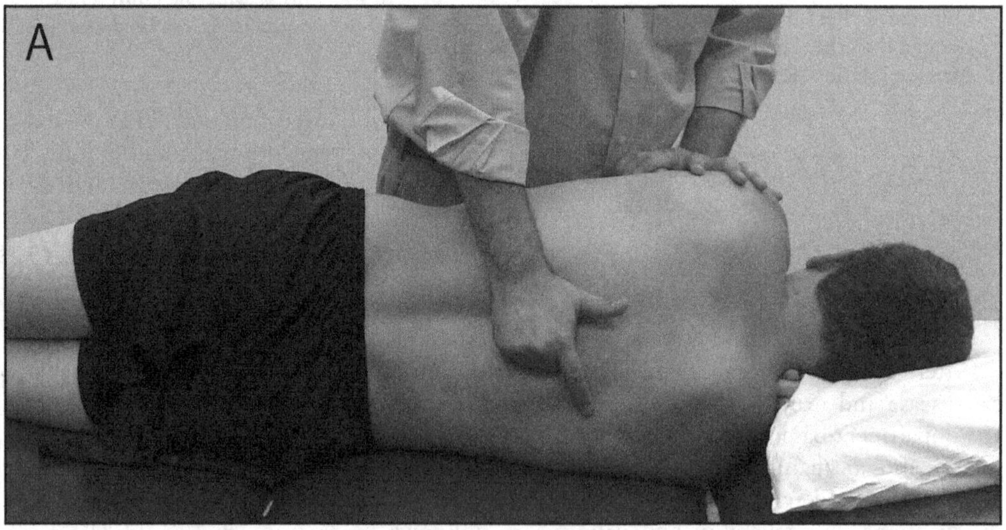

lateral flexion AROM to the left after supine mid-thoracic (T3 to T8) AP thrust manipulation (Figures 5-38 and 5-39), seated thoracic spine thrust manipulation (Figure 5-40), and prone, unilateral PA rib manipulation (Figure 5-41).[208] In 2 controlled trials of healthy volunteers, central PA mobilization (see Figure 5-27) 2 times per week for 3 weeks resulted in no change in thoracic spine mobility[209] and PA thrust manipulation to T4-T5 resulted in no change in PA stiffness compared to controls.[210]

In 30 subjects ages 16 to 55, 47% male and 53% female with mechanical thoracic pain, Schiller[211] compared the effects of thoracic spinal manipulation (TSM) to detuned ultrasound for a maximum of 6 treatments up to 3 weeks. Four undescribed manipulation techniques were used. Outcome measures were ROM, ODI, the McGill Pain Questionnaire (MPQ), and the Numeric Pain Rating Scale-101 Questionnaire (NPRSQ) with follow-up after final treatment and 30 days later. Statistically significant results ($P \leq .025$) were noted for the NPRSQ and for right and left lateral flexion favoring the TSM group after the final treatment. Final treatment results were maintained at the 1-month follow-up. The placebo group showed

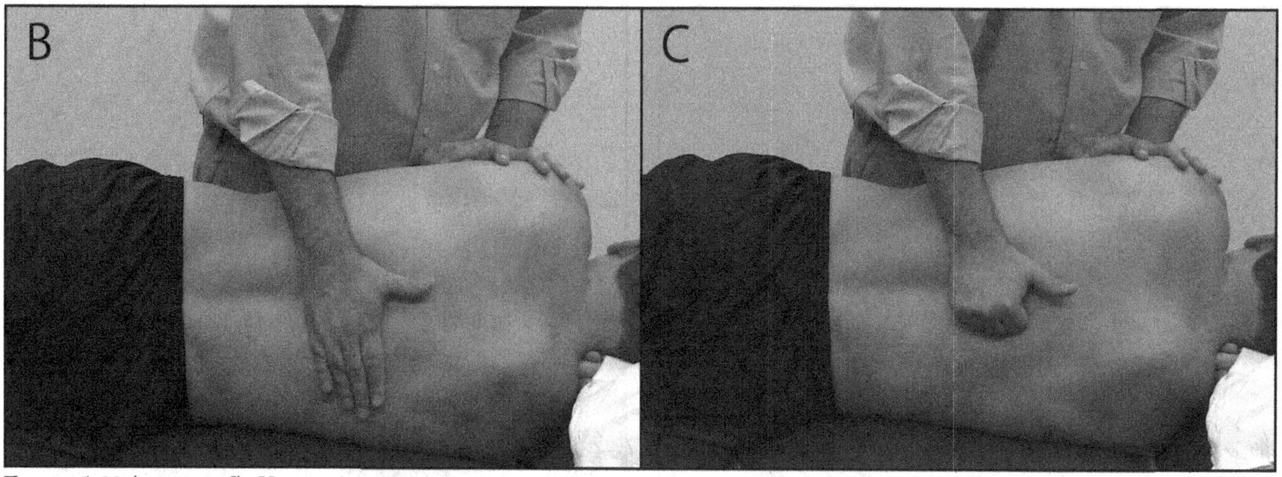

Figure 5-39 (continued). Various hand positions to stabilize the inferior segment (ie, TPs) and localize forces: (B) open hand and (C) closed fist.

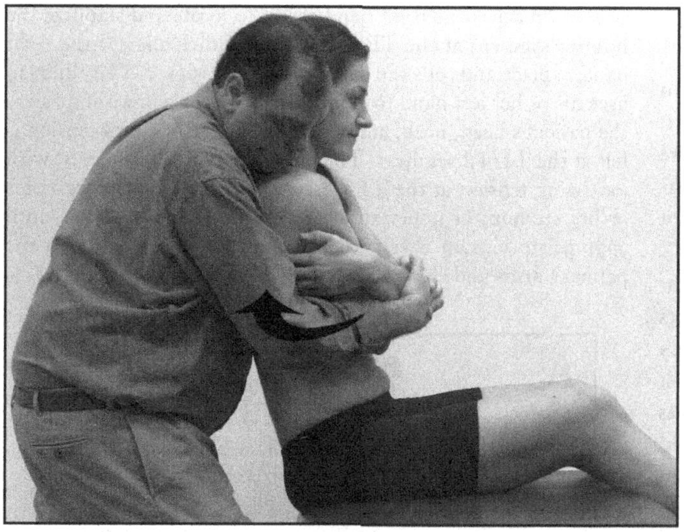

Figure 5-40. Seated mid-thoracic spine distraction thrust manipulation at T5/T6. The patient is sitting with the arms crossed over the chest or hugging the upper body. The clinician is standing in a walk stance knees flexed position and uses the sternum, a mobilization wedge, or towel as a fulcrum against the SP of T6 or mid-thoracic spine. The clinician grasps the patient's elbows and passively brings the patient backwards while maintaining a compressive force at T6 and a distraction force through the patient's arms. As tension is achieved, the clinician applies a high-velocity low amplitude distraction force through his or her hands in an upward direction against the T6 SP or mid-thoracic region using the sternal contact.

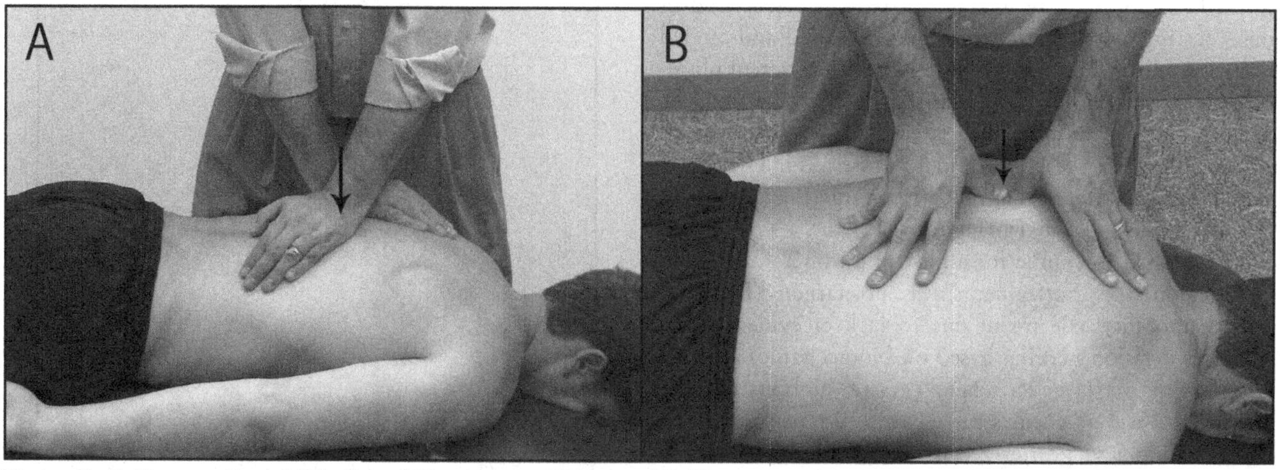

Figure 5-41. Prone unilateral PA rib mobilization/manipulation. (A) The patient is in prone with head and neck in a comfortable position and arms at the sides while the clinician in standing. The clinician reaches across to locate rib 5 as it articulates with the T5 TP using a pisiform or hypothenar eminence contact. The other hand stabilizes T5 to T6 segment on the opposite side. A PA force is applied using the clinician's body weight toward the end of available range until appropriate tension is felt at the costotransverse joint, and he or she applies a high-velocity low amplitude thrust against the rib using the minimum amount of force necessary. This technique is also used as a rib mobilization or nonthrust manipulation. (B) An alternate hand position for mobilization is to use the pads of the thumbs to mobilize just lateral to the TP. *(continued)*

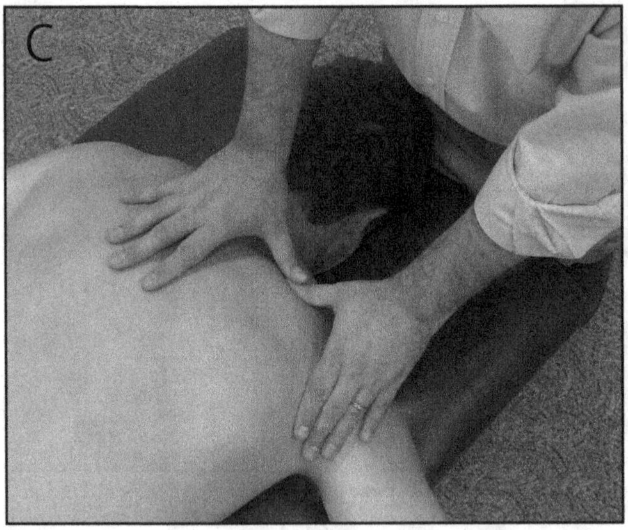

Figure 5-41 (continued). Prone unilateral PA (PA) rib mobilization/manipulation. (C) Rib 2 PA mobilization.

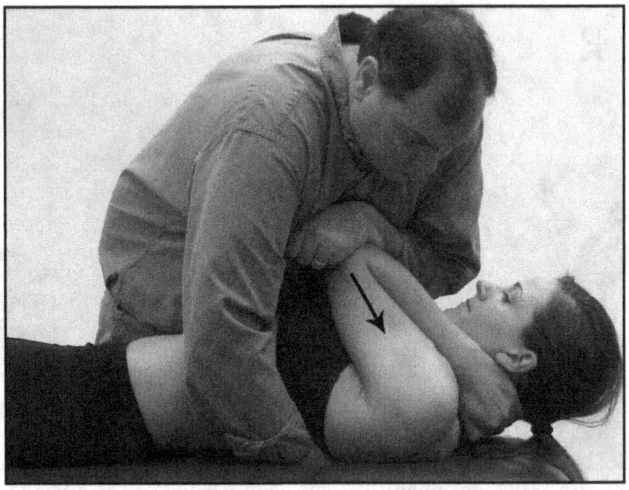

Figure 5-42. Supine upper thoracic spine end-range AP thrust manipulation. With the patient in supine, hands behind neck, and elbows together, the clinician stands on the patient's right side and reaches the right hand across to locate and stabilize the inferior segment at the TP of T2. The clinician keeps the right hand in place and rolls the patient back into supine. The clinician uses his or her left hand to control the patient's elbows and flexes the patient's head, neck, and upper thoracic spine until tension is felt at the T1/T2 segment. The patient may bridge to assist with localizing tension at the T1/T2 segment. The clinician rests his or her sternum or upper abdomen on the patient's elbows until appropriate tension is felt, then applies AP thrust through the patient's arms and chest toward the T1/T2.

a statistically significant improvement in sensory pain only between the first treatment and the final treatment. Sample size was small. No between-group differences were observed in the MPQ and ODI at any follow-up, suggesting that both approaches were effective related to patient experiences in disability and sensory dimensions.[211]

Cleland et al[212] compared the effects of TSM with that of nonthrust manipulation or mobilization in 60 patients ages 18 to 60 years with a primary complaint of neck pain. Outcomes measured at baseline and 48 hours post intervention were the NDI, NPRS, Fear-Avoidance Beliefs Questionnaire, and GROC. The nonthrust group received central PA mobilization on the SP (see Figure 5-27) of T1 to T6 at a grade III or IV for 30 seconds at each segment.[212] Central PA mobilization (see Figure 5-27) is performed exactly the same as central passive accessory movement testing. Mobilization may be progressed and angled in various directions and/or combined with different physiological positions. For example, the mobilization may be performed with the patient in lateral flexion or in flexion with a pillow or towel rolled under the sternum. The thrust group received thrust manipulation targeting the upper thoracic spine at T1 to T4 (Figure 5-42) and T5 to T8 (see Figure 5-38A) in supine for a maximum of 2 attempts at each region. Specific segments were not targeted based on passive mobility assessment due to lack of evidence that supports decision making based on biomechanical theory. Both groups performed a general cervical mobility exercise (Figure 5-43) 3 or 4 times per day for 10 repetitions. The thrust group had greater reductions in disability with a between-group difference of 10% (95% CI: 5.3 to 14.7) and with a between-group difference in pain of 2.0 (95% CI: 1.4 to 2.7). The thrust group also had significantly higher scores on the GROC scale.[212]

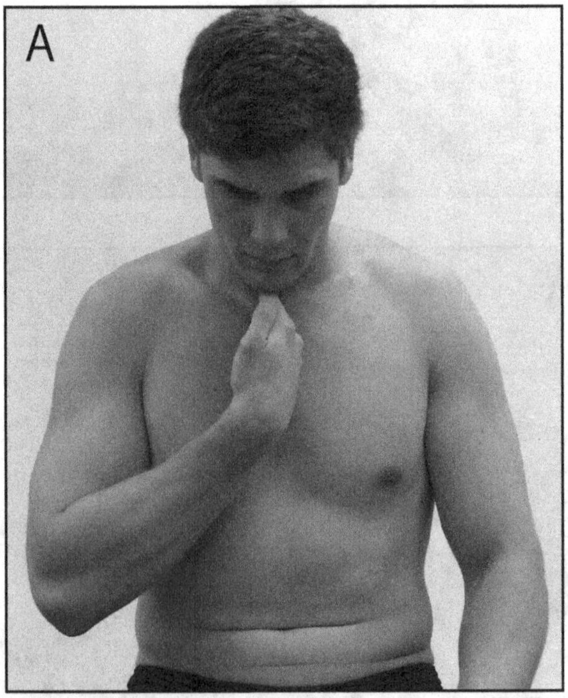

Figure 5-43. Cervical AROM exercise: (A) starting position with all 5 digits over manubrium and chin on the fingers. The exercise alternates as far as possible right and left within pain tolerance and returning to neutral. Initially, 5 digits are used. Then, as mobility increases, the patient progresses to 4, 3, 2, and 1 finger placed over the manubrium. *(continued)*

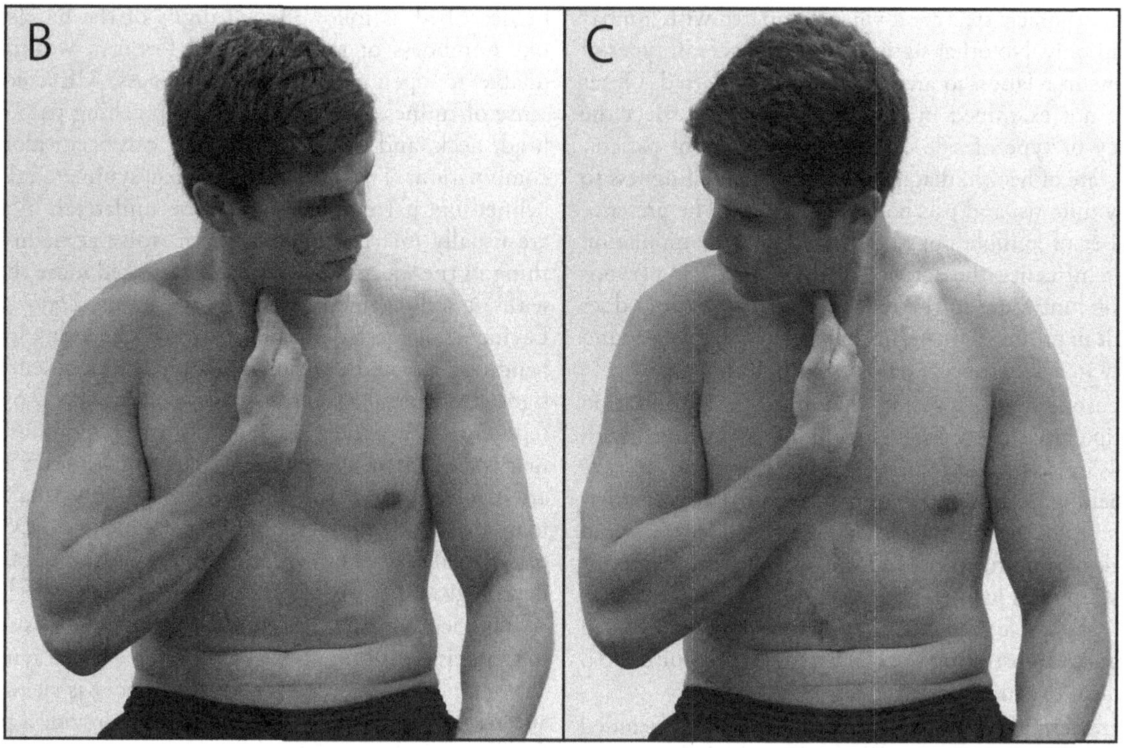

Figure 5-43. Cervical AROM exercise: (B) active rotation to the left; (C) active rotation to the right. The exercise alternates as far as possible right and left within pain tolerance and returning to neutral. Initially, 5 digits are used. Then, as mobility increases, the patient progresses to 4, 3, 2, and 1 finger placed over the manubrium.

The underlying mechanisms (biomechanical, placebo, biological, and neurophysiological) that most likely explain the effects of mobilization and manipulation to the thoracic spine are unknown but theoretically similar to those presented for the lumbopelvic region. Lumbar spine SMT is associated with immediate reduction of temporal sensory summation (TSS), a short-lasting aspect of central sensitization of the nervous system that occurs in the dorsal horn of the spinal cord as well as in the pain processing and behavior areas of the cerebral cortex. Research efforts continue to explain the clinical effectiveness for pain modulation using SMT in some patients. Bishop et al[213] investigated whether or not regional pain modulation occurs as a result of thoracic SMT. Healthy volunteers (n = 90) were randomly assigned to 1 of the following 3 groups:

1. High-velocity low amplitude (HVLA) AP thrust manipulation to the upper thoracic region
2. Upper cervical flexion exercise in supine for 10 repetitions with 5-second holds
3. Resting quietly for 5 minutes

Pain sensitivity measures of cervical and lumbar innervated areas were collected before and immediately after the intervention. In healthy subjects and subjects with LBP, reduction of TSS occurred only in the lower extremities but not the UEs after lumbar SMT. The results of Bishop et al[213] also demonstrated a reduction of TSS in both the lower and UEs. The authors speculate that an intervention that reduces TSS such as SMT may reduce the potential for central sensitization to maintain musculoskeletal pain or may prevent the progression to centrally sensitized pain states.[213]

Contraindications to spinal manipulation and mobilization as presented in Chapter 4 apply to patients for whom manual treatments are considered to the thoracic spine. Patients should be informed of possible side effects. Cleland et al[212] reported similar side effects for nonthrust and thrust manipulation with onset reported within 24 hours of intervention and resolution within 24 hours or less. The nonthrust group reported aggravation of symptoms, muscle spasm, headache, and radiating symptoms in 9 out of 30 subjects, while the thrust group reported aggravation of symptoms, muscle spasm, and headache in 10 out of 30 subjects. Cleland et al[212] reported lower rates for both thrust and nonthrust manipulation of the thoracic spine in comparison to reported side effects for the entire spine.[214,215] However, in reviewing 4712 treatments to the spine Senstad et al[216] reported that the greatest number of reactions per area treated was for the thoracic spine and the lowest number was for the lumbar spine. Where only one area was treated, thoracic and cervical spine treatment resulted in significantly more reactions than treatments to the lumbar spine: 39%, 32%, and 23%, respectively. Headache was somewhat more commonly reported after cervical or thoracic treatment when compared with lumbar treatment only. No other significant differences in types of symptoms in relation to area treated were reported. Other variables not examined in this study that may affect the frequency or type of side effects include type of patient, general state of health, diagnosis, chronicity, willingness to report symptoms, and psychological state.[216] The presence or number of audible pops after a thoracic manipulation does not influence the activity of the autonomic nervous system or contribute to the reduction in pain[217] and does not result in greater short-term changes in pain, ROM, and disability in a subgroup of patients with neck pain.[218]

Liebenson[219,220] suggested that thoracic mobilization or manipulative procedures should be augmented with postural exercises, soft tissue techniques, and muscle strengthening. Vanti et al[221] promoted a balance of interventions from the physical therapist who identifies and treats relevant dysfunction and the patient who maintains mobility, optimal load transfer, and movement patterns as the best strategy for rehabilitation. These authors reported no studies demonstrating the effectiveness of a multimodal approach in the thoracic spine.[221]

In a review of the literature, Vanti et al[221] concluded that studies examining the effects of manual therapy on nonspecific thoracic pain resulted in no firm conclusions. Clinical short-term effects of manipulation included reduction of symptoms, increased muscle activation, and increased ROM. Studies did not differentiate between acute or long-term disorders. Manual therapy appears to be more effective than no treatment, other treatments, or placebo, but no treatment technique was deemed more effective than another. No studies were found on the effectiveness of education, active and home exercise programs, work hardening, and back school for mechanical TSP.[221]

Upper Thoracic Hypomobility With Upper Extremity Referred Pain[13]

Olson[13] equated this disorder to a common clinical condition called *T4 syndrome.* The presentation is similar to the previous description for thoracic hypomobility but specific to the upper thoracic spine with referral of symptoms to the UE. The cervical spine is not considered a source of the UE symptoms.

Evidence for Thoracic Mobilization and Manipulation in Patients With Thoracic Hypomobility and Upper Extremity Pain

T4 syndrome is a poorly defined clinical pattern, not a diagnosis. As described by Grieve,[222] the clinical presentation involves bilateral or unilateral UE symptoms with or without upper thoracic, neck, and/or head symptoms. The UE pain and paresthesia pattern is glove-like with distal symptoms often worse at night and relieved by hanging the arm out of the bed. The paresthesia experience may be described as follows in all digits of the hands, glove-like numbness of the hands and forearm, weakness (eg, unable to open jars), hand clumsiness, UE coldness, a sense of fullness, tightness, and deep aching pain.[223] The head, neck, and thoracic symptoms can occur alone or in combination. The headache is often symmetrical with a helmet-like pattern, but it may be unilateral. Symptoms are usually intermittent and often worse at night or first thing in the morning. Women are affected more than men without well-defined predisposing factors. DeFranca and Levine[224] suggested that repetitive occupations involving bending or seated positions may predispose. Neurological signs are absent. Central passive accessory movements reproduce the patient's symptoms and hypomobility primarily in T3 to T5 segments, but sometimes T2 to T7 are involved.[222,225] Radiographic imaging is usually unremarkable. Differential diagnosis must include TOS, cervical spine dysfunction, carpal tunnel syndrome, cardiac or neurological disease, or other serious pathology.[222,224]

Thoracic somatic dysfunction of the joint or surrounding soft tissue is thought to be the source of the symptoms, although scientific evidence for this theory is lacking. The autonomic nervous system is thought to provide a pathway for the referral of symptoms to the head, neck, and UEs as a result of thoracic spine dysfunction. The close proximity of the sympathetic chain ganglia to dysfunctional thoracic segments may result in mechanical irritation.[226] As discussed earlier, the sympathetic neurons to the head and neck arise from T1 to T4, the UE from T1 to T9, and the thorax from T3 to T6. Other theories suggest that the thoracic joints are not the cause. Sustained or extreme postures may lead to sympathetic nerve ischemia or ischemia in other tissues associated with a sympathetic vasoconstrictor network.[225] A sympathoexcitatory pain mechanism may present with sudomotor changes such as cold extremities and increased sweating and vasomotor changes such as blanching of the skin.[227] Consistent with a sympathoexcitatory pain mechanism, UE coldness has been reported in T4 syndrome.[223]

Thoracic mobilization or manipulation are options for treatment in addition to postural correction and therapeutic exercise.[222] The management of a patient with T4 syndrome over 6 sessions as described by Conroy and Schneiders[228] included grade III central PA mobilization of T4 in prone progressing into thoracic flexion to restore mobility of the T4/T5 segment and postural education exercises. Joint manipulation, while also an option, was not used for this patient because of anxiety and irritability of the disorder. However, DeFranca and Levine[224] reported good results with a central PA to the SP as a grade IV mobilization (see Figure 5-27), prone PA manipulation on the same segment (Figure 5-44), supine AP manipulation (see Figure 5-38 or 5-42) of the dysfunctional upper thoracic spine (T3 to T5), postural stretching, and strengthening exercises in 2 cases of patients with T4 syndrome.

In an attempt to explain the effects of mobilization in T4 syndrome, Jowsey and Perry[229] examined the effects of a T4 mobilization technique on the sympathetic activity in the hands of healthy subjects compared to a validated placebo intervention. A grade III rotatory PA intervertebral mobilization (see Figure 5-44) was used. This technique involves using a pisiform placement of 2 hands adjacent to either side of a single thoracic vertebral segment at T4 and is thought to produce localized joint glide at the costovertebral, costotransverse, intervertebral, and facet joints of the thoracic spine. At the limit of available range, the treatment consisted of 30 oscillations per minute for 3 sets of 1 minute with a 1-minute rest between sets to influence skin conductance in the hand.[230] The placebo was performed in the same manner except that the pressure was maintained statically for 1 minute and repeated for 3 sets with 1-minute intervals. A grade III PA rotatory technique produced a side-specific sympathoexcitatory increase in skin conductance in the right hand postintervention ($F = 4.888$, $df = 35$, $P = .034$) with a trend towards a statistically significant bilateral effect ($F = 4.072$, $df = 35$, $P = .052$). The results support a theoretical link between thoracic mobilization and the SNS.

Invasive procedures include intramuscular injections. Two patients thought to have T4 syndrome were successfully treated with intramuscular injections of bupivacaine at T4.[223] Additionally, gabapentin was prescribed to both patients. In addition to the intramuscular injections, one patient received 3 cervical epidural injections and another patient received osteopathic thoracic spinal mobilization and undefined PT treatment.[223]

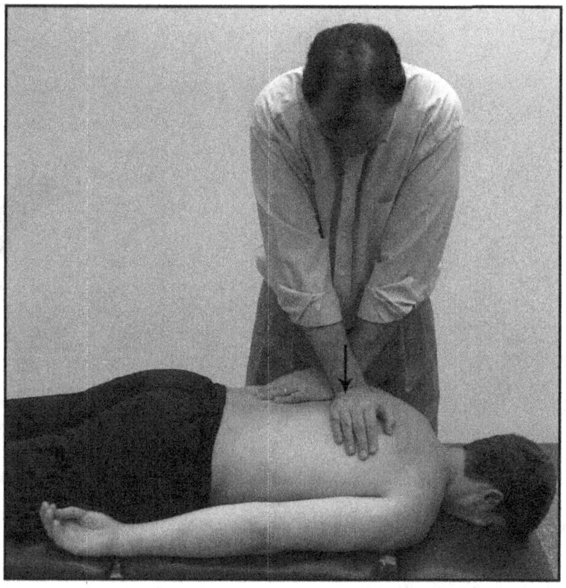

Figure 5-44. Prone PA mobilization/manipulation on the same segment. The patient is prone with the head and neck in a comfortable neutral position. The clinician is at the patient's left side. Using a cross-hand technique at the T4/T5 segment, the clinician places the left hypothenar eminence of the left hand on the left TP of T5 and the right hypothenar eminence on the right TP of T5. The clinician obtains a skin lock, leans his or her body weight over the hands, applies a PA force to achieve tension toward the end of available range, and applies an HVLA thrust against the TP using the minimum about of force necessary. This procedure is also used as a mobilization.

Thoracic Hypomobility With Neck Pain

Patients presenting with neck pain who have mid- and upper thoracic segmental hypomobility have been shown to benefit from thoracic manipulation. Several authors have reported improved outcomes with TSM in patients with mechanical neck pain with or without radiculopathy.[130,231-244] Examination and intervention for identified impairments associated with the cervical spine should also be considered.

Evidence for Thoracic Spinal Mobilization and Manipulation in Patients With Thoracic Hypomobility and Neck Pain

Recent focus of research related to TSM considers the concept of regional interdependence, specifically the use of TSM for patients with neck and/or shoulder pain. Based on low quality evidence, a Cochrane review of mobilization or manipulation for neck pain suggested that TSM may be beneficial for decreasing pain and improving function.[245] Clinical practice guidelines recommend TSM as an intervention strategy for this population.[246] Walser et al[231] concluded that sufficient evidence exists to support the use of TSM for the management of neck conditions for subgroups of patients for short-term benefit of up to 4 weeks, but long-term studies are needed. Only 2 of the most current studies are presented here to support the use of TSM for patients with neck spine without contraindications to manipulation.

Cleland et al[130] examined the results of a clinical prediction rule to identify a subgroup of patients with neck pain likely to benefit from TSM. Patients ($n = 140$) ages 18 to 60 years with a primary report of neck pain with or without unilateral UE symptoms were randomly assigned to an exercise only group consisting of 5 sessions of stretching/strengthening exercise or a manipulation plus exercise group consisting of 2 sessions of TSM and cervical AROM exercise followed by 3 sessions of stretching and strengthening exercise. Outcomes for pain and disability were obtained at baseline, 1 week, 4 weeks, and 6 months.[130]

The exercise only group received manual stretching (Figure 5-45) to the upper trapezius, scalenes, sternocleidomastoid, levator scapulae, and pectoralis major and minor muscles and a home exercise stretching program (Figure 5-46). Each stretch was held for 30 seconds for 2 repetitions. Deep neck flexor training, cervical isometrics, and middle and lower trapezius and serratus anterior muscle exercises were performed for 10 repetitions with

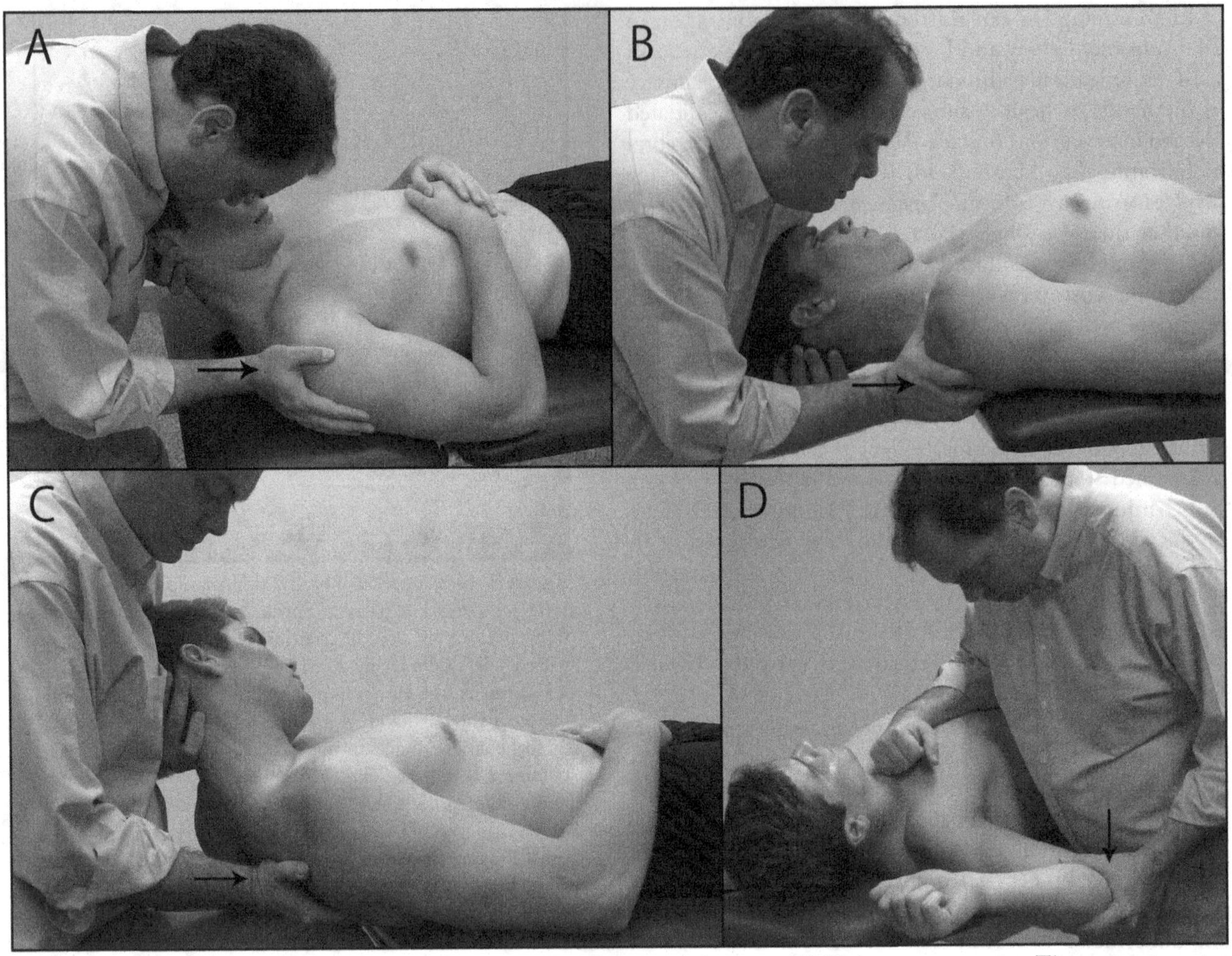

Figure 5-45. Manual muscle lengthening using postisometric relaxation techniques. (A) Right upper trapezius. The patient is supine with the clinician at the head of the table. The clinician passively flexes the head and neck and then adds lateral flexion to the left and rotation to the right. While stabilizing the head and neck in this position, the clinician depresses the shoulder girdle at the right acromion process to the point where stiffness is felt at the end range of available muscle length. The patient is asked to move the shoulder up against the clinician's hand for a 6-second isometric hold. The patient then relaxes completely. The clinician gains further muscle length by depressing the shoulder girdle through the newly gained range. The procedure is repeated 5 to 6 times. The clinician then performs a reassessment and prescribes an exercise program to augment clinical gains or retrain neuromuscular control of the newly gained range. (B) Right anterior scalenes and sternocleidomastoid. The patient is supine with the clinician at the head of the table. The clinician passively performs cervical retraction and then adds lateral flexion to the left and rotation to the right. While stabilizing the head and neck in this position, the clinician depresses the first rib posteriorly to the point where stiffness is felt at the end range of available muscle length. The patient is asked to move the shoulder up against the clinician's hand for a 6-second isometric hold. The patient then relaxes completely. The clinician gains further muscle length by depressing the first rib through the newly gained range. The procedure is repeated 5 to 6 times. The clinician then performs a reassessment and prescribes an exercise program to augment clinical gains or retrain neuromuscular control of the newly gained range. (C) Right levator scapulae. The patient is supine with the clinician at the head of the table. The clinician passively performs cervical flexion and then adds lateral flexion to the left and rotation to the left. While stabilizing the head and neck in this position, the clinician depresses and upward rotates the scapula by placing the thenar eminence of the right hand at the superior medial angle of the scapula to the point where stiffness is felt at the end range of available muscle length. The patient is asked to move the shoulder up against the clinician's hand for a 6-second isometric hold. The patient then relaxes completely. The clinician gains further muscle length by depressing and upwardly rotating the scapula through the newly gained range. The procedure is repeated 5 to 6 times. The clinician then performs a reassessment and prescribes an exercise program to augment clinical gains or retrain neuromuscular control of the newly gained range. (D) Pectoralis major and minor. Performance of this technique is likely contraindicated in glenohumeral instability, limited shoulder mobility, or a painful shoulder. With the patient in supine, the clinician stands on the side to be tested facing the patient and stabilizes the thorax through the sternum using one hand or the forearm. The clinician flexes the externally rotated arm to 90 or 120 degrees and then lowers the arm into horizontal abduction toward the table until stiffness is felt at the end of available range of muscle length. The clinician resists horizontal adduction for a 6-second isometric hold. The patient then relaxes completely. The clinician gains further muscle length by lowering the arm further into horizontal abduction through the newly gained range. The procedure is repeated 5 to 6 times. The clinician then performs a reassessment and prescribes an exercise program to augment clinical gains or retrain neuromuscular control of the newly gained range. Different regions of the pectoral muscles are assessed by changing the range of humeral elevation.

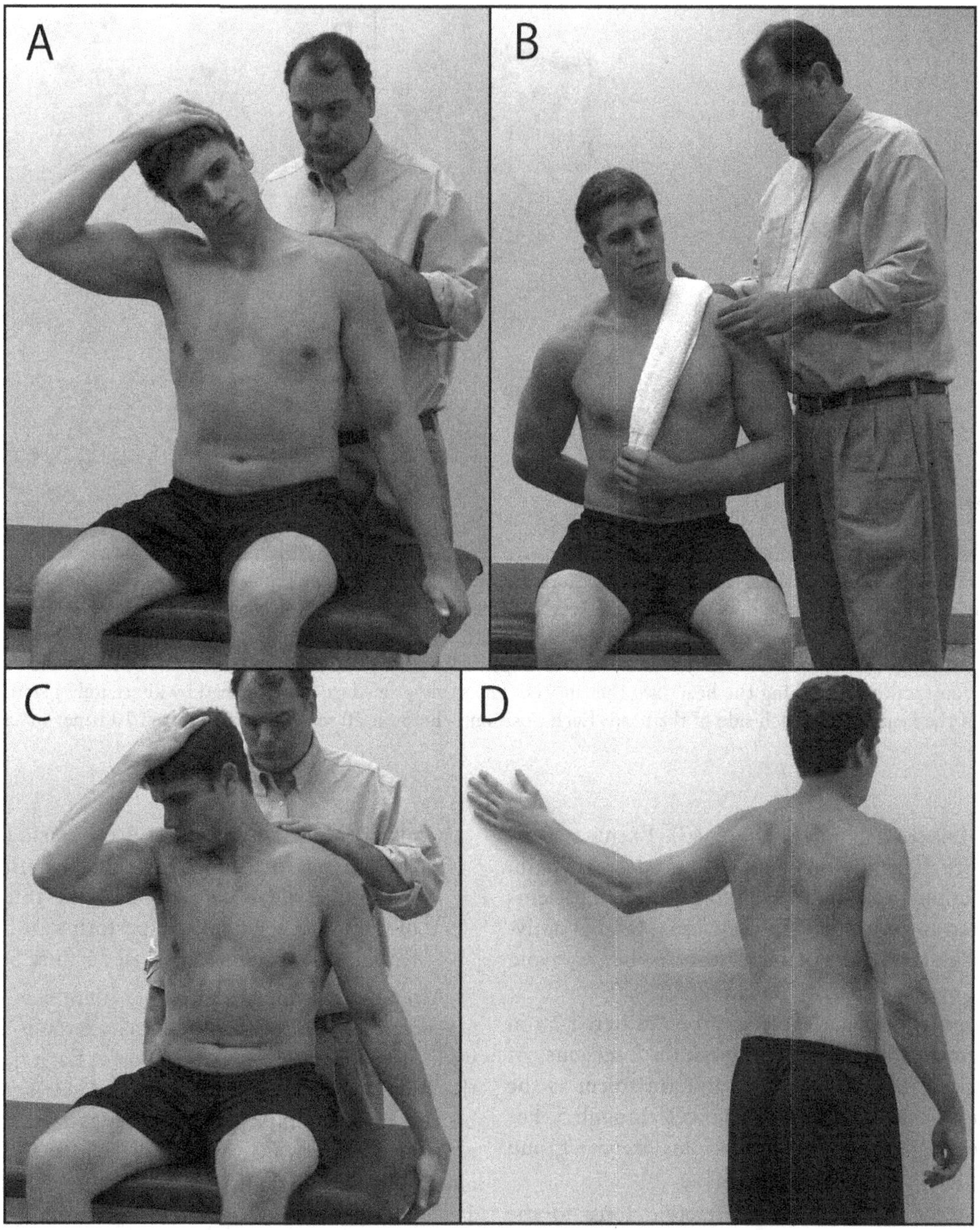

Figure 5-46. Home exercise self-stretching program. (A) Left upper trapezius. In upright sitting, the patient bends the head and neck forward, side bends to the right, rotates to the left, and stabilizes the head with the right hand but does not pull on the head. The patient then grasps the side of the chair with the left hand and leans toward the right until a stretch is felt in the appropriate area. (B) Left scalene and sternocleidomastoid. In upright sitting, the patient uses the right hand or a towel to hold the left shoulder down. The patient then performs a chin tuck and, while holding the chin tuck, side bends to the right and rotates to the left until a stretch is felt in the appropriate area. (C) Left levator scapulae. In upright sitting, the patient bends the head and neck forward, side bends to the right, rotates to the right, and stabilizes the head with the right hand but does not pull on the head. The patient then grasps the side of the chair with the left hand and leans toward the right until a stretch is felt in the appropriate area. (D) Left pectoralis major and minor. In standing, the patient stands facing a wall with the left arm outstretched against the wall and the elbow flexed. The patient first holds the scapula down and back and slowly rotates the body to the right until a stretch is felt in the left chest area. Performance of this technique is likely contraindicated in glenohumeral instability, limited shoulder mobility, or a painful shoulder. (Exercises as described by Cleland JA, Mintken PE, Carpenter K, et al. Examination of a clinical prediction rule to identify patients with neck pain likely to benefit from thoracic spine thrust manipulation and a general cervical range of motion exercise: multi-center randomized clinical trial. *Phys Ther.* 2010;90:1239-1250.)

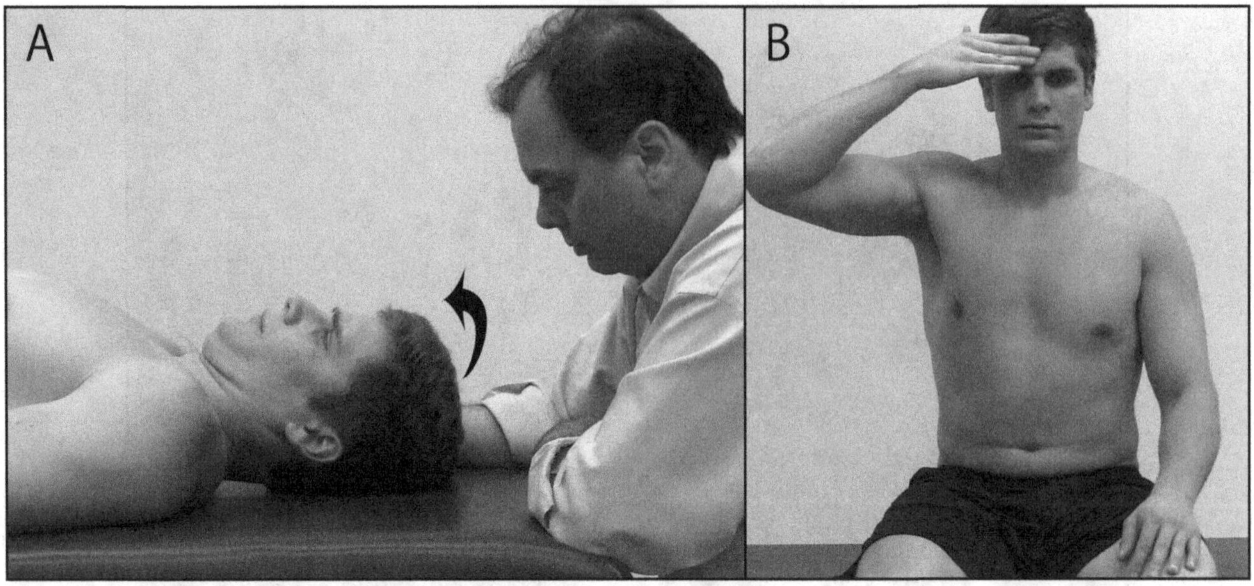

Figure 5-47. Strengthening exercises. (A) Deep neck flexors. In supine with the knees bent with or without a pillow under the head and neck, the patient is asked to nod as if to indicate "yes" and hold this position. The patient also palpates the superficial neck muscles to monitor for excessive use during this exercise. The exercises are stopped if the superficial muscles are felt to be dominant or over working. (B) Cervical isometrics. In neutral sitting, the patient places the fingers against the forehead and performs an isometric contraction by pushing the head into the fingers. The same procedure is performed by alternately placing the fingers on the back of the head and on each side of the head. Each position is held for 10 seconds and repeated 10 times in each direction. *(continued)*

a goal of a 10-second hold (Figure 5-47). Exercises were performed once daily as a home program to decrease pain, improve function, and reduce disability.[247,248] Patients were instructed to continue with their usual level of activity for activities that did not increase pain, but to avoid activities that aggravated symptoms.[249,250]

The manipulation plus exercise group differed from the exercise group only for the first week for 2 sessions. At the third session, they received the same treatment as the exercise group—exercise only for sessions 3 through 5. For the first 2 sessions, the manipulation plus exercise group received 3 different manipulations[130]:

1. A high-velocity, midrange, distraction force to the mid-thoracic spine on the lower thoracic spine in a sitting position. The therapist places his or her upper chest at the level of the patient's mid-thoracic spine and grasps the patient's elbows to perform a seated mid-thoracic spine distraction thrust manipulation (see Figure 5-40).
2. A high-velocity, end-range, AP force applied through the elbows to the upper thoracic spine on the mid-thoracic spine in cervicothoracic flexion. With the patient in supine, the therapist uses his or her manipulative hand to stabilize the inferior vertebra of the targeted segment and performs an HVLA thrust through the patient's arms (see Figure 5-42).
3. A high-velocity, end-range, AP force applied through the elbows to the middle thoracic spine on the lower thoracic spine in cervicothoracic flexion. With the patient in supine, the therapist uses his or her manipulative hand to stabilize the inferior vertebra of the target segment and performs an HVLA thrust through the patient's arms (see Figure 5-38).

After the manipulation, each patient was instructed in a general cervical AROM mobility exercise[251] for patients with neck pain (see Figure 5-43). Each patient places the fingers over the manubrium and starts with the chin on the fingers rotating to one side as far as possible and returning to neutral. Rotation is performed to both sides alternately within pain tolerance 3 to 4 times daily for 10 repetitions to each side. The patient progresses from 5, 4, 3, 2, and 1 finger as mobility increases. Patients were instructed to maintain usual activities that did not increase symptoms and to avoid activities that aggravated symptoms. The results of Cleland et al[130] did not support the validity of the clinical prediction rule. However, the results demonstrated that the manipulation plus exercise group had significantly greater improvements in disability at both short- and long-term follow-up and in pain at the 1-week follow-up compared with the exercise only group. The results suggest that patients with no contraindications to manipulation and a primary condition of mechanical neck pain may benefit from thoracic manipulation and exercise.[130] Though outcomes improve in patients with mechanical neck pain who receive TSM, impairments of the cervical spine must also be addressed.

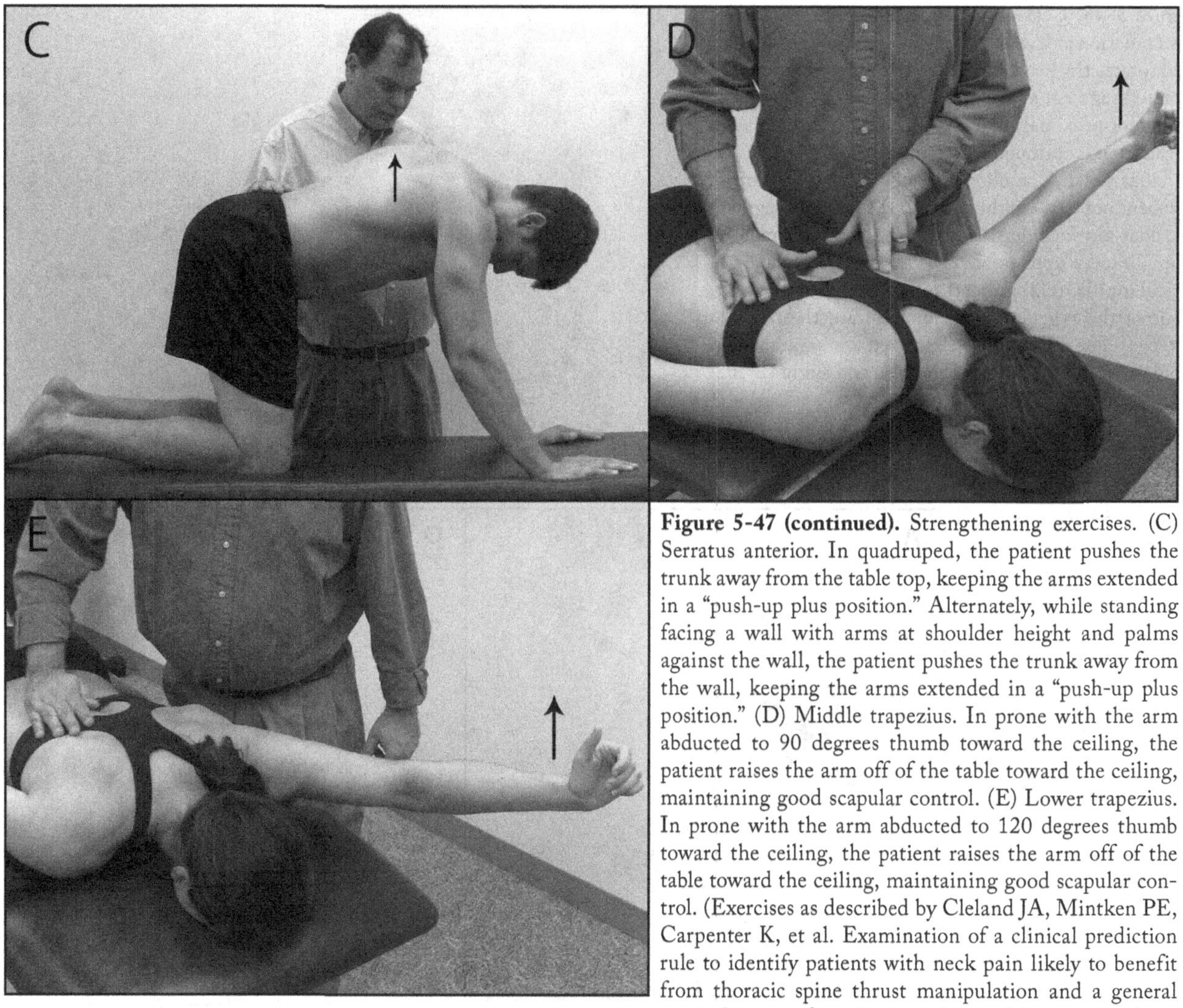

Figure 5-47 (continued). Strengthening exercises. (C) Serratus anterior. In quadruped, the patient pushes the trunk away from the table top, keeping the arms extended in a "push-up plus position." Alternately, while standing facing a wall with arms at shoulder height and palms against the wall, the patient pushes the trunk away from the wall, keeping the arms extended in a "push-up plus position." (D) Middle trapezius. In prone with the arm abducted to 90 degrees thumb toward the ceiling, the patient raises the arm off of the table toward the ceiling, maintaining good scapular control. (E) Lower trapezius. In prone with the arm abducted to 120 degrees thumb toward the ceiling, the patient raises the arm off of the table toward the ceiling, maintaining good scapular control. (Exercises as described by Cleland JA, Mintken PE, Carpenter K, et al. Examination of a clinical prediction rule to identify patients with neck pain likely to benefit from thoracic spine thrust manipulation and a general cervical range of motion exercise: multi-center randomized clinical trial. *Phys Ther.* 2010;90:1239-1250.)

Puentedura et al[243] randomly assigned 24 patients ages 18 to 60 with a primary complaint of neck pain with or without unilateral UE symptoms to either a thoracic group that received TSM and cervical ROM for 2 sessions followed by a standard exercise program for 3 sessions, or a cervical group that received cervical thrust manipulation and the same exercise sessions. The authors excluded patients with any serious pathology such as neoplasm, a diagnosis of cervical spinal stenosis by patient report or bilateral UE symptoms, evidence of central nervous system involvement, 2 or more positive neurologic signs consistent with nerve root compression (ie, changes in sensation, myotomal weakness, or decreased deep tendon reflexes), pending legal action regarding neck pain, a recent history of whiplash injury within 6 weeks of the examination, any history of cervical spine surgery, rheumatoid arthritis, osteoporosis, osteopenia, or AS. Outcomes were measured at 1 week, 4 weeks, and 6 months. The TSM group received 3 techniques (see Figures 5-38, 5-40, and 5-42), the same as used in the Cleland et al[130] study. The cervical group received an HVLA rotational thrust manipulation to both sides (Figure 5-48). The standard exercise routine[243] (Figure 5-49) for both groups included the following:

- Three-finger exercise for cervical rotation (see Figure 5-43A)
- Bilateral shoulder shrug and scapular retractions against gravity
- Bilateral horizontal adduction and abduction with hands clasped behind the head
- Upper cervical flexion and extension with hands behind the head and elbows held together (ie, the elbows are stationary with the head moving into the forearms
- Lower cervical flexion and extension with hands behind the head and elbows together (ie, the upper cervical spine is stationary with the elbows moving up toward the ceiling and floor)

Figure 5-48. Cervical HVLA left rotational thrust manipulation at C2/C3. Using a cradle hold, the clinician rotates the head slightly to the left and locates the targeted segment at the articular pillar of C2 with the middle or proximal phalanx of the right index finger. Rotation is continued until resistance is felt at the articular pillar. The clinician adds a small amount of side bending to the right down to the targeted segment but does not include this segment to localize motion. The clinician applies an HVLA thrust to the right articular pillar (C2) into left rotation upward along the plane of the zygapophyseal joint toward the patient's left eye. The HVLA is performed by simultaneous rapid pronation of the right forearm and slight supination of the left forearm and wrist.

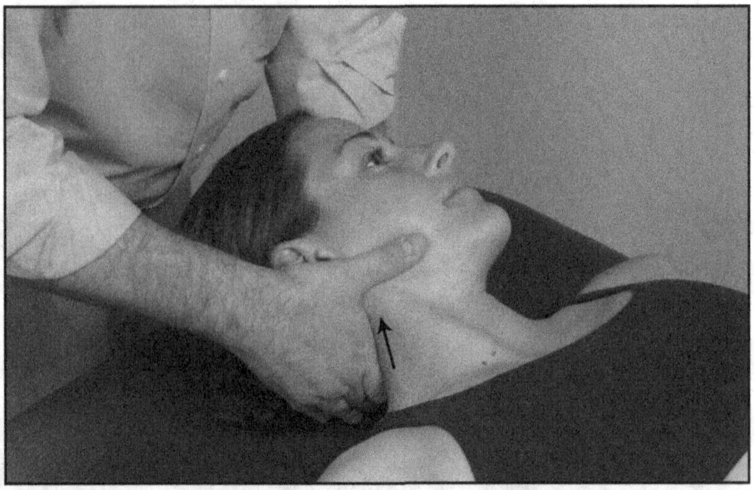

Figure 5-49. Standard exercises as described by Puentedura et al[244]: (A) bilateral shoulder shrug and scapular retractions against gravity; (B) bilateral horizontal adduction and abduction with hands clasped behind the head; and (C) upper cervical flexion and extension with hands behind the head and elbows held together. *(continued)*

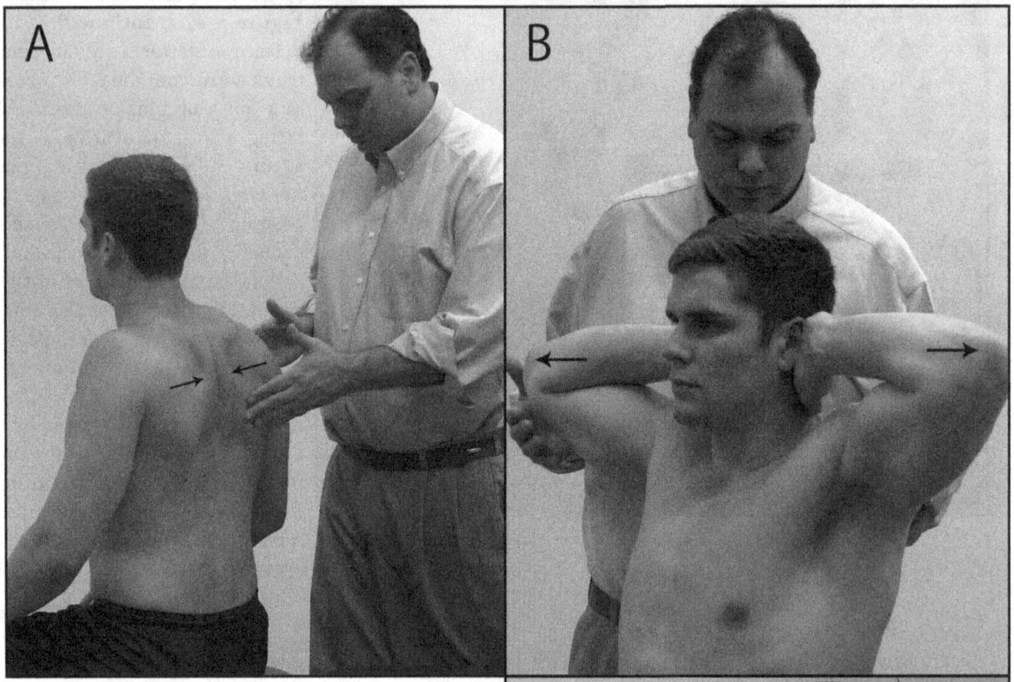

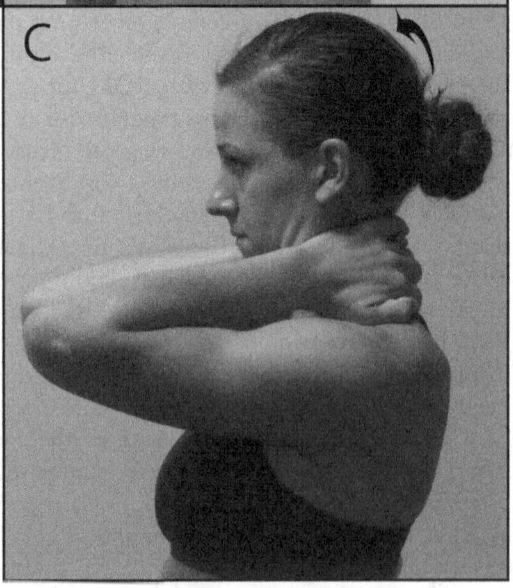

- Elastic band rows with moderate (green) resistance
- Lateral pull downs with moderate (green) resistance[243]

Exercises were performed for 3 sets of 10 repetitions in the clinic and 3 to 4 times per day within pain tolerance. Patients in the cervical group had greater improvements in the NDI ($P \leq .001$) and NPRS ($P \leq .003$) at all follow-up time periods. A statistically significant improvement in the Fear-Avoidance Beliefs Questionnaire with physical activity at all follow-ups was also observed for the cervical group ($P \leq .004$). Number needed to treat to avoid an unsuccessful overall outcome was 1.8 at 1 week and 1.6 at 4 weeks and also at 6 months. The cervical group also experienced less transient posttreatment side effects.[243]

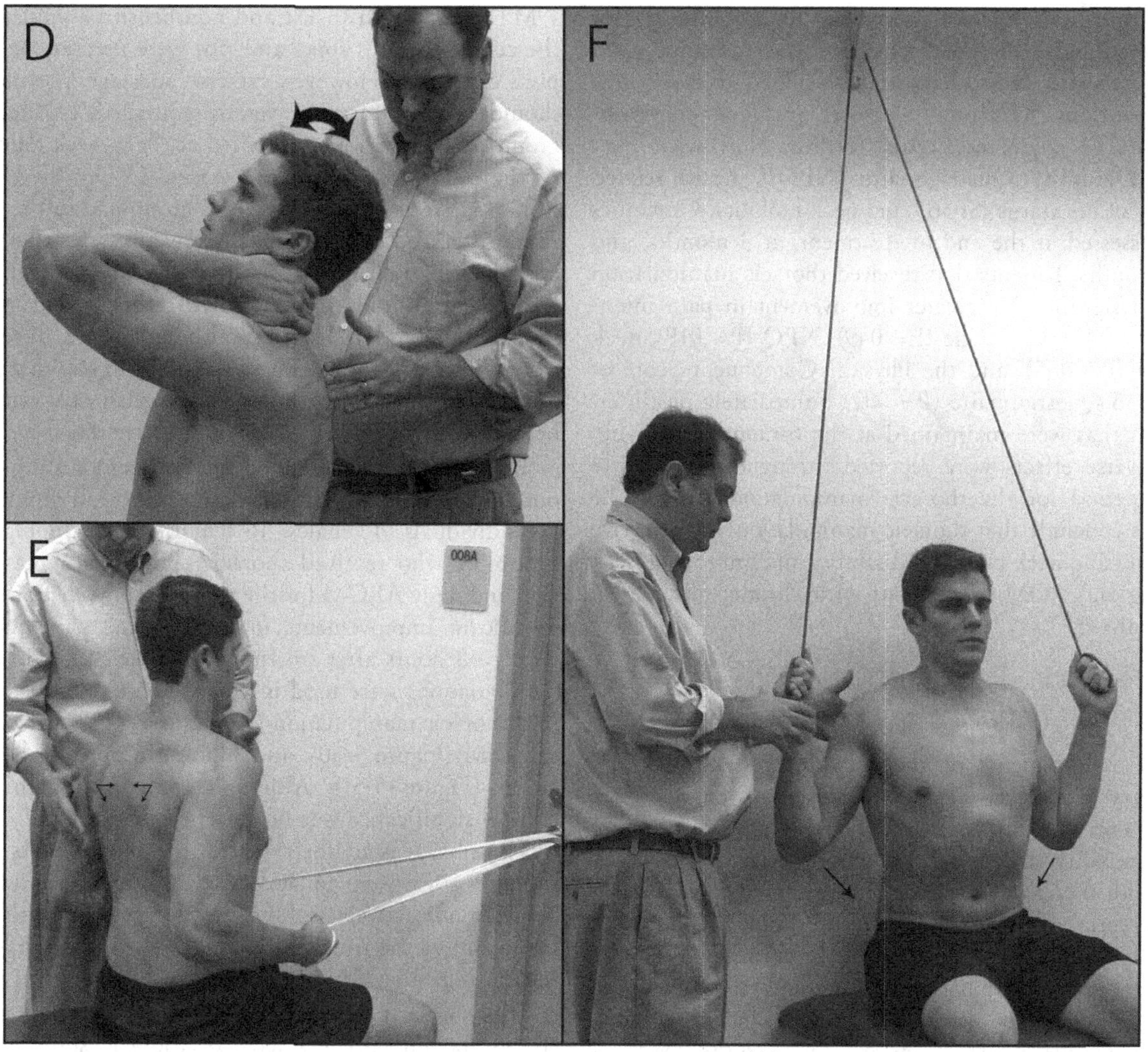

Figure 5-49 (continued). Standard exercises as described by Puentedura et al[244]: (D) lower cervical flexion and extension with hand behind the head and elbow together (upper cervical spine is stationary with the elbows moving up toward the ceiling and toward the floor); (E) low rows with moderate resistance; and (F) lateral pull downs with moderate resistance.

Thoracic manipulation was used in the PT management of 11 patients mean age 51.7 (SD 8.2 years) with a diagnosis of cervical radiculopathy.[233] Subjects were included based on a test item cluster for cervical radiculopathy. The presence of 4 positive examination findings (Spurling's test A, upper limb tension test A [median nerve bias], cervical distraction test, and <60 degrees cervical rotation toward the symptomatic side) were associated with a +LR of 30.3 for detecting cervical radiculopathy when compared to a neurodiagnostic testing reference standard.[252] Exclusion criteria were any medical red flags, bilateral UE symptoms, central nervous system involvement (ie, present Hoffman's sign), or prior cervicothoracic surgery. Intervention was standardized and provided in the order listed: cervical lateral glide mobilization in an upper limb neurodynamic position, thoracic spine mobilization/manipulation, strengthening exercises of the deep neck flexors and scapulothoracic muscles, and mechanical traction. Thoracic manual therapy was based on segmental mobility assessment and directed at hypomobile segments of the upper and mid-thoracic spine (see Figures 5-38 and 5-42). Following a mean of 7.1 (SD 1.5 sessions), 10 of 11 patients (91%) had clinically meaningful improvements in pain and function at the final session and at the 6-month follow-up.[233]

Lau et al[244] assessed the effectiveness of thoracic manipulation (see Figure 5-38) on patients with chronic neck pain for greater than 3 months. Patients (n = 120) ages 18 to 55 years were randomly assigned to 2 groups: an experimental group that received thoracic manipulation and infrared radiation therapy (IRR) and a control group (IRR only). Both groups were treated for 8 sessions 2 times per week and received standardized education and exercises. Daily exercises included cervical AROM of 10 repetitions in all directions; cervical isometrics for stabilization for 5-second holds, 10 repetitions; postural education; and upper trapezius and scalene stretching for 5 to 8 seconds, 10 repetitions. Outcome measures included craniovertebral (CV) angle, neck pain (NPRS, Northwick Park Neck Disability Questionnaire [NPQ]), health-related quality of life status (SF36), and neck mobility. Outcomes were assessed at the end of treatment, at 3 months, and at 6 months. Patients that received thoracic manipulation showed significantly greater improvement in pain intensity (P = .043), CV angle (P = .049), NPQ (P = .018), neck flexion (P = .005), and the Physical Component Score of the SF36 Questionnaire (P = .002) immediately postintervention that were maintained at the 6-month follow-up. No adverse effects were reported throughout the entire study period for the thoracic manipulation group. The authors conclude that thoracic manipulation was effective in decreasing neck pain and disability and improving neck posture and ROM for patients with chronic mechanical neck pain.[244]

Thoracic Hypomobility With Shoulder Impairments

The requirements of thoracic posture and mobility necessary to achieve full shoulder elevation were discussed in the examination section. Deficits in posture, thoracic spine mobility, and/or soft tissue mobility may be associated with increased demands on the shoulder girdle with the potential to contribute to painful shoulder conditions. Several authors have demonstrated improved outcomes using thoracic manipulation in subgroups of patients with painful shoulder conditions.[253-257] Studies include cervicothoracic manual interventions in addition to the treatment of primary impairments of the shoulder girdle.[253,258]

At least 40% of patients with primary complaints of shoulder pain may have impairments of the cervicothoracic spine and rib cage as potential contributors to shoulder complaints.[259] Several investigations[260-262] found a significant association between decreased thoracic spine mobility and patient complaints of neck and shoulder pain. Cervicothoracic spine and rib cage impairments are predictors of poor outcome and triple the risk for developing shoulder conditions.[253,259-262]

Evidence for Thoracic Mobilization and Manipulation in Patients With Thoracic Hypomobility and Shoulder Impairments

Bergman et al[253] randomly assigned subjects with primary shoulder pain to receive either usual medical care (UMC) from their primary care physicians or usual care plus manipulative therapy (UMC + MT) targeting the cervicothoracic spine and rib cage for 6 sessions over 12 weeks. The UMC group could receive oral analgesics, NSAIDs, up to 3 corticosteroid injections, and referral for PT if symptoms lasted longer than 6 weeks. For the UMC + MT group, both thrust and nonthrust manipulation to the cervicothoracic spine and ribs were used at the therapist's discretion. However, exercise, massage, posture, and shoulder joint treatment were discouraged. No between-group differences were identified at the 6-week follow-up. At the end of treatment or 12 weeks, 43% of the UMC + MT group and 21% of the UMC group had full recovery. A consistent between-group difference in severity of main complaint, shoulder pain and disability, and general health favored the addition of manipulative therapy during both intervention and follow-ups, although these differences were not significant.[253] These findings suggest that a subgroup of patients with shoulder pain may exist who may benefit from the addition of manipulative therapy.

Boyles et al[255] conducted an exploratory study without a control group or randomization and found that 56 individuals (40 males, 16 females) with impingement syndrome who received thoracic spine thrust manipulation and daily AROM for the thoracic spine demonstrated significant improvements in self-reported pain and disability 48 hours after treatment. Thoracic and rib thrust manipulations were used in this study: seated distraction mid-thoracic manipulation (see Figure 5-40); seated cervical TSM (Figure 5-50); and supine rib opening manipulation (Figure 5-51). Although statistically significant, clinical significance was not reached for pain and disability. Possible reasons for this are that impairments at the shoulder girdle were not addressed and that these individuals were not actively seeking care for a primary shoulder complaint at the time of the study.[255] A cause-and-effect relationship should not be considered based on this study.

In a similarly designed study, Strunce et al[256] reported on the immediate effects of thoracic spine and rib manipulation in 21 subjects with shoulder pain. Inclusion criteria were primary unilateral shoulder pain, ages 18 to 65, decreased shoulder ROM, and pain reproduced with either the Hawkins-Kennedy or Neer impingement tests. Exclusion criteria were systemic disease such as rheumatoid arthritis or infection, tumor, fracture, rotator cuff tear, adhesive capsulitis, cervical radiculopathy, fear, osteoporosis, or other serious spinal pathology. The type and number of manipulations performed were based on examination findings. Up to 4 thrust manipulations (see Figures 5-38, 5-44, 5-50, and 5-51) could be performed at the discretion of the therapist. No adverse effects were reported. Within session, posttreatment effects showed a 51% (VAS 32 mm) decrease in shoulder pain, increase in ROM (30 to 38 degrees), and a mean GROC of 4.2 (median 5). The results support a clinically relevant relationship between the thoracic spine, rib cage, and shoulder regions. Within session, improvements in pain and shoulder motion as a result of thoracic manipulation may provide useful for clinical reasoning and decision making for evaluation and treatment.[256]

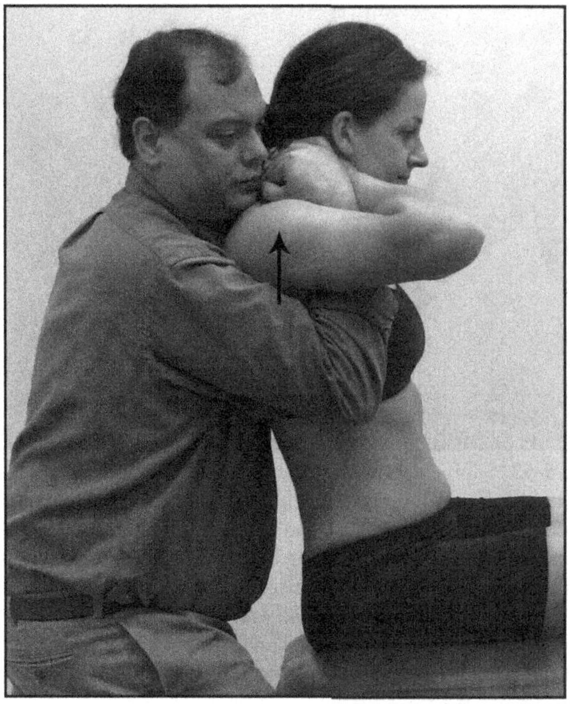

Figure 5-50. Seated cervicothoracic spine distraction manipulation. The clinician is in a walk stance position with knees slightly flexed. The patient is seated and reclined against the clinician's trunk with the hands interlaced behind the neck. The clinician reaches between the patient's elbows to purchase the C7 SP with his or her hands. The clinician's forearms are compressed against the anterior shoulders of the patient. The patient is reclined slightly so that cervical spine is oriented perpendicular to the floor. At the end of exhalation with the patient relaxed, the clinician applies an HVLA thrust using his or her legs to provide a distraction force against gravity.

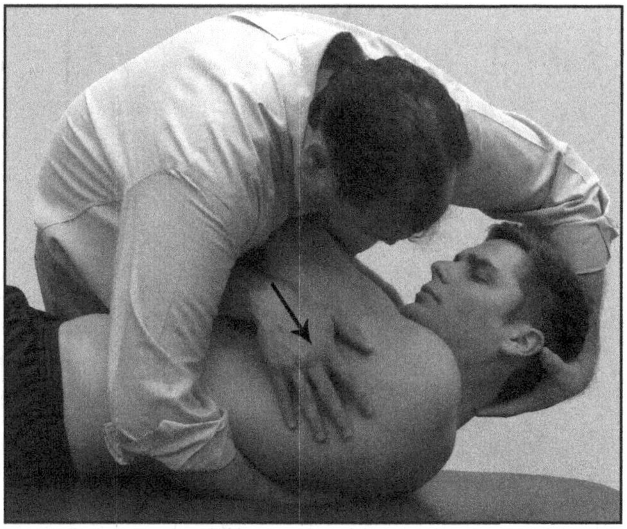

Figure 5-51. Supine unilateral rib opening mobilization/manipulation. Patient is supine with arms folded across the chest, positioned as close to the edge of plinth as possible. The clinician stands on the side opposite the pain, rolls the patient toward the clinician, places the thenar eminence in a skin lock just lateral to the costotransverse joint and medial to the rib angle, and rolls the patient supine over the fulcrum of the thenar eminence. The patient is flexed to the motion barrier via ipsilateral lateral flexion and rotation added for localization. The patient takes a deep breath and relaxes naturally. At the end of exhalation, the clinician applies an HVLA force through the patient's arms to further rotation over the fulcrum created by the thenar eminence. This technique may also be performed as a mobilization.

Mintken et al[257] examined findings in 80 subjects ages 18 to 65 from the history and physical examination to determine prognostic factors that allow clinicians to identify individuals with shoulder pain who are likely to benefit in the short-term from cervical TSM. All subjects received the same treatment regardless of the examination findings: one lateral translation nonthrust mobilization to the lower cervical spine at C5 to C7 for 6 bouts of 30 seconds to each side (Figure 5-52), and 5 different thrust manipulation techniques (see Figures 5-38, 5-40, 5-42, 5-44, and 5-53) targeting the cervical and thoracic regions performed twice for a total of 10 manipulations per treatment session. The shoulder was not treated. Following the manual therapy, 2 exercises were performed: the 3-finger cervical ROM exercise (see Figure 5-43) and a supine general thoracic extension exercise (Figure 5-54). Both exercises were performed 3 to 4 times daily for 10 repetitions. Subjects received a maximum of 3 sessions. No adverse events were reported with only 3/80 reporting a worsening of symptoms. Sixty-one percent (49/80) reported a successful outcome (31 after the first session; 18 after the second session).

Five preliminary factors that best predicted success include the following:

1. Pain free shoulder flexion < 127 degrees
2. Shoulder internal rotation < 53 degrees
3. A negative Neer test
4. Not taking medications
5. Symptoms < 90 days[257]

If 3 or more factors are present, the chance of dramatic success with manipulation improves from 61% to 89% (+LR 5.3; 95% CI: 1.7, 16.0).[257] Results of this study have not been validated.

Thoracic Hypomobility With Low Back Pain

The concept of regional interdependence suggests that thoracic spine hypomobility may place increased loads on the lumbar spine, possibly due to pain and an overactive superficial system, compensation for an underactive deep muscle system, or increased demands for lumbar movement in the presence of stiffness of the thoracic spine. Evaluation of at least the lower thoracic spine is recommended in patients with LBP. Thoracic hypomobility impairments, if identified, are prioritized as needed for intervention in addition to the treatment of the low back.

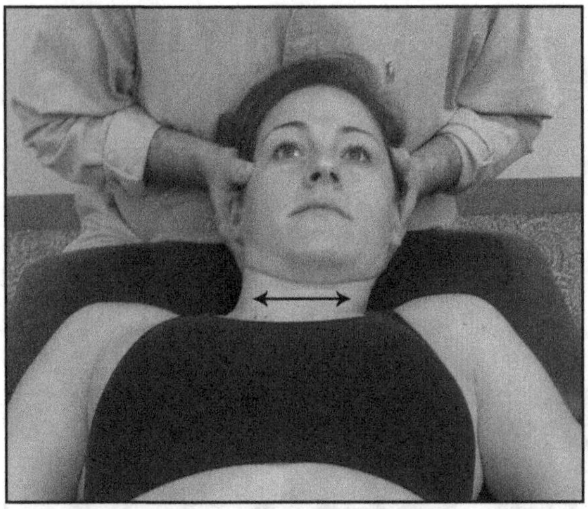

Figure 5-52. Cervical lateral translation. Supine cervical lateral translation to the right and left. The clinician cradles the patient's head, contacting the articular pillars with the lateral aspect of the MCP joints or proximal interphalangeal joints of the index fingers bilaterally from C5 to C7. Translation is performed at each segment in neutral and flexion at C5 to C7 grades III and IV for 6 bouts of 30 seconds.

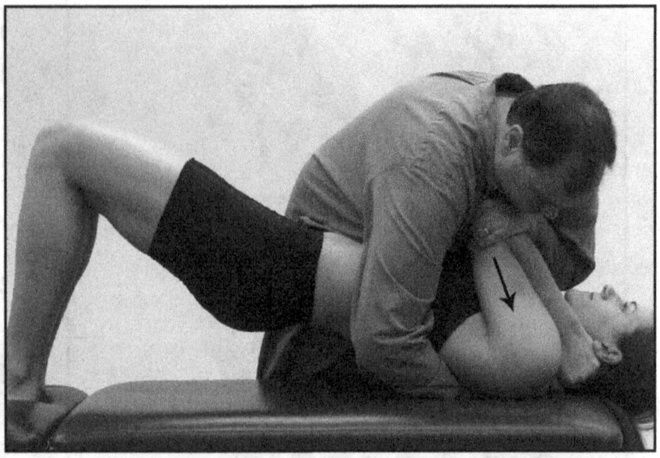

Figure 5-53. Supine cervicothoracic AP manipulation. The patient is supine with hands interlocked behind the neck. The clinician rolls the patient toward the clinician and places the thenar eminence in a skin lock at the T1 segment, pulling the segment inferiorly. With the patient in supine, the clinician localizes motion to the C7 to T1 segment through the patient's arms and asks the patient to bridge until weight shifts onto the stabilizing hand. The patient takes a deep breath and relaxes naturally. At the end of exhalation, the clinician applies an HVLA force through the patient's arms.

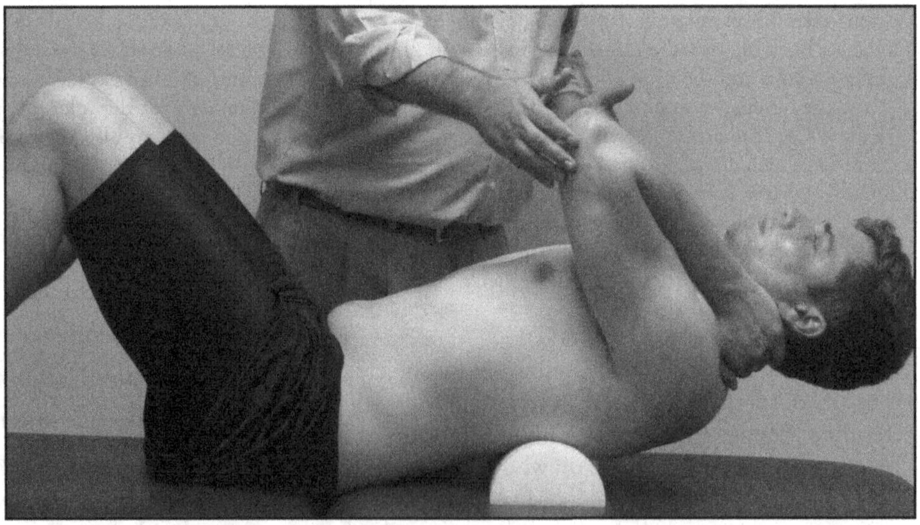

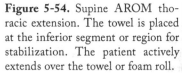

Figure 5-54. Supine AROM thoracic extension. The towel is placed at the inferior segment or region for stabilization. The patient actively extends over the towel or foam roll.

Evidence for Thoracic Mobilization and Manipulation in Patients With Thoracic Hypomobility and Low Back Pain

The association between impaired joint mobility and impaired muscle performance is often unclear because the two are so closely related. An obvious example is quadriceps inhibition that occurs with asymptomatic knee osteoarthritis, referred to as *arthrogenous muscle inhibition* and possibly due to altered afferent input from the dysfunctional joint.[263,264] The clinical question might be, "Is the joint dysfunction a result of poor muscle performance or is poor muscle performance a result of joint dysfunction?" Another common example in the presence of limited lower thoracic extension and lower trapezius weakness, "Is the lower trapezius inhibited and weak due to the loss of thoracic extension?" Clinical observations often lead to speculation that mechanical dysfunction or joint motion restrictions may lead to inhibition of the muscle. Restoration of normal joint motion is often necessary before therapeutic exercise is completely effective. In other words, a joint must have normal mobility in order for its muscles to work efficiently.[265]

Weakness of the lower trapezius is a common clinical finding often associated with the UCS, excessive thoracic kyphosis, and various shoulder disorders. Excessive thoracic kyphosis or limited thoracic extension is thought to inhibit the lower trapezius, resulting in weakness with strength testing. Liebler et al[265] examined the effects of grade IV, central PA mobilization to the lower thoracic spine (T6 to T12) on lower trapezius muscle strength in asymptomatic subjects. The experimental group received 30 seconds of grade IV on each segment, while the control group received grade I mobilization to each segment. The results demonstrated a statistically significant difference between groups with a 6.0% increase in the experimental group versus 0.2% increase in the control. In some patients, weakness may be secondary to apparent joint hypomobility. Mobilization and reassessment of muscle performance may improve clinical decision making and enhance the effectiveness of therapeutic exercise by reducing the neurophysiological inhibition. Findings of muscle weakness provide rationale for examination of joint mobility.

Cleland et al[266] performed the same study as Liebler et al,[265] but used a supine, mid-thoracic, AP thoracic manipulation with an extension bias (Figure 5-55) instead of a grade IV mobilization. Manipulation was performed at restricted thoracic segments based on clinical examination. A percentage increase of lower trapezius strength (ie, 14%) following thoracic manipulation was significantly greater compared to mobilization (ie, 6%). The authors suggested that both mobilization and/or manipulation may be beneficial prior to neuromuscular re-education of the lower trapezius.[266]

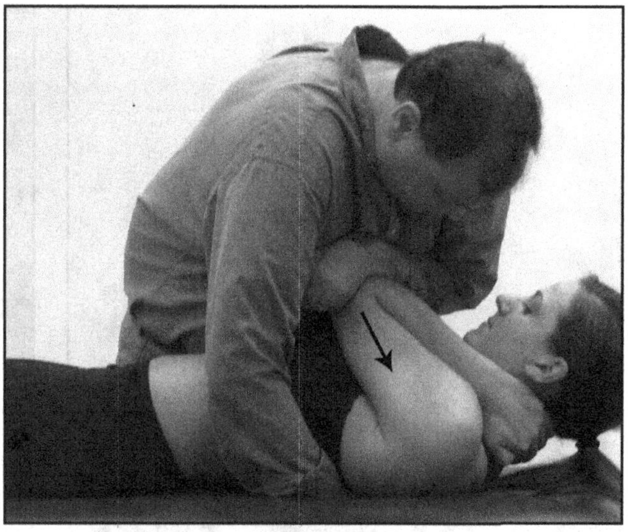

Figure 5-55. Supine mid-lower thoracic AP thrust manipulation with an extension bias. With the patient in supine, hands behind neck or arms hugging the upper body and/or a towel with the away arm on top forming a "V," the clinician stands on the patient's right side and reaches the lower hand across to locate and stabilize the inferior segment at the TP of T5. Keeping the right hand in place, the clinician rolls the patient back into supine. To bias toward unilateral extension, the clinician supports the neck and upper thoracic spine and laterally flexes and rotates toward the side of restriction until tension is felt at the T4 to T5 segment. The clinician rests his or her sternum or upper abdomen on the patient's elbows and apply AP thrust through the patient's arms and chest toward T4 to T5. If a bilateral extension restriction is present, the clinician can perform the exact procedure without lateral flexion and rotation.

Few studies have examined the regional interdependence between the thoracic and lumbar spine or described interventions related to hypomobility of the lower thoracic spine. Whitman et al[267] compared 2 PT treatment programs for patients with lumbar spinal stenosis. One program included manual PT, body weight-supported treadmill walking, and exercise, and the other consisted of lumbar flexion exercises, a treadmill walking program, and subtherapeutic ultrasound. The manual therapy was based on identified impairments and included a variety of techniques such as both thrust and nonthrust manipulation of the thoracic and lumbar spine, pelvis, and lower extremity; manual stretching; and muscle strengthening exercises. Improvement in patient satisfaction, disability, and treadmill walking tests favored the manual therapy and exercise group at 6 weeks, 1 year, and longer-term follow-up.[267]

Sebastian[268] presented a case report describing a patient who experienced LBP with referral to the right gluteal area. Symptoms improved with soft tissue mobilization and muscle energy techniques to the lumbosacral region, but gluteal pain persisted with some recurrence of the LBP. A motion restriction of flexion, left rotation, and left lateral flexion at the T12 motion segment was identified and treated with a supine, AP HVLA to the T12 to L1 motion segment. Based on the patient's response to the thoracolumbar manipulation, decreased pain, and improved function, the authors concluded that the thoracolumbar junction motion restriction was a dominant contributor to the patient's problem. Assessment and treatment of the primary complaint of LBP included the lower thoracic spine. Thoracic manipulation was one component of a multimodal plan of care that included lumbosacral muscle energy techniques, soft tissue mobilization, lumbopelvic stabilization exercise, electrotherapy, and strengthening of the gluteal muscles. The author discussed the anatomical and biomechanical considerations associated with the thoracolumbar junction and LBP.[268] Figures 5-56 and 5-57 show commonly used unilateral manipulation techniques for the thoracolumbar junction.

Horton[269] described the PT management of a patient with acute left-sided back pain at the level of the T8 to T9 motion segment. Onset was 2 days prior to presenting for PT and after a manipulation by a medical practitioner was unsuccessful. The patient presented in a flexed and right laterally flexed posture with complaints of severe pain on attempts to extend, left laterally flex, or rotate. Right side-lying was a position of ease. PAIVM reproduced pain and stiffness on the left at T8 to T9. PPIVM was limited and painful at the same level into left rotation.[269] Due to

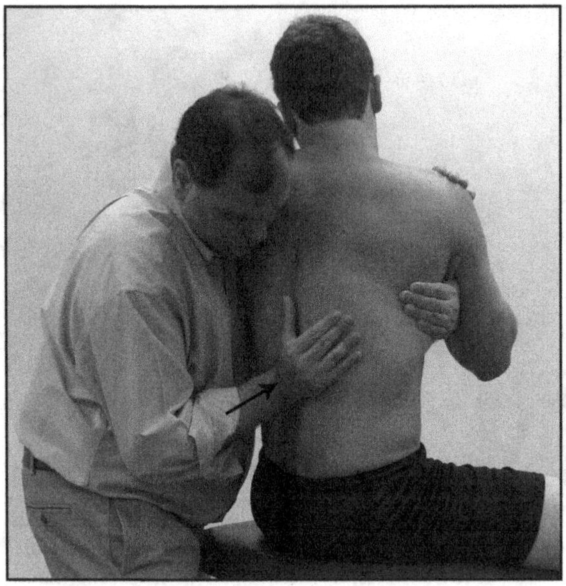

Figure 5-56. Seated thoracolumbar junction left rotation manipulation. With the patient seated, arms folded across the chest, and straddling the table for pelvic stability, the clinician on the patient's left side grasps the patient's trunk under the axilla of both arms to control trunk motion. Using the right hypothenar eminence, the manipulation hand is placed at the right T12 TP using a skin lock with an anterior and superior force. The clinician introduces a translation to the right to produce lateral flexion to the left and rotation to the left with minor flexion and extension adjustments until tension is felt at T12. The clinician then applies an HVLA manipulation through the right hand in a superior direction into rotation using the trunk and legs to produce the manipulation.

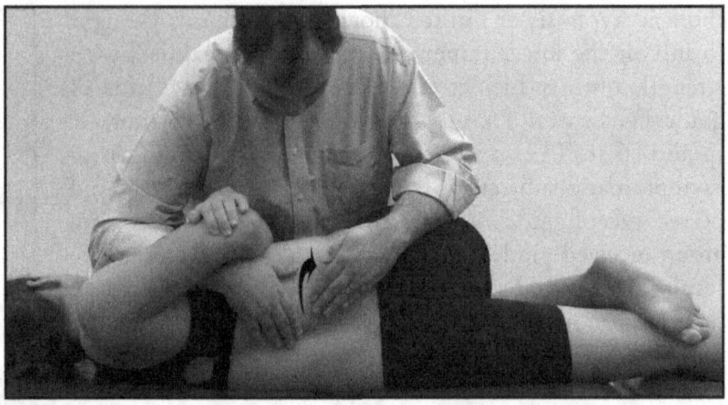

Figure 5-57. Side-lying thoracolumbar junction right rotation thrust manipulation. With the patient in left side-lying, the clinician flexes the upper leg and places the foot in the popliteal fossa, maintaining a neutral lumbar spine. Right rotation down to T12 is introduced by the clinician pulling the left arm superiorly and toward him- or herself. The left forearm is placed on the buttock between the gluteus maximus and medius. The right forearm introduces right rotation through the pectoral and rib cage regions as the left forearm rotates the pelvis and lumbar spine until motion is felt at the T12-L1 segment. The clinician maintains the setup and rolls the patient toward him- or herself. He or she applies a quick, minimal-force rotational HVLA thrust through the pelvis with the left forearm down toward the table.

the severity, irritability, and pain, the therapist chose to use a central sustained natural apophyseal glide (SNAG) as described by Mulligan.[270] A SNAG is a passive accessory glide performed on a patient who is simultaneously actively moving through the painful or restricted range of movement. The technique itself should be painless.[271] The SNAG was performed in a cephalad direction to the SP of T8 with the ulnar border of the therapist's hand while supporting the trunk and assisting movement into the upright posture (Figure 5-58). The SNAG was sustained in the corrected position and repeated 3 times. The patient was able to remain upright. Tape was used to support this position until follow-up the next day. The patient was 95% improved and treated with large amplitude unilateral PA mobilization on the left at T8 to T9 over the zygapophyseal joint (see Figures 5-29 and 5-59). Reassessment revealed full ROM. The patient was discharged.[269] Mechanisms by which a SNAG is believed to be effective are the same as described for mobilization and manipulation. Additional research related to the SNAG concept is available.[272] Austin and Benesky[273] included self-SNAGs for extension (Figure 5-60I) and rotation and (Figure 5-60J) in the management of a collegiate runner with thoracic pain.

Summary of the Proposed Mobilization and Manipulation Classification for Thoracic Spinal Pain With Mobility Deficits and Matched Intervention

Clinicians should adhere to a careful examination, minimum force in technique, an evidence-based approach, treatment guided by assessment and reassessment throughout the plan of care, and careful analysis in the presence of a deterioration of signs and symptoms. PT management includes strategies guided by the patient's examination and impairments to improve mobility. In addition to the thoracic region, management often includes examination and intervention for regions above and below the main complaint, such as the cervicobrachial and lumbopelvic regions as noted in many of the case reports. Various strategies include thoracic spine and/or rib mobilization or manipulation, instrumented soft tissue techniques, self-mobilization, therapeutic exercise, postural exercises, muscle energy techniques, and motor control exercise. Selected manual techniques for the thoracic region have been presented as related to cited research. A wide variety of manual procedures are used clinically with no approach or technique known to be superior to another. While intervention targeting a specific direction and motion of the hypomobile segment is often a goal in using manual techniques, a high level of segmental accuracy is not

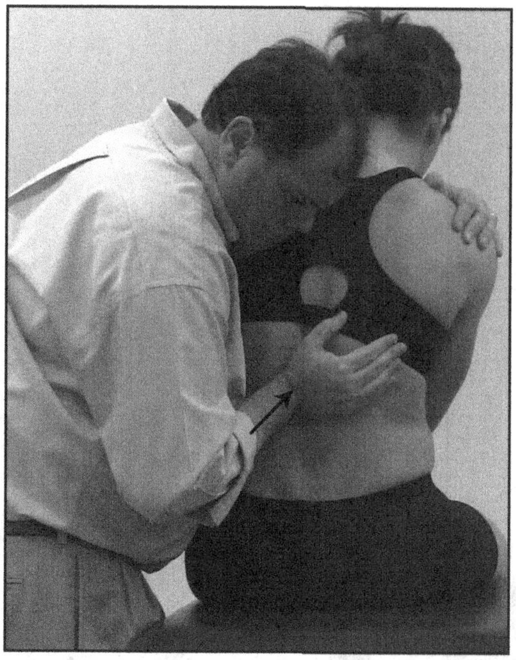

Figure 5-58. Central SNAG. The clinician uses the ulnar border of the hand to perform a sustained glide in a cephalad direction to the SP while supporting the trunk and assisting movement into the upright posture.

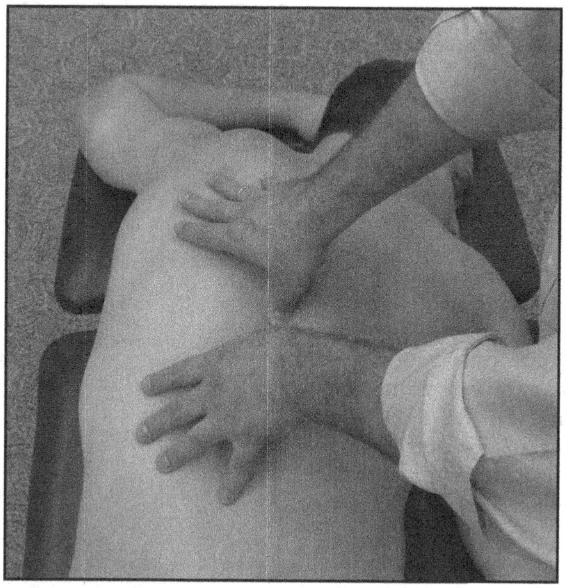

Figure 5-59. Unilateral PA mobilization over the right articular pillar. Mobilization may be angled in various directions and/or combined with different physiological movement positions. For example, a right unilateral PA can be performed with the patient positioned in right lateral flexion.

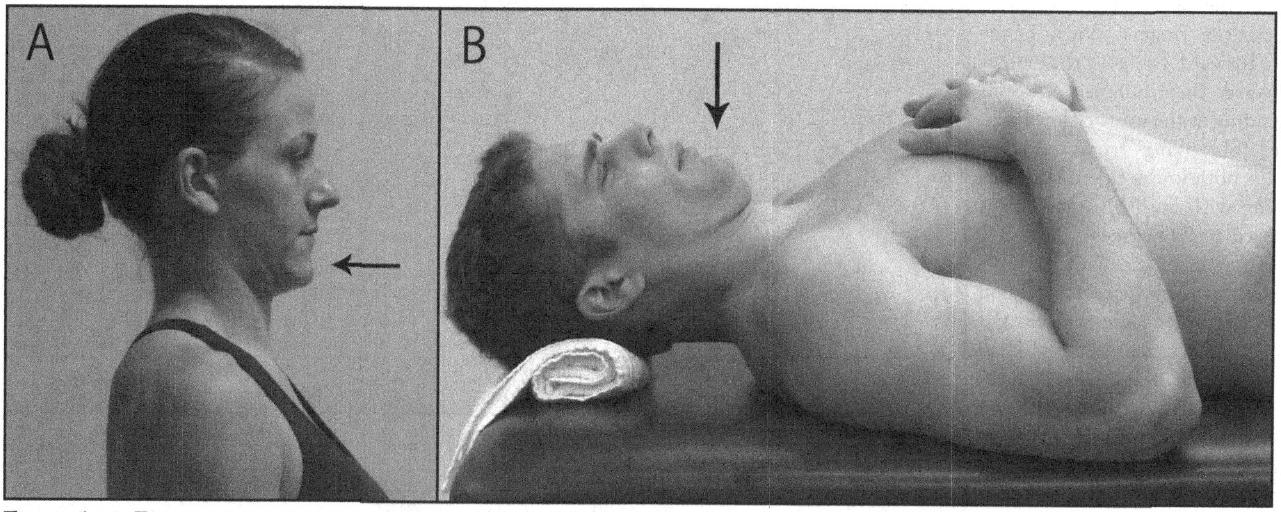

Figure 5-60. Exercises to augment manual interventions. (A) Cervical retraction in sitting; facilitates lower cervical and upper thoracic extension. (B) Cervical retraction in supine. *(continued)*

always possible. However, consideration of a regional focus (upper, mid-, or lower) may be more appropriate based on neurophysiological mechanisms related to effectiveness. Generally, thoracic spine hypomobility is treated prior to rib hypomobility as the thoracic spine is thought to be the driver of rib movement. If impairment of rib mobility remains after treatment of the thoracic spine, then intervention is directed to the rib cage. Manual techniques are usually followed by postural exercises, self-mobilization, and therapeutic exercise to retrain optimal motor control strategies. Exercise is used to augment or maintain clinical gains in mobility, to train neuromuscular control of newly gained ROM, and address functional activity limitations. Additional exercises to augment manual procedures are presented in Figure 5-60.

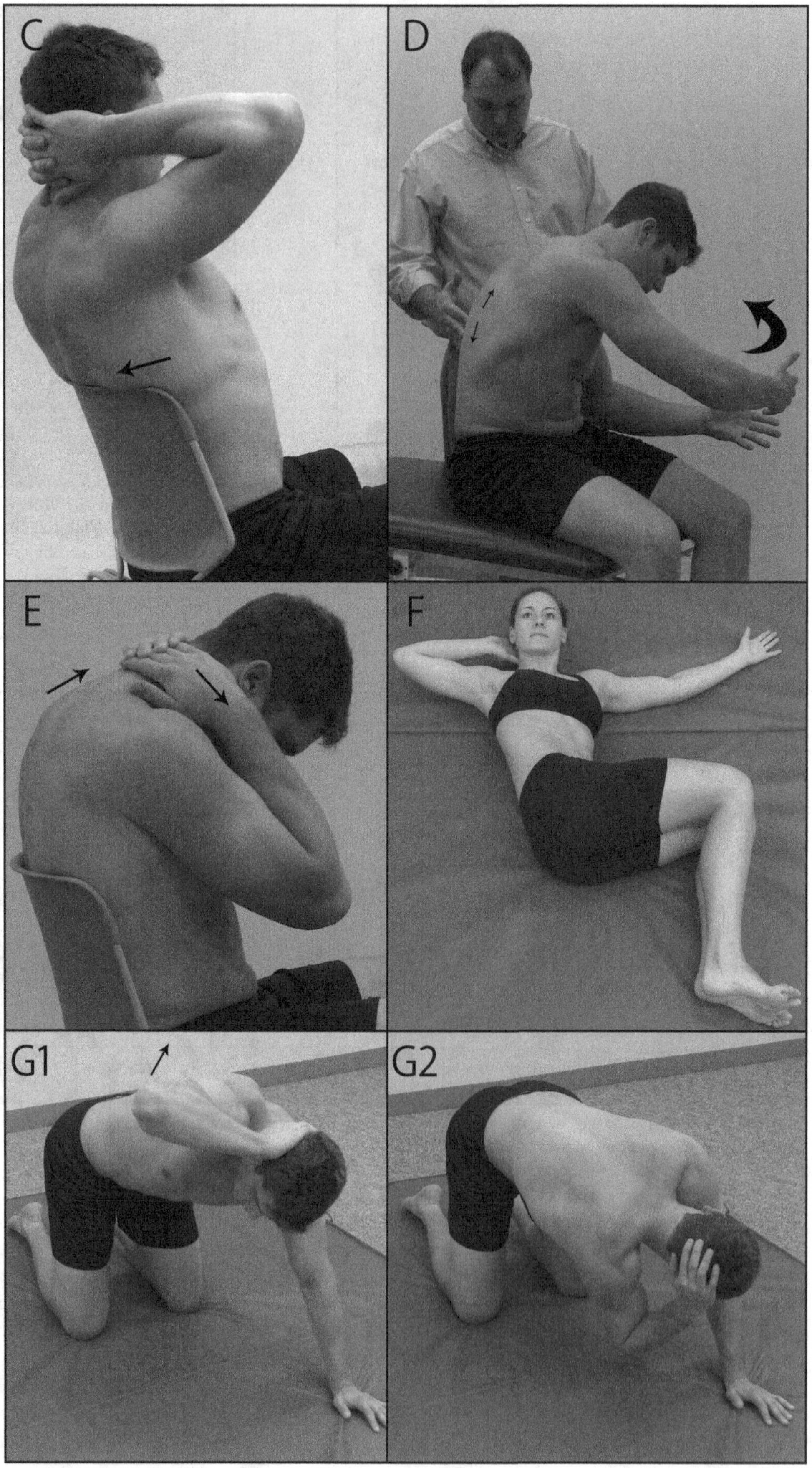

Figure 5-60 (continued). Exercises to augment manual interventions. (C) Seated thoracic extension over chair. In sitting with fingers interlocked behind the head, elbows together, and cervical spine in neutral, the patient uses the back of the chair as a fulcrum to stabilize the area below the chair and lean backwards to self-mobilize the thoracic spine into extension. The patient must not lift the chin or look up toward the ceiling. (D) Ball hug facilitates unilateral thoracic flexion and/or lateral flexion/rotation in the mid-thoracic region. In sitting, the patient holds or imagines holding a large ball and tries to get his or her arms around it. To stretch the right side of the mid-back, the patient turns to the right, reaching more with the right arm to get his or her arms around the ball. (E) Upper thoracic flexion. In sitting, the patient places his or her hands bend the lower neck and interlocks the fingers, slowly bending forward, bringing the elbows toward the abdomen without bending at the waist or low back. (F) Side-lying trunk rotation with both knees flexed. In side-lying with both hips and knees flexed to 90 degrees to stabilize the low back and with the bottom arm resting comfortably on the floor, the patient places the top arm in a hand-behind-head position, inhales, and moves the top arm back toward the floor while exhaling. Moving the hips higher toward the chest (ie, greater than 90 degrees) produces more rotation in the upper thoracic spine. With the hips less than 90 degrees, rotation occurs in the whole spine. The head and neck are kept in a neutral position. (G) Unilateral thoracic rotation in quadruped. For unilateral trunk rotation in quadruped, the patient places the right hand behind the head, inhales, and brings the right elbow up toward the ceiling (1) and then exhales and brings the right elbow down and to the left through available range (2). The cervical spine must be kept in neutral to emphasize motion in the thoracic spine. *(continued)*

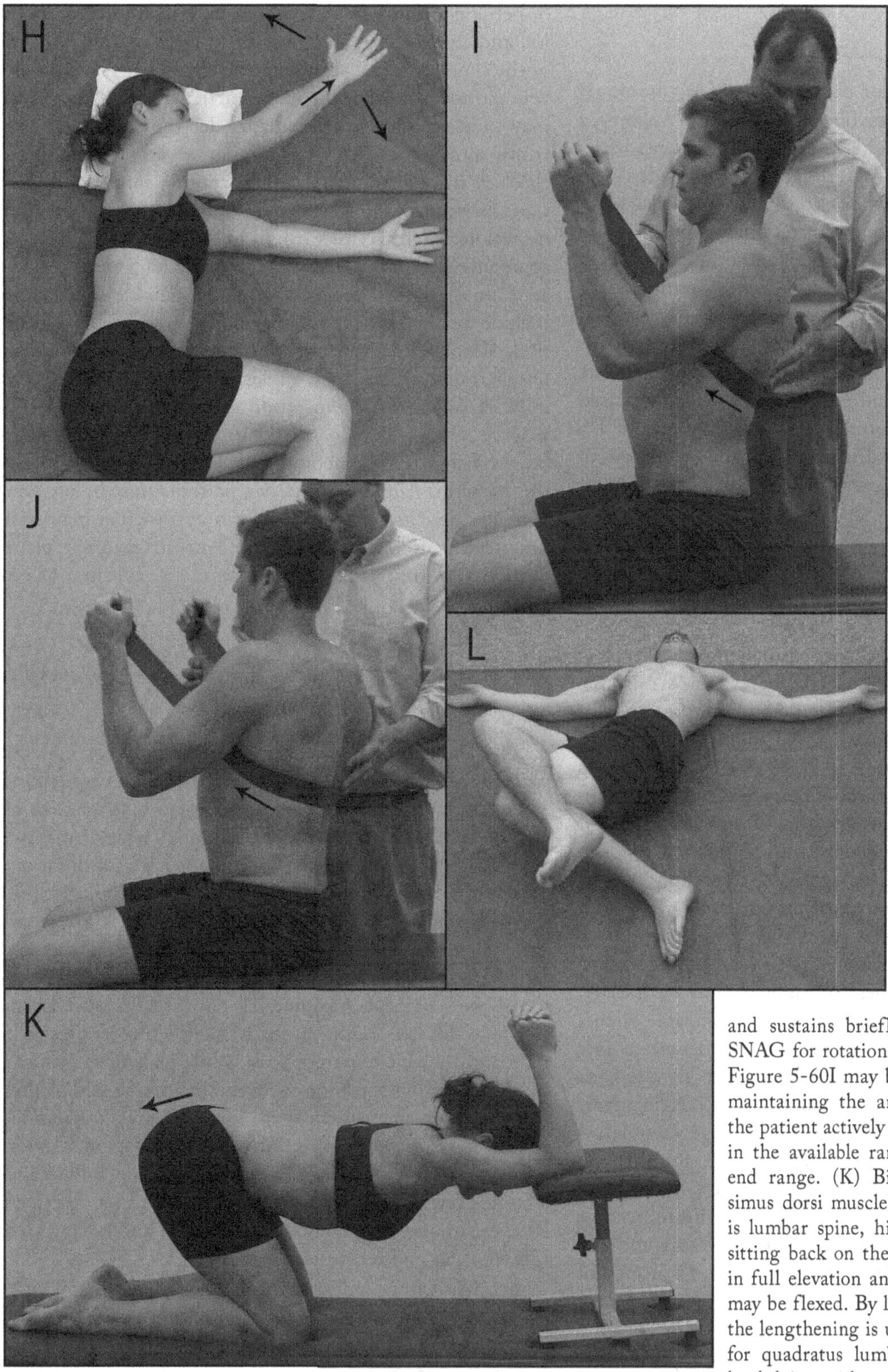

Figure 5-60 (continued). Exercises to augment manual interventions. (H) Side-lying shoulder circles. Side-lying shoulder circles are a combined thoracic and UE movement performed around a 360-degree perimeter as a general mobility exercise. In a side-lying neutral spine posture with the involved side up and hips and knees flexed, the patient reaches in a circular arc of movement both clockwise and counterclockwise keeping the hand in contact with the mat surface. Reaching in various directions focuses the exercise to specific regions of the thorax. Inhalation and exhalation may be used to facilitate rib cage movement. The shoulder girdle must be capable of mobility and stability in the intended directions. (I) Self-SNAG for extension. In sitting, the patient uses a thin towel or belt at the appropriate thoracic segment, pulling anteriorly and superiorly at about a 60-degree angle from the horizontal. While maintaining the pull, the patient actively extends and sustains briefly at end range. (J) Self-SNAG for rotation. The same technique as in Figure 5-60I may be used for rotation. While maintaining the anterior and superior glide, the patient actively performs pain-free rotation in the available range and sustains briefly at end range. (K) Bilateral or unilateral latissimus dorsi muscle lengthening. The position is lumbar spine, hips and knees fully flexed, sitting back on the heels with both shoulders in full elevation and external rotation; elbows may be flexed. By laterally flexing to one side, the lengthening is unilateral. (L) Lengthening for quadratus lumborum muscle. In supine, hook-lying with arms abducted to 90 degrees, head and neck in neutral, the patient crosses one leg over the other, pulling the lower spine into rotation. The position is maintained or a contract and relax muscle energy technique is added. The position also encourages thoracolumbar rotation.

Rib Cage Hypomobility and Anterior Chest Wall Symptoms

Musculoskeletal anterior chest wall pain is commonly called CWS, but poorly described. Verdon et al[274] observed 672 cases of chest pain, and 300 or 44.6% patients had a diagnosis of CWS affecting all ages with a gender ratio of 1:1. History and palpation were the keys for diagnosis. Tender sites included muscular or tendinous insertions on the bone, on cartilage, or at costochondral junctions. Pain is often acute, moderate, well-localized, continuous, or intermittent over a number of hours to days or weeks and aggravated by position or movement. Eighty-eight patients had several painful sites, and 210 patients had a single site most frequently in the midline or left-sided. Pain caused anxiety and cardiac concern, especially when acute. CWS coexisted with coronary disease in 19 and neoplasm in 6 patients. Outcome at 1 year was favorable even though CWS recurred in 50% of patients. CWS is common and benign, but it leads to anxiety and often reoccurs. Because the majority of chest wall pain is left-sided, the possibility of coexistence with coronary disease needs careful examination.[274]

Other names for CWS are costochondritis, atypical chest pain, and musculoskeletal chest pain syndrome. Costochondritis is a form of inflammation in the cartilage of the costochondral or costosternal joints commonly of ribs 2 through 5, attaching to the sternum and causing localized pain and tenderness. The general course is self-limiting, but symptoms often recur. Onset is insidious or related to minor overuse trauma and aggravated by deep breathing or trunk movements.[275] Costochondritis is often referred to as *Tietze's syndrome*, but these are distinct diagnoses. The main difference is that Tietze's syndrome is characterized by nonsuppurative (ie, absence of pus) edema and swelling, redness, tenderness, and warmth,[276] whereas localized swelling, erythema, or palpable edema are not present in costochondritis. A sedimentation rate or C-reactive protein test may be positive in Tietze's's syndrome but normal in costochondritis.[275] A relatively uncommon cause of lower anterior rib cage complaints is slipping rib syndrome associated with the 8th, 9th, or 10th ribs anteriorly at the costal cartilages. Damage to the costal cartilage may allow the cartilage tips to become hypermobile and slip under the superior adjacent rib, causing irritation of the intercostal tissues in the area. For additional reading, Udermann et al[277] presented a case report on the management of slipping rib syndrome in a collegiate swimmer.

Rib Cage Hypomobility and Posterior Symptoms

Examination findings suggestive of rib cage mobility deficits with or without thoracic spinal and/or anterior chest wall symptoms but usually without referral to the UE include limited AROM, limited PROM, no centralization or peripheralization with repeated movements, hypomobility, and/or pain provocation with PPIVM and/or PAIVM of the thoracic spinal segments and the ribs (ie, costotransverse/costovertebral or intercostal articulations). Symptoms may increase with cough, sneeze, deep breathing, and/or trunk movements. Onset is similar to other mechanical thoracic disorders and related to trauma, prolonged postures, awkward movements, or overhead work. Postural deviations such as forward head posture and excessive or reduced kyphosis may be present along with associated muscle imbalances in the region. Muscle imbalances include weakness of the middle and lower trapezius or deep neck flexors and short pectoral muscles, latissimus dorsi, upper trapezius, scalenes, or levator scapulae. Intercostal muscles or iliocostalis insertion sites of the involved ribs may be tender to palpation. Painful hypermobility may be present after thoracotomy or surgical procedures to the sternum. Altered respiratory patterns may be present. Mobility deficits associated with rib dysfunction may exist unilaterally or bilaterally in some or all cardinal plane motions or functional combinations of cardinal plane motions.

Evidence for Mobilization and Manipulation in Patients With Rib Hypomobility

The evidence supporting manual therapy for patients with rib dysfunction exists only at the level of case report. Kelley and Whitney[278] described the PT management of a 16-year-old athlete with nontraumatic onset of diffuse, right mid-back and lower rib pain of 4 weeks duration. Symptoms were produced with running and kicking, deep inhalation, and thoracic lateral flexion, and central PAIVM at T5 to T8 were hypomobile and painful. ES musculature on the right at T5 to T8 and intercostal spaces 6 to 8 were painful. A supine AP nonthrust manipulation at T5 to T6 (see Figure 5-38) was chosen to address the pain and thoracic hypomobility. While placing the patient in the nonthrust position, a cavitation was heard. Upon reassessment, the patient had full pain-free inhalation, improved chest expansion, symmetrical lateral flexion motion, and pain reduced by 2 points. Postural advice and a home exercise program were prescribed but not described by the authors. Telephonic follow-up at 1 month revealed full recovery and return to sports.[278]

Brismée et al[279] described the PT management of a 42-year-old right-handed female with chronic 10-year history of unilateral neck pain right greater than left, upper trapezius pain, and upper limb paresthesia. Upper trapezius pain and paresthesia began 4 years ago after a left-sided impact motor vehicle collision. The main physical examination findings were as follows:

- +CRLF test in left rotation
- Hypomobile elevated first rib on right with reduced inferior glide

- A positive elevated arm stress test on right at 45 seconds that reproduced paresthesia
- Right lateral flexion PPIVM at C4 to C5 that was hypomobile and painful in the neck only
- A positive ulnar nerve tension test on the right for fourth and fifth finger paresthesia and right upper trapezius pulling

PT consisted of postural education for sleep and computer work, mobilization to improve right C4 to C5 lateral flexion, first rib mobilization, neurodynamic mobilization, thoracic spine mobilization and manipulation, and a home exercise program. The first rib mobilization occurred in supine (see Figure 5-23) sustained for 40 seconds each in an inferior, lateral, and ventral direction followed by an inferior, medial, and ventral direction, and an HVLA thrust manipulation. Manual therapy was followed by a right scalene stretching exercise combined with an inferior right first rib mobilization with the head positioned in left lateral flexion and slight right rotation to stabilize the cervical spine held for 40 seconds for 5 repetitions performed 2 times per day.[279] A detailed plan of care and clinical reasoning are discussed in the case report. After 8 weeks and 6 PT sessions, the patient was symptom free.[279]

TOS was part of the differential diagnosis for this patient.[279] However, since TOS is often a diagnosis of exclusion and little agreement exists for diagnosis or conservative management, the topic is not discussed in this reference. Two excellent papers are recommended for review of the classification, varied clinical presentations, and a conservative treatment approach for TOS.[280,281] The main focus of impairment-based management for TOS rehabilitation includes the shoulder girdle through restoration of scapular control, restoration of humeral head control, isolated strengthening of weak shoulder muscles, taping, and other manual therapy strategies to aid in decompressing the thoracic outlet.[280,281] Based on examination findings, cervical, thoracic, and first rib mobilization techniques; soft tissue mobilization; and scalene and pectoral muscle lengthening may have a role in treating the various subgroups of TOS.[282]

The clinical presentation of costochondritis was discussed earlier. When other serious causes of anterior chest wall pain have been ruled out, conservative management is initiated. Aspegren et al[283] described the management of a female athlete with pain of 8 months' duration of the right fifth costicartilage, right chondrosternal joints of ribs 2 to 5, and stiffness of the mid-thoracic region. Motion assessment revealed hypomobility from the fifth through ninth costovertebral, costotransverse joints, and intervertebral segments. Treatment consisted of thoracic manipulation in prone using a prone PA HVLA, Graston Technique[284] to the chondrosternal joints, and KinesioTaping (Kinesio USA)[285] over the chondrosternal joints and fifth costocartilage. The patient was 70% improved after 4 sessions over 2 weeks but continued with an additional 12 sessions. Extended treatment included 2 months of rest from volleyball and weight-lifting. At 6-month follow-up after discharge, no further care was needed.[283]

Graston Technique[284] is a form of soft tissue mobilization that uses hand-held stainless steel instruments and allows clinicians to treat scar tissue and fascial restriction. The instruments are purported to be like tuning forks that resonate in the clinician's hand and allow isolation of adhesions and greater precision in treatment. The metal instruments seemingly do not compress the tissues in the same manner as the pads of the fingers, so deeper adhesions can be located and treated. Current research is available at their Web site.[284] No research is available related to thoracic pain, but a randomized control trial is in progress.[286]

Rabey[287] described the following 2 cases:

1. The management of a 29-year-old female with a 10-week history of insidious onset of central and right chest pain without posterior thoracic pain. Symptoms were worse with lifting, pushing, and deep breathing. MRI scan was normal.
2. A 33-year-old female with insidious onset of left chest pain and pain at the left medial border of the scapula for 18 months. Aggravating factors were sitting at the computer for 1 hour or running for 20 minutes. X-rays were normal.

Both patients were referred with a diagnosis of costochondritis. Patient #1 had painful right lateral flexion and limited thoracic rotation. T1 to T2 and T2 to T3 PPIVM and rib 3 motion palpation were hypomobile. Resisted right external rotation and flexion were weak and painful. Right serratus anterior was weak. Manual treatment initially consisted of unilateral PA mobilization to the T3 articular pillar (see Figure 5-29) and the third rib angle (see Figure 5-30). Due to improvement, the same treatment was repeated at the second and third session. At the third session, an HVLA to T2 to T3 was performed in supine followed by a SNAG over the third rib angle while the patient was turning into right rotation. This treatment was repeated 1 week later. Eventually, scapular motor control exercises were prescribed and the patient was discharged symptom free. Patient #2 had similar examination findings on the left at the T4 to T5 motion segment and ribs 4 and 5. The patient responded to mobilization and HVLA manipulation to the hypomobile regions and motor control exercise for scapular control. In both of these patients, no intervention was applied to the costochondral joints; only to the posterior thoracic articulations. The authors speculate a neuropathic contribution to the anterior chest wall pain mediated by the neurophysiological effects of the manual intervention.[287] Gijsbers and Knaap[288] present a similar case report on a female patient with Tietze's's syndrome. Management included HVLA chiropractic manipulation of the posterior thoracic joints, activator technique to the anterior chest wall, and self-care cryotherapy for 6 sessions over 3 weeks.[288]

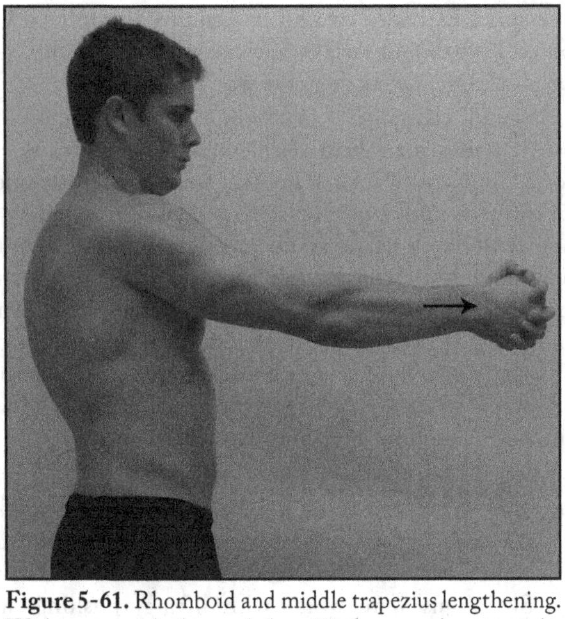

Figure 5-61. Rhomboid and middle trapezius lengthening. With outstretched arm below 90 degrees elevation, the patient reaches forward until a stretch is felt between the shoulder blades.

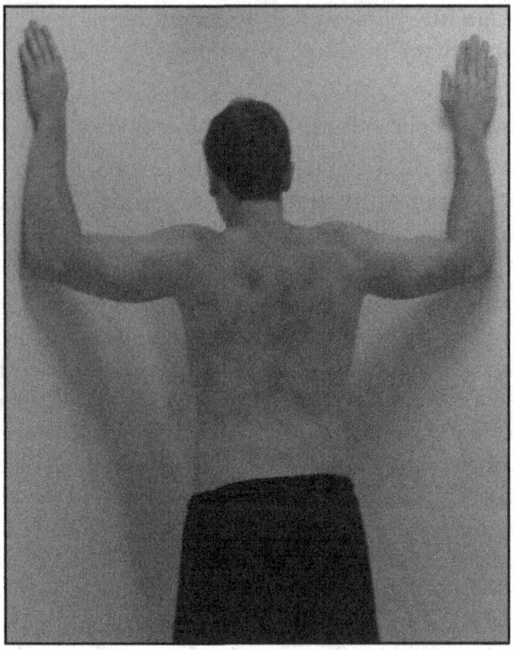

Figure 5-62. Pectoralis major corner stretch.

Fruth[289] described the differential diagnosis and clinical decision-making process for a patient with a 4-month history of right posterior upper thoracic pain that occasionally spread to the anterior chest, a burning sensation between the scapula and the spine, and a knotted feeling under the scapula. Aggravating factors were trunk or UE movements, coughing, sneezing, and changing positions in bed. The examination revealed pain and limited AROM of the trunk, shoulder, and cervical spine. PA PAIVM were hypomobile and painful T2 to T6 and for right ribs 3 to 6. AP accessory motion test of the chondrosternal joints were hypomobile and painful at right ribs 3 to 6. Strength testing of the shoulder girdle was painful and not graded. Palpation revealed periscapular muscle tenderness and active trigger points in right rhomboids, middle trapezius, and medial scapular border. Since passive accessory rib motion testing was not tolerated well, intervention began with ischemic compression[290] to the active trigger points held up to 1 minute or until minimal to no pain with further pressure, followed by middle trapezius and rhomboid stretching. Due to reduced pain, grade II PA mobilization to ribs 3 to 6 cervicothoracic and CV joints and AP mobilization to ribs 3 to 6 chondrosternal joints (see Figure 5-22) were performed in prone and supine, respectively. Home exercise included rhomboid and middle trapezius stretching (Figure 5-61) and prone on elbows positioning to improve thoracic extension (see Figure 5-24).[289] At the second session, the intervention was repeated, adding a superior glide to the rib mobilization and pectoralis major muscle corner stretch (Figure 5-62). Additional sessions included continued ischemic compression; rib mobilization; scapular retraction exercises; and middle trapezius, lower trapezius, and serratus anterior strengthening. The patient returned to full function after 7 visits over 4 weeks.[289]

Second rib syndrome as a single entity is a rarely reported cause of shoulder pain, commonly diagnosed as shoulder impingement and/or rotator cuff partial tear. Grieve[291] described this syndrome by reports of a useless or heavy limb, the inability to grip efficiently with or without shoulder pain, and referred pain to the head from upper cervical dysfunction, but the glenohumeral and clavicular joints appear unaffected. Boyle[292] presented 2 cases of patients thought to have second rib syndrome but presenting with a primary complaint of shoulder pain and no pain in the area of the second rib. The first case involved a 21-year-old male football player presenting immediately 1 day after a sporting collision with an unclear mechanism of injury. Shoulder impingement tests were positive and rotator cuff muscle tests were weak and painful. Passive accessory motion testing at the angle of rib 2 in a PA direction was hypomobile and painful. Two treatment sessions of grade III prone PA rib mobilization (see Figure 5-41C) of 3 repetitions of 60 seconds resulted in complete resolution of symptoms. The second patient had anterior, posterior, and central shoulder pain with referral to the upper arm as a result of pulling weeds in the garden. Symptoms were present for 5 months despite 2 cortisone injections. Shoulder AROM was limited and painful and impingements tests were positive. Passive mobility restrictions were noted at C6 and C7 and ribs 2 and 3. Seventy percent improvement was noted after 2 sessions of second rib mobilization as described previously and soft tissue mobilization to the posterior scalene and levator scapulae muscles. Additional interventions included third rib mobilization, postural re-education, scapula repositioning, AP grade III mobilization of C7, and lower trapezius strengthening for a total of 7 sessions and complete resolution of signs and symptoms. The author recommended palpation of the angle of the second rib in all patients presenting with shoulder pain.[292]

Proposed Stabilization Classification for Thoracic Spinal Pain With Movement Coordination Impairments

Thoracic Clinical Instability

Stabilization exercises are most commonly prescribed for persons with TSP who demonstrate deficits in trunk muscle performance thought to be associated with excessive thorax mobility or instability. In this instance, improvements in trunk muscle function that lead to reduced pain and disability are credited to improved motor control of spinal segments during movement. A gold standard for identifying patients with thoracic instability or movement coordination impairments has not been established, thereby making such a diagnosis difficult and poorly defined. A patient's need for stabilization exercises is necessarily based on clinical examination findings with or without radiographic images.

Olson[13] reported that thoracic clinical instability may be associated with systemic hypermobility, severe postural abnormalities such as scoliosis, thoracotomy, or thoracic laminectomy and after trauma such as motor vehicle accidents. Examination findings include achiness with sustained upright postures, easing with recumbent positions, aberrant movements with AROM, and hypermobility with PPIVM or PAIVM testing. Patients may report difficulty with static or dynamic tasks involving the UE or neck such as lifting, pushing, or pulling. Strength, endurance, and motor control deficits may be noted for the superficial or deep systems. Failed load transfer during AROM rotation, SAL test, or PAL test may also suggest a motor control deficit or clinical instability. Intervention includes postural training, corrective stabilization exercise, mobilization and manipulation for segmental restrictions, and activity or ergonomic modification.[13]

Evidence for a Proposed Stabilization Classification for Thoracic Spinal Pain With Movement Coordination Impairments

Lee and Lee[153] proposed an integrated model that provides the basis for assessment and treatment of TSP with the goal of regaining optimum function of the thorax. These authors define optimum function of the thorax as a balance of stability and mobility altered according to the demands (ie, load, predictability, and threat value) of the task at hand while maintaining normal intra-abdominal pressure and respiratory function. Nonoptimal function results in failure of load transfer between the upper and lower body, requiring assessment of form closure, force closure, motor control strategies, and emotional contributors to determine potential causes of load failure.[153]

As discussed in the previous section, some patients have a primary problem of thoracic hypomobility or stiffness and require manual techniques of mobilization, muscle energy or manipulation, and therapeutic exercise to augment clinical gains and restore functional movement patterns. Other patients may have a primary impairment of thoracic segmental control during movement and require stabilization exercises to address motor control deficits using the same concepts for retraining the superficial and deep muscular systems as discussed for the lumbar spine. However, most patients have more than one problem in more than one region, requiring multimodal interventions for mobility and stability. Interventions are based on the patient's examination findings, current evidence, clinical reasoning, and within and between session reassessment. In general, impairments of hypomobility are addressed prior to restoring muscle function and motor control. If not addressed, the hypomobility has the potential to result in the development of poor motor control patterns.

Research related to the global and superficial muscle stabilizing systems of the thorax was discussed in the physical examination section on muscle performance. Very little is known about the requirements for neuromuscular control of the thorax to meet daily functional demands of mobility and stability. In comparison to the lumbar spine musculature, few studies have investigated the control of the deep system (ie, multifidus, intercostals, levator costarum, diaphragm, transverse abdominis, pelvic floor) and superficial thoracic musculature (ie, ES, rectus abdominis, internal and external oblique, trapezius, rhomboids, levator scapulae, serratus anterior, latissimus dorsi).

Only one study examined the effects of stabilization exercise. El-Ansary et al[293] used a randomized crossover study to examine the effects of 6 weeks of trunk stabilization exercises (Figure 5-63) on 9 subjects with a chronic 4-year history of sternal instability due to cardiac surgery. Outcomes were sternal separation measured by ultrasound, pain during 9 daily tasks, and the quality performance of 2 tasks of moving from supine lying to sitting and reaching in sitting. A daily, 15-minute stabilization program focused on contraction of the transverse abdominis using ultrasound imaging in a progressive manner and variety of positions such as supine, side-lying, sitting, and sitting with unilateral and bilateral arm elevation with and without resistance as described by Lee.[10] Each subject performed exercises in supine supported on an inverted "U" noodle that provided sternal stability so that exercises could be performed with less pain. Overall, sternal separation decreased during trunk stabilization by 6.2 mm (95% CI: 3.5 to 8.9). Pain with everyday tasks decreased 14 mm (95% CI: 5 to 23), but overall task performance during the

Figure 5-63. Six-week trunk stabilization program for sternal instability.[293] Exercises are performed twice a day. Exercises for weeks 1 to 3 activate abdominal muscles to assist in stabilizing the chest wall. The exercises are gentle, require control, and should not be painful. Only the exercises for each week should be performed. The patient holds each exercise for 10 seconds, repeating 10 times while making sure to not hold his or her breath. *(continued)*

Week	Exercises	Image
1	**Lying on your back, a pillow under your knees.** **a. Abdominal exercise.** Use your fingers to feel your abdominal muscles at waist level. At the end of breathing out, gently and slowly draw your abdomen away from your fingers. Imagine you are drawing your two pelvic bones together.	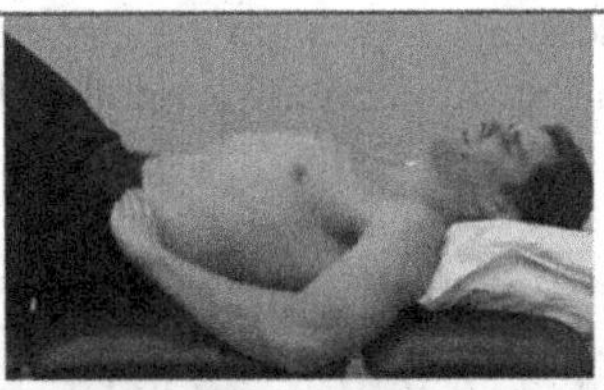
	b. Breathing exercise. Place your hands on the outer part of your lower ribs. Imagine your ribs are like an umbrella. When you breathe in, the bottom of the umbrella goes out. Relax and let your chest and sternum go heavy to the floor as you breathe out.	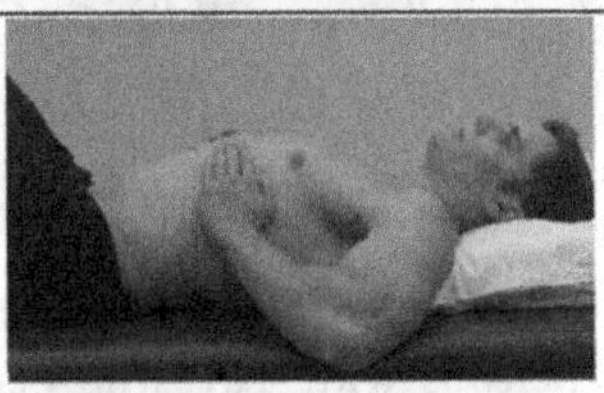
2	**Lying on your side, a pillow between your legs and a rolled towel under your waist.** **a. Repeat exercise 1a (abdominal)**	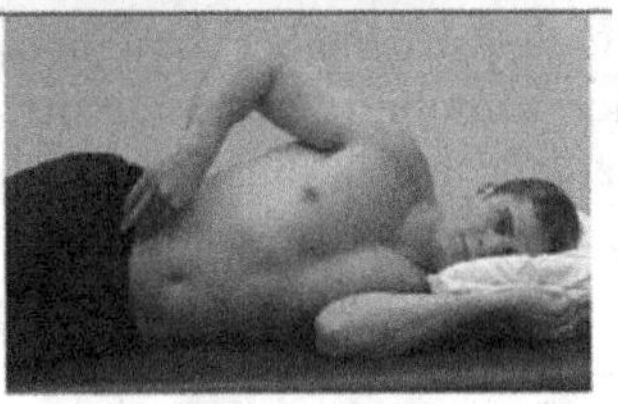
	b. Repeat exercise 1b (breathing)	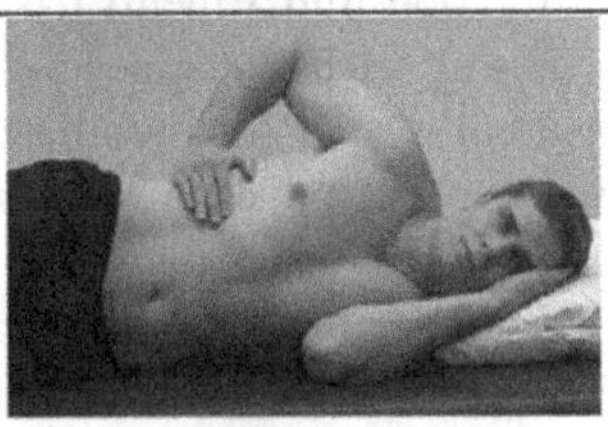
3	**Sit on a chair with feet on the floor and knees below the level of your hips to ensure that you maintain a neutral spine curve in your low back.** **a. Neutral Spine.** Imagine that a string attached to your mid-back is gently pulled up to make you taller and the sternum is lifted up. Maintain for 3 minutes and breathe normally.	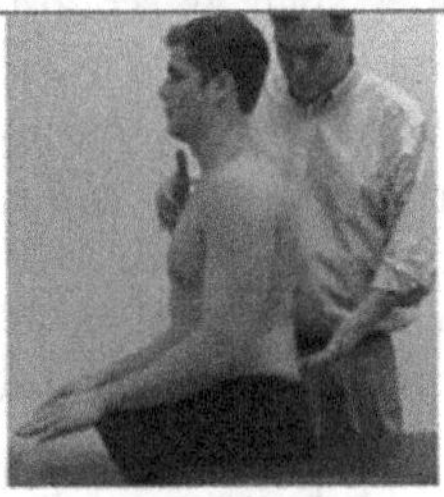
	b. Breathing exercise. While sitting in a neutral spine position, repeat exercise 1b (breathing).	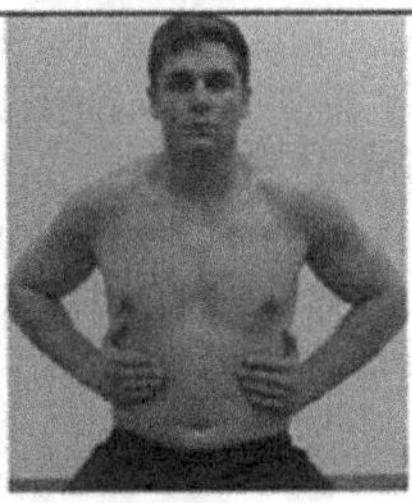
	c. Repeat exercise 1a (abdominal) in sitting.	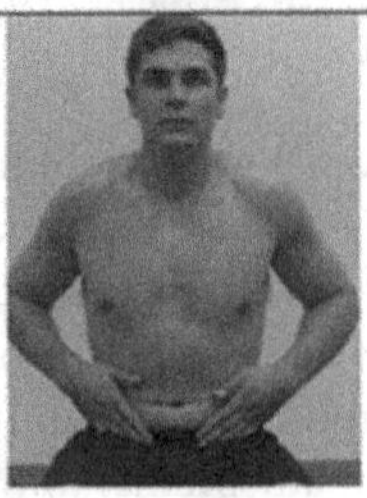

4	**Sit on a chair of medium height, feet on the floor and neutral spine.** **a. Trunk-arm dissociation exercise (both arms – flexion/extension control and one arm – rotational control). At the end of breathing out,** slowly and gently contract your abdominal muscles and raise both arms up overhead.	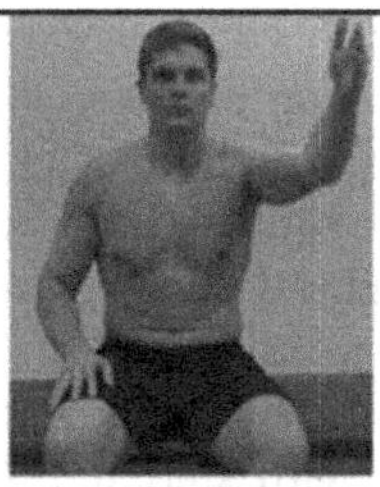
	b. Trunk-leg dissociation exercise: At the end of breathing out, gently lift one knee up from the floor (approx. 2 cm) while slowly and gently contracting your abdominal muscles.	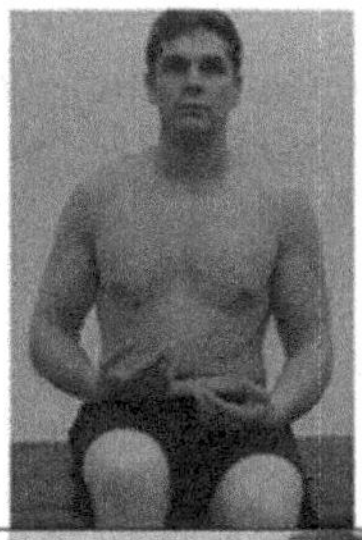
5	**Standing or sitting, ensure that you maintain a neutral spine curve in your low back.** **a. Trunk-arm dissociation exercise (both arms – flexion/extension control).** At the end of breathing out, slowly and gently contract your abdominal muscles and raise both arms up overhead. **Arm reaching:** At the end of breathing out, lift one arm to reach across your body for a glass that is on a table opposite your other shoulder while slowly and gently contracting your abdominal muscles.	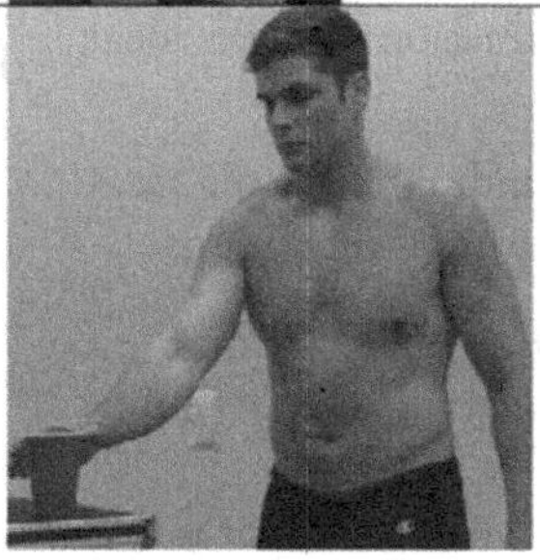
	b. Trunk-leg dissociation exercise. At the end of breathing out, gently lift one leg up from the floor (approx. 2 cm) while gently and slowly contracting your abdominal muscles.	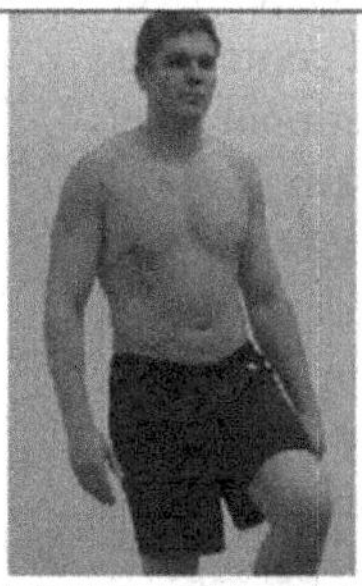
6	**While standing or sitting with an additional (optional) load.** **a. Trunk-arm dissociation exercise with load – flexion (using an elastic band or small hand weight).** After breathing out, gently and slowly contract the abdominal muscles, while lifting one arm overhead.	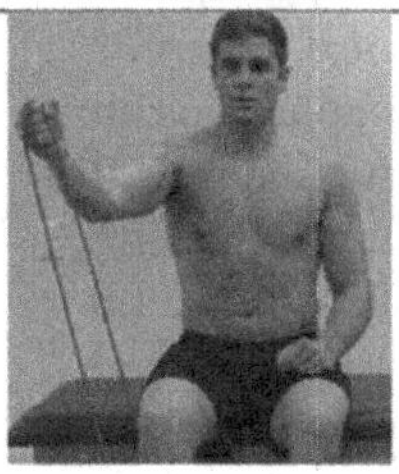
	b. Trunk-arm dissociation exercise with load – diagonal pattern (using an elastic band or small hand weight). At the end of breathing out, gently and slowly contract your abdominal muscles while pulling your arm up and across your body. Maintain a neutral spine.	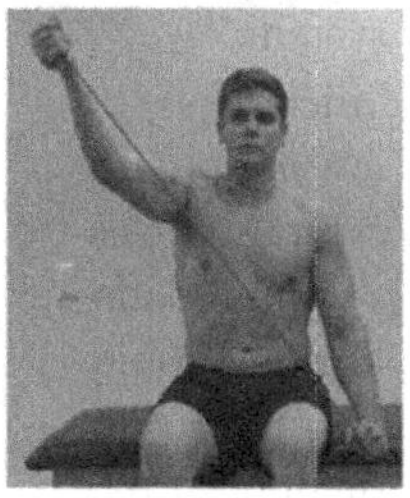

Figure 5-63 (continued). Six-week trunk stabilization program for sternal instability.[293] Exercises are performed twice a day. Exercises for weeks 1 to 3 activate abdominal muscles to assist in stabilizing the chest wall. The exercises are gentle, require control, and should not be painful. Only the exercises for each week should be performed. The patient holds each exercise for 10 seconds, repeating 10 times while making sure to not hold his or her breath.

trunk stabilization exercises did not improve. A clinically meaningful reduction in pain was noted during 3 tasks (side-lying, swinging the arms, and trunk rotation), but no reduction in pain was noted with coughing, sudden loss of footing, or reaching above shoulder height. Driving, sitting to standing, and supine to sitting trended toward a decrease in pain. The authors concluded that trunk stabilization should be included in subjects with sternal instability.[293]

The program for stabilization and motor control of the thorax used by El-Ansary et al[293] is based on a model[10,153] using stabilization concepts similar to the lumbopelvic region. The program[10] involves several steps, as indicated by patient exam:

- Reduction of trunk rigidity or an overactive global system
- Isolation of independent contraction of the local system
- Development of precision and endurance of the local system through 10 second holds of 10 repetitions
- Coordination of the local and global systems

Each step is discussed briefly with detailed information available as presented by Lee.[10]

Reduction of Trunk Rigidity or an Overactive Global System[10]: based on personal experience, Lee[10] believes the first goal of stabilization is isolated contraction of the deep, segmental muscles at the dysfunctional levels in the thorax. However, if the superficial system is dominant or overactive, this overactivity must be addressed first because it inhibits the ability to recruit the local system. The local stabilizers of the lumbopelvic region should be assessed and treated as needed in conjunction with or prior to retraining the thoracic spine. Neutral spine postures and diaphragmatic breathing are used to reduce superficial muscle activity prior to activating the local system.[10] Reduced or absent lateral or posterolateral costal expansion during breathing may result in either excessive abdominal excursion or excessive upper chest breathing. Excessive bracing with the superficial abdominals and thoracic ES limits lower rib cage expansion, and retraining of lateral costal expansion helps to maintain mobility gained from manual intervention, aids in facilitating the deep system, and assists in reducing the overactive global system.[10]

To retrain lateral costal expansion, the clinician places his or her hands on the lateral aspect of the lower rib cage for feedback and to monitor inspiration and expiration (see Figure 5-6). At the end of expiration, gentle compression is applied to focus the patient on where expansion should occur while allowing expansion to occur during inspiration and monitoring for excessive upper chest or abdominal breathing. The patient should practice focused breathing 2 to 3 times per day for several minutes using his or her own hands on the lower rib cage for relaxed and deeper breathing. The patient should monitor breathing patterns throughout the day during sitting, standing, or walking.[10]

The process of assessing sitting posture and the analysis of lumbopelvic upright, thoracic upright, and slump sitting postures on muscle activation patterns is detailed in Chapter 3. With the patient's feet supported and hips at 80 degrees of flexion, the clinician observes posture and corrects as needed to assess the effect on symptoms and determine the patient's ability to find a neutral spine. Variation exists regarding which region of the spine should be corrected first. The clinician uses manual and/or verbal cues to assist the patient in finding a neutral spine posture. Maintaining the lumbar spine in neutral, the patient monitors the sternum and pubic symphysis alignment while the clinician assists manually or verbally. Gentle anterior and superior manual cues are used to correct or maintain lumbar neutral. For areas of increased thoracic kyphosis, the clinician might ask the patient to "imagine that your sternum is being gently lifted" or "imagine that the distance from your sternum to belly button is decreasing as you let your chest go heavy" for areas of decreased thoracic kyphosis.[10] The clinician uses the sternum for inferior and posture manual cueing to gently increase thoracic kyphosis and the posterior thorax for superior and slightly anterior cueing to decrease areas of thoracic kyphosis.[10] Additional cueing options are discussed elsewhere.[10] Achieving a neutral spine posture does not involve excessive contraction of the ES. Weight is evenly distributed or centered over the ischial tuberosities and the manubrium aligns with the pubic bone vertically. Upper chest breathing results in thoracolumbar extension and is corrected through establishing a lateral costal expansion respiratory pattern. Additional corrections for rotational and side-bending thoracic asymmetry are discussed elsewhere.[10] Maintenance of a neutral spine posture and the ability to move in and out of the posture are also conducted in standing, in UE weightbearing against a wall, or in quadruped.[10] When a neutral spine posture is achieved in any of these positions with a normal respiratory pattern, voluntary contraction of the thoracic and lumbopelvic deep stabilizers is begun.[10]

Isolation of an Independent Contraction of the Local System[10]: according to Lee,[10] a neutral spine is a key position to facilitating the deep system and usually started in prone or sitting and progressed as follows. In prone, a towel vertically oriented along the sternum assists with promoting thoracic kyphosis, if needed. The clinician palpates bilaterally adjacent to the SP at the appropriate level to provide tactile feedback in conjunction with verbal cues. Slow, deepening pressure with the fingers in a slightly superior direction reinforces the idea of the spine being suspended by a tent or guy wires. All verbal cues provide the image of supporting wires or connecting strings equal on each side that create a feeling of the spine being suspended.[10] Various cues are possible. For example, while

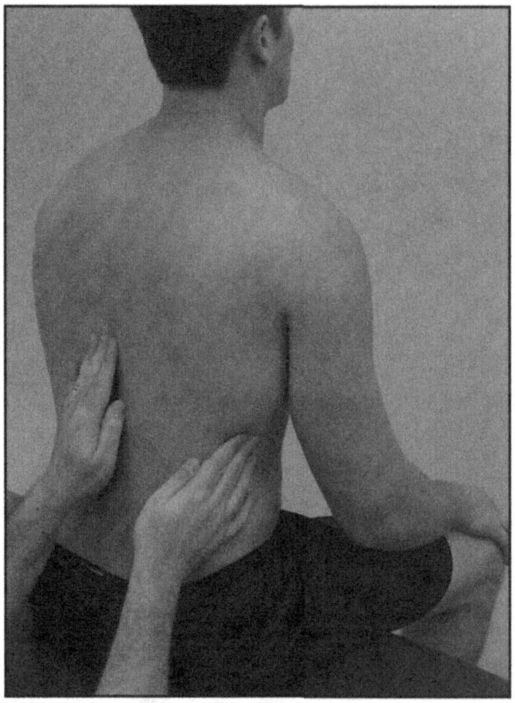

Figure 5-64. Facilitation of the deep thoracic stabilizers.[10] The clinician palpates adjacent to the SP and uses the midaxillary line for a manual or verbal cue. The clinician asks the patient to breathe in, breathe out, and "imagine drawing the ribs in toward the center of your spine, holding the contraction for 10 seconds with normal breathing, neutral spine, and without recruitment of the superficial muscles."

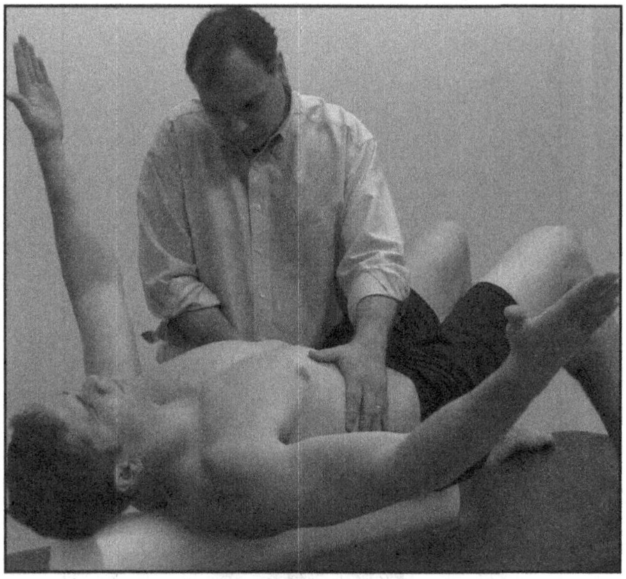

Figure 5-65. Supine trunk-arm dissociation on an unstable surface.[10] The patient is asked to maintain a neutral spine through cocontraction by adding limb loading in a slow, controlled manner starting in supine on a flat surface and progressing to a foam roll. Arms are flexed to 90 degrees, bilaterally or unilaterally, to challenge flexion/extension control or rotation control of the thorax, respectively. All planes of motions and combined movement patterns are also used. Weights of 1 to 5 lb can be added to increase the challenge.

palpating adjacent to the SP and using the midaxillary line for manual or verbal cues, ask the patient to breathe in, breathe out, and "imagine drawing the ribs in toward the center of your spine, holding the contraction for 10 seconds with a normal breathing pattern, a neutral spine, and without recruitment of the superficial muscles" (Figure 5-64).[10] An optimal activation response is a deep, gradual contraction or increase in tension of the muscle. A rapid recruitment or sense that your fingers are being pushed off of the back suggests recruitment of the superficial system, ES, or scapular muscles.[10]

Development of Precision and Endurance of the Local System[10]: similar to training strategies for lumbopelvic stabilization, a goal of 10-second holds and 10 repetitions is set for each patient. Exercises are done frequently throughout the day for short sessions based on the patient's ability for control with optimal strategies. Voluntary deep muscle activation is encouraged during daily activities. Positions are varied from supported in prone or sitting to standing or UE weightbearing against a wall. Excessive superficial activation, breath holding, and loss of neutral postures are signs of nonoptimal strategies suggesting fatigue or that the position or task is too demanding.[10]

Coordination of the Local and Global Systems[10]: when the goals for isolated contraction are met, the next step is to maintain cocontraction of the deep system in the thoracic and lumbopelvic regions while maintaining position and controlling movements that require low load superficial muscle activation.[10] This section generally follows guidelines presented in Chapter 4 for the lumbopelvic region. For upper and middle thoracic regions, arm movements are integrated. For middle and lower thoracic regions, leg movements are incorporated.

For trunk-arm dissociation, the patient is asked to maintain a neutral spine through cocontraction by adding limb loading in a slow, controlled manner, starting in supine on a flat surface and progressing to an unsupported surface such as a foam roll (Figure 5-65). Arms are flexed to 90 degrees, bilaterally or unilaterally, to challenge flexion and extension control or rotational control of the thorax, respectively. Abduction, extension, or diagonal patterns are also used. Weights of 1 to 5 lb can be added to increase the challenge. The challenge is further progressed in sitting or sitting on an unstable surface with or without elastic resistance. Pulling up or down requires flexion or extension control of the thorax, respectively, while unilateral or diagonal patterns require rotational control (Figure 5-66). Similar concepts are applied to the standing position, lunge stance, standing on one leg, in

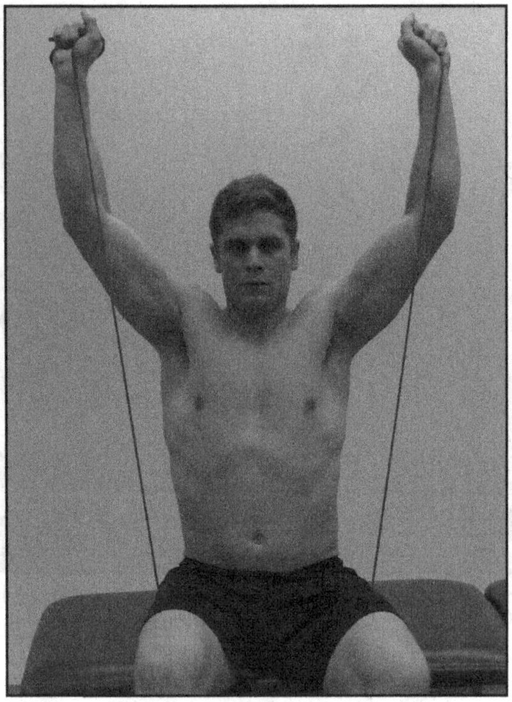

Figure 5-66. Sitting trunk–arm dissociation on a stable surface.[10] Sitting on a stable or unstable surface with or without elastic resistance, the patient is asked to pull up or down against elastic resistance, which challenges flexion or extension control of the thorax, respectively. Unilateral or diagonal patterns challenge rotational control.

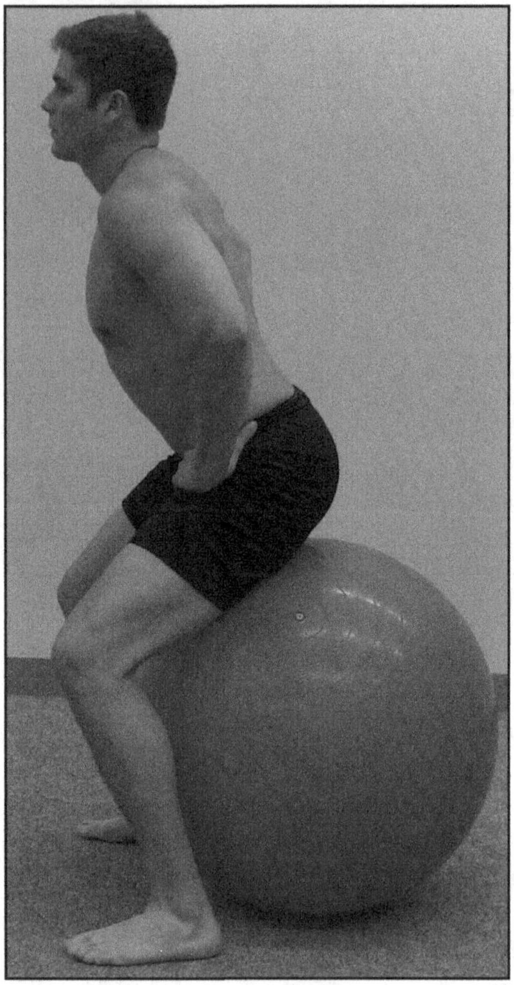

Figure 5-67. Progression in sitting and standing.[10] The patient performs the exercises by moving the trunk on the pelvis or moving the legs under the trunk. In neutral spine with sufficient hip flexion to allow the pelvis to flex over the femoral heads, the patient brings the trunk forward by hinging at the hips and maintaining a neutral spine posture and progresses from sit to stand.

UE weightbearing positions, leaning against a wall, in quadruped over a ball, or in quadruped raising one arm as progressions for rotational control challenges. For all new positions and movements, begin with quality contraction of the deep system, ensure breathing, and focus on low load and control of movements. Movement control exercises should also be related to the patient's functional needs such as raising one arm, pushing, pulling, or lifting.[10]

For trunk-leg dissociation, the same procedure is used. The patient maintains a neutral spine through cocontraction and adds limb loading in a slow, controlled manner starting in supine on a flat surface as described for the lumbopelvic stabilization in Chapter 4. For thoracic stabilization, the focus is on segmental control within the thorax and maintaining a neutral spine between the lumbopelvic and thoracic regions by adding leg movement.[10] Sitting and standing progressions are presented as described by Lee.[10] In sitting, the exercises are performed by moving the trunk on the pelvis or moving the legs under the trunk. Beginning in neutral spine with sufficient hip flexion to allow the pelvis to flex over the femoral heads, the patient brings the trunk forward by hinging at the hips and maintaining a neutral spine posture (Figure 5-67) with progression to sit to stand. Alternately, unilateral hip flexion or knee extension is performed by the patient while maintaining neutral posture and optimal breathing and without excessive superficial muscle activity. Both of these exercises can be performed on an unstable surface such as a ball or wobble board. Supported standing in neutral involves a ball placed to support the lumbar lordosis against a wall with equal weight distribution, hips in neutral, knees under hips, and middle of the patella in line with the second toe of each foot (Figure 5-68). From this position, the patient is asked to squat as if sitting in a chair and maintain a neutral spine. Progressions include squat on an unstable surface, unilateral squat, or a lunge position with the rear leg moving into hip flexion.[10]

The final step is functional movement retraining, control of movement in and out of neutral spine, or intrathoracic movement. Intrathoracic movement is segmental control or the ability to flex, extend, laterally bend, and rotate without loss of segmental or regional control.[154] An example of intrathoracic or segmental movement is flexion or rotation or combined flexion and rotation performed in sitting. From neutral spine, the patient is asked to move segmentally starting with cervical flexion through thoracic flexion and return in a segmental fashion starting at the thoracic region. Functional movement training is directed by the patient's work or recreational needs and has requirements of movement and control through several regions and joints. These higher level movements must be broken down and practiced in parts followed by practicing whole movements. All exercises begin with quality contraction of the deep system, maintenance of normal breathing, and focus on segmental control.[154] Not all patients go through all steps as described or start at the first step. Examination findings guide the exercise prescription. The patient's response and reassessment guides the exercise progression.

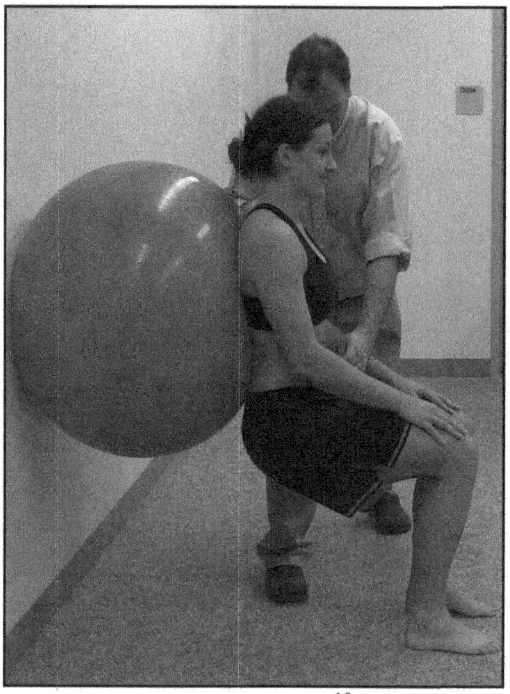

Figure 5-68. Supported standing.[10] A ball against the wall supports the lumbar lordosis with equal weight distribution, hips in neutral, knees under hips, and middle of the patella in line with the second toe of each foot. The patient performs a squat as if sitting in a chair and maintains a neutral spine with progressions to squat on an unstable surface, unilateral squat, or lunge positions.

Neurodynamics and the Thoracic Spine

Altered Neurodynamics and Intervention

In the absence of randomized controlled trials supporting the use of neurodynamic mobilization Nee and Butler[294] proposed that conservative management incorporating neurobiology education, intervention for nonneural tissue impairments, and neurodynamic techniques can be effective in addressing musculoskeletal presentations of altered neurodynamics. Patient education involves a discussion of the role of the nervous system in movement and pain related to mechanical loading. Interventions such as joint or soft tissue mobilization or training motor control to regain optimal function may reduce mechanical forces on sensitive neural tissues. Treatment of nonneural impairments should be followed by reassessment of subjective complaints and positive neurodynamic tests. Absence of improvement related to nonneural techniques suggests a need for neurodynamic mobilization procedures. As discussed by Nee and Butler,[294] a conservative management approach incorporating neurodynamic mobilization requires sound clinical reasoning using the concept of assess, treat, and reassess within and between sessions. The goals of neurodynamic mobilization are to reduce neural tissue mechanosensitivity and restore its movement capabilities.[294]

The SST or long sit slump test were discussed earlier in this chapter as an examination procedure. The SST is considered a positive test when the patient's symptoms are reproduced, asymmetry is noted when compared to the uninvolved side, and a positive sensitizing maneuver is present (ie, movement at site distant to the area of complaint alters the patient's symptoms). Butler[174] recommended assessing the response to the slump test and SST in patients presenting with clinical symptoms of TOS, T4 syndrome, and thoracic nerve root syndrome. When the test is positive, the SST is one component of a multimodal approach. Research is scarce related to the use of SST for examination or intervention.

In addition to mobilization or manipulation of the relevant thoracic segment for a nonirritable thoracic nerve root syndrome, Butler[174] suggested placing the patient in a long sit slump position, overpress the thoracic component, and laterally flex and rotate away from the painful side using rotation or lateral flexion as the treatment followed by reassessment. When indicated, a similar position is suggested using the slump test or SST while performing a PA pressure on the thoracic segment or over the rib at the costotransverse joint, theoretically to influence the SNS (Figure 5-69).[174]

Cleland and McRae[176] described the PT management of a patient presenting with CRPS I 8 weeks after open reduction internal fixation for a right tibia and fibula fracture. The patient's history and physical examination satisfied the criteria for CRPS I with a positive slump test on the right. The patient was treated for 10 sessions over

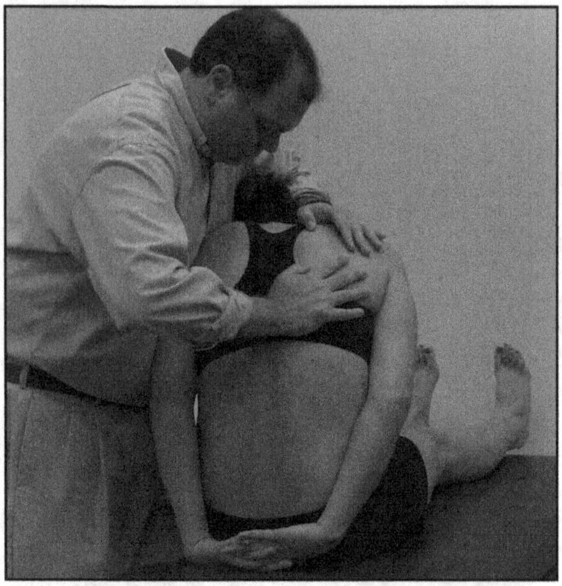

Figure 5-69. Costotransverse mobilization in sympathetic slump position. A grade IV PA mobilization to the right costotransverse joints is performed in the long sit position with thoracic rotation and lateral flexion to the left or away from the painful side.

3 months with desensitization, progressive weightbearing, thoracolumbar mobilization, and neurodynamic mobilization in the long sit slump position. The patient presented in a wheelchair unable to bear weight on the right lower extremity with 10/10 burning pain and severe allodynia (ie, unable to wear a sock or shoe). Desensitization, edema control, activity modification and AROM exercise produced no change after 2 sessions. At the third session, central PA grade III and IV joint mobilizations were added due to hypomobility with no change. At the fourth visit 4 weeks later, grade IV PA mobilization for 30 seconds each to right ribs 10 to 12 at the costotransverse joints was performed in the long sit position with thoracic rotation and lateral flexion to the left (ie, away from the painful side to tension the sympathetic trunk; see Figure 5-69). Immediately after treatment, pain was reduced to 7 to 8 out of 10 and weightbearing in the seated position was tolerated. Costotransverse mobilization in the long sit position was continued on subsequent visits with continued improvement in pain and function. By the 10th session, the patient was using a standard cane for long distances only with pain at 2 to 3 out of 10. Since no improvement in pain or function were noted until treatment in the long sit slump position, the authors hypothesized that long sit slump neurodynamic mobilization was an integral component leading to a successful outcome and recommended that a thorough evaluation be performed to determine an accurate differential diagnosis, list of impairments, and effective management strategies.[176]

Miscellaneous Disorders of the Thorax

Complex Regional Pain Syndrome[295]

CRPS is a chronic pain disorder thought to be associated with altered peripheral or central nervous system function. CRPS I results from tissue injury rather than nerve. CRPS II is associated with a nerve injury. Both CRPS I and II present with a variety of symptoms usually affecting the feet, hands, arms, or legs and often spreading to areas not involved in the original injury. Symptoms include intense burning pain; allodynia; increased skin sensitivity, sweating, and swelling; altered skin color; temperature changes; and changes in nail and hair growth patterns resulting in decreased ability to use the affected extremity. With no known cure, a variety of interventions, medication, PT, sympathetic nerve block, cognitive behavioral therapy, graded exposure,[296] or sympathectomy are available to manage CRPS, which usually requires an interdisciplinary approach.[295] Three nonvalidated stages of CRPS are described as follows[295]:

1. Stage 1 lasts about 1 to 3 months with severe, burning pain, muscle spasm, joint stiffness, rapid hair growth, and changes in skin color and temperature
2. Stage 2 lasts from 3 to 6 months with increasing pain, allodynia, edema, decreased hair growth, brittle/cracked nails, soft bones, stiff joints, and muscle weakness
3. Stage 3 progresses to where skin and bone changes are not reversible.

Pain becomes continuous and may involve the entire limb or affected area with marked atrophy, limited mobility, and disability. Clinical practice guidelines for treatment of CRPS are available.[297]

Related to manual therapy intervention directed to the thoracic spine, Menck et al[298] described the PT management of a patient with UE CRPS I (stage 2) as a result of a trauma (ie, carpal and metacarpal fractures and extensor tendon repair) to the left hand. Using the framework of regional interdependence and the association of the thoracic spine and the SNS, the authors incorporated thoracic manipulation into the overall management. The authors described the PT treatment that occurred 5 months after the initial injury for 36 sessions over 12 weeks. At the start of PT, the patient did not have functional use of the left UE. During the first session, gentle active and passive wrist and finger ROM, edema management, and desensitization were initiated because the patient was unwilling to move the arm. The second session involved thoracic manipulation to T3 to T4, which resulted in a significant decrease in signs and symptoms: normalization of temperature, decreased allodynia, improved thoracic mobility, and increased shoulder flexion. The patient response to manipulation allowed the patient to use the left UE in functional rehabilitation activities. Other interventions included additional thoracic manipulation, aerobic conditioning, neurodynamics, edema management, stress loading of the arm,[299] progressive stretching, and strengthening exercises. The patient was discharged to vocational rehabilitation because of continued anxiety when using the left hand, but with return to full use of the left UE for activities such as cooking, cleaning, driving, and writing.[299] Details of all sessions and clinical reasoning are beyond the scope of this reference, but review of this article is recommended.

Ankylosing Spondylitis

Exercise is considered a key component of PT for patients with AS, a chronic inflammatory rheumatic disease. A systematic review[300] demonstrated that an individual home-based or supervised exercise program is better than no intervention for improved mobility and functional outcomes. Supervised group PT is better than home exercises. Combined inpatient spa exercise therapy and group therapy is better than group PT alone. No combination of exercises or exercise approaches is known to be definitively better than another. Regular home-based exercise therapy is recommended 5 times per week with at least 30 minutes per session.[301] Exercise, spa therapy (ie, exercise in mineral or thermal waters), manual therapy, and electrotherapeutic (ie, infrared radiation) modalities are also supported as effective interventions for AS.[302]

Ince et al[303] examined the effects of a 12-week exercise program in patients (n = 30; 18 male, 12 female) with AS compared to a control group of no exercise. Both groups received routine medical management. The exercise program consisted of 50 minutes of aerobics, stretching, and pulmonary exercises 3 times per week. After 3 months, chest expansion, chin-to-chest distance, Modified Schober Flexion Test, and occiput-to-wall distance were significantly better than the control group. Spinal motion measurements improved significantly for the exercise group with no significant change in the control group. While physical work capacity and vital capacity values improved in the exercise group, the control group values decreased. A multimodal approach is beneficial in the short-term for patients with AS.[303]

Fernández-de-las-Peñas et al[304] examined a 4-month, 15-session rehabilitation program versus conventional exercises for patients with AS (n = 45). The conventional group performed 20 motion and flexibility exercises for the cervical, thoracic, and lumbar spine; strengthening exercises; stretching of shortened muscles; and chest expansion exercises. The experimental group received treatment of the shortened muscle chains in these patients according to the Global Posture Re-education (GPR) method. GPR uses specific strengthening and flexibility exercises in which the shortened muscle chains are stretched and strengthened. The exercise details are listed in the original article.[304]

Changes in activity, mobility, and functional capacity were evaluated using scores from the Bath group. The Bath Ankylosing Spondylitis Metrology Index (BASMI) consists of tragus to wall distance, modified Schober's test , cervical rotation, lumbar side flexion, and intermalleolar distance; the Bath Ankylosing Spondylitis Disease Activity Index (BASDAI); and the Bath Ankylosing Spondylitis Functional Index (BASFI). Both groups showed an improvement in all outcome measures, mobility measures of the BASMI, and BASFI and BASDAI. In the control group, the improvement in tragus to wall distance ($P = .009$) and in lumbar side flexion ($P = .02$) were statistically significant. Although other outcomes improved, they did not reach significance. In the experimental group, improvement in all BASMI clinical measures ($P < .01$) and in the BASFI ($P = .003$) was statistically significant. Between-group comparisons show that the experimental group obtained a greater improvement than the control group in all clinical measures of the BASMI except in tragus to wall distance and in the BASFI. The authors concluded that the GPR method showed promising results in the short-term management of patients with AS.[304] The same authors[304] reported on 12-month follow-up that suggested that patients with AS who received the GPR exercise maintained a greater proportion of their clinical improvement than those patients receiving conventional exercises.[305]

To determine the effects on pulmonary function, Durmuş et al[306] compared the same exercise protocols of GPR and conventional exercise[304] over 12 weeks of daily exercise and a control group of normal activities and routine treatment for AS. Fifty-one patients completed the study. Both exercise groups demonstrated significant improvements in pulmonary function, pain, functional capacity, and disease activity, but the GPR group showed greater improvement in forced vital capacity, forced expiratory volume in 1 second, and peak expiratory flow parameters. In this study, pain scores significantly decreased in both exercise groups but not in the control group.[306]

Karapolat et al[307] compared the effects of conventional exercise, swimming, and walking on pulmonary function; aerobic capacity; quality of life; psychological symptoms; and the Bath group indices. Forty-five subjects with AS were randomized to 3 groups: conventional exercise plus swimming, conventional exercise plus walking, and conventional exercise only for 18 sessions over 6 weeks. All patients performed conventional exercise of flexibility exercises for the cervical, thoracic, or lumbar spine; stretching of major muscle groups (ie, ES, hamstrings, quadriceps, hip flexors, shoulder muscles); and respiratory exercises of pursed-lip breathing, expiratory abdominal augmentation, and synchronization of thoracic and abdominal movement for 30 minutes 6 days per week. The other conventional exercise groups performed either walking for 30 minutes or swimming performed free-style for 30 minutes per day for 6 weeks. The results showed improved pulmonary function and quality of life in all groups, but aerobic capacity increased (ie, pVO_2 and 6-meter walk test) only in the walking and swimming groups. Chest expansion was improved only in the swimming group.[307]

Widberg et al[308] evaluated the effects of self- and manual mobilization on chest expansion, vital capacity, posture, and mobility in a randomized trial (n = 32) comparing active treatment or no treatment for 8 weeks. The PT intervention included soft tissue warm-up to the back muscles using a vibrator and mobility exercises followed by active angular and passive mobility exercises in all planes for the spinal column in sitting, prone, and side-lying positions. Passive mobilization consisted of angular movement and specific, translatory movements. No additional details or images of the techniques were provided. Soft tissue techniques included contract-relax and massage. A home exercise consisted of 3 individually adjusted exercises to be performed 2 to 3 times per day. Patients were treated for 1 hour twice a week. The no treatment group continued normal exercises for 8 weeks and were then offered the same program as the treatment group. In the treatment group, chest expansion measured at the xiphoid process increased ($P < .01$) with no difference in vital capacity compared with the control group. Cervical and thoracic posture improved. Thoracolumbar spine flexion improved ($P < .01$). The BASMI total scoring improved ($P < .001$) in the treatment group compared with the control group. At 4 months' follow-up, cervical spine posture, lumbar flexion, and BASMI were still improved in the treatment group.[308]

Osteoporosis and Vertebral Compression Fractures and Exercise

Li et al[309] examined the effect of exercise therapy on quality of life in postmenopausal women with osteoporosis or osteopenia with or without fractures. This systematic review and meta-analysis included 4 randomized controlled trials[310-313] for a total 256 subjects. Compliance in these studies was greater than 80%. All exercise groups showed significant improvements in physical function, pain, physical role, and vitality ($P < .05$). Intervention with combined exercise of stretching, strengthening, balance, and posture programs had greater effects in all domains of quality of life (ie, physical function, pain, and vitality domains) than controls. Group exercise with more social interaction and support resulted in greater improvement in these 3 domains. Shorter duration exercise of less than 12 weeks produced more improvement in physical function, physical role, and vitality but not pain, whereas a long-duration exercise program of greater than 12 to 25 weeks resulted in greater improvement in physical function and pain domains. Exercise protocols were not standardized, making it difficult to recommend exercise parameters of frequency, type, intensity, and duration.[309]

A review[314] of 9 studies summarized the effects of therapeutic exercise for persons with osteoporotic vertebral fractures. Evidence was inconclusive for exercise leading to pain reduction but supported that exercise will not lead to increased pain or increased analgesic use and can be assumed safely for this population. Significant improvements in favor of the exercise group were found, but in general, the evidence was conflicting that exercise has an overall beneficial effect on quality of life or psychological distress. The data are inconclusive as to an effect for exercise on functional mobility or daily functional level. Modest evidence is present to support exercise to increase strength, but it is unclear which type of strength training is most beneficial.[314] Exercise may be beneficial in improving balance but insufficient to draw conclusions about the effects on ROM. Prone back extension exercises are considered safe to perform.[315-318] A range of adverse effects were reported for 5 studies with 15 out of 185 individuals (8.1%) reporting exercise-related muscle soreness to rib fracture.[314] Preliminary findings suggest potential beneficial effects of exercise as an intervention for persons with osteoporotic vertebral fractures. The specific dosage (ie, intensity, frequency, type, and duration) of exercise intervention has not been determined.

Papaioannou et al[319] found no change in BMD in a 6-month home-based exercise study. Exercises included stretching, strengthening, and aerobic exercise. The exercise group demonstrated significantly more improvement in pain, emotion, leisure, and social domains in the Osteoporosis Quality of Life Questionnaire. Change in BMD was less than the minimal detectable difference of 5.6%, possibly because the intervention was not a high-intensity strength training prescription, which is possibly not appropriate for this population.[319] To have a favorable effect on BMD, exercise programs should have a duration of at least 1 year and include aerobic activities, strength training, and weightbearing exercises. Strength training should be done at least 2 to 3 times per week. In postmenopausal women, power training is considered safe and may have more favorable effects on BMD when compared to strength training.[320,321] de Kam et al[322] suggested that improving balance, muscle strength, and BMD could reduce fall-related fracture and the risk of falling in persons with low BMD. More research is needed to determine optimal exercise parameters.

In a single-group pretest-posttest design, Katzman et al[323] studied the effects of a 12-week group exercise intervention in women 65 years and older (72 + 4.2 years) with a kyphosis of 50 degrees or more; the ability to decrease the kyphosis by 5 degrees in standing; and the ability to walk 0.4 km (0.25 mile) without an assistive device and climb a flight of stairs independently. Subjects were excluded for serious or other chronic medical conditions that would

TABLE 5-6. EXERCISE INTERVENTION AND EXTENSION STRENGTHENING EXERCISES

EXERCISE	*DOSAGE*
Warm-up: AROM shoulder, chest, upper back	5 minutes, 10 repetitions
Strengthening	20 minutes
a. Prone trunk lift to neutral: "W" position, arms at sides, elbows flexed, hands by ears (see Figure 5-70)	a. 3 sets, 8 repetitions
b. Quadruped arm and leg lift: ankle and wrist cuff weights (see Figure 5-71)	b. 0 to 5 lb (0 to 2.3 kg) or elastic band
c. Bilateral shoulder flexion supine on foam roller using elastic bands (see Figure 5-72)	c. 0 to 5 lb (0 to 2.3 kg) or elastic band
d. Side-lying thoracic rotation	
ROM exercises	15 minutes, passive 30-second hold
a. Chest stretching and diaphragmatic breathing, supine on foam roller (see Figure 5-73)	a. Combine with shoulder flexion exercises
b. Prone hip extension bilaterally	b. Passive × 1 with stretch strap
c. Supine straight leg raise	c. Passive × 1 with stretch strap
d. Quadruped thoracic extension and chest stretch	d. Passive × 3
Postural alignment	15 minutes
a. Postural correction	a. Active, standing eyes open, eyes closed
b. Neutral spine: sit-to-stand seated on ball	b. Seated on gym ball (10 repetitions)
c. Home postural correction	c. At least 3×/day
Cool-down	5 minutes
a. Wall push-ups (see Figure 5-74)	a. Body weight resistance × 10
b. Overhead arm wall slides	b. Lift arms from wall end range × 10
c. Calf stretching at wall	c. Passive 30-second hold × 1

Exercises as described by Katzman WB, Sellmeyer DE, Stewart AL, Wanek L, Hamel KA. Changes in flexed posture, musculoskeletal impairments, and physical performance after group exercise in community-dwelling older women. *Arch Phys Med Rehabil.* 2007;88:192-199.

not allow participation in the study or for a VCF within the past 6 months and had to be cleared for a moderate intensity exercise program by a primary care physician. Subjects participated 2 times per week for 12 weeks in a group exercise intervention (Table 5-6; Figures 5-70 through 5-74) supervised by a physical therapist along with a daily posture correction program. Specific exercises were thoracic extension, shoulder flexion and hip extension stretching, trunk extension and scapular muscle strengthening, transversus abdominis stabilization, and postural alignment training. Strengthening consisted of high-intensity, progressive resistive exercise with stretching incorporating foam rollers. Weight in 0.45-kg (1-lb) increments or elastic band resistance of yellow to red to green to blue was increased when a subject could perform 3 sets of 8 repetitions with proper form and without pain or discomfort. No subjects were injured. Significant improvements were noted in kyphosis, extensor strength, popliteal angle, modified physical performance test, and the jug test (ie, time to move five 1-gallon jugs from a low to high self). Posture and physical performance can be improved with group exercise.[323]

In 80 postmenopausal women with osteoporosis, Hongo et al[317] examined the effects of a home-based low-intensity exercise on back extensor strength, spinal mobility, and quality of life. Subjects were excluded with a history or current diagnosis of malignancy, chronic hepatitis, renal disease, chronic digestive disorders, rheumatoid arthritis, parathyroid dysfunction, hyperthyroidism, or diabetes mellitus. Additional exclusions were vertebral fractures within the last 6 months, lack of independence in ADL, acute or severe chronic back pain that could interfere with evaluations of strength, inability to lie in prone position,

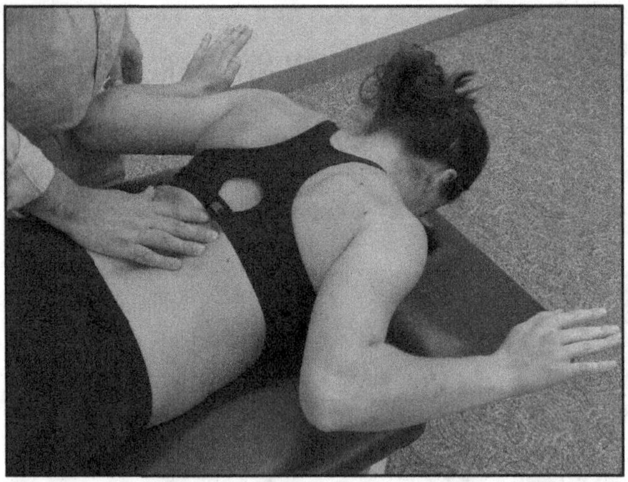

Figure 5-70. Prone trunk lift to neutral: "W" position, arms at sides, elbows flexed, hands by ears.

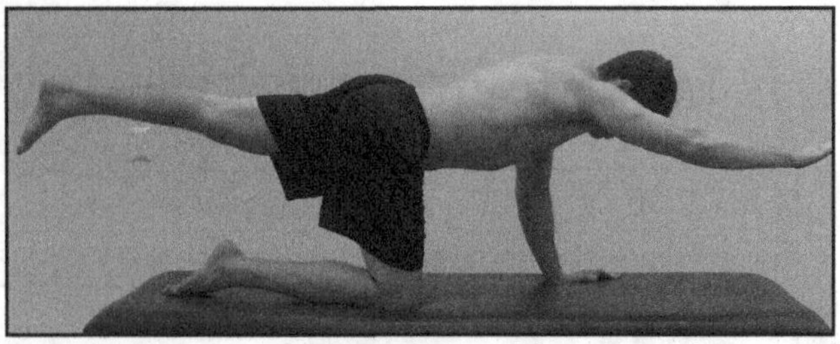

Figure 5-71. Quadruped arm and leg lift: ankle and wrist cuff weights.

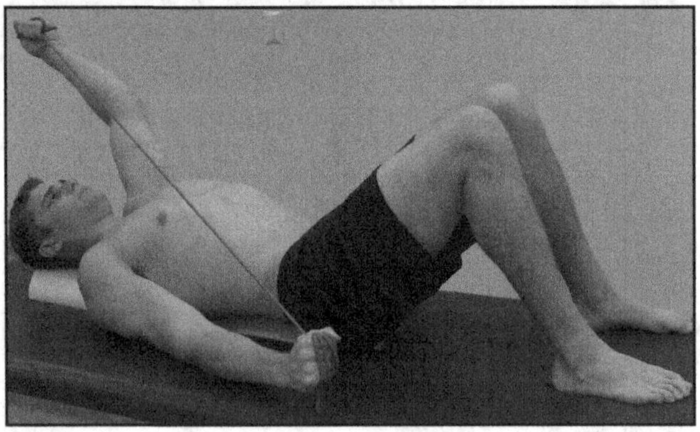

Figure 5-72. Bilateral shoulder flexion supine on foam roller using elastic bands.

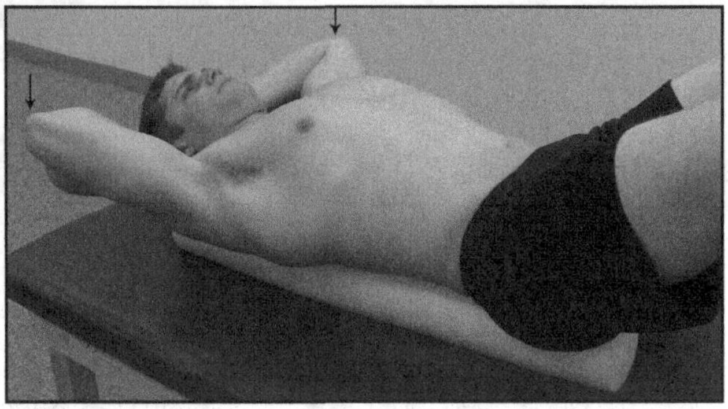

Figure 5-73. Chest stretching and diaphragmatic breathing, supine on foam roller.

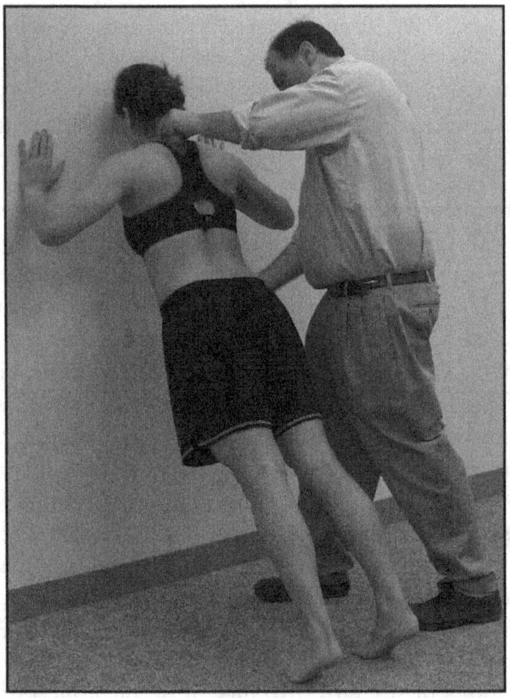

Figure 5-74. Wall push-up.

and history of the medication of bisphosphonate or vitamin D supplements within the last 1 year.

Subjects were randomized to treatment or no treatment groups. The intervention consisted of instruction to lie in a prone position on a bed with a pillow under the abdomen so that the spine was slightly flexed. A warm-up exercise involved slowly extending the spine with the aid of both arms 10 times. Then, the subjects were to lift the upper trunk off the bed with arms at the side toward a neutral position for 5 seconds with a 10-second interval between the contractions, repeated 10 times daily and 5 days per week without supervision. The exercise ranged from 3 to 5 minutes. All subjects kept a diary and were asked to maintain a regular diet and avoid new athletic activities throughout the study. Three subjects reported back pain during the strengthening exercises; all resolved with rest. No new vertebral fractures were reported. Spinal mobility did not change, but back extensor strength significantly increased both in the exercise group (26%) and the control group (11%). Quality of life increased in the exercise group (7%), but did not change in the control group. A low-intensity home program may have beneficial effects of back extensor strength and quality of life.[317]

Chien et al[313] examined a 12-week home-based trunk strengthening program for osteoporotic and osteopenic postmenopausal women (n = 28) without fracture in a single-blind randomized controlled study. Control subjects ages 58.6 + 9.3 years maintained usual activities, diet, and medication. Exercise for the intervention group ages 61.7 + 9.0 included 3 sessions per day 7 days per week. Compliance was defined as 70% completion rate by diary. All exercises were selected by a physical therapist based on the person's abilities. The following exercises were included:

- In supine:
  - Isometric abdominal contraction
  - Gluteal setting and bridging
  - Pelvis raising with legs crossed
  - Pelvis raising with single-leg raise
- In prone:
  - Chin retraction with head and thorax extension progressing to arms at sides, behind head, and overhead
  - Leg raise to extend the spine alternate legs initially, then both
  - Alternate arm-leg raise, and then all 4 limbs together
- In quadruped position:
  - Alternate arm raises
  - Alternate leg raises
  - Opposing arm and leg

All exercises were performed in a posterior pelvic tilt and began with a warm-up and ended with stretching of target muscles. Each movement was held for 3 seconds initially, progressing to a maximum of 10 seconds for 3 sets of 10 repetitions. Subjects exercised and progressed at their own pace. The control group did not change on any outcome measures. The exercise group improved in spinal ROM, motion velocity of isokinetic trunk extensor strength ($P < 0.05$), and the ODI ($P < 0.05$). Better satisfaction was observed in physical role, pain, and mental health domains of the SF36 quality of life questionnaire ($P < 0.05$). The authors concluded that the 12-week home exercise program was somewhat effective for improving spinal ROM and motion velocity, reducing ODI measures and improving quality of life in a population of osteoporotic and osteopenic postmenopausal women without fractures. Future studies are warranted.[313]

Sinaki et al[324] studied the effect of a spinal weighted kypho-orthosis and a specific back extension and gait program on the risk of falls in ambulatory community-dwelling persons older than 60 with osteoporosis-kyphosis: 25 women, 12 with a thoracic kyphosis of 50- to 65-degree Cobb angle and 13 healthy, matched controls of less than 35 to 40 degrees. None of the subjects used an assistive device for walking, but they had been advised to use a cane due to the potential for falls. After baseline evaluations, the kyphotic group received 2 sessions of supervised training in a 4-week spinal proprioceptive extension exercise dynamic program. The daily home program consisted of wearing the weighted kypho-orthosis while performing 10 repetitions of back extension exercises for reduction of kyphosis without increasing lumbar lordosis. Specific proprioceptive exercises were performed for 10 minutes twice daily to improve balance. The weighted kypho-orthosis consisted of a fitted harness with 1 kg of weight suspended between T10 to L4 of the spine and was worn daily for one-half hour in the morning and one-half hour in the afternoon. Compliance was documented with a diary. After 4 weeks, the kyphotic group showed a significant change in balance ($P = .003$); mean height improved ($P < .001$); and several gait parameters ($P < .05$) of forward velocity, cadence, total support time, swing phase, and single support improved. Mean back extensor strength improved significantly from baseline (144.0 ± 46.5 N) to follow-up (198.6 ± 55.2 N). Lower extremity muscle did not change significantly except for improved left ankle plantar flexors ($P = .02$). Back pain decreased significantly ($P = .001$).[324] Sinaki et al[325] reported that the objective of exercise in osteoporosis is to improve axial stability through improved muscle strength. Persons with osteopenia may begin with a more strenuous exercise program than those with osteoporosis, but a specific exercise prescription must be individualized to increase muscle strength safely, decrease complications due to immobility, and prevent falls and fractures.[325]

Manual Therapy and Exercise

In a randomized, single-blind controlled pilot trial, Bennell et al[315] investigated the effectiveness of a manual therapy and exercise program in persons ($n = 20$) ages 53 to 90 with a history of painful osteoporotic vertebral fracture. Subjects were allocated to 2 groups: intervention or control with no treatment. Female subjects were included if they were:

- Equal to or more than 5 years postmenopause
- Greater than 50 years old with primary osteoporosis (ie, DEXA T score < −2.5 at either the spine or proximal femur) with at least one painful vertebral fracture sustained between 3 months and 2 years, previously defined as anterior height reduced by greater than or equal to 20% compared with its posterior height and the posterior height of the adjacent superior or inferior vertebra
- On a stable medication for osteoporosis for at least 6 months
- Community dwelling and able to attend treatment
- English speaking

Exclusion criteria were as follows:

- Secondary causes of bone loss
- Comorbidities that would prevent participation in exercise
- Acute vertebral fracture within the past 3 months

TABLE 5-7. PHYSIOTHERAPY AND HOME EXERCISE PROGRAM

WEEKS	EXERCISE AND DOSAGE
1 only	1. Postural taping: anterior shoulder on each side to opposite rib cage (worn full time) 2. Supine over towel placed lengthwise to promote thoracic extension (5 to 10 minutes daily)
2 only	1. Quadruped, activation of transverse abdominis (8 to 10 reps × 2, 5-second hold, 3×/week)
1 to 2 only	1. Half squats: in front of a chair, squat down to touch the chair with buttocks and stand up. Progress to handheld weights (8 to 10 reps × 2, 3×/week) 2. Bridging in supine; knees bent, feet on the ground lift back and pelvis off ground (5- to 10-second hold × 5; 3×/week
1 to 10	1. Soft tissue massage in prone: upper trapezius, rhomboids, ES (5 minutes) 2. Central passive accessory PA vertebral mobilization (5 oscillations per segment × 2 starting at T1 down to 2 levels below the painful regions, grade 2 to 3) 3. Sitting without back support, transverse abdominis activation (10-second hold, 5 reps, daily) 4. Trunk AROM in sitting, rotation, and lateral flexion (5 reps each direction, daily) 5. Chin retraction against wall in standing, towel roll behind head, heels against wall (10-second hold, 5 reps, daily) 6. Standing wall push-ups (8 to 10 reps × 2, 3×/week) 7. Seated row with hand weights: pull hands up toward chest by bending elbows and then lower (8 to 10 reps × 2, 3×/week)
2 to 10	1. Standing corner stretch: face corner, both hands at chest height on wall elbows flexed to 90 degrees; allow chest to move slowly toward the corner to stretch anterior chest (10- to 30-second hold, 3 reps, daily)
3 to 10	1. Walking hand up the wall in standing: face wall, walk hands ups until arms are extended, then hold hands off the wall (5-second hold, 5 reps daily) 2. Shoulder flexion in supine: holding a cane, take arms overhead to hold at end range (10-second hold, 5 reps daily) 3. Seated overhead dumbbell press: elbows bent and at the side, press straight up until arms are extended (3 to 10 reps × 2, 3×/week) 4. Hip extension in prone: raise one leg off the ground then the other (8 to 10 reps × 2, 3×/week) 5. Step-ups: progress to holding hand weights: step up and down a 10-cm step. Alternate legs (8 to 10 reps × 2, 3×/week) 6. In quadruped, one arm and leg lift; begin with one arm, add opposite leg lift (8 to 10 reps × 2; 3×/week
2 to 3 only	1. Prone lying with arm elevation: arms at shoulder height, elbows bent. Retract scapula then lift arms off floor (5- to 10-second hold × 5, 3×/week)
4 to 10	1. Prone trunk extension: retract chin, then left head and shoulders off floor (5- to 10-second hold × 5, 3×/week)

Reprinted from Bennell KL, Matthews B, Greig A, et al. Effects of an exercise and manual therapy program on physical impairments, function and quality of life in people with osteoporotic vertebral fracture: a randomised, single-blind controlled pilot trial. *BMC Musculoskelet Disord.* 2010;11:36. http://www.biomedcentral.com/1471-2474/11/36. © 2010 Bennell et al; licensee BioMed Central Ltd.

- Radicular signs or symptoms
- Back pain radiating into the lower limb
- Previous participation in a formal program for back pain
- Back pain in the past 6 months
- Allergy to the use of adhesive tape

Intervention included standardized weekly, 45-minute sessions (Table 5-7) over 10 weeks with dosage of manual treatments adjusted based on patient assessment. Postural taping to promote retracted scapulae and thoracic extension was worn full-time for the first week. At each session, central PA mobilization to the thoracic spine and soft tissue massage were performed. The home exercise addressed posture, daily ROM, and strengthening and trunk control exercises 3 times per week. The intervention group showed significant reductions in pain during movement and at rest. Significant improvements were also noted in the Qualeffo-41[326] physical function domain and the Timed Loaded Standing test (ie, amount of time to hold a 2-lb dumbbell in each hand with the arms at 90 degrees shoulder flexion).[327] The TUG (ie, the time to rise from a standard arm chair, walk around a cone on the floor 3 m away, return to the chair, and sit down)[328] and thoracic kyphosis did not differ between groups. Perceived change in back pain over the 10 weeks was rated as "much better" in 82% of the intervention subjects and only 11% in the controls. Manual therapy and exercise appear to be beneficial in persons with a history of osteoporotic vertebral fracture. Six (55%) of the intervention group reported adverse events such as shoulder pain, flare up of a wrist injury, sore knee, sore waist, and skin irritation from tape. All complaints settled after removing the offending activity.[315]

In a similar study, Bautmans et al[329] investigated the effects of manual mobilization, postural taping, and exercises for postural correction on the severity of thoracic kyphosis, back pain, and quality of life in frail, elderly postmenopausal patients with osteoporosis. Subjects with Paget's disease, rheumatoid arthritis, AS, cancer, and cognitive or physical inability to understand and/or participate in the test procedures were excluded. X-ray images of the thoracic and lumbar spine taken within 3 months were available for all subjects. Evidence of a low-impact vertebral fracture was not an exclusion. However, subjects with recent vertebral fractures of less than 3 months and/or symptomatic vertebral fractures were not eligible. Forty-eight subjects with a mean age of 76 ± 7 years and with a diagnosis of osteoporosis (t-score < −2.5) were randomized to 18 sessions of rehabilitation over 3 months or a wait-listed control status. Manual treatment (Figure 5-75) occurred in the seated position. The patient had both hands on the neck or crossed on the shoulders and resting on the therapist's mobilizing arm. The therapist's other hand was placed at the thoracolumbar junction for stabilization. Gentle whole thoracic spine angular mobilizations were performed toward thoracic extension and combined extension with lateral flexion and/or rotation for 10 to 15 passive movements and within the available range of movement. No muscle guarding or pain was provoked.[329] When possible, end-range positions were maintained for up to 5 seconds without added force or thrust. Two methods of tape application (Figure 5-76), V-taping and longitudinal taping, were alternately applied once per week and worn continuously for 3 days. V-taping was applied bilaterally from the acromion to the T12 SP. Longitudinal taping was applied from T1 to the deepest point of the lumbar lordosis. Five basic exercises were performed under therapist supervision and for home exercise. Exercises consisted of a daily 15- to 20-minute session under supervision or at home. The exercises included the following:

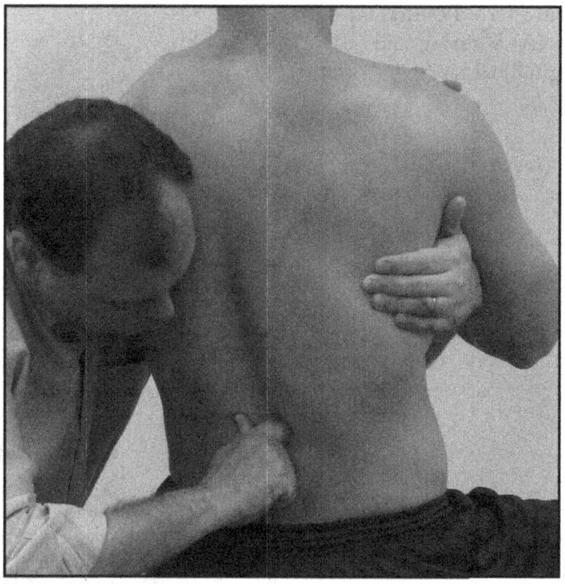

Figure 5-75. Seated manual passive thoracic extension mobilization.

- In sitting lifting both hands together above the head for 3 sets of 10 to 15 movements using a dumbbell as needed
- In sitting or standing with the back against a wall straightening the back as far as possible for 3 sets of 10 to 15 repetitions maintaining upright for 3 to 10 seconds
- While seated on a chair with both hands on the neck or crossed on the shoulders, lifting the arms and extending the upper back without compensation in the hips or lumbar spine for 3 sets of 10 to 15 repetitions maintaining upright for 3 to 10 seconds
- Standing in front of a wall scrolling with both hands as high as possible over the wall for 3 sets of 10 to 15 repetitions, maintaining upright for 3 to 10 seconds
- Lying on the back in hook-lying with a small rolled-up towel under the fifth to seventh thoracic vertebrae perpendicular to the spinal processes, stretching the thoracic spine for 30 to 180 seconds depending on the patient's tolerance without compensation of the lumbar spine or eliciting back pain[329]

Adverse events included skin irritation from the tape, pain during mobilization, and pain with lifting the arms above the head during exercise. In the treatment group, thoracic kyphosis improved significantly after rehabilitation compared with controls (intention-to-treat analysis, P = .017). Compliance was a concern in the treatment group, but thoracic kyphosis improved in patients who were compliant (n = 15) compared with those who were not compliant (P = .002) and controls (P = .001). Mental health worsened slightly in the treatment group, but the worsening was not significant compared with controls. Quality of

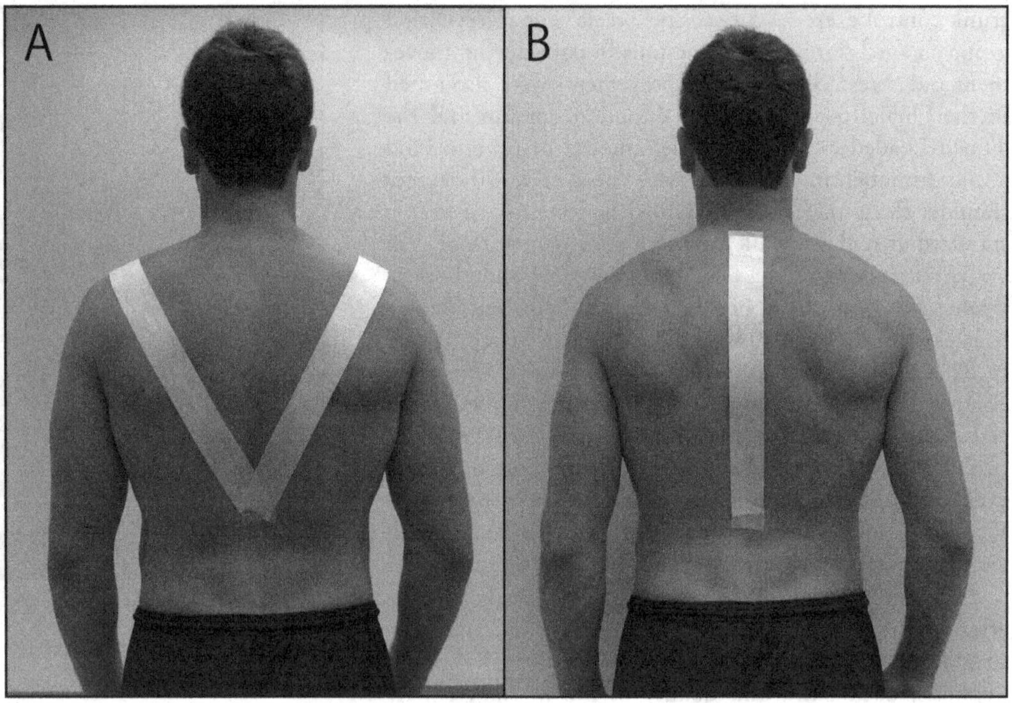

Figure 5-76. Postural taping: (A) V-taping and (B) longitudinal taping.

life or back pain as measured by the Qualeffo-41 did not change.[329]

Clinical Practice Guidelines for the Management of Osteoporosis

Clinical practice guidelines have been established for the diagnosis and management of osteoporosis in Canada.[330] Clinical recommendations and levels of evidence related to exercise and falls include the following:

- Resistance training appropriate for the individual's age and functional ability and/or weightbearing aerobic exercises for persons with osteoporosis or at risk for osteoporosis (grade B)
- Core stabilization exercises to compensate for weakness or postural deviations of persons who have had vertebral fractures (grade B)
- Balance exercises and gait training should be considered for persons at risk for falls (grade A)
- Hip protector use should be considered for older persons in long-term care facilities who are at high risk for fracture (grade B)[331]

Osteoporosis and vertebral fractures, a possible consequence of osteoporosis, lead to an increased risk of future fractures and result in an increased thoracic kyphosis and loss of overall height. Individuals with vertebral fractures are more likely to develop increased disability, reduced spinal ROM, slower gait, impaired pulmonary function, loss of independence, self-esteem issues, fear of further fractures and nearly double the mortality risk compared with age-matched controls.[332] The use of manual therapy and/or exercise with or without other current treatments for individuals with osteoporotic fractures could provide a conservative approach to improving ADL, reducing pain, and improving quality of life. However, high-quality consistent research on the effects of exercise and the type, amount, frequency, and duration of exercise for persons with vertebral fractures is lacking.[314] Physical therapists must closely examine patients with osteopenia, osteoporosis, or the potential to develop osteoporosis to determine an individualized exercise prescription based on the patient's relevant impairments, overall health status, and current fitness levels. Current treatments for persons with these types of fractures include conservative care such as exercise, back bracing, analgesic use, nutrition, antiresorptive (ie, biophosphonates, hormone therapy) pharmacological agents,[333] and surgical procedures such as vertebroplasty and kyphoplasty.[334]

Chronic Thoracic Spinal Pain

Because research is lacking related to chronic pain in this region, the section on chronic LBP in Chapter 4 may be applicable to patients with chronic pain related to the thorax. Chronic pain is a complex problem, is different for each person, is resistant to intervention, and requires a multidimensional approach to management.[335,336] The biopsyhosocial framework is the recommended approach to understanding and managing chronic pain. This perspective focuses on both disease and illness, with illness being viewed as the complex interaction of biological factors (ie, impairments of body structure and functions), psychological factors (ie, beliefs, emotions, activity limitations), and social factors (culture, work, participation restrictions) and refers to how a person and family members live with and respond to chronic pain disability.[337] The current approach for chronic spinal pain supports an interdisciplinary model based on the biopsychosocial model including pain education, cognitive behavioral training, graded exercise and graded exposure, spinal manual therapy techniques, and exercise training.

Interventional Radiology and Surgical Management of Thoracic Disorders

Surgical Intervention for Vertebral Compression Fractures

Surgical intervention for VCFs that require fixation such as spinal decompression and fusion procedures is usually indicated with evidence of spinal instability or burst fractures, with neurological impairment, or in some patients who do not respond to adequate conservative management. The advanced age of the individual, comorbidities in this population, and the difficulty in achieving fixation in weakened bone are considerations. Consequently, a conservative nonoperative approach is usually recommended initially. In the presence of intractable pain, minimally invasive procedures are considered as alternative options. Inpatient care is generally not required for VCFs unless neurologic impairment has occurred or other medical conditions warrant it. Traditionally, pain medication, bed rest, and bracing are recommended. The side effects of narcotics, constipation, mental status changes, and respiratory suppression in the elderly must be considered. Prolonged bed rest may lead to deconditioning, further bone loss, and increased risk of deep vein thrombosis. Ice, heat, positioning, or gentle back massage are considered for pain relief. Gradual mobilization with a wheeled walker or cane is introduced, along with education to prevent falls, use of proper body mechanics, and work simplification. Use of a spinal orthosis may aid in pain relief and promote a more upright posture.[338] As symptoms diminish, the patient is evaluated for therapeutic exercise such as back extensor muscle strengthening, muscle stretching, balance exercises, stabilization exercises, weightbearing exercises and cardiovascular fitness. Generally, two-thirds of patients with acute symptomatic VCF improve over 4 to 6 weeks but have persistent pain.[339]

Vertebral Augmentation Procedures—Kyphoplasty and Vertebroplasty

VCFs refractory to nonoperative care, associated with osteoporosis or metastatic disease, are sometimes treated with vertebroplasty or kyphoplasty. However, the use of these vertebral augmentation procedures is controversial. Vertebroplasty is performed with the patient in prone. A needle is advanced through the pedicle to the vertebral body under fluoroscopy guidance. Polymethylmethacrylate (PMMA) cement is then injected into the fracture site. The PMMA cures in situ. The patient is allowed to perform activities as tolerated.[340] Balloon kyphoplasty is a similar minimally invasive procedure in which an inflatable bone tamp is placed into the vertebral body, inflated, and removed. The space within the vertebral body is then filled with PMMA cement.

In small nonrandomized studies, both procedures have shown promise in reducing pain and improving function.[341-350] Additionally, kyphoplasty is proposed to restore fracture height by about 50%, but consistent results have not been achieved.[346,351] Several randomized controlled studies question the results of previous studies. Comparisions[352,353] of vertebroplasty to a sham procedure found no difference in pain reduction or restoration of function. Patient selection bias and patient crossover casts doubt on the validity of the outcomes, leaving mixed results for the value of vertebral augmentation related to osteoporosis. In a randomized controlled trial comparing balloon kyphoplasty to nonsurgical management in patients with cancer who had 1 to 3 VCFs, kyphoplasty was safe and effective, rapidly reducing pain and improving function at 1-month follow-up.[354]

Complications of Vertebral Augmentation

Both procedures are associated with potential extrusion of PMMA cement through fracture lines, vascular channels, lytic lesions, or hemangiomas.[346,355,356] The cement extrusion can be benign or result in pulmonary embolus[356] or neurologic compromise.[357,358] Rarely, the vertebral body may collapse with potential force of bone into the spinal canal.[358] Subsequent VCFs have occurred 2 to 3 months after the augmentation at adjacent or remote spinal segments.[359-361] A common complaint is a transient increase in pain at the injected site that usually resolves with NSAIDs within 48 hours.[362] Other complications include acute radiculopathy, rib fracture, pneumothorax, spinal cord compression, and infection. Reports of pulmonary embolism and death are rare.

Indications for Vertebral Augmentation

In a small sample (n = 11) of patients with VCF and pain refractory for up to 3 months to medical therapy,

Masala et al[363] reported that indications for kyphoplasty include VCF due to osteoporosis, myeloma, metastasis, and vertebral angioma with no neurological symptoms. Contraindications include coagulation disorders, unstable fractures or complete vertebral collapse, spinal canal compromise greater than 20%, epidural tumor extension, myelopathy, inability to lie prone, allergy to cement or radio-opaque dye, and infection.[362,363] All patients showed an increase in vertebral body height and partial or complete pain relief.[363] Indications for vertebroplasty are similar to kyphoplasty. Failure of medical therapy is defined by the following[364]:

- Pain persisting at a level that prevents ambulation despite 24 hours of analgesics in a nonambulatory patient
- PT is intolerable with pain persisting despite 24 hours of analgesics
- Side effects such as excessive sedation, confusion, or constipation due to the analgesics necessary to reduce pain to a tolerable level

Esses et al[365] reported clinical practice guidelines approved by the American Academy of Orthopedic Surgeons based on a systematic review on the treatment of symptomatic osteoporotic VCF in adults older than 18 years of age who are neurologically intact. The initial recommended treatment for patients who are neurologically intact with clinical signs and symptoms of an acute (ie, 0 to 5 days) VCF is calcitonin for 4 weeks. Calcitonin is a nonsteroidal hormone usually administered in nasal form that inhibits osteoclasts with mild dizziness as a side effect. Due to inconclusive evidence, no recommendation was made for or against the use of opioids/analgesics, bed rest, complementary or alternative medicine, supervised or unsupervised exercises, or electrical stimulation in patients with osteoporotic VCF who are neurologically intact. The authors did not recommend vertebroplasty for this population, but did recommend kyphoplasty as an option possibly due to long-term (ie, up to 12 months) clinically important outcomes. The final recommendation is neither for nor against a specific treatment for individuals with osteoporotic VCF and neurological compromise due to an absence of studies for procedural effectiveness. The authors concluded that the lack of good quality of research limits the strength of the recommendations.[365]

Evidence for Postvertebral Augmentation Care and Rehabilitation

Patients are on bed rest with oral analgesics and muscle relaxants as needed for 1 to 2 hours or as determined by their medical status.[366] Discharge criteria are variable. After 1 hour of bed rest, the patient is discharged when able to ambulate.[367] McGraw et al[368] progressed from 1 hour in supine to 1 hour in sitting, and then allowed standing. Chen et al[369] discharged within 24 hours with a thoracolumbar support. Upon discharge, systemic osteoporosis management is provided by the patient's primary care physician.[366] In 2004, 23 000 vertebral augmentation procedures were performed as inpatient procedures across the United States. Mean length of stay for kyphoplasty was 3.7, and 7.3 days for vertebroplasty. The discharge ratio for home versus a medical facility such as nursing home or rehabilitation was 50:50 and 99:23 for vertebroplasty and kyphoplasty, respectively.[370] Evidence-based guidelines have not been developed for rehabilitation after vertebral augmentation. However, exercises for spinal extension are recommended as pain allows.[371] PT does not appear to be a standard intervention after a vertebral augmentation procedure.[372]

Thoracic Spine Surgery and Evidence for Rehabilitation

Surgical procedures for disorders related to the thoracic spine range from minimally invasive endoscopic to open thoracotomy procedures and are beyond the scope of this reference. Open procedures are associated with significant morbidity. Anterior approaches are related to shoulder girdle dysfunction, impaired ventilation, intercostal neuralgia, and increased postoperative pain.[373-375] A posterior midline approach is associated with extensive muscle denervation,[376-380] extensor atrophy, scarring, weakness, increased intramuscular pressure, ischemia, and persistent, pain.[381-385] However, thoracoscopic procedures also have complications such as atelectasis, pneumothorax, pleural effusion, and hemothorax.[386-388] Thoracic spine procedures appear to be technically demanding and associated with potential significant morbidity. The equivalence or superiority of minimally invasive procedures to open procedures needs further assessment.[389] Indications for thoracic spine surgical intervention include but are not limited to radiculopathy, myelopathy, fractures or fracture dislocations, herniated disc, and scoliosis. Thoracic fusion may be indicated for pathologies such as traumatic instability, scoliotic deformity, tumor, and osteomyelitis.

Evidence-based guidelines for PT after thoracic spine surgery are not available. No randomized controlled trial or case reports were found. Most likely, postsurgical guidelines are developed at each facility in coordination with and approval by the surgeon and individualized to each patient based on sound clinical reasoning, continual assessment, and reassessment. Precautions to movement must be identified and adhered to as dictated by the surgical procedure, surgeon preference, and patient capabilities.[390] Schenk and Wise[390] advocate for a 3-phase PT postsurgical intervention based on the time frame from the surgery to the initial PT visit: phase 1 (0 to 3 weeks); phase 2 (4 to 6 weeks); and phase 3 (7 to 9 weeks). General characteristics[390] of each phase are briefly described. Dependent on the surgical procedure, tissue healing, level of irritability, and PT diagnosis, the authors suggested that most patients will benefit from aerobic conditioning, soft tissue mobilization, neuromobilization, and spinal stabilization exercise.[390] As determined by the patient's response to examination, some patients may benefit from a mobility approach (ie, feel better with movement) or a stability approach (ie, feel better when not moving).[390]

Phase 1—Mobility and Stability (0 to 3 Weeks)

As described by Schenk and Wise,[390] the key points of this phase include education regarding postoperative complications, activity and movement modification as dictated by the procedure, postural advice, and use of modalities for pain control and postsurgical inflammation. Some patients are prescribed a thoracolumbar orthosis and some are not. Based on the severity and irritability of the patient's symptoms, respect for tissue healing, and response to examination, interventions may include pain-free ROM exercise for the thoracic spine. Gentle activation of the deep muscle system of the trunk in neutral position may be initiated with low intensity and in a pain-free manner. Neuromobilization techniques are considered and, if initiated, should be nonprovocative. As indicated, aerobic activity might include ambulation, aquatic therapy, UE, or bicycle ergometry.[390]

Phase 2—Stability and Flexibility Phase (4 to 6 Weeks)

Continual assessment of active ROM is necessary with impairments addressed gradually when safe and as movement restrictions to protect healing tissues are removed. Quality, quantity, and symptom response are important for assessment of movement patterns. Stabilization exercises may be progressed with upper or lower extremity movements when the patient can tolerate additional low-intensity challenges in a pain-free manner with neuromuscular control and optimal breathing patterns. Neuromobilization may or may not be indicated based on reassessment. When the surgical incision is healed, soft tissue mobility should be assessed and treated as indicated.[390]

Phase 3—Functional Stability Phase (7 to 9 Weeks)

As indicated, soft tissue mobilization, progression to weightbearing stabilization, or therapeutic ball exercises are performed. Balance exercises, lunges, squats, diagonal movements, aerobic training, ergonomics, and return to work activities may be continued, added, or progressed as tolerated. Patient progression through each phase and to the final phase is highly variable.[390]

Little evidence is available to guide PT decision making and improve outcomes after thoracic spine surgery. Precautions to movement must be identified and adhered to as dictated by the surgical procedure, surgeon preference, and patient capabilities.[390] Postoperative management is likely to vary considerably from surgeon to surgeon, ranging from no PT postsurgical intervention to standardized postsurgical intervention. Rehabilitation should be individualized to each patient based on sound clinical reasoning, continual assessment and reassessment, and close communication with the patient's surgeon related to precautions, contraindications, and surgeon preference. A time-based approach of postsurgical guidelines is recommended for continued study.[390] As with all postsurgical rehabilitation, communication with the surgeon is important to know the surgical procedure, precautions and guidelines for progression, follow-up surgical appointments, expected outcomes from the surgeon's perspective, and the appropriate evaluation for the patient. The outpatient evaluation process is the same as discussed earlier in this chapter, keeping in mind precautions and contraindications to movement; stage of tissue healing; severity, irritability, nature, stage, and stability of the patient's presentation; and the patient's response to examination.

Spinal Fusion in Adolescent Idiopathic Scoliosis

Adolescent idiopathic scoliosis (AIS) occurs in patients between 10 and 18 years of age with no identifiable cause.[157] Any lateral curve greater than 10 degrees is considered scoliosis as measured on standing AP and lateral radiographics. AIS may not cause pain or neurological compromise, but it progresses rapidly during the growth period of the patient. Generally, treatment options include observation for small degree curves of less than 25 degrees if still growing or less than 50 degrees if done growing; bracing for curves 25 to 45 degrees to prevent further progression; and surgical intervention for curves greater than 45 degrees and still growing or >50 degrees and no longer growing, which is performed to prevent curve progression and obtain some curve correction.[157] Following spinal fusion for AIS, the inpatient stay is about 5 to 7 days. Regular daily activities and return to school occur within 3 to 4 weeks. Participation in recreational and sports activities is individually determined by the surgeon between 3 and 6 months after surgery.[157]

The following inpatient guidelines are adapted from and described in additional detail by Amoroso and Sindle.[194] During the inpatient phase of postoperative rehabilitation for AIS, PT is usually performed 2 times per day. Initial intervention includes education on spinal precautions such as no flexion or rotation, no lifting greater than 8 to 10 lbs, use of brace if prescribed, incentive spirometry, isometric lower extremity exercises, ankle pumps, and log-rolling for supine to sit transfers. As tolerated, patients are progressed from sit-to-stand to assisted ambulation with a rolling walker. Discharge goals are independent ambulation without an assistive device, minimal to no assist for transfers, and stair climbing using one hand rail. Progressive ambulation to improve endurance is encouraged as home exercise.[194]

Postoperative outpatient rehabilitation usually begins 1 to 6 months postsurgery according to surgeon preference. Spinal precautions are strictly adhered to for tissue healing until removed by the surgeon. The key focus is to assess for postural deviation and relevant impairments during this phase to improve, where indicated, posture, strength, trunk stabilization, lower extremity strength, upper and lower extremity flexibility, and general conditioning. Progression emphasizes spinal precautions and preparatory exercises for return to higher level activities necessary to achieve the patient's functional goals.[194]

Summary

In comparison to LBP and cervical pain, research related to thoracic back pain is scarce. The thorax can be a significant source of local pain and symptoms and referred pain from visceral structures, cervical spine structures, and thoracic spine and rib somatic structures posing significant challenges for the clinician. In addition to protection of vital organs, the thorax serves as a transitional zone for transfer of load or forces between the upper and lower halves of the body that is functionally related to the lumbopelvic, cervical, and shoulder girdle regions. Since these regions are interdependent, the thoracic spine must be examined in persons presenting with LBP and neck and shoulder complaints, as well as in those presenting with a primary complaint of thoracic pain.

The medical diagnostic model based on a pathoanatomical source is the most common classification for persons with symptoms related to the thorax or TSP. Neuromusculoskeletal sources of pain include but are not limited to degenerative disc disease, disc herniation, spinal stenosis, fracture or dislocation of the vertebra or ribs, muscle strain, rib syndromes, costochondritis, osteoarthritis, intercostals neuralgia, TOS, trigger points, and scoliosis. Similar to LBP, a precise anatomical tissue cannot be reliably identified as the cause or pain generator for mechanical TSP.

A thoracic spine classification system with strong current evidence to support its use and ability to improve patient outcomes is not available, but it is likely that persons with nonspecific thoracic pain can be classified into subgroups based on patterns of signs and symptoms. To assist the clinician with matching a patient's clinical presentation to an appropriate intervention, a proposed impairment-based classification system for subgroups of thoracic pain is presented, integrating current best research, concepts used in the classification of LBP, and a clinical reasoning process to guide decision making toward best treatment strategies. In an impairment-based approach, the clinician identifies relevant physical impairments such as limited ROM, joint or muscle stiffness or hypermobility, and/or muscle coordination deficits. Evidence-based PT interventions are selected to target the prioritized impairments to address activity limitations or functional deficits important to the patient.

The Appendix section provides case studies for each region (see Appendices F and G) to illustrate the clinical reasoning framework. Each case study allows for practice taking a history and planning a physical examination. The data from the history and physical examination are then synthesized using current best evidence to determine appropriate diagnostic classification, prognosis, and initial management strategies. The case study process provides an opportunity to practice using clinical reasoning and an evidence-based framework.

References

1. Leboeuf-Yde C, Nielsen J, Kyvik KO, Fejer R, Hartvigsen J. Pain in the lumbar, thoracic or cervical regions: do age and gender matter? A population-based study of 34902 Danish twins 20-71 years of age. *BMC Musculoskelet Disord.* 2009;10:39.
2. Briggs AM, Smith AJ, Straker LM, Bragge P. Thoracic spine in the general population: prevalence, incidence and associated factors in children, adolescents and adults. A systematic review. *BMC Musculoskelet Disord.* 2009;10:77.
3. Wedderkopp N, Kjaer P, Hestbaek L, Korsholm L, Leboeuf-Yde C. High-level physical activity in childhood seems to protect against low back pain in early adolescence. *Spine J.* 2009;9:134-141.
4. Grimmer K, Nyland L, Milanese S. Repeated measures of recent headache, neck and upper back pain in Australian adolescents. *Cephalgia.* 2006;26:843-851.
5. El-Metwally A, Salminen JJ, Auvinen AA, Macfarlane G, Mikkelsson M. Risk factors for development of non-specific musculoskeletal pain in preteens and early adolescents: a prospective 1-year follow-up study. *BMC Musculoskelet Disord.* 2007;8:46-54.
6. Dionne CE, Bourbonnais R, Frémont P, et al. Determinants of "return to work in good health" among workers with back pain who consult in primary care settings: a 2-year prospective study. *Eur Spine J.* 2007;16:641-655.
7. Wood KB, Garvey TA, Gundry C, et al. Magnetic resonance imaging of the thoracic spine. Evaluation of asymptomatic individuals. *J Bone Joint Surg Am.* 1995;77:1631-1638.
8. Wood KB, Blair JM, Aepple DM, et al. The natural history of asymptomatic thoracic disc herniations. *Spine.* 1997;22:525-530.
9. Matsumoto M, Okada E, Ichihara D, et al. Age-related changes of thoracic and cervical intervertebral discs in asymptomatic subjects. *Spine.* 2010;35:1359-1364.
10. Lee D. *The Thorax. An Integrated Approach.* White Rock, BC, Canada: Diane G. Lee Physiotherapist Corporation; 2003.
11. McKenzie R, May S. *The Lumbar Spine Mechanical Diagnosis and Therapy.* Vol 2. Raumati Beach, New Zealand: Spinal Publications; 2004.
12. Hefford C. McKenzie classification of mechanical spinal pain: profile of syndromes and directions of preference. *Man Ther.* 2008;13:75-81.

13. Olson KA. *Manual Physical Therapy of the Spine.* St Louis, MO: Saunders; 2007.
14. Lee LJ, Lee D. Integrated, multimodal approach to the thoracic spine and ribs. In: Magee DJ, Zachazewski JE, Quillen WS, eds. *Pathology and Intervention in Musculoskeletal Rehabilitation.* St Louis, MO: Saunders; 2009:306-337.
15. Goodman CC, Snyder TEK. *Differential Diagnosis for Physical Therapists. Screening for Referral.* 4th ed. St Louis, MO: Saunders; 2007.
16. Verdon F, Burnand B, Herzig L, Junod M, Pécoud A, Favrat B. Chest wall syndrome among primary care patients: a cohort study. *BMC Fam Pract.* 2007;8:51.
17. Goodman C. Origins of thoracic pain. In: Cervical and Thoracic Pain: Evidence for Effectiveness of Physical Therapy. Independent Study Course 21.1.2. Orthopaedic Section: APTA, Inc; 2011:15-27.
18. Raiszadeh R, Rhines LF. Management of thoracic spine infections. *Oper Tech Neurosurg.* 2005;7(4):199-205.
19. Karnath B, Holden MD, Hussain N. Chest pain: differentiating cardiac from noncardiac causes. *Chest Pain.* 2004;38:24-27.
20. Deyo RA, Diehl AK. Cancer as a cause of back pain: frequency, clinical presentation, and diagnostic strategies. *J Gen Intern Med.* 1988;3:230-238.
21. Henschke N, Maher CH, Refshauge KM. Screening for malignancy in low back pain patients: a systematic review. *Eur Spine J.* 2007;16(10):1673-1679
22. Brihaye J, Ectors P, Lemort M, Van Houtte P. The management of spinal epidural metastases. *Adv Tech Stand Neurosurg.* 1988;16:121-176.
23. Siemionow K, Ilaslan H, Steinmetz M, McLain RF, Bell G. Identifying serious causes of back pain: cancer infection, fracture. *Cleve Clin J Med.* 2008;75:557-566.
24. Kass SM, Williams PM, Reamy BV. Pleurisy. *Am Fam Physician.* 2007;75(9):1357-1364.
25. Henschke N, Maher CG, Refshauge KM. A systematic review identifies "red flags" to screen for vertebral fracture in patients with low back pain. *J Clin Epidemiol.* 2008;61:110-118.
26. Deyo RA, Rainville J, Kent DL. What can the history and physical examination tell us about low back pain? *JAMA.* 1992;268:760-765.
27. Reiter GT, Wyler AR. Vertebral fracture. *Medscape Reference.* http://emedicine.medscape.com/article/248236-overview#a0101. Updated April 29, 2013. Accessed April 28, 2011.
28. Melton LJ III. Epidemiology of spinal osteoporosis. *Spine.* 1997;22(24 suppl):2S-11S.
29. Melton LJ III, Kan SH, Frye MA, Wahner HW, O'Fallon WM, Riggs BL. Epidemiology of vertebral fractures in women. *Am J Epidemiol.* 1989;129:1000-1011.
30. Resch A, Schneider B, Bernecker P, et al. Risk of vertebral fractures in men: relationship to mineral density of the vertebral body. *Am J Roentgenol.* 1995;164:1447-1450.
31. Old JL, Calvert M. Vertebral compression fractures in the elderly. *Am Fam Physician.* 2004;69:111-116.
32. Silverman SL. The clinical consequences of vertebral compression fracture. *Bone.* 1992;13(suppl 2):S27-S31.
33. Malanga GA, McLean JP, Alladin I, Tai Q, Andrus SG, Smith R. Thoracic discogenic pain syndrome. *Medscape Reference.* http://emedicine.medscape.com/article/96284-overview. Updated December 14, 2011. Accessed July 29, 2010.
34. McInerney J, Ball PA. The pathophysiology of thoracic disc disease. *Neurosurg Focus.* 2000;9(4): e1. http://www.medscape.com/viewarticle/405642_4. Accessed April 30, 2011.
35. O'Connor RC, Andary MT, Russo, RB, DeLano M. Thoracic radiculopathy. *Phys Med Rehabil Clin N Am.* 2002;13:623-644.
36. Wang K, Chen X. Thoracic cord compression caused by continuous multilevel ossification of ligamentum flavum in Chinese patients. *Chin J Traumatol.* 2007;10:213-217.
37. Yngve D. Abdominal reflexes. *J Pediatr Orthop.* 1997;17:105-108.
38. Pearce JM. Beevor's sign. *Eur Neurol.* 2005;53:208-209.
39. Moon JE, Dronen SC. Herpes zoster. *Medscape Reference.* http://emedicine.medscape.com/article/218683-overview. Updated February 26, 2013 Accessed April 29, 2011.
40. Feise RJ, Menke JM. Functional Rating Index: a new valid and reliable instrument to measure the magnitude of clinical change in spinal conditions. *Spine.* 2001;26:78-87.
41. Feise RJ, Menke JM. Functional Rating Index: literature review. *Med Sci Monit.* 2010;16(2):RA25-RA36.
42. Childs JD, Piva SR. Psychometric properties of the Functional Rating Index in patients with low back pain. *Eur Spine J.* 2005;14:1008-1012.
43. Stewart M, Maher CG, Refshauge KM, Bogduk N, Nicholas M. Responsiveness of pain and disability measures for chronic whiplash. *Spine.* 2007;32:580-585.
44. Briggs AM, Bragge P, Smith AJ, Govil D, Straker LM. Prevalence and associated factors for thoracic spine pain in the adult working population: a literature review. *J Occup Health.* 2009;51:177-192.
45. Roelen CAM, Schreuder KJ, Koopmans PC, Grothoff JW. Perceived job demands relate to self-reported health complaints. *Occup Med.* 2008;58:58-63.
46. Sik EC, Batt ME, Heslop LM. Atypical chest pain in athletes. *Curr Sports Med Rep.* 2009;8(2):0-6.
47. Dreyfuss P, Tibiletti C, Dreyer SJ. Thoracic zygapophyseal joint pain patterns: a study in normal volunteers. *Spine.* 1994;19:807-811.
48. Fukui S, Ohseto K, Shiotani M. Patterns of pain induced by distending the thoracic zygapophyseal joints. *Reg Anesth.* 1997;22:332-336.
49. Young B, Gill H, Wainner R, Flynn T. Thoracic costotransverse joint pain patterns: a study in normal volunteers. *BMC Musculoskelet Disord.* 2008;9:140.
50. Dwyer A, Aprill C, Bogduk N. Cervical zygapophyseal joint pain patterns. I: a study in normal volunteers. *Spine.* 1990;15:453-457.
51. Aprill C, Dwyer A, Bogduk N. Cervical zygapophyseal joint pain patterns. II: a clinical evaluation. *Spine.* 1990;15:458-461.
52. Slipman CW, Plastaras C, Patel R, et al. Provocative cervical discography symptom mapping. *Spine J.* 2005;5:381-388.
53. Schellhas KP, Smith MD, Gundry CR, Pollei SR. Cervical discogenic pain. Prospective correlation of magnetic resonance imaging and discography in asymptomatic subjects and pain sufferes. *Spine.* 1996;21:300-312.
54. Hassett G, Barnsley L. Pain referral from the sternoclavicular joint: a study in normal volunteers. *Rheumatology.* 2001;40:859-862.
55. Ostelo RWJG, de Vet HCW. Clinically important outcomes in low back pain. *Best Pract Res. Clin Rheum.* 2005;19:593-607.
56. Ostelo RWJG, Deyo RA, Stratford P, et al. Interpreting change scores for pain and functional status in low back pain. Toward international consensus regarding minimal important change. *Spine.* 2008;33:90-94.
57. Maitland GD. *Vertebral Manipulation.* 6th ed. Woburn, MA: Butterworth-Heinemann; 2002.
58. Goodman CC, Fuller KS. *Pathology. Implications for the Physical Therapist.* 3rd ed. St Louis, MO: Saunders; 2009.
59. Boissonnault WG. Patient health history including identification of health risk factors. In: Boissonnault WG, ed. *Primary Care for the Physical Therapist. Examination and Triage.* Philadelphia, PA: Saunders; 2005:70.

60. Idler EL, Benyamini Y. Self-rated health and mortality: a review of twenty-seven community studies. *J Health Soc Behav.* 1997;38:21-37.
61. Idler EL, Russell LB, Davis D. Survival, functional limitations, and self-rated health in the NHANES I Epidemiologic Follow-up Study 1992; First National Health and Nutrition Examination Survey. *Am J Epidemiol.* 2000;9:874-883.
62. Kopec JA, Schultz SE, Goel V, Williams JI. Can the Health Utilities Index measure change? *Medical Care.* 2001;39:562-574.
63. Kopec JA, Sayre EC, Esdaile JM. Predictors of back pain in a general population cohort. *Spine.* 2004;29:70-77.
64. Hagen KB, Tambs K, Bjerkedal T. A prospective cohort study of risk factors for disability retirement because of back pain in the general working population. *Spine.* 2002;27:1790-1796.
65. Rubin DL. Epidemiology and risk factors for spine pain. *Neurol Clin.* 2007;25:353-371.
66. US Department of Health and Human Services. *How Tobacco Smoke Causes Disease: The Biology and Behavioral Basis for Smoking-Attributable Disease. A Report of the Surgeon General.* Atlanta, GA: US Department of Health and Human Services, Centers for Disease Control and Prevention, National Center for Chronic Disease Prevention and Health Promotion, Office on Smoking and Health; 2010.
67. US Department of Health and Human Services. *The Health Consequences of Smoking: A Report of the Surgeon General.* Atlanta, GA: US Department of Health and Human Services, Centers for Disease Control and Prevention, National Center for Chronic Disease Prevention and Health Promotion, Office on Smoking and Health; 2004.
68. Vismara L, Menegoni F, Zaina F, Galli M, Negrini S, Capodaglio P. Effect of obesity and low back pain on spinal mobility: a cross sectional study in women. *J Neuroeng Rehabil.* 2010;7:3.
69. Billek-Sawhney B, Sawhney R. Cardiovascular considerations in outpatient orthopedic physical therapy [abstract]. *J Orthop Sports Phys Ther.* 1998;27:57.
70. Scherer SA, Noteboom JT, Flynn TW. Cardiovascular assessment in the orthopaedic practice setting. *J Orthop Sports Phys Ther.* 2005;35:730-737.
71. Chou R, Huffman LH. Medications for acute and chronic low back pain: a review of the evidence for an American Pain Society/American College of Physicians Clinical Practice Guideline. *Ann Intern Med.* 2007;147:505-514.
72. Luo X, Pietrobon R, Curtis LH, Hey LA. Prescription of nonsteroidal anti-inflammatory drugs and muscle relaxants for back pain in the United States. *Spine.* 2004;29:E531-E537.
73. Luo X, Pietrobon R, Hey L. Patterns and trends in opioid use among individuals with back pain in the United States. *Spine.* 2004;29:884-890; discussion 891.
74. Bernstein E, Carey TS, Garrett JM. The use of muscle relaxant medications in acute low back pain. *Spine.* 2004;29:1346-1351.
75. Verbeek J, Sengers M, Riemens L, Haafkens J. Patient expectations of treatment for back pain. *Spine.* 2004;26:2504-2513.
76. Wilson IB, Dukes K, Greenfield S, Kaplan S, Hillman B. Patients' role in the use of radiology testing for common office practice complaints. *Arch Intern Med.* 2001;16:256-263.
77. Ash LM, Modic MT, Obushowski NA, Ross JS, Brant-Zawadzki MN, Grooff PN. Effects of diagnostic information, per se, on patient outcomes in acute radiculopathy and low back pain. *Am J Neuroradiol.* 2008;29:1098-1103.
78. Gilbert FJ, Grant Am, Gillan MG, et al. Low back pain: influence of early MR imaging or CT on treatment and outcomes—multicenter randomized trial. *Radiology.* 2004;231:343-351.
79. Kendrick D, Fielding K, Bentley E, Kerslake R, Miller P, Pringle M. Radiography of the lumbar spine in primary care patients with low back pain: randomized controlled trial. *BMJ.* 2001;322:400-405.
80. Kerry S, Hilton S, Dundas D, Rink E, Oakeshott P. Radiography for low back pain: a randomized controlled trial and observational study in primary care. *Br J Gen Pract.* 2002;52:469-474.
81. Lurie JD, Birkmeyer NJ, Weinstein JN. Rates of advanced spinal imaging and spine surgery. *Spine.* 2003;28:616-620.
82. Bussieres AE, Taylor JA, Peterson C. Diagnostic imaging practice guidelines for musculoskeletal complaints in adults—an evidence-based approach—part 3: spinal disorders. *J Manipulative Physiol Ther.* 2008;31(1):33-88.
83. The North American Menopause Society (NAMS). Management of osteoporosis in postmenopausal women: 2010 position statement of The NAMS. *Menopause.* 2010;17(1):25-54.
84. World Health Organization. WHO fracture risk assessment tool. *FRAX.* http://www.shef.ac.uk/FRAX. Accessed May 6, 2011.
85. Deyo RA, Diehl AK. Lumbar spine films in primary care: current use and effects of selective ordering criteria. *J Gen Intern Med.* 1986;1:20-25.
86. Atlas SJ, Deyo RA. Evaluating and managing acute low back pain in the primary care setting. *J Gen Intern Med.* 2001;16:120-131.
87. Refshauge KM, Maher CG. Low back pain investigations and prognosis: a review. *Br J Sports Med.* 2006;40:494-498.
88. Mondloch MV, Cole DC, Frank JW. Does how you do depend on how you think you'll do? A systematic review of the evidence for a relation between patients' recovery expectations and health outcomes. *Can Med Assoc J.* 2001;165(2):174-179.
89. Myers SS, Phillips RS, Davis RB, et al. patient expectations as predictors of outcome in patients with acute low back pain. *J Gen Intern Med.* 2007;23(2):148-153.
90. American Academy of Orthopaedic Manual Physical Therapists. *Orthopaedic Manual Physical Therapy. Description of Advanced Clinical Practice.* Tallahassee, FL: Author; 2009.
91. Rubinstein SM, van Tulder M. A best-evidence review of diagnostic procedures for neck and low back pain. *Best Pract Res Clin Rheum.* 2008;22:471-482.
92. Bombardier C. Outcomes assessment in the evaluation of treatment of spinal disorders: summary and general recommendations. *Spine.* 2000;225:3100-3103.
93. Zuberbier OA, Kozlowski AJ, Hunt DG, et al. Analysis of convergent and discriminant validity of published lumbar flexion, extension, and lateral flexion scores. *Spine.* 2001;26:472-478.
94. Fritz J, George S. Identifying psychosocial variables in patients with acute work-related low back pain: the importance of fear-avoidance beliefs. *Phys Ther.* 2002;82:973-983.
95. Tubach F, Leclerc A, Landre M, Pietri-Taleb F. Risk factors for sick leave due to low back pain: a prospective study. *J Occup Environ Med.* 2002;44:451-458.
96. Smith M, Russell A, Hodges P. Disorders of breathing and continence have a stronger association with back pain than obesity and physical activity. *Aust J Physiother.* 2006;52:11-16.
97. Roussel N, Nijs J, Truijen S, Vervecken L, Mottram S, Stassijns G. Altered breathing patterns during lumbopelvic motor control tests in chronic low back pain: a case-control study. *Eur Spine J.* 2009;18:1066-1073.
98. Chaitow L. Breathing pattern disorders, motor control, and low back pain. *J Osteopath Med.* 2004;7:34-41.
99. Miner JR, Heegaard W, Plummer D. End-tidal carbon dioxide monitoring during procedural sedation. *Acad Emerg Med.* 2002;9:275-280.

100. Lee D, Lee LF. *The Pelvic Girdle. An Integration of Clinical Expertise and Research.* 4th ed. Philadelphia, PA: Churchill Livingstone; 2011.
101. Hodges PW, Gurfinkel VS, Brumagne S, et al. Coexistence of stability and mobility in postural control: evidence from postural compensation for respiration. *Exp Brain Res.* 2002;144:293-302.
102. Hodges PW, Eriksson AE, Shirley D, et al. Intra-abdominal pressure increases stiffness of the lumbar spine. *J Biomech.* 2005;38:1873-1880.
103. Hodges PW, Gandevia S. Activation of the human diaphragm during a repetitive postural task. *J Physiol.* 2000;522(pt 1):165-175.
104. Maitre B, Similowski T, Derenne JP. Physical examination of the adult patient with respiratory diseases: inspection and palpation. *Eur Respir J.* 1995;8:1584-1593.
105. Cahalin LP, Braga M, Matsuo Y, et al. Efficacy of diaphragmatic breathing in persons with chronic obstructive pulmonarydisease: a review of the literature. *J Cardiopulm Rehabil.* 2002;22:7-21.
106. Allison GT, Kendle K, Roll S, et al. The role of the diaphragm during abdominal hollowing exercises. *Aust J Physiother.* 1998;44:95-102.
107. Comerford MJ, Mottram SL. Functional stability retraining: principles and strategies for managing mechanical dysfunction. *Man Ther.* 2001;6:3-14.
108. 1Van der Hulst M, Vollenbroek-Hutten MM, Rietman JS, Hermens HJ. Lumbar and abdominal muscle activity during walking in subjects with chronic low back pain: support of the "guarding" hypothesis? *J Electromyogr Kinesiol.* 2010;20:31-38.
109. Saunders SW, Coppeiters M, Magarey M, Hodges PW. Low back pain and associated changes in abdominal muscle activation during human locomotion. Paper presented at: Australian Conference of Science and Medicine in Sport; October 6-9, 2004; Alice Springs, Australia.
110. Saunders SW, Rath D, Hodges PW. Postural and respiratory activation of the trunk muscles varies with mode and speed of locomotion. *Gait Posture.* 2004;20:280-290.
111. Silverman SL. The clinical consequences of vertebral compression fracture. *Bone.* 1992;13:S27-S31.
112. Nevitt MC, Ettinger B, Black DM, et al. The association of radiographically detected vertebral fractures with back pain and function: a prospective study. *Ann Intern Med.* 1998;128:793-800.
113. Sinaki M, Brey RH, Hughes CA, et al. Balance disorder and increased risk of falls in osteoporosis and kyphosis: significance of kyphotic posture and muscle strength. *Osteoporos Int.* 2005;16:1004-1010.
114. Cook DJ, Guyatt GH, Adachi JD, et al. Quality of life issues in women with vertebral fractures due to osteoporosis. *Arthritis Rheum.* 1993;36:750-756.
115. Cortet B, Roches E, Logier R, et al. Evaluation of spinal curvatures after a recent osteoporotic vertebral fracture. *Jt Bone Spine.* 2002;69:201-208.
116. Ensrud KE, Black DM, Harris F, et al. Correlates of kyphosis in older women. *J Am Geriatr Soc.* 1997;45:682-687.
117. Lynn SG, Sinaki M, Westerlind KC. Balance characteristics of persons with osteoporosis. *Arch Phys Med Rehabil.* 1997;78:273-277.
118. Liu-Ambrose T, Eng JJ, Khan KM, et al. Older women with osteoporosis have increased postural sway and weaker quadriceps strength than counterparts with normal bone mass: overlooked determinants of fracture risk? *J Gerontol A Biol Sci Med Sci.* 2003;58:862-866.
119. Greig AM, Bennell KL, Briggs AM, Wark JD, Hodges PW. Balance impairment is related to vertebra fracture rather than thoracic kyphosis in individuals with osteoporosis. *Osteoporos Int.* 2007;18:543-551.
120. Schenkman M, Shipp KM, Chandler J, et al. Relationships between mobility of axial structures and physical performance. *Phys Ther.* 1996;76:276-285.
121. Ryan SD, Fried LP. The impact of kyphosis on daily functioning. *J Am Geriatr Soc.* 1997;45:1479-1486.
122. Balzini L, Vannucchi L, Benvenuti F, et al. Clinical characteristics of flexed posture in elderly women. *J Am Geriatr Soc.* 2003;51:1419-1426.
123. Hirose D, Ishida K, Nagano Y, et al. Posture of the trunk in the sagittal plane is associated with gait in community-dwelling elderly population. *Clin Biomech.* 2004;19:57-63.
124. Katzman WB, VIttinghoff E, Ensrud K, Black DM, Kado DM. Increasing kyphosis predicts worsening mobility in older community-dwelling women: a prospective cohort study. *J Am Geriatr Soc.* 2011;59:96-2011.
125. Greendale GA, Nili NS, Huang MH, Seeger L, Karlamangla AS. The reliability and validity of three non-radiological measures of thoracic kyphosis and their relations to the standing radiological Cobb angle. *Osteoporos Int.* 2011;22(6):1897-1905.
126. Page P, Frank C, Lardner R. *Assessment and Treatment of Muscle Imbalance. The Janda Approach.* Champaign, IL: Human Kinetics; 2010.
127. Janda V. Muscles and cervicogenic pain syndromes. In: Grant R, ed. *Physical Therapy of the Cervical and Thoracic Spine.* New York, NY: Churchill Livingstone; 1988:159-161.
128. Murray PM, Weinstein SL, Spratt KF. The natural history and long-term follow-up of Scheuermann kyphosis. *J Bone Joint Surg Am.* 1993;75:236-248.
129. Di Bari M, Chiarlone M, Matteuzzi D, et al. Thoracic kyphosis and ventilator dysfunction in unselected older persons: an epidemiological study in Dicomano, Italy. *J Am Geriatr Soc.* 2004;52:909-915.
130. Cleland JA, Mintken PE, Carpenter K, et al. Examination of a clinical prediction rule to identify patients with neck pain likely to benefit from thoracic spine thrust manipulation and a general cervical range of motion exercise: multi-center randomized clinical trial. *Phys Ther.* 2010;90:1239-1250.
131. Lau KT, Cheung KY, Chan KB, Chan MH, Lo KY, Chiu TTW. Relationships between sagittal postures of thoracic and cervical spine, presence of neck pain, neck pain severity and disability. *Man Ther.* 2010;15:457-462.
132. Bullock MP, Foster NE, Wright CC. Shoulder impingement: the effect of sitting posture on shoulder pain and range of motion. *Man Ther.* 2005;10:28-37.
133. Lewis JS, Wright C, Green A. Subacromial impingement syndrome: the effect of changing posture on shoulder range of movement. *J Orthop Sports Phys Ther.* 2005;35(2):72-87.
134. Griegel-Morris P, Larson K, Mueller-Klaus K, Oatis CA. Incidence of common postural abnormalities in the cervical, shoulder, and thoracic regions and their association with pain in two age groups of healthy subjects. *Phys Ther.* 1992;72:425-432.
135. Fon GT, Pitt MJ, Thies AC. Thoracic kyphosis: range in normal subjects. AJR Am J Roentgenol. 1980;134:979-983.
136. Cobb RJ. Outline for the study of scoliosis. *Am Acad Orthop Surg.* 1948;5:261-275.
137. Bartynski WS, Heller MT, Grahovac SZ, Rothfus WE, Kurs-Lasky M. Severe thoracic kyphosis in the older patient in the absence of vertebral fracture: association of extreme curve with age. *AJNR Am J Neuroradiol.* 2005;26:2077-2085.

138. Cleland JA, Childs JD, Fritz JM, Whitman JM. Interrater reliability of the history and physical examination in patients with mechanical neck pain. *Arch Phys Med Rehabil.* 2006;87:1388-1395.
139. Chow RK, Harrison JE. Relationship of kyphosis to physical fitness and bone mass on post-menopausal women. *Am J Phys Med.* 1987;66:219-227.
140. Kado DM, Huang M-H, Barrett-Connor E, Greendale GA. Hyperkyphotic posture and poor physical functional ability in older community-dwelling men and women: the Rancho Bernardo Study. *J Geront A.* 2005;60:633-637.
141. Greendale GA, Huang M-H, Karlamangla AS, Seeger L, Crawford S. Yoga decreases kyphosis in senior women and men with adult-onset hyperkyphosis: results of a randomized controlled trial. *J Am Geriatr Soc.* 2009;57:1569-1579.
142. MacIntyre JN, Bennett L, Bonnyman AM, Stratford PW. Optimizing reliability of digital inclinometer and flexicurve rule measures of spine curvatures in postmenopausal women with osteoporosis of the spine: an illustration of the use of generalizability theory. *ISRN Rheumatol.* 2011;2011:571698.
143. Lewis JS, Valentine RE. Clinical measurement of the thoracic kyphosis. A study of the intra-rater reliability in subjects with and without shoulder pain. *BMC Musculoskelet Disord.* 2010;11:39.
144. Theodoridis D, Ruston S. The effect of shoulder movements on thoracic spine 3D motion. *Clin Biomech (Bristol Avon).* 2002;17:418-421.
145. Crosbie J, Kilbreath SL, Hollmann L, York S. Scapulohumeral rhythm and associated spinal motion. *Clin Biomech (Bristol Avon).* 2008;23:184-192.
146. Crawford HJ, Jull GA. The influence of thoracic posture and movement on range of arm elevation. *Physiother Theory Pract.* 1993;9:143-148.
147. Stewart S, Jull GA, Ng JK-F, Willems JM. An initial analysis of thoracic spine movement during unilateral arm elevation. *J Man Manip Ther.* 1995;3:15-20.
148. Edmonston SJ, Singer KP. Thoracic spine: anatomical and biomechanical considerations for manual therapy. *Man Ther.* 1997;2:132-143.
149. Moll JMH, Wright V. An objective clinical study of chest expansion. *Ann Rheum Dis.* 1972;31:1-8.
150. Bennett PH, Burch TA. New York symposium on population studies in the rheumatic diseases: new diagnostic criteria. *Bull Rheum Dis.* 1967;17:453-458.
151. Bockenhauer SE, Haifan C, Julliard KN, Weedon J. Measuring thoracic excursion: reliability of the cloth measure technique. *J Am Osteopath Assoc.* 2007;107(5):191-196.
152. Hsu CH, Change YW, Chou WY, Chiou CP, Change WN, Wong CY. Measurement of spinal range of motion in healthy individuals using an electromagnetic tracing device. *J Neurosurg Spine.* 2008;8:125-142.
153. Lee LJ, Lee D. Integrated, multimodal approach to the thoracic spine and ribs. In: Magee DJ, Zachazewski JE, Quillen WS, eds. *Pathology and Intervention in Musculoskeletal Rehabilitation.* St Louis, MO: Saunders Elsevier; 2009:306-337.
154. Lee LJ. Is it time for a closer look at the thorax? *MPA in Touch.* 2008;1:13-16.
155. Lee LJ, Coppieters MW, Hodges PW. Differential activation of the thoracic multifidus and longissimus thoracis during trunk rotation. *Spine.* 2005;30:870-876.
156. Lee CN, Robbins DP, Roberts HJ, et al. Reliability and validity of single inclinometer measurements for thoracic spine range of motion. *Physiother Can.* 2003;55(2):73-78.
157. Scoliosis Research Society. Adolescent idiopathic scoliosis. *Scoliosis Research Society (SRS).* http://www.srs.org/professionals/conditions_and_treatment/adolescent_idiopathic_scoliosis/index.htm. Accessed June 22, 2011.
158. Magarey ME. Examination of the cervical and thoracic spine. In: Grant R, ed. *Physical Therapy of the Cervical and Thoracic Spine.* 2nd ed. New York, NY: Churchill Livingstone; 1994:125.
159. McKenzie R, May S. *The Cervical and Thoracic Spine Mechanical Diagnosis and Therapy.* Vol 2. Raumati Beach, New Zealand: Spinal Publications; 2006.
160. McKenzie R, May S. *The Cervical and Thoracic Spine. Mechanical Diagnosis and Therapy.* Vol 1. Raumati Beach, New Zealand: Spinal Publications; 2006.
161. Edwards BC. Combined movements of the lumbar spine: examination and clinical significance. *Aust J Physiother.* 1979;25:147-152.
162. Lee LJ. A clinical test for failed load transfer in the upper quadrant: how to direct treatment decisions for the thoracic spine, cervical spine, and shoulder complex. Paper presented at: 2005 Orthopaedic Symposium of the Canadian Physiotherapy Association; October 28-30, 2005; London, ON, Canada.
163. Kibler WB, Sciascia A. Shoulder injuries in athletes. Current concepts: scapular dyskinesis. *Br J Sports Med.* 2010;44:300-305.
164. Lee LJ, Coppieters MW, Hodges PW. Anticipatory postural adjustments to arm movement reveal complex control of paraspinal muscles in the thorax. *J Electromyogr Kinesiol.* 2009;19:46-54.
165. Maitland G, Hengeveld E, Banks K, English K. *Maitland's Vertebral Manipulation.* 6th ed. Boston, MA: Butterworth-Heinemann; 2002.
166. Bourdillon JF, Day EA, Bookhout MR. *Spinal Manipulation.* 5th ed. London, England: Butterworth-Heinemann; 1992.
167. Brismée JM, Gipson D, Ivie D, et al. Interrater reliability of a passive physiological intervetebral motion test in the mid-thoracic spine. *J Manipulative Physiol Ther.* 2006;29:368-373.
168. Christensen HW, Vach W, Vach K, et al. Palpation of the upper thoracic spine: an observer reliability study. *J Manipulative Physiol Ther.* 2002;25:285-292.
169. Haas M, Raphael R, Panzer D. Reliability of manual end-play palpation of the thoracic spine. *Chiropr Tech.* 1995;7:6786-6792.
170. National Institute of Neurological Disorders and Stroke. NINDS complex regional pain syndrome information page. *National Institute of Neurological Disorders and Stroke.* http://www.ninds.nih.gov/disorders/reflex_sympathetic_dystrophy/reflex_sympathetic_dystrophy.htm. Updated June 26, 2013. Accessed May 27, 2011.
171. Slater H. Sympathetic nervous system and pain: a reappraisal. In: Grant R, ed. *Physical Therapy of the Cervical and Thoracic Spine.* 3rd ed. St Louis, MO: Churchill Livingstone; 2002:295-319.
172. Slater H, Vicenzino B, Wright A. "Sympathetic slump": the effect of a novel manual therapy technique on peripheral sympathetic nervous system function. *J Man Manip Ther.* 1994;2(4):156-162.
173. Butler DS, Slater H. Neural injury in the thoracic spine: a conceptual basis for manual therapy. In: Grant R, ed. *Physical Therapy of the Cervical and Thoracic Spine.* 3rd ed. New York, NY: Churchill Livingstone; 1994:313-338.
174. Butler DS. *The Sensitive Nervous System.* Adelaide, Australia: NOI Publications; 2000.
175. Cleland J, Durall C, Scott SA. Effects of slump long sitting on peripheral sudomotor and vasomotor function: a pilot study. *J Man Manip Ther.* 2002;10(2):67-75.
176. Cleland J, McRae M. Complex regional pain syndrome I: management through the use of vertebral and sympathetic trunk mobilization. *J Man Manip Ther.* 2002;10(4):188-199.

177. Slater H, Wright A. An investigation of the physiological effects of the sympathetic slump on the peripheral sympathetic nervous system function in patients with frozen shoulder. In: Shacklock M, ed. *Moving in on Pain*. Adelaide, Australia: Butterworth-Heinemann; 1995:174-184.
178. Lindfren K-A, Leino E, Hakola M, Hamberg J. Cervical spine rotation and lateral flexion combined motion in the examination of the thoracic outlet. *Arch Phys Med Rehabil.* 1990;71:343-344.
179. Lindgren KA, Leino E, Manninen H. Cervical rotation lateral flexion test in brachialgia. *Arch Phys Med Rehabil.* 1992;73:735-737.
180. Lindgren KA, Leino E, Manninen H. Cineradiography of the hypomobile first rib. *Arch Phys Med Rehabil.* 1989;70:408-409.
181. Boissonault WG. *Primary Care for the Physical Therapist. Examination and Triage.* 2nd ed. St Louis, MO: Elsevier Saunders; 2011.
182. Christensen HW, Vach W, Manniche C, Haghfelt T, Hartvigsen L, Høilund-Carlsen PF. Palpation of muscular tenderness in the anterior chest wall: an observer reliability study. *J Manipulative Physiol Ther.* 2003;26:469-475.
183. Arroyo JF, Jolliet P, Junod AF. Costovertebral joint dysfunction: another misdiagnosed cause of atypical chest pain. *Postgrad Med J.* 1992;68:655-659.
184. Menck JY, Requejo SM, Kulig K. Thoracic spine dysfunction in upper extremity complex regional pain syndrome type I. *J Orthop Sports Phys Ther.* 2000;30:401-409.
185. Cleland JA, Mintken PE, Carpenter K, et al. Examination of a clinical prediction rule to identify patients with neck pain likely to benefit from thoracic spine thrust manipulation and a general cervical range of motion exercise: multi-center randomized clinical trial. *Phys Ther.* 2010;90:1239-1250.
186. Gregory PL, Biswas AC, Batt ME. Musculoskeletal problems of the chest wall in athletes. *Sports Med.* 2002;32:235-250.
187. Fritz JM, Whitman JM Childs JD. Lumbar spine segmental mobility assessment: an examination oof validity for determining intervention strategies with low bac pain. *Arch Phys Med Rehabil.* 2005;86:1745-1752.
188. Heiderscheit B, Boissonnault W. Reliability of joint mobility and pain assessment of the thoracic spine and rib cage in asymptomatic individuals. *J Man Manip Ther.* 2008;16:210-216.
189. Nomden JG, Slagers AJ, Bergman GJD, Winters JC, Kropmans TJB, Dijkstra PU. Interobserver reliability of physical examination. *Man Ther.* 2009;14:152-159.
190. Smedmark V, Wallin M, Arvidsson I. Inter-examiner reliability in assessing passive intervertebral motion of the cervical spine. *Man Ther.* 2000;5(2):97-101.
191. Lee LJ, Coppieters MW, Hodges PW. En bloc control of deep and superficial thoracic muscles in sagittal loading and unloading of the trunk. *Gait Posture.* 2011;33:588-593.
192. Moseley GL, Hodges PW, Gandevia SC. External perturbation of the trunk in standing humans differentially activates components of the medial back muscles. *J Physiol.* 2003;547(pt 2):581-587.
193. Lee LJ, Coppieters MW, Hodges PW. Differential activation of the thoracic multifidus and longissimus thoracis during trunk rotation. *Spine.* 2005;30:870-876.
194. Amoroso L, Sindle K. Spinal fusion in adolescent idiopathic scoliosis. In: Cioppa-Mosca J, Cahill JB, Cavanaugh JT, Corradi-Scalise D, Rudnick H, Wolff AL. *Postsurgical Rehabilitation Guidelines for the Orthopedic Clinician. Hospital for Special Surgery.* Department of Rehabilitation. St Louis, MO: Mosby, Inc; 2006.
195. Shin S, Yoon D, Yoon KB. Identification of the correct cervical level by palpation of spinous processes [abstract]. *Anesth Analg.* 2011;112:1232-1235.
196. Holmaas G, Frederiksen D, Ulnik A, Vingsnes SO, Østgaard G, Nordli H. Identification of thoracic intervertebral spaces by means of surface anatomy: a magnetic resonance imaging study. *Acta Anaesthesiol Scand.* 2006;50:368-373.
197. Robinson R, Robinson HS, Bjørke G, Kvale A. Reliability and validity of a palpation technique for identifying the spinous processes of C7 and L5. *Man Ther.* 2009;14:409-414.
198. Mitchell FL, Moran PS, Pruzzo NA. *An Evaluation and Treatment Manual of Osteopathic Muscle Energy Procedures.* Valley Park, MO: Mitchell, Moran & Pruzzo, Assoc; 1979.
199. Geelhoed MA, Viti JA, Brewer PA. A pilot study to investigate the validity of the rule of threes of the thoracic spine. *J Man Manip Ther.* 2005;13:23-25.
200. Geelhoed MA, McGaugh J, Brewer PA, Murphy D. A new model fo facilitate palpation of the level of the transverse processes of the thoracic spine. *J Orthop Sports Phys Ther.* 2006;36:876-881.
201. Cornwall J, Mercer S. Thoracic zygapophysial joint palpation. *J Physiother.* 2006;34(2):56-59.
202. Fryer G, Morris T, Gibbons P. The relation between thoracic paraspinal tissues and pressure sensitivity measured by a digital algometer. *Int J Osteopath Med.* 2004;7(2):64-69.
203. Fryer G, Morris T, Gibbons P, Briggs A. The electromyographic activity of thoracic paraspinal muscles identified as abnormal with palpation. *J Manipulative Physiol Ther.* 2006;29:437-447.
204. Haas M, Raphael R, Panzer D. Reliability of manual end-play palpation of the thoracic spine. *Chiropr Tech.* 1995;7:120-124.
205. Christensen HW, Vach W, Manniche C, Hagfelt T, Hartvisger L, Hoilund-Carlsen PF. Palpation of the upper thoracic spine: an observer reliability study. *J Manipulative Physiol Ther.* 2002;25:285-292.
206. American College of Radiology. ACR appropriateness criteria. *ACR—American College of Radiology.* http://www.acr.org/Quality-Safety/Appropriateness-Criteria. Accessed June 4, 2011.
207. Haas M, Panzer D, Peterson DC, Raphael R. Short term responsiveness of manual thoracic end-play assessment to spinal manipulation: a randomized controlled trial of construct validity. *J Manipulative Physiol Ther.* 1995;18:582-589.
208. Gavin D. The effect of joint manipulation techniques on active range of motion in the mid-thoracic spine of asymptomatic subjects. *J Manual Manipulative Ther.* 1999;7:114-122.
209. Lee M, Latimer G, Maher C. Manipulation: Investigation of a proposed mechanism [abstract]. *Clin Biomech.* 1993;8:302-306.
210. Kessler TJ, Brunner F, Kunzer S, Crippa N, Kissling R. Effects of Maitland's manual mobilization on the thoracic spine [abstract]. *Rehabilitation.* 2005;44:361-366.
211. Schiller L. Effectiveness of spinal manipulative therapy in the treatment of mechanical thoracic spine pain: a pilot randomized clinical trial. *J Manipulative Physiol Ther.* 2001;24:394-401.
212. Cleland JA, Glynn P, Whitman JM, Eberhart SL, MacDonald C, Childs JD. Short-term effects of thrust versus nonthrust mobilization/manipulation directed at the thoracic spine in patients with neck pain: a randomized clinical trial. *Phys Ther.* 2007;87:431-440.
213. Bishop MD, Beneciuk JM, George SZ. Immediate reduction in temporal sensory summation after thoracic spinal manipulation. *Spine J.* 2011;11(5):440-446.
214. Senstad O, Leboeuf-Yde C, Borchgrevink C. Frequency and characteristics of side effects of spinal manipulative therapy. *Spine.* 1997;22:435-440.
215. Cagnie B, Vinck E, Beernaert A, Cambier D. How common are side effects of spinal manipulation and can these side effects be predicted? *Man Ther.* 2004;9:151-156.

216. Senstad O, Leboeuf-Yde C, Borchgrevink C. Predictors of side effects to spinal manipulative therapy. *J Manipulative Physiol Ther.* 1996;19:441-445.
217. Sillevis R, Cleland J. Immediate effects of the audible pop from a thoracic spine thrust manipulation on the autonomic nervous system and pain: a secondary analysis of a randomized clinical trial. *J Manipulative Physiol Ther.* 2011;34:37-45.
218. Cleland J, Flynn T, Childs JD, Eberhart S. The audible pop from thoracic spine thrust manipulation and its relation to short-term outcomes in patients with neck pain. *J Man Manip Ther.* 2007;15:143-154.
219. Liebenson C. Self-treatment of mid-thoracic dysfunction: a key link in the body axis—part one. *J Bodyw Mov Ther.* 2001;5:90-98.
220. Liebenson C. Self-treatment of mid-thoracic dysfunction: a key link in the body axis—part two. Treatment. *J Bodyw Mov Ther.* 2001;5:191-195.
221. Vanti C, Ferrari S, Morsillo F, Tosarelli D, Pillastrini P. Manual therapy for non-specific thoracic pain in adults: review of the literature. *J Back Muscloskelet Med.* 2008;21(3):143-152.
222. Grieve GP. Thoracic musculoskeletal problems. In: Boyling J, Palastanga N, eds. *Grieve's Modern Manual Therapy.* 2nd ed. Edinburgh, Scotland: Churchill Livingstone;1994.
223. Mellick GA, Mellick LB. Clinical presentation, quantitative sensory testing, and therapy of 2 patients with fourth thoracic syndrome. *J Maipulative Physiol Ther.* 2006;29:403-408.
224. DeFranca CG, Levine LJ. The T4 syndrome. *J Man Manip Physiol Ther.* 1995;18:34-37.
225. Evans P. The T4 syndrome: some basic science aspects. *Physiotherapy.* 1997;83(4):186-189.
226. Menck JY, Requejo SM, Kulig K. Thoracic spine dysfunction in upper extremity complex regional pain syndrome type I. *J Orthop Sports Phys Ther.* 2000;30:401-409.
227. Siddall PJ, Cousins MJ. Spinal pain mechanisms. *Spine.* 1997;22:98-104.
228. Conroy JL, Schneiders AG. The T4 syndrome. *Man Ther.* 2005;10:292-296.
229. Jowsey P, Perry J. Sympathetic nervous system effects in the hands following a grade III posteroanterior rotator mobilization technique applied to T4: a randomized placebo-controlled trial. *Man Ther.* 2010;15:248-253.
230. Chiu TW, Wright A. To compare the effects of different rates of application of a cervical mobilisation technique on sympathetic outflow to the upper limb in normal subjects. *Man Ther.* 1996;1:198-203.
231. Walser RF, Meserve BB, Boucher TR, et al. The effectiveness of thoracic spine manipulation for management of musculoskeletal conditions: a systematic review and meta-analysis of randomized clinical trials. *J Man Manip Ther.* 2009;17:237-246.
232. Cleland JA, Childs JD, McRae M, Palmer JA, Stowell T. Immediate effects of thoracic manipulation in patients with neck pain: a randomized clinical trial. *Man Ther.* 2005;10:128-135.
233. Cleland JA, Whitman JM, Fritz JM, Palmer JA. Manual physical therapy, cervical traction, and strengthening exercises in patients with cervical radiculopathy: a case series. *J Orthop Sports Phys Ther.* 2005;35:802-811.
234. Cleland JA, Childs JD, Fritz JM, Whitman JM, Eberhart S. Development of a clinical prediction rule for guiding treatment of a subgroup of patients with neck pain: use of thoracic spine manipulation, exercise, and patient education. *Phys Ther.* 2007;87:9-23.
235. Carpenter KJ, Mintken P, Cleland JA. Evaluation of outcomes in patients with neck pain treated with thoracic spine manipulation and exercise: a case series. *N Z J Physiother.* 2009;37:71-80.
236. Fernández-de-las-Peñas C, Fernández-Carnero J, Fernández AP, Lomas-Varga R, Miangolarra-Page JC. Dorsal manipulation in whiplash injury treatment: a randomized controlled trial. *J Whiplash Rel Disord.* 2004;3(2):55-72.
237. Fernández-de-Las-Peñas C, Palomeque-del-Cerro L, Rodríguez-Blanco C, Gómez-Conesa A, Miangolarra-Page JC. Changes in neck pain and active range of motion after a single thoracic spine manipulation in subjects with mechanical neck pain: a case series. *J Manipulative Physiol Ther.* 2007;30:312-320.
238. Browder DA, Erhard RE, Piva SR, et al. Intermittent cervical traction and thoracic manipulation for management of mild cervical compressive myelopathy attributed to cervical herniated disc: a case series. *J Orthop Sports Phys Ther.* 2004;34:701-712.
239. Pho C, Godges JJ. Management of whiplash-associated disorder addressing thoracic and cervical spine impairments: a case report. *J Orthop Sports Phys Ther.* 2004;34:511-523.
240. Walker MJ, Boyles RE, Young BA, et al. The effectiveness of manual physical therapy and exercise for mechanical neck pain. A randomized clinical trial. *Spine.* 2008;33:2371-2388.
241. Costello M. Treatment of a patient with cervical radiculopathy using thoracic spine thrust manipulation, soft tissue mobilization, and exercise. *J Man Manp Ther.* 2008;16(3):129-135.
242. González-Iglesias J, Fernández-de-las-Peñas C, Cleland JA, Gutiérrez-Vega MR. Thoracic spine manipulation for the management of patients with neck pain: a randomized clinical trial. *J Orthop Sports Phys Ther.* 2009;39:20-27.
243. Puentedura EJ, Landers MR, Cleland JA, Mintken PE, Huijbregts P, Fernández-de-Las-Peñas C. Thoracic spine thrust manipulation versus cervical spine thrust manipulation in patients with acute neck pain: a randomized clinical trial. *J Orthop Sports Phys Ther.* 2011;41:208-220.
244. Lau H, Wing Chiu TT, Lam TH. The effectiveness of thoracic manipulation on patients with chronic mechanical neck pain—a randomized controlled trial. *Man Ther.* 2011;16(2):141-147.
245. Gross A, Miller J, D'Sylvia J, et al; the Children's Oncology Group. Manipulation or mobilization for neck pain: a Cochrane Review. *Man Ther.* 2010;15:315-333.
246. Childs JD, Cleland JA, Elliott JM, et al. Neck pain: clinical practice guidelines linked to the International Classification of Functioning, Disability and Health from the Orthopedic Section of the American Physical Therapy Association. *J Orthop Sports Phys Ther.* 2008;38:A1-A34.
247. Brosseau L, Tugwell P, Wells G. Philadelphia Panel evidence-based clinical practice guidelines on selected rehabilitation interventions for neck pain. *Phys Ther.* 2001;81:1701-1717.
248. Sarig-Bahat H. Evidence for exercise therapy in mechanical neck disorders. *Man Ther.* 2003;8:10-20.
249. Bergstrom G, Bodin L, Bertilsson H, Jensen IB. Risk factors for new episodes of sick leave due to neck or back pain in a working population. A prospective study with an 18-month and a three-year follow-up. *Occup Environ Med.* 2007;64:279-287.
250. Chiu TTW, Lam T-H, Hedley AJ. A randomized controlled trial on the efficacy of exercise for patients with chronic neck pain. *Spine.* 2005;30:E1-E7.
251. Erhard RE. *The Spinal Exercise Handbook: A Home Exercise Manual for a Managed Care Environment.* Pittsburgh, PA: Laurel Concepts; 1998.
252. Wainner RS, Fritz JM, Irrgang JJ, Boninger ML, Delitto A, Allison S. Reliability and diagnostic accuracy of the clinical examination and patient self-report measures for cervical radiculopathy. *Spine.* 2003;28:52-62.

253. Bergman G, Winters JC, Groenier KH, et al. Manipulative therapy in addition to usual medical care for patients with shoulder dysfunction and pain: a randomized controlled trial. *Ann Intern Med.* 2004;141:432-439.
254. Bang D, Deyle G. Comparison of supervised exercise with and without manual physical therapy for patients with shoulder impingement syndrome. *J Orthop Sports Phys Ther.* 2000;30(3):126-137.
255. Boyles RE, Ritland B, Miracle BM, et al. The short term effects of thoracic spine thrust manipulation on patients with shoulder impingement syndrome. *Man Ther.* 2009;14:375-380.
256. Strunce JB, Walker MJ, Boyles RE, Young BA. The immediate effects of thoracic spine and rib manipulation on subjects with primary complaints of shoulder pain. *J Man Manip Ther.* 2009;17:230-236.
257. Mintken PE, Cleland JA, Carpenter KJ, Bieniek ML, Keirns M, Whitman JM. Some factors predict successful short-term outcomes in individuals with shoulder pain receiving cervicothoracic manipulation: a single-arm trial. *Phys Ther.* 2010;91(1):26-42.
258. Winters JC, Sobel JS, Groenier KH, Arendzen HJ, Meyboom-de Jong B. Comparison of physiotherapy, manipulation, and corticosteroid injection for treating shoulder complaints in general practice: randomize, single blind study. *BMJ.* 1997;314:1320-1325.
259. Sobel JS, Winters JC, Groenier K, et al. Physical examination of the cervical spine and shoulder girdle in patients with shoulder complaints. *J Manipulative Physiol Ther.* 1997;20:257-262.
260. Norlander S, Aste-Norlander U, Nordgren B, Sahlstedt B. Mobility in the cervicothoracic motion segment: an indicative factor of musculoskeletal neck-shoulder pain. *Scand J Rehabil Med.* 1996;28:183-192.
261. Norlander S, Gustavsson BA, Lindell J, Nordgren B. Reduced mobility in the cervicothoracic motion segment: A risk factor for musculoskeletal neck-shoulder pain: a two-year prospective follow-up study. *Scand J Rehabil Med.* 1997;29:167-174.
262. Norlander S, Nordgren B. Clinical symptoms related to musculoskeletal neck shoulder pain and mobility in the cervicothoracic spine. *Scand J Rehabil Med.* 1998;30:243-251.
263. Hurley MV, Newham KJ. The influence of arthrogenous muscle inhibition on quadriceps rehabilitation or patient with early, unilateral osteoarthritic knees. *Br J Rheumatol.* 1993;32(2):127-131.
264. Hurly MN, Jones DW, Newham DJ. Arthrogenic quadriceps inhibition and rehabilitation of patients with extensive traumatic knee injuries. *Clin Sci.* 1994;86:305-310.
265. Liebler EJ, Tufano-Coors L, Douris P, et al. The effect on thoracic spine mobilization on lower trapezius strength testing. *J Man Manip Ther.* 2001;9:207-212.
266. Cleland JA, Selleck B, Stowell T, et al. Short term effects of thoracic manipulation on lower trapezius strength. *J Man Manip Ther.* 2004;12:82-90.
267. Whitman JM, Flynn TW, Childs JD, et al. A comparison between two physical therapy treatment programs for patients with lumbar spinal stenosis. *Spine.* 2006;31:2541-2549.
268. Sebastian D. Thorocolumbar junction syndrome: a case report. *Physiother Theory Pract.* 2006;22:53-60.
269. Horton SJ. Acute locked thoracic spine: treatment with a modified SNAG. Case report. *Man Ther.* 2002;7(2):103-107.
270. Mulligan BR. *Manual Therapy "NAGS," "SNAGS," MWMs, etc.* 4th ed. Wellington, New Zealand: Plane View Services; 1999.
271. Wilson E. The Mulligan concept: NAGS, SNAGS and mobilizations with ovement. *J Bodyw Mov Ther.* 2001;5(2):81-89.
272. Mulligan Concept. Publications on the Mulligan Concept. *Mulligan Concept.* http://www.bmulligan.com/research/research.html. Updated June 11, 2013. Accessed June 12, 2011.
273. Austin GP, Benesky WT. Thoracic pain in a collegiate runner. *Man Ther.* 2000;7:168-172.
274. Verdon F, Burnand B, Herzig L, Junod M, Pécoud A, Favrat B. *BMC Fam Pract.* 2007;8:51.
275. Flowers LK, Brenner BE. Costochondritis. *Medscape Reference.* http://emedicine.medscape.com/article/808554-overview. Updated April 13, 2012. Accessed April 28, 2011.
276. Fam AG, Smythe HA. Musculoskeletal chest wall pain. *CMAJ.* 1985;133:379-389.
277. Udermann BE, Cavanaugh DG, Gibson MH, Doberstein ST, Mayer JM, Murray SR. Slipping rib syndrome in a collegiate swimmer: a case report. *J Athl Train.* 2005;40(2):120-122.
278. Kelley JL, Whitney SL. The use of nonthrust manipulation in an adolescent for the treatment of thoracic pain and rib dysfunction: a case report. *J Orthop Sports Phys Ther.* 2006;36:887-892.
279. Brismée J, Phelps V, Sizer P. Differential diagnosis and treatment of chronic neck and upper trapezius pain and upper extremity paresthesia: a case study involving the management of an elevated first rib and uncovertebral joint dysfunction. *J Man Manip Ther.* 2005;13(2):79-90.
280. Watson LA, PIzzari, Balster S. Thoracic outlet syndrome part 1: clinical manifestations, differentiation and treatment pathways. *Man Ther.* 2009;14:586-595.
281. Watson LA, Pizzari T, Balster S. Thoracic outlet syndrome part 2: conservative management of thoracic outlet. *Man Ther.* 2010;15:305-314.
282. Mackinnon SE, Novak CB. Thoracic outlet syndrome. *Curr Probl Surg.* 2002;39:1070-1145.
283. Aspegren D, Hyde T, Miller M. Conservative treatment of a female collegiate volleyball player with costochondritis. *J Manipulative Physiol Ther.* 2007;30:321-325.
284. Graston Technique. About Graston Technique. *Graston Technique.* http://www.grastontechnique.com/AboutUs/ASynopsis.html. Accessed June 16, 2011.
285. Kinesio Taping Association International. Kinesio Taping. *Kinesio.* http://www.kinesiotaping.com. Accessed June 16, 2011.
286. Crothers A, Walker B, French SD. Spinal manipulative therapy versus Graston Technique in the treatment of non-specific thoracic spine pain: design of a randomized controlled trial. *Chriopr Osteopat.* 2008;16:12.
287. Rabey MI. Costochondritis: are symptoms and signs due to neurogenic inflammation. Two cases that responded to manual therapy directed towards posterior spinal structures. *Man Ther.* 2008;13:82-86.
288. Gijsbers E, Knaap SF. Clinical presentation and chiropractic treatment of Tietze's syndrome: a 34-year-old female with left-sided chest pain. *J Chiropr Med.* 2011;10:60-63.
289. Fruth SJ. Differential diagnosis and treatment in a patient with posterior upper thoracic pain. *Phys Ther.* 2006;86:254-268.
290. Travell JG, Simons GS. *Myofascial Pain and Dysfunction: The Trigger Point Manual.* Baltimore, MD: Williams & Wilkins; 1983.
291. Grieve GP. *Common Vertebral Joint Problems.* 2nd ed. Edinburgh, Scotland: Churchill Livingstone; 1988.
292. Boyle JJW. Is the pain and dysfunction of shoulder impingement lesion resally second rib syndrome in disguise? Two case reports. *Man Ther.* 1999;4:44-48.

293. El-Ansary D, Waddington G, Adams R. Trunk stabilization exercises reduce sternal separation in chronic sternal instability after cardiac surgery: a randomized cross-over trial. *Aust J Physiother.* 2007;53:255-260.
294. Nee RJ, Butler D. Management of peripheral neuropathic pain: integrating neurobiology neurodynamics, and clinical evidence. *Phys Ther Sport.* 2006;7:36-49.
295. National Institute of Neurological Disorders and Stroke. Complex regional pain syndrome fact sheet. *National Institute of Neurological Disorders and Stroke.* http://www.ninds.nih.gov/disorders/reflex_sympathetic_dystrophy/detail_reflex_sympathetic_dystrophy.htm. Updated June 26, 2013. Accessed June 16, 2011.
296. De Jong JR, Vlaeyen JW, Onghena P, Cuypers C, Den Hollander M, Ruijgrok J. Reduction of pain-related fear in complex regional pain syndrome type I: the application of graded exposure in vivo. *Pain.* 2005;116:264-275.
297. National Guideline Clearinghouse. Complex regional pain syndrome/reflex sympathetic dystrophy medical treatment guidelines. *Agency for Healthcare Research and Quality.* http://www.guideline.gov/content.aspx?id=38440. Accessed July 2, 2013.
298. Menck JY, Requejo SM, Kulig K. Thoracic spine dysfunction in upper extremity complex regional pain syndrome type I. *J Orthop Sports Phys Ther.* 2000;30:401-409.
299. Dzwierzynski WW, Sanger JR. Reflex sympathetic dystrophy. *Hand Clin.* 1994;10:29-44.
300. Daqfinrud H, Kvien TK, Hagen KB. Physiotherapy interventions for ankylosing spondylitis. *Cochrane Database Syst Rev.* 2008;(1):CD002822.
301. Aytekin E, Caglar NS, Ozgonenel L, Tutun S, Demiryonatar DY, Demir SE. Home-based exercise therapy in patients with ankylosing spondylitis: effecs on pain, mobility, disease activity, quality of life and respiratory functions. *Clin Rheumatol.* 2012:31(1):91-97.
302. Passalent LA. Physiotherapy for ankylosing spondylitis: evidence and application. *Curr Opin Rheumatol.* 2011;23(2):142-147.
303. Ince G, Sarpel T, Durgun B, Erdogan S. Effects of a multimodal exercise program for people with ankylosing spondylitis. *Phys Ther.* 2006;86:924-935.
304. Fernández-de-las-Peñas C, Alonso-Blanco C, Morales-Cabezas M, Miangolarra-Page JC. Two exercise interventions for the management of patients with ankylosing spondylitis: a randomized controlled trial. *Am J Phys Med Rehabil.* 2005;84:407-419.
305. Fernández-de-las-Peñas C, Alonso-Blanco C, Morales-Cabezas M, Miangolarra-Page JC. One-year follow-up of two exercise interventions for the management of patients with ankylosing spondylitis: a randomized controlled trial. *Am J Phys Med Rehabil.* 2006;85:559-567.
306. Durmuş D, Alayli G, Uzun O, et al. Effects of two exercise interventions on pulmonary functions in the patients with ankylosing spondylitis. *Joint Bone Spine.* 2009;76:150-155.
307. Karapolat H, Eyigor S, Zoghi M, Akkoc Y, Kirazli Y, Keser G. Are swimming or aerobic exercise better than conventional exercise in ankylosing spondylitis patients? A randomized controlled study. *Eur J Phys Rehabil Med.* 2009;45:449-457.
308. Widberg K, Karimi H, Hafström I. Self- and manual mobilization improves spine mobility in men with ankylosing spondylitis—a randomized study. *Clin Rehabil.* 2009;76(2):150-155.
309. Li WC, Chen YC, Yang RS, Tsauo JY. Effects of exercise programmes on quality of life in osteoporotic and osteopenic postmenopausal women: a systematic review and meta-analysis. *Clin Rehabil.* 2009;23:888-896.
310. Liu-Ambrose TYL, Khan KM, Eng JJ, Lord SR, Lentle B, McKay HA. Both resistance and agility training reduce back pain and improve health related quality of life in older women with low bone mass. *Osteoporos Int.* 2005;16:1321-1329.
311. Carter ND, Khan KM, McKay HA, et al. Community-based exercise program reduces risk factors for falls in 65- to 75-year-old women with osteoporosis: randomized controlled trial. *CMAJ.* 2002;167:997-1004.
312. Devereux K, Robertson D, Briffa NK. Effects of a water-based program on women 65 years and over: a randomized controlled trial. *Aust J Physiother.* 2005;51:102-108.
313. Chien MY, Yang RS, Tsauo JY. Home-based trunk-strengthening exercise for osteoporotic and osteopenic postmenopausal women without fracture—a pilot study. *Clin Rehabil.* 2005;19:28-36.
314. Dusdal K, Grundmanis J, Luttin K, et al. Effects of therapeutic exercise for persons with osteoporotic vertebral fractures: a systematic review. *Osteoporos Int.* 2011;22:755-769.
315. Bennell KL, Matthews B, Greig A, et al. Effects of an exercise and manual therapy program on physical impairments, function and quality of life in people with osteoporotic vertebral fracture: a randomised, single-blind controlled pilot trial. *BMC Musculoskelet Disord.* 2010;11:36.
316. Gold DT, Shipp KM, Pieper CF, Duncan PW, Martinez S, Lyles KW. Group treatment improves trunk strength and psychological status in older women with vertebral fractures: results of a randomized, clinical trial. *J Am Geriatr Soc.* 2004;52:1471-1478.
317. Hongo M, Itoi E, Sinaki M, et al. Effect of low-intensity back exercise on quality of life and back extensor strength in patients with osteoporosis: a randomized controlled trial. *Osteoporos Int.* 2007;18:1389-1395.
318. Malmros B, Mortensen L, Jensen MB, Charles P. Positive effects of physiotherapy on chronic pain and performance in osteoporosis. *Osteoporos Int.* 1998;8:215-221.
319. Papaioannou A, Adachi JD, Winegard K, et al. Efficacy of home-based exercise for improving quality of life among elderly women with symptomatic osteoporosis-related vertebral fractures. *Osteoporos Int.* 2003;14:677-682.
320. Stengel SV, Kemmler W, Pintag R, et al. Power training is more effective than strength training for maintaining bone mineral density in postmenopausal women. *J Appl Physiol.* 2005;99:181-188.
321. Stengel S, Kemmler W, Kalender WA, Engelke K, Lauber D. Differential effects of strength versus power training on bone mineral density in postmenopausal women: a 2-year longitudinal study. *Br J Sports Med.* 2007;41:649-655.
322. de Kam D, Smulder E, Weerdesteyn V, Smits-Engelman BCM. Exercise interventions to reduce fall-related fractures and their risk factors in individuals with low bone density: a systematic review of randomized controlled trials. *Osteoporos Int.* 2009;20:2111-2125.
323. Katzman WB, Sellmeyer DE, Stewart AL, Wanek L, Hamel KA. Changes in flexed posture, musculoskeletal impairments, and physical performance after group exercise in community-dwelling older women. *Arch Phys Med Rehabil.* 2007;88:192-199.
324. Sinaki M, Brey R, Hughes C, Larson D, Kaufman K. Significant reduction in risk of falls and back pain in osteoporotic-kyphotic women through a spinal proprioceptive extension exercise dynamic (SPEED) program. *Mayo Clin Proc.* 2005;80:849-855.
325. Sinaki M, Pfeifer M, Preisinger E, et al. The role of exercise in the treatment of osteoporosis. *Curr Osteoporos Rep.* 2010;8(3):138-144.

326. Lips P, Cooper C, Agnusei D, et al. Quality of life in patients with vertebral fractures: validation of the Quality of Life Questionnaire of the European Foundation for Osteoporosis (QUALEFFO). Working party for Quality of life of the European Foundation for Osteoporosis. *Osteoporos Int.* 1999;19(2):150-160.
327. Shipp KM, Purse JL, Gold DT, et al. Timed loaded standing: a measure of combined trunk and arm endurance suitable for people with vertebral osteoporosis. *Osteoporos Int.* 2000;11:914-922.
328. Podsiadlo D, Richardson S. The timed "Up & Go": a test of basic functional mobility for frail elderly persons. *J Am Geriatr Soc.* 1991;39(2):142-148.
329. Bautmans I, Van Arken J, Van Mackelenberg M, Mets T. Rehabilitation using manual mobilization for thoracic kyphosis in elderly postmenopausal patients with osteoporosis. *J Rehabil Med.* 2010;42:129-135.
330. Papaioannou A, Morin S, Cheung AM, et al; Scientific Advisory Council of Osteoporosis Canada. 2010 Clinical Practice Guidelines for the Diagnosis and Management of Osteoporosis in Canada: summary. *CMAJ.* 2010;182:1864-1873.
331. Papaioannou A, Morin S, Cheung AM, et al; Scientific Advisory Council of Osteoporosis Canada. Appendix 1: Background materials for 2010 Clinical Practice Guidelines for the Diagnosis and Management of Osteoporosis in Canada. http://www.cmaj.ca/cgi/data/cmaj.100771/DC1/1. Accessed June 17, 2011.
332. Lau E, Ong K, Kurtz S, et al. Mortality following the diagnosis of a vertebral compression fracture in the Medicare population. *J Bone Joint Surg Am.* 2008;90:1479-1486.
333. Cummings SR, Karpf DB, Harris F, et al. Improvement in spine bonedensity and reduction in risk of vertebral fractures during treatment with antiresorptive drugs. *Am J Med.* 2002;112:281-289.
334. Legroux-Gerot I, Lormeau C, Boutry N, Cotten A, Duquesnoy B, Cortet B. Long-term follow-up of vertebral osteoporotic fractures treated by percutaneous vertebroplasty. *Clin Rheumatol.* 2004;23:310-317.
335. O'Sullivan P. Diagnosis and classification of chronic low back pain disorders: maladaptive movement and motor control impairments as underlying mechanism. *Man Ther.* 2005;10:242-255.
336. McCarthy C, Arnall F, Strimpakos N, Freemont A, Oldham J. The Biopsychosocial classification of non-specific low back pain: a systematic review. *Phys Ther Rev.* 2004;9(1):17-30.
337. Gatchel RJ, Peng YB, Peters ML, Fuchs PN, Turk DC. The biopsychosocial approach to chronic pain: scientific advances and future directions. *Psychol Bull.* 2007;133:581-624.
338. Pfeifer M, Begerow B, Minne HW. Effecs of a new spinal orthosis on posture, trunk strength, and quality of life in women with postmenopausal osteoporosis: a randomized trial. *Am J Phys Med Rehabil.* 2004;83(3):177-186.
339. Lieberman I, Reinhardt MK. Vertebroplasty and kyphoplasty for osteolytic vertebral collapse. *Clin Orthop Rel Res.* 2003;415(suppl):176-186.
340. Zampini JM, Kimball M, Patel K. Percutaneous augmentation of vertebral compression fractures. *Semin Spine Surg.* 2011;23:40-44.
341. Mathis JM, Petri M, Naff N. Percutaneous vertebroplasty treatment of steroid-induced osteoporotic compression fractures. *Arthritis Rheum.* 1998;41:171-175.
342. Barr JD, Barr MS, Lemley TJ, McCann RM. Percutaneous vertebroplasty for pain relief and spinal stabilization. *Spine.* 2000;25:923-928.
343. Cortet B, Cotten A, Boutry N, et al. Percutaneous vertebroplasty in the treatment of osteoporotic vertebral compression fractures: an open prospective study. *J Rheumatol.* 1999;26:2222-2228.
344. Garfin SR, Yuan HA, Reiley MA. New technologies in spine: kyphoplasty and vertebroplasty for the treatment of painful osteoporotic compression fractures. *Spine.* 2001;26:1511-1515.
345. Mehbod A, Aunoble S, LeHuec JC. Vertebroplasty for osteoporotic spine fracture: prevention and treatment. *Eur Spine J.* 2003;12:S155-S162.
346. Lieberman IH, Dudeny S, Reinhart MK, Bell G. Initial outcome and efficacy of "kyphoplasty" in the treatment of painful osteoporotic vertebral compression fractures. *Spine.* 2001;26:1631-1637.
347. Garfin SR, Buckley RA, Ledlie J. Balloon kyphoplasty for symptomatic vertebral body compression fractures results in rapid, significant, and sustained improvements in back pain, function, and quality of life for elderly patients. *Spine.* 2008;31:2213-2220.
348. Kasperk C, Hillmeier J, Noldge G, et al. Treatment of painful vertebral fractures by kyphoplasty in patients with primary osteoporosis: a prospective nonrandomized controlled study. *J Bone Miner Res.* 2005;20:604-612.
349. Crandall D, Slaughter D, Hankins PJ, Moore C, Jerman J. Acute versus chronic vertebral compression fractures treated with kyphoplasty: early results. *Spine J.* 2004;4:418-424.
350. Grafe IA, DaFonseca K, Hillmeier J, et al. Reduction of pain and fracture incidence after kyphoplasty: 1-year outcomes of a prospective controlled trial of patients with primary osteoporosis. *Osteoporos Int.* 2005;16:2005-2012.
351. Voggenreiter G. Balloon kyphoplasty is effective in deformity correction of osteoporotic vertebral compression fractures. *Spine.* 2005;30:2806-2812.
352. Buchbinder R, Osborne RH, Ebeling PR, et al. A randomized trial of vertebroplasty for painful osteoporotic vertebral fractures. *N Engl J Med.* 2009;361:557-568.
353. Kallmes DF, Comstock BA, Heagerty PJ, et al. A randomized trial of vertebroplasty for osteoporotic spinal fractures. *N Engl J Med.* 2009;361:569-579.
354. Berenson J, Pflugmacher R, Jarzem P, et al. Balloon kyphoplasty versus non-surgical fracture management for treatment of painful vertebral body compression fractures in patients with cancer: a multicentre randomized controlled trial. *Lancet Oncol.* 2011;12:225-235.
355. Jensen ME, Evans AJ, Mathis JM, Kallmes DF, Cloft HJ, Dion JE. Percutaneous polymethylmethacrylate vertebroplasty in the treatment of osteoporotic vertebral body compression fractures: technical aspects. *Am J Neuroradiol.* 1997;18:1897-1904.
356. Truumees E, Hilibrand A, Vaccaro AR. Percutaneous vertebral augmentation. *Spine J.* 2004;4:218-229.
357. Chen JK, Le HM, Shih JT, Hung ST. Combined extraforaminal and intradiscal cement leakage following percutaneous vertebroplasty. *Spine.* 2007;32:E358-E362.
358. Patel AA, Vaccaro AR, Martyak GG, et al. Neurologic deficit following percutaneous vertebral stabilization. *Spine.* 2007;32:1728-1734.
359. Fribourg D, Tang C, Sra P, Delamarter R, Bae H. Incidence of subsequent vertebral fracture after kyphoplasty. *Spine.* 2004;29:2270-2276.
360. Harrop JS, Prpa B, Reinhardt MK, Lieberman I. Primary and secondary osteoporosis' incidence of subsequent vertebral compression fractures after kyphoplasty. *Spine.* 2004;29:2120-2125.

361. Mudano AS, Bian J, Cope JU, et al. Vertebroplasty and kyphoplasty are associated with an increased risk of secondary vertebral compression fractures: a population-based cohort study. *Osteoporos Int.* 2009;20:819-826.
362. McGraw JK, Cardella J, Barr JD, et al. Society of Interventional Radiology quality improvement guidelines for percutaneous vertebroplasty. *J Vasc Interv Radiol.* 2003;14:311-315.
363. Masala S, Fiori R, Massari F, Simonetti G. Kyphoplasty: indication, contraindications and technique [abstract]. *Radiol Med.* 2005;110:97-105.
364. ACR-ASNR-ASSR-SIR-SNIS Practice Guideline for the Performance of Vertebral Augmentation. Revised 2012. http://www.asnr.org/sites/default/files/guidelines/Vertebral_Augmentation.pdf. Accessed July 2, 2013.
365. Esses SI, McGuire R, Jenkins J, et al. The treatment of symptomatic osteoporotic spinal compression fractures. *J Am Acad Orthop Surg.* 2011;19:176-182.
366. Singh MK, Siegal JA. Percutaneous vertebroplasty. *Medscape Reference.* http://emedicine.medscape.com/article/1145447-overview#a1. Updated June 26, 2012. Accessed June 21, 2011.
367. Evans AJ, Jensen ME, Kip KE, et al. Vertebral compression fractures: pain reduction and improvement in functional mobility after percutaneous polymethylmethacrylate vertebroplasty—retrospective report of 245 cases. *Radiology.* 2003;226:366-372.
368. McGraw JK, Lippert JA, Minkus KD, Rami PM, Davis TM, Budzik RF. Prospective evaluation of pain and relief of 100 patients undergoing percutaneous vertebroplasty: results and follow-up. *J Vasc Interv Radiol.* 2002;13:883-886.
369. Chen LH, Niu CC, Yu SW, Fu TS, Lai PL, Chen WJ. Minimally invasive treatment of osteoporotic vertebral compression fracture. *Chang Gung Med J.* 2004;27:261-267.
370. Lad SP, Patil CG, Lad EM, Hayden MG, Boakye M. National trends in vertebral augmentation procedures for the treatment of vertebral compression fractures [abstract]. *Surg Neurol.* 2008;71:580-584.
371. Spivak JM, Johnson MG. Percutaneous treatment of vertebral body pathology. *J Am Acad Orthop Surg.* 2005;13:6-17.
372. Cahoj P, Cook J, Robinson B. Efficacy of percutaneous vertebral augmentation and use of physical therapy intervention following vertebral compression fractures in older adults: a systematic review. *J Geriatr Phys Ther.* 2007;30:31-40.
373. Faciszewski T, Winter RB, Lonstein JE, Denis F, Johnson L. The surgical and medical perioperative complications of anterior spinal fusion surgery in the thoracic and lumbar spine in adults. A review of 1223 procedures. *Spine.* 1995;20:1592-1599.
374. Landreneau RJ, Hazelrigg SR, Mack MJ, et al. Postoperative pain-related morbidity: video-assisted thoracic surgery versus thoracotomy. *Ann Thorac Surg.* 1993;56:1285-1289.
375. McDonnell MF, Glassman SD, Dimar JR II, Puno RM, Johnson JR. Perioperative complications of anterior procedures on the spine. *J Bone Joint Surg Am.* 1996;78:839-847.
376. Kawaguchi Y, Matsui H, Tsuji H. Back muscle injury after posterior lumbar spine surgery. A histologic and enzymatic analysis. *Spine.* 1996;21:941-944.
377. Kawaguchi Y, Matsui H, Tsuji H. Back muscle injury after posterior lumbar spine surgery. Part 1: histologic and histochemical analyses in rats. *Spine.* 1994;19:2590-2597.
378. Kawaguchi Y, Matsui H, Tsuji H. Back muscle injury after posterior lumbar spine surgery. Part 2: histologic and histochemical analyses in humans. *Spine.* 1994;19:2598-2602.
379. Kawaguchi Y, Yabuki S, Styf J, et al. Back muscle injury after posterior lumbar spine surgery. Topographic evaluation of intramuscular pressure and blood flow in the porcine back muscle during surgery. *Spine.* 1996;21:2683-2688.
380. Styf JR, Willén J. The effects of external compression by three different retractors on pressure in the erector spine muscles during and after posterior lumbar spine surgery in humans. *Spine.* 1998;23:354-358.
381. Jackson RK. The long-term effects of wide laminectomy for lumbar disc excision. A review of 130 patients. *J Bone Joint Surg Br.* 1971;53:609-616.
382. Macnab I, Cuthbert H, Godfrey CM. The incidence of denervation of the sacrospinalis muscles following spinal surgery. *Spine.* 1977;2:294-298.
383. Mayer TG, Vanharanta H, Gatchel RJ, et al. Comparison of CT scan muscle measurements and isokinetic trunk strength in postoperative patients. *Spine.* 1989;14:33-36.
384. Rampersaud YR, Annand N, Dekutoski MB. Use of minimally invasive surgical techniques in the management of thoracolumbar trauma: current concepts. *Spine.* 2006;31(11 suppl):S96-S104.
385. Rantanen J, Hurme M, Falck B, et al. The lumbar multifidus muscle five years after surgery for a lumbar intervertebral disc herniation. *Spine.* 1993;18:568-574.
386. Dickman CA, Rosenthal D, Karahalios DG, et al. Thoracic vertebrectomy and reconstruction using a microsurgical thoracoscopic approach. *Neurosurgery.* 1996;38:279-293.
387. Huang TJ, Hsu RW, Sum CW, Liu HP. Complications in thoracoscopic spinal surgery: a study of 90 consecutive patients. *Surg Endosc.* 1999;13:346-350.
388. McAfee PC, Regan JR, Zdeblick T, et al. The incidence of complications in endoscopic anterior thoracolumbar spinal reconstructive surgery. A prospective multicenter study comprising the first 100 consecutive cases. *Spine.* 1995;20:1624-1632.
389. Smith JS, Ogden AT, Fessler RG. Minimally invasive posterior thoracic fusion. *Neurosurg Focus.* 2008;25(2):E9.
390. Schenk RJ, Wise, CH. Cervical and Thoracic Spine: Postoperative Management. In: Independent Study Course 21.1.6. Cervical and Thoracic Pain: Evidence for Effectiveness of Physical Therapy. Orthopaedic Section, APTA, Inc; 2011.

Please visit www.routledge.com/9781556429323 to access additional material.

Chapter 6

Evidence-Based Physical Therapy Practice for Neck Pain

Introduction

Neck pain is a commonly reported area of pain and disability. In fact, most people will experience some neck pain in their lifetime.[1] Twelve-month prevalence estimates, or the number of people in a given population who have neck pain at a specific point in time, range from about 22% to 70% in the general population[2-6] and 27% to 48% in workers.[1] Fortunately, for most individuals, neck pain will not seriously interrupt daily activity.[1] With 54% of the population reporting pain in the last 6 months, only 10% to 20% will report neck pain that is currently affecting their lives.[2,3,7-9] Neck pain is more prevalent among those performing repetitive static or demanding physical work, those with previous neck trauma, and those with comorbidities such as depression, headache, and low back pain (LBP). Patients with neck pain make up about 25% of all patients seen in outpatient physical therapy (PT).[10]

Similar to LBP, the etiology of neck pain and associated risk factors are multifactorial and both physical and psychosocial in nature.[1] Neck pain increases in incidence with age, peaking in the middle years and declining with older age.[1] Headache associated with neck pain also increases with age.[11] Fourteen to 18% of chronic headaches are cervicogenic in origin.[12] Age, a history of neck pain, and genetics are considered nonmodifiable risk factors for neck pain.[13] Haldemen et al[1] reported a general physical exercise program, exposure to environmental tobacco, and smoking as modifiable or preventative risk factors. In the working environment, sedentary positions, repetitive or precision work, high job quotas, and low social support are risk factors for the development of neck pain.[1]

Neck pain often coexists with other problems, such as LBP, headache, and poor self-rated health. In patients with neck pain, poor psychological health, poor general health, prior neck pain, and other musculoskeletal complaints are prognostic factors of poor outcome.[14] Common cervical spine degenerative changes found on imaging are not a risk factor and have not been shown to be associated with neck pain.[1] Age greater than 40, coexisting LBP, a longer duration of neck pain, worrisome attitude, poor quality of life, less vitality, bicycling as a regular activity, and loss of strength in the hands are reported as factors predisposing to chronic neck pain.[15] A better prognosis is associated with younger age, optimism, a self-assured coping style, and a reduced need to socialize.[1,14]

The Course of Neck Pain

Generally, functional outcomes for patients are positive,[10,16] but some individuals suffer a high recurrence rate and persistent pain.[14,17,18] A synthesis of best evidence suggests that 50% to 75% of individuals who report neck pain at some point in time will also report neck pain 1 to 5 years later.[14] Studies demonstrate that 37% have pain for at least a year while 14% have pain for at least 6 months, and 5% are disabled.[2,7] Thirty percent of patients with neck pain eventually develop chronic pain.[2] People with work-related neck complaints have similar recurrences. Pransky et al[19] report that 42% of patients with cervical pain missed more than one week of work with a 26% recurrence

Stetts DM, Carpenter JG. *Physical Therapy Management of Patients With Spinal Pain: An Evidence-Based Approach (pp 447-587).*

rate in one year. In patients with whiplash-associated disorder (WAD), 14% to 42% develop persistent symptoms and 10% develop chronic disabling pain.[20] At a mean follow-up of 17 years, 55% of patients (n = 108) with WAD have persistent disability and neck pain, headache, and radiating pain associated with the original trauma.[21] Individuals with persistent symptoms and potential psychosocial issues contribute significantly to healthcare costs. In the United States, the annual management of neck pain is second only to LBP in worker's compensation costs, resulting in a burden not only to the patient, but also to the health care system.[22]

Diagnosis

Similar to low back pain, many potential sources of cervical pain have been identified, but a precise anatomical tissue is not easily or reliably identified as the cause or pain generator in most patients. A pathoanatomical diagnosis of cervical pain is common and consists of labels such as osteoarthritis, degenerative disc or facet disease, and disc herniation or muscle strain, but standardized diagnostic criteria have not been described or validated, and the pathophysiological mechanisms remain unclear. Even with technological advances, degenerative abnormalities on radiographic imaging are not definitive in all cases.

Cervical disc pathology and spinal cord or nerve root impingement may be considered as normal, age-related changes, or the cause of symptoms.[23] A range of abnormalities and degenerative changes on imaging studies are present in asymptomatic individuals. In 30 asymptomatic volunteers, Ernst et al[24] reported that 11 individuals had annular tears at one or more levels (37%), of which 94% enhanced after contrast injection. Four patients (13%) had medullary compression. The prevalence of a bulging disk, focal disk protrusion, and extrusion was 73%, 50%, and 13%, respectively.[24] In subjects ages 45 to 54, Teresi et al[23] reported disc protrusion (ie, herniation or bulge) in 5 of 25 (20%) and in 24 of 42 (57%) subjects older than 64 years. Posterolateral protrusions occur most frequently in subjects over age 64 in only 9 of 100 patients. Impingement of the spinal cord due to disc protrusion was noted in 9 of 58 (16%) subjects less than 64 years of age, and in 11 of 42 (26%) over 64 years of age. The area of spinal cord compression, with an average of 7%, did not exceed 16%.[23] Because degenerative abnormalities are relatively easy to identify on imaging studies, and widely present in the absence of symptoms, pathology itself may be of limited use for determining the cause of the patient's symptoms or the best intervention. Labeling all patients with neck pain by using specific anatomical diagnoses also is not likely to improve outcomes. Yet, specific diagnoses are relevant in many instances such as cancer, infection, cervical myelopathy (CM), and inflammatory or systemic disease. When a pathoanatomical diagnosis of neck pain cannot be made, neck pain and related symptoms are categorized as nonspecific or mechanical neck pain (MNP), and often treated as a homogenous group that excludes medical disease and neurological compromise.

In the development of an evidence-based approach to neck pain management, the assumption that all persons with MNP are equally likely to respond to a particular intervention is not valid. Most clinicians and researchers now recognize that persons with MNP can be classified into subgroups based on patterns of signs and symptoms and/or pathophysiological mechanisms underlying the disorder. Preliminary evidence suggests classifying people with MNP into subgroups with similar characteristics and then, matching those subgroups to the best management strategies result in better PT outcomes when compared to unmatched strategies.[25]

Classification Systems

The Bone and Joint Decade 2000-2010 Task Force on Neck Pain found over 300 definitions for neck pain.[26] MNP, as described by Bogduk[27] over 30 years ago, is pain that may or may not have an identifiable or specific etiology, but that can be provoked by neck movements or provocative tests. One or more of the following signs may be present: pain in the area of the cervical and/or upper thoracic regions, paresthesia or other changes in cutaneous sensation of spinal origin located in the upper thoracic, shoulder, or arms, or possible alterations in reflexes or loss of motor function in the upper extremities originating from the spine.[15] Many factors, such as trauma, injury, stress, or poor posture are thought to either cause or contribute to a diagnosis of MNP.

Bogduk and McGuirk[28] suggested that neck pain may be divided into upper and lower cervical spinal pain with the defining line above or below C4. Pain from upper cervical segments can often refer to the head. From lower cervical segments, pain is often referred to the scapular region, anterior chest wall, shoulder, or upper extremity. These authors also defined suboccipital (SO) pain as located between the superior nuchal line and C2, an area thought to be the source of cervicogenic headache (CGH). The subgrouping of pain into upper and lower cervical regions may be an important aspect for diagnostic classification.[28]

Neck pain and related areas of symptoms of the head, face, trunk, or extremities may be classified based upon duration of symptoms, pathoanatomical structures, clinical patterns, movement impairment, and/or biopsychosocial factors.[15,26,29,30] The neck pain clinical practice guidelines, described by Childs et al[15] and linked to the International Classification of Functioning, Disability, and Health (ICF) by incorporating ICF impairments of body function terminology, suggest the following subgroup classifications with key characteristics (located in summary tables):

TABLE 6-1. NECK PAIN AND MOBILITY DEFICITS CLASSIFICATION SUMMARY

DIAGNOSTIC CLASSIFICATION	*KEY EXAM FINDINGS*	*FACTORS AGAINST*	*INTERVENTION*
Neck pain with mobility deficits ICD-10 terms: • Cervicalgia • Pain in the thoracic spine	• Recent onset of symptoms due to unguarded/awkward movement or position • Unilateral/local neck symptom with or without referred symptoms in the upper quarter o No radicular symptoms • No peripheralization with active/repeated movements • Limited cervical ROM • Pain at end-ranges of AROM/PROM • Restricted cervical and thoracic segmental mobility • Symptoms provoked with cervical and/or thoracic PAIVM and/or PPIVM • Regional impairments: o Mobility o Muscle performance/ length • No signs of nerve root compression • Altered neurodynamics	• Contraindications or precautions to mobilization or manipulation to the cervical or thoracic spine • Peripheralization or centralization of symptoms with active or repeated motion testing • Signs and symptoms of nerve root compromise • Patient expectations	• Thoracic mobilization or manipulation • Cervical mobilization or manipulation • AROM/PROM to augment mobilization/ manipulation • Muscle lengthening exercises • Muscle performance: endurance, coordination, strengthening exercise • Neural mobilization • Address regional and functional/activity limitations

ICD-10 indicates International Classification of Diseases, 10th edition; ROM, range of motion; AROM, active range of motion; PROM, passive range of motion; PAIVM, passive accessory intervertebral movement; PPIVM, passive physiological intervertebral movements.

- Neck pain with mobility deficits (Table 6-1)
- Neck pain with headaches (Table 6-2)
- Neck pain with movement coordination impairment (Table 6-3)
- Neck pain with radiating pain (Table 6-4)

WAD (Tables 6-5 and 6-6) is not included in the clinical practice guidelines.

The classification approach described in this reference pursues an evidence-based strategy by integrating clinical expertise, current best practice guidelines, clinical reasoning, unique patient circumstances related to subgroups of patients with neck pain, and the importance of clinical characteristics which are most likely to respond to optimal PT interventions and improve outcomes. The key characteristics obtained during the history and tests and measures are used to place a patient into a diagnostic classification of neck pain[15,31] and/or the ICF impairment-based category[15] that initially guides PT intervention.

General Overview of the Clinical Manifestations of Neck Pain

Disability and pain noted with MNP vary from a nuisance status with minimal disability to very high disability levels with significant loss of function. Whether

TABLE 6-2. NECK PAIN WITH HEADACHE CLASSIFICATION SUMMARY

DIAGNOSTIC CLASSIFICATION	KEY EXAM FINDINGS	FACTORS AGAINST	INTERVENTION
Neck pain with headache Subtypes (see also Table 6-11): • Cervicogenic • Headache • Tissue-tension headache ICD-10 terms • Headache and cervicocranial syndrome	• Unilateral headache associated with neck/suboccipital area symptoms aggravated by neck movements or positions • Headache produced or aggravated with provocation of the ipsilateral/involved posterior cervical soft tissue and motion segments • Restricted cervical ROM • Upper cervical motion segment dysfunction above C4 (PAIVM, PPIVM) • DNF and upper quarter strength, endurance, and coordination deficits • + Cervical flexion rotation test • Poor performance of the CCFT • Upper quarter muscle flexibility deficits • Active trigger points • Altered neurodynamics	• Headache associated with nonmusculoskeletal cause • Signs of nerve root compression • Patient expectations • Reproduction or worsening of symptoms • Cervical disorders that cannot withstand loading associated with therapeutic exercise	• Cervical spine manipulation or mobilization • Specific motor control • Exercises • Strengthening exercises for upper quarter impairments of strength and endurance • Spinal posture education • Muscle lengthening or soft tissue procedures • Trigger point therapy • Muscle energy techniques

ICD-10 indicates International Classification of Diseases, 10th edition; ROM, range of motion; PAIVM, passive accessory intervertebral movement; PPIVM, passive physiological intervertebral movements; DNF, deep neck flexors; CCFT, craniocervical flexion test.

neck pain is due to microtrauma or macrotrauma, such as WAD, an inflammatory response sets off a series of events that influence both peripheral and central pain processing mechanisms and potentially lead to altered motor, sensory, and autonomic nervous system outputs. The clinical presentation resulting from the body's response to injury varies by stage (ie, acute, subacute, or chronic), mode of onset (ie, insidious or traumatic), and type form (ie, MNP alone, neck pain with upper extremity-related symptoms, or neck pain with CGH).

Altered Sensory Processing

Local cervical mechanical hyperalgesia or a decreased pressure pain threshold has been found in chronic idiopathic neck pain,[32] acute WAD,[33-35] chronic WAD,[36] and CGH.[37] The theoretical cause of the local cervical hyperalgesia may be due to sensitized peripheral nociceptors in cervical structures, or due to central sensitization of nociceptive pathways.[32] In patients who recover or have mild symptoms, local mechanical hyperalgesia resolves, but in moderate to severe WAD with persistent symptoms, local mechanical hyperalgesia continues unchanged at 6 months and 2 years postinjury.[35] Widespread mechanical hyperalgesia may occur in the upper and lower extremities even without complaints in those areas in patients with acute and chronic WAD and cervical radiculopathy (CR) but not in neck pain of insidious onset.[35,38] The widespread sensitivity is probably due to altered nociceptor processing within the central nervous system. Patients with WAD and persistent moderate to severe symptoms have widespread mechanical and thermal (heat and cold) sensory hypersensitivity and heightened responses to neurodynamic testing of the upper extremity soon after injury.[35] This same population of WAD in some cases demonstrates cold hyperalgesia and altered peripheral vasoconstrictor activity, suggesting sympathetic nervous system dysfunction and peripheral nerve injury may be contributors.[35] Cold hyperalgesia does not seem to be a feature of idiopathic neck pain.[36] Early assessment of sensory function

Table 6-3. Neck Pain With Movement Coordination Impairments Classification Summary

DIAGNOSTIC CLASSIFICATION	*KEY EXAM FINDINGS*	*FACTORS AGAINST*	*INTERVENTION*
Neck pain with movement coordination impairments ICD-10 terms: • Sprain and strain of the cervical spine	• Neck pain and neck-related (referred) upper extremity pain • Symptoms may be linked to, or precipitated by, trauma or whiplash and may be of longer duration (>12 weeks) • No centralization or peripheralization • Absence of nerve root compression • Neck pain with mid-range motion that worsens with end range movements or positions • DNF and upper quarter strength, endurance, and coordination deficits • Neck and neck-related upper extremity pain reproduced with provocation of the involved cervical segments • Poor performance of the CCFT and DNF endurance test • Upper quarter muscle flexibility deficits • Difficulty with repetitive activities • Somatosensory dysfunction	• Signs of nerve root compression • Patient expectations • Centralization or peripheralization with active/repeated movements • Reproduction or worsening of symptoms • Cervical disorders that cannot withstand loading associated with therapeutic exercise	• Specific motor control exercises • General exercises for upper quarter impairments of strength and endurance • Spinal posture education • Muscle lengthening exercises • Task-specific training for endurance, coordination, and strengthening to address activity limitations • Sensorimotor control exercises

ICD-10 indicates International Classification of Diseases, 10th edition; DNF, deep neck flexors; CCFT, craniocervical flexion test.

is recommended because cold hyperalgesia and impaired peripheral vasoconstriction, high pain intensity and disability, older age, reduced range of motion (ROM), and posttraumatic stress symptoms are predictive of poor outcome at 6 months[39] and 2 years, with the exception of sympathetic nervous system dysfunction.[40]

The existing literature provides no consensus for optimal testing procedures or intervention for altered sensory processing. Clinically, manual examination is used to assess mechanical hyperalgesia, but pressure algometry can be used to quantify mechanical pain thresholds. Tests for the presence of allodynia with light tactile stimulation may be used clinically. Local mechanical neck hyperalgesia alone suggests peripheral sensitization of cervical spine tissues which may respond to manual therapy (MT) and specific exercise targeting muscle recruitment.[41-44] Clinical findings of widespread sensory hypersensitivity and/or cold hyperalgesia require careful application of nonprovocative MT and exercise. Optimal intervention strategies are not clear. Provocative manual intervention may facilitate neuropathic pain or hypersensitivity through ongoing peripheral nociceptive input.[45,46] Gentle MT, specific exercise, and advice may be effective in some patients with widespread sensitivity,[47] but the effectiveness is unknown. Those with cold hyperalgesia or complex sensory impairments may not respond as well and may require the addition of pharmacological management.[47]

TABLE 6-4. NECK PAIN WITH RADIATING PAIN CLASSIFICATION SUMMARY

DIAGNOSTIC CLASSIFICATION	*KEY EXAM FINDINGS*	*FACTORS AGAINST*	*INTERVENTION*
Neck pain with radiating pain ICD-10 terms: • Cervical spondylosis with radiculopathy • Cervical disc disorder with radiculopathy	• Neck pain with associated radiating or referred pain in the involved UE that may be somatic, neuropathic in origin, or both • UE paresthesia, numbness, and weakness may be present • Centralization or peripheralization with active/repeated movements • Neck and neck-related radiating pain reproduced with o Cervical extension, lateral flexion, and rotation toward the involved side (Spurling's test) o ULNDT • Neck and neck-related radiating pain with neck distraction • May have UE sensory, strength, or reflex impairments associated with the involved nerve(s) • Symptoms provoked with cervical and/or thoracic PAIVM and/or PPIVM • Regional impairments: o Mobility o Muscle performance/length • Signs of nerve root compression • Altered neurodynamics	• Contraindications or precautions to mobilization or manipulation to the cervical or thoracic spine • Patient expectations	• Thoracic mobilization or manipulation • ICT • Cervical mobilization or manipulation, MET • Repeated movements that centralize symptoms • AROM/PROM to augment mobilization/manipulation • Muscle lengthening exercises • Muscle performance: endurance, coordination, and strengthening exercise • Gentle neural mobilization • Address regional and functional/activity limitations

ICD-10 indicates International Classification of Diseases, 10th edition; UE, upper extremity; ULNDT, upper limb neurodynamic tests; PAIVM, passive accessory intervertebral movement; PPIVM, passive physiological intervertebral movements; ICT, intermittent cervical traction; MET, muscle energy technique; AROM, active range of motion; PROM, passive range of motion.

Altered Motor Performance

Both cervical physiological and segmental motion can be reduced[48-50] or excessive[50-52] in patients with neck pain when compared to healthy individuals. Decreased functional cervical ROM is a physical factor common to most individuals with neck pain. Reduced ROM of at least a 25% loss, compared with normal subjects, is predictive of chronicity in persons with WAD with persistent symptoms.[48] In addition, neck pain patients, of insidious or traumatic origin and with CGH, may demonstrate muscle performance deficits; strength and endurance are compromised in the cervical extensors,[53,54] cervical flexors,[55,56] and upper cervical flexors.[57,58]

Neck pain is associated with reduced activity[41,47,58,59-63] of the deep cervical flexors (ie, longus capitis and colli) and increased activity of the superficial system, sternocleidomastoid (SCM) and scalenes.[64] These motor control changes are assessed clinically, using the craniocervical flexion test (CCFT).[61] Greater coactivation of the superficial extensors and flexors may be found in patients with chronic headache,[65] and office workers during typing,[66] increasing compressive forces and suggesting an altered motor control strategy resulting in poor segmental support. The upper trapezius (UT), SCM, and scalenes are also involved in patients with neck pain, but their role is not fully understood. Increased UT activity has been noted in prolonged computer activity.[67] Along with the SCM and

TABLE 6-5. QUEBEC TASK FORCE CLASSIFICATION

CLASSIFICATION	*CLINICAL FINDINGS*
0	No complaints about the neck; no physical signs
I	No complaint of neck pain, stiffness or tenderness only; no physical signs
II	Neck complaint; musculoskeletal signs including decreased range of movement; point tenderness; no neurological signs
III	Neck complaint; musculoskeletal signs; neurological signs including decreased/absent deep tendon reflexes, muscle weakness, and sensory deficits
IV	Neck complaint and fracture or dislocation

Data adapted from Spitzer WO, Skovron ML, Salmi LR et al. Scientific monograph of the Quebec Task Force on Whiplash-Associated Disorders: redefining "whiplash" and its management. *Spine.* 1995;20:1S-73S.

TABLE 6-6. PROPOSED ADAPTATION TO THE QUEBEC TASK FORCE WAD II CLASSIFICATION

PROPOSED CLASSIFICATION FOR WAD II	*CLINICAL PRESENTATION*
IIA	• Neck pain; no neurological signs • Decreased ROM and altered muscle recruitment on the craniocervical flexion test • Local cervical mechanical hyperalgesia
IIB	• The same as WAD IIA • Psychological impairment with elevated psychological distress as demonstrated on the General Health Questionnaire-28 and the Tampa Scale of Kinesiophobia
IIC	• Neck pain; no neurological signs • Decreased ROM and altered muscle recruitment on the craniocervical flexion test • Increased joint position error • Local cervical mechanical hyperalgesia • Generalized sensory hypersensitivity (mechanical, thermal, and neural tissue) • Some sympathetic nervous system disturbances • Psychological impairment with elevated psychological distress as demonstrated on the General Health Questionnaire-28 and the Tampa Scale of Kinesiophobia • Symptoms of acute posttraumatic stress as identified by the Impact of Event Scale

WAD indicates whiplash-associated disorder; ROM, range of motion.

Data adapted from Sterling M. A proposed new classification system for whiplash associated disorders: implications for assessment and management. *Man Ther.* 2004;9:60-70.

scalenes[55,64] the UT has shown a decreased ability to relax after activation.[64,68]

In pain-free individuals, the neck muscles are activated in a preplanned or feedforward manner prior to onset of an arm movement independent of direction,[69,70] presumably to control segmental motion occurring in the neck. However, in individuals with neck pain, both the superficial and deep neck muscles are delayed,[70] suggesting an altered motor control strategy during upper extremity tasks. Individuals with neck pain consistently have delayed activation of the deep neck muscles with a related increase in the superficial muscles during low load activity.[63,64] Poor motor control is believed to result in loss of control of joint movement and repeated tissue stress from microtrauma that may then lead to pain.[51,52] However, the reverse may also be true. Pain may be the initial event that changes motor control.[64,67]

Experimentally induced pain in normal subjects can be used to assess changes in muscle performance in the absence of changes in muscle properties. Experimental muscle pain inhibits the painful muscle, specifically the muscle acting as the agonist,[71-73] and influences the coordination of synergists and/or antagonists[71,74,75] in order to minimize the use of the injured muscle. Similar changes in motor control strategies have been observed in persons with neck pain. Nociceptors projecting to the sensorimotor cortex are likely to result in decreased motor neuron output, but changes in motor planning also occur in patients with neck pain as evidenced by muscle activation patterns during rapid arm movements becoming direction specific, reflecting changes in central strategies.[74]

Changes in muscle properties,[76-78] such as fatty infiltration or muscle fiber type proportions (ie, slow twitch fibers change to fast twitch fibers), have been identified and may be due to nerve injury or changes in motor strategies from disuse.[79] Change in muscle fiber type proportions is consistent with decreased muscular endurance in patients with neck pain.[53,57,80] Atrophy and fatty infiltrate of the deep SO muscles and multifidus has been observed in patients with chronic WAD[81] and in chronic neck pain.[79,82-84]

Recommended therapeutic exercises for persons with chronic neck pain and impaired motor control strategies are specifically designed to address both the altered neural input (ie, central processes) and muscle properties (ie, peripheral mechanisms).[78,85] Training of the deep cervical flexors through a low load exercise program increases the muscle activation,[86] improves speed of activation, and aids in maintenance of upright sitting posture.[87] A high load training program does not produce similar outcomes,[87] but remains important to reduce deficits in strength and endurance.[88] Early (and pain-free) rehabilitation of impaired neck muscle performance is recommended to address early onset of altered motor control.[89] Motor control changes are present in patients who no longer have symptoms[86] and in patients reporting full recovery from whiplash.[39,89] Theoretically, the presence of motor control deficits may play a role in the high recurrence rate of neck pain.[77]

Altered Sensorimotor Control

Altered sensorimotor function includes deficits in balance, eye movement control, and proprioceptive acuity. The large amounts of mechanoreceptors in the joints and muscle of the cervical spine, and the connections from the cervical afferents to the vestibular, visual, and postural control systems suggest that the neck provides important somatosensory input that affects control of postural stability, head orientation, and eye movement.[90] In persons with insidious onset neck pain and WAD, abnormal afferent input from the somatosensory, visual, or vestibular systems can lead to altered sensory motor control and present as dizziness, unsteadiness in upright postures, and reduced ability to control head and eye movement.[91-94] Potential mechanisms that can alter proprioceptive input include trauma or impaired muscle function,[91] chemical mediators that alter muscle spindle sensitivity,[95,96] pain that alters mechanoreceptor function at the spinal cord and centrally,[97-99] and the effects of stress on muscle spindle activity.[100]

Dizziness associated with neck pain and disability has a 33% incidence that correlates with duration, higher intensity neck pain and disability scores, and a history of neck trauma.[101] Chronic WAD patients show a 74% incidence of dizziness and unsteadiness[102] that is also common in CGH.[103] In WAD, vertebral artery insufficiency, minor brain trauma, vestibular disorder, medication, and anxiety must be ruled out before cervical joint and muscle mechanoreceptors can be implicated as the cause of dizziness.[91,104-107] Screening for cervicogenic dizziness is discussed under Screening for Red Flags.

Clinical measures of altered sensorimotor control, postural stability, cervical joint position error (JPE), and eye movement control are found in both chronic, insidious onset neck pain and WAD, occurring to a greater extent in WAD and persons with dizziness. However, no relationship exists among the 3 measures,[108] meaning each can occur independently of the other.

Impaired postural stability has been demonstrated by an inability to maintain tandem stance for 30 seconds with eyes closed.[109,110] Elderly persons with neck pain have greater balance deficits than healthy controls.[111] Deficits in cervical JPE are tested by a patient's ability to relocate the head to a natural posture or to a preset target during rotation with eyes closed.[112] Reduced accuracy is ascribed to abnormal afferent cervical input during slow movement with the vestibular system below threshold.[113] As described by Jull et al,[114] eye movement control involves 3 systems: smooth-pursuit, saccadic, and optokinetic. Smooth-pursuit confirms stable images of a moving target with slow eye follow. Using the saccadic system allows rapid eye movements to change a point of visual fixation. The optokinetic system allows visual fixation of a target during movement. Dysfunction of eye control on smooth-pursuit and/or saccadic eye movement soon after whiplash injury is prognostic for persistent disability at 8 months, while normal eye movement soon after whiplash injury is predictive of full recovery or minor disability.[115] Altered smooth-pursuit eye movement control during the smooth-pursuit neck torsion (SPNT) test[107] is present in persons with WAD, but not vestibular disorders,[107,116,117] and is attributed to altered afferent input from cervical structures. In WAD, the SPNT test is correlated with cognitive difficulties, such as reading.[106]

Jull et al[114] recommended a multimodal rehabilitation program that includes MT to address painful and impaired cervical joints and muscle function and specific programs targeting neck JPE, gaze stability, balance, and eye-head coordination to address the potential causes of altered cervical somatosensory input. Selected interventions are discussed later in this chapter with detailed references.[116]

Evaluation

History and Diagnostic Triage

As discussed in Chapter 2, most diagnoses or diagnostic hypotheses emerge during the patient interview and the rest during the physical examination.[118] The process of diagnostic triage for persons with MNP is the same as for LBP (covered in Chapter 4) and begins with ruling out serious underlying pathology or nonspinal pathology. In this first stage, the clinician determines if the patient is appropriate for PT, if a medical referral is needed, or whether a referral is needed in conjunction with PT. The components of the subjective examination are the same as discussed in Chapter 1 and listed in Table 4-1 for LBP. Specific review of the section on medical screening assists in identifying systemic disease or illness that can mimic neuromusculoskeletal symptoms or conditions. The likelihood of serious cervical spine pathology is low, but a missed or delayed diagnosis is costly, often resulting in prolonged illness and sometimes mortality. Serious conditions, such as cancer and infections, are estimated to account for less than 0.4% of cases of neck pain.[119] Most medical red flags are symptoms and can be obtained prior to the physical examination, but clinical signs may add to the diagnostic accuracy for identifying serious pathology and are presented here as part of the differential diagnosis. Serious underlying pathology in neck pain is associated with key clinical findings. Nordin et al[120] recommend consideration of the following in nonemergency clinical assessment:

- Spontaneous or pathologic fractures following minor trauma
- Neoplasm in the presence of a previous history of cancer, unexplained weight loss, constitutional symptoms, and failure to improve with a month of therapy
- Systemic inflammatory diseases (eg, ankylosing spondylitis [AS] and inflammatory arthritis)
- Infection
- CM
- Previous cervical spine or neck surgery or open injury

Screening for Red Flags

Screening for Cancer

Cervical spine tumors are either primary bone tumors or metastatic tumors. Primary bone tumors in the lumbar and thoracic area have a higher occurrence rate than in the cervical area; the percentage of occurrence for neoplastic tumors is less than 1% in the cervical area.[121] Less than 5% of all primary bone neoplasms above the sacrum are in the cervical area and generally occur in the older person.[122] Metastatic disease of the spine occurs in 30% to 70% of patients with a known cancer.[123] In the cervical spine, metastatic disease occurs in 8% to 20% of patients with known metastatic disease and is relatively uncommon.[124] Cervical spine metastasis occurs more frequently in cancers of the breast, lung, prostate, and melanoma.[125,126] Pain is the presenting symptom, often with insidious onset, unrelieved by rest, worse at night, and unchanged with movement.[121] However, the clinical pattern of symptoms is widely variable from neck pain alone to neck pain and associated symptoms.

A Pancoast tumor is located in the upper lobe of the lung representing 5% to 25% of all lung tumors.[127] Men (ages 50 years or older and with a history of tobacco use) are affected more than women. Due to tumor location, the upper quarter region can be affected, resulting in a variety of clinical findings. In addition to altered pulmonary function, radiation of pain occurs in the arms and hands along the C8, T1, and T2 dermatomes and ulnar nerve distribution in the axilla, shoulder, and subscapular regions, and up to the head and neck.[128] Atrophy of the intrinsic muscles of the hand and Horner's syndrome, enophthalmos (ie, receding of the eyeball), ptosis, and a unilaterally constricted pupil are additional signs.[128]

Table 4-2 lists the likelihood ratios for the diagnostic accuracy of clinical findings that assist the clinician in determining the need for medical referral and further testing. Henschke and colleagues[129] concluded that only 4 features, when used alone, significantly raise the posttest probability of cancer:

1. A previous history of cancer (+LR 23.7)
2. An elevated ESR (+LR 18.0)
3. Low hematocrit (+LR 18.2)
4. Clinician judgment (+LR 12.1)

Deyo and Diehl[130] reported 4 clinical findings with the highest positive likelihood ratios (+LR) for detecting the presence of metastatic cancer in LBP:

1. Previous history of non-skin cancer (+LR 14.7)
2. Failure of conservative management in past month (+LR 3.0)
3. Age > 50 years (+LR 2.7)
4. Unexplained weight loss of more than 4.5 kg in 6 months (+LR 2.7)

The absence of all 4 of these clinical findings essentially rules out cancer (Sn 1.0, Sp 0.6) in the lumbar spine. Specific research has not addressed these findings for patients with neck pain.

Screening for Infection

Infection in the cervical region is rare. Cervical vertebral osteomyelitis is a type of bacterial infection inclusive of diskitis, spondylitis, and spondylodiscitis, making up about 3% to 10% of all vertebral osteomyelitis, or 1 per 100,000 annually.[131] Tuberculosis, urinary and respiratory tract infections, and intravenous drug use are common sources of cervical osteomyelitis, with occurrences in up to 27% of intravenous drug users.[131] Invasive procedures, such as tracheotomy and tonsillectomy, may be direct sources of the cervical spine infection. Other risk factors are diabetes, renal insufficiency, heart or liver disease, alcoholism, and chronic immunosuppression.[131]

Initial presentation may be one of vague nonspecific neck pain, but as pain progresses, dysphagia or severe torticollis may occur.[131,132] Neurological deficits may not occur initially, but have been reported in 44% to 60% of all cases.[132] Most cases are reported between C5 to C6, with the least reported cases between C2 to C5. Fever may not be present early, but may develop in up to 66% of cases as the infection. Weight loss has also been reported.[133] Laboratory tests, such as white blood cell count, erythrocyte sedimentation rate, and C-reactive protein levels are recommended. Erythrocyte sedimentation rate is 70% to 100% sensitive for spinal infection, but lacks specificity.[131,134] For imaging, radiographs may detect end plate erosion 2 to 4 weeks after onset, but false positive results may occur due to degenerative changes with sensitivity (82%), specificity (57%), and accuracy (73%). MRI has been proven to be the gold standard with sensitivity (96%), specificity (94%), and accuracy (94%).[131,135]

Screening for Spinal Fracture

Fractures in the cervical spine are rare with prevalence estimated at less than 0.4% in population surveys.[136,137] A prevalence of 3.5% ± 5% is representative of fractures among patients presenting to emergency departments with cervical trauma.[119] Mechanisms of injury are trauma-related, resulting from a fall, motor vehicle collision (MVC), or sports injury, which account for 20%, 50%, and 15%, respectively, of cervical spine injuries related to interpersonal violence. About half of the fractures occur at C6 or C7 and one-third at C2.[138] The rate of neurological dysfunction is between 20% and 40%.[139]

Use of the Canadian C-spine rule[140,141] (CCR; Figure 6-1) is recommended to determine who would benefit from radiographic evaluation prior to initiating PT. The CCR is for use in alert (ie, Glasgow Coma Scale 15) and stable (ie, normal vital signs) trauma patients with immediate concern of a cervical spine fracture. Patients were excluded in these studies if under 16 years of age, had a penetrating neck trauma or acute paralysis, or were injured more than 48 hours previously, had vertebral disease, or were pregnant. The rule, as described by Stiell et al,[140] is made of 3 main questions (see Figure 6-1):

1. Are any high-risk factors present, such as: age greater than or equal to 65 years, a dangerous injury mechanism, or paresthesia in extremities, a dangerous injury mechanism includes a fall from a height of 3 or more feet or 5 stairs, an axial load to the head, a high-speed MVC greater than 62 mph or with ejection or roll over, and a bicycle or motorized recreational vehicle collision? If a high risk factor is present, radiographs are mandatory.
2. Are any low-risk factors present that allow safe assessment of ROM, such as a simple rear-end motor vehicle collision, able to assume sitting in the emergency department, able to ambulate at any time since injury, a delay in onset of neck pain, or absence of midline cervical spine tenderness? A simple rear-end vehicle collision does not include a rollover, being hit by a high-speed vehicle, being pushed into oncoming traffic, or hit by a bus or large truck. If there are no low-risk factors present that allow assessment of active range of motion (AROM), then radiographs are mandatory.
3. Is the patient able to actively rotate the neck 45 degrees to the left and right? If the patient is unable to perform this amount of AROM, then radiographs are mandatory.

The CCR had 100% sensitivity (95% CI: 98% to 100%) and 42.5% specificity (95% CI: 40% to 44%) for identifying 151 clinically important cervical spine injuries.[140]

Screening for Cervical Arterial Dysfunction

Screening for adverse neurovascular events, such as ischemic stroke related to management of patients presenting with neck pain and headache, has been an ongoing concern of physical therapists. The current terminology of cervical arterial dysfunction (CAD) describes potential adverse events involving both the vertebrobasilar system supplying the hindbrain (ie, pons, brainstem, vestibular apparatus, cerebellum, medulla oblongata) and the internal carotids supplying the cerebral hemispheres and retina.

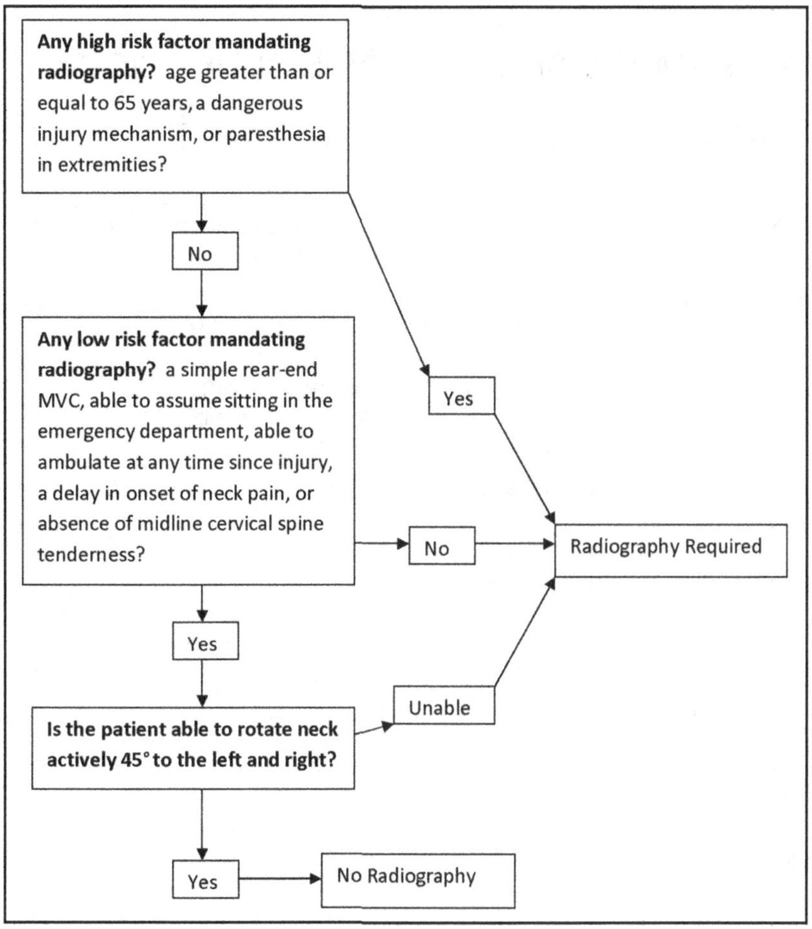

Figure 6-1. Canadian C-spine rule.[140,141]

The internal carotids supply about 80% of the blood to the brain, as compared to 20% by the vertebral arteries. Since the patient with CAD in the early stages may present with the same complaints of neck pain and/or headache as a patient with MNP, the therapist must be aware of, and alert to, the difficulties of a differential diagnosis. The prevalence of patients presenting to therapists with CAD is unknown, but thought to be very low. The uncertainty related to limited knowledge and current guidelines warrants a comprehensive approach to clinical decision making for each patient.[142]

CAD may take the form of stenotic, occlusive, or dissecting aneurysms[143-145] as a result of a tear to the intimal lining of the arterial wall and subsequent hemorrhaging. Internal carotid artery (ICA) dissection is associated with cervical rotation and extension movements that compress the artery against the transverse process of the upper cervical vertebra.[145] Vertebral artery (VA) dissection is associated with contralateral cervical rotation that stretches or compresses the artery between the first 2 cervical vertebra.[146] Spontaneous CAD has been linked to genetic predisposition (ie, vessel abnormalities, connective tissue disease, or gene mutations), and environmental factors, such as infection or oral contraceptive use, trauma, and atherosclerosis.[147] CAD has been reported following major trauma such as whiplash, or minor trauma, such as sport or recreational activities, sustained or repeated neck movements, carrying a heavy load, coughing and sneezing, MT, and pregnancy and delivery.[145,148] Zetterling et al[149] reported arterial dissection following yoga, star gazing, painting the ceiling, and visits to the hairdresser.

Clinically, the presentation of CAD varies considerably. Patients may initially present with no pain, head and neck pain, or transient ischemic attack and stroke as the dissection progresses from the nonischemic to the ischemic phase. During the nonischemic phase of CAD, pain may be the only symptom and may last from minutes to weeks before ischemic responses occur. Reported clinical presentations of CAD[142,150,152] are presented in Table 6-7. CAD does not usually present with only one sign or symptom.[150] Neck pain is usually sudden, severe and sharp ipsilaterally in the upper posterior to middle cervical spine, with or without occipital headache alone during VA dissection[143,152-156] (Figure 6-2). Ipsilateral frontotemporal headache, upper/mid-cervical or anterolateral neck pain or facial pain are described during ICA dissection[152,156] (Figure 6-3). Neck pain occurs in 34% to 46% of symptomatic VA dissection patients and 9% to 20% of patients with symptomatic ICA dissection.[143,152,156] Facial pain is usually not present in VA dissection, but is present in

TABLE 6-7. REPORTED CLINICAL PRESENTATIONS OF CERVICAL ARTERIAL DYSFUNCTION

	NON-ISCHEMIC SIGNS AND SYMPTOMS	*ISCHEMIC SIGNS AND SYMPTOMS*
Vertebral artery dissection	• Ipsilateral posterior neck pain • Occipital headache • Rarely C5-C6 nerve root impairment	• Hindbrain transient ischemic attack, dizziness, diplopia, dysarthria, dysphagia, drop attacks, nausea, nystagmus, facial numbness, ataxia, vomiting, hoarseness, loss of short-term memory, limb (arm/leg) weakness, anhidrosis, hearing difficulties, malaise, vagueness, perioral dysesthesia, photophobia, papillary changes, clumsiness and agitation • Hindbrain stroke (also known as Wallenberg syndrome) • Cranial nerve palsies
Internal carotid dissection	• Neck pain • Head pain • Horner syndrome • Cranial nerve palsies (CN IX to XII) • Pulsatile tinnitus Less commonly • Ipsilateral carotid bruit • Scalp tenderness • Neck swelling • Orbital pain and facial dryness • CN VI palsy	• Transient ischemic attack • Ischemic stroke (middle cerebra artery) • Retinal infarction • Amaurosis fugax (ie, temporary partial or total vision loss)

34% to 53% of patients with ICA dissection.[152,157] During VA dissection, headaches are usually reported as an ipsilateral, constant ache in the occipital or parieto-occipital regions, and in the frontotemporal or hemicranial regions during ICA dissection.[156] Overall, headaches occur in 67% to 72% of patients with symptomatic CAD.[143,156,157] Neck pain as the only presenting feature for internal carotid artery dissection occurs in about 6% of cases.[156,158] In 17% of cases, headache occurs in combination with neck pain.[158] Other symptoms are listed in Table 6-7. The classic signs and symptoms related to VA insufficiency include dizziness, drop attacks, diplopia, dysarthria, dysphagia, ataxia, nausea, numbness of the unilateral face, nystagmus, and ataxia.[159] Strict use of the classic signs and symptoms may be misleading and lead to a poor understanding of the patient's presentation.[150]

No consensus or evidence-based guidelines exist as to the best way to assess for CAD or the possibility of an adverse event related to examination, and/or treatment of a patient presenting with neck pain, and/or related symptoms. A comprehensive approach to assess for potential CAD begins with a careful history and includes review of cardiovascular risk factors, such as hypertension, hypercholesterolemia, coagulation abnormalities, direct vessel trauma, diabetes mellitus, a history of smoking, bacterial infection and family history of cardiovascular disease (CVD). Other pertinent information includes a history of trauma (ie, MVC, fall, lifting or coughing), recent cervical spine surgery, nerve blocks, radiation therapy, intubation, central venous catheterization, or connective tissue disorders. Obtaining a clear picture of the patient's presenting symptoms and their progression may alert the therapist to an early hypothesis of an underlying vascular pathology.[150] In fact, Cassidy et al[160] suggested that some patients with an arterial dissection in progress may be referred to or seek PT. Therapists should develop a high index of suspicion with acute onset of neck and head pain described as "unlike any other," and consider the signs and symptoms associated with the nonischemic and ischemic phases of CAD[150] (see Table 6-7).

Key procedures for the physical examination, as recommended by Kerry and Taylor,[142,150] included blood

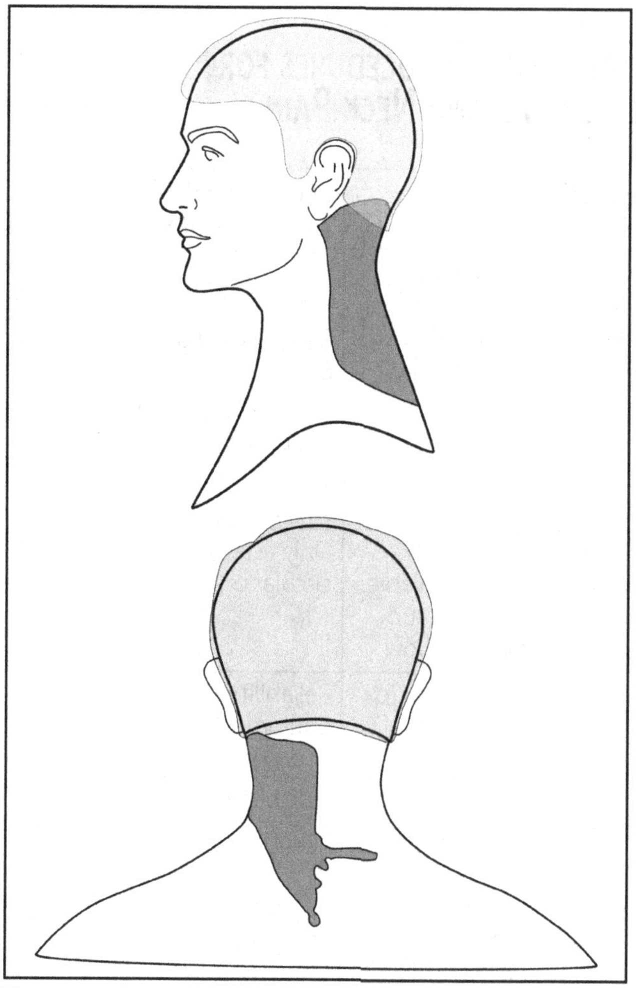

Figure 6-2. Pain patterns related to vertebral artery dissection. (Redrawn from *Man Ther*, 11(4), Kerry R, Taylor AJ, Cervical arterial dysfunction assessment and manual therapy, 243-253, Copyright 2006, with permission from Elsevier.)

pressure examination, cranial nerve examination, eye examination, handheld Doppler ultrasound, and functional positional tests of cervical rotation and extension (Table 6-8). Functional positioning tests actively or passively place the cervical spine in sustained end-range positions for the purpose of compromising blood flow in the vertebral arteries to screen for otherwise unapparent VA pathology that may present a premanipulation risk. Extension, rotation, combined extension and rotation or a premanipulative test position are commonly used to monitor for symptoms associated with CAD. The Australian Physiotherapy Association[161] suggests a 10-second sustained hold of rotation, and a patient-reported movement or position, as a minimum requirement to establish whether or not vertebral artery insufficiency is present. If manipulation is considered as treatment, a premanipulative test is recommended. If symptoms are reproduced, the test is considered positive, contraindicates continued treatment, and warrants medical referral.[161]

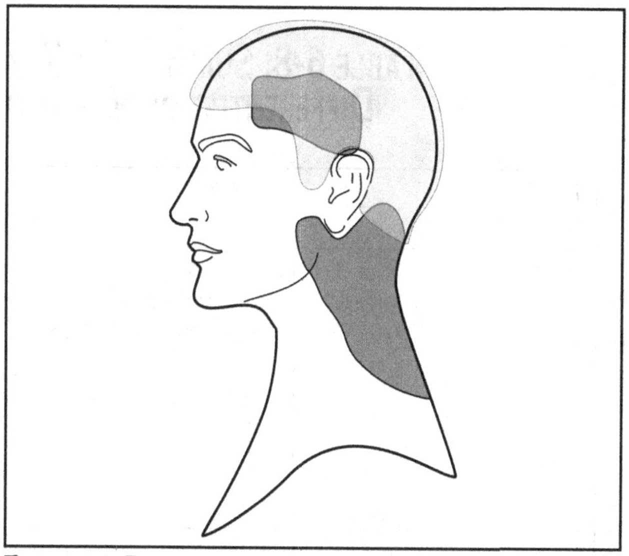

Figure 6-3. Pain patterns related to internal carotid artery dissection. (Redrawn from *Man Ther*, 11(4), Kerry R, Taylor AJ, Cervical arterial dysfunction assessment and manual therapy, 243-253, Copyright 2006, with permission from Elsevier.)

If the index of suspicion is high, based on the patient's history, end range provocative testing is not indicated and the patient is referred appropriately.[162] Sound clinical reasoning should determine whether the benefits outweigh the risks when performing a functional positional test that may place the patient in test positions of potentially greater risk than the intended examination or treatment procedures.[162] In general, functional positioning tests have poor diagnostic utility as predictors of risk and will not assist the clinician with decision making related to the presence or absence of CAD.[150,163] Kerry et al reported that "the real risk of arterial complications following MT is unknown and impossible to estimate based on existing data."[163(p45)] The use of functional positional tests prior to performing spinal manipulative therapy remains controversial.

Additionally, the Australian Physiotherapy Association[161] prudently recommends assessing for the presence of symptoms and signs associated with VBI during 4 stages: the history, physical examination, during treatment, and following cervical spine treatment. Further decisions on management and treatment selection are based on continued reevaluation of outcomes.[161] Thiel and Rix[164] made the following recommendations:

> Practitioners must assess the patient thoroughly through careful history taking and physical examination for the possibility of vertebral artery dissection. It is important to note that vertebral artery dissection (VAD) may present as pain only and may not be associated with symptoms and signs of brainstem ischemia. If there is a strong likelihood of VAD, provocative premanipulation tests should not be performed and the patient must be referred appropriately. In the patient presenting with symptoms of

Table 6-8. Summary of Key Examination Procedures for Differentiation Vasculogenic Head and Neck Pain

TEST	PURPOSE	EVIDENCE STATUS	LIMITATIONS AND ADVANTAGES
Functional positional test—Cervical rotation	Affects flow in contralateral vertebral artery Limited effect on internal carotid artery	Poor sensitivity, variable specificity Blood flow studies support effect on VA flow	Only assesses posterior circulation Results should be interpreted with caution Recommended by existing protocols Cannot predict propensity for injury
Functional positional test—Cervical extension	Affects flow in internal carotid arteries. Limited effect on vertebral arteries	No specific diagnostic utility evidence available. Blood flow studies support effect on ICA flow	Only assesses anterior circulation
Blood pressure examination	Measure of cardiovascular health	Correlates to ICA atherosclerotic pathology	Reliability dependent on equipment, environment, and experience
Cranial nerve examination	Identifies specific cranial nerve dysfunction, resulting from ischemia or vessel compression	No specific diagnostic utility evidence available	Reliability dependent on experience
Eye examination	Assists in diagnosis of possible neural deficit related to ICA dysfunction	No specific diagnostic utility evidence available	Eye symptoms may be early warning of serious underlying pathology
Hand-held Doppler ultrasound	Direct assessment of blood flow velocity	Limited manual therapy specific evidence Existing studies suggest good to excellent reliability. Validity requires further study	Reliability dependent on equipment, environment, and experience

Reprinted from *Man Ther,* 11(4), Kerry R, Taylor AJ, Cervical arterial dysfunction assessment and manual therapy, 243-253, Copyright 2006, with permission from Elsevier.

brainstem ischemia due to nondissection, stenotic vertebral artery pathologies, provocative testing is very unlikely to provide any useful additional diagnostic information. In the patient with unapparent vertebral artery pathology, where spinal manipulative therapy is considered as the treatment of choice, provocative testing is very unlikely to provide any useful information in assessing the probability of manipulation induced vertebral artery injury.[164(p157)]

Some MT interventions have inherent risk if performed in the presence of CAD. Therefore, the clinician must take a comprehensive and reasoned approach to early identification. During the reasoning process of provocative testing, the clinician should ask whether the test will add any further benefit to the screening process. The clinician is responsible for performing a prudent examination and clearly documenting that screening was performed. The clinician must make the best decision based on the uncertainties inherent in the clinical presentation and current limitations of screening procedures to decide when a referral for additional testing and medical opinion is needed. With the growth of evidence to support spinal manipulative therapy in persons with neck pain,[165] a detailed understanding of CAD is necessary.[142-164]

Screening for Dizziness

Clinically, dizziness has a wide range of descriptions and causes, making differential diagnosis challenging. The cause may be cardiovascular, neurological, metabolic, psychiatric, vestibular or cervicogenic.[166] The complaint of dizziness may be described as light-headedness, faintness, heavy headedness, falling, waving, imbalance, swimming sensations, floating, unsteadiness or spinning.[167] Dizziness caused by cardiovascular or metabolic disorders may result in precautions or contraindications to PT and require medical referral, whereas dizziness related to the cervical spine, musculoskeletal impairments, and the vestibular system may be appropriate for PT intervention.[166,168] A discussion of pathophysiology of vestibular, presyncope, and other dizziness subtypes is beyond the scope of this reference.

Dizziness has been classified into 4 subtypes: vestibular, presyncope, dysequilibrium, and other dizziness.[169,170] Vertigo is usually defined as a spinning sensation of either the body or environment suggesting vestibular dysfunction,[171] whereas patients with presyncopal dizziness complain of lightheadedness, impending faintness, or tiredness resulting from altered blood supply, oxygen, or glucose.[171] After 1 minute of standing, preceded by 5 minutes of sitting, normative values for blood pressure drop are 1.2 ± 9.8 mm Hg. A drop in systolic blood pressure of more than 20 mm Hg has a specificity of 0.97 for detecting orthostatic hypotension and warrants referral in the presence of presyncopal dizziness.[172] Another test for orthostatic hypotension involves the blood pressure response when moving from lying to a standing position, in which orthostatic hypotension is indicated by a drop of at least 20 mm Hg of systolic blood pressure or 10 mm Hg of diastolic blood pressure within 3 minutes of standing.[173] Patients with dysequilibrium complain of unsteadiness, imbalance and weakness, and a sense that a fall will occur, often associated with visual impairment, peripheral neuropathy, or musculoskeletal disturbances.[170,171] The subtype of "other" dizziness includes reports of floating, anxiety, depression, and fatigue, suggesting a psychiatric disorder.[171] Symptoms of presyncopal and other dizziness may indicate the need for referral.[166,168] This classification serves as an initial guide, but patients often have more than one system involved, as often seen in older adults.

Cervicogenic dizziness (CD) is considered a diagnosis of exclusion.[167] When all other causes of dizziness have been ruled out, CD is considered. Therefore, a thorough history and physical examination are necessary to identify patients with CD, musculoskeletal impairments, and vestibular disorders appropriate for PT. Cervicogenic dizziness is defined as "a specific sensation of altered orientation in space and dysequilibrium originating from abnormal afferent activities from the neck."[168] The proposed mechanism for CD is a sensory mismatch between somatosensory information from the neck and input from the visual and vestibular systems.[167] In other words, cervical spine dysfunction results in altered afferent input from the articular mechanoreceptors and proprioceptors[174] often related to trauma, degenerative processes, inflammation, or mechanical disorders.[174] Cervical spondylosis, nerve root compression, WAD, and temporomandibular disorders have been reported as a cause of dizziness.[175] Dizziness is reported with CAD, CD, and vestibular disorders. The nature of the dizziness may assist with differentiating a vascular versus a nonvascular cause.[175] Distinct vertigo is not typically present with VA insufficiency, although it has been reported.[176] Dizziness that occurs with rotation and does not improve with sustained movement is likely vascular in nature. A nonvascular vestibular dizziness is different from vascular dizziness, in that it may improve with repeated movement and has a short latency.[175]

A diagnosis of CD is associated with the following findings: pain or discomfort in the neck (often posttrauma), persistent occipital headache, jaw pain and/or upper extremity radicular symptoms, limited cervical ROM, and dizziness of short duration.[174,177] The dizziness is not usually described as vertigo. The severity of the dizziness can be relative to the severity of pain, stiffness and numbness.[174] Vidal and Huijbregts[168] described the following signs and symptoms for CD:

- Intermittent dizziness precipitated by head and neck movement
- Onset of symptoms is immediate with the provoking position
- Duration may be brief, or minutes to hours, but is fatigable with motion
- Associated signs and symptoms include neck pain, SO headache, and occasional paresthesia in the trigeminal distribution
- A medical history of cervical spine trauma and degeneration
- Upper cervical mobility deficits on AROM and passive physiological intervertebral movements (PPIVM) testing
- A positive neck torsion test for nystagmus and reproduction of dizziness

Patients with CD also complain of, or present with, balance problems.[167] Specific components of the history and physical examination related to testing for CD are covered later in this chapter and further discussed in the literature.[168,178]

Screening for Cervical Spine Ligamentous Instability

The diagnosis of cervical spine instability is controversial and once again presents a diagnostic challenge due to its often subtle clinical presentation. Cervical spine instability (CSI) may be a life-threatening instability appreciated with imaging, as is often related to the transverse ligament in rheumatoid arthritis (RA), AS, Down's syndrome, Klippel-Feil syndrome, congenital absence of an immature dens leading to compression of neurovascular structures,[179] or described as a minor nonradiographic clinical instability. A minor clinical CSI is considered a movement impairment with subtle clinical features theorized to involve the active and neural stabilizing systems without disruption of the passive system, as described by Panjabi.[51,52] Clinical CSI may be a feature of osteoarthritis,[180] segmental degeneration,[181] RA,[182] CGH,[183,184] and whiplash.[182,185] Mechanisms thought to injure the cervical spine-stabilizing structures include genetic predisposition,[186] surgery,[51,52] disk degeneration,[187] and trauma.[188,189] The clinical examination may reveal subtle findings and imaging studies for instability may be normal.[190] Radiographic imaging to assess segmental mobility exhibits poor correlation between the images of excessive mobility and the clinical symptoms.[179] Cook et al[190] reported that reliable and valid clinical or diagnostic tests and standard identifiers have not been described to assist with diagnosis. Anecdotally, cardinal symptoms of upper cervical instability and associated cervical cord compression have been described as any of the following reproduced by active or passive head or neck movements: drop attacks, facial or lip paresthesia, bilateral or quadrilateral limb paresthesia, or nystagmus.[191]

In a survey of Australian manipulative physiotherapists, Niere and Torney[192] descriptively reported the following responses as either very important or vitally important to the diagnosis of minor CSI:

- A history of major trauma
- Complaints of neck catching, locking, or giving way
- Poor muscular control
- Signs of hypermobility on x-ray
- Excessively free end-feel on passive motion testing and unpredictability of symptoms[192]

Cook et al[190] reported on the findings of a Delphi expert consensus survey to describe symptoms and examination findings for clinical CSI. The symptoms with the highest consensus were intolerance to prolonged static postures, fatigue and inability to hold head up, better with external support (including hands or collar), "frequent need for self-manipulation, "feeling of instability, shaking, or lack of control, "frequent episodes of acute attacks," and "sharp pain, possibly with sudden movements."[190] The highest consensus on examination findings were poor coordination/neuromuscular control, including poor recruitment and dissociation of cervical segments with movement, abnormal joint play, motion that is not smooth throughout ROM (including segmental hinging, pivoting, or fulcruming), and "aberrant movement."[190] Patient reports may assist the clinician in identifying the patient with clinical CSI. Specific details of the history and physical examination related to testing for CSI, such as ligamentous stability tests are covered later in this chapter.

Screening for Rheumatic Disease

Rheumatoid Arthritis

RA is a chronic systemic inflammatory disorder. Of more than 100 rheumatic diseases, RA is the most common inflammatory disease that affects the cervical spine,[128,193] with a prevalence between 43% and 86%[194-197] and an etiology that remains unknown. The synovial tissues of diarthrodial joints are primarily affected, but extraarticular features manifest in the skin, eyes, lungs, and nervous system, emphasizing the systemic nature of the disease.[128] Risk factors for RA cervical disease and its progression are male gender, seropositive rheumatoid factor, rheumatoid nodules, early bone erosion, long-standing disease, and prolonged use of steroids.[193,198] Cervical involvement progresses early in the course of the disease and is associated with the degree of systemic involvement.[199]

The pathophysiology of joint destruction is synovial proliferation and inflammation. Fibroblastic inflammatory granulation tissue forms within the synovium and proliferates to form a pannus that invades the hyaline cartilage, resulting in periarticular inflammation and enzymatic destruction of cartilage, subchondral bone, ligaments, and tendons that may lead to joint instability and subluxation.[193,199,200] The synovial articulations of the upper cervical spine are targets of the rheumatoid process. However, the C2 to C7 intervertebral joints, uncovertebral, apophyseal joints, and annulus fibrosus are also susceptible to pannus infiltration. Pressure on the spinal cord or brainstem may result from static or dynamic subluxation of the spine, or by direct pressure from the pannus.[201] The most common subluxation in the cervical spine is at the atlantoaxial (AA) articulation, with 75% of cases occurring when C1 slips forward on C2 due to disruption of the transverse ligament, possibly leading to spinal cord compromise or CM.[193,199] Typical progression of the disease leads to superior migration of the odontoid. In the mid to lower cervical spine, radiographic attention is focused on millimeters of vertebral slip of one vertebra on the other and its potential for spinal cord compression.[193]

The incidence of neck pain has been reported at 40% to 88%, with cervical subluxation noted in 43% to 86% on radiographic imaging. However, neurological deficits have been reported in only 7% to 34%.[202,203] In a RA population that showed 80% radiographic cervical instability, only 36% had neurological compromise.[203] In other studies,[193,204] only 50% with radiographic instability were symptomatic, demonstrating that a subgroup of patients with RA and radiographic instability have minimal to no pain and no neurological deficit, but still may be at risk.

Clinical signs and symptoms of RA vary among patients, but also over the course of the disease. Common reports include morning stiffness (lasting longer than 45 minutes) and neck pain.[128] Pain described as a deep ache is typically located at the SO region and may be associated with occipital headache. Compression of C2 sensory fibers may result in migraine, mastoid, ear, or facial pain. Cervical ROM is reduced. Weakness, gait ataxia, and loss of hand dexterity and paresthesia suggest myelopathy, with a reported prevalence of 11% to 58%.[193,202,205] Symptoms related to vertebrobasilar insufficiency (VBI) may also be present.[199] Weakness, disuse atrophy, joint subluxation, and motion limitations pose a challenge to performing and interpreting a neurological examination.[199] In patients with neck pain, a thorough history screening for RA and careful examination is important in light of the need for early disease management and the potential for cervical instability and life-threatening neurological compromise.

Ankylosing Spondylitis

The diagnostic accuracy of history and physical examination for early diagnosis of AS, before radiographic abnormalities, is discussed in Chapter 4. Although AS primarily affects the sacroiliac and lumbar spine regions, progression to the thoracic and cervical spine occurs with time, age, and severity with cervical radiographic findings demonstrated in 82% of patients.[206,207] Neck pain can become more of a complaint than pain in the low back area in those individuals who are generally older and have had the disease longer.[208] Due to bony ankylosis and osteoporosis, the cervical spine is at increased risk of spinal fracture.[209,210] Low-energy falls, such as trips and slips involving hyperextension, may result in neurological deficit from these unstable fractures.[209,210]

Screening for Acute Coronary Syndrome

Goodman and Snyder[128] described substernal or retrosternal chest, neck and/or arm pain or discomfort, palpitations, dyspnea, syncope, cough, diaphoresis, fatigue, and cyanosis as common key symptoms of cardiac disease. Chest pain of cardiac or noncardiac origin may radiate to the neck, jaw, UT, upper back, and shoulder or arms (left more often than right) along the ulnar nerve distribution. The heart supplied by the C3 to T4 spinal segments can refer visceral symptoms to corresponding somatic regions.[128] Associated symptoms include pallor, nausea, and vomiting.[128] Nonmodifiable risk factors include age, male gender, family history, race (ie, African American women), and menopausal women. Modifiable risk factors include physical inactivity, cigarette smoking, elevated serum cholesterol, and high blood pressure. Obesity, response to stress, personality, peripheral vascular disease, hormonal status, and alcohol consumption are contributing factors.[128]

Acute coronary syndrome (ACS), caused by insufficient blood supply to the myocardium, is a spectrum of clinical presentations, ranging from unstable angina to myocardial infarction with non-ST segment elevation, or ST segment elevation.[211] Increased myocardial oxygen and nutrition requirements relating to exertion, emotional stress or physiological stress, such as dehydration, blood loss, and infection or surgery, can lead to ACS. Angina is a typical symptom of myocardial ischemia often described as a sensation of substernal or retrosternal chest pressure, squeezing, or heaviness during exertion of 70% to 90% incidence, but only 33% or less complain of chest pain.[211] Some patients present with neck, jaw, ear, arm, or epigastric discomfort. Diabetic or elderly persons may have no pain, but do report complaints of weakness, light-headedness, shortness of breath, diaphoresis, or nausea and vomiting, and may have altered mental status. Stable angina lasts 5 to 15 minutes when provoked by a predictable level of activity or emotional stress, and is relieved by rest or nitroglycerin. A lag time of 5 to 10 minutes for onset of angina after exertion, stress, a large meal or cold exposure is common.[128] Patients with unstable angina, characterized by abrupt changes in intensity or frequency not relieved by rest or nitroglycerin, are at risk for adverse cardiac events.[128,212] Neck pain is more common in unstable angina (15% to 31%) as compared to acute MI (11% to 13%).[213,214]

The presentation of ACS in women and men differs, with women experiencing more subtle symptoms in the absence of traditional angina and chest pain (Figure 6-4).[128] A key sign of ACS in women is unexplained severe, episodic fatigue that interferes with performing daily activities. Weakness, fatigue, trouble sleeping, and nausea may occur up to a month prior to an acute MI. Less common warning signs of heart attack, especially in women, include the following:

- Unusual chest pain quality and location (ie, burning, heaviness; left chest), and stomach or abdominal pain
- Continuous midthoracic or interscapular pain
- Continuous neck or shoulder pain
- Isolated right biceps pain
- Pain relieved by antacids
- Pain unrelieved by rest or nitroglycerin
- Nausea and vomiting
- Flu-like manifestations without chest pain/discomfort
- Unexplained intense anxiety, weakness or fatigue, breathlessness, and dizziness[128]

Common signs that warn of heart attack include the following:

- Prolonged uncomfortable pressure, fullness, squeezing, or pain in the center of the chest
- Pain that spreads to the throat, neck, back, jaw, shoulders, or arms
- Chest discomfort with lightheadedness, dizziness, sweating, pallor, nausea, or shortness of breath
- Prolonged symptoms unrelieved by antacids, nitroglycerin, or rest[215]

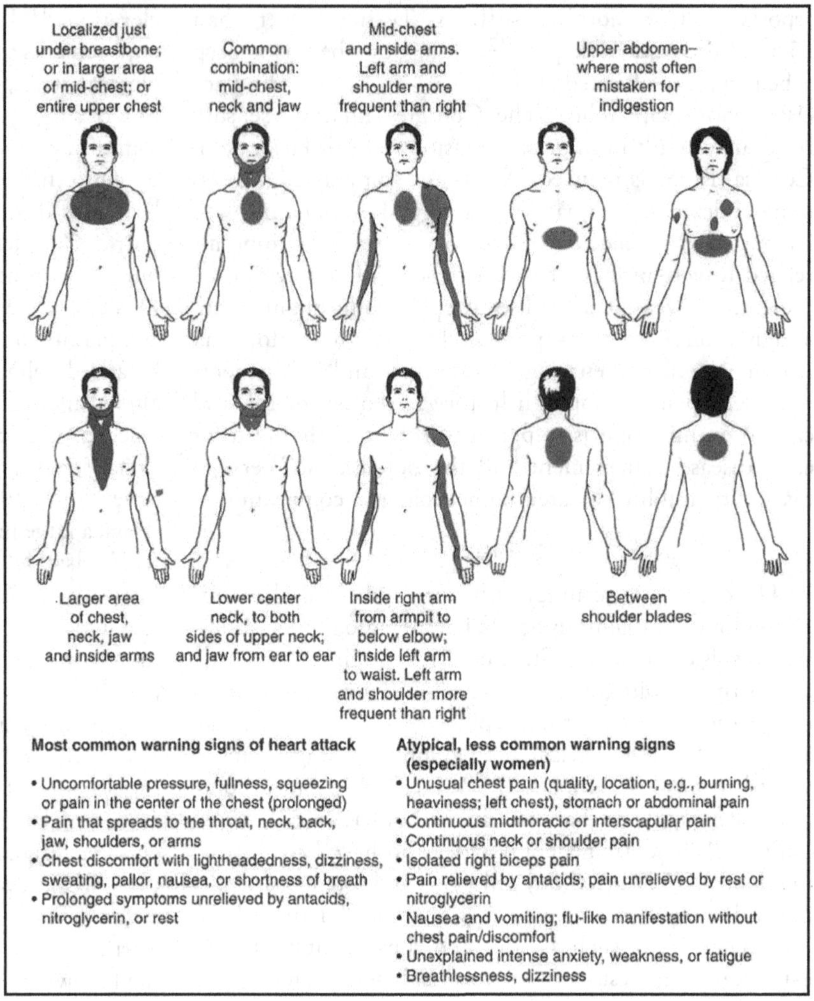

Figure 6-4. Early warning signs of a heart attack. (Reprinted with permission from This figure was published in *Differential Diagnosis for Physical Therapists. Screening for Referral* by Goodman CC, Snyder TEK, Copyright Saunders, an imprint of Elsevier, 2007.)

Patients with atypical symptoms are more likely to be diagnosed with a musculoskeletal, neurological or gastrointestinal problem.[214,216] Careful pursuit of symptoms and related activities are important for differential diagnosis. As the index of suspicion for acute coronary syndrome rises, assessment of vital signs and appropriate medical referral are warranted.

Screening for Neurological Impairment

Persons with MNP and neurological impairment are more likely to have slower recovery rates, recurrent episodes, and an increased risk for surgery when compared to individuals without neurological involvement. Early identification of neurological disorders is critical to reducing the potential for permanent motor or sensory loss and progression to a chronic pain status. Neurological involvement is classified as CM or radiculopathy, but some individuals may present with both conditions (called myeloradiculopathy).

Both CM and radiculopathy are associated with progressive degenerative changes in the cervical spine known collectively as cervical spondylosis. Degenerative changes include cervical disc herniation, facet and uncovertebral joint hypertrophy, osteophytes and spurring, and ossification or thickening of the ligamentum flavum, or posterior longitudinal ligament. The spondylotic changes result in narrowing of the spinal canal, compressing the spinal cord (ie, myelopathy) and/or in the lateral recess, and neuroforamen compressing the nerve root (ie, radiculopathy). Differential diagnosis includes other neurological or disease processes, such as multiple sclerosis, syringomyelia, or tumor.

Clinical Features of Cervical Myelopathy

The natural history of CM is mixed, presenting as a slow stepwise decline or long periods of quiescence.[217] CM is the most common spinal cord dysfunction in persons over 55 years of age[218] and present in 90% of persons 70 years or older,[219] affecting most often persons of Asian descent[220] and males.[221] The clinical features of CM are varied, making early diagnosis difficult. The lower extremities may be involved first with weakness and spasticity, or hyperreflexia affecting gait,[222,223] often producing a wide-based gait and balance problems. Upper extremity changes present as weakness, atrophy, and problems with finger fine motor control.[223,224] Additional manifestations include neck stiffness or pain, pain in the upper quarter region (shoulder, scapula), widespread numbness, paresthesia in both arms or hands, and sensory and ataxic changes of the lower extremities.[225] Sensory changes, although inconsistent, may occur later rather than early in the upper extremities and more than in the lower extremities, but upper extremity symptoms have also been an early presentation. Advanced CM findings may include paraparesis, quadriparesis,[220] and bowel and bladder changes.[226]

Both clinical and imaging findings are used to diagnosis CM.[227] Clinical tests include deep tendon reflex testing,[228] Babinski's,[228] the hand withdrawal reflex test,[228] Hoffmann's test,[229] clonus,[230] inverted supinator sign,[231] and suprapatellar quadriceps reflex testing.[232] Hoffman, Babinski's, clonus, and deep tendon reflexes associated with hyperreflexia are more specific than sensitive, and therefore considered better tests for ruling in CM. The inverted supinator sign (ie, finger flexion or elbow extension during the brachioradialis reflex test) may be the most sensitive test for ruling out CM.[233] Cook et al[234] identified 5 findings to assist in the diagnosis of CM:

1. Age > 45 years
2. Positive Babinski's sign
3. Positive inverted supinator sign
4. Positive Hoffman
5. Gait dysfunction described as spastic, wide-based gait, or ataxic

Absence of a positive finding, or the presence of 1 of 5 tests, resulted in a sensitivity of 0.94, a -LR of 0.18 (95% CI: 0.12 to 0.42), and provides a moderate level of confidence that the patient does not have CM, whereas 3 of 5 positive test findings resulted in a +LR of 30.9 (95% CI: 5.5 to 181.8) and a posttest probability of 94%, thereby assisting with ruling in CM.[234] If CM is suspected, based on history and clinical examination, a referral for additional testing is warranted. Magnetic resonance imaging is the most accurate imaging procedure for CM because it conveys the amount of compression on the spinal cord[235] and demonstrates relatively high sensitivity 0.79% to 0.95%, specificity 0.82 to 0.88, +LR = 4.39 to 7.92, and -LR = 0.06 to 0.27 in identifying abnormalities, such as disk herniation and ligamentous ossification.[235] MRI findings that demonstrate spinal cord related findings are not definitive of CM since other diseases, such as multiple sclerosis or syringomyelia, present with similar symptoms. In addition to a clear compression of the spinal cord at an appropriate symptomatic level on MRI, a detailed history and examination findings are required to make a diagnosis.[227]

Clinical Features of Cervical Radiculopathy

A diagnosis of CR involves a lesion or disease of the dorsal root ganglion, or cervical spinal nerve root at or near the cervical intervertebral foramen.[236] CR is most commonly caused by inflammation, cervical spondylosis, a disk herniation, or other space-occupying lesion, such as a tumor, resulting in neurological deficit of some combination of sensory loss, motor loss, or impaired reflexes in a segmental distribution.[119,225,237] Cervical spondylosis accounts for approximately 68% of confirmed CR, and disk protrusions for 22%. Peak incidence occurs in the fourth or fifth decade of life.[238] The C7 nerve root is most commonly involved, followed by C6 and C8 (in 46%, 18%, and 6% of cases, respectively), with multilevel involvement of C5, C6 and C6, and C7 also reported.[238] The etiology of CR is compromise or direct compression of the cervical spinal nerve or its roots, causing ischemia and a block of conduction along the affected axons. Radicular pain is not attributed to compression of axons. Production of pain is due to compression of the dorsal root ganglion.[119]

Symptoms of CR vary based on the affected nerve root or dorsal root ganglion and may exist in the neck, scapular or shoulder regions, upper arm or forearm, or hand.[225] Patient descriptions are inconsistent and expressed as a severe burning, shooting, stabbing, or lancinating pain traveling distally into the extremity to a dull ache in the neck and upper extremity. Pain located in the medial border of the scapula or shoulder may radiate or refer into the ipsilateral arm and hand along a dermatomal distribution.[239] However, absence of symptoms radiating in a dermatomal distribution does not rule out a CR.[240] Henderson et al[241] reviewed clinical findings in more than 800 patients with CR and found arm pain was in 99.4%, sensory deficits in 85.2%, neck pain in 79.7%, reflex deficits in 71.2%, motor deficits in 68%, scapular pain in 52.5%, anterior chest pain in 17.8%, headaches in 9.7%, anterior chest and arm pain in 5.9%, and left-sided chest and arm pain in 1.3%.[241]

In a population undergoing nerve root decompression, Tanaka et al[242,243] reported an early history of neck and scapular pain in 70% of CR cases that were present for a week or more prior to the onset of classic reports of upper extremity radicular symptoms. Suprascapular pain was noted in 82% of cases for C5 and C6 CR, interscapular or scapular pain always for C7 or C8 CR, and subscapular pain was commonly reported for C8 CR. Lateral (C6), posterior (C7), or medial (C8) arm pain was frequently associated with the ascribed nerve root. For severe finger paresthesia or sensory deficit involving the thumb, index, long finger, or the little finger, the nerve root indicated was C6, C7 or C8, respectively. Patterns of sensory and motor involvement were variable, but when the weakest muscle was deltoid, biceps or wrist extensors, wrist flexors or triceps, or intrinsics, the nerve root indicated was C5, C6, C7, or C8, respectively. Tanaka et al[242,243] concluded that the sites of the neck and arm pain are important for the diagnosis of CR, but only severe finger paresthesia supports the diagnosis. Predictable patterns of motor loss and sensory and reflex changes may be demonstrated for specific nerve root levels. Chapter 3 discusses the diagnostic accuracy of the traditional upper quarter neurological screening examination consisting of motor function, sensibility changes, and deep tendon reflexes.[244]

In patients with suspected CR, diagnostic accuracy of 34 clinical examination items was examined,[245] demonstrating that at least two thirds of these items had at least fair or better reliability and 12 had likelihood ratio point estimates above 2 or below 0.50. The 12 items were the upper limb tension test A (ULTT A), cervical rotation to the involved side less than 60 degrees, cervical flexion less than 55 degrees, reduced or absent biceps deep tendon reflex, the distraction test, MMT of the involved biceps, Valsalva's test, Spurling test A, shoulder abduction test, involved C5 dermatome sensation and 2 questions: "Where are your symptoms most bothersome?" and "Do your symptoms improve with moving or positioning your neck?"[245] No abnormal findings for the triceps or brachioradialis DTRs were recorded in this population. Although 12 tests had +LRs, a test item cluster of 4 variables formed a clinical prediction rule (CPR) with a high +LR:

1. ULTT A (most useful test when used alone for ruling out CR)
2. Cervical rotation less than 60 degrees to the involved side
3. Distraction test
4. Spurling test A[245]

If 3 items are positive, the +LR was 6.1 (95% CI: 2.0 to 18.6), specificity was 0.94 (95% CI: 0.88 to 1.0), and the probability of CR increases to 65%. If all 4 items are present, the probability of CR increases to 90% with a +LR 30.3 (95% CI: 1.7 to 538.2).[245] The test item cluster produces larger posttest probability changes for the diagnosis of CR than any single test item. Due to wide 95% confidence intervals for all individual items and the test item cluster, additional validation is required.[245]

In other research examining the clinical usefulness of tests for CR, Rubinstein et al[246] found that a positive Spurling's test, manual traction, and the Valsalva's maneuver had low to moderate sensitivity and high specificity useful for ruling in a CR. The ULTT test was found to have high sensitivity and low specificity useful for ruling out a CR. The shoulder abduction test showed low to moderate sensitivity and moderate to high specificity useful for ruling in CR. Based on the quality of available evidence in this systematic review, the authors are unable to make any strong recommendations on the use of these tests, especially in primary care.[246] Patients with neurological findings consistent with CR should be referred for additional testing. Special tests related to diagnosis of CR are covered in the Physical Examination section of this chapter.

Screening for Yellow Flags

In addition to red flag screening, the clinician should also assess for the presence of yellow flags, or psychosocial risk factors, predictive for chronic disability and pain. Accurate identification of patients with risk factors that interfere with the normal recovery process guides appropriate physical, cognitive, and behavioral management strategies to address factors that can be modified to influence outcomes.

The role of psychosocial or psychological factors in the transition from acute to chronic neck pain has not been studied as extensively as LBP and is controversial. Nederland[247] examined the value of fear-avoidance variables such as pain catastrophizing and kinesiophobia, or fear of movement in predicting chronic neck pain disability in posttraumatic neck pain at 24 weeks' follow-up. Using a combination of a baseline Neck Disability Index (NDI) cutoff score of 15 or more and Tampa Scale of Kinesiophobia cutoff score of 40 or more, the posttest probability of a chronic disability outcome is 83.3% (95% CI: 70.3% to 91.3%), potentially identifying posttraumatic neck pain patients that should be offered early intervention to prevent chronicity.[247]

Bot et al[248] described the 12-month course for a cohort of patients (n = 423) with neck and shoulder pain followed by their general practitioner (GP) in an effort to identify predictors of recovery. At 3 months, the probability of recovery was reduced by the presence of more intense pain at baseline, longer duration of symptoms before presenting to the GP, a history of neck or shoulder symptoms, frequent discomfort, more resting, and being less vital. At the 12 month follow-up, the following conditions significantly reduced the probability of recovery: a longer duration of symptoms before presenting to the GP, a history of neck or shoulder symptoms, both shoulder involvement, numbness in hand and fingers, multiple musculoskeletal complaints, and more worrying.[248] However, more fear-avoidance predicted a larger reduction in pain at 3 and 12 months, and functional disability at 3 months, which contrasts with the fear-avoidance model. The authors state the effects were small and that this finding may be random. More research is recommended.[248]

In addition to a primary complaint of neck pain, psychosocial and physical features are also important prognostic indicators. In WAD, a systematic review[249] concludes that prognosis is multifactorial, integrating physical and psychosocial features. Biological features, such as higher NDI scores and reduced motion,[40,251] are predictive of poor outcome following WAD, and are useful for classification purposes.[40,252,253] Physical factors of motor and sensory impairments may have a stronger association with chronic pain and disability levels than psychosocial or workplace dimensions,[254] but psychosocial factors, such as fear-avoidance beliefs, fear of movement, or reinjury and coping strategies, have a role in the transition from acute to chronic neck pain.[255]

Several studies suggest that the relationship between neck pain disability and fear-avoidance beliefs may not be as strong as the association in persons with LBP. George et al[256] examined pain intensity, disability, and fear-avoidance beliefs in patients with neck pain and LBP. In general, patients with neck pain had a weaker association among the variables than patients with LBP, weaker FABQ subscale scores, and lower correlations between FABQ scores and concurrent pain and disability measures.[256] In a prospective study of acute WAD, high fear of movement and injury scores were not associated with a poor outcome at 6-month follow-up.[257] The results of this study show that all patients who suffer WAD display initial psychological distress that decreases in those patients who recover. Individuals who have persistent symptoms at 6 months are characterized with a moderate posttraumatic stress reaction and sustained psychological distress.[257] Posttraumatic stress symptoms are associated with poor functional recovery, greater severity of complaints, and greater pain and disability.[257,258]

Kamper et al[259] also examined the role of fear as a mediator between initial pain and later disability in WAD, demonstrating that the Fear-Avoidance Model explained 20% to 40% of the relationship between initial pain and later disability in patients with WAD. The authors note that while the contribution of fear influences disability, other factors, such as severity of anatomical injury, comorbid physical and psychological disorders, and sociocultural indicators are also involved in this complex relationship.

Several studies have looked at coping strategies and how they relate to neck pain prognosis. In patients with WAD, Buitenhuis et al[260] investigated coping styles and the duration of neck complaints[260] and found that patients who sought symptom relief through distraction activities, such as drinking or smoking, had a significantly longer duration of symptoms at 12-month follow-up. Patients who shared concerns through a social support network had a shorter duration of symptoms.[260] Similarly, Carroll et al[261] found that passive coping strategies resulted in slower recovery. A passive coping style may also be a risk factor for chronic neck pain of insidious onset.[262,263] Passive coping strategies are examples of prognostic indicators that are modifiable through continued assurance and education.

The relationship between physical and psychosocial factors and initiation and maintenance of chronic neck disability seems to be complex, unclear, and may be different than the factors associated with LBP. Persistent neck pain regardless of mechanism of onset, is associated with psychological distress.[264] WAD may also include anxiety, depression, behavioral alterations, passive coping styles, and posttraumatic stress reactions.[257,264,265] Persistently high pain levels and motor and sensory impairments appear to influence psychological stress, and vice versa. In a review of late WAD (eg limited motion and other symptoms > 6 months that prevent return to normal activities) and 21 psychological risk factors, most findings were inconclusive due to poor methodology, with no association found between late WAD and personality traits, general psychological distress, well being, social support, life control, and psychosocial work factors.[255] Further study is needed, but clinicians should recognize and assess the presence and individual effects of psychological and psychosocial stress and fear-avoidance beliefs through the use of appropriate self-report questionnaires.

Outcomes Measures

Common functional measures (Table 6-9) used for patients with neck pain are the NDI,[266] Patient Specific Functional and Pain Scale (PSFS),[267] the Global Rate of Change Scale (GRC),[268] Fear-Avoidance Belief Questionnaire (FABQ),[269] the Numeric Pain Rating Scale (NPRS), the Impact of Event Scale (IES),[270] the Dizziness Handicap Inventory,[271] Tampa Scale of Kinesiophobia (TSK),[272] and, to investigate neuropathic pain state, the self-report version of the Leeds Assessment of Neuropathic Symptoms and Signs (S-LANSS) questionnaire.[273] The S-LANSS is discussed in Chapter 4.

Neck Disability Index

The NDI (Figure 6-5) was developed by Vernon and Mior,[266] using the Oswestry Low Back Pain Index as a template. The index consists of 10 items: 4 are related to pain intensity, headache, concentration and sleep, 4 inquire about lifting, work, driving, and recreation, and 2 are about personal care and reading activities. Each item is scored from 0 to 5 and the total score is expressed out of 50 or as a percentage (ie, total score divided by 50 × 100). If 1 item is left blank, the score is expressed out of 50. Occasionally, the "driving" item or "work" items are not applicable to a person's life and may be left blank. The work item may be interpreted as "work at a job or housework." If 3 or more items are missing, the score may not be valid. Retesting is recommended at 2-week intervals throughout the episode of care.[274] Higher percentages indicate higher perceived disability. A nonvalidated interpretation of scores is: no disability (0 to 4); mild disability (5 to 14), moderate disability (15 to 24), severe disability (25 to 34); and complete disability (more than 35).[266] In patients with WAD, Sterling et al[275] defined recovery as less than 4 (18%), mild disability as 5 to 14 (10% to 28%), and moderate to severe disability as more than 15 (30%).

Table 6-9. Summary of Outcome Measures

OUTCOME	RELIABILITY	SCORE (POINTS)
Neck Disability Index	High[266]	• MDC = 5 neck pain WAD I/II[276] • MDC = 10 cervical radiculopathy and WAD III • MCID = 7 points[276] • MDC = 10.25[277] • MDC = 10.2; MCID = 10 with and without UE symptoms[277] • MDC = 13.4; MCID = 8.5 for cervical radiculopathy[278]
Patient Specific Functional Scale	Acceptable[267] High[281]	• MDC = 2 for mean of 3 activity ratings[267] • MDC = 2.1; MCID = 2 for cervical radiculopathy[280] • MDC = 3.3; MCID = 2.2 for cervical radiculopathy[278]
Global Rate of Change	ICC 0.90 on 11-point scale[281]	• MCID ≥5 on a 15-point scale for mechanical neck[282,284]
Fear-Avoidance Belief Questionnaire (PA) = Physical activity (W) = Work subscale	Test-retest reliability for the FABQ-PA (0.85 95% CI: 0.77, 0.90) and the FABQ-W (0.93 95% CI: 0.89, 0.96)[286]	• MDC, MCID unknown • Recommended cutoff scores: FABQ-Total = 48, FABQ-W > 18, FABQ-PA > 15, and NDI ≥ 15 at risk for prolonged neck-related disability; NDI was the best predictor[287]
Impact of Event Scale	Good[270]	Measures trauma-related distress • 0 to 8 (subclinical range) • 9 to 25 (mild range) • 26 to 43 (moderate range) • 44+ (severe range) *26 or above within a month of WAD injury is a strong predictor of poor outcome at 6 and 12 months = moderate or severe impact[251,275]; may indicate the need for psychological referral
Numeric Pain Rating Scale (0 to 11 scale)	Moderate reliability[324]	• MDC = 2.1 (95% CI: 1.6 to 2.6); MCID of 1.3 for MNP with or without upper extremity symptoms[324] • MDC = 4.1; MCID 2.2[324]

ICC indicates intraclass correlation coefficient; FABQ, Fear-Avoidance Belief Questionnaire; CI, confidence interval; MDC, minimal detectable change; WAD, whiplash-associated disorder; MCID, minimal clinically important difference; UE, upper extremity; NDI, Neck Disability Index; MNP, mechanical neck pain.

The NDI has acceptable content validity and retest reliability in both acute and chronic neck pain populations with a musculoskeletal or neural source of symptoms of traumatic or nontraumatic origin.[276]

Based on a systematic review of the NDI by MacDermid et al,[276] consider the following recommendations:

- The NDI should be scored out of 50.
- The minimal detectable change (MDC) is 5 points (10%) or up to 10 points (20%) for CR.
- The MDC is 5 points minimum for WAD I and II, and 10 points for WAD III for short-term therapy (2 weeks).
- The minimal clinically important difference (MCID) is approximately 7 points.
- Scores of 40 to 50 and 0 to 10 approach a ceiling and floor effect, respectively in which case use of the PSFS should be considered.

Other studies suggest slightly different values for interpreting the NDI. In a population with neck pain (with

Neck Disability Index

This questionnaire is designed to help us better understand how your **neck pain** affects your ability to manage everyday -life activities. Please mark in each section the **one box** that applies to you. Although you may consider that two of the statements in any one section relate to you, please mark the box that **most closely** describes your present -day situation.

Section 1 - Pain Intensity

- ☐ I have no neck pain at the moment.
- ☐ The pain is very mild at the moment.
- ☐ The pain is moderate at the moment.
- ☐ The pain is fairly severe at the moment.
- ☐ The pain is very severe at the moment.
- ☐ The pain is the worst imaginable at the moment.

Section 2 - Personal Care

- ☐ I can look after myself normally without causing extra neck pain.
- ☐ I can look after myself normally, but it causes extra neck pain.
- ☐ It is painful to look after myself, and I am slow and careful.
- ☐ I need some help but manage most of my personal care.
- ☐ I need help every day in most aspects of self -care.
- ☐ I do not get dressed. I wash with difficulty and stay in bed.

Section 3 – Lifting

- ☐ I can lift heavy weights without causing extra neck pain.
- ☐ I can lift heavy weights, but it gives me extra neck pain.
- ☐ Neck pain prevents me from lifting heavy weights off the floor but I can manage if items are conveniently positioned, ie. on a table.
- ☐ Neck pain prevents me from lifting heavy weights, but I can manage light weights if they are conveniently positioned.
- ☐ I can lift only very light weights.
- ☐ I cannot lift or carry anything at all.

Section 4 – Reading

- ☐ I can read as much as I want with no neck pain.
- ☐ I can read as much as I want with slight neck pain.
- ☐ I can read as much as I want with moderate neck pain.
- ☐ I can't read as much as I want because of moderate neck pain.
- ☐ I can't read as much as I want because of severe neck pain.
- ☐ I can't read at all.

Section 5 – Headaches

- ☐ I have no headaches at all.
- ☐ I have slight headaches that come infrequently.
- ☐ I have moderate headaches that come infrequently.
- ☐ I have moderate headaches that come frequently.
- ☐ I have severe headaches that come frequently.
- ☐ I have headaches almost all the time.

Section 6 – Concentration

- ☐ I can concentrate fully without difficulty.
- ☐ I can concentrate fully with slight difficulty.
- ☐ I have a fair degree of difficulty concentrating.
- ☐ I have a lot of difficulty concentrating.
- ☐ I have a great deal of difficulty concentrating.
- ☐ I can't concentrate at all.

Section 7 – Work

- ☐ I can do as much work as I want.
- ☐ I can only do my usual work, but no more.
- ☐ I can do most of my usual work, but no more.
- ☐ I can't do my usual work.
- ☐ I can hardly do any work at all.
- ☐ I can't do any work at all.

Section 8 – Driving

- ☐ I can drive my car without neck pain.
- ☐ I can drive my car with only slight neck pain.
- ☐ I can drive as long as I want with moderate neck pain.
- ☐ I can't drive as long as I want because of moderate neck pain.
- ☐ I can hardly drive at all because of severe neck pain.
- ☐ I can't drive my car at all because of neck pain.

Section 9 – Sleeping

- ☐ I have no trouble sleeping.
- ☐ My sleep is slightly disturbed for less than 1 hour.
- ☐ My sleep is mildly disturbed for up to 1-2 hours.
- ☐ My sleep is moderately disturbed for up to 2-3 hours.
- ☐ My sleep is greatly disturbed for up to 3-5 hours.
- ☐ My sleep is completely disturbed for up to 5-7 hours.

Section 10 – Recreation

- ☐ I am able to engage in all my recreational activities with no neck pain at all.
- ☐ I am able to engage in all my recreational activities with some neck pain.
- ☐ I am able to engage in most, but not all of my recreational activities because of pain in my neck.
- ☐ I am able to engage in only a few of my recreational activities because of neck pain.
- ☐ I can hardly do recreational activities due to neck pain.
- ☐ I can't do any recreational activities due to neck pain.

Patient Name ______________________ Date ____________

Score ________ [50]

Figure 6-5. The Neck Disability Index. (Reprinted with permission from Howard Vernon. Copyright VERNON H & HAGINO C, 1991.)

or without upper extremity symptoms), the MCID was 7.5 points and the MDC 10.2. The authors recommend the use of a 10-point change for the MCID because the MCID was within the bounds of measurement error.[277] In a cohort of patients with CR,[278] the NDI has fair test-retest reliability. The MDC for the NDI was 13.4 and the MCID 8.5—slightly different than the recommendations by MacDermid et al.[276] Relative to the ICF categories, the Neck Bournemouth Questionnaire and the NDI demonstrate a well-balanced distribution of items.[279]

Patient-Specific Functional and Pain Scale

The PSFS (discussed in Chapter 4; see Figure 4-12) is related to LBP. Acceptable reliability and validity have also been reported in the neck pain population.[267] Westaway et al[267] reported a MDC of 2 points (for a mean of 3 activity ratings), meaning patients that truly have not changed will report a change of less than 2 points on reassessment.[267] In a small group of patients with CR, Cleland et al[280] reported high test-retest reliability was for the PSFS (ICC 0.82; 95% CI: 0.54 to 0.93). The MDC for the PSFS is 2.1. The MCID for the PSFS is 2.0. When compared with the NDI, the PSFS had superior reliability, construct validity, and responsiveness in this population.[280] In contrast, Young et al[278] reported poor reliability in patients with CR as compared to the NDI and NPRS, but adequate responsiveness in all 3 measures: MDC (NDI 13.4; PSFS 3.3; NPRS 4.1) and MCID (NDI 8.5; PSFS 2.2; NPRS 2.2).

Global Rate of Change Scale

The GRC (discussed in Chapter 4; see Figure 4-13) is related to LBP. Although it hasn't been studied in patients with neck pain, the scale is also used to quantify a patient's improvement or worsening over time to determine the effect of an intervention or plan of care, and to guide management decisions. Test-retest reliability for LBP is ICC 0.90 on an 11-point scale.[281] Arbitrary cutoff values of meaningful improvement, or deterioration as >5 or <5 on a 15-point scale, have been used in clinical research related to neck pain.[282-284] The MCID for the GROC has been reported as a 3-point change from baseline.[269] Kamper et al[285] provided a detailed overview of the strengths and weaknesses of GRC scales used in clinical work and research.

Fear-Avoidance Belief Questionnaire

The FABQ (see Figure 4-14) is discussed in Chapter 4 along with the fear-avoidance model in LBP. The same form is used with the word "neck" substituted for the word "back" as appropriate, but research is limited for its use with neck pain. The FABQ values for LBP cannot be used for neck pain. The relationship between fear-related behavior and pain, and disability among patients with neck pain is weaker than among LBP.[286] Much controversy exists as to the amount of fear-avoidance beliefs involved in the initiation and development of chronic neck pain.

Landers et al[287] recruited 79 subjects with acute, subacute, and chronic neck pain from outpatient physiotherapy clinics to determine if fear-avoidance beliefs and nonorganic behavior, signs and symptoms associated with distress and illness behavior are predictive of disability. A 12-week NDI score > 15 was operationally defined as prolonged disability. The FABQ-Physical Activity Scale (PA), initial NDI, and cervical nonorganic sign (CNOS) score accounted for 67.5% of the variance in the 12-week NDI scores. The initial NDI (ie, 56.0% of the variance in 12-week NDI) was the best predictor of 12-week NDI scores followed by FABQ-PA (ie, additional 6.2% of the variance) and CNOS (ie, additional 5.3% of the variance). The authors assert that the presence of prolonged disability in patients with neck pain is at least partially related to fear-avoidance beliefs and recommend cutoff scores of FABQ-Total = 48, FABQ-Work Scale = 18 and FABQ-PA = 15. In this study initial NDI was the best predictor of neck-related disability, but the FABQ-PA and CNOS were also predictive.[287]

Other studies also support a smaller role of fear-avoidance beliefs as contributors of neck-related disability. In a cohort of outpatients with MNP, with or without upper extremity symptoms, and a NDI greater than 10%, Cleland et al[286] examined the psychometric properties of the FABQ and the TSK. No differences were noted in test-retest reliability between the FABQ-PA and the FABQ-W. The FABQ-PA did not significantly correlate with the concurrent pain or disability (r = 0.19 and 0.07, respectively), but the FABQ-W did significantly correlate with concurrent measures of pain and disability (r = 0.34 and 0.25, respectively). Although significant correlations exist between the TSK, FABQ-PA, and FABQ-W, the relationship is fair and supports the theory that fear about work and physical activities is a separate construct than fear about movement and reinjury (TSK). The result of this study and George et al[256] suggested that the FABQ-PA is not significantly related to concurrent measures of pain or disability in patients with chronic neck pain, but the FABQ-W has fair but statistically significant correlations with concurrent measures of pain and disability. The authors suggest a weaker relationship between fear and avoidance beliefs and pain/disability among patients, with mechanical neck pain with physical and psychosocial factors more likely to play a role in chronic disability.[256]

Impact of Event Scale

The IES (Figure 6-6) is a self-report measure designed to assess current subjective distress for any specific life event.[270] The IES demonstrated good reliability[270] and validity in studies of the acute emotional response to trauma[288] and measuring trauma-related distress. However, the IES cannot be used by itself to diagnose posttraumatic distress disorder.[289] Sterling et al[290] used the IES in subjects with WAD.

The IES instrument consists of 15 items suitable for repeated measurement to monitor progress over time.[291] Seven items measure intrusive symptoms, such as troubled dreams, intrusive thoughts or strong feelings about the incident, 5 cover acute intrusive symptoms while awake, and 2 cover symptoms such as nightmares and insomnia during sleep. Eight items measure avoidance of feelings, situations, or ideas and awareness of emotional numbness. Patients are asked to rate each item on a 4-point scale as to how often each symptom occurred over the past 7 days: 0 (not at all); 1 (rarely); 3 (sometimes), and 5 (often). Scores range from 0 to 35 for intrusion, 0 to 40 for avoidance, and 0 to 75 for the total IES.[270] Subjects in the original study[270] scored a mean total stress score of 39.5 (SD = 17.2, range 0 to 69), a mean intrusion subscale score from items 1, 4, 5, 6, 10, 11, 14 of 21.4 (SD = 9.6, range 0 to 35), and a mean avoidance subscale score from items 2, 3, 7, 8, 9, 12, 13, 15 of 18.2 (SD = 10.8, range 0 to 38). The total score is interpreted as follows: 0 to 8 (subclinical range), 9 to 25 (mild range), 26 to 43 (moderate range), 44+ (severe range). A suggested cutoff point is 26, above which a moderate or severe impact is indicated.

A criticism of the IES is the absence of items relating to persistent hyperarousal, the third major symptom cluster of posttraumatic stress disorder.[292] Therefore, the Impact of Event Scale-Revised (IES-R) was published to include the content area of hyperarousal along with minor

On ______________________ you experienced a motor vehicle accident.

Below is a list of comments made by people after stressful life events. Please check each item, indicating how frequently these comments were true for you DURING THE PAST SEVEN DAYS. If they did not, occur during that time please mark the 'NOT AT ALL' column.

	Frequency			
1. I thought about it when I didn't mean to	Not at all	Rarely	Sometimes	Often
2. I avoided letting myself get upset when I thought about it or was reminded of it	Not at all	Rarely	Sometimes	Often
3. I tried to remove it from memory	Not at all	Rarely	Sometimes	Often
4. I had trouble falling asleep or staying asleep because pictures or thoughts about it came into my mind	Not at all	Rarely	Sometimes	Often
5. I had waves of strong feelings about it	Not at all	Rarely	Sometimes	Often
6. I had dreams about it	Not at all	Rarely	Sometimes	Often
7. I stayed away from reminders about it	Not at all	Rarely	Sometimes	Often
8. I felt as if it hadn't happened or it wasn't real	Not at all	Rarely	Sometimes	Often
9. I tried not to talk about it	Not at all	Rarely	Sometimes	Often
10. Pictures about it popped into my mind	Not at all	Rarely	Sometimes	Often
11. Other things kept making me think about it	Not at all	Rarely	Sometimes	Often
12. I was aware that I still had a lot of feelings about it but I didn't deal with them	Not at all	Rarely	Sometimes	Often
13. I tried not to think about it	Not at all	Rarely	Sometimes	Often
14. Any reminder brought back feelings about it	Not at all	Rarely	Sometimes	Often
15. My feelings were kind of numb	Not at all	Rarely	Sometimes	Often

Scoring: Not at all = 0; Rarely = 1; Sometimes = 3; Often = 5; Total = total the scores.
Intrusive subscale: sum of items 1, 4, 5, 6, 10, 11 and 14.
Avoidance subscale: sum of items 2, 3, 7, 8, 9, 12, 13 and 15.
Total score: 9–25 (mild range); 26–43 (moderate range); 443 (severe range).

Figure 6-6. Revised Impact of Event Scale (IES). (Reprinted with permission from Horowitz M, Wilner N, Alvarez W. Impact of event scale: a measure of subjective stress. *Psychosomatic Medicine.* 1979;41:209-218.)

modifications of the original IES.[293] Higher scores on both scales indicate more symptoms of posttraumatic stress.

Since whiplash injury is a traumatic event, the psychological stress related to the collision may play a role in the development of persistent symptoms. Sterling et al[290] measured psychological distress using the General Health Questionnaire 28 (GHQ-28), fear of movement and reinjury using the TSK, acute posttraumatic stress using the IES, and general health and well being using the Short Form-36 (SF-36) in 76 whiplash subjects within 1 month of injury, and then at 2, 3, and 6 months' follow-up. At 6 months, subjects were classified as recovered (NDI < 8), mild pain and disability (NDI 10-28), or moderate to severe pain and disability (NDI > 30). All groups showed psychological distress to some degree at 1 month, but the scores for the recovered and mild symptom groups returned to normal by 2 months, along with reduced pain and disability. Scores for the moderate to severe group remained elevated. TSK scores decreased by 2 months in the mild symptoms group and by 6 months in the persistent moderate to severe group. At 6 months, the persistent moderate to severe symptom group continued to have elevated psychological distress and a moderate posttraumatic stress reaction (as indicated by elevated IES scores). IES scores were significantly higher (29.12 ± 3.1 at less than 1 month) for the moderate to severe group. The total score was above the score of 26, suggesting a moderate posttraumatic stress reaction (PTSR). At 6 months the IES score was reduced to 23.13 ± 1.5, and considered a mild PTSR state. A moderate PTSR within a month of injury is a strong predictor of poor outcome at 6 months and 12 months postinjury.[39,40] A cutoff IES score of 26 or above may indicate the need for a psychological referral. The optimal time frame for referral is debatable. Forbes et al[294] suggested monitoring the trauma-related symptoms for 2 weeks prior to referring for psychological intervention. The IES is also a component of the proposed classification of WAD.[295]

Components of the Patient's History

A patient's experience of neck pain is multifactorial, consisting of individual occupational and psychological or psychosocial factors. The relative contribution of each of these factors varies with each patient as they relate to the development and persistence of MNP. However, the goals and process related to obtaining a relevant history during the patient interview are unchanged (as discussed in Chapter 2). During the interview the clinician reflects on the patient responses and the context in which the patient presents as potential key factors to developing a preliminary PT diagnosis, prognosis, and plan for the physical examination. The information obtained through the interview guides decision making throughout the episode of care. Nordin et al[120] found no acceptable studies demonstrating the diagnostic accuracy of the history in patients with neck pain.

Demographic Profile Considerations for Patients With Mechanical Neck Pain

The relationship between physical spinal loads and psychosocial factors as potential causes or contributors to the development or persistence of neck pain and associated symptoms is complex. For most individuals, the impact of one factor alone is likely to be small. As part of the history, clinicians should gain awareness and understanding of the potential risk and prognostic factors for each patient.

Age, Gender, Race, and Ethnicity Considerations

General Population

A best evidence synthesis[13] reported that age as a risk factor for incident neck pain is varied. Neck pain prevalence increases with age, but age is a weak predictor. The prevalence of neck pain peaks at middle ages of 35 to 49 and declines later in life, with younger persons having a better prognosis.[14] Gender as a risk factor and predictor of recovery is equivocal.[14,296] Poor psychological status is a risk factor for neck pain and a predictor for poor outcome.[297] No studies have examined the influence of cultural factors.[13]

Whiplash Associated Disorders

A best evidence synthesis[297] reported that younger age persons have a slightly higher risk for WAD, compared to 55 years and older. Generally, the evidence related to gender is inconsistent, but females may be at slightly greater risk for WAD than males. Neither age nor gender plays a major role in recovery.[298] No studies have examined psychosocial or cultural factors in the onset of WAD. Hospital visits related to WAD have increased over the past 30 years.[297]

Worker Populations

Another best evidence synthesis[299] reported that older workers are more likely to develop neck pain,[300,301] but age is not a prognostic factor for outcome.[302] Gender as a prognostic indicator is variable, with women reporting slightly more persistent or recurrent symptoms.[302] The evidence related to the influence of marital status and education is inconsistent. Income is not associated with risk of neck pain. A history of headaches is linked with an increased risk of neck pain. Workers who are depressed have a higher risk of developing neck pain, but psychological factors are not predictors of poor outcome.[302] At least 5% of workers may develop persistent neck symptoms and, depending on occupation, up to 10% have at least one episode that limits activities. A single risk factor is insufficient to cause neck pain in workers.[302] Current evidence indicates that specific workplace or job demands are not associated with recovery from neck pain, but collar workers take fewer sick leaves than blue-collar workers. Changing jobs has a favorable outcome for assembly workers.[302]

Occupational, Leisure, Sport Activity, and Socioeconomic Considerations

General Population

Employment status, income, and home ownership are not risk factors, except that the incidence of neck pain is higher in those who are not working due to ill health or disabilitiy.[13] Participation in exercise and physical activity varies in its association as a risk factor for neck pain.[13] General physical acitivty does not appear to be associated with prognosis in the general population, except for bicycling which is associated with a poorer prognosis.[14]

Whiplash Associated Disorders

Preliminary evidence supports the efficacy of whiplash head restraint devices in rear-end collisions.[297] The effect of occupation type and preinjury physical fitness or exercise programs has not been studied.[298]

Worker Population

A best evidence synthesis[299] reports that the type of occupation and low-to-moderate physical performance capacity of the neck and shoulder muscles is a risk factor for neck pain. Workers who participate regularly in exercise or sports have as similar incidence of neck pain as those who do not. Likewise, time spent on hobbies is not associated with the development of neck pain. Several factors in the workplace are associated with increased risk: psychological job stress, low coworker support, job insecurity, working in static positions for prolonged periods, repetitive or precision work, working with the neck in flexion of 20 degrees or more 70% of the time, working with hands above shoulder level, carrying or lifting heavy loads, working in awkward positions, head and neck posture, use of a telephone shoulder rest, keyboard position that causes an elbow angle greater than 121 degrees, and a computer mouse position that causes more than 25 degrees of shoulder flexion.

Use of chairs with arm rests lowers the risk of neck pain, but modifying workstations and workers' posture do not reduce the incidence of neck pain.[299]

Chief Complaint, Description, and Assessment of Presenting Symptoms

Synthesis of the patient's description of symptoms (ie, intensity, quality, nature, and relationship) initiates the process of understanding the underlying mechanisms. The patient should be adequately undressed so that the clinician is able to precisely note the area and extent of symptoms. When the patient points to the area of pain, the clinician confirms an understanding of the location by placing a hand on the patient and tracing the distribution. In persons presenting with a primary complaint of neck pain, the clinician should clear areas that the patient has not reported as symptomatic. Certain areas should be routinely questioned:

- Neck circumferentially and thoracic spine
- Chest and abdomen
- Both upper extremities, circumferentially
- Head and face
- If not offered by the patient, specifically ask for numbness, tingling, other sensory symptoms (ie, cold, heaviness, dizziness, unsteadiness, nausea, and visual disturbances), or areas that do not feel normal

Pain patterns may be classified as nonmusculoskeletal, musculoskeletal, or have components of both disorders. The patient's description and pattern of pain or other symptoms often form the initial impression or working diagnosis, which in turn focuses the rest of the history and identifies areas for further questioning and clarification.

Nonmusculoskeletal Pain or Viscerally Referred Pain

Viscerally referred pain to the neck, arms, and trunk is most likely the result of pulmonary, cardiovascular, or gastrointestinal disease.[303] Visceral referred pain patterns that may mimic musculoskeletal patterns in persons with neck pain and associated symptoms are depicted in Chapter 2 (see Figure 2-3). The pulmonary system can refer pain to the neck and shoulders usually with concomitant features of coughing, dyspnea, sore throat, and hoarseness. The cardiovascular system, as a referral source to the neck and upper extremity, is discussed under Acute Coronary Syndrome. Within the gastrointestinal system, esophagitis or peptic ulcer refer pain to the upper and mid-abdomen, mid-thoracic region, anterior chest, neck, and bilateral shoulders. The usual referral pattern for the liver and pancreas is the right upper and mid-thoracic spine or upper abdominal and thoracolumbar regions. However, if the diaphragm is irritated with these conditions, neck and shoulder pain may occur. The liver can refer to the right side of the neck, anteriorly, posteriorly, and laterally.[303] If the pain pattern generates an initial hypothesis for a nonmusculoskeletal disorder, clinicians should question for clusters of symptoms, such as eating, swallowing, breathing, persistent cough, heartburn, or relief with antacids or eating, and signs that may suggest a particular system is involved. Visceral symptoms or symptoms of systemic disease may indicate the need for medical referral, or provide contraindications or precautions to PT management, or affect prognosis.

Musculoskeletal Pain or Somatic Referred Pain

Neck pain, by definition, is located in an area bound by the T1 spinous process, the superior nuchal line, and laterally by the lateral margins of the neck.[304] However, persons with neck pain report symptoms from the inferior border of the scapula to the head and face, with or without referral to the upper extremities and trunk. The presentation may include local symptoms with or without associated upper extremity complaints, pain in the upper extremity alone, pain in the chest, face, throat, or as a headache. Pain from the cervical somatic structures (ie, ligament, facet, muscle, intervertebral disc) of the cervical spine can be local to the neck or referred into the thorax, head, face, or upper extremity. Somatic referred pain is perceived in an area that shares the same segmental innervation as its source. Patients describe somatic referred pain as deep, dull aching and expanding into wide areas that are difficult to localize. The perception of pain from a particular structure is not the same among individuals, but it is similar in distribution. Somatic referred pain does not involve spinal nerve or nerve roots, so neurological signs are absent.[305]

Many studies using healthy subjects demonstrate local pain and somatic referred pain patterns from the experimental stimulation of muscle,[306,307] facet joints,[308-310] and the intervertebral disc.[311-314] Pain from the cervical zygapophyseal joints is depicted in Figure 5-5, as follows:

- C2 to C3 refers superiorly to the head.
- C3 to C4 and C4 to C5 referral is primarily over the posterior neck.
- C5 to C6 spreads across the supraspinous fossa of the scapula with C6 to C7 spreading more inferiorly over the scapula.[119]

The atlantooccipital and AA joints can produce neck pain in the SO region and headache.[315] For patients with headache, a description of the quality of pain may prove helpful for early classification. A tension-type headache is described as band-like with a pressing or tightening quality of mild to moderate intensity. A headache of throbbing pulsating pain building to a severe intensity suggests migraine,

Table 6-10. Referred Pain Patterns From the Cervical Zygapophysial Joints

LEVEL	PAIN PATTERN
C1 to C2	Posterior view: suboccipital region cephalad to occiput and vertex or caudad into neck Lateral view: over the vertex and in the upper forehead in the region of the ear and orbit; rarely encompassed the temporoparietal region and supraorbital forehead
C2 to C3	Posterior view: similar to C1 to C2 anywhere within a band from the occiput to the vertex; less focus on the suboccipital or occipital region; more often extended over the lateral occiput toward the mastoid region Lateral view: extended from the occiput across the parietal and upper temporal regions to end in the forehead or in the orbit; the typical forehead pain was lower than C1 to C2; C2 to C3 did not encompass the ear
C3 to C4	Limited data from this level: pain could occur anywhere over the suboccipital and occipital regions, cranially in the vertex or forehead, or caudally along the posterolateral neck
C4 to C5	Tended to be focal and centered over the lower posterior quadrant of the neck; could spread laterally into the uppermost and proximal region of the shoulder girdle and to the suboccipital region; no pain was reported in the head
C5 to C6	Typically centered over the base of the neck and the top of the shoulder girdle; it could spread toward the suboccipital region or across the outer margin of the shoulder girdle and arm; infrequently, pain spread inferiorly over the scapular region or into the posterior arm; no pain was reported in the head
C6 to C7	Similar focus to C5 to C6 but typically spread inferiorly and medially into or around the central or medial aspect of the scapula; pain did not spread into the lateral arm or into the head

Adapted from Cooper G, Bailey B, Bogduk N. Cervical zygapophysial joint pain maps. *Pain Medicine.* 2007;8(4):344-353.

while an aching quality suggests CGH. Classification of headache as cervicogenic, migraine, or tension-type is discussed in the Diagnosis section of this chapter.

In contrast to pain patterns from normal volunteers, Cooper et al[316] investigated referred pain patterns from patients with cervical zygapophysial joint pain via diagnostic blocks. In general, pain patterns varied widely, but segmental patterns were identified. The most symptomatic levels were C2 to C3 (36%), followed by C5 to C6, then C6 to C7 (35% and 17%), respectively. C1 to C3, C3 to C4, and C4 to C5 were symptomatic in less than 5% of cases. Table 6-10 lists the common pain patterns of the cervical zygapophysial joints as described by Cooper et al.[316]

Similar patterns of pain have been demonstrated for cervical intervertebral (IV) disc by mechanical stimulation.[311-313] Slipman et al[317] generated pain referral maps for 10 patients undergoing cervical discography and 10 asymptomatic subjects. Symptoms were provoked about equally unilaterally or bilaterally between groups. The following is a summary of results:

- The C2 to C3 through C7 to T1 IV discs produced posterior or posterior inferior neck pain.
- C2 to C3 through C6 to C7 IV discs produced head and/or face symptoms.
- C3 to C4 through C6 to C7 IV discs produced trapezius and shoulder symptoms.
- C3 to C4 through C6 to C7 IV discs produced extremity symptoms.
- C4 to C5 and C5 to C6 IV discs produced anterior chest wall symptoms.
- CV 3 to C4 through C7 to T1 IV discs produced interscapular pain.
- C7 to T1 IV discs produced midline pain extending from the posterior cervical spine to the midthoracic distribution.[317]

The authors conclude that cervical internal disc disruption can produce both axial and peripheral symptoms.[317] Bogduk[119] reported that it is the nerve supply, and not the structure, that determines the pain pattern. Clinically, zygapophysial joint pain and IV disc pain are impossible to differentiate, but the pain pattern may serve as a guide to the segmental level[119] or reflect the innervations of the source.[316]

Radicular Pain

Radicular pain is described under Screening for Neurological Impairment. As described by Bogduk,[119] radicular pain is shooting, stabbing, or electric in nature, spreading distally into the involved extremity and commonly associated with paresthesia. Radicular pain is perceived in the extremity, not in the neck. Based on intentional provocation of cervical spinal nerves with needles,[318] pain is typically reported as deep, spreading through the shoulder girdle and throughout the length of the upper limb, but not in a dermatomal pattern. Radicular pain from C5 tends to remain in the arm, but C6, C7, and C8 pain extends into the forearm and hand. These patterns indicate that the pain is not restricted to skin afferents, but also involves afferents from deep tissues, such as muscles and joints.[119] Bogduk[119] contended that, because segmental innervation of deep tissues (ie, muscle and joint) are not the same as the skin, radicular pain cannot be distributed in a dermatomal pattern. Bogduk[119] suggested that the segmental innervation of muscle is a better guide to the pattern of radicular pain than are the dermatomes. Dermatomes are important for the neurologic signs of radiculopathy, but have little to do with the distribution of radicular pain.[119] Dermatomes and segmental innervations of the upper quarter are presented in Chapter 2 (see Figures 2-4 and 2-5) and Chapter 3 (see Tables 3-6, 3-8, and 3-9).

Altered Sensation

In addition to pain, sensory complaints, such as numbness and tingling, are common in patients with neurological impairments. Due to the subjective and multifactorial nature of these specific symptoms, the evaluation is challenging in both acute and chronic presentations of spinal pain. In addition to determining the exact location of complaints of altered sensation, such as numbness and/or tingling, the clinician must ask the patient to further describe the altered sensation. Patients may report one or more of the following features:

- Absence of sensation or decrease of sensation (anesthesia or hypoesthesia)
- An abnormal skin sensation (paresthesia) frequently described as a tingling or prickling sensation
- An unpleasant abnormal sensation (dysesthesia), such as burning or a hypersensitivity, or allodynia (ie, a painful response to a normally nonpainful stimulus)[319]

Loss of sensation or allodynia may suggest involvement of the nervous system. The location or pattern of symptoms may lead to early hypothesis generation, such as a peripheral nerve or nerve root distribution, or, if loss is to one side of the body, a central nervous system disorder. Associated symptoms such as headache, visual problems, and unsteadiness are also sought at this time. Additional questions about onset, progression, or provocative or easing factors may be pursued at this time or later in the history.

Neuropathic Pain

Neuropathic pain develops as a result of lesions or disease affecting the somatosensory nervous system either peripherally or centrally.[320] Common conditions associated with neuropathic pain include painful polyneuropathy, postherpetic neuralgia, and trigeminal neuralgia. Clinically, neuropathic pain can present as spontaneous ongoing and/or shooting pain with amplified pain responses after noxious or non-noxious stimuli.[320] Patient reports of widespread pain over large areas of the neck, shoulder girdle, and extremities, or in other presumably uninjured areas may be representative of a neurophysiological disturbance or altered pain processing mechanism in the peripheral or central nervous systems resulting in widespread hypersensitivity.[321,322] Widespread hypersensitivity is common in some patients with WAD and chronic musculoskeletal pain. Increased, widespread responsiveness to a variety of stimuli, such as mechanical pressure, heat, cold, light, or sound is commonly reported by patients.[323] Additional symptoms, such as fatigue, concentration difficulties, and sleep disturbances provide clues to heighten the suspicion of altered pain processing mechanisms.[323]

A detailed description of the patient's complaints may guide early hypothesis formation and focus to the rest of the history. Specifically, the body chart, pain patterns, and distribution and quality of abnormal symptoms, such as altered sensation, assist in determining the extent of the neurological examination and differentiating visceral, somatic, and neuropathic pain. The significant overlap of referred pain from several sources and different segments requires careful interpretation and synthesis with additional information from the history.

Pain Intensity Outcomes

Numeric Pain Rating Scale or Visual Analogue Scale

The NPRS and VAS are discussed in Chapter 4. The psychometric properties as examined by Cleland et al[324] in a cohort of patients with MNP (with or without upper extremity symptoms) found moderate reliability (ICC 0.76; 95% CI: 0.51 to 0.87), MDC of 2.1 (95% CI: 1.6 to 2.6), and an MCID of 1.3 on the 0 to 11 NPRS scale. If a patient's rating decreases by at least 1.3, meaningful improvement has occurred from the patient's perspective. The NPRS is defined as the intensity of the current, best, and worst levels of pain over the past 24 hours, ranging from 0 (no pain) to 10 (worst pain imaginable), with the average representing the patient's level of pain over the past 24 hours. In a population with CR, NPRS had fair test-retest reliability. The MDC was reported as 4.1 and the MCID as 2.2, which was consistent with what the MCID reported for the MNP population.[324] Change between sessions can be measured using the NPRS or the global rating of change scale.

History of the Current Episode

The clinician should elicit the most recent chronological details about the manner of onset (ie, macro- or microtraumatic, insidious, or nontraumatic), date of onset, progression of each symptom, all treatments to date and their effects, and the overall progression of the problem or stability. Details of the current episode help to determine a musculoskeletal or nonmusculoskeletal nature, stage (ie, acute, subacute, or chronic), and stability or the patient's perception as to whether the problem is getting better, worse, or staying the same. In the presence of trauma, such as a fall or motor vehicle collision, the clinician must pursue details of the injury along with initial treatment, initial symptoms, and the progression of those symptoms. For insidious onset neck pain, information about contributing factors, such as illness or unusual activity, is sought. Knowledge of the problem over time provides insight into whether the problem is getting better, worse, or remaining the same, and may prove useful for prognosis or provide clues to a progressive nature. Information about previous treatment provides data on what treatment has been effective, not effective, or not utilized. When the most recent episode of symptoms is not the patient's first episode, the quickest way to obtain relevant data is to start with the present episode.

Predictive Factors Associated With History

In the general population, initial pain intensity, duration of symptoms, and pain-related difficulties with performing activities is modestly predictive of the presence pain and/or greater intensity at follow-up.[325] Most WAD studies indicate that collision-related factors (ie, awareness of collision, direction of collision, and head position) are not prognostic of recovery.[298] Persons with grade III WAD recover more slowly than grade I WAD.[298] Diagnostic classification of WAD is present in the Diagnosis section of this chapter. Approximately 55% of persons injured in motor vehicle collisions have some degree of persistent symptoms at 12 months with projected patterns of poorer recovery depending on initial levels of mild, moderate, or severe pain and disability.[326] Increased initial symptom severity such as intensity, greater number of symptoms, more areas of pain, and more activity limitation is prognostic of a poorer outcome.[298] The greater the initial symptom severity, the more likely recovery was to be slow and less complete.[298]

History of Previous Episodes of Neck Pain

Between half and three quarters of people who experience neck pain at some initial point will report neck pain 1 to 5 years later.[14] Due to the recurrent nature of neck pain, the history of previous episodes begins with the question, "Have you had this problem before?" If the patient is not sure, the clinician should ask if the past symptoms are similar to the current ones. With a long history of recurrence, the clinician chronologically determines the initial manner of onset, severity, previous treatment and effects, frequency of recurrences, time to recover, level of recovery, and status between episodes.

The initial onset and mechanism of injury should be described in detail. Frequency and duration of episodes, and level of recovery from the last episode or between episodes may affect the potential for recovery. The clinician looks for a pattern or activity related to each onset. For example, if each episode of neck pain is associated with prolonged sitting at work, an important aspect of management and prevention should address activities in this environment. Previous treatment and effects and level of recovery provide context to the present episode, help to establish reasonable goals for treatment and likelihood of recurrence, and provide data on the stability of the problem over time. If the symptoms are easier to provoke, last longer with each episode, and full recovery does not occur between episodes, then the clinician infers a progressive nature with a poorer prognosis for recovery.

Predictive Factors Associated With Previous History

A prior history of neck pain or injury predicts greater presence and/or greater intensity of neck pain at follow-up based on modest effects. In patients with WAD, a prior history of neck pain was a strong predictor of neck pain at 1 year postinjury. Persons with prior neck pain and headaches are about 3 times more likely to have CGHs one year after injury when compared to persons without a prior history.[327] Passive coping strategies or interventions predict a poorer outcome.[14] In the presence of depression, passive coping strategies at 6 weeks are a strong and independent predictor of a slower recovery.[328] Prior self-reported musculoskeletal pain and/or sick leave predicts a poor outcome in workers with neck pain. For some workers with neck pain, changing jobs is predictive of a better outcome.[14]

Symptom Behavior

Aggravating Factors

MNP varies in intensity as related to the patient's daily activity. Symptoms provoked by mechanical loads increase the likelihood of a mechanical disorder. The patient can usually identify the exact posture or movement and amount (ie, time, distance, or repetitions) it takes to produce or increase each symptom and how long it takes for the provoked symptom or symptoms to ease. For some patients, describing aggravating and easing factors is not so straightforward. Common aggravating factors for neck pain include the following:

- Static postures of sitting, standing, or bending
- Reaching, lifting, or carrying
- Reading or driving
- Computer or office work
- Daily care or household activities
- Looking up, looking down, or looking over the right or left shoulder

Additional aggravating factors may be obtained from self-report measures, such as the NDI. These activities should be analyzed to determine the general requirements for motion and stability of the neck and shoulder girdle and associated regions. Daily activity limitations and participation restrictions at work or recreation should be documented at baseline. The baseline aggravating factors are then used to set functional goals and reassessed to evaluate intervention effectiveness. Analysis of the aggravating movements or posture also provides guidance for the selection of specific tests and measures or interventions.

The patient's response to mechanical loads also presents information about the status of pain processing. For example, when high levels of pain are perceived with minimal movement, the clinician should consider an acute condition, altered central pain processing, or neuropathic pain. The presence of severe and irritable symptoms or sensitization of the nervous system requires examination and intervention procedures that are nonprovocative. A nonsevere, nonirritable presentation, in which symptoms are provoked consistently with mechanical load and relieved when the stress is removed, is likely to indicate a peripheral nociceptive mechanism. A detailed, provocative examination is generally indicated. A patient's description and reaction to symptoms and limitations also provide insight into psychological status, such as fear-avoidance, poor coping, or anxiety.

Visceral pathology may present with symptoms that are not mechanical or partially mechanical. Gastrointestinal symptoms are often associated with eating, or relieved by eating or taking antacid medication. Positioning or moving the trunk may relieve or increase symptoms with abdominal organ distension, such as acute gall bladder or pancreatic pain.

Easing Factors

The clinician should seek easing factors, such as movement, positions, medication, or other treatments for all symptoms because they may serve as a factor in the initial intervention or as self-management strategies. For patients who have good days and bad days, knowing what movements or positions create good days is equally as important as determining the aggravators on bad days. The patient with a chronic problem and a central sensitization component may require a multidisciplinary approach with a focus on resolving activity limitations rather than resolution of pain.

24-Hour Behavior

Pain at night is typical of mechanical problems when the patient reports an inability to lie on the involved side or reports waking with symptoms that are simply relieved by a change of position and return to sleep. If the pain is the most intense at night and the patient is unsure of what wakes her, reports she must get up and walk around, and has difficulty returning to sleep, the clinician should consider the possibility of an active inflammatory component or more serious pathology, such as neoplasm.[329] If night pain is a primary mechanical complaint, the clinician should determine the frequency, the provocative position, and symptoms produced. This information is helpful to reassess at subsequent sessions as one way to determine treatment effectiveness.

Most musculoskeletal problems are better in the morning, eased by rest. Some degenerative joint disorders are better and less painful in the morning, but patients often report stiffness that is eased with movement within 30 to 60 minutes. Systemic inflammatory disorders, such as AS, are usually better with rest, but present with the greatest stiffness first thing in the morning, usually lasting longer than 60 minutes.[329] Symptoms that are worse in the morning may be due to poor sleeping posture. Symptoms that are unchanged in the morning may be nonmechanical or minor mechanical problems. Symptoms that are improved in the morning and remain better with movement throughout the day are likely mechanical in nature and a good prognostic indicator. Symptoms that are improved in the morning, but worsen with activities of the day, are mechanical and may have a limited prognosis. Follow-up questions should identify those activities for intervention and as potential barriers to recovery. Symptoms that do not vary with daily activities are minor mechanical problems or suggestive of a more serious pathology.

Review of Medical Screening Questionnaire and General Medical History

Reviewing the medical screening questionnaire (see Table 2-5) with the patient is a limited discussion of general health, a systems review, and an evaluation of past medical, surgical, medication, and diagnostic test histories. This review screens for systemic disease that may mimic musculoskeletal conditions and requires referral to another medical provider or may identify precautions or contraindications related to PT intervention. Synthesis of this information helps the clinician to understand the patient's neck pain within the context of general health in order to formulate a diagnosis, prognosis, plan of care, and safely select interventions.

The clinician must be alert for the presence of red or yellow flags during the history and physical examination.

Screening for red flags (ie, cancer, infection, CAD, fracture, instability, headache, dizziness, rheumatic disease, and neurological involvement) was discussed earlier. Chapter 2 (see Tables 2-7 and 2-8) reviews fear-avoidance beliefs and behaviors and the characteristics of systemic disease. The following discussion is a brief review of general health factors that may influence the examination or management of patients with neck pain referred to PT.

General Health Status Considerations

General health factors to include comorbid LBP and self-perceived poor general health are prognostic of neck pain outcomes in the general population.[14] Persons with poor general health due to comorbidities are likely to progress slowly with rehab and are at risk for delay in the normal healing process. Good psychological health and better social support are predictive of better outcome in primary care and general populations with initial neck pain. Individuals with passive coping strategies may suffer a poorer outcome.[14] Poor psychological health is a risk factor for new episodes of neck pain.[14] In the general worker population, health status is not associated with neck pain recurrence, but self-reported prior musculoskeletal pain and having little perceived influence over ones own work situation are predictive of poorer outcomes.[302] Identification of prognostic factors assists with developing realistic expectations for recovery and selection of interventions when the prognostic factors are modifiable. However, prognosis for neck pain is determined by a combination of individual factors, with more research needed before firm conclusions are possible.[14,302]

Smoking, Obesity, and Cardiovascular Considerations

Preliminary findings suggest an association between metabolic syndrome and neck pain.[330] Males and females with metabolic syndrome have an increased prevalence of neck pain that is higher in females but with a stronger association in males. Waist circumference and body mass index (BMI) are higher in males with neck pain. Yet, in women, BMI and waist circumference, with or without neck pain, was similar. Males with neck pain have higher cholesterol and triglyceride levels and a higher BMI when compared with females. The authors hypothesize that stress and physical inactivity are 2 factors related to both neck pain and metabolic syndrome.[330] As previously discussed, smoking is related to increased degenerative spinal changes, increased risk for osteoporosis, and decreasing bone density and may also be an indicator of other health risk factors, such as CVD.[331] Billek-Sawhney and Sawhney[332] report that 62% of patients examined in an orthopaedic PT practice have CVD. To minimize the risk of an adverse cardiac event related to physical activity or exercise, baseline screening should determine if CVD exists or if CVD risk factors are present.[333] Cardiovascular screening is recommended to identify individuals with medical precautions or contraindications to physical activity and exercise.

Medication Usage

With little evidence to support the effectiveness of medication for neck pain, drug treatment considerations are revisited from the LBP literature.[334] Douglass and Bope[334] suggest first-line drugs include acetaminophen, cyclooxygenase 2-specific inhibitors, or nonsteroidal anti-inflammatory drugs (NSAIDs). Muscle relaxants may be used short term. If other treatments are ineffective, opioids are used and continued if improved function outweighs impairment. Adjuvant antidepressants and anticonvulsants are used in chronic or neuropathic pain. Epidural steroids are considered only in radiculopathy. In a best evidence synthesis, Hurwitz et al[335] reported that studies are available to evaluate the effectiveness of commonly used analgesics, including acetaminophen, NSAIDs, and narcotics, or studies of muscle relaxants and antidepressant medications in WAD. Medications were commonly used in several studies with usual care protocols.[335] Two studies related to WAD report that corticosteroid injections are not effective with chronic zygapophyseal joint pain. However, in acute WAD, infusion of methylprednisolone results in fewer sick days and less disabling pain over 6 months.[336,337] Although commonly prescribed for musculoskeletal symptoms and associated with increased risk of cardiovascular or gastrointestinal side effects, evidence for the effectiveness of NSAIDs is scarce.[338,339] A thoroughly documented history related to medication use may reveal comorbidities, adverse effects, drug interactions, effectiveness, or symptoms that mimic musculoskeletal or systemic pathology. No evidence exists to support superiority of one medication over another for neck pain.[340] Consensus guidelines are not available to guide the use of medication in the management of neck pain.

Imaging or Other Diagnostic Test Results

The results of radiographic imaging or other diagnostic tests should be documented and reviewed in the context of the patient's history. A synthesis of best evidence by Guzman et al[340] summarized the following clinical recommendation for neck pain: for patients with blunt trauma to the neck, screening protocols using the Canadian C-spine rule and National Emergency X-radiography Utilization Study[341] (NEXUS) are very effective at identifying low-risk patients who do not require imaging. The NEXUS criteria describe low risk criteria, suggesting a C-spine x-ray is not required when all of the following are present:

- Absence of posterior midline cervical spine tenderness
- No evidence of intoxication
- A normal level of alertness and consciousness
- Absence of focal neurological deficit
- Absence of any distracting injuries[341]

In persons with nontraumatic neck pain, the radiographic findings may have little to do with neck pain.[340] For example, degenerative changes found on MRI are common in asymptomatic subjects, increase with age, and are not well correlated with neck pain.[342-344] Related to laboratory findings, Guzman et al[340] reported that routine blood tests do not add additional information in the absence of red flags. Use of electrodiagnostic testing is not supported in patients with neck pain without suspected radiculopathy. The traditional role of imaging has been to provide accurate diagnostic anatomic information that guides the treatment decision-making process. However, even with extensive testing, a pathological cause for neck pain and related symptoms is not always identifiable.

Patient Expectations or Goals

An expectation is defined as a strong belief that something will happen in the future[345] and thought to be learned from cultural and prior knowledge. Patients with higher expectations for a quick recovery are likely to show more rapid improvement than those who are unsure if they will recover. Patients with limited expectations of recovery may take longer to recover or be at risk for developing a chronic problem. Establishing patient goals and expectations provides an opportunity to target interventions to recovery of specific functional needs.[346]

Clinicians often ask, "What are your goals for physical therapy?" Perhaps additional questions, such as the following, will reveal more about the patient's expectations:

- How much benefit do you expect to get from physical therapy?
- What treatments are you expecting?
- How will you fit physical therapy into your daily routine?[347]

Answers to these questions may provide areas for the clinician to address through simple communication of reassurance, advice to remain active, discussion about realistic expectations for recovery, and instilling confidence for self-management. More research is needed to fully understand why some patients recover and others do not and the best intervention strategies for patients with low expectations for recovery.

Interview Summary

At the end of the formal interview, the clinician should ask, "Are there any other problems or concerns that you would like to tell me about or that we have not discussed?" The clinician then presents a brief summary of the key findings from the interview and discusses the plan for the physical examination.

Components of the Physical Examination

At the end of the formal interview, clinicians briefly review the subjective data and begin planning the physical examination based on the working hypotheses. For the novice and experienced clinician, this reflection is a challenge to identify anatomical and biomechanical relationships, movement impairments, pain patterns, activity limitations, and risk and prognostic factors that guide the physical examination and may inform intervention strategies. A deliberate approach allows for a systematic review of the important points of the history, provides a database that initially prioritizes the focus and comprehensiveness of the physical examination, and provides a baseline that can be used in the reassessment of the patient's progress. As a clinician gains experience and more easily recognizes patterns emerging from the history, this process occurs with less deliberation; however, this reflective process is always a useful exercise with any patient, the complex patient, or a patient that is not responding as expected.

The process of planning the examination is discussed in Chapter 2. A planning the examination form (see Table 2-9) assists the clinician with analyzing the information gained from the history and planning appropriate tests and measures to increase the probability of performing an efficient and appropriate examination. To plan the extent and vigor of the physical examination, the clinician considers the severity, irritability, nature, stage, and stability of the patient's symptoms or problem.[348] The clinician also considers risk factors associated with the development of persistent neck pain or other factors contributing to the condition, such as posture, ergonomics, conditioning, depression, job requirements, body awareness and sensorimotor integrity, trauma, previous episodes, and other medical problems. The end result of this process is to generate a working diagnostic classification or working hypothesis of the patient's MNP and a plan to test the working hypotheses through the physical examination and continued reassessment. The clinician should establish a clear plan of what needs to be examined at the first session and over the next 1 to 2 visits. Two sample case studies using the clinical reasoning guide to plan the examination form are provided in the Appendix section.

Summary of Diagnostic Triage and Subjective Examination

The etiology of neck pain and associated risk factors are multifactorial (both physical and psychosocial in nature). Neck pain and headaches increase as one ages, peaking in the middle years and declining with older age.[1] In the working environment, sedentary positions, repetitive or precision work, high job quotas, and low social support are risk factors for the development of neck pain.[1] Poor psychological health, poor general health, prior neck pain, and other musculoskeletal complaints are prognostic factors of poor outcome.[14] Common cervical spine degenerative changes found on imaging are not a risk factor and have not been shown to be associated with neck pain. Age greater than 40, coexisting LBP, a longer duration of neck pain, worrisome attitude, poor quality of life, less vitality, bicycling as a regular activity, and loss of strength in the hands are factors predisposing to a chronic neck pain condition.[15] A better prognosis is associated with younger age, optimism, a self-assured coping style, and a reduced need to socialize.[1,14]

Many potential sources of cervical pain have been identified, but a precise anatomical tissue is not easily or reliably identified as the cause or pain generator in most patients. Labeling patients with neck pain by using specific anatomical diagnoses may not improve outcomes. Yet, specific diagnoses are relevant in many instances, such as cancer, infection, CM, and inflammatory or systemic disease. The process of diagnostic triage for persons with MNP begins with ruling out serious underlying pathology or nonspinal pathology. In this first stage the clinician determines whether the patient is appropriate for PT, if a medical referral is needed, or whether a medical referral is needed in conjunction with PT.

When a pathoanatomical diagnosis of neck pain cannot be made, neck pain and associated symptoms that exclude medical disease and neurological compromise are categorized as nonspecific or MNP, and often incorrectly treated as a homogenous group. The subjective examination seeks to identify key information from all patients with the context and details specific to the patient's presenting problems. This early information provides the basis to form initial diagnostic hypotheses and subgroup classifications, which then guide the focus and comprehensiveness of the physical examination. Obtaining accurate, relevant data from the patient history aids in diagnostic triage, planning the physical examination, and implementing an effective management strategy.

At the end of the history, the clinician determines the severity of the patient's symptoms, irritability and stage of the disorder, a working hypothesis or competing hypotheses, and an initial prognosis. The physical examination continues the process of diagnostic triage and diagnostic classification of MNP and/or associated symptoms seeking to confirm or refute an underlying serious pathological condition, any condition resulting in neurological compromise, or other competing medical disease. Basic components and general procedures of the physical examination are discussed in Chapter 3. Table 6-11 is an outline of commonly used tests and measures sequenced by patient position (standing, sitting, supine, prone, and side-lying) to assist with organization of the physical examination. The sequence varies according to patient and condition, but not all tests and measures are performed on every patient. Initially, the history assists with prioritizing the tests and measures that are conducted at the first session.

A basic premise of diagnostic triage and classification of individuals with MNP is that subgroups can be identified from key history and clinical examination findings. The physical examination is a continuation of the history designed to test hypotheses generated by the subjective examination. Data from the history and examination are then used to place a patient into a specific subgroup or subgroups designed to guide and initiate intervention.

Selection of tests and measures is based on the best evidence that supports the test's ability to significantly increase the probability of making a correct diagnosis and selecting the best intervention. Cook and Hegedus[349] examined the clinical utility of diagnostic tests for the spine and determined that 4 cervical tests are good screening tools (ie, highly sensitive and low negative LRs) and one is good for confirming a diagnosis (ie, high specificity and high positive LR). The tests included the upper limb neurodynamic tests (ULNDT; ie, median and radial nerve biased), palpation side glide, a posterior-to-anterior (PA) passive accessory test, and Spurling's test. With the exception of the ULNDT (radial nerve bias) and the palpation side glide at C5 to C6, all tests served as effective screening tools whereas only the palpation side glide at C2 to C3 served as a diagnostic test. No studies met the inclusion criteria for testing the thoracic spine.[349] Little evidence is available to validate most of the tests and measures for the cervical spine. However, it is the clinician's decision to perform a test as determined by the clinical reasoning process.

Considerations for Ligamentous Stability and Vertebral Artery Testing

Based on a detailed history, review of systems, available medical testing, diagnostic imaging, and index of suspicion for fracture, ligamentous instability, and/or VBI, additional tests may be indicated to continue the clinical reasoning process of ruling in or ruling out a serious underlying pathology that requires immediate medical referral or consultation in conjunction with PT. If red flags are present, additional testing may be indicated prior to initiating the PT examination, such that ligamentous instability testing, vertebrobasilar tests, and AROM would not be performed and the patient would be referred for appropriate management. In patients with recent trauma, the Canadian C-spine rule[140,141] or the NEXUS[341] is recommended to determine who would benefit from radiographic evaluation prior to initiating PT. The criteria for these guidelines are discussed in screening for cervical spine fracture.

Table 6-11. Cervical Spine Examination Outline

STANDING

- General observation, baseline vital signs, and gait assessment
- Static posture
- Balance
- Functional activity analysis
- Shoulder girdle, upper extremity, and temporomandibular joint screen

SITTING

- Static seated posture
- Peripheral joint screen: elbow, wrist, and hand, as indicated
- Neurological exam: MMT, DTR, and sensation; UMN, as needed
- AROM, and AROM with overpressure
- Special tests: neck torsion test, and Dix-Hallpike maneuver
- Thoracic spine screen
- Repeated movements: retraction and retraction with OP; retraction/extension and flexion/protrusion
- Combined movements as needed
- Special tests: compression, distraction, Spurling's test, and shoulder abduction test
- Cervical rotation lateral flexion test
- Segmental mobility testing (T1 to T4)—positional testing
- Special tests: thoracic outlet syndrome
- Sensorimotor control

SUPINE

- Ligamentous stability tests
- Repeated movements
- Anterior cervical palpation
- First rib mobility—caudal glide
- Passive segmental motion testing
- Muscle performance
  - Muscle length tests
  - Deep neck flexor endurance test
  - Craniocervical flexion test
- Upper limb neurodynamic tests

PRONE

- PAIVMs: central and unilateral PA, cervical and thoracic
- Scapular holding test
- MMT: middle and lower trapezius, cervical flexor and extensors
- Cervical extensor control
- Closed-chain scapular stability test

MMT indicates manual muscle test; DTR, deep tendon reflexes; UMN, upper motor neuron; AROM, active range of motion; OP, overpressure; PAIVM, passive accessory intervertebral movement; PA, posterior-to-anterior.

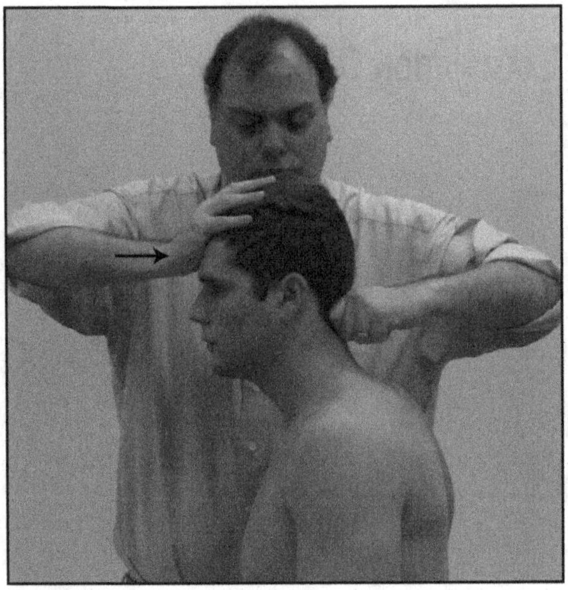

Figure 6-7. Sharp-Purser test.

Screening for cervical ligamentous stability is discussed under Screening for Red Flags. With the exception of the Sharp-Purser test (Figure 6-7), ligamentous stability tests are provocative tests with little known about their diagnostic accuracy. They are designed to challenge the structural integrity of the osteoarticular and ligamentous systems, and have inherent risks associated with their performance.[350] With little data available to support or refute the validity of these tests, and with the potential risks as provocative tests, ligamentous stability tests should be used judiciously. In the presence of signs and symptoms consistent with cervical instability and specific patient populations, such as rheumatoid arthritis, the clinician should be cautious about performing these screening procedures and refer for medical management. In patients with neck pain secondary to trauma or with signs and symptoms suggesting clinical cervical spine instability, Leal and Dennison[351] suggested that ligamentous instability should be assessed prior to cervical AROM testing. These authors recommend screening tests for those patients in whom ligamentous injury is suspected given the potential serious consequences of missing a transverse ligament or alar ligament injury. Leal and Dennison[351] also proposed that ligamentous stability screening procedures be considered as the standard level of care for screening potential upper cervical spine ligamentous injuries. Negative tests should be interpreted with caution since a negative test does not rule out ligamentous injury or instability.[351] Test procedures for ligamentous stability tests are discussed in the supine examination sequence.

Screening for CAD is discussed under Screening for Red Flags. Similar to the clinical reasoning process for ligamentous stability testing, if red flags are present, it suggests vertebral artery or internal carotid artery dysfunction, and the performance of provocative screening procedures may be unsafe and clinically unnecessary. The patient should be referred for medical evaluation.[350]

Several screening procedures have been advocated to identify patients at risk for VBI, but no studies have demonstrated that these procedures effectively identify patients with vascular insufficiency or those at risk of a cerebrovascular accident. The tests and measures portion should include routine physical assessment using incrementally greater movements and loads on the cervical spine.[162] During the physical examination, treatment, and after treatment, the clinician should constantly assess for signs and/or symptoms suggesting an underlying vascular pathology related to head and neck pain. Screening procedures are highly variable. At a minimum, key procedures listed in Table 6-8, as described by Kerry and Taylor,[142,150] are recommended for the physical examination. Premanipulative test procedures are discussed in the intervention section. The uncertainty related to limited knowledge and current guidelines warrants a comprehensive approach to clinical decision making for each patient, prudent assessment, and documentation of screening exam procedures.[142,162]

Physical Examination of the Cervical Spine (Includes Upper Thoracic Spine)

Examination Procedures in Standing

- General observation and baseline vital signs
- Gait
- Static standing posture
- Balance
- Analysis of functional activity
- Shoulder girdle, upper extremity, and temporomandibular (TMD) joint screen

General Observation and Baseline Vital Signs

General observation, such as willingness to move and facial expression, observation of respiratory patterns, and obtaining data related to vital signs are discussed in Chapters 3, 4, and 5. At the start of the physical examination, baseline symptoms should be documented and then monitored as the examination continues. Establishing resting symptoms prior to each test and during each test or measure enables the clinician to document an accurate response to posture, movement, and activity, and to ensure the symptoms are not getting worse. Observation requires adequate exposure of the upper half of the body, including the spine and upper extremities.

Gait

General guidelines for analysis of gait and gait speed are discussed in Chapter 3. Abnormalities in gait have been linked to CM, cervical dizziness, and cervical stenosis.[167,224,227,352] Functional deficits in walking ability are a common initial feature of patients with CM. In comparison to normal subjects, persons with CM characterized by mild lower extremity spasticity and 4 out of 5 muscle strength had lower gait velocity, decreased step and stride length, and increased double limb support time. Using a 10-m walk test and a battery of balance tests, gait speed and balance deficits were revealed in older adults (ie, females ages 65 to 82) with neck pain.[353] In comparison to age-matched controls, older adults with neck pain had a slower self-selected gait speed and cadence when walking while turning their head from side to side, and a significantly longer gait cycle duration both with and without head turns, potentially placing them at greater risk for falls.[353] Gait and balance deficits related to neck pain may be due to altered cervical somatosensory input, such as impaired cervical muscle activity, joint proprioception, and integration with the postural control system.[354] Questions related to gait or balance difficulties should be asked routinely during the patient interview with appropriate follow-up and assessment during the physical examination.

Static Standing Posture

General concepts of postural assessment in both sitting and standing are discussed in Chapter 3 and include the position of the pelvis, shape of the spinal curves, position of the head on neck, neck on trunk, shoulder girdles, and muscle symmetry. Typical postural deviations include forward head, increased or decreased upper thoracic kyphosis, anterior translation of the cervical spine, and protracted, elevated or depressed scapulae possibly affecting all movements of the cervical spine and upper extremity. While static postures vary considerably, a common postural abnormality thought to be associated with neck pain is the forward head posture. Forward head posture may be due to anterior translation of the head, lower cervical spine, or both, and may result in upper cervical extension. The cause of neck pain related to forward head posture may be due to an increase in compressive force on the cervical zygapophyseal joints[355,356] and altered muscle activation because of lengthening of anterior neck muscles and shortening of posterior neck muscles.[357,358] However, results do not reveal a strong association between forward head posture and neck pain or neck pain and headache.[57,359] Some studies support a relationship[360,361] and others do not.[362,363] Reliability of postural assessment in patients with neck pain revealed a k value between moderate and substantial, with the exception of forward head posture, which exhibited a k value of −0.1 (agreement less than chance) and a prevalence of 90%.[364] Similarly, Silva et al[365] reported that assessment of head posture by observation and qualitative descriptors using a 4-category scale showed poor reliability and validity in patients with neck pain.

Continued study of forward head posture and neck pain involves objective measures, such as digitized video. Silva et al[366] found a significantly smaller angle between C7, the tragus of the ear, and the horizontal, resulting in a greater forward head posture in subjects with chronic nontraumatic neck pain as compared to pain-free subjects, although the difference was too small (neck pain, mean ± SD, 45.4 ± 6.8 degrees; pain-free, mean ± SD, 48.6 ± 7.1 degrees) to be clinically meaningful. The results of Lau et al[367] showed that photographic measurement is a reliable tool to assess sagittal postures of the thoracic and cervical spine. Subjects with neck pain had a greater upper thoracic angle (UTA) and a smaller craniovertebral (CV) angle. The UTA (ie, sagittal posture) was measured as an angle between a horizontal line and a line drawn between the seventh cervical spinous process and the seventh thoracic spinous process. The CV angle (ie, sagittal posture) of the cervical spine was measured as an angle between lines drawn from the tragus of the ear to the seventh cervical vertebra and the horizontal.[367] Both the CV and the UTA are predictors of neck pain, but the UTA was a better predictor for the presence of neck pain. Sagittal postures of the cervical and thoracic spine correlate with neck pain severity and disability. Essentially, the greater the forward head posture, the more likely the presence of neck pain.[367] Yip et al[368] also reported that a smaller CV angle in neck pain subjects as compared to normal subjects correlates with greater FHP and greater disability.

Considering the paucity of convincing research, the clinician must determine the relevance of postural findings to the patient's presentation and postural demands reported during the interview. Observed postural deformities should be corrected passively by the clinician or actively by the patient to note any change in the patient's symptoms and assist in establishing a provocative or easing link between the posture and the patient's problem. Provocative postures require further assessment of mobility, muscle activation patterns, and dynamic motor control. The patient must have sufficient ROM to correct deviations from normal. Posture should be comfortable and maintained with minimal activity of the superficial trunk muscles. The patient should be able to easily move in and out of functional postures as required by activities of daily living, work, or recreation.

Balance

Postural control is required for all daily activities. Optimal postural control should result in bilateral or unilateral maintenance of the normal standing posture on the weight-bearing side with minimal effort and normal breathing patterns. Head, spinal curves, pelvis, and lower extremities should remain stable in all planes, with loss of control in any plane or region suggesting the need for further examination of the neuromuscular system. Treleaven et al[369] showed that subjects with whiplash-associated disorders who do and do not complain of dizziness have standing balance deficits likely due to altered postural control mechanisms and not due to medications, anxiety, or compensation status. Compared to controls, patients with idiopathic and whiplash-induced neck pain have deficits in standing balance, with both groups significantly less likely to complete the eyes closed tandem test for 30 seconds.[110] Chapter 3 discusses the clinical examination for standing balance in persons with neck pain.[114]

Problems with static balance may contribute to difficulties in dynamic and functional balance tests.[370] Forty subjects with persistent pain associated with WAD and complaints of dizziness were compared to healthy controls during the following tests: single leg stance with eyes open and closed, the step test, Fukuda stepping test, tandem walk on a firm and soft surface, Singleton test with eyes open and closed, a stair walking test, and the timed 10-m walk test with and without head movement. Preliminary results suggest that subjects with WAD had significant deficits in single leg stance with eyes closed, the step test, tandem walk on a firm and soft surface, stair walking, and the timed 10-m walk with and without head movement when compared to the control subjects.[370] Assessment of balance in patients with neck pain using functional balance tests should be considered.

Analysis of Functional Activity

Functional movements are assessed by asking the patient to perform a movement (such as looking up), an activity (such as reaching), or a position (such as sitting) that reproduces or eases symptoms. Often, this provocative or easing test can be analyzed biomechanically or altered actively or passively to assist in determining the source or cause of the change in symptoms. If easing, the movement may assist in management. If provocative, the movement is reassessed within and between sessions to determine a treatment effect. Jull et al[114] recommended observing key elements of the patient's functional activity during work, sport, or daily movements. Key elements include spinal posture, changes in posture over time, and orientation of the spine and scapula during arm movements to assess for provocative factors, or perpetuators of neck pain or associated symptoms.[114]

Occupations requiring static low load and repetitive movements have a high prevalence of work-related neck and shoulder disorders.[358] Yet, evidence is limited to support modifying workstations and worker's posture to reduce the incidence of neck pain.[299] Szeto et al[371] found that during a 1-hour typing trial, workers had increased forward neck flexion compared to relaxed sitting, with 13% more neck flexion in symptomatic persons than asymptomatic persons. The increased neck flexion is associated with significantly higher activity in the UT and lower cervical extensors[372] (CE) in the subgroup with neck and shoulder discomfort independent of ergonomic setup. The authors[372] suggested that the altered motor activity in the UT and CE is a maladaptive response to greater extensor demand of the forward neck flexion, resulting in increased compressive loads on the cervical spine, which implicates poor sitting posture in the development and continuation of neck symptoms. Assessment during movement allows for observation of dynamic postural control strategies and assessment of mobility in adjacent regions. For example, a provocative activity that requires looking up or reaching may reveal a pattern of limited mobility in the upper thoracic spine, resulting in increased demands for mobility in the lower cervical spine. This information may focus the examination and guide initial intervention to address hypomobility in the upper thoracic spine and impaired motor control strategies in the cervical spine.

Shoulder Girdle, Upper Extremity, and Temporomandibular Screen

Shoulder Girdle: Full motion of the cervical spine and shoulder girdle require adequate mobility of the upper thoracic spine. Considering the regional interdependence among the cervical spine, thoracic spine, and upper extremity (ie, shoulder, elbow, wrist, and hand) and the potential for referred or radicular symptoms to the upper extremity, a shoulder girdle examination is often indicated. The focus and extent of the shoulder girdle examination at the initial session varies according to the patient history and presentation. Patients who have symptoms in the area of the shoulder or complain of neck and/or shoulder symptoms when using the upper extremity for reaching, lifting, or carrying activities require a more detailed examination to assist with differential diagnosis. Shoulder symptoms related to an activity such as reaching may be related to the cervical spine, thoracic spine and/or shoulder. A standard examination for the shoulder girdle does not exist, but the exam should adequately determine whether a primary shoulder problem exists or reveal any secondary sources of symptoms. The shoulder girdle, upper extremity, and TMD may also be assessed in sitting.

Static postural assessment of the upper extremity and shoulder girdle includes observation of muscular symmetry, bony symmetry of clavicle, acromioclavicular joint, sternoclavicular joint, humeral position, and scapular position. Laterally, the line of gravity goes through the humeral head with approximately one third of the humeral head anterior to the acromion process. The optimal position at rest or during elevation of the scapula is not agreed upon since variability between asymptomatic individuals is common. Scapular rest position is observed when the patient is asked to assume a neutral lumbopelvic upright posture. A kyphosis is present in the thoracic spine with a neutral head on neck and neck on trunk posture. The scapulae should be flat against the thoracic wall. At rest, the superior angle of the scapula, spine of the scapula, and inferior angles are about level with T2 to T3, T3 to T4, and T7 to T9 spinous processes, respectively.[373] The medial borders are parallel to the spine or in 2 to 3 degrees of upward rotation. The scapula lies in 30 degrees of internal rotation (ie, scapular plane) with respect to the frontal plane and 8 degrees of anterior tilt.[374] Occasionally, altered scapular rest position may be protective in nature such as noted in the presence of increased nervous tissue mechanosensitivity, perhaps related to a painful CR.

Observation of shoulder girdle motion is important in patients with neck pain because of the muscular attachments to the cervicothoracic spine and scapula, and because of the neurovascular structures that course through the region. A discussion of the biomechanics and examination of this region is beyond the scope of this reference. However, the importance of scapular stabilization is reviewed here as it relates to patients presenting with neck and shoulder pain. Optimal scapular stabilization is needed for functional scapulohumeral motions. During elevation in the plane of the scapula, the scapula upwardly rotates, posteriorly tilts, and externally rotates.[375,376] These motions occur with scapular retraction and elevation, and clavicular elevation, retraction, and posterior rotation.[374,376,377] The amount of muscular activity of the trapezius, serratus anterior, levator scapulae, and rhomboids is task dependent, however muscular activation is the main scapular stabilizer. Altered muscle activation patterns have been associated with muscle length, weakness, poor activation and/or timing impairments during elevation or upper extremity use, resulting in a nonspecific response to a painful shoulder, commonly referred to as scapular dyskinesis.[378] The response is classified by altered scapular resting position, altered scapular motion—visualized by decreased upward rotation, decreased external rotation, and/or decreased posterior tilt—and altered muscle activation patterns that can be asymptomatic or symptomatic and can either be the cause or effect of a problem.[378]

To determine the relevance of an altered scapular position during movement, the clinician manually corrects, or the patient actively corrects, the scapular position. The patient then repeats the movement and compares the symptoms with and without scapular correction. An immediate decrease in neck or shoulder symptoms or change in available motion suggests that poor scapular stabilization is relevant to the patient's problem and serves to educate the patient and direct further examination and intervention. A study on the effects of passive correction of scapular position in patients with neck pain confirms this strategy.[379] The findings of 15 patients with a bilateral scapular rest position of downward rotation suggest that passive correction of scapular position results in decreased neck pain,[380] improved neck rotation ROM, and proprioception.[379]

A minimal examination of the shoulder girdle in standing involves observing the quality, quantity, and symptom response of active ROM and resisted isometric contractions. Spinal posture and scapular orientation during movement are observed for loss of postural or scapular control. Specific loading of the patient's upper extremity with resistance or specific aggravating activities may be necessary to reveal poor scapular or cervicothoracic control. Resisted isometric shoulder testing (Figure 6-8) may also reveal poor scapular control. Observation of poor scapular stabilization strategies that produce or increase the patient's neck and/or shoulder symptoms directs the clinician to additional tests of muscle performance (ie, length, strength, endurance, and timing).

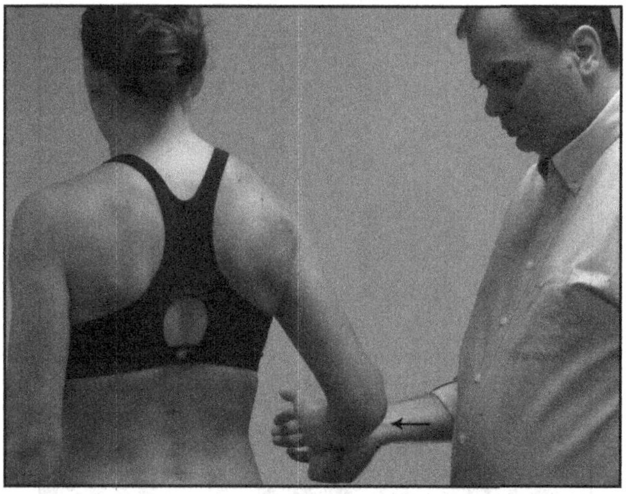

Figure 6-8. Resisted isometric external rotation with poor scapular control.

Temporomandibular Joint Region: In some patients with neck pain, symptoms are reported in the TMD region necessitating some level of TMD examination based on working hypotheses. A close biomechanical relationship exists between the cervical spine and the TMD region. Mandibular opening and closing are linked to craniocervical extension and flexion, respectively; alterations in movement and motor control in either region may affect this coordination and create disorders of one or both areas.[381]

ROM of the TMD joint may be reliably measured with a hand-held millimeter ruler.[382] Walker et al[382] examined 6 TMJ motions (ie, opening, left excursion, right excursion, protrusion, overbite, and overjet) measured by 2 therapists. Opening was the only measurement to discriminate between subjects with and without TMD joint disorders (mean 36.2 ± 6.4 versus 43.5 ± 6.1 mm). The error of measurement varied from 0.2 to 2.5 mm. Intrarater reliability coefficients (ICC 3, 1) and interrater reliability coefficients (ICC 2, 1) varied from 0.70 to 0.99 and 0.90 to 1.0, respectively. Mouth opening is recommended as a screening procedure to implicate the TMJ and assist in discriminating between patients with and without a TMJ disorder. Additional resources are available related to evaluation and management of TMD disorders.[383,384]

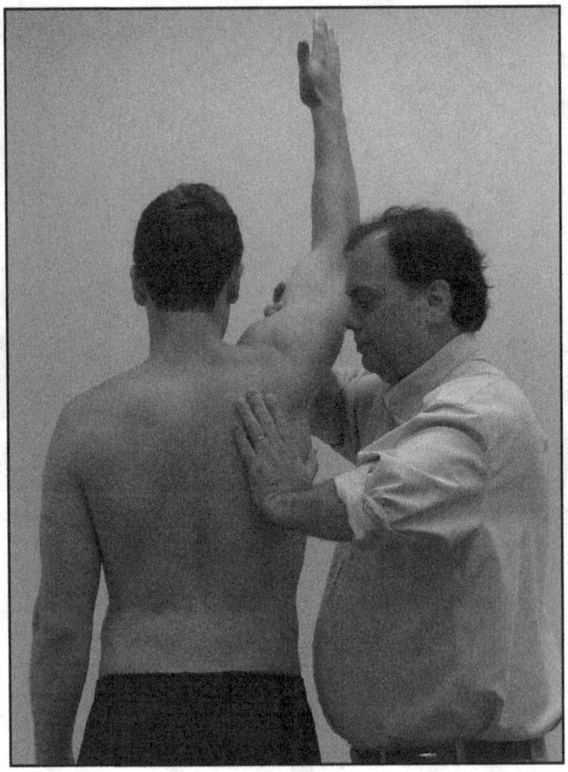

Figure 6-9. Shoulder flexion with overpressure.

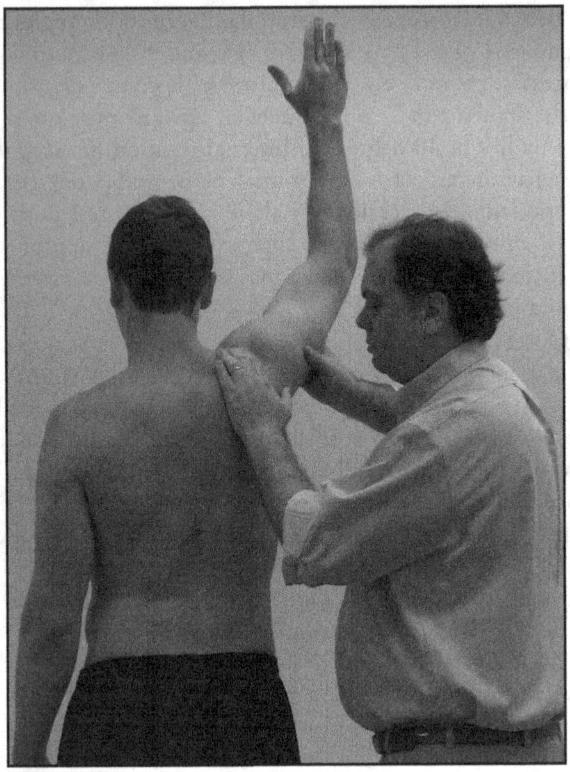

Figure 6-10. Shoulder abduction with overpressure.

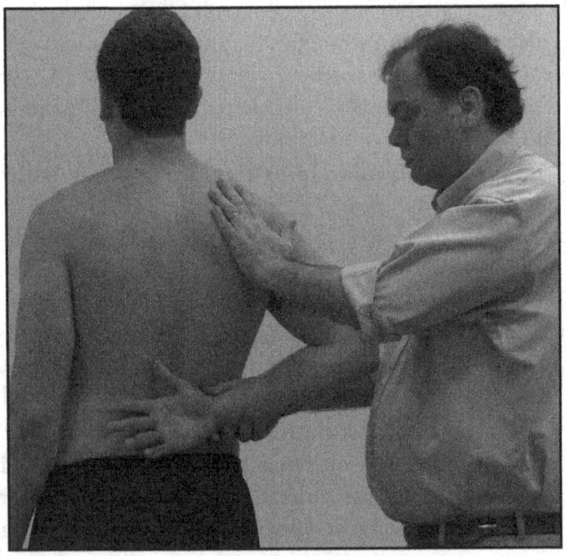

Figure 6-11. Hand behind back with overpressure.

Test Procedures for Upper Extremity Active Range of Motion

Flexion, abduction, combined movements of hand behind back (HBB) and hand behind head (HBH), elbow and wrist flexion and extension, and opening and closing of the hand are performed as indicated. Quality, quantity, and symptom response are noted. If the patient has full AROM with good control and no symptoms, overpressure (OP) is applied.

Flexion, Overpressure

The examiner stabilizes the scapula and trunk with one hand and gradually moves the proximal humerus into flexion, noting the end feel quality, quantity and symptom response (Figure 6-9).

Abduction, Overpressure

The examiner stabilizes the scapula and trunk with one hand and gradually moves the proximal humerus into abduction, noting the end feel quality and symptom response (Figure 6-10).

Hand Behind Back, Overpressure

HBB is a combined movement of extension, adduction and internal rotation (Figure 6-11). While stabilizing the scapula, and with the patient's hand behind the back, the examiner gently grasps the distal forearm and gradually moves the upper extremity into extension, adduction, and finally internal rotation to the end of available range.

Hand Behind Head, Overpressure

HBH is a combined movement of elevation and external rotation as the patient places the hand behind the head (Figure 6-12). To apply overpressure, the examiner stabilizes the scapula and trunk and gradually moves the humerus further into elevation and external rotation.

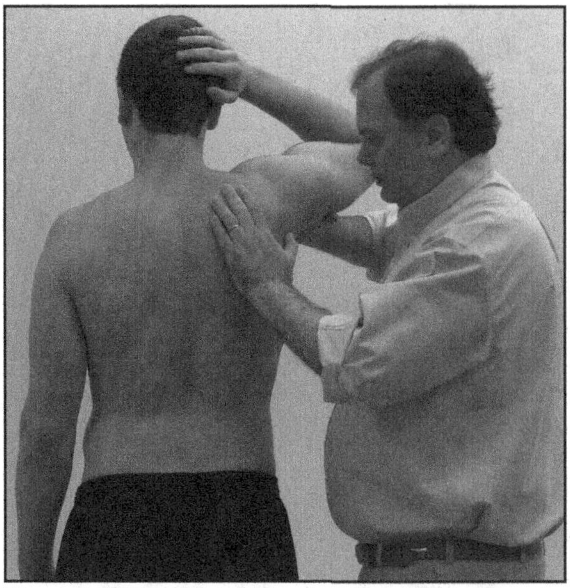

Figure 6-12. Hand behind head with overpressure.

Test Procedures for Resisted Isometric Testing

Resisted isometric shoulder motions, such as flexion, abduction, external rotation, or internal rotation may reveal poor scapular (see Figure 6-8) or postural control and weakness, or pain in the shoulder and neck regions. Jull et al[114] suggested that resisted isometric shoulder abduction, flexion, and external rotation may reveal deficits in maintaining scapular upward rotation, posterior tilt, and external rotation, respectively. Apparent weakness, pain, and observation of poor scapular control should be followed by the scapular retraction test[385] (Figure 6-13) or reposition test.[386] These tests require the clinician to manually reposition the scapula, repeat the test, and reassess any change in symptoms or strength. A positive test alters the patient's symptoms and requires additional testing of the scapular muscles followed by intervention to address deficits.

Examination Procedures in Sitting

- Static seated posture
- Peripheral joint screen
- Neurological exam
- AROM and AROM with overpressure
- Special tests: neck torsion nystagmus test, and Dix-Hallpike maneuver
- Thoracic spine screen
- Repeated movements: retraction, and retraction w/ OP; retraction/extension, and flexion/protrusion
- Combined movements as needed

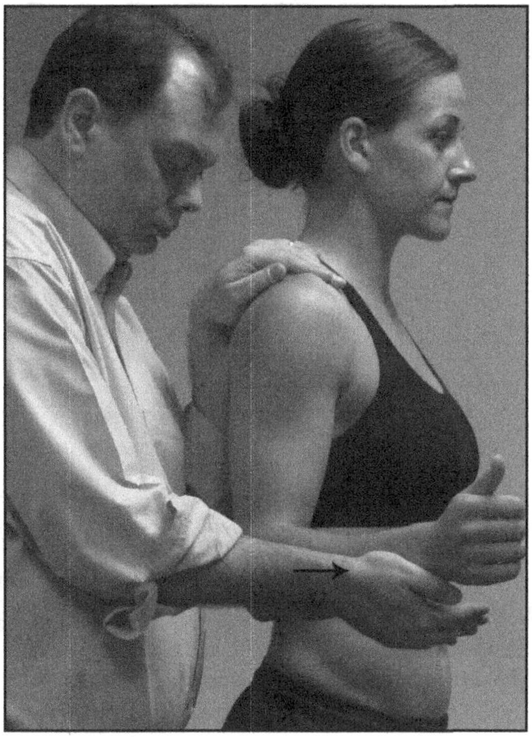

Figure 6-13. Scapular retraction test. If apparent weakness is noted with resisted external rotation, the clinician manually repositions the scapula and notes any change in strength. A positive test results in improved strength, suggesting a deficit of muscles that control the scapula. Additional testing of scapular stabilizers is indicated.

- Special tests: compression, distraction, Spurling's test, and shoulder abduction test
- Cervical rotation lateral flexion test
- Segmental mobility testing (T1 to T4)—positional testing
- Thoracic outlet syndrome tests
- Sensorimotor control

Posture in Sitting

Diagnostic Utility

The role of sitting posture in the development and continuation of neck pain remains controversial, but increasing knowledge in this area has demonstrated altered motor control strategies in a subgroup of individuals who sit during work. Changes in cervical and thoracic posture during a 10-minute computer task were examined in persons with and without chronic nonsevere neck pain.[87] Subjects with neck pain demonstrated a progressive change during the task consistent with more forward head posture while no change was observed for control subjects. The authors suggest that increased forward head posture may reflect a reduced ability, such as impaired endurance, to maintain an upright neutral posture.[87] In the same study,

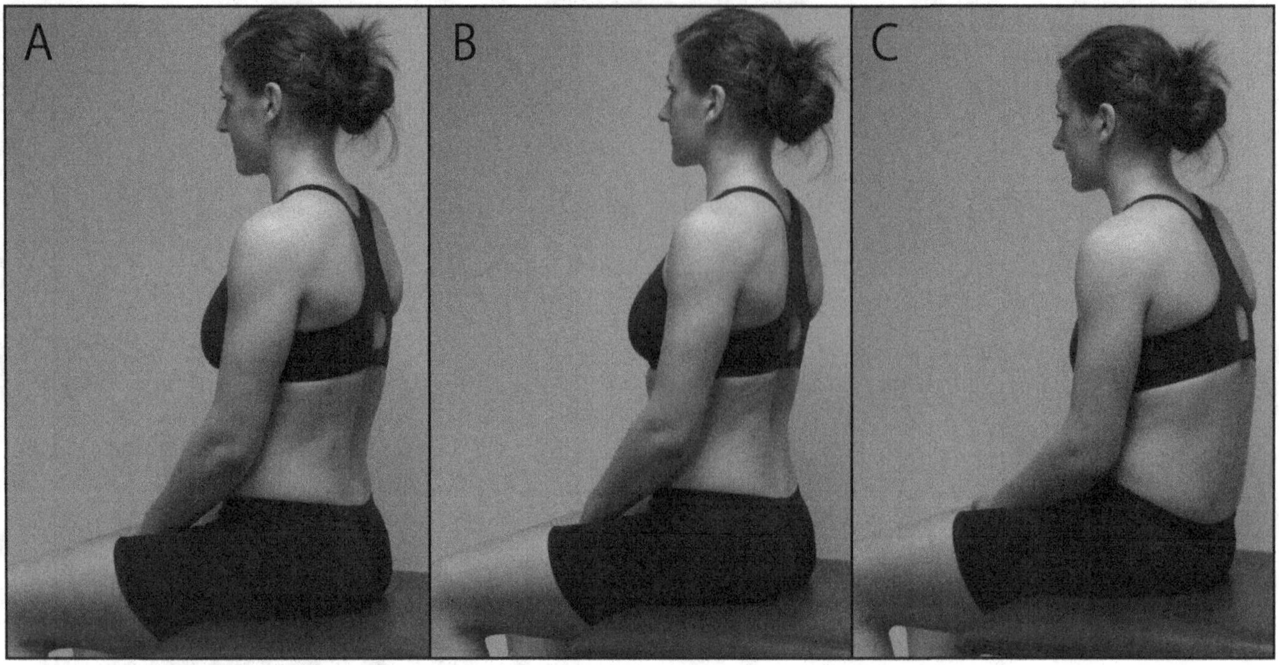

Figure 6-14. Sitting posture: (A) lumbopelvic upright, (B) thoracic upright, and (C) slump sitting.

Falla et al[87] then randomized the subjects with neck pain to receive either training of the deep craniocervical flexors (CCF) or a 6-week endurance - strength training program. Only the CCF group improved the ability to maintain an upright neutral posture during the same 10-minute task.[87] The authors suggest that poor head control in sitting may be a functional consequence of deep cervical muscle impairment and report that further research is necessary to determine the clinical relevance related to management and prevention of recurrent neck pain.[87]

To demonstrate a link between thoracolumbar posture, head and neck posture, and muscle activity, Caneiro et al[387] examined muscle activity of the cervicothoracic region and altered head and neck kinematics during 3 upright sitting postures (Figure 6-14). As expected, slump sitting results in greater head and neck flexion, anterior head translation, and increased cervical erector spinae (CES) activity compared to thoracic and lumbopelvic sitting. Thoracic upright sitting showed increased activity of the thoracic erector spinae (TES) compared to lumbopelvic and slump postures. The favored posture for sitting is the lumbopelvic posture, resulting in a relatively neutral head and neck alignment and diminished CES and TES as compared to slump sitting.[387] These findings are consistent with research that demonstrated increased deep neck flexor and lumbar multifidus activity in a therapist facilitated lumbopelvic posture compared to nonfacilitated thoracic upright sitting postures.[87,388]

Similarly, Edmonson et al[389] examined the influence of whole body sitting posture on cervicothoracic posture, mechanical load, and extensor muscle activity in 23 asymptomatic subjects. Head and neck posture and gravitational load moment measurements were taken in a slouched posture and lumbopelvic neutral posture. Sagittal head translation, upper cervical extension, and load moment were significantly greater in the slouched posture with cervical extensor activity 40% higher in the slouched posture. The authors conclude that more neutral sitting decreases the demand for cervical extensor activity and alters the relative contribution of the cervical and thoracic extensors to control head and neck posture. Facilitating postures that promote optimal patterns of muscular activity may reduce the loads on the cervical spine and posture-related neck pain.[389]

Test Procedure

Jull et al[114] described the following process of assessing upright sitting posture in patients with neck pain. First, the patient's unsupported sitting posture is observed with the feet flat on the floor and hips in 80 degrees of flexion. As needed, the clinician manually and verbally assists lumbopelvic upright posture rather than simply telling the patient to "sit up straight" (ie, the thoracic upright posture). Anterior rotation of the pelvis restores the normal low lumbar lordosis and thoracic kyphosis with a slight sternal lift or depression for adjustment; scapulae should sit flush on the thoracic wall. The head-on-neck posture is adjusted with a gentle occipital lift away from cervical extension to result in a neutral spine posture.[114] The scapulae are manually repositioned as needed and discussed above in standing. The patient is asked to actively maintain this position.[114] Effect of any postural correction on the patient's symptoms is assessed to determine relevance. Symptoms may increase, decrease, or remain the same, or patients may have difficulty assuming the desired position perhaps due to spinal mobility deficits. Occasionally, a lateral or rotational deviation of the head and neck is visible, which can be habitual or protective and correctable. In acute onset of severe neck pain for a small number of patients, any attempt at correction of a lateral deviation is very painful and often referred to as a wry neck or torticollis.

Static postural alignment varies greatly among individuals and not all deviations from what is considered normal or ideal should be considered pathological. However, observed postural deformities should be corrected passively by the clinician or actively by the patient to note any change in the patient's symptoms and assist in establishing a provocative or easing link between the posture and the patient's problem. Provocative postures require further analysis of mobility, muscle activation patterns, and dynamic motor control. The patient must have sufficient ROM to correct deviations from normal. The posture should be comfortable, maintained with minimal activity of the superficial trunk muscles, and allow ease of movement during functional activities as required by activities of daily living, work, or recreation.[390]

Neurological Examination

The neurological examination aids in identifying signs consistent with upper motor neuron (UMN) pathology, such as CM, or lower motor neuron (LMN) pathology, such as radiculopathy or peripheral neuropathy. LMN pathology presents as reduced or absent DTRs, diminished or absent sensation to light touch or pin prick in an appropriate area, and corresponding muscle weakness. UMN pathology presents with hyperreflexia of the upper and lower extremities or clonus, sensory changes in a nondermatomal or nonperipheral nerve distribution often bilaterally in the hands and/or feet, clumsiness in gait, general weakness below the level of the lesion, and a positive Babinski's or Hoffman response. A neurological examination is required for all patients who exhibit cervicothoracic pain with symptoms extending into the extremities, weakness, numbness, paresthesia, anesthesia, radicular pain, referred pain to the head, face, thorax, chest wall or abdomen, a history of neurological deficit or for any patient with symptoms of an unknown origin. Details from the history should indicate the need for an UMN, LMN, or cranial nerve examination. The neurological screening examination is discussed in Chapter 3.

Cervical Spine Movement Testing

Review of Cervical Spine Function

Function of the cervical spine is closely linked to motion in the thoracic spine, shoulder girdle, and TMD regions. The cervical spine is typically divided into an upper cervical (ie, craniocervical or occiput-C1 and C1 to C2 segments) and lower cervical or typical cervical region (C2 to C7) with C2 to C3 identified as a transitional

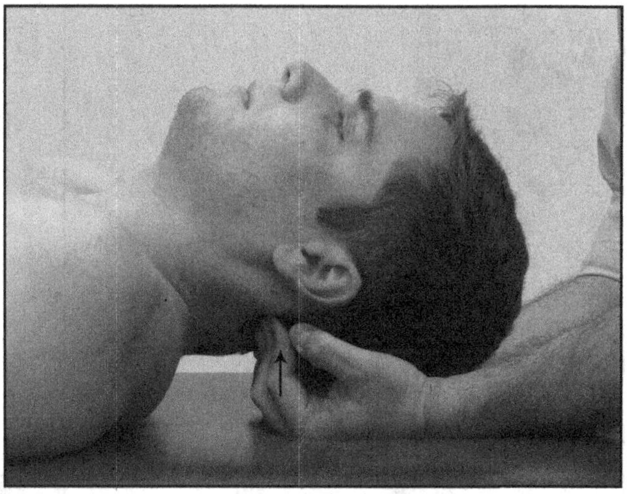

Figure 6-15. Transverse ligament anterior shear test.

segment. The primary motion at occiput-C1 occurs in the sagittal plane while C1 to C2 allows primarily rotation in the transverse plane. The upper cervical spine accounts for about one third of sagittal plane motion and one half of transverse plane motion of the available cervical spine motion. The lower cervical spine permits flexion and extension with lateral flexion and rotation coupled to the same side.[391,392] Clinically, accepted values for AROM are flexion (80 to 90 degrees), extension (70 degrees), lateral flexion (20 to 45 degrees), and rotation (70 to 90 degrees).[393]

Control of the cervical spine is complex. Daily functional activities of orienting the head and neck in space can be achieved with a variety of motor control strategies and movement patterns.[392,394] Muscular control is achieved by the interaction of deep[395-397] and superficial muscle[398,399] groups. The requirements of the cervicothoracic and axioscapular muscles are task-specific and patient-specific. Flexion and extension of the head and neck begins and ends in the lower cervical spine (C4 to C7) with the middle and upper cervical regions contributing during the middle phase.[391,400] During extension, the upper cervical spine reaches its maximum at the end of extension.[391,400] Flexion of the cervical spine and return to neutral requires eccentric control followed by concentric control of the cervical extensors while extension requires eccentric followed by concentric control of the cervical flexor muscles.[401] Assessment of muscle function begins with observation of dynamic postural control of the head and neck during AROM and functional activity.

Based on patient history, ligamentous stability testing (see Figures 6-7 and 6-15 through 6-18) and/or CAD testing may be indicated prior to AROM testing. If dizziness is a symptom, differentiation among vestibular, cervicogenic, arterial, or neurogenic etiology is indicated. In general, active motion tests assess the patient's willingness to move or fear of movement and the articular, muscular, vascular,

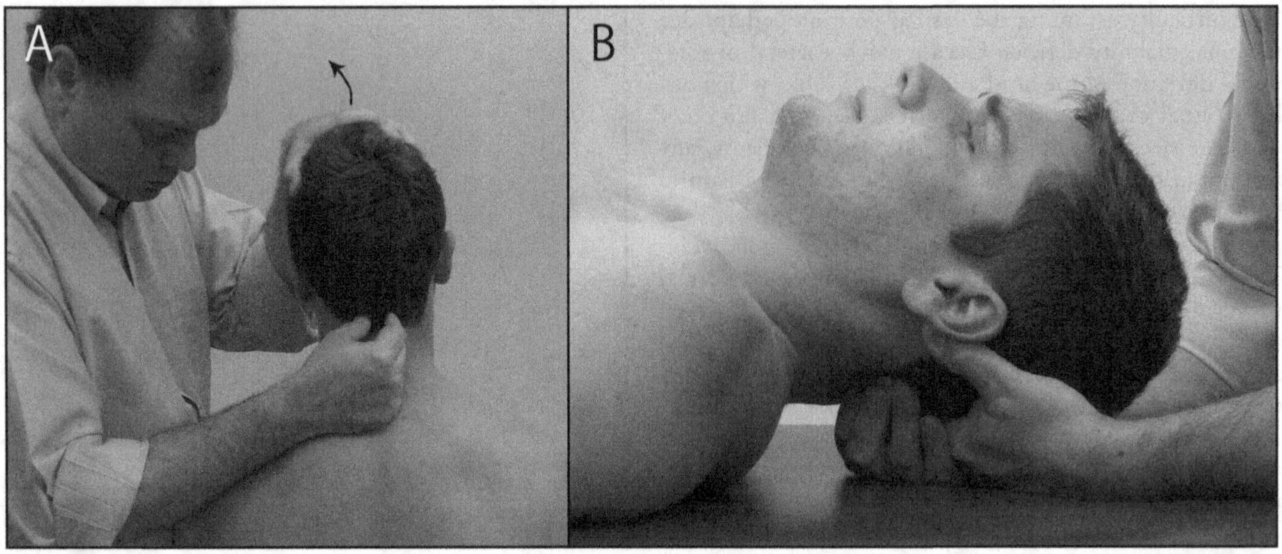

Figure 6-16. Alar ligament test. (A) For demonstration purposes the alar ligament test is shown in sitting. The right hand is monitoring the C2 spinous process while the clinician gently side bends the occiput to the left. A normal response is immediate movement of the C2 spinous process to the right. (B) The procedure is typically performed in supine.

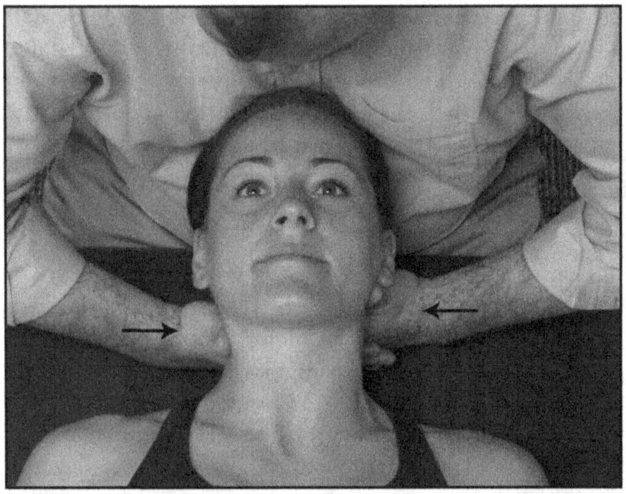

Figure 6-17. Transverse or lateral shear for atlantoaxial complex.

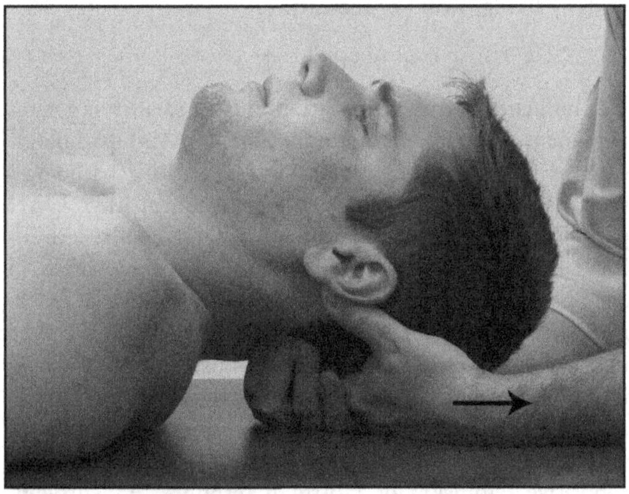

Figure 6-18. Longitudinal traction.

and neural control systems. Therefore, mobility deficits found on AROM testing may be due to impairments in any of these systems. Further testing is needed to determine the cause of reduced mobility. Limited mobility assists with the diagnostic classification of neck pain with mobility deficits and CGH[15] and is predictive of chronicity in persons with WAD.[48] Cervical AROM fits the ICF category of measurement of impairment of body function and mobility of several joints. A symptom response to movement, such as end range pain and the presence or absence of centralization or peripheralization, also aids in diagnostic classification, confirms the cervical spine as the origin of symptoms, and guides the type of intervention and dosage associated with patterns of restriction and intensity of pain. Clinicians frequently target mobility deficits as part of the overall intervention, but it remains unclear as to whether changes in impairments explain concurrent improvements in function. However, targeting specific impairments may result in reduced disability.

Impairments of reduced AROM are common. Cervical AROM has been shown to differentiate between asymptomatic individuals and patients with neck disorders (cervicogenic headache and WAD).[34,48,402,403] However, AROM measures do not correlate highly with function or disability in chronic neck pain,[404-406] but a gain or loss from baseline in pain-limited AROM often indicates a positive or negative response to treatment. Therefore, the quality and symptom response may be more important than the gross available range. Pain-limited AROM is recorded to determine a baseline response, reveal impairments, or reveal a direction-specific preference for movement.

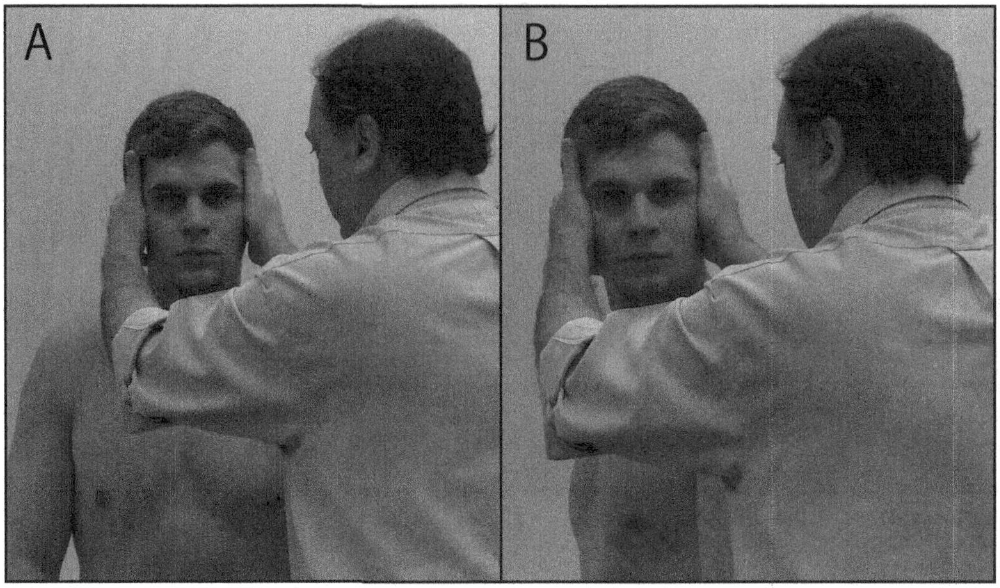

Figure 6-19. Neck torsion test: (A) part 1 and (B) part 2.

Dizziness With Active Range of Motion

In addition to pain, dizziness may be reported with neck movements during the history. Dizziness and vertigo as symptoms of a red flag disorder were discussed earlier and have been associated with CAD, cervicogenic dizziness, and vestibular disorders. When all other causes (ie, neurologic, vascular, or vestibular) of dizziness have been ruled out, cervicogenic dizziness is considered. Therefore, a thorough history and physical examination are necessary to identify patients with cervicogenic dizziness, musculoskeletal impairments, and vestibular disorders appropriate for PT. Dizziness produced with active cervical rotation or other neck motions may be due to cervicogenic dizziness, CAD, or a vestibular disorder. No definitive tests are available to assist with differentiation.

The Neck Torsion Nystagmus Test

The neck torsion nystagmus test (Figure 6-19) is considered by some to assist with detecting cervicogenic dizziness.[407,408] However, diagnostic utility of this test is unknown. To perform the test, the head is held stationary while the neck and trunk are rotated. If symptoms are provoked, cervicogenic dizziness is considered because keeping the head still minimizes the vestibular system while stimulating the neck structures (somatic and vascular). However, specificity of this test for cervicogenic dizziness has not been demonstrated. In 262 patients with WAD, 64% had nystagmus during this maneuver[409] and up to 50% of normal subjects also have nystagmus.[408,410] If dizziness and/or nystagmus are not produced with the neck torsion test, the vestibular system or vascular system is implicated. To further implicate the vestibular system using rotation as the provocative movement, the vestibular system is biased by moving the head and trunk en bloc. Rotation of the head occurs, but the cervical spine does not, stimulating only the vestibular system. Provocation of symptoms suggests a vestibular component since the cervical spine is maintained in neutral (ie, rotation is not allowed). Additional tests of the vestibular system are warranted.[411]

The evaluation and management of vestibular disorders are beyond the scope of this reference. An in depth discussion is available by Clendaniel.[412] As discussed earlier, a comprehensive history and appropriate examination may reveal additional signs and symptoms to help with the differential diagnosis and expedite consultation with a physical therapist that specializes in vestibular rehabilitation as needed.

Vertebrobasilar Insufficiency Tests

Symptoms related to CAD are discussed under Diagnostic Triage as well as the uncertainty and decision-making process related to identifying patients at risk for VBI. In patients with dizziness or positional vertigo and neck pain, differentiating between a vestibular disorder such as benign paroxysmal positional vertigo (BPPV) and VBI can also be a challenge. BPPV is relatively common compared to VBI. However, it is unlikely that VBI would present with an isolated symptom of dizziness or the nystagmus associated with BPPV. VBI (see Table 6-7) is associated with weakness, slurred speech, and mental confusion in addition to nystagmus and vertigo. BPPV is not associated with neurological symptoms such as weakness, slurred speech, and mental confusion. Screening procedures for VBI are discussed under Diagnostic Triage.

BPPV is an inner ear disorder characterized by repeated episodes of positional vertigo.[413] Positional vertigo is a spinning sensation produced by changes in head position relative to gravity regardless of the position of the spine. Symptoms related to VBI are brought on by the position of the cervical spine regardless of head position

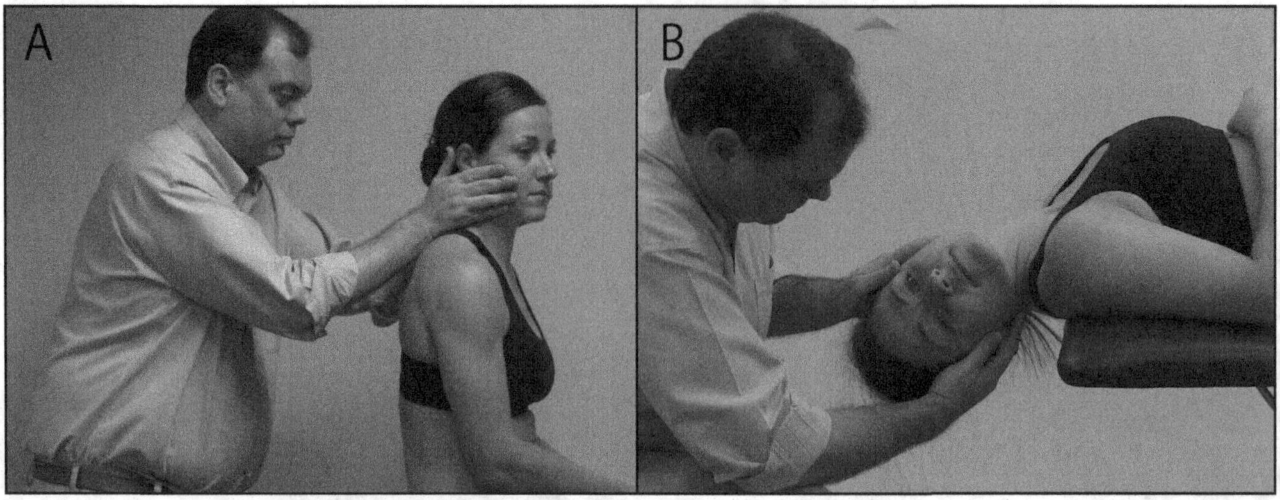

Figure 6-20. Dix-Hallpike maneuver: (A) part 1 and (B) part 2.

relative to gravity.[411] The provocative diagnostic tests for VBI and BPPV (ie, Dix-Hallpike maneuver) use similar test positions of cervical rotation and extension. VBI tests commonly involve full extension and rotation whereas Dix-Hallpike involves 45 degrees of rotation and 20 degrees of extension.[411]

The Dix-Hallpike Maneuver[413]

The patient should be informed that this test (Figure 6-20) is provocative and may produce vertigo and nystagmus. With the patient seated upright and legs extended on a table, the examiner rotates the patient's head 45 degrees to the side to be tested. While maintaining the head and neck position, the examiner quickly moves the patient into supine and then slightly extends the patient's neck about 20 degrees below the horizontal plane. The patient's chin points slightly upward with the eyes open and head hanging off the edge of the table supported by the examiner. While observing the eyes, the examiner notes the presence or absence of nystagmus and vertigo and notes the duration, latency, and direction if nystagmus is present. In most cases, nystagmus and vertigo are produced in a few seconds. However, the response is delayed in some patients. The test should be held for at least 30 seconds. The nystagmus observed is normally a rotational-vertical movement of the eyes and usually lasts under 20 seconds. Any vertigo and nystagmus should be allowed to resolve before returning the patient to upright. If the nystagmus does not resolve, the patient is returned to the upright position and allowed to resolve. The test is repeated on the other side.[43] Because the Dix-Hallpike test is the gold standard for posterior canal BPPV, determining reliability and validity is difficult.[413,414] Halker et al[414] estimated Sn 0.79 (95% CI: 0.65 to 0.94), Sp 0.75 (95% CI: 0.33 to 1.0), +LR 3.17 (95% CI: 0.58 to 17.50), and –LR 0.28 (95% CI: 0.11 to 0.69). Another position to assist with differentiating BPPV and VBI places the cervical spine in a position identical to the Dix-Hallpike position without changing the orientation of the head relative to gravity. In sitting, the patient is asked to flex at the hips, move the trunk toward the thighs and, at the same time, extend and rotate the neck, placing the neck in the same position as the Dix-Hallpike test and VBI test, but the head remains unchanged relative to gravity. Therefore, any symptoms provoked may be related to VBI.[411] Diagnostic utility of this procedure is unknown.

For patients unable to move into the Dix-Hallpike test position, alternative test positions in supine and side-lying are available.[414] The examiner must consider the risks versus benefits associated with performing this test in patients with significant vascular disease[415] or with a high risk of VBI. Additional care and precautions are warranted in patients with cervical stenosis, severe kyphoscoliosis, limited cervical ROM, Down's syndrome, severe rheumatoid arthritis, CR, Paget's disease, AS, low back dysfunction, spinal cord injuries, and morbid obesity.[415,416]

Active Range of Motion Measurement—Diagnostic Utility

Lind et al[417] described a wide variation of normal cervical AROM in people between ages 12 and 79:

- Flexion for women/men (mean 68 degrees/76 degrees, range 24 to 114 degrees)
- Lateral flexion for women/men (mean 45 degrees/45 degrees, range 22 to 81 degrees)
- Rotation for women/men (mean 145 degrees/139 degrees, range 80 to 200 degrees).

Youdas et al[418] determined normal values for cervical AROM in healthy subjects spanning 9 decades. In general, females of the same age group had a greater AROM than males for all motions except neck flexion. In both males and females, AROM decreased significantly with

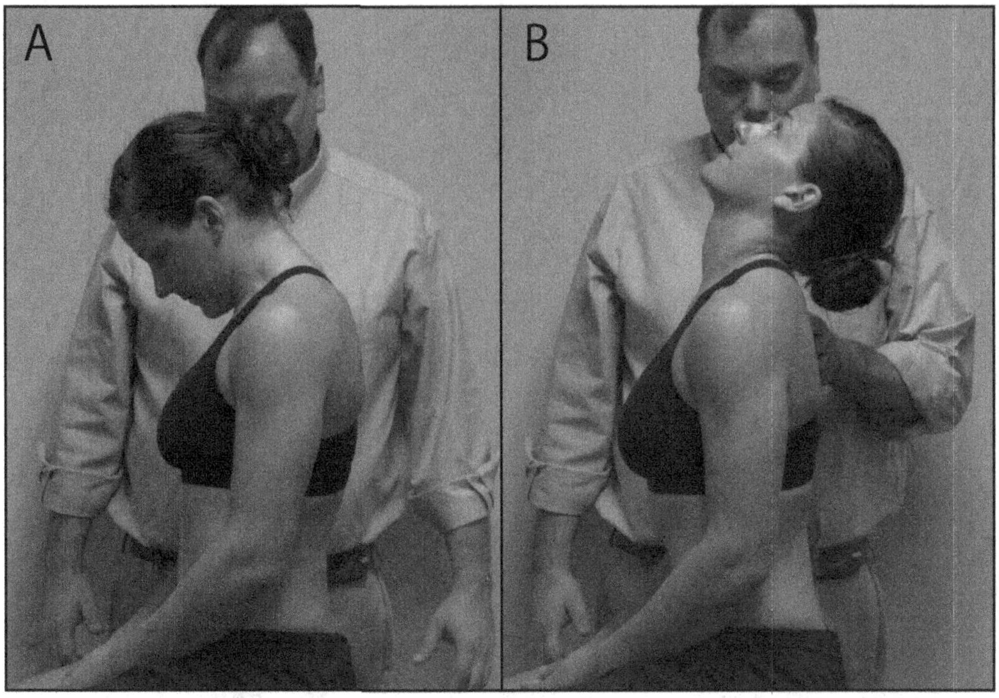

Figure 6-21. Cervical active range of motion: (A) flexion and (B) extension. *(continued)*

age. Systematic review[419] of the clinimetric evaluation of AROM in patients with nonspecific neck pain indicates that the cervical ROM instrument and single inclinometer have acceptable reliability for clinical use. Visual estimate is not reliable and tape measure reproducibility is doubtful. Interrater reliability of the single inclinometer has been reported as good to excellent for all measures of cervical AROM.[245,364,420] The MDC or measurement error provides a threshold for interpreting changes in AROM over time or between sessions. Using a gravity inclinometer, Piva et al[420] report the MDC for flexion (16 degrees), extension (16 degrees), left/right lateral flexion (12 degrees/10 degrees), and left/rotation measured supine (11 degrees/13 degrees). The MDC value for flexion suggests that flexion AROM must change more than 16 degrees to be reasonably confident that true change has occurred beyond that attributable to measurement error. Cleland et al[364] reported the MDC for flexion (19 degrees), extension (13 degrees), left/right lateral flexion (19 degrees/10 degrees), and left/right rotation measured in sitting (14 degrees/14 degrees). The reliability of the assessment of symptom reproduction varies from poor to excellent.[364,420] Accurate measurements before and after initial intervention help to determine patients who will improve between sessions.[421]

Active Range of Motion Test Procedure

Cardinal plane movements of flexion (FLEX), extension (EXT), lateral flexion (LF), and rotation (ROT) are tested observing the quality, quantity, and symptom response (ie, produced, abolished, no effect, increased, decreased, peripheralized, or centralized). Observations cover the upper cervical spine, lower cervical spine, and upper thoracic spine and include ease of movement, quality of the curve, and recovery from motion. Observation of the quality of motion allows for assessment of intersegmental motion and muscle function. Gross range of movement and the behavior of symptoms during movement or at end range are noted along with any change in intensity or location from the rest position and where in the range the symptoms change. Deviations from the expected movement plane either during or at the end of range are corrected to determine relevance. If correction alters the patient's symptoms, then relevance is established. Observations of segmental or intervertebral movement note the presence or absence of a smooth controlled motion, or a fulcrum or sharp angulation that suggests altered (ie, reduced or excessive) segmental mobility. Observations of altered segmental mobility must be confirmed by passive segmental mobility tests and muscle performance tests. Keeping in mind severity and irritability, the patient is asked either to move as far as he or she can or only to the onset or increase of baseline symptoms. The clinician determines which motions should be tested and makes the assessment in a standardized manner.

Flexion

The patient is asked to look down and bring his or her chin to their chest (Figure 6-21). During flexion and extension, observe for initiation of motion from the lower cervical spine. Hypertonicity of cervical extensor muscles may be a protective response to limit flexion or loss of deep cervical extensor control.[114] On return to neutral from flexion, excessive craniocervical extension suggests

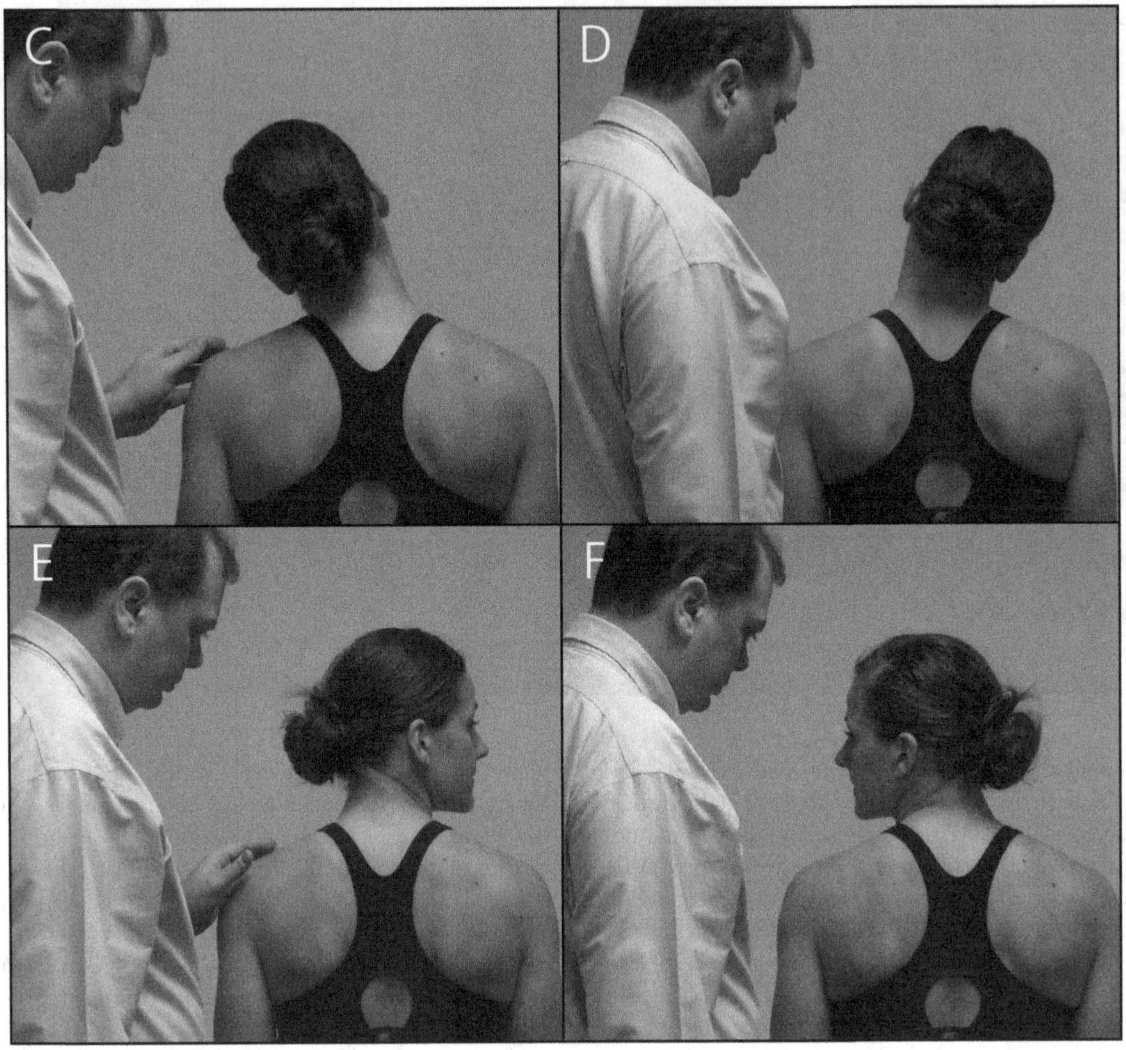

Figure 6-21 (continued). Cervical active range of motion: (C) lateral flexion left, (D) lateral flexion right, (E) rotation right, and (F) rotation left.

dominant superficial extensors and loss of deep craniocervical flexor control.[114]

Extension

The patient is asked to look up to the ceiling and look back along the ceiling with her eyes (see Figure 6-21). A hypothesis of poor eccentric control during extension is determined by unwillingness to allow the head to move posteriorly behind the frontal plane of the shoulders with a dominant upper cervical extension pattern. Another suggestion of poor eccentric control of extension is observed when the head drops or translates backward and may be painful or described as feeling a loss of control.[114] On return from extension, a poor control strategy is initiated by the SCM and anterior scalene muscles, resulting in lower cervical flexion, but not upper cervical flexion. Recovery from extension is poor when upper cervical flexion is absent or delayed.[114]

Lateral Flexion (Left/Right)

The patient is asked to bring her left or right ear toward her shoulder (see Figure 6-21). Restriction of lateral flexion may be due to segmental dysfunction or muscular restriction of several segments often associated with short scalenes or neural tissue sensitivity.[114] In patients with chronic neck disorders, extension and rotation deficits are greater than lateral flexion deficits.[48,62,403]

Rotation (Left/Right)

The patient is asked to look and turn her head to the left or right (see Figure 6-21). Mobility deficits in rotation may occur in the upper cervical, lower cervical or upper thoracic regions. Observation of the quality of motion assists in locating the region. Upper thoracic restrictions may present as a loss of end-range motion. Lower cervical motion loss may be noted when the head turns easily on the neck,

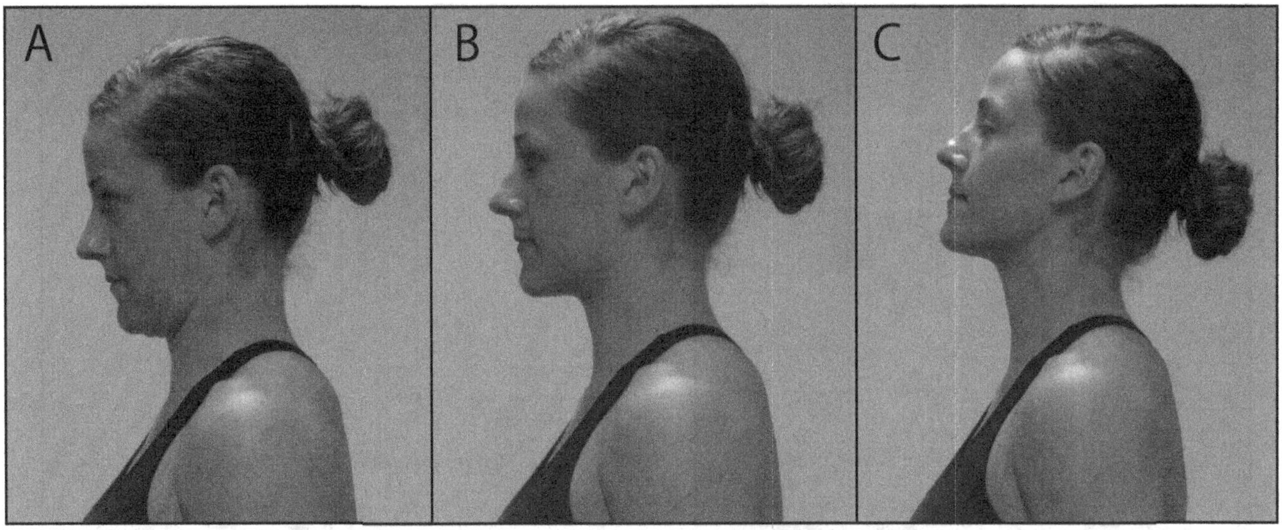

Figure 6-22. Upper cervical active range of motion: (A) flexion, (B) neutral, and (C) extension.

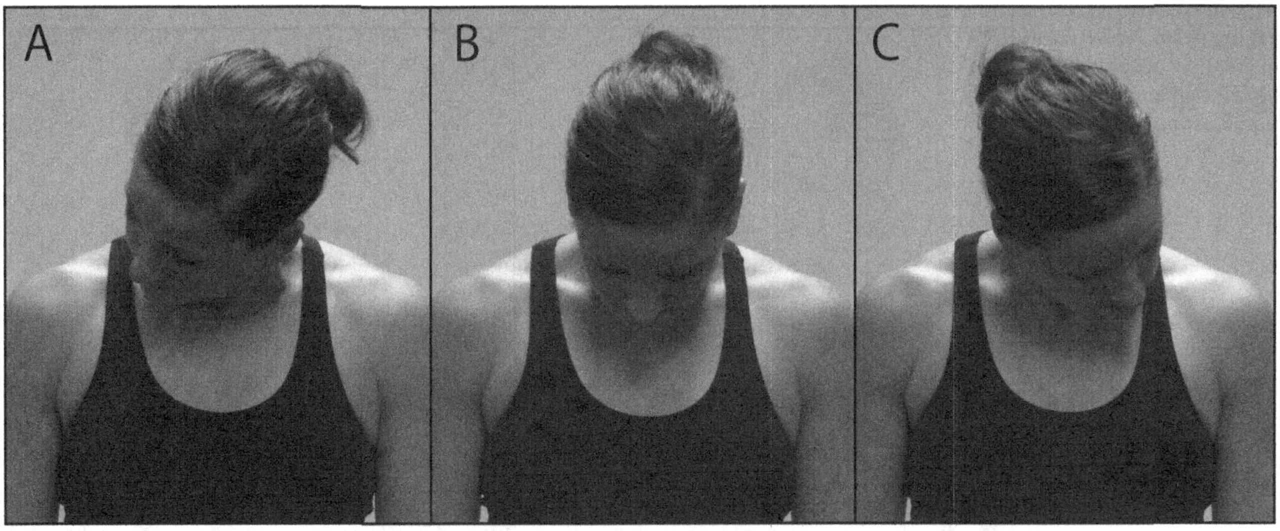

Figure 6-23. Upper cervical rotation active range of motion: (A) rotation right, (B) neutral, and (C) rotation left.

but motion remains limited. Upper cervical motion loss is suspected when rotation occurs mainly through the lower region with little head on neck rotation observed.

Upper Cervical Flexion, Extension, and Lateral Flexion

The patient is asked to perform head nodding or "yes" motions for flexion and extension with the lower cervical spine in neutral (Figure 6-22). For lateral flexion, a similar side-to-side nodding motion is performed with an imaginary axis through the patient's nose.

Upper Cervical Rotation

To actively test rotation occurring primarily at the AA joint, the patient flexes the head and neck, bringing the chin to the chest (Figure 6-23). While maintaining flexion, the patient rotates her head to each side. Quality, quantity and symptom response are recorded.

Retraction and Protrusion

Protrusion is a result of lower cervical flexion and upper cervical extension. Retraction is a result of lower cervical extension and upper cervical flexion.[422] For protrusion (Figure 6-24) in sitting, the patient is asked to poke or extend the chin forward as a far as possible, keeping the head horizontal and return to neutral.[422] For retraction in sitting (Figure 6-25), the patient is asked to slide or draw the head backward while tucking in the chin and keeping the head horizontal or facing forward and return to neutral. Symptom response is noted along with a qualitative assessment of range of movement loss as minor, moderate, or major.[422]

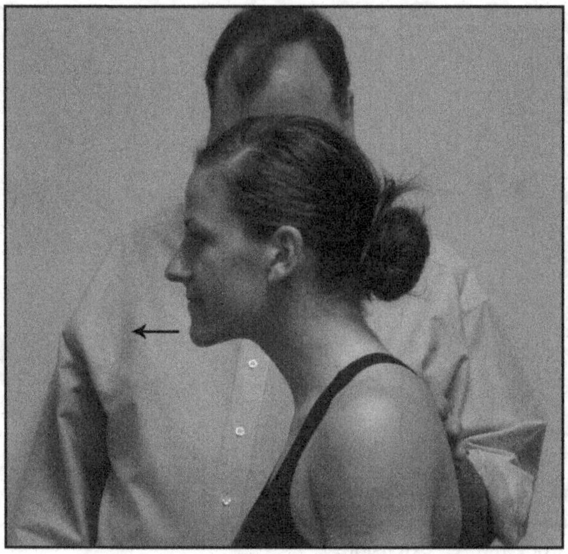

Figure 6-24. Protrusion in sitting.

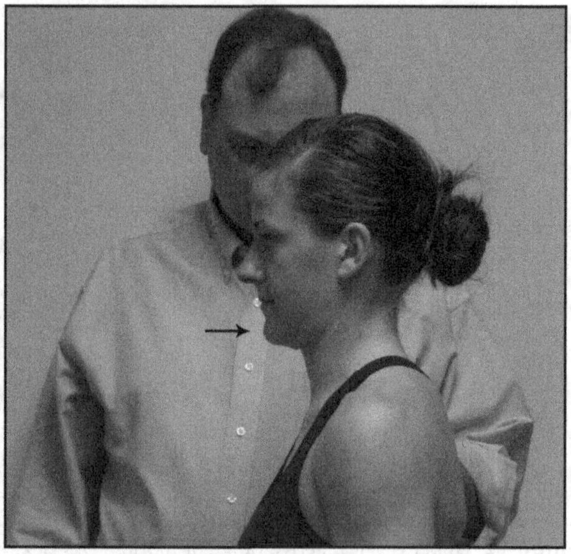

Figure 6-25. Retraction in sitting.

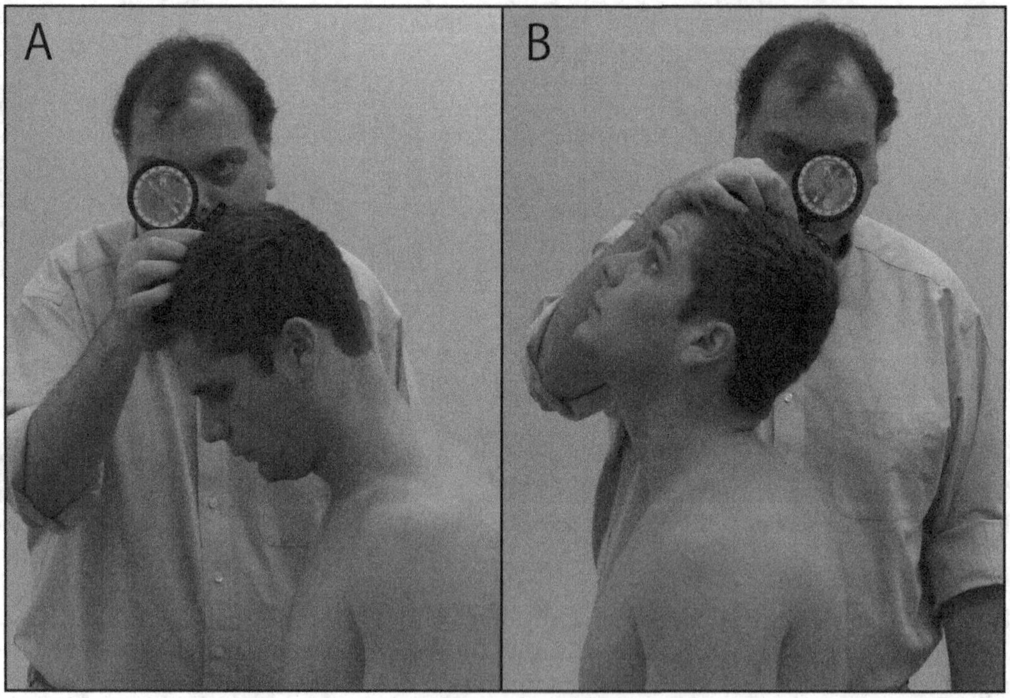

Figure 6-26. Active range of motion measurement: (A) flexion and (B) extension. *(continued)*

Active Range of Motion Measurement

If AROM is limited and painful, single inclinometry measurements are recorded in degrees along with quality and symptom response. The procedure is standardized with the patient adopting the same resting neutral posture in sitting during each measurement. For flexion (Figure 6-26A), the inclinometer is centered on top of the patient's head in line with the external auditory meatus and zeroed. The patient performs flexion and the amount is recorded. For extension (Figure 6-26B), the inclinometer is centered on top of the patient's head in line with the external auditory meatus and zeroed. The patient performs extension and the amount is recorded. For lateral flexion (Figure 6-26C), the inclinometer is placed in the frontal plane on top of the patient's head in line with the external auditory meatus and zeroed. The patient performs lateral flexion and the amount is recorded. For rotation (Figure 6-26D), using a standard goniometer, the stationary arm is in line with the acromioclavicular joint and the movable arm with the nose. The patient rotates and the amount is recorded. For rotation in supine (Figure 6-26E), the inclinometer is centered on the forehead in line with the nose and zeroed. The patient rotates to one side and the amount is recorded.

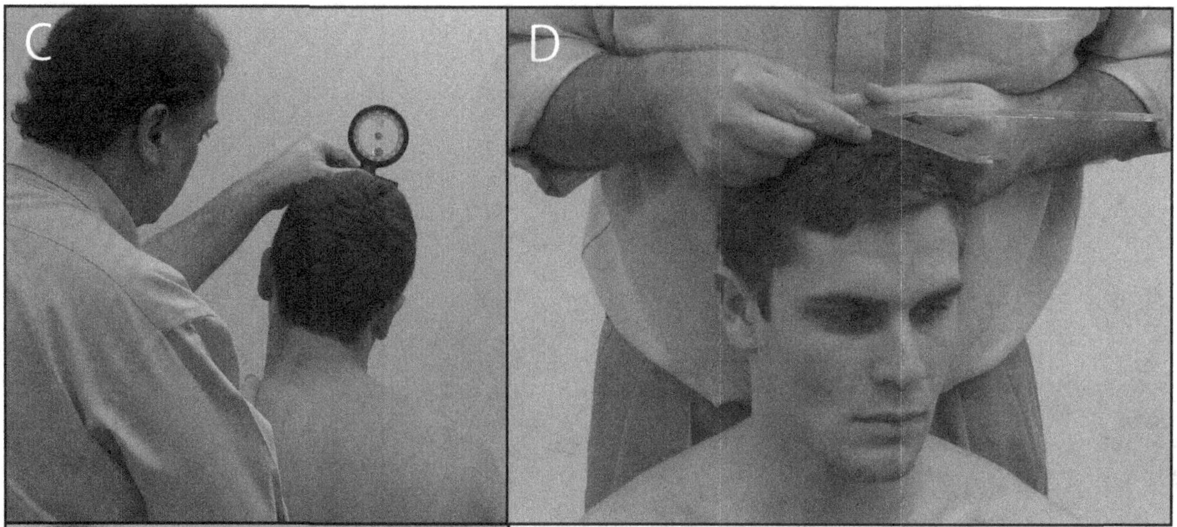

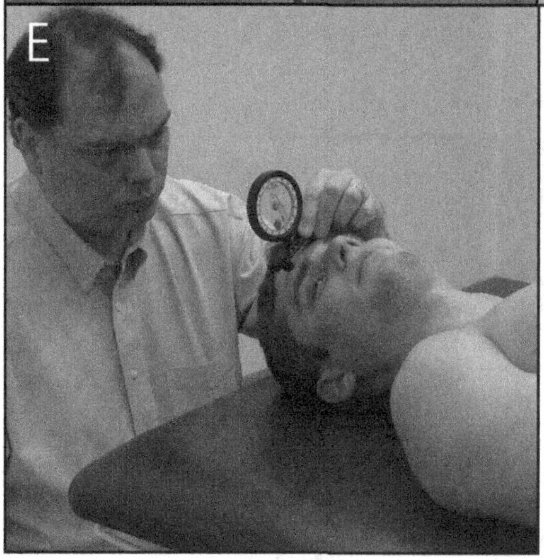

Figure 6-26 (continued). Active range of motion measurement: (C) lateral flexion, (D) rotation in sitting, and (E) rotation in supine.

Active Range of Motion With Overpressure

If AROM is full range, painless, and safe for the patient, passive OP is performed in an oscillatory manner at the limit of the movement to confirm end feel, stress the tissue at end range, and identify the effect on symptoms. For flexion (Figure 6-27A), one hand stabilizes at the cervicothoracic junction while the other hand on the posterior aspect of the head gently guides the cervical spine into flexion, while asking for a change in symptoms. For extension (Figure 6-27B), one hand stabilizes at the cervicothoracic junction while the other hand placed under the mandible gently guides the head and neck further into extension. For lateral flexion (Figure 6-27C), one hand stabilizes the trunk through the acromion process while the other hand placed on the lateral aspect of the head gently guides the head and neck further into right or left lateral flexion. For rotation (Figure 6-27D), the clinician stands on the side of rotation. The forearm stabilizes the trunk while both hands are placed on the lateral side of the head or at the zygoma of the mandible. The hands gently guide the head and neck further into rotation. Symptoms are assessed during overpressure as well as after completion of the procedure. If AROM with OP does not increase or reproduce comparable symptoms, as is common in CGH, additional testing is warranted. Repeated active movements, sustained movements, or combined movements may be necessary to apply additional mechanical load or stress to the cervical spine.

Thoracic Spine

Several studies have found a relationship between upper thoracic mobility and neck or shoulder pain.[423-425] A cross-sectional study of 281 workers evaluated the influence of segmental flexion mobility between C7 and T5 in neck-shoulder pain. Neck-shoulder pain is more frequent among patients with hypomobility at C7 to T1.[423] Reduced relative flexion mobility at C7 to T1 and T1 to T2 predicted neck-shoulder pain and symptom weakness in the hands.[425] The strongest relationship between neck-shoulder pain and segmental mobility was classified as C7 to T1 inverse function, meaning that the mobility at C7 to T1 was equal to or less than T1 to T2.

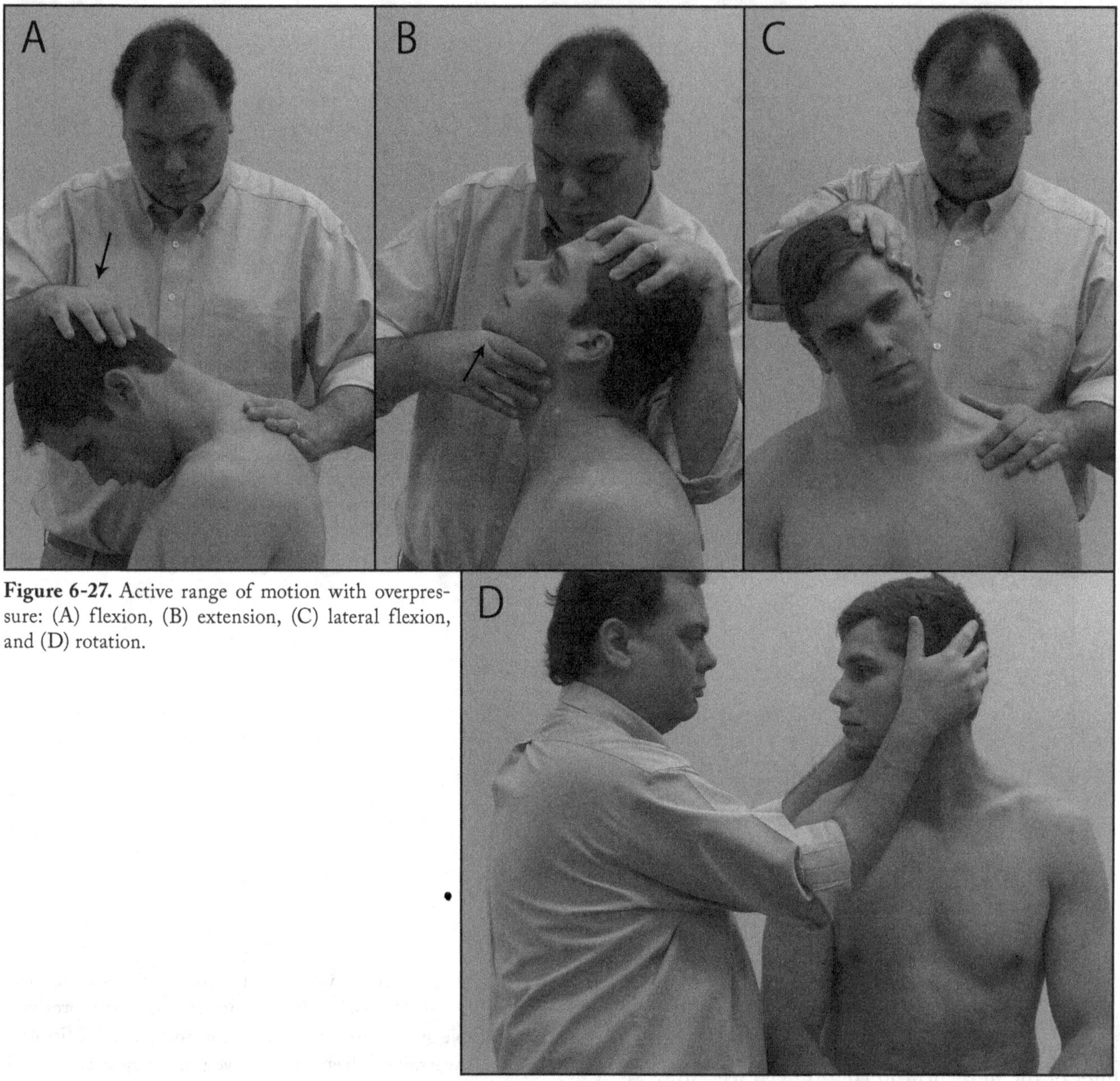

Figure 6-27. Active range of motion with overpressure: (A) flexion, (B) extension, (C) lateral flexion, and (D) rotation.

Reduced mobility explained 14% of the neck-shoulder pain and 15% of a self-report of weakness in the hands.[425] Decreased mobility at C7 to T1 and T3 to T4 was a significant predictor of headache. Mobility at T1 to T2 was significantly reduced for all severe symptoms. At T2 to T3, it was significantly increased compared to subjects without neck-shoulder pain.[425] Cervicothoracic and upper thoracic mobility are significant factors in musculoskeletal neck-shoulder pain.[425] Several studies have evaluated the clinical effectiveness of treating the thoracic spine with thrust manipulation for patients with MNP.[283,426-432]

The thoracic spine is examined as determined by the history, but generally performed for those with neck pain, upper thoracic and chest wall symptoms, or upper extremity symptoms. The working hypotheses and the interdependence between the cervical and thoracic spine dictate the initial focus and extent of the examination in this region. The clinician determines which movements should be tested at the first session. Thoracic rotation (Figure 6-28) is described here to assess the effect on symptoms and assess side-to-side symmetry. In a neutral upright sitting posture with feet supported, the patient crosses the arms, and places hands on the opposite shoulders. Keeping the cervical spine in neutral, the patient rotates the trunk to each side and the symptom response is recorded along with a qualitative description of the movement. Overpressure is performed if the movement is full and painless. Provocation of symptoms is an indication for further examination of the thoracic region.

Repeated Movements

The response to repeated movements is important for subgroup classification of patients with MNP.[422,433-435] Assessment using repeated movements in the cervical spine is the same as used in the lumbar spine. When a patient's symptoms centralize during repeated movements, such as cervical retraction or flexion, the direction that produces the centralization suggests a subgroup classification within the neck pain with radiating pain classification (see Table 6-4) that is likely to respond to repeated movement in the direction that resulted in centralization.[422,433] For example, if centralization occurs with repeated cervical retraction, then repeated retraction is the recommended intervention.

Compared to the lumbar spine, little research is available to describe diagnostic utility of repeated movements in the cervical spine. Childs et al[434] included centralization as 1 of 5 proposed treatment-based classifications for neck pain. For cervical patients, interexaminer reliability for syndrome classification was $\kappa = 0.63$ with 92% and subsyndrome classification was $\kappa = 0.84$ with 88% agreement.[435] Clinicians trained in the diagnostic classification related to repeated movements for neck pain demonstrated moderate agreement for diagnosis ($\kappa = 0.55$, 95% CI: 0.52 to 0.58, 67%), for derangement or direction specific subcategory ($\kappa = 0.47$, 95% CI: 0.44 to 0.50, 63%) and directional preference of treatment ($\kappa = 0.46$, CI: 0.43 to 0.49, $P < .05$; 70%). Schenk et al[436] described the use of repeated cervical end range movements in the examination and treatment of a patient with CR. When a patient centralizes during the initial examination, the repeated cervical movement (protrusion, retraction, flexion, retraction with extension, lateral flexion or rotation) that produces the centralization becomes the initial intervention or management strategy.

Test Procedure

Based on the response to one repetition during AROM in sitting, sagittal plane movements (protrusion, retraction, or retraction with extension, flexion) are tested first. In patients with acute or severe symptoms, testing in the unloaded position or supine is necessary.[422,433] Lateral flexion or rotation is tested toward the side of pain when the response to sagittal plane movement is nonresponsive or inconclusive or with unilateral or asymmetrical symptoms.

Clear communication is necessary to correctly note the response. Repeated movements occur actively by the patient with added patient overpressure as needed. Clinician forces are added only to gain further understanding or to alter the loading strategy of the response to the repeated movements. General concepts related to repeated movement testing according to McKenzie and May[422,433] for the cervical spine are discussed next. A detailed description[422,434] of this approach is available for review. Not all test positions are needed for all patients. The history,

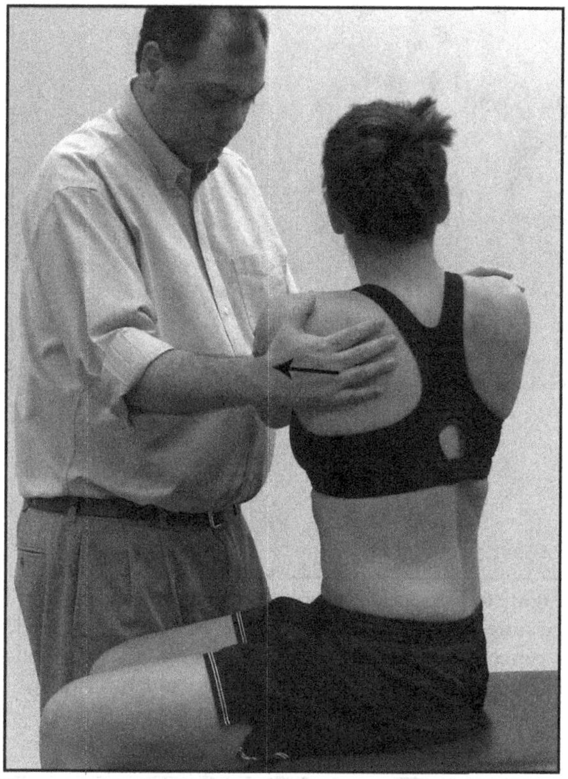

Figure 6-28. AROM thoracic rotation with overpressure.

working hypothesis, and response to one repetition dictate which movements are tested first for each patient. The patient response further dictates which direction of movements are continued, stopped, or added for assessment and appropriate classification. Patients who cannot tolerate repeated movements in sitting or peripheralized may be assessed in lying, as follows:

- Establish baseline resting symptoms and explain the procedure
- Assess the response to one repetition and ask for 10 to 15 repetitions
  - o Repeated protrusion in sitting (see Figure 6-24)
  - o Repeated flexion in sitting (see Figure 6-21A)
  - o Repeated flexion in sitting with patient overpressure (Figure 6-29)
  - o Repeated retraction in sitting (see Figure 6-25)
  - o Repeated retraction in sitting with patient overpressure (Figure 6-30)
  - o Repeated retraction in sitting with clinician overpressure (Figure 6-31)
  - o Repeated retraction and extension in sitting (Figure 6-32)
  - o Repeated lateral flexion in sitting (Figure 6-33)
  - o Repeated rotation in sitting (Figure 6-34)

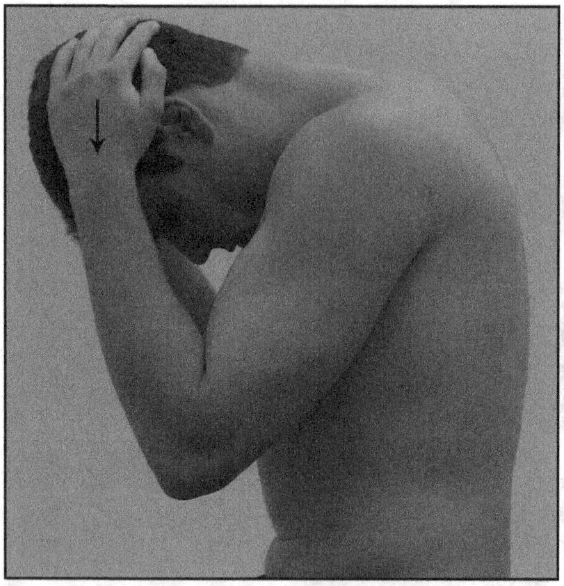

Figure 6-29. Repeated flexion in sitting with patient overpressure. Flexion is not a routine test procedure. If needed, a patient sits slouched and then bends the head and neck forward to place the chin on the chest and returns to neutral. Clinician overpressure is added as needed.

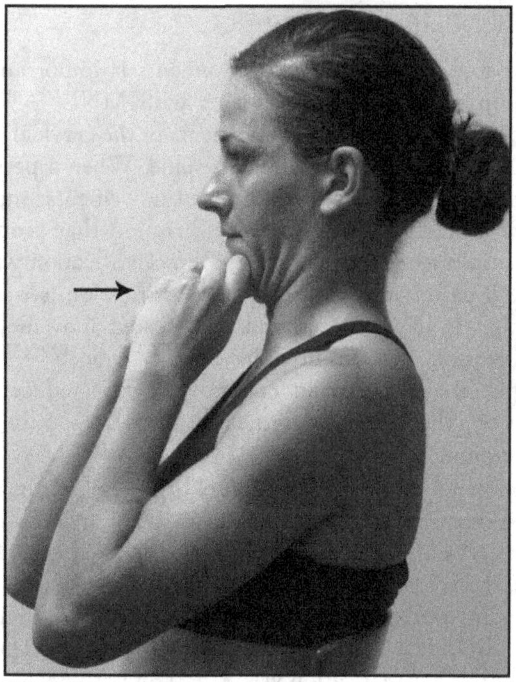

Figure 6-30. Repeated retraction in sitting with patient overpressure. The patient presses the chin with the fingers at the end range of movement. Overpressure may also be performed through the maxilla rather than the mandible to protect the temporomandibular joint.

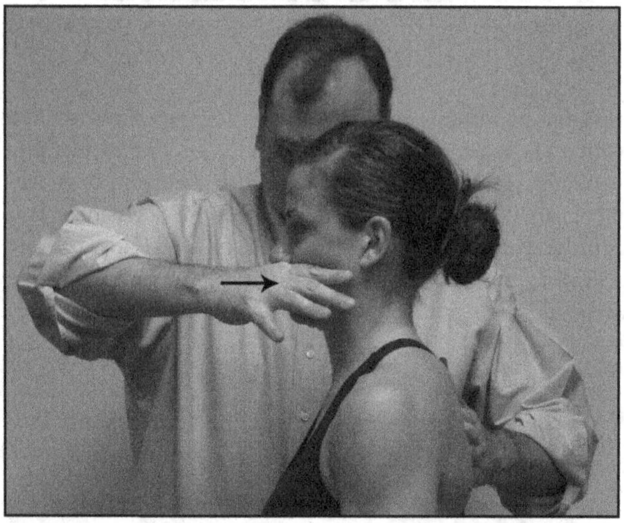

Figure 6-31. Repeated retraction in sitting with clinician overpressure through the maxilla. Overpressure may also be performed through the mandible.

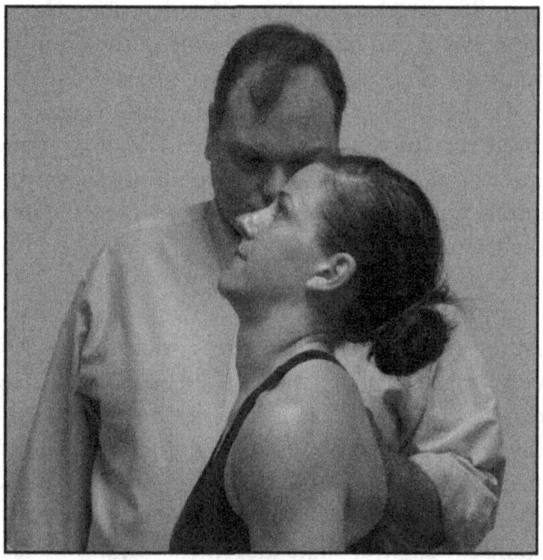

Figure 6-32. Repeated retraction and extension in sitting. The test movement is retraction followed by extension. The patient performs retraction as described above and slowly tips the head back as far as able and returns to neutral.

- During the repeated movements of 10 to 15 repetitions, continually ask the patient about any change in symptom behavior such as location, intensity, symptoms during movement or at end range and note any change in quantity of movement.
- Record the response about 1 to 2 minutes after the movements.
- Potential Responses: centralized, peripheralized, better, no better, worse, no worse, or no effect
- If possible, appropriately classify the patient at this time: neck pain with radiating pain (see Table 6-4) or neck pain with mobility deficits (see Table 6-1).

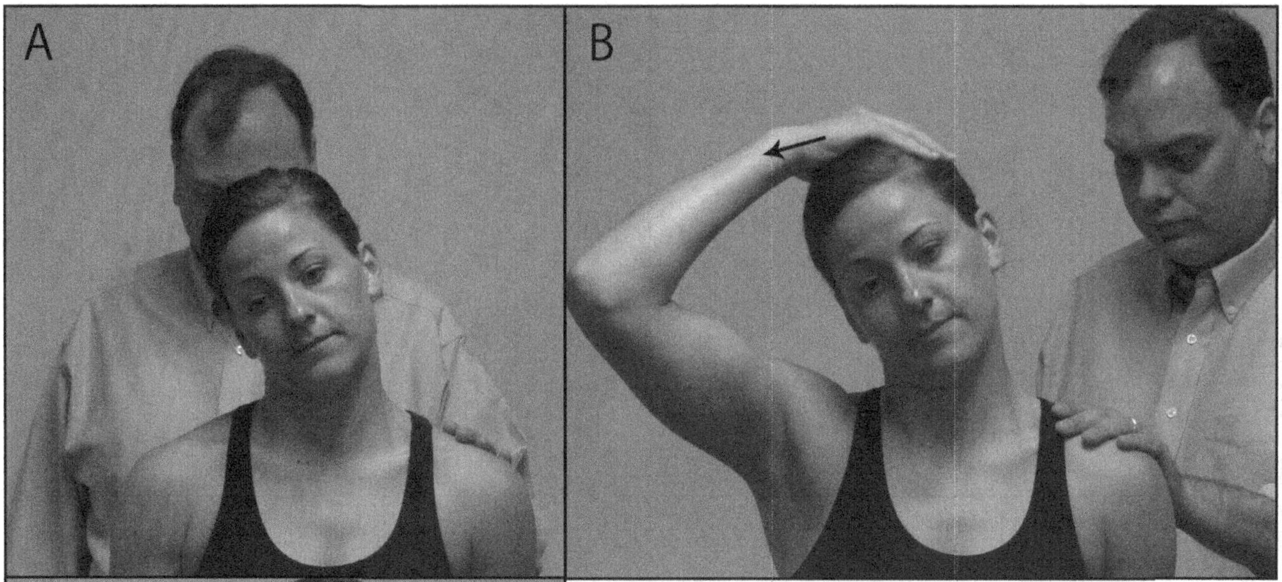

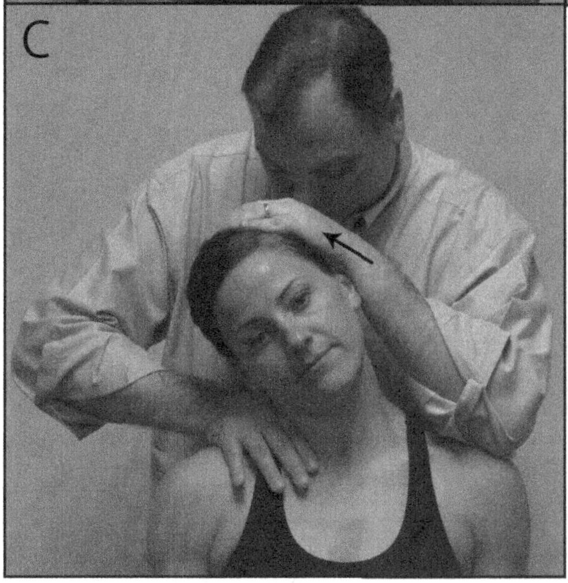

Figure 6-33. Repeated lateral flexion in sitting: (A) The patient first retracts to a neutral position and then performs lateral flexion to the side of pain and returns to neutral. As needed, patient overpressure is added. (B) For left lateral flexion with overpressure, the patient places the left hand over the head with fingers reaching to the ear and the head is gently pulled down to the shoulder. (C) Clinician overpressure is added as needed.

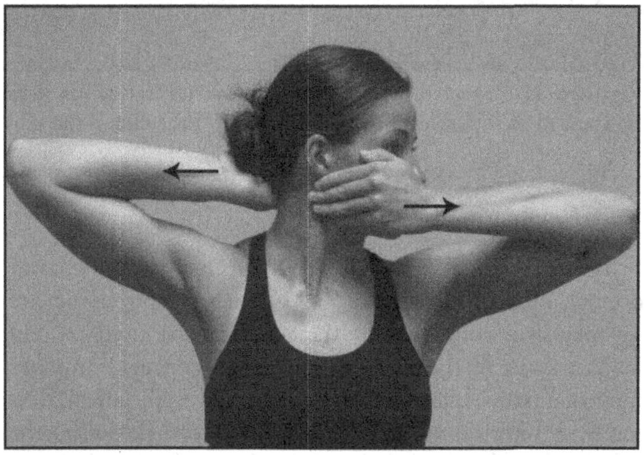

Figure 6-34. Repeated rotation in sitting with patient overpressure. The patient first retracts to neutral and then rotates toward the side of pain and returns to neutral. As needed, patient overpressure is added. The patient places one hand behind the head and one on the chin to provide overpressure. Clinician overpressure is added as needed.

- If a repeated movement decreases, abolishes or centralizes symptoms or a directional preference is obtained, further testing is unnecessary.[422,433]
  - If centralization or DP occur, the clinician proceeds with a matched intervention or loading strategy (ie retraction, flexion, lateral flexion, or rotation).
  - If peripheralized or partially centralized in weight-bearing, the clinician attempts to obtain centralization through repeated movements in unloaded positions such as repeated retraction in lying with pillows as needed, retraction in lying with patient overpressure, and retraction off the end of the table (Figures 6-35).
  - If the response is limited motion and end range pain that is produced, increased, or no worse and with no centralization or peripheralization, further examination is needed; the clinician considers a classification of neck pain with mobility deficits (see Table 6-1) and examines further for information to confirm.

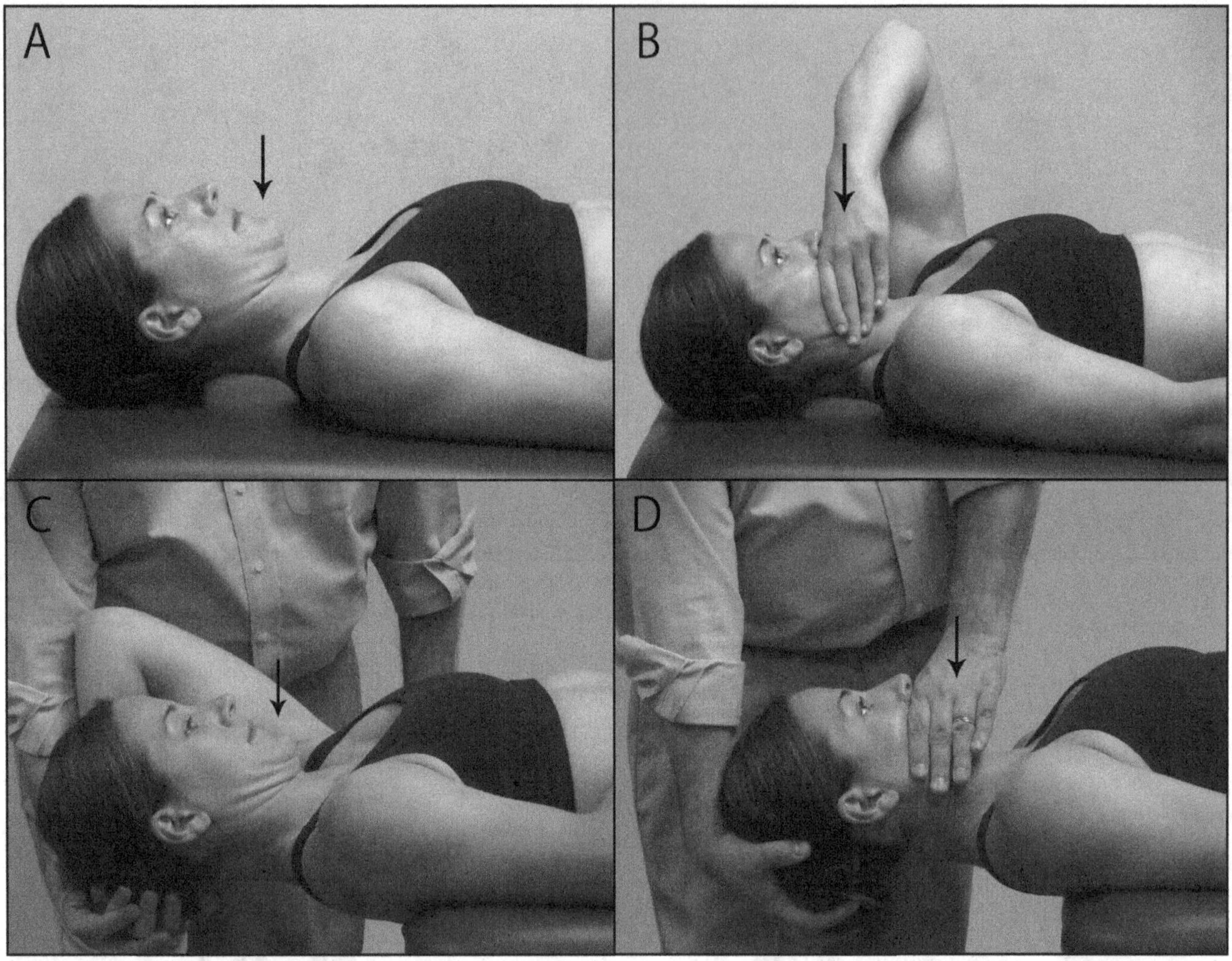

Figure 6-35. Repeated movements in supine: (A) retraction in lying; (B) retraction in lying with patient overpressure; (C) retraction off the end of the table; and (D) retraction off the end of the table with clinician overpressure.

Combined Movement Testing

If AROM and repeated movements are full range and do not increase or produce a patient's symptoms or are inconclusive, combined movements may be used to add load or stress to the cervical spine. This concept combines movements of either flexion or extension with lateral flexion.[437,438] For example, extension and lateral flexion to the left are thought to produce maximal compression forces to the spinal structures on the left. Flexion and lateral flexion to the left are thought to produce maximal tensile stresses to the spinal structures on the right. In addition to being used as a provocative test, combined movements may help to direct positioning during treatment. A detailed discussion of examination and intervention using combined movements in the cervical spine is available for review by McCarthy.[438]

Special Tests

Compression

Compression (Figure 6-36), distraction, and Spurling's test are provocative tests which position the neck to aggravate or relieve symptoms usually associated with cervicobrachial syndrome or CR. With the patient seated, the examiner stands behind the patient and places both hands on top of the head and gradually exerts a downward pressure while assessing for a change in baseline symptoms. In 100 patients with neck and/or shoulder pain, reliability of compression is poor ($\kappa = 0.34$) without knowledge of history and increases to fair ($\kappa = 0.44$) with knowledge of the patient's history.[439]

Traction/Distraction

Axial traction is performed in sitting to decrease symptoms (Figure 6-37). The examiner stands behind the patient and gently lifts the head with the hands under the maxilla and the thenar eminences under the occiput while assessing for change in baseline symptoms. The reliability of traction in sitting is fair without and with knowledge of the patient's history, $\kappa = 0.56$ and $\kappa = 0.41$, respectively.[439]

Distraction is also performed in supine (Figure 6-37B) to reduce symptoms. The examiner grasps the chin and

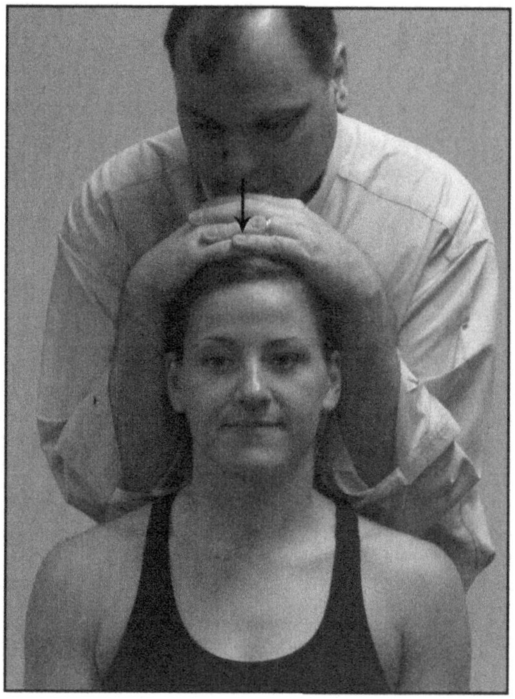

Figure 6-36. Compression.

occiput in slight flexion while applying an unloading force of 14 lbs. The test is positive if symptoms are reduced. In patients suspected of CR or carpal tunnel syndrome, the reliability is substantial: κ = 0.88 (0.64, 1.0).[245] As a single test item, diagnostic accuracy is Sn 0.44 (0.21 to 0.67), Sp 0.90 (0.82 to 0.98), -LR 0.62 (0.40 to 0.90), and +LR 4.4 (1.8 to 11.1). Neck distraction is one variable out of 4 of a test item cluster for the diagnosis of CR.[245] In a systematic review examining diagnostic accuracy of tests for CR, both traction, neck distraction, and Spurling's test demonstrate low to moderate sensitivity and high specificity.[440] Both neck traction and distraction may also result in an increase in symptoms, possibly associated with tensile stress on involved tissues.

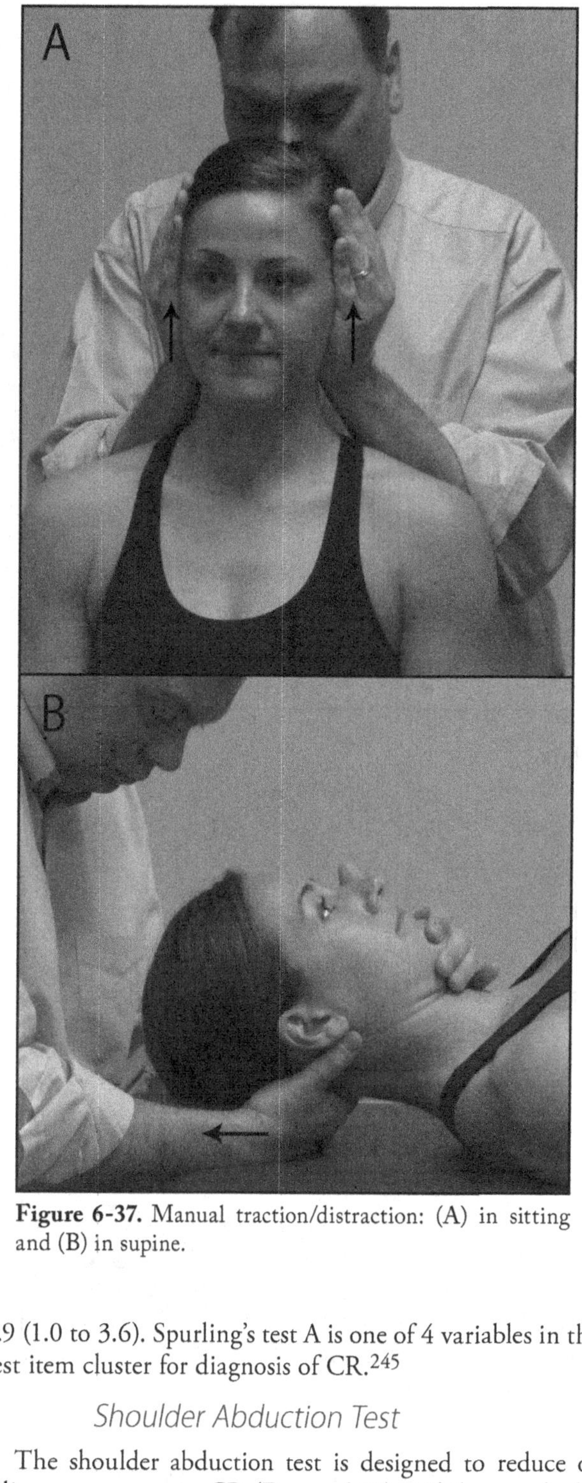

Figure 6-37. Manual traction/distraction: (A) in sitting and (B) in supine.

Spurling's Test

Spurling's test is performed to provoke symptoms associated with CR. The test is described with variations of extension, lateral flexion, and rotation to the same side. The test is presented here as described by Wainner et al[245] with 2 variations, A and B. Spurling's test A (Figure 6-38A) is performed by applying 7 kg of pressure with the patient sitting and neck laterally flexed to the tested side, reliability κ = 0.60 (0.32, 0.87). Spurling's test B (Figure 6-38B) is performed by applying 7 kg of pressure with the patient sitting and the neck extended, laterally flexed and rotated to the tested side, reliability, κ = 0.62 (0.25, 0.99). Diagnostic accuracy for test A is Sn = 0.50 (0.27 to 0.73), Sp 0.86 (0.77 to 0.94), -LR -0.58 (0.36 to 0.94), and +LR 3.5 (1.6 to 7.5). Diagnostic accuracy for test B is Sn = 0.50 (0.27 to 0.73), Sp 0.74 (0.63 to 0.85), -LR -0.67 (0.42 to 1.1), and +LR 1.9 (1.0 to 3.6). Spurling's test A is one of 4 variables in the test item cluster for diagnosis of CR.[245]

Shoulder Abduction Test

The shoulder abduction test is designed to reduce or relieve symptoms in CR (Figure 6-39). While seated, the patient is asked to place the hand of the involved extremity on top of the head. The test is positive if baseline symptoms are reduced. Reliability is poor if κ = 0.20 (0.00 to 0.59). Diagnostic accuracy as reported by Wainner et al[245] is Sn 0.17 (0.0 to 0.34), Sp 0.92 (0.85 to 0.99), -LR 0.91 (0.73 to 1.1), and +LR 2.1 (0.55 to 8.0). Rubinstein et al[440] reported a wide range in sensitivity, ranging from 0.17 to 0.78, due to variation in quality of studies and the reference standard, but report a moderate to high specificity.

Figure 6-38. Spurling's test: (A) test A and (B) test B.

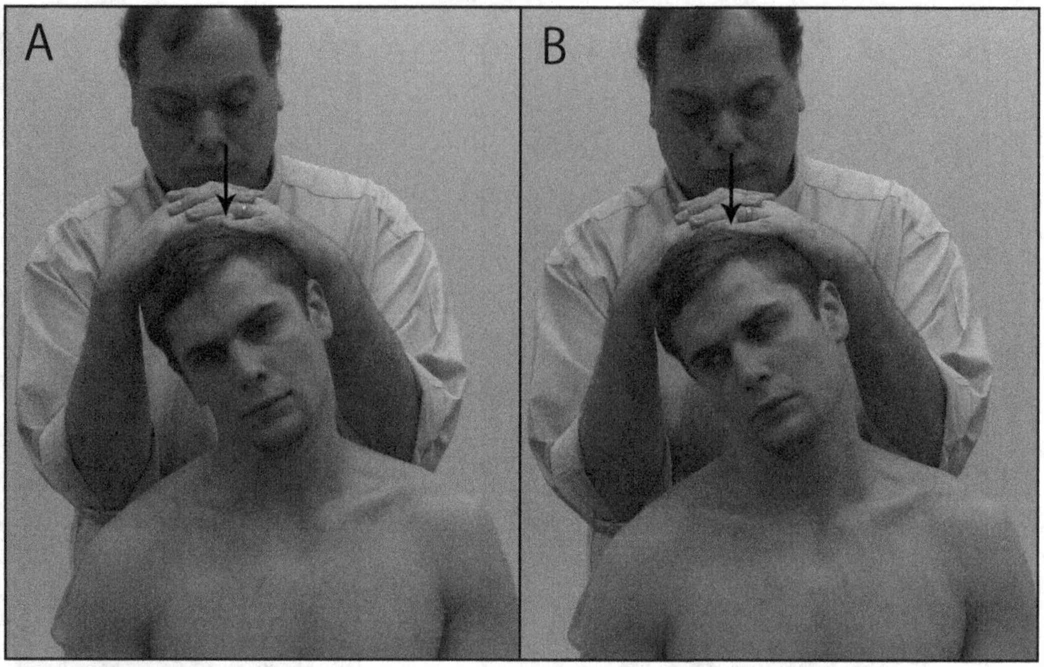

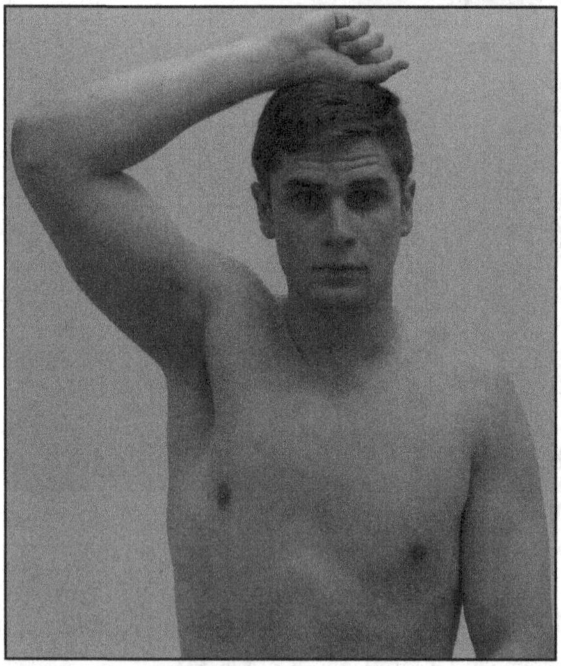

Figure 6-39. Shoulder abduction test.

Cervical Rotation Lateral Flexion Test

The CRLF (see Figure 5-20) is discussed in Chapter 5 as part of the thoracic spine examination. The test is purported to determine the presence of first rib hypomobility in patients with brachialgia and thoracic outlet syndrome and is applicable in patients presenting with neck pain and shoulder or upper extremity symptoms. The first rib may be palpated in sitting, supine or prone. In sitting, the posterior superior aspect of the first rib is palpated bilaterally for tenderness and the relative heights compared. A rib that is more superior compared to the other side suggests an elevated rib on that side and requires additional tests for confirmation. In addition to the CRLF, passive thoracic spine, first rib mobility tests, and scalene muscle length tests may be indicated.

Segmental Motion Testing for T1 to T4

The complex interdependence between the cervical spine and thoracic spine provides rationale for examination of this region in all patients presenting with neck pain and/or associated shoulder and upper extremity symptoms. Segmental motion testing for the upper thoracic spine may be examined in sitting (as described in Chapter 5) or in prone (see Figure 5-17). This method of segmental motion assessment is based upon the biomechanical model of motion in the thoracic spine. Flexion occurs when both inferior facets of superior vertebrae glide upward on the superior facets of the inferior vertebra as the superior vertebral body rolls and glides anteriorly. The reverse occurs during thoracic extension. Central (Figure 6-40) and unilateral PAIVM (Figure 6-41) are assessed in prone.

Thoracic Outlet Syndrome Screening

Thoracic outlet syndrome (TOS) describes the location of a problem, but doesn't actually characterize it. Compromise of the neurovascular bundle within the TOS occurs at one of 3 sites: the interscalene space, costoclavicular space, or sub-pectoralis minor space. Based on a variable clinical presentation, TOS is classified as arterial (ATOS), venous (VTOS), and neurogenic (NTOS). NTOS, described as a brachial plexopathy, is the most common, while ATOS and VTOS are recognized as

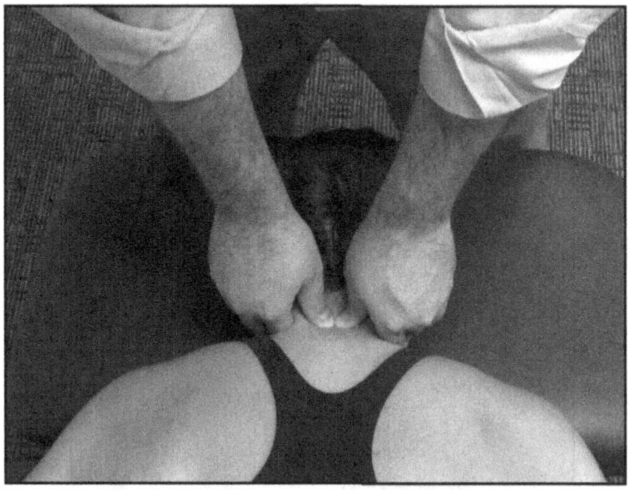

Figure 6-40. Cervical spine central passive segmental mobility tests.

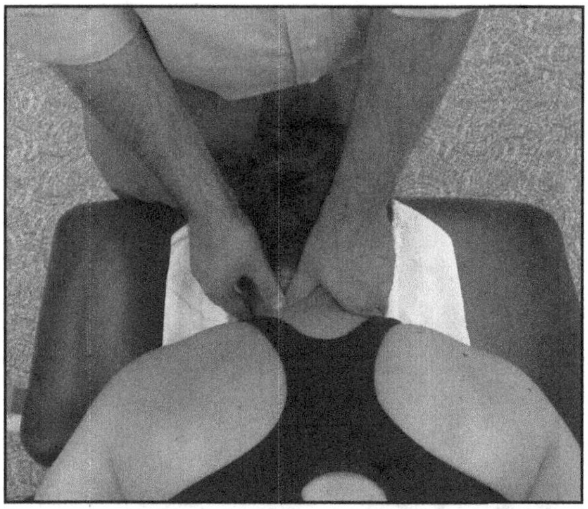

Figure 6-41. Cervical spine unilateral passive segmental mobility tests.

compression of the subclavian artery and subclavian vein, respectively.[441] Patients complain of neck pain, shoulder pain, vague upper extremity pain, paresthesia often of the entire hand or specific digits, a tired, heavy aching sensation, hand and arm weakness, and swelling. Often using the hands or arms in an elevated position produces or exacerbates the symptoms. Considering this wide variation of clinical symptoms, multiple diagnoses must be considered in the differential diagnosis.[441]

Patients with ATOS have true claudication of the arm, especially when elevated, often due to compression of the subclavian artery in the area of the first rib which often develops spontaneously.[442] Physical findings include loss of pulses at rest, coldness, paresthesia and fatigue, and perhaps color changes and ischemic finger tips, but rarely neck or shoulder symptoms.[442] ATOS accounts for 3% to 4% of TOS and is associated with a cervical rib.[441] VTOS accounts for a small number of patients: 2% to 3%. Symptoms are preceded by excessive arm activity, such as throwing, swimming, weight lifting and include swelling, edema, arm discomfort and cyanosis, and distended superficial veins.[442] Neurogenic or NTOS accounts for over 90% of TOS and involves symptoms of the upper plexus (ie, C5, C6, and C7) and the lower plexus (ie, C8 and T1) often associated with a history of neck pain.[442] Neck pain, paresthesia, and weakness in the shoulder, arm, and hand plus occipital headache are classic symptoms of NTOS. Common neuromusculoskeletal disorders, such as CR or ulnar neuropathy, may present similarly and patients may present with more than one problem. Therefore, a careful differential diagnosis is required. In addition to a detailed history, the physical examination includes assessment of the entire upper quarter as related to observation, posture, breathing patterns, muscle imbalance, altered joint mobility, a neurological exam, neurodynamics, and provocative neurovascular tests. The provocative tests attempt to stress the neurovascular structures and produce the patient's symptoms. Provocative test procedures are discussed below. Additional testing such as radiography, angiography, or electrodiagnostic studies may be indicated.

A detailed review of TOS is beyond the scope of this reference. Two excellent papers by Watson et al[443,444] that review the classification, varied clinical presentations, and a conservative treatment approach for TOS are available for review.[443-444] The main focus of these authors for TOS rehabilitation is on the shoulder girdle through restoration of scapular control, restoration of humeral head control, isolated strengthening of weak shoulder muscles, taping, and MT strategies to aid in decompressing the thoracic outlet. Based on examination findings, impairment-based management is indicated and tailored to the patient's individual deficits.[443,444] Cervical, thoracic and first rib mobilization techniques, soft tissue mobilization, scalene and pectoral muscle lengthening may have a role in treating the various subgroups of TOS.[445] TOS is often a diagnosis of exclusion and little agreement exists for diagnosis or conservative management. Surgical management is generally indicated for vascular TOS with true vascular compromise due to the potential for ischemia and for those with NTOS who do not respond to a conservative approach.

Provocative Tests for TOS: Provocative tests have been reported to have a high false positive rate.[244] Wright's test and the elevated arm stress test have the highest reported sensitivity for NTOS and vascular TOS. The ULND, also known as the *upper limb tension test*, has a high sensitivity for provocation of sensitized neural tissue in the cervical spine, brachial plexus, and upper extremity, but is not specific to a problem in one area. Gillard et al[446] examined the diagnostic utility of Adson's test, Wright's test, the elevated arm stress test, hyperabduction test, Tinel's test, and pressure in the supra- and infraclavicular areas. A cluster of 2 provocative tests increased sensitivity to 90%. A cluster

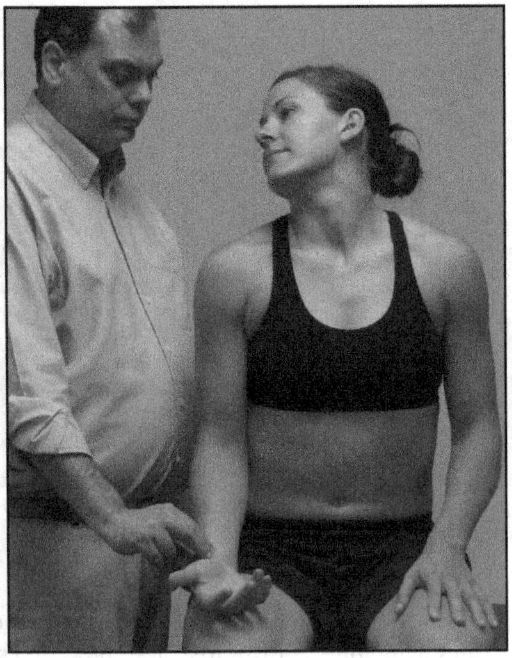

Figure 6-42. Adson's test.

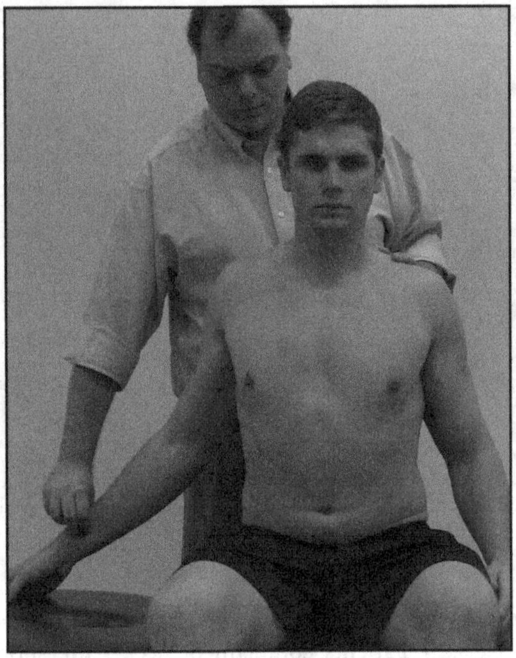

Figure 6-43. Costoclavicular maneuver.

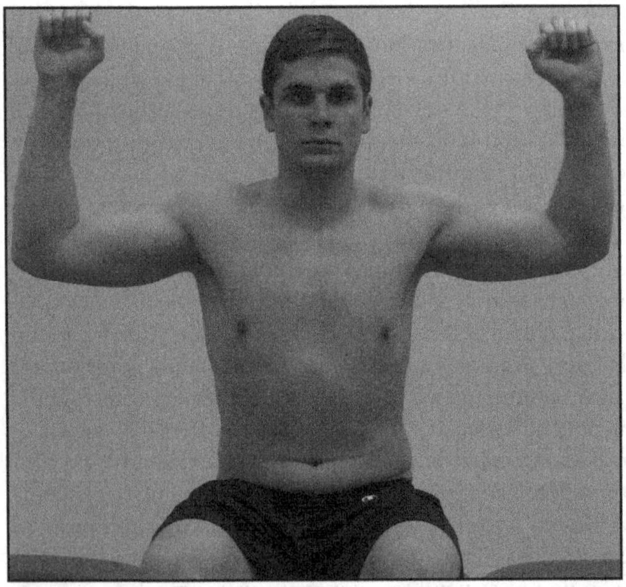

Figure 6-44. Elevated arm stress test.

of 5 provocative tests resulted in Sn 83% and Sp 84%.[446] Common provocative tests for TOS are discussed as follows, but descriptions of how to perform these tests are not standardized throughout the literature:

- *Adson's test* (Figure 6-42): With patient seated and arms resting at the sides, the examiner palpates the radial pulse as the patient inhales deeply, holds his or her breath, extends, and rotates toward the tested side. This test is theorized to address compromise of the brachial plexus through the scalene triangle. A positive test is a change in radial pulse and/or reproduction of symptoms. Diagnostic accuracy is: Sn 0.79, Sp 0.74 to 1.00; +LR 3.29, -LR 0.28. A change in radial pulse has a large percentage of false positives. Therefore, symptom reproduction may be a better indicator of a positive test.[446-451]
- *Costoclavicular maneuver* (Figure 6-43): With the patient seated and arms at the sides, the examiner palpates the radial pulse as the patient retracts and depresses the shoulder girdle to assess tissue compromise by narrowing the costoclavicular space. The position is held for up to 1 minute. A positive test is a change in radial pulse and/or reproduction of symptoms. Specificity ranges from 0.54 to 1.00.[449,451,452]
- *Elevated arm stress test* (Figure 6-44): The patient is seated with arms above 90 degrees of abduction and full external rotation. The head remains in neutral as the patient opens and closes the hand into fists for 3 minutes; the test is timed to onset of symptoms. A positive test is reproduction of symptoms and stopping the test by dropping the arms to relieve symptoms. Diagnostic accuracy is Sn 0.52 to 0.84, Sp 0.30 to 1.00; +LR 1.2 to 5.2, and -LR 0.4-0.53.[449,451,452]
- *Wright's test* (Figure 6-45): With the patient seated with arms at the sides, the examiner palpates the radial pulse and places the patient's shoulder into abduction with the arm above the shoulder and hand above the head. The position is held for 1 to 2 minutes and timed to onset of symptoms. The test purports to compress tissue under the pectoralis minor (Pec Minor). A positive test is a change in radial pulse and/

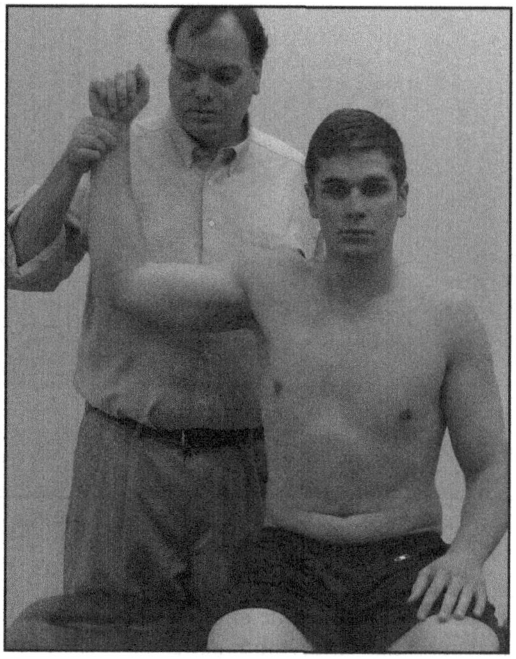

Figure 6-45. Wright's test.

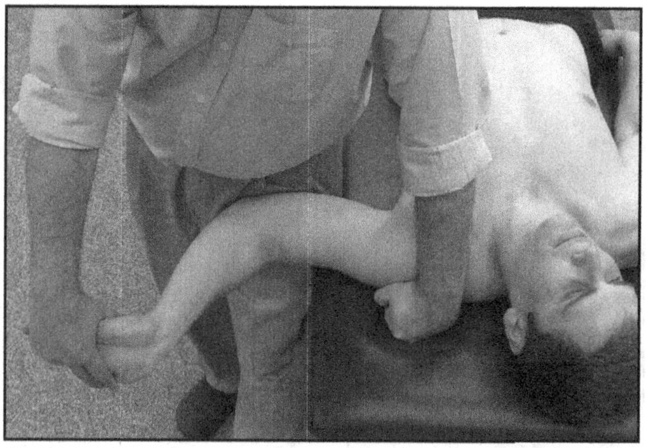

Figure 6-46. Upper limb neurodynamic test 1 (median nerve).

or symptom reproduction. Diagnostic accuracy is: Sn 0.70 to 0.90, Sp 0.29 to 0.53; +LR 1.27 to 1.49, -LR 0.34 to 0.57.[446]

Upper Limb Neurodynamic Test[439,453,454]

The ULNDT, also known as the *upper limb neural tension test* (median nerve bias), is described as a test to challenge movement of the median nerve relative to its surroundings through the neck and upper extremity. The patient is supine with the examiner on the side to be tested. Baseline symptoms are assessed and reassessed after each step in the test procedure. The clinician depresses the shoulder girdle and then abducts the shoulder up to 110 degrees with slight extension keeping the elbow in 90 degrees flexion. The forearm is then maximally supinated and followed by wrist and finger extension. Maintaining all of the previous movements, elbow extension is added. Testing is stopped at onset of symptom reproduction and a sensitizing maneuver is added slowly to determine the effect on the symptoms. The sensitizing maneuver is lateral flexion of the neck to the contralateral side (Figure 6-46). A positive test is reproduction of the patient's symptoms, an increase in symptoms with the sensitizing maneuver, and an asymmetrical response such as limited elbow extension compared to the uninvolved side. Diagnostic accuracy for TOS is: Sn 0.90, Sp 0.38; +LR 1.5, -LR 0.3.[439,453,454] The ULNDTs are discussed in the supine position sequence.

Sensorimotor Control Tests

Altered sensorimotor function includes deficits in balance, eye movement control, and proprioceptive acuity. The large amounts of mechanoreceptors in the joints and muscle of the cervical spine and the connections from the cervical afferents to the vestibular, visual, and postural control systems suggest that the neck provides important somatosensory input that affects control of postural stability, head orientation, and eye movement.[90] In persons with insidious onset neck pain and WAD, abnormal afferent input from the somatosensory, visual, or vestibular systems can lead to altered sensory motor control and manifest as dizziness, unsteadiness in upright postures, and reduced control of head and eye movement.[91-94] Indications for sensorimotor control tests are neck pain, dizziness, unsteadiness, and visual disturbances.

Balance, cervical joint position sense, and oculomotor control are assessed for impairments of sensorimotor control. The clinical examination of static standing balance is discussed in Chapter 3 in persons with neck pain.[102,110,369] Dynamic balance tests[370] could include, but are not limited to, the timed 10-m walk test[457] (with and without head turns[370]) and the Dynamic Gait Index.[11,456]

Cervical joint position sense can be assessed by using a laser pointer mounted to a headband.[94,112] While sitting 90 cm away from a wall, the patient focuses on the natural resting head posture for a few seconds with the laser marked on the wall. With the eyes closed, the patient actively moves the head and tries to return to the resting posture as accurately as possible. The difference between the start position and return position of the laser beam on the wall is measured in centimeters and converted to degrees using the following formula: tan - 1[error distance/90 cm] = angle. A 7.1-cm error distance equals a meaningful joint position error (JPE) of 4.5 degrees. Errors greater than 4.5 degrees suggest impairment in head-neck relocation accuracy.[94,112] JPE can be measured for all directions of active cervical motion. Additional signs of impairment include jerky or altered movement patterns, searching, and overshooting of the position in order to gain additional proprioceptive feedback. Patients may also experience dizziness or unsteadiness with the test.[94,112]

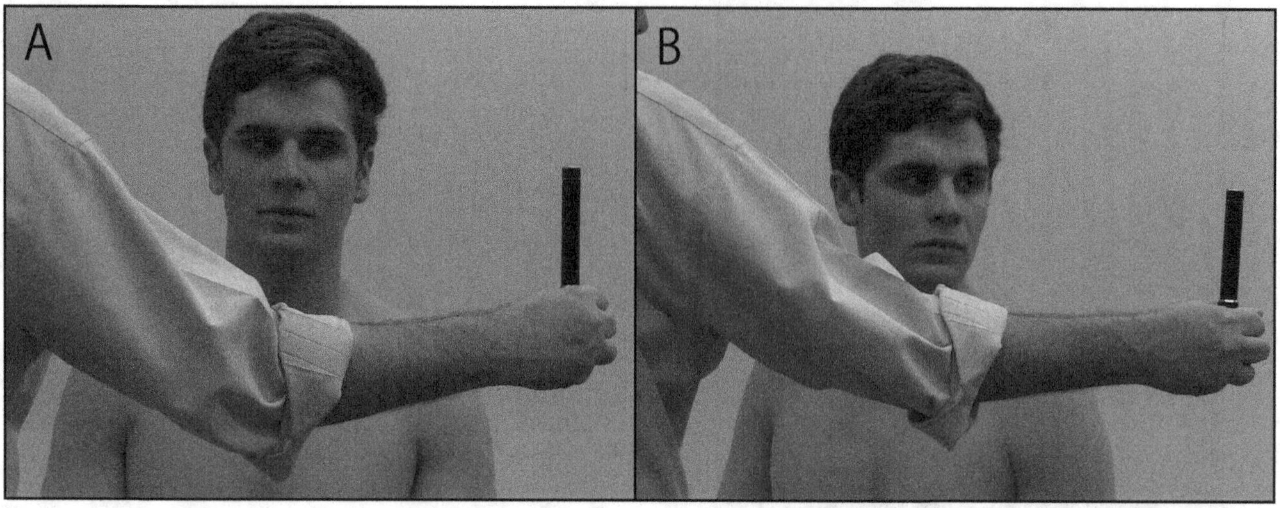

Figure 6-47. Smooth pursuit neck torsion test: (A) neutral and (B) neck and trunk rotated.

Oculomotor control involves assessment of eye movement. The tests include (a) smooth pursuit (a qualitative assessment of eye follow while keeping the head still), (b) gaze stability (head movement while focusing on an object), (c) head and eye movement coordination, and (d) saccades or quick movements of the eyes to refocus. Clinical observation includes quality and control of eye movements as well as symptom reproduction. The tests are used in patients with vestibular and CNS disorders and are not specific to patients with neck pain.[457]

The smooth pursuit neck torsion test (Figure 6-47) is proposed as a test for detecting impaired eye movement control due to altered cervical afferent input, but has not been adequately studied for sensitivity and specificity. The subject keeps their head still and follows a slow moving target with just the eyes through a range of about 30 to 45 degrees to each side of neutral. The difference in smooth pursuit eye movement control with neutral head, neck, and trunk posture is compared to when the neck and trunk are rotated 45 degrees left and 45 degrees right, relative to a stationary head.[458] The trunk is rotated on the neck to avoid vestibular stimulation. When asked to follow a slow-moving target with the eyes at 20 degrees per second while keeping the head still, the desired response is accurate and smooth eye movement. Quick saccadic eye movements in an attempt to catch up to the target suggest impairment.[116] A positive test is a difference in the ability to follow (ie, increased saccades) or symptoms in the neck rotated position compared to the neutral position. The test will be most obvious in WAD and patients with dizziness.[107,116,458] Poor eye movement noted in neutral and unchanged in the neck rotated position suggests a CNS disorder.[457]

Gaze stability is tested by asking the patient to focus on a target and maintain focus while actively moving the head into cervical rotation, flexion, extension, and lateral flexion. A positive test is reproduction of symptoms or inability to keep focus on the target or move as quickly or as far through range as asymptomatic persons.[114,457]

For head and eye movement coordination, the patient is asked to first move the eyes to focus on a point or target and then move the head to that point while maintaining focus. The targets can be left or right or up and down. Asymptomatic individuals can perform isolated eye and head movements and maintain focus. Patients with neck pain may lose focus or be unable to keep the head still while moving the eyes.[459]

Saccadic eye movement involves the patient quickly moving the eyes to fix on targets placed in several different locations. Poor performance is indicated by inability to fix on the target, overshooting, or taking more than 2 eye movements to reach the target. Dizziness or blurred vision may be reported.[457]

In patients where sensorimotor control tests appear inconclusive or do not suggest a cervical origin of symptoms, additional testing of the vestibular or CNS is warranted. In addition to neck pain, other coexisting conditions such as diabetes or simply age as a factor could be causes of altered sensorimotor control.[114]

Examination Procedures in Supine

- Ligamentous stability tests
- Repeated movements
- Anterior cervical palpation
- First rib mobility—caudal glide
- Passive segmental motion testing
- Cervical flexion rotation test
- Muscle performance
    - Muscle length tests
    - Craniocervical flexion test
- ULNDTs

Ligamentous Stability Tests

Ligamentous stability tests are designed to challenge the structural integrity of the osteoarticular-ligamentous system and have inherent risks associated with their performance.[350] With little data available to support or refute the validity of these tests and potential risks as provocative tests, the use of ligamentous stability tests is controversial. In the presence of neurological compromise or signs and symptoms consistent with upper cervical instability, and specific patient populations, such as rheumatoid arthritis, the clinician should refer for medical management. In patients with neck pain with signs and symptoms of ligamentous instability secondary to trauma, and after the need for radiographs has been considered or radiographs are negative, Leal and Dennison[351] suggested that ligamentous instability should be assessed prior to cervical AROM testing. These authors recommend screening tests for those patients in whom ligamentous injury is suspected, given the potential serious consequences of missing a transverse ligament or alar ligament injury. Leal and Dennison[351] also propose that ligamentous stability screening procedures be considered as the standard level of care for screening potential upper cervical spine ligamentous injuries. Provocative tests are not recommended in the presence of symptoms suggestive of neurological insult.[460] Negative tests should be interpreted with caution since a negative test does not rule out ligamentous injury or instability.[351] Screening for cervical ligamentous stability is discussed under screening for red flags.

Sharp-Purser Test

No consensus exists as to sequence of testing, but Aspinall[461] suggested performing the Sharp-Purser test prior to the other tests. In contrast to the other ligamentous stability tests that are provocative in nature, the Sharp-Purser test is an alleviation or relocation procedure rather than a provocation. If the Sharp-Purser test is considered negative (ie, no excessive mobility, no reduction or production of symptoms), then the transverse ligament test is considered.[460] In detecting AA instability in the presence of an atlantodental interval greater than 3 mm, which is considered abnormal in subjects with rheumatoid arthritis, the Sharp-Purser test demonstrated moderate sensitivity (0.69), high specificity (0.96), +LR 17.25, and -LR 0.32.[462,463]

The Sharp-Purser test (see Figure 6-7) assesses the stability of C1 on C2. If the transverse ligament is lax or no longer intact, C1 has the ability to translate forward on C2 in flexion. The patient is in sitting with flexion of the head on neck. The examiner stabilizes the spinous process of C2 with pincer grip while other hand is placed on the forehead. The examiner applies a posterior force through the forehead. A positive test occurs when the head and C1 complex slides posteriorly, hitting the dens, indicating a reduction of the subluxed atlas on axis or when a firm end feel is not appreciated.[461] Symptoms present at baseline may also be relieved.

Transverse Ligament or Anterior Shear Test[461]

To assess the transverse ligament, the patient is in supine while the examiner supports the occiput with both hands, placing the fingers over the posterior arch of the atlas bilaterally (see Figure 6-15). Using the fingers, the examiner translates the atlas and occiput anteriorly on a fixed axis (C2), holding the position for 15 seconds. The patient may be asked to count backwards from 15 with the eyes open. A positive test occurs with reproduction of symptoms (ie, nausea, vertigo, paresthesia, nystagmus, etc) suggestive of upper cervical instability and/or a soft end feel. The validity of this test is unknown. During the anterior shear test in neutral, reliable imaging measurements of the atlantodental interval and displacement of the atlas, with respect to the odontoid process of the axis, demonstrated that the atlas is displaced anteriorly.[464]

Alar Ligament Test

As described by Pettman,[465] the test is performed in head on neck neutral, flexion, and extension to assess the alar ligament fiber orientation (see Figure 6-16). The examiner passively stabilizes the lamina and spinous process of C2 to prevent the axis from rotating and side-bending,. and then passively side-bends the head on neck in all 3 positions. The test is performed to each side. For example, during passive side-bending to the right of head on neck, the left alar is tested. No right side-bending of the head on neck should occur if the ligament is intact.[465] A positive test is excessive side-bending movement in all 3 positions.[465,466] If C2 is not passively stabilized, the test may be performed in supine while the examiner supports the head in one hand and monitors the spinous process of C2 in a pincer grip. The occiput is gently side-bent to each side. The normal response is that the spinous process of C2 immediately moves in the opposite direction to side-bending. During side-bending to the left, the right alar ligament tightens, which pulls C2 immediately into left rotation. The examiner feels the C2 spinous process move immediately to the right.[465] A positive test is a delay in the movement of the C2 spinous process. Validity of this test is unknown. Preliminary evidence using MRI imaging[467] demonstrates that the side-bending stress test and a rotation stress test for the alar ligaments result in an increased length of the contralateral alar ligament. The rotation stress test is not presented here, but available for review.[465,467] Due to imaging limitations, the tests were only performed in neutral. In the presence of a positive side-bending or rotation stress test, Osmotherly et al[467] suggested that the imaging findings support their use in clinical practice and that testing in both directions is not needed to infer instability since a bilateral effect on the alar ligaments was not observed.

Transverse or Lateral Shear Test for Atlantoaxial Complex[461]

This test assesses the integrity of the dens and osseous portion of C1 and its alar attachment (see Figure 6-17). As an example, the head is sidebent on the neck to the left to passively stabilize occiput and C1. Using the index finger MCP, the lateral mass of C1 can be manually stabilized on the right while C2 is then passively translated to the right using the left index finger MCP. The test is performed to each side with the head on neck in neutral, flexion, and extension due to the orientation of the alar ligaments. The test is negative if, in at least one of the test positions, no movement is appreciated. If increased translation is perceived, compromise of the stabilizing structures is possible.[461] The validity of this test is unknown.

Longitudinal Traction or Distraction Test[461]

This test is purported to test the tectorial membrane, a continuation of the posterior longitudinal ligament (see Figure 6-18). With the patient supine, the examiner stabilizes C2 and applies a cephalad traction force through the occiput. The test is repeated with the head in neutral, flexed, or extended. The test is held for 15 seconds. A positive test is excessive movement or reproduction of symptoms. The validity of this test is unknown.[461] During the distraction test in neutral, reliable imaging measurements of the basion-dental interval and tectorial membrane support the theory behind use of this test as a method of assessing tectorial membrane integrity.[467]

Repeated Movements

In patients with acute or severe symptoms, testing in the unloaded position (ie, supine) is often necessary.[422,433] If symptoms peripheralize or are partially centralized in weightbearing, the clinician attempts to obtain centralization through repeated movements in unloaded positions such as repeated retraction in lying, retraction in lying with patient overpressure and retraction off the end of the table (see Figure 6-35), as follows:[422,433]

- Retraction in lying (see Figure 6-35A). Depending upon the amount of thoracic kyphosis and forward head posture, the patient may need to perform retraction in lying into 1 or 2 pillows or towels initially and progress to retraction into the table.
- Retraction in lying with patient overpressure (see Figure 6-35B). Patient overpressure may also be performed into the mandible or maxilla if pressure on the TMD joint must be avoided.
- Repeated retraction off the table (see Figure 6-35C). The patient or clinician supports the patient's head with the head and neck off the treatment table to the level of T3 to T4. The patient first performs repeated retraction. The effect on symptoms is noted.

Anterior Cervical Palpation

Palpation is performed in sitting, supine, or prone, but described here prior to beginning passive segmental mobility tests. The patient should be comfortably positioned as the clinician begins light palpation of temperature and skin texture along the posterior, lateral, and anterior aspects of the neck and areas of symptoms. Soft tissues are palpated to note asymmetry in tissue tension from side-to-side. For example, increased tension is often noted in the scalene muscles possibly for several reasons: (a) compensation for weak deep neck flexors (DNF), (b) a reaction to neural tissue sensitivity, (c) an upper chest breathing pattern, or (d) cervical spine dysfunction.[114] Abnormal soft tissue findings then require additional testing to determine a potential cause. Palpation starts at the posterior occiput, using the external occipital protuberance (ie, inion) as a landmark and moving slightly laterally and distally toward the acromioclavicular joint and superior medial angle of the scapula. Posteriorly, the cervical extensors are palpated bilaterally just lateral to the spinous processes. The SCM is palpated from the mastoid process behind the ear to the clavicle and sternum. As needed, the clavicle, sternoclavicular joints, and first 3 ribs are palpated anteriorly. The ribs may be followed gently laterally and posteriorly, but are difficult to locate as they pass under the clavicle. The superior clavicular fossa is palpated for swelling or lymph nodes, keeping in mind the neurovascular structure in the area. The face, mandible, TMD joints, and head can be palpated at this time also. Lymph nodes lie along the SCM, but are normally palpable only if swollen. The scalenes are posterior to the SCM and the carotid pulse is anterior to the SCM between it and the trachea. The hyoid bone is above the thyroid cartilage anterior to C2 to C3 with the thyroid cartilage anterior to C4 to C5. While palpating the hyoid bone, ask the patient to swallow. The hyoid bone, thyroid cartilage, and first cricoid ring should move superiorly without pain.

To palpate bony structures, begin at the inion in midline and move distally. The first bump palpated is the C2 SP. The C2 to T1 SP are differentiated by moving the neck slightly into flexion and extension. To differentiate between C6 and C7, the clinician should feel the C6 spinous process (SP) move while the C7 SP remains stationary. The facet joints are palpated as firm bony structures through the soft tissue posteriorly located about 0.5 to 1.0 inches lateral to the SP. In between the occiput and the C2 SP and the C2 SP and lateral mass of C1 are the SO muscles overlying the posterior arch of C1. The lateral masses of C1 are located just inferior and anterior to the mastoid process. The transverse processes of the cervical vertebrae are distal to the lateral mass of C1 in the lateral aspect of the neck following the lordotic curve. By locating the T1 SP and corresponding transverse process, the first rib can be palpated where it articulates with the transverse process. Reliability of palpation for tenderness is fair with (κ = 0.49 [SD 0.14]) or without (κ = 0.4 [SD 0.13]) knowledge of the historical findings.[439]

Passive Segmental Motion Testing

PROM in the spine is produced by applying manual examination techniques of either PPIVM or passive accessory intervertebral movements (PAIVM) to the individual motion segments. PPIVM tests involve physiological segmental motion palpation in the same planes as AROM, such as cervical flexion, extension, lateral flexion, and rotation. PAIVM tests involve accessory segmental motion palpation of joint play or gliding motions, such as posterior to anterior gliding centrally over the spinous process or unilaterally over the facet joints. Segmental motion tests are usually graded as normal, hypomobile, or hypermobile with or without a pain response and tested at each segment in a specific direction. Cervical and thoracic segmental mobility tests fit the ICF category of measurement of impairment of body function, mobility of single joints.[15]

Diagnostic Utility

Cleland et al[364] reported the intertester reliability of cervical segmental mobility tests, PAIVM for occiput on C1, C2 to C7, and T1 to T9 and pain provocation for the cervical spine (weighted κ = -0.26 to 0.74, -0.52 to 0.90), respectively. The overall findings for reliability of mobility assessment and pain provocation were highly variable, consistent with other studies.[468,469] Using a lateral glide segmental mobility test to detect only hypomobility, Piva et al[420] also reported variable reliability at different segments. Findings include substantial and moderate reliability for occipital-atlas mobility and symptom provocation of the lower cervical segments. Reliability for C2-C6 segmental motion tests revealed no agreement to fair for mobility (κ = -0.07 to 0.45) and slightly higher for pain provocation (κ = 0.29 to 0.76).[420] In addition, Jull et al[470] found excellent agreement (70%) between examiner pairs when using manual passive segmental examination to determine the presence of painful upper cervical joint dysfunction in 40 subjects with and without neck pain and headaches. In the cervical spine, Jull et al[471] reported a correct diagnosis of symptomatic cervical zygapophysial joint syndromes in 20 patients with Sn = 1.0 and Sp = 1.0, demonstrating excellent validity for PAIVMs and PPIVMs. The reference standard for the symptomatic zygapophysial joint was a radiological-controlled diagnostic nerve block. An examiner blinded to patient condition accurately identified the symptomatic joint in 15 patients and correctly identified 5 patients without joint dysfunction. Despite the challenges with diagnostic utility, manual examination continues to be used in clinical practice to obtain information about physiological and accessory segmental mobility deficits and symptom response to manual provocation. Several approaches to passive segmental mobility testing are available with no approach known to be superior to another.

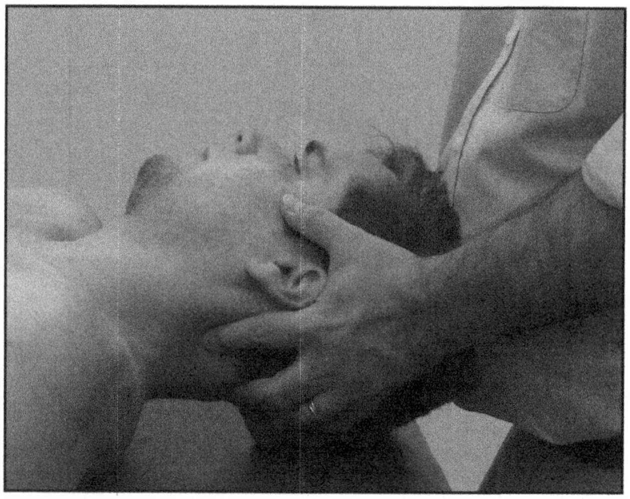

Figure 6-48. Cervical passive physiological intervertebral movement for C2 to C7—right rotation at C2 to C3.

Passive Physiological Intervertebral Movement Tests for C2 to C7

In supine, physiological movement of each cervical segment from C2 to C7 are examined passively in each plane of movement: flexion, extension, lateral flexion, and rotation (Figure 6-48). The examiner cradles the patient's head and palpates at the posterior lateral margin of the zygapophyseal joint using the pad of the index or middle finger. For the C2 to C3 motion segment flexion and extension, the palpation finger will be on the articular pillar at joint line between the 2 segments. The examiner attempts to produce flexion at each segment palpating on both sides, moving only to the end of motion for that segment and not beyond. The cervical spine and each segment are returned to neutral for each segmental test. For lateral flexion, the palpation finger is on the side of the lateral flexion (ie, right side for right lateral flexion) to monitor closing. For rotation, the palpation finger is on the side opposite the rotation (ie, right side for left rotation) to monitor opening of the motion segment.[472] The examiner judges the segment as hypomobile, normal, or hypermobile based on perception of the mobility at each spinal segment relative to those above and below the tested segment and based on the examiner's experience and perception of normal mobility. Additionally, each segment is monitored for reproduction of the patient's pain.

Passive Sidegliding Intervertebral Movement Tests for C2 to C7

The patient is in supine with a cradle hold and the palpating fingers on the articular pillars of the segment of interest (Figure 6-49). In neutral, the examiner passively assesses quality, quantity, and symptom response at each segment beginning at C2 by laterally translating or sidegliding to the left and then to the right and progressing to C7. If translation to one side is reduced compared to the

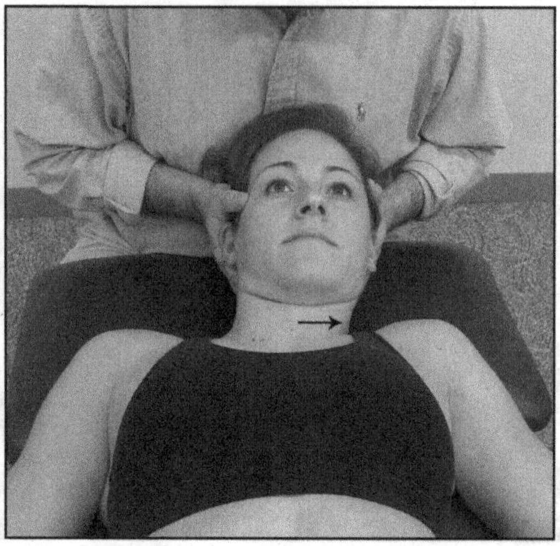

Figure 6-49. Cervical side-gliding to the left passive intervertebral movement tests for C2 to C7.

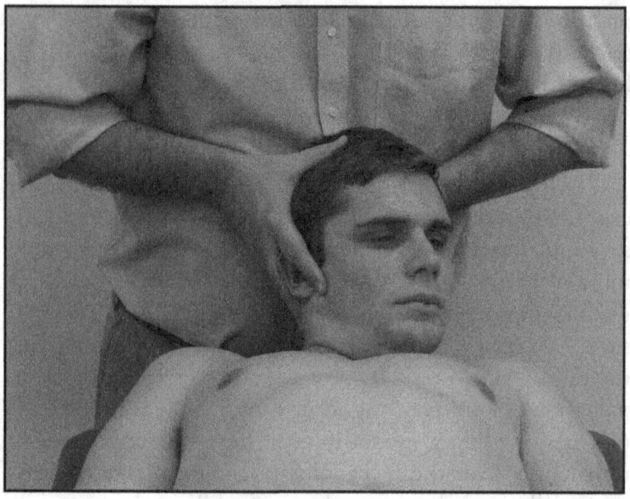

Figure 6-50. Passive mobility tests for atlantoaxial motion segment.

opposite side, the test is considered positive for a mobility deficit at that segment. Lateral translation to each side is also assessed with each segment in extension and flexion in an attempt to further localize the side and direction of mobility deficit.[473] For example, C2 to C3 is placed in extension followed by lateral translation to the left and right. If translation to the left is limited compared to the right, the motion restriction is described as extension, right lateral flexion, and right rotation possibly due to a mobility deficit of closing at the C2 to C3 motion segment on the right. The motion segment is also assessed in flexion. For example, C2 to C3 is placed in flexion followed by lateral translation to the left and right. If translation to the left is limited compared to the right in flexion, the motion restriction is described as flexion, right lateral flexion, and right rotation possibly due to a mobility deficit of opening at the C2 to C3 motion segment on the left. The examiner judges the segment as hypomobile, normal, or hypermobile based on perception of the mobility at each spinal segment relative to those above and below the tested segment and based on the examiner's experience and perception of normal mobility. Additionally, each segment is monitored for reproduction of the patient's pain.

Passive Mobility Test for Atlantoaxial Motion Segment

The primary motion at C1 to C2 is rotation with about half of the total range (45 degrees) to one side occurring at this segment (Figure 6-50). To test AA motion with the patient in supine, the patient's head is cradled by the examiner and flexed passively to end range in an attempt to block rotational motion below C1 to C2. While maintaining end range flexion, the patient's head and neck are rotated first to the uninvolved side and then compared to the involved side. As always, quality, quantity, and symptom response are recorded. A reproduction of the patient's symptoms and/or motion limitation of less than 45 degrees is considered a positive test for a mobility deficit at C1 to C2. This test is also called the flexion-rotation test (FRT) with frequent findings of pain and mobility deficit in patients with CGH.[474-476]

Clinically, the FRT is positive if there is a 10 degree visually estimated loss of mobility on either side and is reliable and valid when compared with goniometry.[477] Excellent intertester and intratester reliability have been reported for immediate retest in asymptomatic subjects and subjects with CGH.[478] In a single-blind comparative group design, Ogince et al[478] tested 23 subjects with CGH, 23 controls, and 12 subjects with migraine with aura. Average ROM for unilateral rotation of the most restricted side for migraine group, asymptomatic, and CGH was 39 degrees (SD 6.9), 39 degrees (SD 6.5), and 20 degrees (SD 11), respectively, demonstrating a significant difference in the CGH group. If the FRT is equal to or less than 32 degrees, the test is positive (Sn 0.91, Sp 0.90).[478] Hall et al[479] reported that the FRT is a reliable tool for measurement of upper cervical ROM in the evaluation of CGH with an MDC of 7 degrees at the 90% confidence interval to be confident a true change in mobility has occurred after intervention.

Passive Mobility Tests for the Occiput-Axis Motion Segment

Several manual procedures have been described to assess mobility at the occiput-axis (OA) motion segment. The primary movements of OA are flexion and extension, which allow for the functional movement of nodding. For flexion, the examiner palpates for opening or increased space between the mastoid process and C1. For extension, the examiner palpates for closing or decreased space between the mastoid process and C1. To perform passive accessory segmental mobility of OA with the patient in supine, the examiner cradles the head and rotates it 30 degrees to the

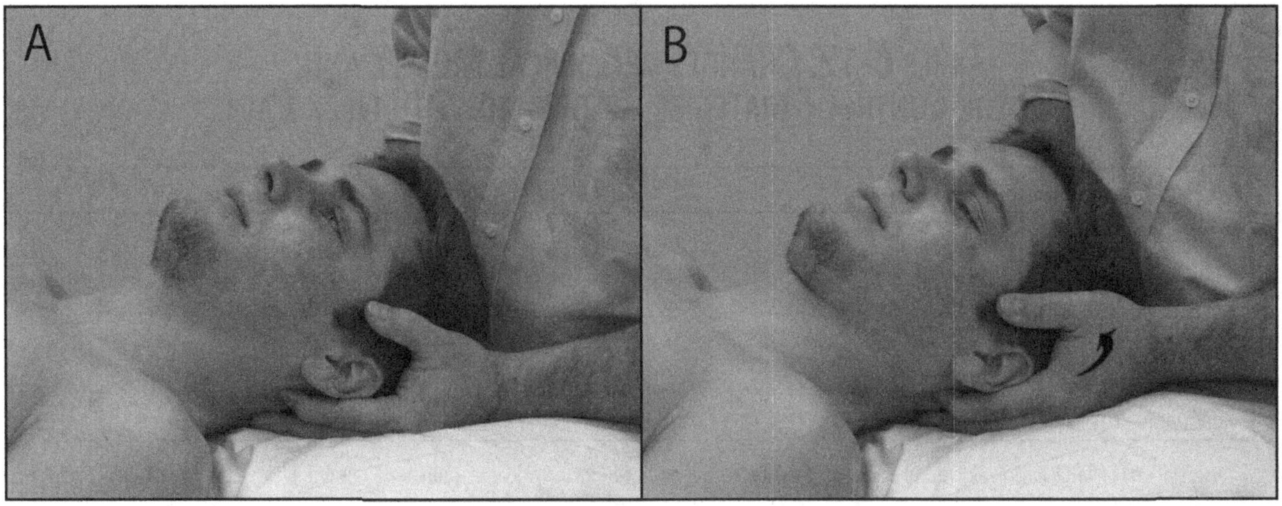

Figure 6-51. Passive physiological mobility tests for occiput-axis motion segment: (A) neutral and (B) flexion.

side to be tested.[473] Anterior glide for extension and posterior glide for flexion of the occiput on C1 are performed assessing the quality, quantity, and symptom response on the uninvolved side and then the involved side. To assess passive physiological motion of flexion and extension at OA (Figure 6-51), the examiner cradles the patient's head and palpates between the mastoid process and the lateral mass of C1.

First Rib Mobility—Caudal or Inferior Glide

Indications for assessing first rib mobility include symptoms in that region, a positive CRLF test, increased tissue tension on palpation of the scalene muscles, an upper chest breathing pattern, cervicobrachial symptoms, or symptoms referred into the upper extremity suggestive of TOS (see Figure 5-23). Inferior glide is assessed in supine or prone. With the patient supine, the examiner places the thumbs or anterolateral aspect of the second MCP on the superior posterior aspect of the first rib and gently oscillates inferiorly to assess quality, quantity, and symptom response. The patient's neck may be placed in slight lateral flexion toward the side to be tested to place the scalenes on slack. An alternate technique for first rib caudal glide is described in Chapter 5.

Muscle Performance

Efficient motor control is necessary for all movement and functional tasks. Efficiency is task-dependent and involves several factors:[114] optimal force generation and timing of muscle activation, minimal extraneous or unnecessary muscle activity, and appropriate muscle relaxation when the task is complete. Current research in patients with neck pain has been related to factors resulting in poor efficiency in motor control. However, more task-specific studies are needed. Altered muscle performance in patients with neck pain is a result of altered neural control and muscle fiber properties thought to contribute to the development or persistence of neck pain.[114]

Panjabi et al[480] estimated that neck muscles provide about 80% of mechanical stability to the cervical spine and the osteoligamentous system contributes about 20%. The superficial flexor and extensor muscles produce greater torque than the deep muscle system and are involved in movement and support of the head.[481] The deep muscle system has segmental attachments, less torque-producing capability, and more muscle spindles to guide and support the cervical motion segments.[482-484] A complex interplay between both systems is necessary for normal function since activation of the superficial system alone results in segmental buckling.[481] Regardless of etiology of neck pain and injury, a muscular imbalance results between systems along with reorganization of motor control strategies.[485]

Changes in muscle properties may be related to injury, pain, disuse, the inflammatory process, and nerve injury.[79,253] In people with chronic neck pain, both widespread atrophy and fatty infiltration of the extensor muscles has been observed more in the deeper (multifidi, rectus capitis major and minor, and longus capitis and colli) than superficial systems,[62,79,486-488] and in WAD with high pain and disability levels,[79] but not in persistent insidious-onset neck pain.[253] In the UT, changes in oxidative metabolism[489,490] and intramuscular microcirculation[490,491] have been observed in patients with neck and arm pain. Altered proportion of fiber types in the cervical flexor and extensor muscles seems to result in loss of muscular endurance due to preferential atrophy of slow-twitch fibers.[492]

Changes in muscle behavior include increased superficial activity of the anterior scalenes (AS) and SCM during upper extremity movements[69] and craniocervical flexion.[64,493] Increased coactivation of the superficial flexors and extensors has been observed during isometric

TABLE 6-12. CHANGES IN CERVICAL MUSCLE AND MOTOR CONTROL STRATEGIES ASSOCIATED WITH NECK PAIN

MUSCLE CHANGES	*ALTERED CONTROL STRATEGIES*
• Muscle atrophy • Muscle fiber/capillary ratio • Fatty infiltration • Muscle fiber type proportions • Muscle fiber contractile properties • Muscle fiber membrane properties	• Reduced deep cervical activity • Increased superficial muscle activity • Delay in feed-forward activation • Reduced resting periods • Lengthened activation after voluntary contraction

Adapted from Falla D, Farina D. Neural and muscular factors associated with motor impairment in neck pain. *Curr Rheumatol Rep.* 2007;9(6):497-502.

activity,[494] experimentally induced neck pain,[495] and in tasks such as typing,[496] possibly resulting in increased loads on the cervical spine. The superficial muscles, AS and SCM[64] and UT,[69,497,498] also take more time to relax after activity. In contrast to the superficial system, deep cervical flexor (ie, longus colli and capitis) activity is less in neck pain patients.[64,69] During rapid arm movements, onset of the deep neck muscles is delayed and direction-specific, which is opposite that of healthy subjects.[69] Alterations in precision[58] and endurance[58,499] have been observed at low and moderate intensities of 20% to 50% of maximum (the amount used in most daily activities). Additionally, disturbed oculomotor control,[116,500] reduced proprioceptive acuity (ie, increased positioning error),[95] and impaired balance have been observed in patients with neck pain.[108,116,369,501] The cause and effect relationship between neck pain and altered motor control presents pain as a cause of altered motor control or altered motor control as a potential cause of pain. Table 6-12 is a list of changes in cervical muscle properties and altered motor control strategies linked to reduced endurance, decreased strength, and altered coordination.

Muscle Performance Assessment

Patients with MNP have a wide range of mobility and muscle performance deficits and often involve impairments and symptoms in the thorax and upper extremity with or without psychological contributors. Each patient has unique strength and endurance needs specific to her occupational and recreational demands. The assessment of muscle performance begins with observation, static and dynamic postural analysis, quality of active movements of neck, thorax, shoulder girdle, upper extremities, and palpation. Procedures related to muscle length, strength and endurance are performed as indicated to provide additional information about cervical muscle function. Tests of muscle strength are not usually performed at the initial evaluation due to the potential to aggravate symptoms or for pain inhibition which alters test results. Few reliable and valid tests are available to assess cervical muscle strength and endurance in patients with neck pain.

Endurance is generally defined as the ability to generate force over a period of time or to sustain forces repeatedly with a higher workload correlated with a shorter endurance time. Endurance or avoidance of fatigue is complex and affected by motivation, muscle fiber type, the type of contraction (ie, concentric, eccentric), intensity, pattern of muscle activation, and speed of the task.[502] Clinical measurements include EMG, perceived exertion, duration of static or dynamic endurance tasks.

Deep Neck Flexor Muscle Endurance Test

The DNF muscle endurance test emphasizes craniocervical flexion. The test has minor variations, but essentially asks the subject to maintain craniocervical flexion in the supine position while holding the back of the head 2.5 cm or 1 inch above the table.[503] This test is also used for diagnostic classification in the impairment-based category for neck pain with movement coordination deficits (see Table 6-3) and neck pain with headache (see Table 6-2).[15]

Test Procedure[504]

With the subject in supine, hook-lying and hands resting on the abdomen, the patient is asked to tuck the chin maximally, hold it, and lift the head and neck about 2.5 cm from the resting position. In this position, the clinician draws an imaginary line across 2 approximated skin folds on the anterior and lateral neck, and then slides the width of the index and middle fingers under the posterior occiput (Figure 6-52). The patient rests the head on the examiner's fingers. The timed portion of the test begins when the subject performs the chin tuck and raises the head to the point

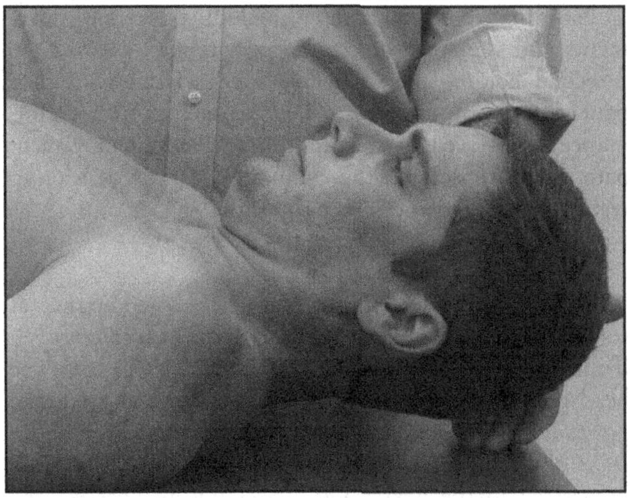

Figure 6-52. Deep neck flexor endurance test.

Table 6-13. Normative Data (Mean + SD in Seconds) for the Deep Neck Flexor Endurance Test

	AGE 20 TO 40 YEARS	AGE 41 TO 60 YEARS	AGE 61 TO 80 YEARS
Women	23.1 ± 12.2	36.2 ± 15.6	28.5 ± 9.8
Men	38.4 ± 26.2	38.1 ± 17.2	40.9 ± 16.0

Data adapted from Domenech MA, Sizer PS, Dedrick GS, McGalliard MK, Brismee JM. The deep neck flexor endurance test: normative data scores in health adults. *PMR.* 2011;3:105-110.

that the back of the head is maintained in contact with the examiner's fingers as a cue for the head test position. The test stops when 1 of 4 movements occur[504]:

1. The edges of the drawn line on the skin folds are no longer approximated due to loss of the chin tuck.
2. The patient rests on the examiner's fingers for more than 1 second.
3. The patient raises the head so that contact is no longer made with the examiner's fingers.
4. The patient is unable to continue.

One deviation from the test position is allowed and corrected. The time is noted for 2 trials and the results averaged with 5 minutes allowed between tests. Normative data for pain free subjects is listed in Table 6-13. Domenech et al[504] reported interrater reliability ICC (2, k), 0.66 (0.34 to 0.86). Variability between subjects was high. Age and activity level did not affect DNF endurance, but men had significantly greater DNF endurance than women.[504] Harris et al[505] demonstrated moderate to good interrater reliability for subjects without neck pain (ICC, 0.82 to 0.91) and moderate (ICC, 0.67 to 0.78) for subjects with neck pain. Mean endurance times are significantly greater in the group without neck pain (38.95 seconds, SD 26.4) than the group with neck pain (24.1 seconds, SD 12.8). In subjects with neck pain, Cleland et al[364] reported an ICC (2,1), 0.57 (0.14 to 0.81), a mean DNF endurance time of 5 ± 4 seconds, SEM (2.3 seconds), and MDC 6.4 seconds.

In an isometric replication of the DNF endurance test (ie, head lift test) and isometric craniocervical flexion using dynamometry at 50% and 20% maximum voluntary contraction,[506] the head lift test required significantly greater activity of the superficial cervical flexor muscles (SCM and AS) than the CCFT, with no differences in the activation of the deep cervical flexors between the 2 tests. The CCFT is considered a more selective test of the DNF.[506]

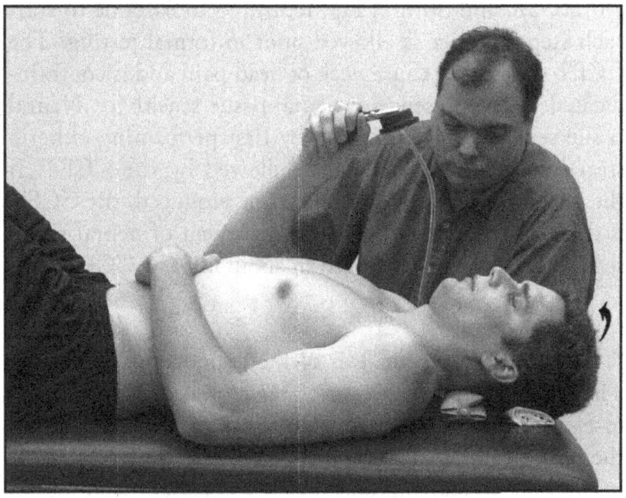

Figure 6-53. Craniocervical flexion test.

Craniocervical Flexion Test

The CCFT (Figure 6-53) indicates impairment in the DNF muscles in patients with neck pain regardless of diagnostic classification or acuity. It fits the ICF category of measurement of impairment of body function, control of simple voluntary movements, and endurance of isolated muscles. The CCFT is able to capture the reduced capacity to maintain isometric craniocervical flexion at 20% to 50% MVIC, an activation level that likely reflects daily activities.[493] The test emphasizes precision and motor control, not strength. Impairments identified using the CCFT become the target of a specific motor control exercise approach that includes training the DNF.[493] Two studies related to WAD and CGH have demonstrated that recovery of impaired neuromuscular control is not automatic even when symptoms resolve.[183,275,507] The CCFT is capable of detecting change related to a DNF training program.[47,183] A specific exercise approach is effective at increasing DNF activation[47] which improves the ability to maintain neck posture during prolonged sitting,[87] but does not restore normal muscle activity during untrained functional upper extremity tasks.[508] The CCFT has 2 stages.

Test Procedure Setup[114,493]

The patient is supine with a line bisecting the neck and the line of the face horizontal to the table. A neutral neck position (without a pillow) is desired, but some patients with excessive cervicothoracic kyphosis may need a towel under the occiput. The uninflated biofeedback pressure unit (Stabilizer, Chattanooga, TN) is placed under the neck and slipped superiorly so that it is next to the occiput and inflated to 20 mm Hg. The pressure should be stabilized. The patient is informed that this is a test of precision and control, not strength, and asked to nod slowly and gently as if to say "yes" and hold the position. The patient should feel the back of the head slide up the table. The nodding action is done in 5 steps from a 20 mm Hg to 22, 24, 26, 28, and 30 mm Hg, returning to baseline to start each step. Practice is allowed prior to formal testing. The CCFT should not cause neck or head pain and is contraindicated in the presence of neural tissue sensitivity. Neural tissue sensitivity is examined by first performing either a straight leg raise or ULNDT followed by the CCFT. If the neck or head pain is increased or produced, the CCFT is delayed and priority given to treatment of neural tissue sensitivity, which is observed in about 10% of CGH.[12,183]

Test Procedure—Stage 1[114,493]

Stage 1 involves analysis of the craniocervical motion. The patient holds the pressure gauge for feedback and nods to elevate the pressure from 20 to 22 mm Hg and holds the position for 2 or 3 seconds before relaxing and returning to neutral starting position. If the patient is an upper chest breather, the nod should be performed during slow exhalation to minimize anterior scalene activity.[509] The same steps are repeated to 30 mm Hg. The clinician analyzes the rotation motion of the head by observation and palpation of the superficial flexors, SCM and AS, which should be negligible until the final 2 test stages. Abnormal movements suggesting poor activation of the DNF include the following[114]:

- The range of head rotation does not increase with progressive steps of the test and becomes more of head retraction than rotation
- The patient lifts the head
- The movement is performed too quickly
- Activity in the superficial flexor or hyoid muscles (ie, jaw clenches or mouth opens) is palpable or visible in the first 3 stages
- The pressure dial does not return to baseline, reading more than 20 mm Hg, suggesting inability to relax the muscles after a contraction or a proprioceptive deficit

Performance is documented, including aberrant movements and the stage of correct performance for a 2- to 3-second hold without palpable superficial activity. The patient does not proceed to stage 2 unless correct performance is observed. If substitution or aberrant movement patterns are observed, these must be corrected prior to testing or training endurance capacity.[114]

Test Procedure—Stage 2[114,493]

Stage 2 involves testing isometric DNF endurance at test stages that the patient is able to perform correctly even if unable to perform all stages. The patient performs the head nod to the first stage of 22 mm Hg and holds the position for 10 seconds. If able to perform at least 3 repetitions of 10-second holds without substitution, the test is progressed to the next stage. The clinician observes the movement for signs of poor endurance. Poor endurance is indicated by: (a) inability to hold the pressure steady, (b) a decrease in pressure, and (c) recruitment of the superficial flexors. The baseline performance is documented as the stage of correct performance pressure and number of 10-second holds without substitution. Training begins at this level. Most asymptomatic individuals can perform at least 20 to 26 and 28 mm Hg.[63,510] Patients with neck pain generally do not reach the first or second stages of the test.[183,510]

Muscle Strength Tests

Since muscle strength is reduced in patients with neck pain, headache, and other cervicobrachial disorders,[59,419,511,526] strength and endurance measures are common in the clinical setting. However, no consensus exists on how best to measure these aspects of muscle performance in patients with neck pain. Debate exists as to the correlations between pain and strength measurements.[514,517] Yet, improvements in neck muscle strength and decreased pain have been reported after training.[80,518,519] When appropriate and safe for the patient to perform, strength measurements may be of clinical value for determining training dosage and documenting treatment effectiveness.

Strength is measured as the maximum force produced during an isometric contraction, the maximum load that can be lifted, or the peak torque during an isokinetic contraction. The isometric contraction is referred to as a maximum voluntary contraction (MVC). Many protocols, manual muscle testing (MMT), hand-held dynamometry (HHD), and isokinetic testing produce a range of strength scores, but no reliable reference values.[520] In the following tests, a general strength output is measured with no differentiation of superficial or deep muscle groups:

- *MMT*: The patient is prone for extension and supine for flexion and rotation strength testing.[521] A grade 3 movement through the test range against gravity is sufficient for most functional activities since the moment developed by the muscles is in excess of the strength required for normal activities.[520] Due to uncertain reliability[419] and low validity, MMT is not recommended for assessment of cervical strength above grade 3. Given the limitations of MMT, a hand-held dynamometer can be used to quantify muscle performance above a grade 3

- *Hand-held dynamometry*: The use of HHD in the cervical spine is limited since the device is unable to measure rotation, reliability, and validity, which are vulnerable to examiner bias.[520] Bohannon[522] reviewed the normative data (obtained using a HHD) in healthy individuals and advised caution when using norms to interpret patient performance. Data were reported only for neck flexion.[523-525] Intrasession and intersession reliability coefficients were >0.85 for all muscles tested using the break test. Using the 5th percentile, the normal lower limit in Newtons for neck flexion with the head raised to 30 degrees with the chin tucked in women is: (a) 20 to 29 years: 82 ± 13; (b) 30 to 39 years: 86 ± 13; (c) 40 to 49 years: 78 ± 14; (d) 50 to 59 years: 72 ± 15; and (e) 60 to 69 years; 66 ± 13. The normal lower limit in Newtons for neck flexion in men is: (a) 20 to 29 years: 144 ± 23; (b) 30 to 39 years: 133 ± 22; (c) 40 to 49 years: 136 ± 21; (d) 50 to 59 years: 118 ± 28; and (e) 60 to 69 years; 114 ± 22.[524] Experimentally, fixed frame dynamometry provides a large range of cervical strength scores.[520] For example, flexion and extension for women and men ranged from 11 to 116 Newton meters and 22 to 139 Newton meters, respectively.[520] Reported values with wide variation limit their clinical use. The results of isometric testing vary with the device used as well as how it is used. When used clinically, reference values must be obtained from the device and methods used[520]
- *Functional lifting tests—the cervical progressive isoinertial lifting evaluation test* (Figure 6-54): The cervical progressive isoinertial lifting evaluation (PILE) test is performed with the patient standing in front of 2 shelves: lower shelf height is 76 cm, or 29.9 inches, and upper shelf height is 137 cm, or 53.9 inches. The patient is asked to lift weights in a plastic box from the lower to upper shelf. For women, the initial weight is 3.6 kg (7.9 lbs) and 5.9 kg (13 lbs) for men. The lift involves a single movement from one level to the next and back again. After every 4 lifts, during approximately 20 seconds, the weight is increased by 2.25 kg (5 lbs) for women, and 4.5 kg (9.9 lbs) for men. The weight lifted during the last single movement is recorded. The test is stopped if the heart rate reaches 85% of the estimated age-adjusted maximum.[526] For the cervical PILE test, intraobserver reliability ICC ranged from 0.88 to 0.96, with an almost perfect interobserver reliability coefficient, ICC = 1.00 (95% CI: 0.99 to 1.0). The intraobserver SEM ranged from 6.10 to 8.28 sec and the interobserver SEM ranged from 0.77 to 1.19 sec (determined over 3 separate sessions).[527] In a group of subjects sick-listed with spinal pain, the cervical PILE test had the highest ability to detect disability in subjects with neck pain.[528] The cervical PILE test is recommended as a measure of muscle endurance during a functional lifting task[528]

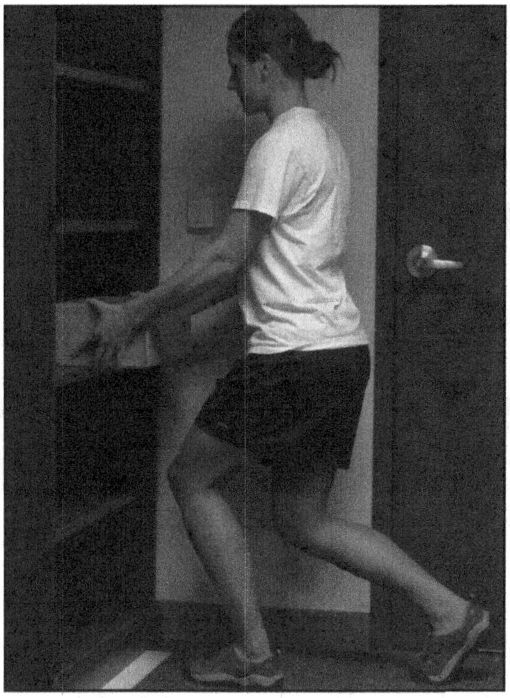

Figure 6-54. Cervical progressive isoinertial lifting evaluation (PILE) test.

In healthy subjects, women are 40% weaker than men, with a significant drop in cervical strength delayed until the seventh decade.[520] Neck extensors can produce higher forces than flexor or lateral flexor muscles. In addition to pain inhibition, a detailed review of factors, such as age, gender, and measurement systems that affect strength testing is recommended.[502]

Muscle Length Tests

Altered muscle length-tension relationships imply that a person has an inadequate balance of mobility and stability during functional movements. A postural and movement analysis of the cervicothoracic spine and scapula may suggest a pattern of muscle imbalance that requires muscle length testing. Muscle length tests are judiciously performed or deferred in patients whose presentation is severe and irritable or when muscle stiffness is related to protecting injured soft tissues or sensitized neural structures. Muscle length testing for the latissimus dorsi (see Figure 4-67) is discussed in Chapter 4 and is relevant to patients presenting with cervicobrachial pain. Altered muscle activity related to neck pain is discussed in the section under

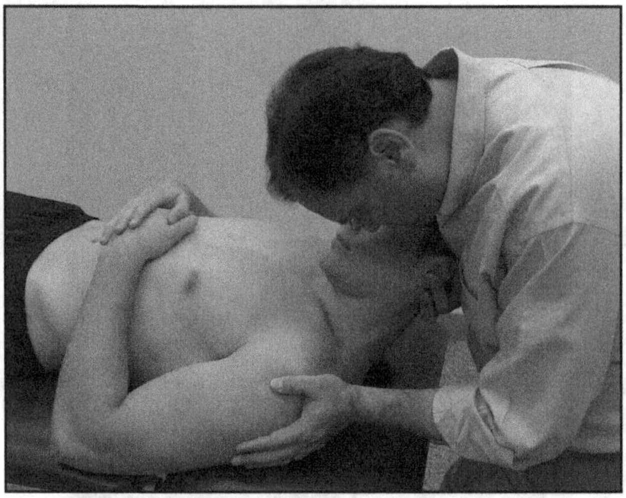

Figure 6-55. Upper trapezius muscle length test.

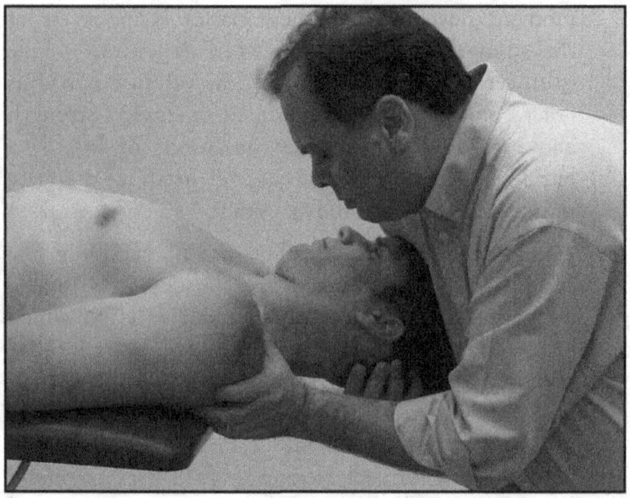

Figure 6-56. Anterior and middle scalenes muscle length test.

Muscle Performance. Patients with MNP and relevant muscle length impairments may benefit from specific interventions targeting these deficits. Muscle length test procedures for the UT, scalenes, levator scapulae, pectoral and SO muscles are as follows:

- *Upper trapezius and sternocleidomastoid*: Based on its attachments and function, a short or stiff UT may result in excessive scapular elevation and inadequate upward rotation along with a weak middle and lower trapezius.[529] Direct compressive effects on the cervical spine due to its attachment to the spinous processes, ligamentum nuchae, and superior nuchal line are also possible. A short UT often results in excessive shoulder girdle elevation before 60 degrees of elevation. Bilaterally, a short UT may limit cervical flexion; unilaterally, a short UT may limit cervical flexion, lateral flexion to the opposite side and rotation to the same side. A short SCM is associated with weak DNF and a forward head posture.
    - Test procedure (Figure 6-55): With the patient in supine, the examiner flexes the patient's head and neck, laterally flexes away from the tested side, and rotates toward the tested side. Maintaining this position, the shoulder girdle is gently depressed through the acromion assessing resistance to motion, end feel, and symptom response. The uninvolved side is tested first and compared to the involved side. The patient should perceive a stretch in the area of the muscle. To facilitate more SCM lengthening, add and maintain a chin nod or upper cervical flexion during the procedure.[473] In 22 patients with MNP, Cleland et al[364] reported kappa values (95% CI), percentage agreement, and prevalence of positive findings for the right UT and left UT as κ = 0.79 (0.52 to 1.0), 90%, 73% and κ = 0.63 (0.31 to 0.96), 82%, 68%. Relevance is based on clinical expertise.
- *Anterior and middle scalenes*: Based on the attachments and function of the scalenes (ie, anterior, posterior, middle), short scalenes may be associated with upper chest breathing patterns, result in an elevated first rib, and limit extension, lateral flexion away, and rotation in varying degrees toward or away. Opinions vary on the degree and direction of rotation to lengthen the scalenes.
    - Test procedure (Figure 6-56): With the patient in supine and head and neck supported off the table, one hand is under the occiput with the shoulder over the patient's forehead. The other hand is placed to stabilize the first and second ribs. The head and neck are retracted or translated posteriorly toward the floor to create extension in the typical cervical spine, keeping the upper cervical spine flexed or in neutral. Maintaining the retracted position, laterally flex away and rotate toward the tested side, assessing resistance to motion, end feel, and symptom response. The uninvolved side is tested first and compared to the involved side. The patient should perceive a stretch in the area of the scalenes or along the SCM.[364,473] Cleland et al[364] reported kappa values (95% CI), percentage agreement, and prevalence of positive findings for the right scalenes and left scalenes as κ = 0.81 (0.57 to 1.0), 90%, 37% and κ = 0.62 (0.29 to 0.96), 81%, 59%. Relevance is based on clinical expertise.
- *Levator scapulae (LS)*: Based on the attachments and function of the levator scapulae, a shortened LS may result in a downwardly rotated and/or elevated scapula and altered scapular movement during elevation. In addition, the vertical orientation of its fibers and attachment to C1 to C4 vertebrae may result in compressive forces on the cervical spine.[114,530] If short bilaterally, the LS may limit cervical flexion;

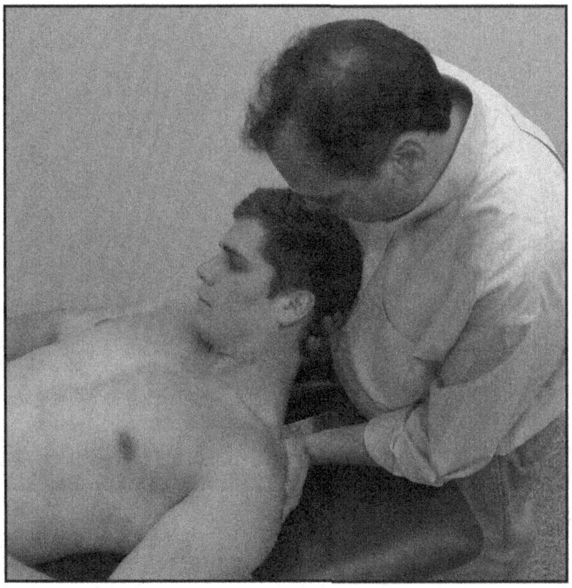

Figure 6-57. Levator scapulae muscle length test.

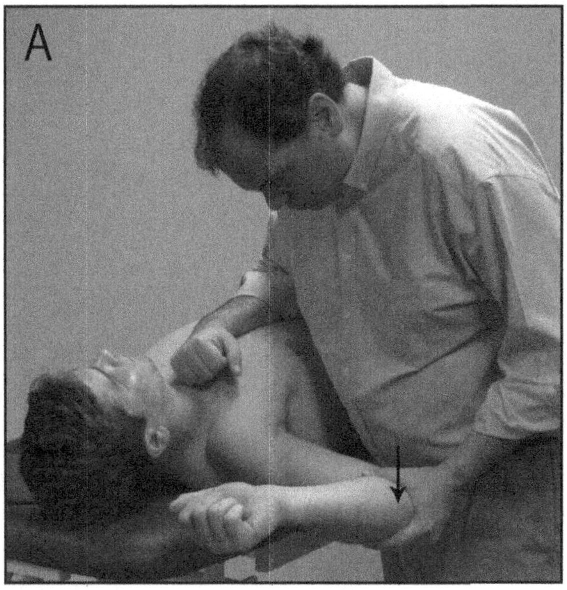

Figure 6-58. Muscle length: (A) pectoralis major midsternal fibers. *(continued)*

unilaterally, a short LS may limit rotation and lateral flexion to the opposite side.

- o Test procedure (Figure 6-57): With the patient in supine, the examiner flexes the patient's head and neck, laterally flexes, and rotates away from the tested side. Maintaining this position, depression and upward rotation is added with the hand at the superior medial angle of the scapula to further lengthen the LS, assessing resistance to motion, end feel, and symptom response. The uninvolved side is tested first and compared to the involved side. The patient should perceive a stretch along the LS. The splenius cervicis and posterior scalenes are most likely also lengthened with the procedure. The test may also be performed in side-lying.[473] Cleland et al[364] reported kappa values (95% CI), percentage agreement, and prevalence of positive findings for the right LS and left LS as κ = 0.61 (0.26 to 0.95), 81%, 32% and κ = 0.54 (0.19 to 0.90), 77%, 45%. Relevance is based on clinical expertise.

- *Pectoralis major (Pec Maj)*: A short pectoralis major muscle may be associated with an internally rotated and adducted humerus that results in an abducted or protracted scapula (often seen with static postural analysis). Biomechanics of the shoulder girdle complex may be altered due to inhibition of antagonist muscles, shoulder external rotators and scapular adductors through reciprocal inhibition.[529]
  - o Test procedure (Figure 6-58A): Page et al[529] described 3 test positions for the different portions of the Pec Maj. With the patient in supine, arm to be tested at the edge of the table, and scapula supported by the table, the examiner stabilizes the sternum with the forearm. Different portions (ie, lower sternal, midsternal, and clavicular) of the Pec Maj are tested by changing the amount of shoulder abduction. Lower sternal fibers are tested by abducting the arm to 150 degrees with slight external rotation. With slight overpressure, the arm should be able to reach the horizontal plane. Inability to reach the horizontal suggests a short Pec Maj and symptoms of stretch or pull in the muscle region should be noted.[529] The midsternal fibers are tested by abducting the arm to 90 degrees with external rotation. Normal length is noted by the arm resting below the horizontal with slight overpressure. The clavicular fibers are tested by placing the arm close to the body and moving into extension. Normal length is observed by the arm resting below the horizontal with slight overpressure.[529] Cleland et al[364] reported kappa values (95% CI), percentage agreement, and prevalence of positive findings for the right Pec Maj and left Pec Maj as κ = 0.90 (0.72 to 1.0), 95%, 41% and κ = 0.50 (0.01 to 1.0), 86%, 23%. Relevance is based on clinical expertise.

- *Pectoralis minor (Pec Minor)*: Because of its attachments to the coracoid process and the superior margins of the third, fourth, and fifth ribs, the Pec Minor muscle tilts the scapula anteriorly and assists in forced inspiration, respectively. Pec Minor tightness contributes to forward shoulder and to an altered scapular position which in turn changes the force couples and muscular balance in the shoulder girdle. Pec Minor shortness may be associated with excessive anterior

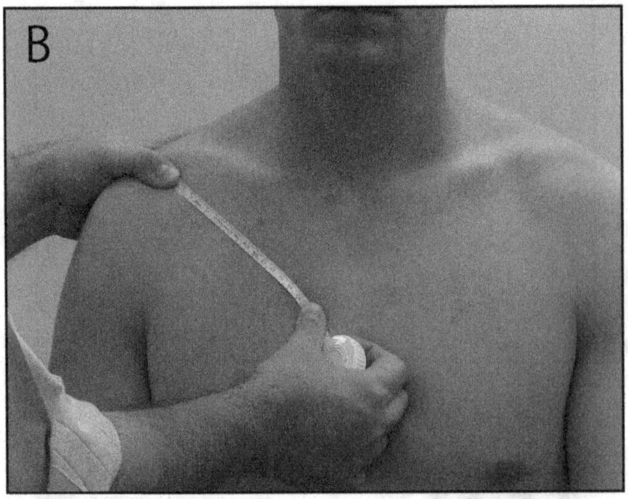

Figure 6-58 (continued). Muscle length: (B) pectoralis minor.

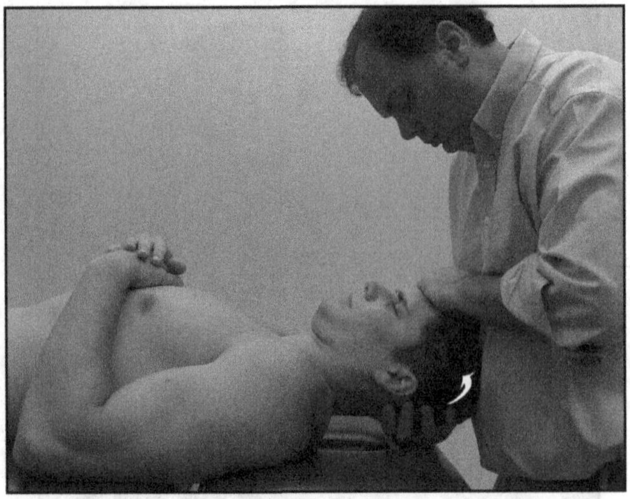

Figure 6-59. SO muscle length test.

tilt and internal rotation of the scapula during arm elevation.

- Test procedure: Pec Minor length is traditionally tested in supine with the patient's arms resting at the sides and elbows flexed. Measurements are taken bilaterally from the posterior aspect of the acromion process to the table top and compared. Normal has been described at 2.6 cm. Comparing normal subjects with symptomatic shoulder subjects, Lewis and Valentine[531] reported excellent reliability (ICC > 0.90) but poor diagnostic accuracy (Sn 100%, Sp 0%). In other words, everyone had a Pec Minor length > 2.6 cm, with a range of 5.9 to 6.5 cm. The findings from this test should be used with caution. Borstad[532] proposed another procedure (Figure 6-58B), validated against direct visualization of the Pec Minor, in fresh donors in a sitting position. The tape measurement is taken in standing from the medial inferior angle of the coracoid process and just lateral to the sternocostal junction of the inferior aspect of the fourth rib, ICC 0.82 to 0.86. The mean for men was 16.8 (0.3) cm and 15.5 (0.3) cm for women. The measurements were normalized to patient height (resting length/height x 100) to develop a pectoralis minor index (PMI). PMI mean = 8.24 (SD = 0.8) cm. A short Pec Minor is defined as less than 7.44 cm (mean PMI ± 1 SD). The author concluded that this procedure may assist with treatment planning and reassessment postintervention.[532]

- *SOs*: Short SO muscles are associated with forward head posture and headache or referred pain to the head. The primary movement of the SO muscles is capital extension and, when short, these muscles limit primarily capital flexion.
  - Test procedure (Figure 6-59): With the patient in supine, the examiner supports the occiput with one hand and provides upper cervical flexion through the forehead with the other hand. Alternatively, with the patient in supine, the examiner supports the occiput with one hand and stabilizes C2 with the other hand, using either a pincer grip on the C2 SP or the anterolateral border of the second metacarpal phalangeal joint or proximal phalanx. The other hand is placed posteriorly on the occiput and the examiner's anterior shoulder is placed on the forehead to lengthen the upper cervical extensors through upper cervical flexion. The SO muscles are biased to one side by rotating the head 30 degrees and adding upper cervical flexion; left rotation lengthens the left SOs.[364] The resistance to motion, end feel, and symptom response are noted. The uninvolved side is tested first and compared to the involved side. The patient should perceive a stretch in the region of the SO muscles. Cleland et al[364] reported kappa values (95% CI), percentage agreement, and prevalence of positive findings for the right and left SOs as κ = 0.63 (0.26 to 1.0), 86%, 23% and κ = 0.58 (0.15 to 1.0), 86%, 18%, respectively. Relevance is based on clinical expertise.

Upper Limb Neurodynamic Tests

Neurodynamics refers to the biomechanical, physiological, and structural functions associated with the nervous system.[533,534] During functional activity, nervous tissue must have the ability to slide, lengthen, and undergo compressive mechanical loads. Inflammation, neural edema, reduced intraneural blood flow, or fibrosis associated with the nerve and/or the tissue it runs through may cause altered neurodynamics.[533,535] Movement in one part of the nervous system causes movement within the system.

For example, during neck flexion the cauda equina moves superiorly.[536,537] The median nerve adapts by lengthening to a 20% increase in the nerve bed length with full elbow and wrist extension.[538] Physiological changes that occur with tension include (a) an 8% or 15% stretch of a peripheral nerve for 30 minutes reduces blood flow by 50% and 80% to 100%, respectively,[539,540] (b) a 6% stretch of a peripheral nerve for 1 hour decreases action potential by 70%,[541] and (c) compression of 20 to 30 mm Hg decreases venous blood flow while intraneural blood flow is blocked with 80 mm Hg of compression.[539,542] Due to the functional loads placed on the nervous system, neural tissue sliding is needed to dissipate tension and distribute forces.[539,542]

Given that the nervous system is subject to various loads during normal movement, a neurodynamic test is designed to challenge its mechanics and/or physiology and produce a response that suggests altered neurodynamics. For example, the ULND 1 (ie, median nerve) test challenges movement of the median nerve relative to its surroundings through the neck and upper extremity. In addition to mechanical responses, changes in intraneural blood flow, axonal transport, action potentials, neural tissue inflammation, or neural tissue sensitivity are possible during the test. The basic concepts related to neurodynamics and contraindications and precautions to testing are discussed in Chapter 3, with research still very limited as to the mechanics and physiology of these procedures. As a reminder, acute nerve root injuries require care and gentle movements, such that ULNDTs may not be indicated. Additionally, patients with central sensitization should be tested cautiously as repeated testing and movements may aggravate the symptoms.[543]

Testing procedures are similar to those described for movement testing. The uninvolved side or least painful side is tested first. Resting symptoms are established prior to starting the series of movements. During each step in the procedure, the clinician notes the quality, range of movement, resistance through the range and at the end of each movement, and the symptom response. The test is considered positive if all or some of the patient's symptoms are reproduced, ROM is limited compared to the uninvolved side, and symptom reproduction occurs with a sensitizing maneuver—movement of a body segment away from the site of symptoms.[543] If symptoms are produced, most likely the patient will be unable to complete all of the test components. A sensitizing maneuver is necessary to assist in structurally differentiating between a somatic and neural source of symptoms. A positive test does not indicate the site of injury, but does suggest increased neural tissue sensitivity.[543]

Nee et al[544] reviewed the validity, plausibility, reliability and definition of the ULNDTs for detecting peripheral neuropathic pain. The plausibility of ULNDTs is supported by biomechanical and experimental pain data. The clinically reliable definition of a positive ULNDT indicates that the patient's symptoms should at least be partially reproduced and structural differentiation should alter these symptoms.[544] Limited evidence suggests that the median nerve test, but not the radial nerve test, helps determine whether a patient has CR, but the median nerve test does not help diagnose carpal tunnel syndrome. The authors report that a cautious interpretation of this data is needed because diagnostic accuracy may be distorted because of variable definitions of a positive ULNDT.[544] Patients with peripheral neuropathic pain who present with increased nerve mechanosensitivity and no conduction loss may be incorrectly classified by electrophysiological testing standards as not having peripheral neuropathic pain. Concurrent validity of the ulnar nerve test is based on a single case study on cubital tunnel syndrome. More research is needed to improve the validity of ULNDTs for prognostic and treatment purposes.[544]

Test Procedures: Four ULNDT[535] involve movements of the neck and upper extremity that are biased to the peripheral nerves of the upper extremity (ie, median, radial, and ulnar). The 4 tests are ULNDT 1 (median nerve), ULNDT 2a (median nerve), ULNDT 2b (radial nerve), and ULNDT 3 (ulnar nerve). The decision to perform a ULNDT is based upon information from the history, tests and measures, a working hypothesis of neurogenic pain in the upper extremity, and aggravating or easing factors that mimic components of the ULNDT. For example, a patient may report and actively demonstrate that reaching the hand behind the back toward the back pocket produces elbow pain, leading the clinician to assess ULNDT (radial nerve) since the movement patterns are similar.

ULNDT 1 (Median Nerve[535]; see Figure 6-46): The patient is supine toward the side of the table with arms by the sides. The examiner faces the patient's head with the near hand pressing into the table, stabilizing—not depressing—the superior aspect of the patient's shoulder and the other hand holds the patient's hand in neutral with the elbow flexed to 90 degrees and supported on the examiner's thigh. The following movements are added sequentially and with care, assessing the response to each component:

- Glenohumeral abduction up to 90 to 110 degrees, if available
- Wrist/finger extension and forearm supination
- Glenohumeral external rotation
- Elbow extension[535]

With the addition of each component, symptoms, ROM, and resistance to motion are assessed and compared to the uninvolved side. With the onset of patient's symptoms or new symptoms, structural differentiation is necessary. If the patient's symptoms of elbow pain are reproduced, contralateral cervical lateral flexion (ie, movement of a body segment away from the site of symptoms) is slowly added (actively or passively). Any change in the elbow pain (usually an increase in symptoms) is a positive differentiation. A decrease in symptoms with ipsilateral cervical lateral flexion is also a positive differentiation, suggesting altered neurodynamics. In 400 asymptomatic individuals, the following responses[545] were observed during the ULNDT 1:

- Deep stretch or ache in the cubital fossa traveling to the anterior radial forearm and radial side of the hand (80%)
- Tingling sensation in the thumb and first 3 fingers (77%)
- Stretch in the anterior shoulder (10%)
- Contralateral cervical lateral flexion increases symptoms (90%)
- Ipsilateral cervical lateral flexion decreases symptoms (70%)[545]

A wide range of normal values related to ROM and symptom response support the clinical practice of not solely evaluating ULNDTs by comparing findings to normative values.[546]

Diagnostic Accuracy: As previously discussed under Screening for CR, Wainner et al[245] examined the reliability of 12 test items, including ULNDT 1 and ULNDT 2b, in patients referred for CR or carpal tunnel syndrome. Interexaminer reliability for ULNDT 1 (median nerve) and ULNDT 2b (radial nerve) were κ = 0.76 (0.51, 1.0) and κ = 0.83 (0.65, 1.0). A test item cluster of 4 variables was identified that includes ULNDT 1, cervical rotation < 60 degrees to the involved side, distraction test, and Spurling test A. For ruling out CR, ULNDT A is the most useful (Sn 0.97 [0.90, 1.0], Sp 0.22 [0.12, 0.33], +LR 1.3 [1.1, 1.5], and -LR 0.12 [0.01, 1.9]). If 3 items are positive, then the positive likelihood ratio is 6.1 (95% CI: 2.0 to 18.6), specificity was 0.94 (95% CI: 0.88 to 1.0) and the probability of CR increases to 65%. If all 4 items are present, the probability of CR increases to 90% with a +LR 30.3 (95% CI: 1.7 to 538.2).[245] The test item cluster produced larger posttest probability changes for the diagnosis for CR than any single examination item. Due to wide 95% confidence intervals for all individual items and the test item cluster, validation is required.[245]

Another study investigated use of the ULNDT 1 in a cohort of patients with neck pain, with or without upper extremity symptoms. Raney et al[547] identified a preliminary CPR that includes ULND 1 to identify patients who might benefit from cervical traction and exercise. The following variables were identified:

- Peripheralization with lower cervical spine (C4-7) PAIVM mobility testing
- Positive shoulder abduction test
- Age > 55
- Positive ULND 1 (median nerve)
- Positive neck distraction test[547]

The presence of at least 3 out of 5 predictors results in a +LR = 4.81 (95% CI: 2.17 to 11.4) and a 79.2% likelihood of success with cervical traction. For at least 4 out of 5 variables, the +LR is equal to 23.1 (2.5 to 227.9) resulting in a posttest probability of success with cervical traction to 94.8%. The CPR may aid the clinicians in identifying patients with neck pain likely to benefit from cervical traction and exercise.[547]

Several studies investigated the diagnostic accuracy of the ULNDT 1 for carpal tunnel syndrome, demonstrating inconsistent results. In a group of 21 subjects with carpal tunnel syndrome (using the results of a nerve conduction study as a reference standard), ULNDT 1 (median nerve) demonstrated Sn (0.82), Sp (0.75), +LR (3.29), and -LR (0.24) and positive prognostic value (PPV = 93%),[548] suggesting a high degree of accuracy on the ability of the ULNDT 1 to detect the presence or absence of nerve conduction delay. In contrast, Wainner et al[245] reported Sn (0.75), Sp (0.13), +LR (0.86) and -LR (1.9) of the ULNDT 1, using a reference standard of clinical findings and abnormal electrophysiologic tests. Vanti et al[549] concluded the diagnostic accuracy of ULNDT1 is not satisfactory for the diagnosis of CTS, based on a positive test defined as the presence of symptoms only in the thumb or lateral 2 fingers, +LR 1.96 (95% CI: 1.28 to 3.01), and -LR 0.75 (95% CI: 0.49 to 1.16). The inconsistent results are likely due to variations in the performance and interpretation of the ULNDT.

ULNDT 2a (Median Nerve[535]; Figure 6-60): The patient is supine, lying in a diagonal with the shoulder just off the edge of the treatment table. The clinician stands at the head of the patient, facing the feet with the thigh in contact with the shoulder and arm in about 10 degrees abduction. One hand supports the elbow in 90 degrees flexion; the other hand maintains the wrist and hand in neutral. The following movements are added sequentially and with care, assessing the response to each component:

- Shoulder girdle depression using the thigh
- Elbow extension
- Whole arm external rotation
- Wrist/finger extension
- Glenohumeral abduction up to 40 degrees, as needed[535]

When symptoms are provoked distally, sensitization or structural differentiation is performed by adding contralateral cervical lateral flexion and ipsilateral cervical lateral flexion. An increase and decrease in symptoms suggests altered neurodynamics. If a median nerve assessment is indicated, the benefits of the ULNDT 2a versus ULNDT 1 are the ability to use shoulder girdle depression as a sensitizing maneuver and in those patients where abduction of the glenohumeral joint is not appropriate or painful.

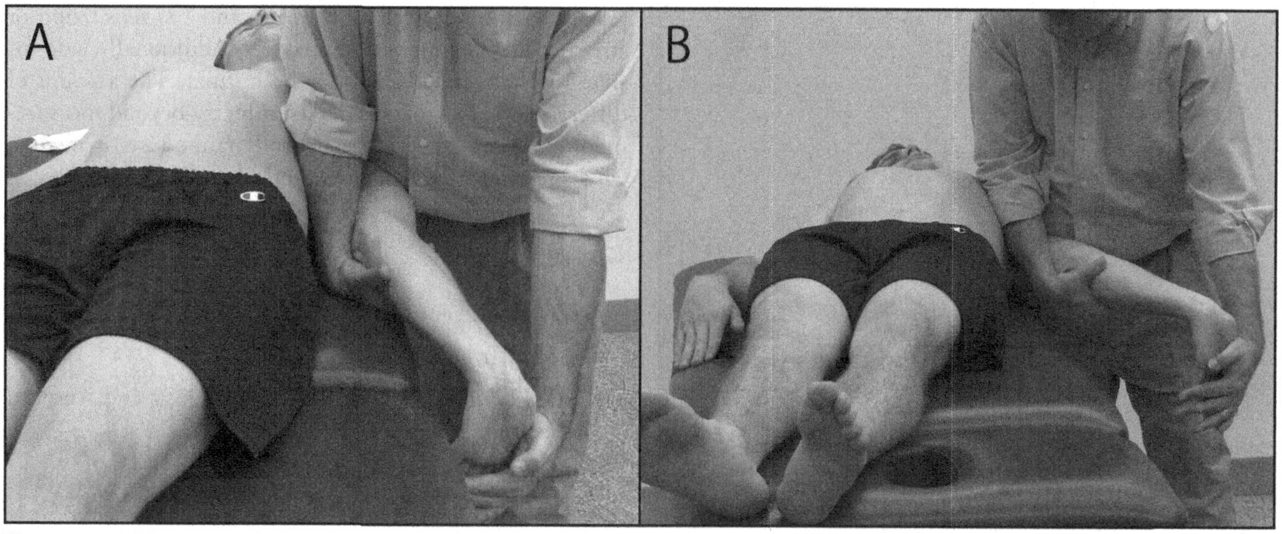

Figure 6-60. Upper limb neurodynamic test 2a (median nerve).

ULNDT 2b (Radial Nerve[535]; Figure 6-61): The position for the ULNDT 2b is with the patient supine, lying in a diagonal with the shoulder just off the edge of the treatment table. The clinician stands at the head of the patient, facing the feet with the thigh in contact with the shoulder and arm in about 10 degrees abduction. One hand supports the elbow in 90 degrees flexion; the other hand maintains the wrist and hand in neutral. The following movements are added sequentially and with care, assessing the response to each component:

- Shoulder girdle depression using the thigh
- Elbow extension
- Whole arm internal rotation
- Wrist/finger flexion with thumb flexion and slight ulnar deviation of the wrist as needed
- Glenohumeral abduction up to 40 degrees, as needed[535]

When symptoms are provoked distally, sensitization or structural differentiation is performed by adding contralateral cervical lateral flexion and ipsilateral cervical lateral flexion. An increase and decrease in symptoms, respectively, suggests altered neurodynamics.

Diagnostic Accuracy: The responses to the ULNDT 2b in 50 asymptomatic subjects ages 18 to 30 years include:

- A strong painful stretch over the radial, proximal forearm (84%)
- A painful stretch in the lateral aspect of the arm (32%), biceps brachii (14%), or dorsal aspect of the hand (12%)[550]

The ULNDT 2b may play a role in differentiating symptoms for patients with neck pain and upper extremity symptoms, specifically lateral elbow pain. Using the ULNDT 2b, responses were recorded in 20 subjects with unilateral symptoms of tennis elbow.[551] The examination findings reveal local muscle and joint signs, in addition to comparable joint signs associated with the cervical spine and first rib. Results reveal that neural tissue in the symptomatic upper extremity was less extensible, indicated by less glenohumeral abduction, average 12.5 degrees, and reproduced the subject's tennis elbow symptoms in 55% (11/20) of the cases. The symptoms were increased by adding contralateral cervical lateral flexion. These results support a preliminary role of altered neurodynamics in some cases of tennis elbow[551] and may be useful in the examination of patients with neck pain and lateral elbow pain.

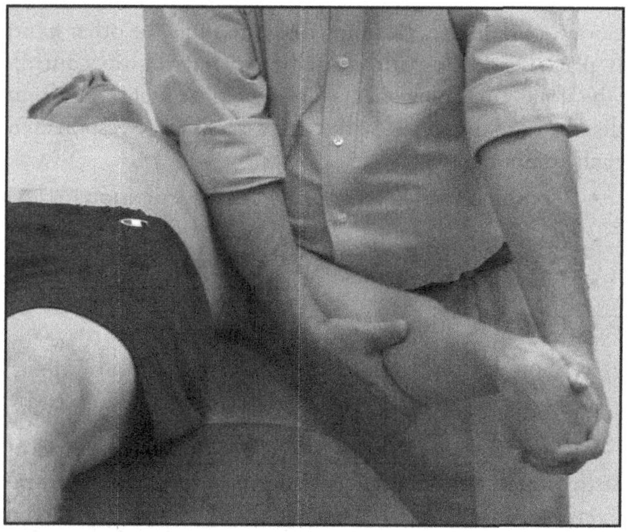

Figure 6-61. Upper limb neurodynamic test 2b (radial nerve).

ULNDT 3 (Ulnar Nerve[539]; Figure 6-62): The patient is supine toward the side of the table with arms by the sides. The examiner faces the patient's head, keeping the patient's arm at the side as much as possible and supporting the

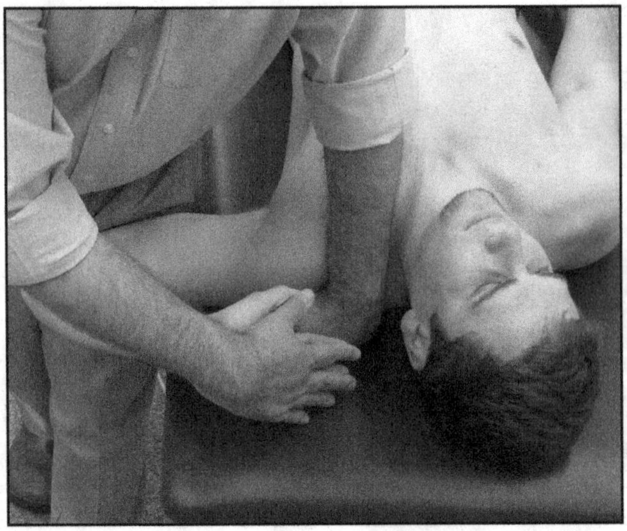
Figure 6-62. Upper limb neurodynamic test 3 (ulnar nerve).

elbow at 90 degrees flexion with one hand. The other hand is placed palm-to-palm with finger and thumb control. The following movements are added sequentially from distal to proximal and with care, assessing the response to each component:

- Combined wrist, finger, and thumb extension
- Pronation
- Elbow flexion
- Lateral rotation
- Shoulder girdle depression
- Abduction[535]

When symptoms are provoked distally, sensitization or structural differentiation is performed by adding contralateral cervical lateral flexion and ipsilateral cervical lateral flexion.

Diagnostic Accuracy: In asymptomatic subjects, symptoms were reported in the hypothenar eminence and medial 2 fingers by 82% of subjects, with 64% reporting pins and needle sensations in the same area.[535,552] Garmer et al[553] also described the symptom responses in 55 asymptomatic volunteers. The test was initiated with scapular depression and then sequenced distal to proximal. Ninety-nine percent reported sensations in the ulnar nerve tract or sensory distribution, with 75% reporting specifically in the ulnar distribution of the hand. Onset of sensation occurred between 18 degrees and 37 degrees of shoulder abduction in 80% of subjects. Most commonly reported sensations are stretch (69%), burning (56%), tingling (39%), and numbness (26%).[553]

While more research is needed in the area of neurodynamic testing, preliminary evidence supports its continued use. Clinicians must be aware of normal responses in asymptomatic subjects. Both symptomatic and asymptomatic individuals may have a variety of sensory responses related to the series of movements and the sensitizing or structural differentiation procedures. Additionally, side-to-side differences in ROM may be normal. The amount of difference needed to consider asymmetry beyond measurement error for each of the neurodynamic tests is median 27 degrees, radial 20 degrees, and ulnar 21 degrees.[554]

Examination Procedures in Prone

- PAIVMs: central and unilateral PA
- Scapular holding test
- MMT: middle and lower trapezius, and cervical flexor and extensors
- Cervical extensor control
- Closed-chain scapular stability test

Passive Segmental Mobility Tests

Prior to performing passive mobility tests, the patient is positioned comfortably in prone so that the cervical spine is in mid-flexion and extension (for each patient with no lateral flexion or rotation). If possible, the patient has the forehead resting on both palms. Alternatively, the patient may be resting in the face hole of the treatment table with their arms at their sides. The head of the table may be flexed to accommodate a forward head posture, or pillows may be placed under the thorax. Temperature and sweating are assessed along with soft tissue mobility over the posterior neck, posterior shoulder girdle, and thorax. Soft tissue is palpated from the superior nuchal line on the occiput moving toward the atlas, comparing soft tissue bilaterally at the base of the occiput for local areas of thickness or tenderness between the occiput and C2. Palpation continues from C2 to T4, as needed, just lateral to the spinous process and over the articular pillars. The spinous processes are located starting at C2 through T4.

Test Procedures[472]

PAIVMs, central PA, and unilateral PA PAIVMs on each side are performed from C2 through T4, as needed. PAIVMs assess both pain provocation and mobility of the cervical segments to identify the relevant symptomatic and/or dysfunctional (ie, hypomobile or hypermobile) segments. A detailed PAIVM procedure and diagnostic utility are described in Chapter 3. A review examining the methodological quality of reliability studies of manual tests for cervical dysfunction concludes that the ability to detect segmental cervical dysfunction based on manual assessment alone is questionable.[555] Inconsistency in reliability, sensitivity, and specificity of manual examination may be a reflection of poor methodology.[556] Most manual physical therapists, however, accept the face validity of manual segmental motion testing when used in combination with the results of other examination procedures. Despite some disagreement and a need for more research, a growing body of evidence supports the use of passive segmental motion tests in clinical decision making for diagnosis and intervention for spinal pain. Cervical and thoracic segmental mobility tests fit the ICF category, measurement of impairment of body function, and mobility of single joints.[15]

Central Posterior-to-Anterior PAIVM (see Figure 6-40): Using pressure through the thumb pads against the spinous process (SP) of the cervical and upper thoracic regions, each segment is gently moved in a PA direction. The elbows are straight, allowing the clinician's sternum to be directly over the SP. Assessment is performed superficial to deep in a progressive oscillatory manner to assess symptom response and quality of movement through range and at end range. The clinician does not push on the spine, but instead leans forward, translating the weight of the trunk through the arms to the spine.

Lee et al[557] examined intervertebral movements of the cervical spine produced by central PA PAIVM in an open interventional magnetic resonance imaging scanner. The responses to central PA mobilization to the fifth cervical vertebra in prone are (a) generally extension produced in the upper motion segments and flexion in the lower segments, (b) middle segments showed inconsistent rotational direction, (c) repeated PA load cycles increased the cervical lordosis, and (d) forces applied to one SP moved the target vertebra and the entire cervical spine. The authors conclude that central PA mobilization should be viewed as a 3-point bending of the cervical spine rather than simple gliding of one vertebra on the other.[557]

Unilateral Posterior-to-Anterior PAIVM (see Figure 6-41): In the same position as described for central PA PAIVM, the clinician uses both thumbs to produce the passive accessory movement in a PA direction over the articular pillar at each level. The thumbs are placed in the area of the zygapophyseal joints, 1.3 to 2.5 cm (0.5 to 1.0 inches) lateral to the SP beginning on the uninvolved side, making side-to-side and level above and below comparisons. Inclination of the CPA or UPA may be varied medially, laterally, superiorly or inferiorly.

Upper Cervical PAIVM: The soft tissue should be palpated closely from the occiput to C2 spinous process and from midline along the atlas to the tip of the transverse process. A PA pressure is gently applied centrally in the region of the posterior arch of the atlas under the occiput and unilaterally along the posterior arch toward the lateral mass of C1. Comparison is made bilaterally. The pressure can be angled in various directions toward the eye. Central and unilateral PA PAIVM tests are applied to the C2 to C3 motion segment. With pain provoked unilaterally on the right articular pillar of C2, the symptoms can be from either the C2 to C3 segment or the C1 to C2 segment or both. To differentiate, the test is repeated with the head rotated about 30 to 40 degrees to the right, effectively increasing motion at C1 to C2. If the pain response is greater with the head rotated to the right, the C1 to C2 joint is implicated. If the pain response is greater with the head in neutral, the C2 to C3 joint is implicated.[572] Diagnostic utility of this differentiation procedure is unknown. Interrater reliability of PAIVM and PPIVM manual examination unilaterally above C4 was determined in 80 subjects (60 with CGH and 20 asymptomatic individuals).[558] After adjustments, the prevalence-adjusted and bias-adjusted kappa coefficients were 0.70 for all segments (occiput to C1, C1 to C2, and C2 to C3). No subjects had a dominant symptomatic C3 to C4 segment.[558]

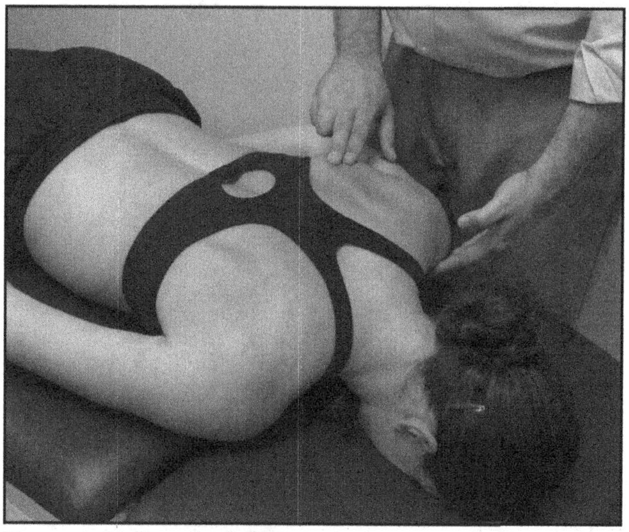

Figure 6-63. Scapular holding test.

Scapular Holding Test[115] (Figure 6-63): The scapular holding test is performed in prone with the arms at the sides. The examiner passively positions the scapula in a neutral position for 10 seconds, repeated up to 5 times.[114] The test position (Figure 6-63) is the mid position between the available range for upward and downward rotation, external and internal rotation, and anterior and posterior tilting.[559] The muscle activity pattern and ability to hold the scapular position are observed for appropriate activation of the trapezius muscle. Common substitutions include (a) scapular depression using the latissimus dorsi, (b) scapular elevation and downward rotation using the rhomboids or levator scapula, and (c) attempts to use external rotation by lifting the elbow using the infraspinatus/teres minor.[114] The scapular holding test is also described as scapula setting or the scapular orientation exercise,[559-560] useful for assessment of scapular dyskinesis, and is taught in a variety of positions.

The muscular activation pattern needed to perform the scapular holding test and elevate the arm has not been widely investigated, and patients find this exercise difficult to perform.[559] In normal subjects (n = 13) relative to the amount of activity used to elevate the arm, all parts of the trapezius were active in maintaining the neutral scapular position, while the latissimus dorsi was not; the serratus anterior was not measured. The authors suggest that

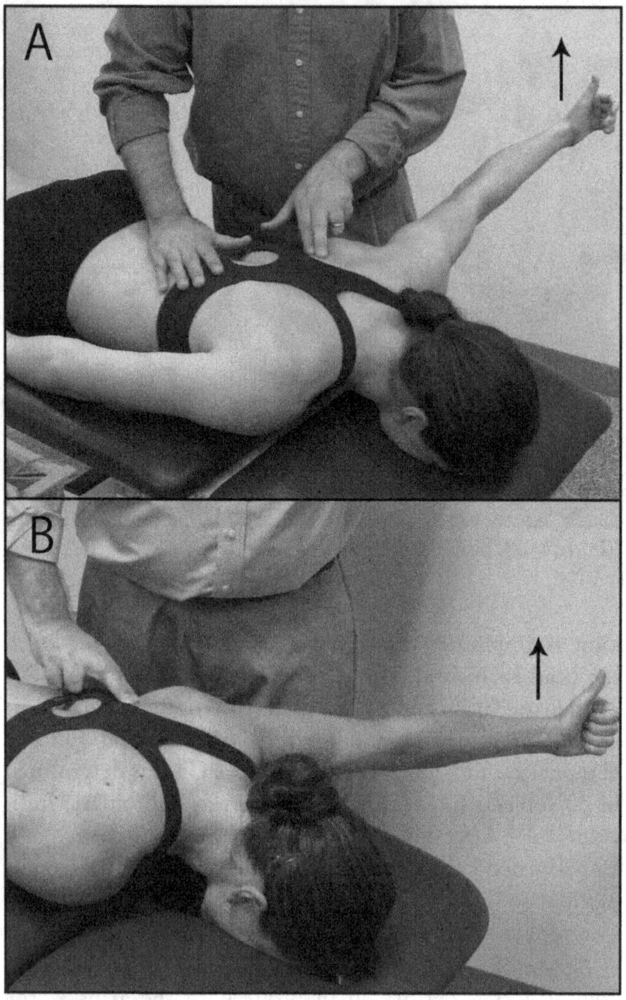

Figure 6-64. Trapezius strength test: (A) middle and (B) lower.

retraining of these muscles may be appropriate in subjects unable to maintain a scapular neutral position. Normal subjects are to reproduce the neutral scapula position after 5 minutes of training.[559]

Additional study of the scapular holding test suggests a beneficial training effect used as a scapular corrective exercise. Wegner et al[561] examined the surface electromyography of the 3 portions of the trapezius in healthy controls (n = 20) compared to a neck pain group with poor scapular posture (n = 18) during a functional typing task. During the typing task, the neck pain group had more activity in the middle trapezius (P = .02) and less activity in the lower trapezius (P = .03) than the control group. A scapular postural correction exercise of holding in a neutral scapular posture was used to correct the poor scapular posture in the neck pain group. After correcting the scapula position, both groups demonstrated similar activity in the middle and lower trapezius. A scapular postural correction exercise may alter the activity in the trapezius to similar levels observed in healthy individuals.[561]

Trapezius Strength Tests: Testing the strength of the middle and lower trapezii is indicated for many reasons. Specifically, if the upper crossed syndrome is present and in the presence of scapular dyskinesia or poor scapular stabilization with upper extremity activity, the middle and lower trapezii are often found to be weak or inhibited. The manual muscle test position is prone with the patient's arm externally rotated and abducted to 90 or 130 degrees (Figure 6-64) for the middle trapezius and lower trapezius, respectively.[562] The scapula should be in a position of upward rotation, external rotation, and posterior tilt without excessive shoulder girdle elevation. The examiner provides stabilization over the opposite scapular region to prevent trunk rotation and applies a downward resistance toward the floor at the distal forearm or distal arm above the elbow. Weakness is identified when the patient is no longer able to hold the scapular position in the test position against the thoracic wall. In 22 subjects with MNP, interrater reliability ranged from no agreement to moderate agreement when dichotomized to normal or reduced when compared with the uninvolved side.[364]

Cervical Extensor Muscle Control: Cervical extension is tested in quadruped or in the prone-on-elbows position, as described by Jull et al.[114] The SO extensors are tested first, with the mid and lower cervical spine in neutral. The patient is asked to perform craniocervical flexion and extension or the nodding "yes" motion with axis through the ear and upper cervical rotation at C1 to C2. The examiner may stabilize C2 to provide feedback for the patient. The test should be performed in a smooth, coordinated manner, maintaining control of the mid and lower cervical spine in neutral.[114]

The second test is thought to bias the deep cervical extensors over the superficial extensors.[115] Cervical extension is performed while maintaining the upper cervical spine in neutral with the axis of motion through the C7 vertebra. The patient is instructed to curl the neck into flexion and back to neutral and then curl the neck into extension, testing eccentric and then concentric control. Maintaining the upper cervical spine in neutral minimizes the action of the superficial extensors. Impaired extensor control—moving from flexion to neutral—occurs with loss of upper cervical neutral. Moving from neutral to extension should occur with minimal upper cervical extension. Impaired extensor control is indicated by excessive upper cervical extension or inability to move toward full extension. If the test provokes pain, the patient should initially perform it in the pain free-range, moving from flexion to neutral.[114]

Closed-Chain Scapular Stability Test[114]: The closed-chain stability test (Figure 6-65) is performed in quadruped as a test of the axioscapular muscles, primarily the serratus anterior.[114] Patients are asked to assume neutral spine posture in quadruped. The first step is to allow the thorax to sink between the scapula and then actively return to a neutral spine position by pushing through the arms to bring the thorax back to a position where the scapulae are flush with the posterior thoracic wall, and hold the position. The patient is then asked to complete the motion to end range of scapular protraction. Winging of the medial scapular border or inability to protract through the full range suggests weakness or poor control.[114] A similar test can be performed in upright with the patient supporting the body in a plank position leaning against a wall. Alternatively, a manual muscle test may be used to assess the strength of the serratus anterior.

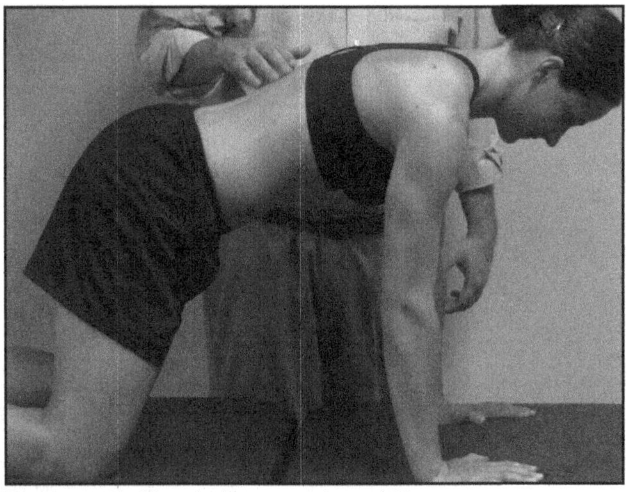

Figure 6-65. Closed-chain scapular stability test.

Imaging Guidelines

At this point in the examination, the clinician may consider whether to recommend diagnostic imaging and/or refer to a medical colleague or subspecialist. The index of suspicion for recommending diagnostic imaging should be high enough that it is likely to change the intervention or alter the treatment threshold. Clinical decision making to use diagnostic imaging requires careful consideration of the history, physical examination, and, if initiated, the response to intervention. Cervical spine imaging for traumatic neck pain, indicated by Canadian C-spine rule[140] or NEXUS[341] clinical criteria, is discussed under Diagnostic Triage and Screening for Red Flags. The American College of Radiology (ACR) has also established appropriateness criteria to assist providers in making the most appropriate imaging decisions.[563] ACR evidence-based guidelines that apply to patients with chronic neck pain regardless of etiology are recommended for review.[563]

Concluding the Physical Examination

At the conclusion of the physical examination, the clinician briefly reflects on whether the goals of the examination have been met. Did the physical examination:

- Reproduce the patient's symptoms in patterns consistent with the information obtained in the patient interview?
- Result in a determination of the impact of posture, movement, work, recreational and psychosocial factors as causes of, contributors to, or perpetuators of the patient's problem?
- Establish the treatment threshold for a diagnostic classification?
- Establish an accurate baseline of outcome measures from which to evaluate and progress treatment?

Review of examination findings should provide data that refines, supports, or negates competing hypotheses to the point where the examination ends and treatment begins. Key history and exam findings are used to place the patient into a diagnostic classification or impairment-based category of MNP with or without upper extremity related symptoms that initially guides PT intervention. An algorithm of the clinical decision-making process is in Figure 6-66.

Diagnostic Classification and Matched Intervention

At this point in the evaluation, the clinician designates a baseline diagnostic classification and decides to proceed with PT intervention. With little evidence to support classification based on a pathoanatomical source, current evidence suggests use of a diagnostic classification system that identifies subgroups of patients who are most likely to respond to specific interventions with the potential to maximize outcomes.

Several classification systems[1,31,434,575] for patients with neck pain have been described with little information available related to validity. Childs et al[434] proposed a treatment-based classification system of patients with neck pain related to cervical and/or upper thoracic dysfunction. This system uses data from the history and physical examination to place patients into treatment subgroups labeled to match the goal of treatment: mobility, centralization, exercise and conditioning, pain control, and reduce headache.[434] In a prospective observational study of 274 patients, ages 44.4 + 16 years (with 74% women), Fritz and Brennan[25] reported that patients with neck pain receiving interventions matched to the appropriate subgroup had better outcomes (ie, pain and disability) than those receiving unmatched interventions. Interrater reliability for classification is high. The most common classification is centralization (34.7%) followed by exercise and conditioning (32.8%) and mobility (17.5%).[25]

Neck pain clinical practice guidelines[15] linked to the ICF by incorporating ICF impairments of body function terminology recommend the following subgroup classifications: (a) neck pain with mobility deficits (see Table 6-1), (b) neck pain with headaches (see Table 6-2), (c) neck pain with movement coordination impairment (see Table 6-3), and (d) neck pain with radiating pain (see Table 6-4).

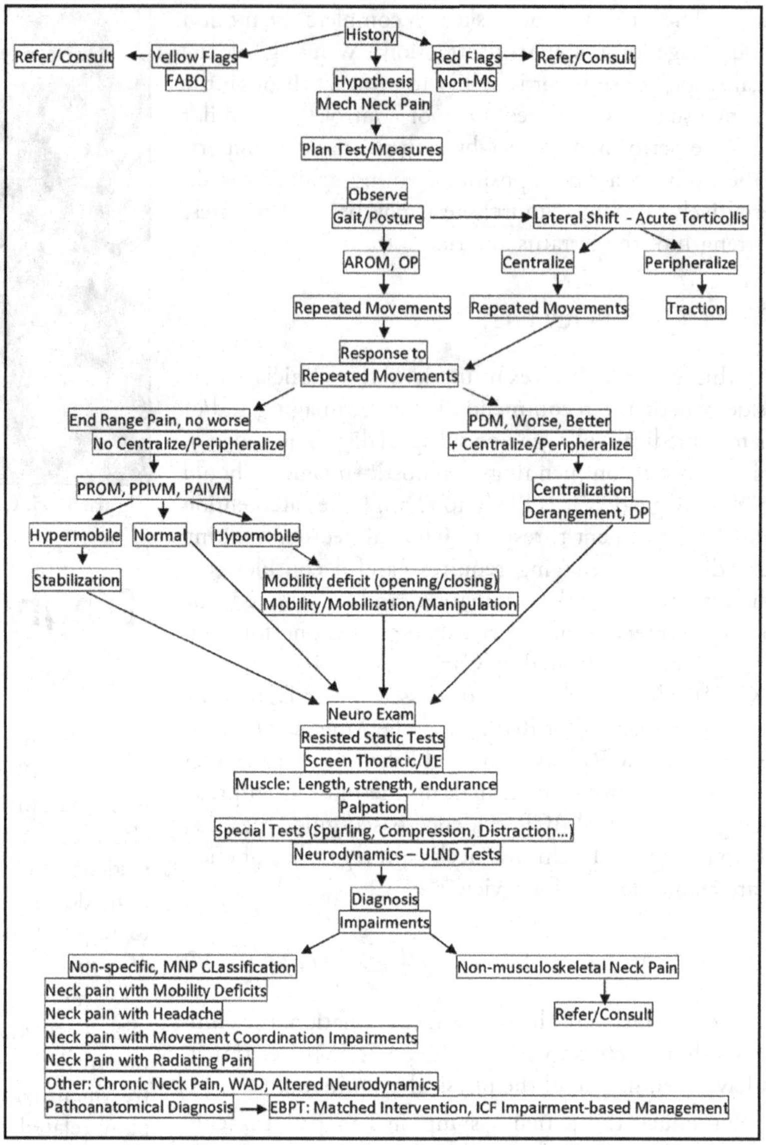

Figure 6-66. Decision-making algorithm.

Whiplash associated disorders (see Tables 6-5 and 6-6) are not included in the clinical practice guidelines.

The classification approach used in this reference pursues an evidence-based strategy integrating current best practice guidelines, clinical expertise, clinical reasoning, and distinctive patient circumstances related to subgroups of patients with neck pain. Each subgroup is characterized by important key findings from the history and physical examination that are used to place a patient into a diagnostic classification[15,31] and/or the ICF impairment-based category of neck pain[15] that initially guides PT intervention. Considering the complex nature of neck pain, patients will often present with criteria from more than one subgroup and most will require multimodal treatment.

Diagnostic classification that guides PT intervention is not a protocol. Not all patients will fit neatly into one classification or may not fit at all into the classification system. Patient presentations will vary even within subgroups. In this situation, clinicians utilize clinical reasoning to prioritize criteria, classification, and relevant impairments in deciding on the best initial treatment or in pursuing an impairment-based approach to management. Continued assessment and reassessment of patient response to treatment provide additional criteria for reclassification and progression of treatment.

Neck Pain With Mobility Deficits Classification

The ICD-10 and related terms for neck pain with mobility deficits are cervicalgia or pain in the thoracic spine. The primary impairment is reduced motion associated with a functional limitation. The ICF category is as follows: (1) measurement of impairment of body function, and mobility of several joints; (2) body structure-cervical vertebral column, and (3) activities and participation specified as moving the head and neck while looking left and right.[15] Common interview findings include age < 50 years old, acute onset of less than 12 weeks possibly related to an unguarded or awkward movement or position, unilateral, local neck pain with or without referred pain to the upper extremity, and complaints of restricted cervical motions.[15,25,282,576,577] Examination findings include limited cervical ROM, with pain at end range of AROM and PROM with or without side-to-side discrepancy, no peripheralization with active ROM, reduced cervical and thoracic segmental mobility, symptoms provoked with cervical and thoracic PAIVM and/or PPIVM, and no signs of nerve root compression, neurovascular compromise or contraindication to mobilization or manipulation.[15] Altered neurodynamics, discussed later in this chapter, can affect cervical mobility and should be examined for and addressed if contributing to the mobility deficit.

The primary goal for intervention for the neck pain with mobility deficit subgroup is to improve functional ROM and to decrease pain and disability. Initial management might include mobilization (nonthrust manipulation) and/or manipulation or high velocity low amplitude (HVLA) thrust to cervical, cervicothoracic, and/or thoracic spine and rib cage dysfunction identified by passive segmental mobility testing. MT is augmented by AROM, self-mobilization, and/or muscle lengthening exercises, motor control, endurance, and strengthening exercises to maintain and improve mobility and functional gains. The evidence to support the use of mobilization (nonthrust manipulation) and manipulation is discussed below. A summary of neck pain with mobility deficits is provided in Table 6-1.[15]

Intervention for Neck Pain With Mobility Deficits Classification

Screening procedures to reduce the risk associated with cervical spine manipulation are discussed under Diagnostic Triage for Cervical Artery Dysfunction (CAD) and Considerations for Ligamentous Stability and Vertebral Artery Testing. Because some MT interventions have inherent risk if performed in the presence of CAD, the clinician must take a comprehensive and reasoned approach to early identification. The clinical reasoning process informs the clinician as to which patients are most likely to benefit and least likely to be harmed as a result of manual intervention. The clinician must make the best decision based on the uncertainties inherent in the clinical presentation and current limitations of screening procedures to decide when a referral for additional testing and medical opinion is needed. The clinician is responsible for performing a prudent examination and clearly documenting that screening was performed.

Before performing a cervical thrust manipulation, a simulated manipulation position (SMP) may be used to screen for patient tolerance to the procedure.[350] The SMP is a premanipulative hold of the cervical spine in the intended HVLA thrust position for 10 to 15 seconds. Theoretically, positional testing may result in reduced blood flow through the ICA or VA and produce symptoms suggestive of diminished cerebral perfusion. The SMP is used as a screening test to assist with identifying patients at risk of neurovascular compromise after cervical manipulation. If symptoms are produced during or immediately after the test, cervical manipulation is contraindicated.[578] The diagnostic accuracy of the SMP is unknown; however, Bowler et al[578] examined blood flow changes bilaterally in the ICA and VA in 14 healthy subjects during a SMP compared to a neutral neck position. The SMP position was held for a C2 to C3 manipulation with the head rotated to one side and laterally flexed to the opposite side. The position was held for 10 seconds or longer to obtain Doppler blood flow measurements approximately at C2 to C3; blood flow was not adversely affected on either side for the ICA and VA in healthy adults.[578]

When using good judgment, thrust techniques are considered important for pain relief and controlling symptoms early in the plan of care.[350] When safety, efficacy, and consent have been determined for the individual patient, the objective is to reduce or eliminate symptoms and/or improve the quantity of available motion.[350] Application of each technique is geared toward as much specificity as possible in applying force that is consistent with the orientation of the facet joint and motion deficit.[350] While a local spinal segmental effect is attempted, a regional effect also occurs. The monograph by Wise and Schenk[350] is recommended for further study. The authors[350] recommend the following when considering the use of cervical thrust manipulation procedures:

- Be well-informed as to the serious and benign risks and educate patients.
- Use premanipulative clinical screening and referral for additional testing, such as radiographic or ultrasound imaging, prior to the use of these techniques.[350]
- Due to inherent risks related to clinical screening procedures, these tests should only be used where thrust procedures are being considered as a viable treatment option.[350]
- Cervical thrust techniques are best used by those who already possess fundamental skills, extensive instruction, and practice in orthopaedic and manual PT[3,50]
- If safety concerns or increased risks are present, evidence supports the use of nonthrust procedures and exercises as successful management strategies.[350]

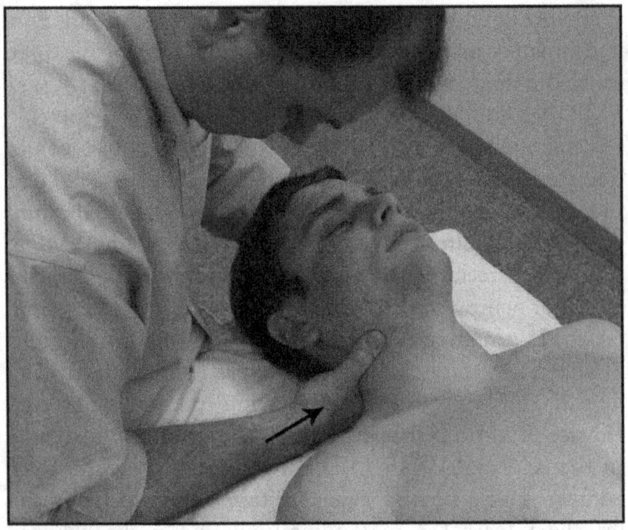

Figure 6-67. Cervical spine (C2 to C7) opening or lateral glide (translation) mobilization or manipulation.

- Due to severity of potential adverse events from cervical thrust procedures, judicious use and care in patient selection are necessary.[350]
- A multimodal approach including exercise and thrust and nonthrust procedures should be considered.[350]
- If appropriate, thoracic thrust procedures should be considered.[350]
- The clinician is advised to use short lever arms, locking techniques to localize forces, and avoid rotational forces.[350]
- Instruction in the first professional PT education should proceed with extreme caution by instructors with experience in these techniques using an appropriate model of instruction that allows for sufficient practice time and feedback.[350]

Considering that current research does not strongly support the use of cervical thrust manipulation in favor of benefits outweighing the risks, the authors[350] suggest that cervical thrust techniques may be a postgraduate skill, reserved for therapists with appropriate knowledge and skills.

In addition to the key interview and examination findings that describe the classification of neck pain with mobility deficits, CPRs may assist in determining who might benefit from cervical spine manipulation. Tseng et al[577] developed a CPR to determine who might benefit from cervical spine manipulation. Vertebral artery testing was performed by placing the subject's head into full extension and then rotating to the end range to each side and holding the position for 10 to 30 seconds. With the patient in supine, the examiner used sidegliding or translation to each side (see Figure 6-49) from the occiput to C7 to identify hypomobile segments. When the hypomobile segment was localized, the examiner flexed and laterally flexed the patient's neck to lock the facet joints of other spinal segments until a barrier was reached. A specific HVLA thrust force was exerted on the hypomobile segment to gap the facet joint; the direction of the thrust was not described. All hypomobile segments were treated with only one thrust to each segment.[577] Although not yet validated, 6 variables make up the CPR:

1. Neck disability index less than 11.5.
2. A bilateral involvement pattern.
3. Not performing sedentary work for more than 5 hours per day.
4. Feeling better while moving the neck.
5. Not feeling worse while extending the neck.
6. A diagnosis of spondylosis without radiculopathy.[577]

If 4 out of the 6 criteria are present with a pretest probability of 60%, a positive immediate response to cervical manipulation is likely 89% of the time (+LR 5.33 [1.72 to 16.54]).[577] A positive response is defined as a 50% reduction in pain, a 4-point change on a 15-point scale of global perceived effect or a report of high satisfaction with treatment.[577] This study examined only the immediate response to cervical manipulation.

Puentendura et al[579] also developed a preliminary CPR rule to improve decision making related to the use of cervical spine manipulation. Four variables were identified:

1. Symptoms less than 38 days.
2. Positive expectation that manipulation will help.
3. A side-to-side difference in cervical rotation ROM of 10 degrees or greater.
4. Pain with PA PAIVM or spring testing of the middle cervical spine.[579]

With at least 3 attributes present (+LR 13.5), a positive response ranged from 39% to 90%, defined as a +5 or quite a bit better on the 15-point Global Rating of Change Scale. Patients were treated for 1 to 2 sessions over about 7 days. A thorough history and physical examination were performed to include screening for VBI and upper cervical spine ligamentous laxity. Each patient received cervical spine manipulation—a rotation or upslope procedure (Figure 6-67) between C3 and C7 to each side of the cervical spine at a level determined by the treating therapist. A maximum of 2 manipulations to each side were allowed. The manipulation was followed by active ROM exercises for 10 repetitions, 3 to 4 times daily. No serious adverse events were reported. Adverse events were defined as moderate to severe symptoms that require the patient to withdraw from the study. However, 12% did report a worsening of symptoms after the first treatment session. Since no control group was used in this study, the authors report it is impossible to know if the improvement was actually due to the treatment.[579] In this study, patients who had only one or none of the predictor variables failed to achieve a successful outcome, suggesting another intervention is appropriate for this group of patients.[579]

Intervention for the neck pain with mobility deficits is provided to decrease pain and disability and improve functional mobility. Initial management might include mobilization and/or manipulation to cervical, cervicothoracic, and/or thoracic spine and rib cage dysfunction identified by passive segmental mobility testing. MT is augmented by AROM, self-mobilization, and/or muscle lengthening exercises, motor control, endurance, and strengthening exercises to maintain and improve mobility and functional gains. Many variations of MT procedures are available with no specific technique known to be superior to another. Selected interventions of mobilization, manipulation, and muscle lengthening procedures for neck pain with mobility deficits are presented below. Clinicians are reminded to reassess after each mobilization or manipulative procedure to determine treatment effectiveness and reclassify as appropriate. AROM, motor control, endurance and strengthening exercises are discussed under the neck pain with movement coordination classification.

Selected Cervical and Thoracic Segmental Mobilization (ie, Nonthrust Manipulation), Manipulation, and Muscle Energy Techniques

Central PA and Unilateral PA PAIVM Mobilization

Central PA (see Figure 6-40) and unilateral PA PAIVM (see Figure 6-41) to hypomobile cervical and thoracic segments are performed in the same manner as the assessment.[472] Variations include central PA mobilization performed with cervical spine in slight flexion or extension. Unilateral PA mobilization can be performed with the cervical spine in lateral flexion or rotation and angled medially, superiorly, or inferiorly.[472]

Cervical Spine Closing (ie, Downglide or Downslope), Mobilization, or Manipulation (C2 to C7; Figure 6-68)[580,581]

With the patient in supine and head in neutral, supported on a pillow, the clinician uses either a cradle or chin hold procedure. For the cradle procedure, both hands support or cradle the posterior occiput and neck. For the chin hold procedure, one hand gently encircles the chin with the forearm, supporting the posterior lateral aspect of the occiput. To perform at the right C5 to C6 segment, the mobilization or manipulation hand contacts the right articular pillar of C5 using the radial border of the proximal or middle phalanx of the index finger. Maintaining

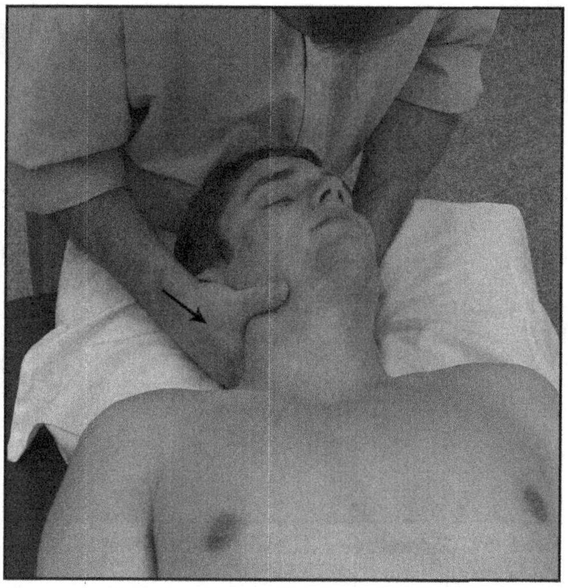

Figure 6-68. Cervical spine (C2 to C7) closing or downglide mobilization or manipulation using a cradle hold.

this position, the clinician gently introduces right lateral flexion of the head and neck until tension is palpated at the right contact point followed by rotation to the left down to C4 to C5, leaving C5 to C6 free to move. Slight adjustments of flexion, extension lateral flexion, rotation, traction, sideglide or downglide are made to achieve a firm tension barrier. A graded oscillation or HVLA thrust is directed along the plane of the facet downward and caudally toward the patient's left shoulder or axilla using the minimum force necessary. If the patient feels pain, alter the hand position or use an alternate procedure. Reassessment is completed after the procedure. Variations for this procedure are available in selected references.[580,581]

Cervical Spine Opening or Lateral Glide Translation Mobilization or Manipulation (C2 to C7; Figure 6-69)[582,583]

With the patient in supine and head on a pillow, the posterior head and neck are cradled while contacting the articular pillars with the lateral aspect of the metacarpophalangeal joints (MCP) or the proximal or middle phalanx of the index finger. The mobilization or manipulation hand and forearm should be directed laterally to apply the translation. For a C2 to C3 left-sided opening motion deficit, a force is applied to the left through the right hand contact on the articular pillar of C2 until a motion restriction or barrier is identified. The craniocervical spine and head move in the same lateral direction. For C2 to C3 left-sided opening motion deficit, a force is applied to the left through the right hand contact on the C2 articular pillar until the motion restriction or barrier is identified. The craniocervical spine and head move in the same lateral direction. When a firm tension barrier is identified, a

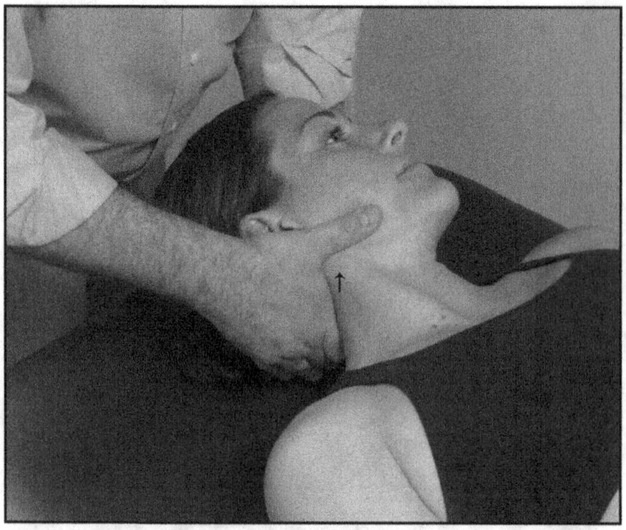

Figure 6-69. Cervical spine (C2-C7) opening or upglide mobilization or manipulation.

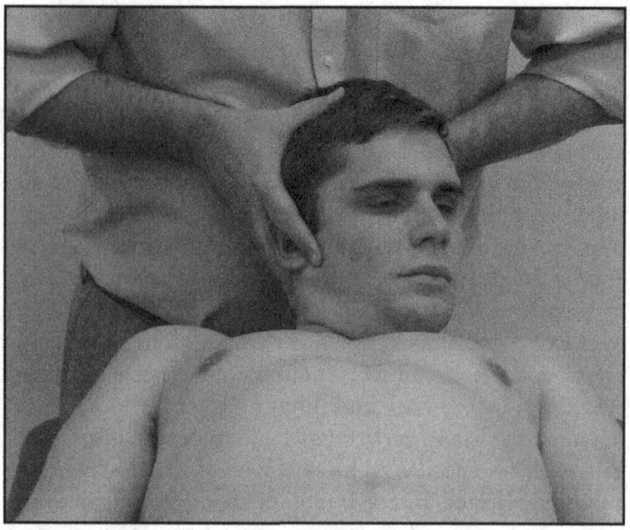

Figure 6-70. Atlantoaxial muscle energy technique.

HVLA thrust or graded oscillation is directed at the target segment in the appropriate right or left lateral translation direction using the minimum force necessary. The procedure can be performed in neutral or slight flexion.[582,583]

Cervical Spine Opening (ie, Upglide or Upslope) Mobilization or Manipulation (C2 to C7; see Figure 6-67)[580,581]

With the patient in supine and head in neutral, supported on a pillow, the clinician uses either a cradle or chin hold procedure. For the cradle procedure both hands cradle the posterior occiput and neck. For the chin hold procedure, one hand gently encircles the chin with the forearm supporting the posterior lateral aspect of the occiput. To perform at the right C5 to C6 segment, the mobilization or manipulation hand contacts the right articular pillar of C5 using the radial border of the proximal or middle phalanx of the index finger. Maintaining this position, the clinician gently introduces right lateral flexion of the head and neck until tension is palpated at the contact point followed by a little rotation to the left down to C4 to C5, leaving C5 to C6 free to move. Slight final adjustments of flexion, extension, lateral flexion, rotation, traction, sideglide, and upglide are made to achieve a firm tension barrier. A graded oscillation or HVLA thrust is directed along the plane of the facet (ie, upwards and toward midline) toward the patient's left eye using rapid pronation of the right forearm and slight supination of the left wrist and forearm. The force is high velocity low amplitude (HVLA) using the minimum force necessary. Reassessment is completed after the procedure. Many variations for this procedure are available in selected references.[580,581]

Atlantoaxial Muscle Energy Technique[473]

A muscle energy technique (Figure 6-70) for AA joint is performed in the same position as the segmental mobility test. With the patient in supine, the clinician cradles the occiput with both hands and flexes the head and neck to end range. For a left rotation motion deficit, left rotation is passively added up to the first barrier or point of motion restriction while maintaining head and neck flexion. The patient is asked to lightly turn the head to the right in an isometric contraction or simply look to the right against controlled resistance by the therapist for 5 seconds. The muscle is then allowed to relax for up to 10 seconds prior to engaging the new barrier. Any slack or increase in length present in the soft tissues following the relaxation is taken up into left rotation to a new barrier. The procedure is repeated 3 to 5 times. Muscle length and cervical mobility are then reassessed to determine if a change in length, tissue texture, or mobility has occurred.[473]

Occipitoatlantal Mobilization Technique

A posterior glide of the occiput on C1 is described as a mobilization procedure (Figure 6-71) to address a flexion mobility deficit unilaterally or bilaterally at the OA joint. For a left OA flexion mobility deficit with the patient in supine, the clinician cradles the occiput in both hands and rotates the head about 30 degrees to the left and adds slight upper cervical lateral flexion to the right. The left hand cups the occiput, using the web formed by the thumb and index finger, along the soft tissue of the posterior SO area. The mobilization hand is placed on the forehead to apply a unilateral anterior-to-posterior graded oscillation at the left OA joint. The reverse procedure addresses flexion mobility deficits at the right OA joint.[583] In supine with the head and neck in neutral, the clinician passively flexes the upper cervical spine to the point of motion restriction using the same hand positions. The mobilization hand applies an anterior-to-posterior glide to simultaneously address both sides.

The same procedure can be used to perform a MET to lengthen the posterior SO muscles and improve upper cervical flexion. In neutral, with one hand cupping the posterior occiput and one hand on the patient's forehead, the clinician introduces upper cervical flexion to the first barrier. The patient is asked either to look up or gently push the occiput isometrically toward the table against a controlled resistance from the therapist for 5 seconds. The muscle is then allowed to relax for up to 10 seconds prior to engaging the new barrier. Any slack or increase in length present in the soft tissues following the relaxation is taken up into flexion to a new barrier. The procedure is repeated 3 to 5 times. Muscle length and cervical mobility are then reassessed to determine if a change in length, tissue texture, or mobility has occurred.[473]

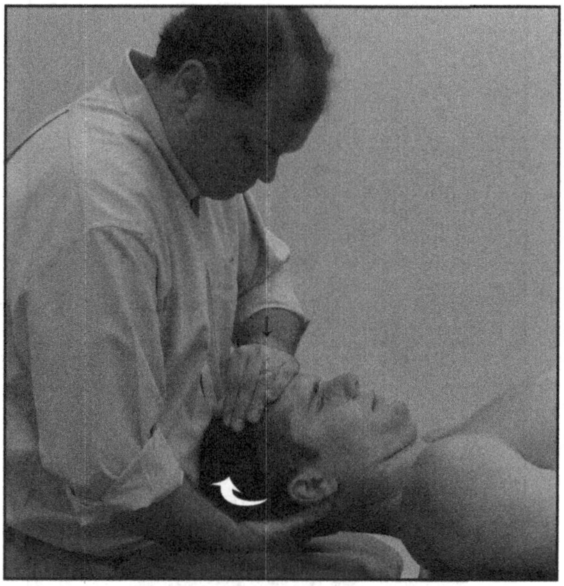

Figure 6-71. Occipitoatlantal posterior glide mobilization.

Selected Thoracic Spine and Rib Mobilization and Manipulation Procedures

Manipulation for the cervicothoracic junction is presented in Chapter 5 in sitting (see Figure 5-50) and supine (see Figure 5-53). Thoracic spine manipulation is presented in Chapter 5 in supine (see Figures 5-38 and 5-55), prone (see Figures 5-37 and 5-44), and seated (see Figure 5-40). First rib mobilization or manipulation supine (see Figure 5-23) and unilateral PA rib mobilization (see Figure 5-41) procedures are presented in Chapter 5.

Muscle Lengthening Manual Procedures (see Figure 5-45)

Muscle energy techniques are applied to lengthen soft tissue[584] of common muscles that tend to tighten, including the posterior SOs, anterior and middle scalenes, long cervical extensors, SCM, levator scapula, and UT. The procedure is performed slowly and carefully with continual feedback from the patient. Symptoms other than a pleasant stretch or pulling sensation in an appropriate area indicate an incorrect procedure that should be stopped. If the muscle is acutely painful, the procedure begins by lengthening the involved muscle lightly to a first resistance barrier perceived by the examiner or from patient feedback. A moderate comfortable stretch is allowed if the muscle is not painful. If the muscle is painful, the patient lightly contracts the involved muscle isometrically against a controlled resistance for 5 seconds. If the muscle is not painful, a moderate isometric contraction is allowed. The muscle is then allowed to relax for up to 10 seconds prior to engaging the new barrier. Any slack or increase in length present in the soft tissues following the relaxation is taken up to a new barrier. The procedure is repeated 3 to 5 times. Muscle length and cervical mobility are then reassessed to determine if a change in length, tissue texture, or mobility has occurred.[584]

Manual lengthening procedures for the anterior and middle scalenes, long cervical extensors, SCM, levator scapula and UT are presented in Chapter 5 (see Figure 5-45). Not covered in Chapter 5 was the muscle lengthening procedure for the Pec Minor and posterior SO muscles which starts with the patient in supine. The examiner stabilizes the sternum with the forearm of one hand while the other hand produces a posterior, superior, and lateral force at the coracoid process and anterior shoulder region until a stretch is felt in the pectoral region. The patient gently pushes the shoulder anteriorly against the examiner's controlled resistance for 5 seconds. After relaxation, the soft tissue slack is taken up by gently lengthening the muscle moving the coracoid process and anterior shoulder region in a posterior, superior, and lateral direction.

Exercises for muscle lengthening are often prescribed as a home program to augment in clinic procedures. In general, exercises for muscle lengthening are performed slowly in a neutral posture, held for 30 seconds, and repeated 3 to 5 times. Exercises to lengthen the posterior SOs, anterior and middle scalenes, long cervical extensors, SCM, levator scapula and UT muscles are presented in Chapter 5 (see Figure 5-46).

Mobility Exercises

Motion gained by MT procedures should be maintained with specific exercise prescription. In the acute stages of neck pain, patients may be instructed in pain-free AROM. Mobility exercises can be performed initially in supine, using a pillow for support. To integrate mobility

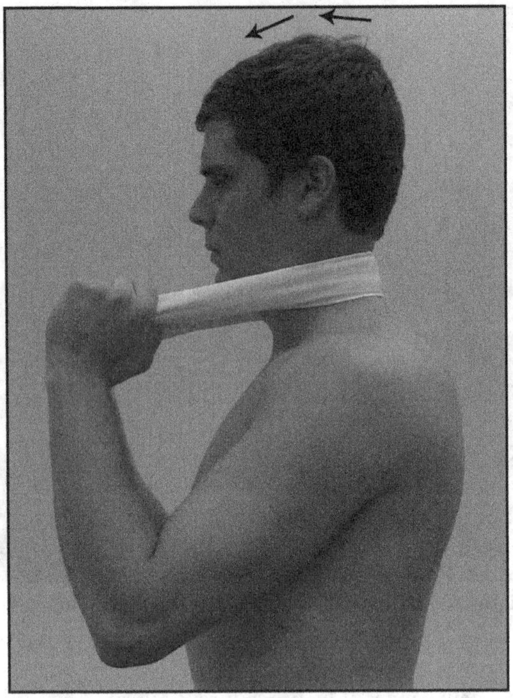

Figure 6-72. Occipitoatlantal flexion self-mobilization exercise.

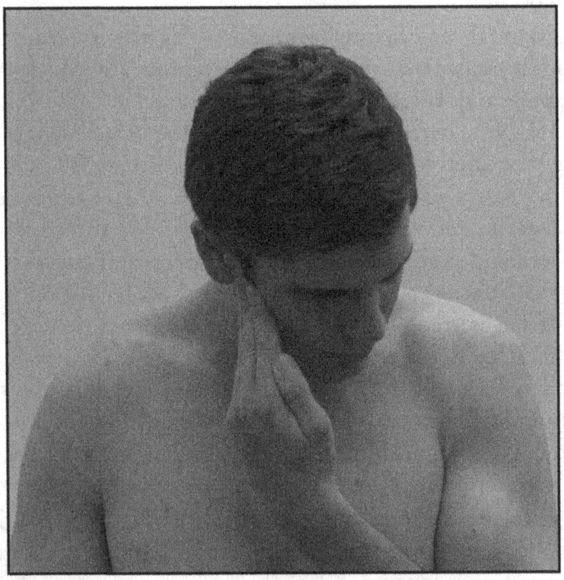

Figure 6-73. Atlantoaxial rotation self-MET.

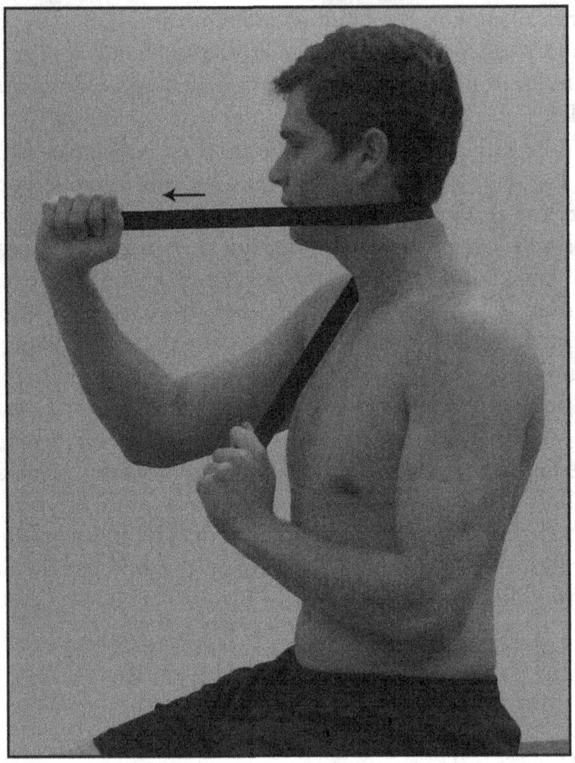

Figure 6-74. Atlantoaxial or C1 to C2 self-sustained natural apophyseal glide (SNAG).

exercises with motor control, emphasis is on quality of movement and practicing correct movement patterns.[585] Segmental joint restrictions are addressed using self-mobilization techniques to augment manual procedures. General cervical AROM exercises are described in Chapter 5 (see Figure 5-43).

OA Flexion

The exercise is similar to the mobilization and muscle energy technique treatment position. To self-mobilize the left OA in supine or sitting, the patient rotates the head about 30 degrees to the left and adds slight upper cervical lateral flexion to the right. A towel, or the fingers clasped behind the neck to stabilize at C2, assists with localizing motion to the upper cervical spine. The patient actively performs upper cervical flexion with an imaginary axis through the external auditory meatus while adding a gentle upper cervical retraction. The reverse procedure addresses flexion mobility deficits at the right OA joint.[583] Keeping the head and neck in neutral, the patient actively performs upper cervical flexion to simultaneously address both sides (Figure 6-72).

AA Rotation

The patient can perform a self-treatment using the same position and procedure for the AA muscle energy technique (Figure 6-73). In sitting, the patient actively flexes the head and neck by moving the chin toward the chest and then rotating to the involved side toward the end of range. The patient then isometrically resists rotation to the opposite side with the hand on the zygoma for 5 seconds. The patient then relaxes for up to 10 seconds prior to engaging the new barrier. Any slack or increase in length present in the soft tissues following the relaxation is taken up to a new rotation barrier. The procedure is repeated 3 to 5 times. An alternate self-mobilization technique is a self-sustained natural apophyseal glide (SNAG)[586] (Figure 6-74). In sitting upright neutral posture for a right rotation

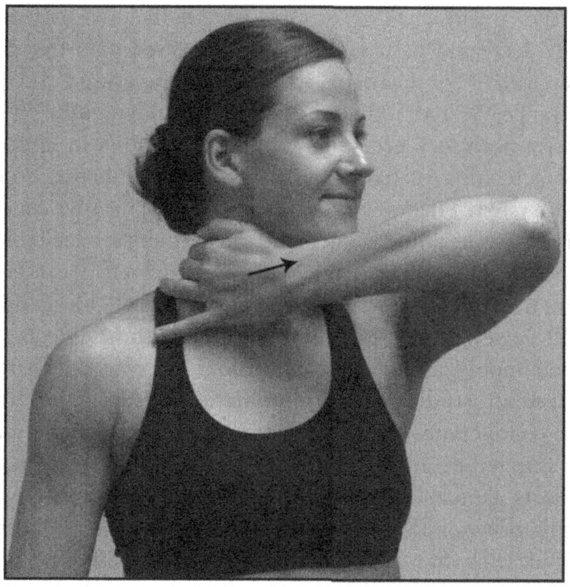

Figure 6-75. C2 to C7 opening self-mobilization.

limitation, the patient places the strap on the posterior aspect of C1 on the left side and pulls horizontally across the face. The strap facilitates rotation at C1 to C2 in the direction that is limited. While pulling horizontally, the head is actively rotated toward the involved side and sustained at end range for 3 seconds. The technique should be performed in the pain-free range with no symptoms other than stretching. The horizontal pull is maintained on the return to neutral position.[586]

C2 to C7 Opening Self-Mobilization[587]

For a right-sided restriction in flexion, left lateral flexion, and left rotation in sitting, the patient hooks the left index or middle finger over the articular pillar of superior vertebra of the involved motion segment on the right and performs active flexion, left lateral flexion, and left rotation (Figure 6-75). The index or middle finger guides motion at the articular pillar and applying overpressure at end of available range. A towel can be used in place of the fingers as needed.[587]

C2 to C7 Closing Self-Mobilization[587]

For a right-sided restriction in extension, right lateral flexion, and right rotation, the patient hooks the left index or middle finger over the articular pillar of the inferior vertebra of the involved motion segment on the right (Figure 6-76). The patient looks up and to the right while applying a slight PA pressure with the left index or middle finger. The patient then performs a gentle chin retraction followed by right rotation and slight extension until a stretch or tension is felt at the motion segment.[587]

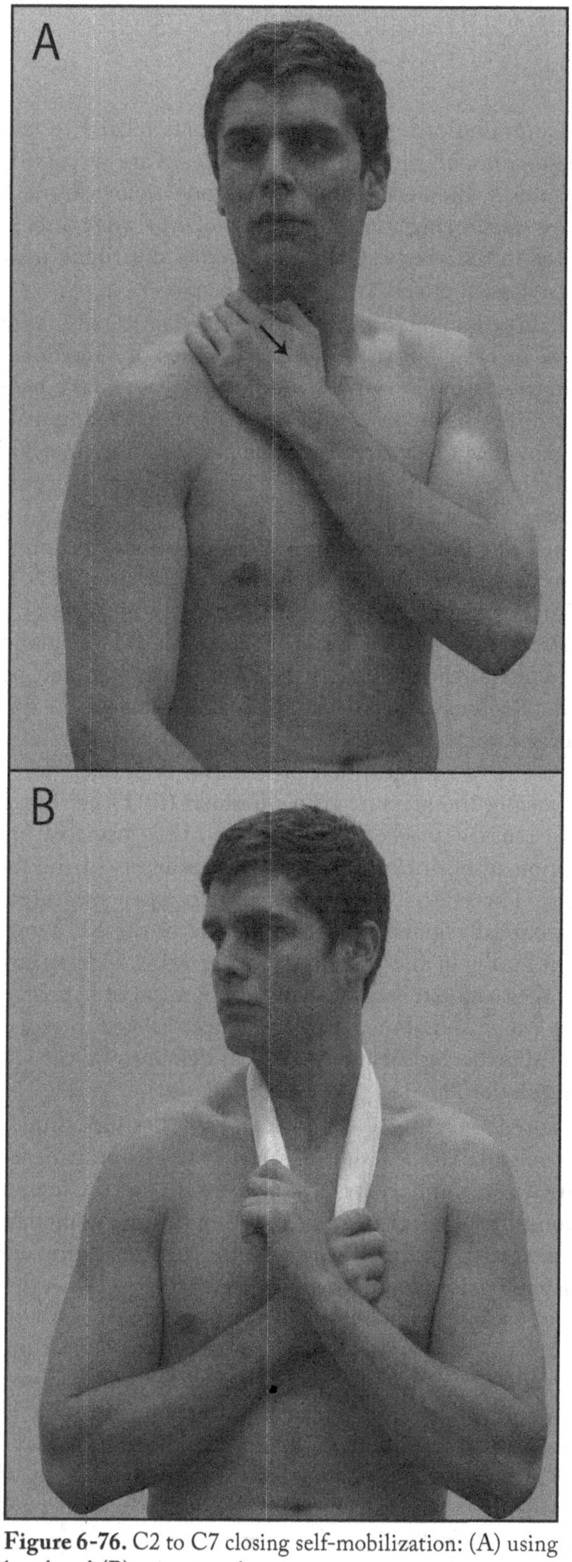

Figure 6-76. C2 to C7 closing self-mobilization: (A) using hand and (B) using towel.

Neurophysiological Effects of Manual Therapy

Contraindications and adverse events related to cervical spine mobilization and manipulation are discussed in Chapter 4. Biomechanical and neurophysiological mechanisms supporting the effectiveness of MT were also presented in Chapter 4. Continued studies describing neurophysiological effects are presented here.

Pain reduction is a primary outcome of spinal manipulative therapy, but the exact mechanisms of alterations in pain processing are largely unknown. A systematic review examined the hypoalgesic effects of spinal manipulative therapy (SMT) alone versus a comparison group in healthy and clinical populations.[588] SMT is defined as high-velocity low-amplitude thrust (HVLAT) manipulation to the spine. The comparison group included sham techniques, exercise, patient education, and/or other forms of MT. The primary outcomes were a pain sensitivity measure or the subject's response to the SMT. The clinical populations were lateral epicondylalgia, LBP, sacroiliac pain and neck pain. Regions targeted for SMT were the cervical spine, thoracic spine, and lumbosacral spine. The results of the meta-analysis suggest that SMT has a favorable effect on increasing the pressure pain threshold (PPT) or reducing pain sensitivity when compared to other forms of intervention in both healthy and clinical subjects in the short term. The effect on PPT was greatest when measured at anatomical regions remote to the site of the SMT rather than locally at the site of SMT, suggesting an interaction between a spinal cord mediated mechanism of hypoalgesia and a supraspinal mediated mechanism related to expectation. Further studies are needed to demonstrate the effect on function.[588]

Based on clinical observations, the lasting effects of hypoalgesia as a result of SMT vary from patient to patient. A summary by Coronado et al[589] of the temporal neurophysiological effects of HVLA thrust manipulation in patients with spinal pain revealed that the lasting effect related to pain modulation of a single session HVLA thrust manipulation without concurrent treatment is short term or absent; temporal changes ranged from no effect up to a maximum of 5 hours, consistent with clinical observation. Immediate and transient changes suggest that long term effects reported in clinical studies[590-593] may be the result of the interaction of thrust manipulation with concurrent treatment such as exercise, increased patient activity, normalization of movement, and/or patient expectations,[589] underscoring the importance of multimodal intervention and patient variables of adherence to exercise and motivation.

Neurophysiological effects of MT occur whether nonthrust manipulation or thrust manipulation are performed. Similarly, alterations in pain processing are found locally at the site of mobilization and at areas remote to the treatment.[594,595] The effects include increased PPT, decreased pain scale rating, increased pain-free grip strength,[596-598] changes in skin temperature,[604] conductance,[599] and inductance with neurodynamics.[601,602] Passive accessory cervical mobilization results in concurrent activation of pain modulation and sympathetic nervous system effects with evidence to support the central nervous system involvement in mediating the mechanical response, but not thermal hypoalgesia which is extrasegmental in nature, lasting up to 24 hours.[603] Hegedus et al[604] reviewed the temporal nature of these effects for spinal mobilization when used alone without concurrent treatment. Studies on asymptomatic subjects found that skin conductance increased lasting, 10 minutes maximum, but skin temperature did not.[604] Studies with symptomatic subjects demonstrated a significant reduction in pain with oscillatory mobilizations to the cervical spine.[605,606] Spinal mobilization has an immediate effect on pain that lasts for up to 24 hours, but other effects last predominantly 5 minutes or less.[604]

Considering that immediate effects on pain can last for up to 24 hours with mobilization, clinicians often choose the most painful segment for a mobilization procedure based on clinical examination findings and experience. Kanlayanaphotporn et al[606] examined the immediate effects of a central PA mobilization (see Figure 6-40) on the most painful segment on neck pain and active cervical ROM compared to a randomly assigned unilateral or central mobilization in 60 patients with central or bilateral MNP. Pain dominant and resistance dominant problems were treated with low-grade and high-grade mobilization, respectively, for two 1-minute repetitions. Patients were reassessed after 5 minutes. Both groups reported a significant reduction in neck pain at rest, but no differences were noted in ROM. The central PA mobilization on the most painful segment showed a greater decrease in neck pain with a mean VAS difference of 10 mm on the most painful movement compared to the group that received the random mobilization,[606] supporting a commonly used clinical decision-making process.

A similar protocol was used to determine the immediate effects on pain and active ROM of a cervical unilateral PA mobilization (see Figure 6-41) technique on the painful side in patients with MNP and unilateral symptoms compared to a randomly selected central or unilateral mobilization technique.[607] Two to 4 spinal levels were mobilized for each group, using two 1-minute repetitions. Ninety percent were treated with grades IV to IV+. No differences were observed between groups, but within-group decreases in neck pain at rest and on the most painful movement and increases in active cervical ROM were significant after mobilization. This study suggests that, in patients with unilateral neck pain, a therapist-selected unilateral PA mobilization technique is as effective as a randomly selected mobilization technique.[607] These results provide support for alternative treatment options for pain reduction in selecting an appropriate motion segment for mobilization, specifically in patients who are unable to tolerate a therapist-selected segment.

In addition to pain modulation, biomechanical theory supports the concept of joint mobilization to improve mobility, but little is known about the specific effects (if any) related to kinematics. Lee et al[608] examined the effects of a central PA at C5 in 119 healthy adults applied in an oscillatory manner for 5 cycles at a grade III. The mobilization produced extension in the upper cervical segments up to C2/C3 and flexion in the lower motion segments up to C7/T1 with the middle segments inconsistent in motion direction. Movement occurred at the target vertebra (C5) and the entire cervical spine, resulting in an increased lordosis.[608] Emerging evidence continues to elucidate the neurophysiological mechanisms by which passive movements through spinal manipulative therapy, thrust, and nonthrust manipulation (mobilization) provide reductions in pain and disability in patients with neck pain with mobility deficits.

Evidence for Cervical Spine Mobilization and Manipulation and Exercise

Systematic Reviews

Mobilization and/or manipulation are often used either alone or concurrently with exercise or other modalities to treat neck pain. While additional research is still needed, current evidence supports the use of MT and exercise for patients with neck pain. Gross et al[6109] reviewed the literature through July 2009 to determine the effects of mobilization or manipulation in adults experiencing neck pain with or without CGH, or radicular findings classified as acute of less than 30 days duration, subacute of 30 to 90 days, and chronic greater than 90 days. The authors concluded the following:

- Cervical manipulation and mobilization produce similar pain relief, functional improvements, and patient satisfaction.
- Cervical manipulation may only provide short-term relief.
- Thoracic manipulation alone, or with electrotherapy, improves pain (NNT 7; 46.6% treatment advantage), function (NNT 5; 40.6% treatment advantage), and immediate pain reduction in chronic neck pain (NNT 5; 29% treatment advantage).
- The best technique and dosage are unknown.[609]
- Miller et al[610] reviewed the literature through July 2009 to determine the effectiveness of MT (mobilization or manipulation), combined with exercise, in adults experiencing neck pain with or without CGH or radiculopathy.

The authors conclude:

- MT and exercise provide greater long-term improvement in pain (NNT 5, treatment advantage 27%) and global perceived effect compared to no treatment for chronic neck pain, subacute and chronic neck pain with CGH, and chronic neck pain with or without radicular findings.
- High quality evidence suggests MT and exercise result in greater short-term pain relief than exercise alone, but no long-term differences across several outcomes for subacute and chronic neck pain with or without CGH.
- Moderate quality evidence suggests that MT and exercise is superior to MT alone for pain reduction and improved quality of life for chronic neck pain. Optimal MT techniques, exercises, and dosage are unknown.[610]

Randomized Controlled Trials

Current research suggests that MT plus exercise is more effective than exercise alone for patients with neck pain. However, it remains controversial whether or not manipulation is more effective than mobilization or a combined approach, or if both are equally effective. Leaver et al[611] investigated whether cervical manipulation provides more rapid and complete recovery from an episode of primary neck pain of less than 3 months than mobilization. Both groups (n = 182; ages 18 to 70 years) received 4 treatments over 2 weeks with selection of manual procedures based on clinical judgment. Exercise and advice to remain active were tailored to the individual patient, but mobilization and manipulation were not combined. No serious neurovascular events were reported with similar minor adverse effects of headache and increased neck pain in both groups. Neck manipulation did not provide more rapid recovery from an episode of neck pain or better outcomes than mobilization.[611]

Using an impairment-based strategy, Walker et al[612] compared a combined MT approach plus exercise to a minimal intervention for patients with MNP with or without unilateral upper extremity symptoms. Both groups were treated 2 times per week for up to 6 sessions. Each treatment consisted of 1 to 3 therapist-selected manual interventions, such as thrust and nonthrust manipulation, muscle energy, or stretching techniques and a standard home exercise program of cervical retraction, DNF strengthening, and cervical rotation ROM exercises plus specific exercises to augment manual procedures.[612] The minimal intervention received general practitioner care, postural advice, advice to maintain neck motion and daily activities, cervical rotation ROM exercise, instructions for continued prescription medication use, and subtherapeutic pulsed (10%) ultrasound at 0.1 W/cm^2 for 10 minutes to the cervical spine. Combined MT and exercise was significantly more effective in reducing neck pain and disability, UE pain scores, and patient-perceived improvement at 3 and 6 weeks and 1-year follow-ups. At 1-year follow-up, patient perceived treatment success in the MT group was 62% (29 of 47) as compared to the minimal intervention group of 32% (15 of 47), who also demonstrated statistically greater healthcare utilization.[612]

Since patients received both thrust and nonthrust manipulation in the Walker et al[612] study, comparisons were made in a secondary analysis between patients who received cervical thrust manipulation and those who received only nonthrust manipulation.[613] The main cervical manipulations used were the cervical opening translation manipulation (see Figure 6-69) and the cervical closing manipulation (see Figure 6-64). Both subgroups demonstrated improvement in short- and long-term pain and disability scores with no between group differences or serious adverse reactions reported, suggesting equal effectiveness of cervical thrust and nonthrust manipulation.[613]

Nonthrust manipulation and manipulation to the cervical spine and thoracic spine are effective in the treatment of patients with neck pain, but controversy exists as to whether cervical or thoracic procedures are more effective. Puentedura et al[614] compared the use of cervical spine manipulation to thoracic spine manipulation (TSM) to treat 24 patients (18 to 60 years) with MNP, with or without UE symptoms of mean duration 15 days, and at least 4 out of 6 CPR criteria.[282] Patients randomly received TSM and cervical ROM for 2 sessions followed by a standard exercise program for 3 sessions or a cervical group who received cervical thrust manipulation (see Figure 6-67) and the same exercise sessions. The manipulation techniques and exercises for this study are presented in Chapter 5 (see Figures 5-38, 5-40, 5-42, 5-43, 5-48, and 5-49). Patients in the cervical group had greater improvements in NDI and NPRS at all follow-up time periods. A statistically significant improvement in the FABQ-PA at all follow-ups was also observed for the cervical group. Number needed to treat to avoid an unsuccessful overall outcome was 1.8 at 1 week and 1.6 at 4 weeks and also at 6 months. The cervical group also experienced less transient posttreatment side effects.[614]

Similarly, Dunning et al[615] compared the outcomes of HVLA thrust manipulation to both the upper cervical (C1 to C2) and upper thoracic (T1 to T2) regions to nonthrust mobilization in the same regions in patients with MNP. Outcome measures included upper cervical rotation ROM, pain, disability, and motor performance of the DNF 48 hours postintervention. Eligible patients included those with a primary complaint of neck pain in the region between the superior nuchal line and first thoracic spinous process of any duration, between 18 and 70 years of age, and having a NDI score of 20% or greater (ie, 10 points or greater on 0/50 scale). Screening questions for cervical artery disease were negative; premanipulative cervical artery testing was not performed. The thrust manipulation group received a single HVLA thrust to C1 to C2 using a primary lever of rotation and a single HVLA thrust directed bilaterally to the T1 to T2 (see Figure 5-53) with the patient in supine. The nonthrust manipulation group received a unilateral PA mobilization bilaterally to C1 to C2 and a central PA mobilization to T1 to T2 for 1 bout of 30 seconds. The thrust manipulation group experienced greater improvements in pain and disability, C1 to C2 ROM, and motor performance in the DNF at a 48-hour reassessment.[615]

While current evidence supports the use of cervical spine MT, evidence is lacking as to the comparative effectiveness of manipulation, medication, and home exercise with advice for acute and subacute neck pain. Bronfort et al[616] examined a cohort of patients (ages 18 to 65 years) with mechanical nonspecific neck pain classified as grades I or II according to the Bone and Joint Decade 2000 to 2010 Task Force on Neck Pain.[617] Symptoms were present for 2 to 12 weeks with a neck pain score of 3 or more on a 0 to 10 scale. Maximum treatment duration was 12 weeks performed by 6 chiropractors. At the provider's discretion, the treatment group received 15 to 20 minutes of manipulation or mobilization of segmental hypomobility, light soft-tissue massage, assisted stretching, hot and cold packs, and advice to stay active or modify activity. At the physician's discretion, the medication group received first line acetaminophen, nonsteroidal anti-inflammatory drugs, or both. Second line intervention included narcotics. Muscle relaxants were also used along with advice to stay active or modify activity. The home exercise with advice group had two 1-hour sessions 1 to 2 weeks apart, emphasizing self-mobilization, controlled exercise of the neck and shoulder (including neck retraction, extension, rotation, lateral bending motions), and scapular retraction with no resistance. The exercise dosage was 5 to 10 repetitions up to 6 to 8 times per day. The authors conclude that SMT was more effective for pain reduction than management with medication alone in both the short and long term. A supervised home exercise and advice strategy resulted in similar outcomes at most time points.[616]

Similar to the previous study,[616] Hoving et al[576] examined whether short-term effects at 13 weeks favoring MT were retained in the 1-year follow-up of a previous study[618] using 3 treatment strategies. Patients (n = 183) were 18 to 70 years old with a primary complaint of MNP and/or stiffness for at least 2 weeks. The 3 treatment groups seen over 6 weeks were (a) MT with patients seen 1 time per week for 45 minutes for nonthrust manipulation or mobilization and coordination or stabilization exercises and home exercises, (b) PT with patients seen for 30 minutes, twice a week for active, passive, postural, stretching, relaxation, and functional exercises, and manual traction and massage with no manual mobilization techniques included, and (c) general practitioner (GP) visits of 1 time per week for analgesics, advice, self-care, education, self-care of heat and exercise, and ergonomic advice.[576] Outcomes at 1 year are as follows:

- Maximum MT group improvement occurred after the intervention at 13 weeks
- No major improvement was seen at 13 weeks in the PT group
- The GP group improved after the 13 weeks and continued to improve up to 52 weeks
- Higher improvement scores were noted for MT for all outcomes (ie, NDI, pain, perceived recovery) followed by PT and then GP care[618]

During the course of one year, MT was more effective than GP care and slightly more effective than PT. Differences between PT and GP care were not significant. Almost twice as many patients in the PT and GP groups received additional treatments compared with MT. The MT group recovered earlier, but the GP and PT groups caught up in the long term.[618] In the Hoving et al[618] study, the total costs of MT were about one third of the costs of PT and GP care. The differences were significant for MT versus PT and MT versus GP care and GP care versus PT. In this study, MT plus exercise was less costly and also more effective than PT or GP.[619]

In patients with chronic neck pain, MT plus exercise is favored over MT alone or exercise alone, but in some patients with chronic neck pain, MT plus high dose supervised exercise or high dose supervised exercise alone may result in similar outcomes. Two randomized controlled trials[620,621] determined that cervical and thoracic spinal manipulation, combined with low tech supervised exercise and high tech supervised exercise alone, resulted in significantly reduced pain at one and 2 year follow-ups compared to spinal manipulation alone in patients with chronic neck pain of longer than 12 weeks. Similarly, Evans et al[622] examined the effectiveness of three 12-week treatment strategies for chronic neck pain (n = 270): (a) spinal manipulation (SMT) and high dose supervised strengthening exercise (SMT + ET), (b) high dose supervised strengthening alone (ET), and (c) low dose home exercise and advice (HEA). Subjects had a mean duration of neck pain of 9.4 years, moderate in severity (5.6/10), and 72% were women. The ET group received one-on-one supervision of 20 1-hour sessions with emphasis on high numbers of repetitions and progressively increased loads. With the patient lying on the table, wearing headgear with 1.25 to 10 pound attachments guided by a pulley, the patient performed 3 sets of 15 to 25 repetitions of dynamic neck extension, flexion, and rotation. Upper body strengthening was included with a 5-minute aerobic and stretching warm-up. The SMT + ET group received 20 sessions of SMT + ET, using HVLA thrust techniques to the cervical and thoracic spine at the examiner's discretion and light soft tissue massage. HEA consisted of two 1-hour sessions of gentle self-mobilization of the neck and shoulders with no resistance for neck retraction, extension, flexion, rotation, and lateral flexion. Patients performed 5 to 10 repetitions of each exercise up to 6 to 8 times per day as tolerated. Advice, ergonomics and postural education were also provided. Patients had similar expectations for recovery, with lower expectations reported for the HEA group.[622] The authors conclude that high dose ET, with or without SMT, resulted in greater short term pain reduction, satisfaction, and global perceived effect than home exercise for nonspecific chronic neck pain. The differences between the SMT + ET and the ET group were not significant, suggesting that SMT is of little benefit to ET in chronic neck pain.[622] The most important outcome identified by patients was pain severity in 55% of subjects. All 3 groups showed a reduction in pain, but more patients in the 2 supervised exercise groups (ie, 65% to 74% at 12 weeks and 51% to 57% at 52 weeks) reported a 2.5/10 reduction in pain compared to the HEA group (42% at 12 weeks, 41% at 52 weeks).[622]

The decision to use MT and exercise in patients presenting with neck pain is tailored to each patient based on key interview and physical examination findings, appropriate diagnostic classification or impairment-based classification, and clinical reasoning related to application of the current best evidence and patient expectations. Within and between session reassessments of patient response are keys to differential diagnosis for appropriate classification, a thorough examination, and treatment progression. Self-treatment strategies, exercises to augment MT sessions and address patient-specific impairments and activity limitations complement a multimodal PT approach.

Evidence for Thoracic Spine Mobilization/Manipulation and Exercises for Cervical Pain

Patients presenting with neck pain have been shown to benefit from thoracic manipulation and exercise and combined thoracic spine and cervical mobilization and manipulation and exercise. Several authors report improved outcomes with thoracic spine manipulation in patients with MNP with or without radiculopathy.[282,283,431,582,591,612,614,623-641] The results of the Cleland et al[432] study suggested that patients with no contraindications to manipulation and a primary condition of MNP may benefit from thoracic manipulation and exercise. Lau et al[633] concluded that TSM is effective in decreasing neck pain and disability, improving neck posture, and ROM for patients with chronic MNP. The thoracic manipulation techniques and supporting evidence are discussed in Chapter 5.

Electrotherapy for Neck Pain

Modalities such as electrotherapy are often widely used for patients with neck pain, even with little to no evidence to support their use over MT and exercise. A systemic review by Kroeling et al[634] concluded that very low quality evidence suggests pulsed electromagnetic field therapy, repetitive magnetic stimulation, and transcutaneous electrical nerve stimulation (TENS) are more effective than placebo, and that modulated galvanic current, iontophoresis and electric muscle stimulation are not more effective than placebo. The quality of evidence is low or very low for all studies. In acute neck pain, TENS possibly relieves pain better than electrical stimulation, but is not superior to MT and ultrasound and not as good as exercise. Electrotherapy provides no added benefit when used with infrared, hot packs and exercise, physiotherapy, or combined use of a neck collar, exercise and pain medication. For acute WAD, iontophoresis is no more effective than no treatment, interferential current or combined traction, exercise, and massage for relieving neck pain with headache. For patients with chronic neck pain, TENS possibly relieves pain better than placebo and electrical stimulation, but is not superior to MT and ultrasound and not as good as exercise, and infrared. Pulsed electromagnetic field is possibly better than placebo, galvanic current, and electrical stimulation. Electrical stimulation results in no additional benefits when added to either mobilization or manipulation.[634]

Effectiveness of Patient Education Strategies

Patient education is a very important part of a multimodal PT approach that includes advice to remain active, skills to cope with stress and pain, neuroscience of pain education, and self care; however, patient education strategies in the absence of other interventions are unlikely to be effective for most patients. Gross et al[635] examined 15 RCTs through July 2010. Only one trial favored the use of an education video for acute WAD when compared to no treatment. Advice to remain active, advice on stress-coping skills, workplace ergonomics, and self care (as treatment strategies alone) are not supported by strong evidence in this review.[635]

Summary of Neck Pain With Mobility Deficits Classification

Recommendations of the neck pain clinical practice guidelines (CPG)[15] include the following (see Table 6-1): combined cervical mobilization and manipulation with exercise are more effective in decreasing neck pain, headache, and disability than mobilization or manipulation alone; and thoracic spine manipulation can be used for patients with primary complaints of neck pain and for decreasing pain and disability in patients with neck pain and associated arm pain.[15] In addition, systematic review[610] on the effectiveness of MT and exercise for neck pain suggests that, compared to no treatment, MT and exercise result in clinically important long-term improvements in pain, function, and global perceived effect, MT and exercise provide greater short-term pain relief than exercise alone, but not in the long-term for all outcomes in subacute and chronic neck pain with or without CGH, and MT and exercise is superior to MT alone for reducing pain and improving quality of life for chronic neck pain. Evidence related to MT and exercise for radiculopathy is limited.

Neck Pain With Radiating Pain

According to the neck pain clinical practice guidelines (CPG),[15] 2 ICD diagnoses, cervical spondylosis and cervical disc disorder are associated with the classification "neck pain with radiating pain." ICF categories include body function and radiating pain in a segment or region, body structure and spinal nerves, and activities and participation and reaching.[15] Symptoms with this classification include neck pain with an associated radiating or narrow band of lancinating pain in the involved upper extremity, upper extremity paresthesia, and related numbness and weakness.[15] Clinical findings that assist with diagnostic classification are upper extremity symptoms, radicular or referred pain produced or aggravated with Spurling's test, ULNDTs, and decreased with neck distraction, decreased cervical rotation of less than 60 degrees to the involved side, signs of nerve root compression (ie, sensory, strength, or reflex deficits), and success in reducing upper extremity symptoms using initial examination and intervention procedures, such as distraction.[15] Recommended interventions include upper quarter and nerve mobilization techniques, cervical traction, and thoracic mobilization and manipulation.[15] Although not part of the neck clinical practice guidelines, the subgroup of patients with radiating pain could include patients with cervicobrachial pain, demonstrating the centralization phenomenon or symptoms associated with neuropathic pain mechanisms.

Cervicobrachial pain is the presence of upper quadrant symptoms associated with neck pain described with a variety of characteristics such as a dull, poorly localized ache, burning, weakness, paresthesia, and hyperesthesia. Jull et al[114] reported several structures as pathological causes of cervicobrachial symptoms, including somatic structures of the cervical spine, peripheral nerve tissue such as irritation or sensitization of nerve tissue or CR, neurovascular structures, or nonmusculoskeletal causes. A variety of potential pain mechanisms and symptom descriptors support the hypothesis that cervicobrachial pain is a heterogeneous

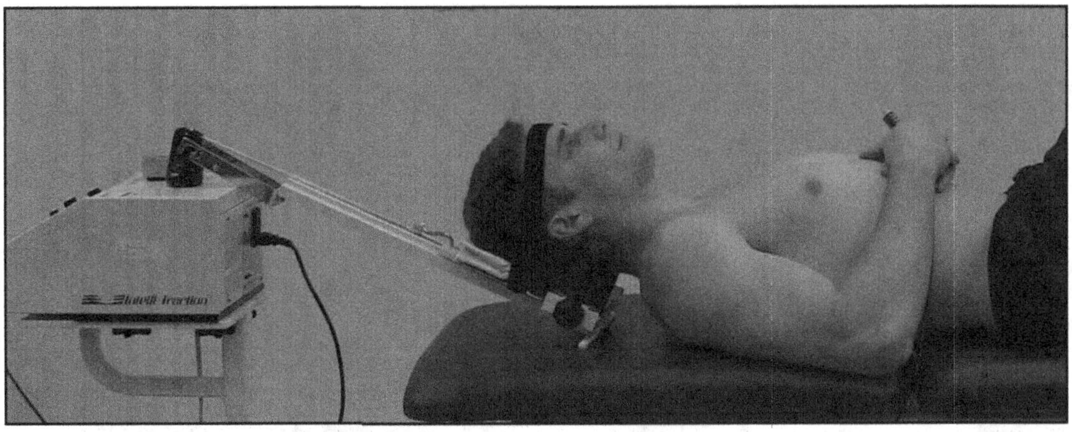

Figure 6-77. Intermittent cervical traction.

population that requires careful differential diagnosis and management. Therefore, determining the presence of a neuropathic component during the initial session is important because it will guide patient management. A neuropathic component could present as a range of conditions from mechanosensitive neural tissue to CR in the acute, subacute, or chronic stages.[114]

Evidence to Support Noninvasive Management of Cervicobrachial Pain and Cervical Radiculopathy

The clinical presentation of CR was discussed earlier in this chapter under Diagnostic Triage. Many noninvasive interventions used to treat patients with CR include traction, mobilization and manipulation to the cervical and thoracic spine, therapeutic exercise, and various pain modalities. However, few studies have examined the effectiveness of these interventions. Salt et al[636] systematically reviewed 10 articles, to January 2010, on noninvasive management of cervicobrachial pain defined as upper quadrant pain with cervical spine pain. Overall, general physiotherapy (PT) exercise or traction was not more effective in reducing pain compared to other interventions, with only MT and exercise trending to a favorable response, but without statistical significance. The effects of noninvasive management on function and disability were mixed.[636] The neck pain clinical practice guideline[15] recommends consideration of mechanical intermittent cervical traction (ICT; Figure 6-77) combined with other interventions, such as MT and exercise, to reduce pain and disability in patients with cervicobrachial pain.

Additional studies since the Salt et al[636] review provided more support for MT and exercise. Boyles et al[637] reviewed 4 studies through February 2011 on the effectiveness of manual PT in the treatment of CR. The MT techniques included muscle energy techniques, nonthrust manipulation, thrust manipulation and mobilization of the cervical and/or thoracic spine, soft-tissue mobilization, and neural mobilization. MT was either used alone or in combination with therapeutic exercise and often a form of cervical traction. The authors conclude that MT plus therapeutic exercise is promising with regard to improving function, AROM, pain, and disability levels.[637]

Similarly, a multimodal approach of cervical, thoracic, and neurodynamic mobilization techniques plus exercise may be more effective than MT or exercise alone. The effects of MT, exercise, and a combination of MT and exercise for treatment of CR were studied in 30 subjects who had 4 examination findings (previously described by Wainner et al[245]) to indicate a diagnosis of CR.[638] Patients were seen 3 times per week for 3 weeks. The MT group received (a) cervical lateral glides (see Figure 6-67) toward the side of symptoms grades III-IV for 30 to 45 seconds at each segment of the cervical spine (C2 to C7), (b) thoracic central PA mobilization (see Figure 5-27) grades III-IV targeting hypomobile segments for 30 to 45 seconds each, and (c) neurodynamic techniques for the median nerve (Figure 6-78) using a sliding technique and progressing to a tension technique (Figure 6-79). The exercise group received (a) DNF strengthening for 10 repetitions of 10-second holds (see Figure 6-53), (b) lower and middle trapezius strengthening in prone (see Figure 5-47D-E), and (c) serratus anterior strengthening against the wall (Figure 5-47C). The combined MT and exercise group received both protocols.[638] All 3 groups demonstrated significant improvements in pain (NPRS) and function (NDI), with the MT and exercise group showing significantly greater results. All patients demonstrated similar statistically significant improvements in cervical ROM. The author concludes that a multimodal treatment approach is superior to either MT or exercise alone.[638]

In the treatment of CR, cervical traction is a traditionally used modality either alone or as a multimodal approach including MT and exercise, but either conflicting or little-to-no evidence is available to support its use over MT and exercise alone. The effectiveness of MT and

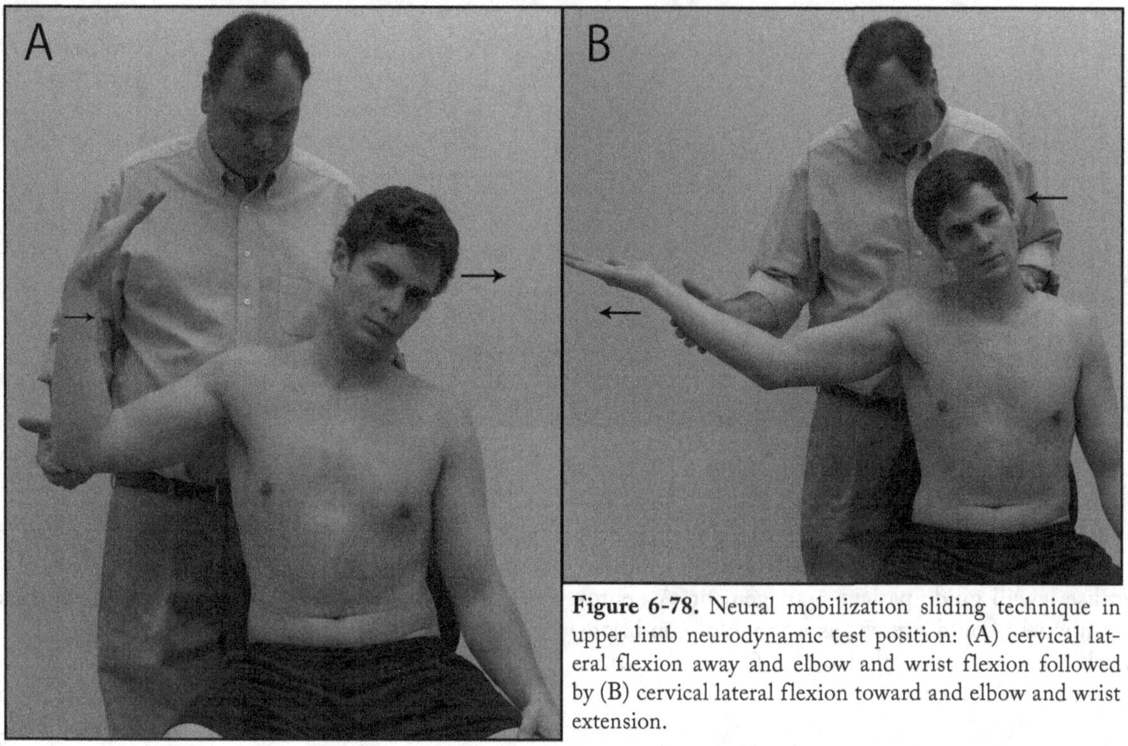

Figure 6-78. Neural mobilization sliding technique in upper limb neurodynamic test position: (A) cervical lateral flexion away and elbow and wrist flexion followed by (B) cervical lateral flexion toward and elbow and wrist extension.

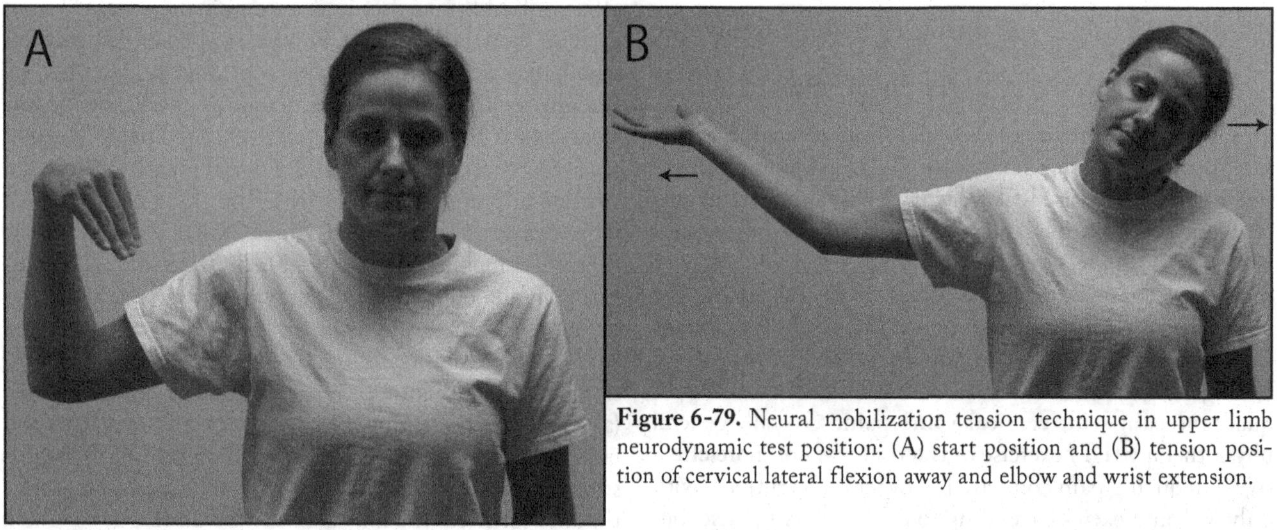

Figure 6-79. Neural mobilization tension technique in upper limb neurodynamic test position: (A) start position and (B) tension position of cervical lateral flexion away and elbow and wrist extension.

exercise with or without ICT on pain, function, and disability was examined by Young et al[639] in patients (n=81; ages 18 to 70) with CR diagnosed using the 3 out of 4 criteria established by Wainner et al.[245] Patients were treated 2 times per week for an average of 7 visits over 4.2 weeks. Both groups received MT and exercise, including posture education, mobilization or manipulation in prone, supine, or sitting (see Figures 5-37, 5-38, 5-40, 5-50, and 5-53) to hypomobile segments of the upper- and mid-thoracic spine based on therapist preference, and (c) after treatment of the thoracic spine, cervical spine mobilization could include retraction in supine with clinician overpressure (Figure 6-80), rotations, lateral glide in the ULNDT 1 (median nerve) position (Figure 6-81), and cervical PA glides for at least 1 set of 30 seconds or 15 to 20 repetitions (techniques were chosen based on centralization or reduction in symptoms). They also received exercise that augmented the manual procedures and could include retraction, extension, DNF strengthening, and scapular strengthening (at least one exercise was used at each treatment session) and ICT or sham traction. ICT (see Figure 6-77) was performed in supine at an angle of 15 degrees flexion beginning at 9.1 kg (20 lbs), or 10% of patient's body weight, whichever was less, and increased 0.91 to 2.25 kg

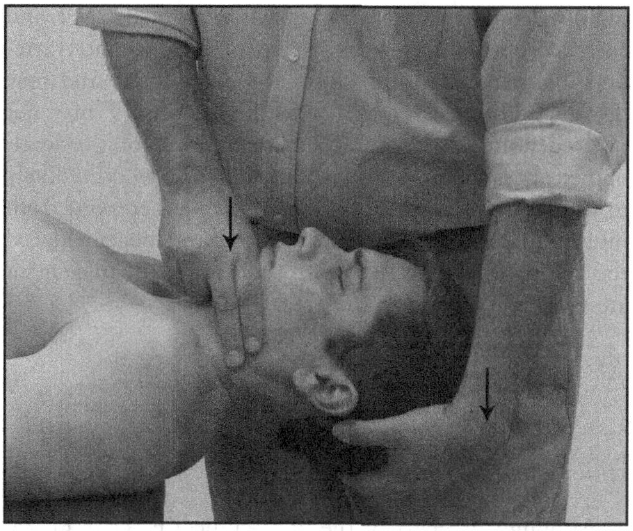
Figure 6-80. Retraction in lying with clinician overpressure.

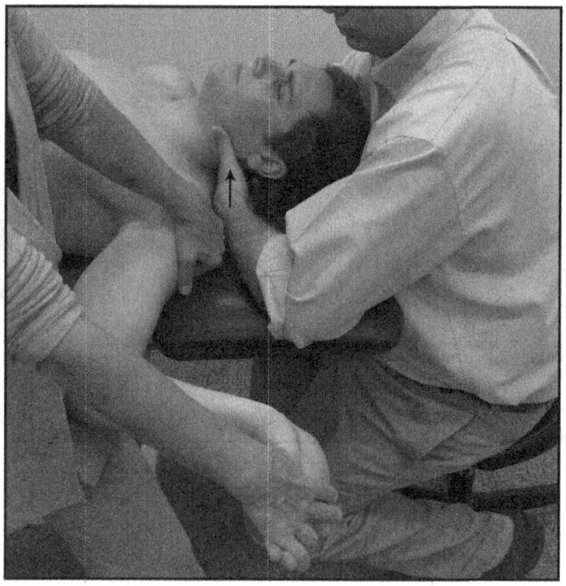
Figure 6-81. Contralateral glide in upper limb neurodynamic median nerve position.

(2 to 5 lbs) every session based on centralization or reduction of symptoms. Maximum force was 15.91 kg (35 lbs). The on/off cycle was 50/10. Sham traction was identical except for the force with only 2.27 kg (5 lbs) or less of force applied.[639] At 4 weeks, significant improvement occurred in both groups in pain, function, disability, and symptom distribution, suggesting the addition of ICT to MT and exercise provides no additional benefit.[639]

While more robust research is needed to resolve controversy on the effectiveness of cervical traction, results are promising based on this case series[624] of 11 patients (age 51.7 years; SD 8.2) with CR. A similar standardized treatment protocol[631] of MT, cervical traction, and exercise included: (a) cervical lateral glides, grades III and IV, away from the symptomatic side from C2 to C7 in the ULND position (see Figure 6-81), (b) upper and mid-thoracic spine manipulation targeting hypomobile segments, (c) DNF and scapulothoracic strengthening for serratus anterior and middle and lower trapezius, and (d) ICT in 25 degrees of flexion for 15 minutes per session beginning at 8.2 kg (18 lbs) and increased to a maximum of 0.5 to 0.9 kg (1 to 2 lbs) per session, depending on patient response and adjusted to produce centralization or reduction of the patient's symptoms. The on/off cycle time was set to a ratio of 30:10 seconds with the off force set at 5.4 kg (12 lbs). Ten of the 11 patients (91%) reported clinically meaningful improvement in pain and function after a mean of 7.1 (SD, 1.5) PT sessions and at the 6-month follow-up.[624]

Another study showing the benefits of a multimodal approach for management of CR is a retrospective case series by Forbush et al.[640] Subjects included 10 older adults (ages 65 or older [mean 74.9 years and range of 67 to 82]) with advanced cervical spondylarthrosis with radiculopathy of symptom duration for more than 6 months. All patients had limited cervical lateral flexion ROM, a positive Spurling's test, and neck distraction test. Nine out of 10 had a positive ULNDT. A multimodal intervention consisted of soft tissue mobilization of the upper thoracic and cervical spine in a seated position, manual traction of the upper cervical spine, and deep pressure to the UT. Additionally, HVLA thrust manipulation was performed to any cervical or thoracic segments with a soft capsular restricted end feel and the upper ribs as needed, MET on segments with a nondistinct or hard capsular end feel, long-axis lengthening of all cervical musculature, and ICT. Home exercises included DNF activation and general ROM.[640] All 10 patients had substantial improvement in pain and disability. Gains were maintained at 6 months with the mean pain score less than 1/10 (baseline 5.7) and the mean NDI score 6/50 (baseline 27.4) at discharge.[640]

Absence of an identified subgroup of individuals who are likely to respond to cervical traction is one possibility for limited evidence to support its effectiveness. Cleland et al[641] identified a subset of predictor variables to identify persons with CR who are most likely to achieve short-term success at 4-week follow-up with PT intervention. The variables are as follows: age < 54 years, dominant arm not affected, looking down does not increase symptoms, and multimodal treatment including MT, ICT, and DNF strengthening for at least 50% of sessions. When 3 out of 4 variables or 4 out of 4 variables are present, the +LR was 5.2 (95% CI: = 2.4, 11.3) and 8.3 (95% CI: 1.9, 63.9) and posttest probability of success was 85% and 90%, respectively.[641]

Identifying the key characteristics of a subgroup of patients with CR is likely to assist with improved outcomes and clinical decision making related to use of

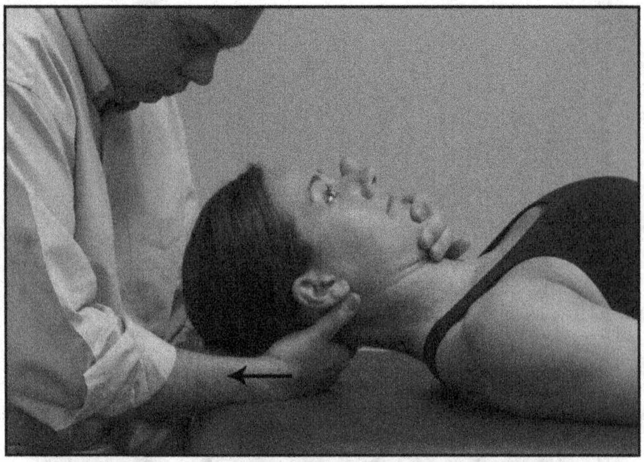

Figure 6-82. Manual distraction/traction supine.

cervical traction as part of multimodal management. A CPR was developed by Raney et al[547] to identify patients with neck pain likely to benefit from cervical mechanical traction and exercise. Patients (n = 68) received 6 sessions of ICT, starting with 4.5 to 5.4 kg (10 to 12 lbs) for 15 minutes. Over 3 weeks, the force was adjusted upward to a maximum 40 lbs based on centralization of symptoms. Exercise included holding a neutral sitting posture 2 times for 10 seconds every hour and supine DNF training for 10 repetitions of 10-second holds twice daily. The study found 5 variables that suggest a patient with neck pain is likely to benefit from traction and exercise:

1. Age > 55 years
2. Positive shoulder abduction sign
3. Relief of symptoms with manual distraction—an axial traction force applied until symptoms decrease or centralize (Figure 6-82)
4. Peripheralization with lower cervical spine (C4 to C7) mobility testing
5. Positive ULNDT using the median nerve bias with shoulder to 90 abduction[547]

Thirty out of 68 patients achieved a successful outcome. The presence of 3 out of 5 predictors resulted in a +LR equal to 4.81 (95% CI: 2.17 to 11.4), increasing the likelihood of success with cervical traction and exercise from 44% to 79.2%. With 4 of 5 variables present, the +LR was equal to 23.1 (2.5 to 227.9), increasing the posttest probability of improvement with ICT traction to 94.8%. A comparison group was not utilized in the development of this preliminary CPR and additional studies are needed for validation.[547]

Overall, the literature supports a multimodal, nonsurgical approach, consisting of MT, ICT, and exercise for patients with CR. Optimal MT techniques and dosage are unknown. Langevin et al[642] present a protocol for patients with CR, comparing a standardized MT (ie, cervical mobilization) and exercise approach to a specific MT and exercise approach targeting the opening of the intervertebral foramen. The study[642] is now in progress and may provide additional information. The use of ICT may not be needed in all cases of CR. Further research on the development of a subgroup of patients with CR who are likely to achieve success with cervical traction either alone or in multimodal program is needed. Surgical management and the comparative effectiveness to nonsurgical management are discussed later in this chapter.

Neck Pain with Radiating Pain Classification—Cervicobrachial Pain and Repeated Movements

Although not part of the neck clinical practice guidelines, in addition to patients with cervicobrachial pain related to neuropathic pain mechanism, the subgroup of patients with neck pain and radiating pain could also include patients with cervicobrachial pain and a response of centralization to repeated movement. The response to repeated movements is important for classification of patients with MNP into subgroups[422,433-435] who preferentially respond to exercises in a specific direction. If a repeated movement decreases, abolishes or centralizes symptoms, further testing is not necessary because an initial treatment threshold is reached. The matched intervention for the subgroup is the use of repeated active or sustained end-range movements (ie, protrusion/flexion, cervical retraction/extension, lateral flexion right/left, and rotation right/left) in the direction that caused the centralization during assessment.[422,433] If peripheralization or partial centralization occurs in weight-bearing, unloaded positions are attempted to begin intervention. If the response is limited motion and end range pain (ie, produced, increased, or no worse) with no centralization or peripheralization, further examination is needed. The clinician considers a classification of neck pain with mobility deficits (see Table 6-1). Additional examination is warranted for diagnostic classification.

Evidence to Support Direction-Specific Exercise of Repeated Movements for the Neck Pain With Radiating Pain Classification

Evidence supporting a repeated movement approach for management of patients with cervical pain or cervicobrachial pain is scarce and based primarily on clinician observation, experience, and a favorable prognosis of the centralization phenomenon.[643] In a randomized controlled trial, 77 patients with neck pain and CR were assigned to general exercise, a repeated movement treatment approach[422,433] or a control group.[644] At 12 months, all groups had significant improvement in pain and NDI with no significant difference among groups. The repeated movement group was favored over the control group for more rapidly reduced pain at 3 weeks, reduced pain at 24 weeks, and for reduced postintervention NDI with a tendency for fewer health care visits for additional healthcare. All 3 groups had similar recurrence rates: overall, 79% were better or had complete symptom resolution while 51% continued with constant or daily pain.[644]

Similarly, only minimal clinically important outcomes were achieved comparing a repeated movement approach to a cognitive behavioral approach, which included patients with chronic neck and back pain. A cohort of 315 patients with neck or back pain longer than 3 months were randomized to a brief physiotherapy cognitive behavioral approach (CBA) or repeated movements approach[422] with or without an educational booklet.[645] Outcomes between groups were not statistically different, except the CBA group relied less on health professionals. The repeated movements group had slightly more improvement on activity avoidance and greater satisfaction. Both interventions resulted in modest improvements over time (ie, 50% reduction) on the Roland Disability Questionnaire Scores and Northwick Park Neck Pain Scores. The repeated movement approach provides higher patient satisfaction overall, but the cognitive behavioral group is more cost-effective due to fewer (ie, 3 versus 4) treatment sessions.[645]

While further research is needed to determine the effectiveness of repeated movements in this classification, a multimodal strategy incorporating this concept may result in better outcomes. Schenk et al[436] described the use of repeated end range movements in the diagnosis and successful management of a patient with CR. Based on a directional preference and a goal of centralization, repeated movements were used in combination with exercises for cervical spine stabilization and neural mobilization.[436]

Extensive details of the diagnostic classification and management of persons with neck pain classified based solely on the patient's response to repeated end range movements are available from McKenzie and May.[422,433] General characteristics of subgroups (ie, extension and flexion) within the neck pain with radiating pain classification are presented below as an overview of the history and examination findings and matched intervention strategies based on the response to repeated movements.[433]

Repeated Movements—Extension Exercise Subgroup Classification

The clinical presentation for patients who have a directional preference or respond to extension-oriented loading strategies ranges from acute to chronic—with intermittent or constant symptoms and central or symmetrical symptoms—around the lower cervical spine. Patients may also have unilateral or asymmetrical symptoms in the neck with or without radiating pain into the scapula or upper arm. Some patients may have symptoms that extend below the elbow with or without paresthesia[422,433] that are aggravated by flexion activities such as prolonged sitting and eased with movement away from a flexed position or an activity such as walking. Sitting posture usually reveals a decreased lumbar lordosis and forward head. Extension ROM is limited; lateral flexion may be reduced bilaterally. Repeated protrusion or flexion (see Figures 6-21 and 6-24) increases, peripheralizes, or worsens symptoms, whereas repeated retraction and/or retraction extension (see Figures 6-25, 6-29, 6-30, 6-31, and 6-32) decrease, centralize, or improve symptoms and increase ROM. The response to examination procedures determines the appropriate initial intervention or loading strategy.[433] The majority of patients respond to sagittal plane (ie cervical retraction) procedures assessed and performed in sitting with more acute or severe presentations requiring a supine (see Figure 6-35) or an unloaded position. If the response to sagittal plane procedures is not obvious, or symptoms worsen in extension, lateral procedures (see Figures 6-33 and 6-34) are assessed.[433] Commonly prescribed extension exercises, patient and therapist assisted, are provided below as an introduction to progressive loading strategies. All patients do not progress through each level. The starting point is determined by the clinician with preference to patient procedures augmented by clinician procedures, as needed. The progression is determined by patient response.[433] Selected procedures are provided next. McKenzie and May[422,433] provided specific details and procedures for exercise progressions and management.

Intervention guidelines and end range exercises[422,433] for patients with central and symmetrical pain patterns include retraction in sitting (see Figure 6-25), retraction in sitting with patient overpressure (see Figure 6-30), retraction in sitting with clinician overpressure (see Figure 6-31), retraction and extension in sitting (see Figure 6-32), and postural correction and education. If the response to retraction in sitting is peripheralization, or the patient is unable to perform, similar procedures (see Figure 6-35) are performed in supine: retraction in supine with pillow as needed, retraction in supine with patient overpressure, retraction off the table, and retraction off the table with clinician overpressure. Exercises are performed 10 to 15 repetitions every 2 to 3 hours as long as symptoms do not peripheralize or get worse. Symptoms may initially increase centrally as part of the centralization process. All patients may need to be taught how to maintain retraction when moving from a lying position to sitting.[422,433]

Patients with unilateral symptoms may respond to sagittal plane procedures alone or may peripheralize. If sagittal plane procedures in sitting result in peripheralization, the next step is to perform sagittal plane procedures in supine.

If the response to sagittal plane procedures is not obvious, or symptoms worsen, lateral procedures (ie, lateral flexion or rotation) are performed.[433] Lateral movements are performed toward the side of pain. If the response is not positive, then movements to the opposite side are assessed. The suggested order for lateral movements is[433] repeated rotation or lateral flexion in sitting (see Figures 6-33 and 6-34) and repeated rotation or lateral flexion with patient or clinician overpressure in sitting (see Figures 6-33 and 6-34). Patients who do not have a positive response in sitting should be assessed in supine with repeated rotation or lateral flexion and patient overpressure as needed. The intervention is the movement direction that decreases, abolishes, or centralizes symptoms. These same exercises may be appropriate for cervical and upper thoracic extension mobility deficits.

A patient who presents with a lateral deviation, or shift of the head and neck to one side in either flexion, lateral flexion or rotation, or a combined deviation, usually have a lateral component sometimes called acute torticollis or wry neck.[433] Onset of the postural deformity is associated with neck pain. The patient is unable to bring the head and neck back to neutral due to pain. Any attempt to actively correct results in an increase in pain and either centralization or peripheralization of symptoms. If able to correct to midline, the patient typically cannot sustain the position. Symptoms may resolve in 3 to 4 days, but, if present longer, may require intervention.[433] If the patient peripheralizes with active motion testing or sagittal plane repeated movements, procedures in supine are attempted with careful monitoring of symptoms. Retraction, lateral flexion, or rotation in supine are assessed and progressed based on patient response. Patients presenting with lateral deviation of the head and neck may fit either classification of neck pain with mobility deficits or neck pain with radiating pain with the patient's response guiding the initial intervention.

Repeated Movements—Flexion Exercise Subgroup Classification

A flexion subgroup presentation is not common.[422,433] Patients may have anterior and posterior neck pain with or without swallowing problems. Examination findings include limited flexion, but full pain-free extension. Management involves exercises for repeated flexion in sitting and repeated flexion in sitting with patient overpressure (see Figure 6-29) repeated 10 to 15 times every 2 to 4 hours.

Not all patients who have a directional preference or initially centralize with repeated end-range movements have a favorable outcome. An increase or worsening of symptoms possibly suggests a poor prognosis for noninvasive management or additional testing is necessary for diagnostic classification and appropriate management. Patients with constant, cervicobrachial pain and nerve root signs and symptoms generally do not respond to a repeated movement strategy[433] and, as discussed earlier, may require a trial of some combination of MT, exercise, and/or ICT. If the response is inconclusive, additional testing or a brief trial of repeated movements may be needed to assign a diagnostic classification. Though clinical observation supports the continued use of repeated end movement for diagnosis and management, additional research is needed to determine the extent of its effectiveness in patients with neck pain.

Neck Pain with Radiating Pain Classification—Cervicobrachial Pain and Neuropathic Pain

Physical therapists must be able to differentiate between somatic referred and neuropathic pain (ie, sensitized peripheral nervous tissue), presenting as neck pain that is spreading down the arm. The differentiation of somatic referred pain from neuropathic pain begins with hypothesis generation during the history and continues through the examination until a treatment threshold has been met. While overlap exists between somatic and neuropathic complaints, the nature of the patient's symptoms and descriptors, such as the inclusion of burning pain, electric shocks, cold pain, itching, paresthesia, numbness, and tingling may raise the likelihood of neuropathic pain. When neuropathic pain is suspected, the self-report version of the Leeds Assessment of Neuropathic Symptoms and Signs (S-LANSS),[273] as discussed in Chapter 4, should be utilized. Jull et al[114] proposed the following signs and symptoms of sensitized peripheral nervous tissue:

- An antalgic posture to protect or de-tension sensitized nervous tissue, such as shoulder girdle elevation, adduction, and elbow flexion
- Active and passive movements that lengthen neural tissue, such as cervical lateral flexion away from the painful side
- Mechanical allodynia to palpation of neural tissue
- Provocative tests that suggest a local cause of the irritated neural tissue such as the ULNDT
- Clinical neurological examination including manual muscle testing, reflexes, sensibility to pinprick, light touch, vibration, and neural tissue palpation

Electromyography and nerve conduction studies may be useful. Jull et al[114] proposed that a clinical hypothesis can be made that a patient's arm pain is due to somatic referral when no evidence supports the presence of nerve conduction loss or mechanosensitive peripheral nerve tissue. Clinically, it is more likely that cervicobrachial pain may have varying components of neuropathic pain where the neuropathic component may be minor or subtle in some cases and very clear in other cases, rather than an all-or-none situation.[646] The physiological mechanisms of neuropathic pain are speculative, and further research and classification of the effectiveness management strategies are needed.[114]

Although CR is included in this population, studies examining the effectiveness of PT treatment for a mechanosensitive neural tissue component are limited, but promising. Coppieters et al[598] compared immediate effects of cervical mobilization and therapeutic ultrasound in 20 patients with subacute peripheral neurogenic cervicobrachial pain. Mobilization consisted of a contralateral glide mobilization of grades 1 to 4 sustained and low or high frequency at 1 or more cervical motion segments, including the level of segmental hypomobility in various positions of the ULNDT at therapist discretion. Outcomes were elbow extension ROM, symptom distribution, and pain intensity during the ULND median nerve test. For the mobilization group, elbow extension increased from 137.3 degrees to 156.7 degrees, area of symptom distribution decreased by 43.4%, and pain intensity decreased from 7.3 to 5.8. Differences were significant between groups and the ultrasound group showed no significant improvements.[598]

Another study using similar MT neural tissue techniques demonstrated short term improvement in pain versus no treatment. Allison et al[647] compared the effects of MT with neural tissue techniques (NT group) to MT of the thoracic spine and glenohumeral (GH) joint (MT indirect group) and a control (no MT or exercise) group in 30 patients with chronic cervicobrachial pain. Both MT groups had a home exercise component. The NT group received neural tissue techniques performed before the onset of pain that included the contralateral lateral glide technique in various ULNDT positions (see Figure 6-81), shoulder girdle oscillations in prone, and contract relax techniques into shoulder abduction and external rotation. Home exercises were contralateral cervical lateral flexion with the shoulder in abduction, and external rotation resting on the table in a flexed position up to 10 repetitions 1 to 3 times daily. Active shoulder abduction and external rotation movements were performed in supine. The MT indirect group received PA GH mobilization in neutral and increased positions of shoulder abduction in supine. Unilateral PA thoracic mobilization at T2 to T5 on the side of the pain was performed and progressed in grade, repetitions, and number of thoracic spine levels. Home exercises included pendulum, active-assisted wand exercises for external rotation in supine to first onset of pain, anterior and posterior shoulder stretches, and resistance band exercises into abduction and external rotation to first onset of pain. Both intervention groups had significant improvements in pain and disability, with the NT group having a significantly lower VAS score at 8 weeks.[647]

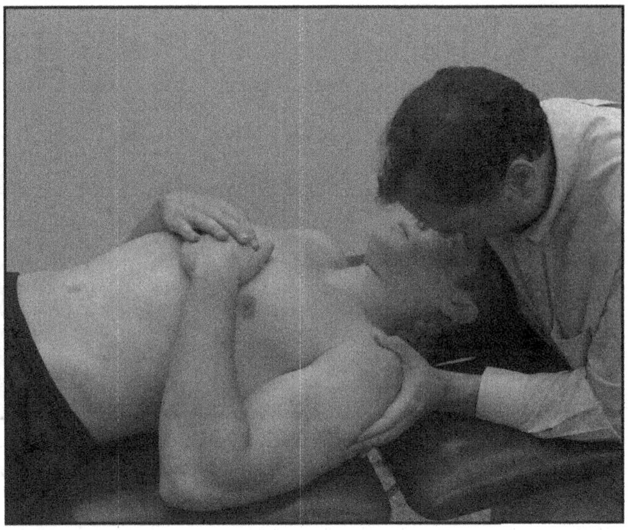

Figure 6-83. Contralateral cervical lateral glide to the right.

Initial outcomes for MT and neural tissue management of neuropathic neck and arm pain are positive, but how does neural tissue management alone compare to simple advice to remain active? Nee et al[648] randomized 60 participants with nontraumatic nerve-related neck and unilateral arm pain to an experimental (n = 40) or control (n = 20) group. The experimental group received education, MT, and nerve gliding exercises in 4 sessions over 2 weeks. Both groups were advised to continue usual activities. The MT group received a contralateral cervical lateral glide (C4 to C7; Figure 6-83), and a shoulder girdle oscillation combined with active craniocervical flexion to lengthen the posterior cervical spine (Figure 6-84) while attempting to glide the cervical nerve roots within the intervertebral foramina and spinal canal to reduce mechanosensitivity. A home program of neural mobilization, consisting of 10 to 15 repetitions 3 times daily on days they did not have treatment, included both sliding and tension techniques for cervical nerve roots and the median nerve. An example of a sliding procedure in standing in the ULNDT position is elbow and wrist flexion countered by cervical lateral flexion (see Figure 6-78). A sample tension procedure in the ULNDT position is elbow and wrist extension with contralateral cervical lateral flexion (see Figure 6-79). The procedures did not provoke the patient's symptoms. Only a gentle stretch or pulling sensation that resolved immediately after the exercise was allowed. The neural tissue management program related to progression and dosage is described in Nee et al.[649] Follow-up at 3 to 4 weeks after baseline was as follows: NNT favored the neural tissue group for participant-reported improvement (2.7, 95% CI: 1.7 to 6.5), neck pain (3.6, 95% CI: 2.1 to 10), arm pain (3.6, 95% CI: 2.1 to 10), NDI (4.3, 95% CI: 2.4 to 18.2), and Patient-Specific Functional Scale (3.0, 95% CI: 1.9 to 6.7). Adverse events of worsening in the

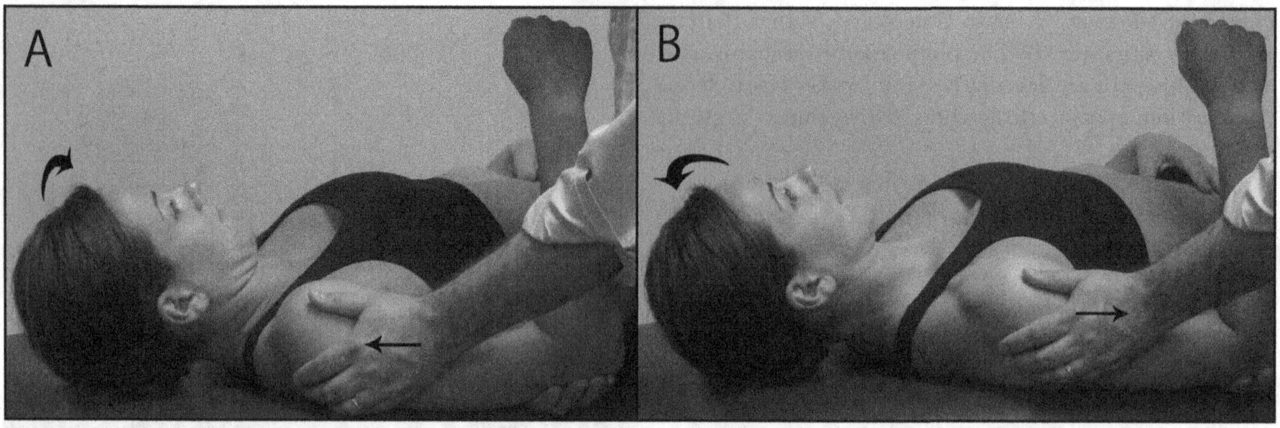

Figure 6-84. Shoulder girdle oscillation combined with active craniocervical flexion: (A) passive shoulder girdle elevation with active craniocervical flexion and (B) passive shoulder girdle depression as the patient return to neutral resting position.

experimental (13%) and control (20%) groups were not different and did not reduce the chance of improving with manual intervention (RR = 1.03, 95% CI: 0.58 to 1.84).[648] The authors conclude that physical therapists can inform patients that neural tissue management provides immediate clinically relevant benefits over advice to remain active with no harmful effects.[648,649]

Summary of Neck Pain With Radiating Pain Classification (see Table 6-4)

Current evidence reviewed the effects of MT, neural tissue management, exercise, and ICT for patients with cervicobrachial pain of somatic origin or neuropathic origin including CR. Evidence related to use of a repeated end range movement strategy is limited, but supported through clinical observation. The neck pain clinical practice guideline[15] recommends consideration of mechanical ICT combined with other interventions, such as MT and exercise, to reduce pain and disability in patients with cervicobrachial pain. Evidence since publication of the neck pain clinical practice guidelines[15] suggests that, in some patients, ICT provides no additional benefits to MT and exercise. A preliminary CPR provides support for a subgroup of patients with cervicobrachial pain likely to respond to ICT and exercise alone. In patients identified with chronic nerve-related neck and arm pain, preliminary evidence supports a 2-week, specific neural tissue management approach as effective in reducing neck pain and disability and improving function compared to advice to remain active in the short term.[649]

Neck Pain With Movement Coordination Impairments Classification

The neck pain with movement coordination impairment (MCI) classification is associated with the ICD, sprain, and strain of the cervical spine.[15] ICF categories are as follows: body functions—control of complex voluntary movement, body structure—ligaments and fascia of head and neck regions, and activities and participation—maintaining a body position, specified as maintaining alignment of the head, neck and thorax—such that the cervical motion segments function in a neutral or mid-range position.[15]

In order to classify a neck pain patient with MCI, information from the history includes neck pain and neck-related or referred upper extremity pain often precipitated by trauma or whiplash and symptoms of greater than 12 weeks.[15,25] Examination findings included the following[15,25]:

- Poor performance of the CCFT
- Poor performance of the deep flexor endurance test
- Coordination, strength, and endurance deficits of the neck and upper quarter muscles
- Flexibility deficits of upper quarter muscles
- Difficulty with performance of repetitive activities

Additional findings include absence of signs of nerve root compression and no centralization or peripheralization. ICF impairment terminology includes the following:

- Neck pain with mid-range motion that worsens with end range movements or positions
- DNF strength, endurance, and coordination deficits
- Neck and neck-related upper extremity pain reproduced with provocation of the involved cervical segments
- Cervical clinical instability may be present; however, muscle spasm adjacent to the involved cervical segment(s) may prohibit accurate testing[15]

Common interventions include general exercises for upper quarter impairments of strength, endurance, and specific motor control exercises. Two clinically used exercise regimes address impaired cervical flexor muscle performance: general strengthening exercises or head lift exercises[620,650] and a low-load program designed to focus on motor control and coordination between the superficial and DNF muscles and the quality of the craniocervical flexion movement.[114] The low load craniocervical program aims to improve DNF activation of the longus capitis and longus colli with minimal activation of the SCM and anterior scalene (AS; which flex the neck but not the head). The general strengthening or high-load program emphasizes activation of all muscles to produce a head lift.[508] Both the low-load and high-load exercises elicit similar EMG activation of the DNF when tested isometrically as a maximum voluntary contraction (MVC) and at 20% and 50% of MVC, but the high-load strategy elicits higher SCM and AS activation.[651] Most patients with neck pain, regardless of the initial classification, require assessment and intervention for muscle performance deficits for optimal recovery.

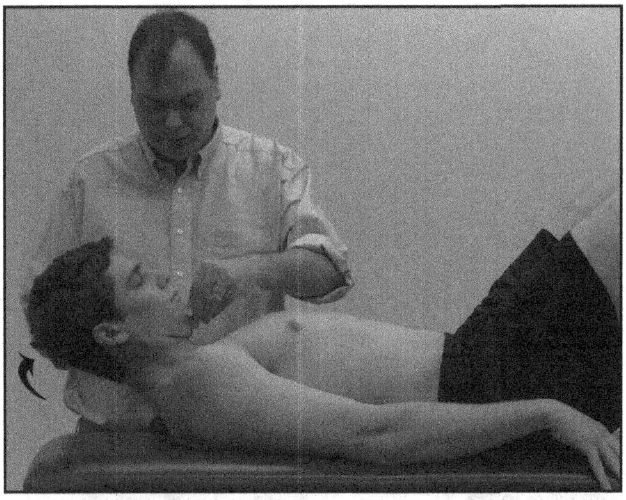

Figure 6-85. Neck flexion progression moving through full range of motion in supine.

Evidence to Support Therapeutic Exercise for Neck Pain With Movement Coordination Deficits

Retraining the DNF has been shown to decrease neck pain,[83,518] increase DNF performance during the CCFT,[87] and may enhance the ability to maintain an upright cervical spine posture.[89] Patients with neck pain tend to move into a forward head posture when distracted.[372] Falla et al[87] compared the effects of a low-load craniocervical flexion training program to a conventional neck flexor endurance-strength training program on functional control of head and neck posture (ie performing a 10-minute computer task) in 58 people with chronic neck pain with a NDI less than, or equal to, 15/50). Subjects ages 37.9 (SD = 10.2) years had symptoms more than 3 months (mean 7.9 years, SD = 6.4 years) and poor performance on the CCFT (ie inability to reach 24 mm Hg). Following baseline measures of posture, subjects were randomized to 2 exercise groups for training 1 day per week over 6 weeks. The low load group performed exercises twice per day, no longer than 10 to 20 minutes per day, and targeted the DNF over the superficial neck flexors using pressure biofeedback (Stabilizer) and progressively increased to 10-second holds for 10 repetitions at each level.[87] The neck flexor endurance-strength group performed a progressive resistance exercise program for neck flexion. Subjects maintained a neutral upper cervical spine while moving through a full ROM in supine (Figure 6-85). For the first 2 weeks, subjects performed 12 to 15 repetitions with a 12-repetition maximum weight followed by 4 weeks of progressing, as tolerated in 0.5 kg increments for 3 sets of 15 repetitions one time per day. If unable to perform the required repetitions, the subject was inclined up from the horizontal to allow the repetitions. After 6 weeks, average pain intensity and perceived disability were significantly improved for both groups. Only the low load craniocervical flexion group showed a significant improvement in ability to maintain an upright cervical spine posture. Possible associations between recurrent neck pain and posture over time warrant further research that may prevent neck pain in office workers.[87]

Exercise to retrain cervical spine muscle performance is effective in the long term for alleviating neck pain.[183,651] Ylinen et al[651] evaluated the efficacy of an intensive isometric neck strength training program compared to a lighter endurance training program on pain and disability in women with chronic neck pain. Female office workers, ages 25 to 53 years (n = 180), were randomly assigned to either 2 training groups (ie, endurance or strength) or to a control group. Over a 2-week period, each training session lasted for 45 minutes for 5 days per week, followed by a home exercise program. The endurance training group performed dynamic neck exercises, which included lifting the head up from the supine and prone positions for 3 sets of 20 repetitions. The strength training group performed high-intensity (ie, 80% of maximum) isometric neck strengthening and stabilization exercises with an elastic band in sitting for 15 repetitions forward, backward, and obliquely to the right and left. Both training groups performed dynamic exercises for the shoulders and upper extremities with dumbbells, including shrugs, presses, curls, bent over rows, flyes, and pullovers for 3 sets of 20 repetitions with a pair of 2 kg dumbbells and 1 set for each exercise with the highest possible individual load for 15 repetitions. All groups were advised to do aerobic and stretching exercises and squats, sit-ups, and back extension exercises regularly, 3 times a week. Both groups also received 4 sessions of massage, mobilization to decrease pain and improve ability to perform exercises, and behavioral support to reduce fear of pain and improve exercise motivation. The control group was advised to perform aerobic exercise and the same stretching exercises for 20 to

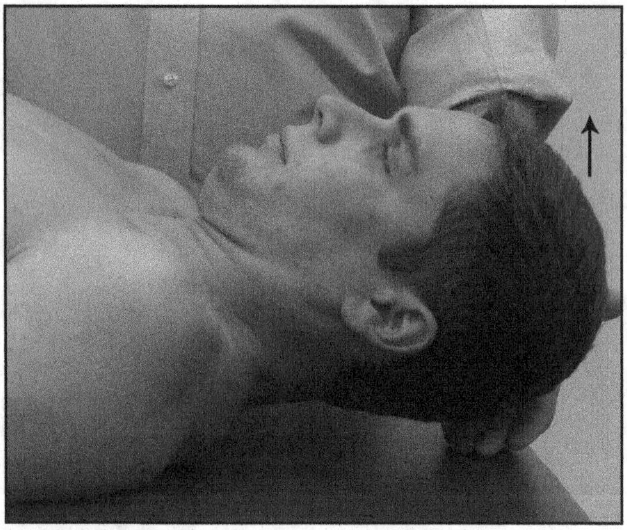

Figure 6-86. Head lift in supine.

30 minutes 3 times per week. Patients were followed at 2 months, 6 months, and 1 year. Disability and pain were significantly lower in the 2 training groups compared to the control with no between group differences. Analgesic use and health care visits also declined. Considerable or complete relief from pain was obtained by 73% in the strength training group, 59% in the endurance group, and 21% in the control group, with only 3% reporting a worsening due to training.[664] At 3-year follow-up, neck pain and disability, strength, ROM, and pressure pain threshold were statistically unchanged compared to the 12-month follow-up.[652]

Exercises targeting the DNF may also provide immediate changes in pain in patients with chronic neck pain.[518] O'Leary et al[518] examined the effects of 2 specific cervical flexor muscle exercise protocols on immediate cervical spine pain in persons with chronic neck pain of more than 3 months duration. Subjects (n = 48) were randomized to a craniocervical flexion (ie trains DNF) group or a cervical flexion endurance (ie trains all cervical flexors) group. The craniocervical flexion (DNF) group performed craniocervical flexion to a targeted, biofeedback level for 10 repetitions of 10-second holds (see Figure 6-53). The flexion endurance group performed a head lift in supine with the craniocervical spine in neutral no more than 2 cm above the support surface for 3 sets of 12 repetitions of 3-second holds (Figure 6-86). Immediately after 1 session of exercise, local pressure pain threshold (PPT) at the neck increased by 21% for craniocervical flexion group and 7.3% for craniocervical flexion endurance group (d = 0.61 to 0.88 and 0.14 to 0.47, respectively) with no changes in local thermal pain threshold and no changes in the leg. Only the CCF (ie DNF) exercise demonstrated a small, significant improvement in VAS ratings which was not clinically meaningful perhaps because baseline pain was only 1.4 to 1.6 on a 10 cm VAS. Targeting the DNF through craniocervical flexion exercise may provide immediate localized hypoalgesia to the neck with some perceived pain relief on movement in patients with chronic neck pain.[518]

Another study in patients with chronic neck pain supports the benefits of combined exercise of DNF and strength training. A comparison (of 145 patients randomly assigned to a 6-week exercise [n = 67]) and a nonexercise group (n = 78) was used to determine the efficacy of neck exercise in patients with chronic neck pain.[653] The exercise group received infrared irradiation, advice, and exercises, including DNF activation and dynamic strengthening, for 6 weeks. The control group received infrared irradiation and advice. The exercise group had significantly more improvement in disability score, subjective report of pain, and isometric neck muscle strength in most directions. At 6-month follow-up, significant differences between the 2 groups were maintained only in report of pain and patient satisfaction.[653]

Improvements in muscle function following exercise training seem to be task-specific and directly related to the type of exercise: low-load craniocervical flexion versus high-load endurance and strength training of all cervical flexors.[83,654] For example, after 6 weeks of low-load CCF muscle training, patients with neck pain showed a significant increase in DNF electromyographic (EMG) amplitude during a CCFT, a decrease in SCM EMG amplitude, and increase in craniocervical flexion ROM,[654] resulting in improved craniocervical test performance. Despite similar reductions in pain and disability between the 2 groups, patients who performed cervical flexor strength training did not demonstrate a similar improvement in CCFT performance.[654] After 6 weeks of cervical flexor endurance and strength training, Falla et al[88] report reduced SCM fatigue and an increase in cervical flexion strength in persons with chronic pain, whereas low load training had no effect on SCM fatigue or cervical flexion strength. In contrast, O'Leary et al[518] examined 2 6-week, 6-session exercise programs: specific DNF exercise and cervical flexion exercise using the head lift to compare the effectiveness in improving craniocervical flexion isometric performance in persons with mild neck pain and disability. Isometric craniocervical muscle performance can be retrained with either a specific craniocervical flexion exercise (ie DNF) protocol or a conventional craniocervical flexion exercise (ie. head lift) program in patients with more than 3 months of mild levels of reported neck pain and disability (NDI between 10 and 28/100). These results may not apply to patients with higher pain levels and disability.[548]

To further examine specificity of exercise training, Falla et al[508] compared low-load and high-load cervical muscle training using a similar protocol to Falla et al[71] to determine whether either training program changes muscle activation during a functional task in patients with chronic neck pain. After 6 weeks of training, EMG of the SCM was measured during a repetitive upper limb task. Both groups demonstrated reduced pain intensity, but no change in SCM activation, during the functional task. The authors recommend training the cervical muscles in functional postures and tasks important to the patient.[508]

Low-load training of the DNF is considered a specific motor control exercise designed theoretically to improve coordination between the superficial and deep systems and to improve the timing of DNF activation during functional movements. To determine the effects of low-load craniocervical flexion and neck flexor strengthening exercises on spatial and temporal characteristics of DNF activation, Jull et al[655] examined EMG activity during a neck movement task and a task challenging cervical postural stability. Forty-six subjects with chronic neck pain participated in a low-load or higher load program for 6 weeks. EMG activity was recorded from the DNF, SCM, and anterior scalene (AS) muscles pre- and postintervention during the CCFT and rapid, unilateral shoulder arm movements. The low-load program increased DNF EMG amplitude and decreased SCM and AS EMG amplitude across all stages of the CCFT. No change occurred in DNF EMG amplitude following high-load training. No significant between group difference was observed pre to post intervention in relative latency of DNF, but a greater proportion of the low-load group shortened the relative latency (ie DNF speed was enhanced) between the activation of the deltoid and the DNF during rapid arm movement compared to the strength group. Specific low-load CCF exercise changes spatial and temporal characteristics of DNF activation, which may partially explain its efficacy in rehabilitation. Both exercise groups had similar pain reduction.[655]

In addition to impairments in cervical muscle function, deficits in somatosensory function have been identified in patients with neck pain. Jull et al[656] compared the effects of proprioceptive training and craniocervical flexion (CCF) training on cervical joint position error (JPE) in patients with persistent neck pain. Joint position error is discussed in the examination section under Sensorimotor Control Tests. Sixty-four female subjects with persistent neck pain and deficits in JPE were randomized into 2 exercise groups: proprioceptive or CCF training for 6 weeks, 1 time per week. The CCF group performed low-load training of the DNF, as described by Jull et al.[86] Proprioceptive exercises included head relocation practice, gaze stability, eye following, and eye and head coordination. Relocation involves relocating the head back to the natural head posture and to predetermined positions within active ranges first with eyes open, then eyes closed, using feedback from a laser pointer (Figure 6-87) attached to the head.[112] Oculomotor exercises begin with eye movement with the head stationary and progressing to movements of the head with visual fixation on a target.[112] Eye and head coordination exercises

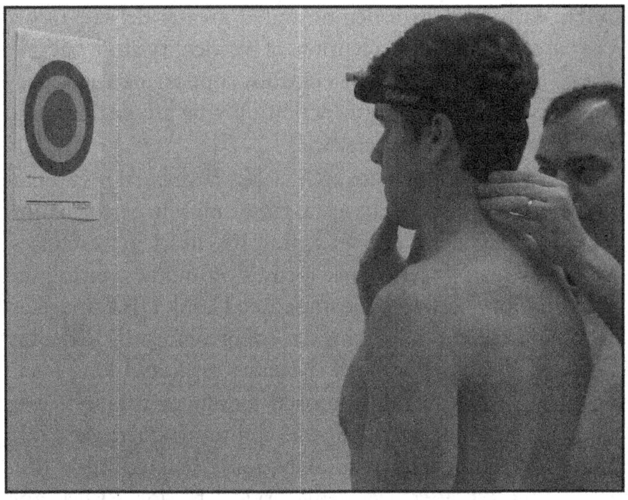

Figure 6-87. Proprioceptive exercises—head relocation.

begin with rotation of the eyes and head to the same side in both left and right directions. The patient practices leading with the eyes first to a target, followed by the head keeping the eyes focused on the target. As a progression, the eyes are moved first, then the head, to look between 2 targets positioned horizontally or vertically. Finally, the eyes and head are rotated to the opposite side in both the left and right directions and progressed by increasing the speed and range of movements and/or alteration of the visual target. Both groups demonstrated significant decreases in JPE, neck pain intensity, and perceived disability. Only the proprioceptive group training had a greater reduction in JPE from right rotation with no other significant differences observed between groups. The authors theorize that improved proprioceptive acuity may be due to improved quality of cervical afferent input or by addressing input through direct training of relocation sense.[656]

Abnormal afferent input from the somatosensory, visual, or vestibular systems can lead to altered sensory motor control and manifest as dizziness, unsteadiness in upright postures, and reduced control of head and eye movement.[91,94] To determine whether deficits in somatosensory function (ie balance, eye movement control, and proprioception) are present in elderly patients with neck pain, Uthaikhup et al[657] tested sensorimotor function in 20 elders with neck pain and 20 healthy elders, ages 65 years and older. Clinical tests included cervical joint position sense (JPS), computerized rod-and-frame test (RFT), smooth pursuit neck torsion test (SPNT), standing balance with eyes open, eyes closed on firm and soft surfaces in comfortable stance, step test, and the 10-m walk test (with and without head movement). Elders with neck pain had greater deficits in the SPNT, RFT (frame angled at 108 and 158 anticlockwise), standing balance (amplitude of sway)—eyes open on a firm surface in the mediolateral direction and total number of steps on the step test for both left and right sides.

Elders with neck pain demonstrated greater deficits in eye movement control, perception of verticality and balance when compared to healthy controls, supporting the theory that cervical afferent dysfunction may be a contributor to sensorimotor disturbances.[657]

In summary, 2 exercise approaches have been investigated to address impaired cervical flexor muscle performance: a high-load general strengthening (ie, head lift exercises) and a low-load strategy that focuses on motor control and coordination between the superficial and DNF muscles. Both approaches have similar effectiveness in reducing pain and disability in both the short term and long term. The low, load exercise approach enhances the ability to maintain upright posture, the ability to increase DNF EMG amplitude, decrease SCM and AS amplitude during the CCFT, increase craniocervical flexion ROM, and improve sensorimotor function. Cervical flexor strength and endurance training does not demonstrate a similar improvement in CCF test performance, but does reduce SCM fatigue and increase cervical flexion strength in persons with chronic pain, whereas low-load CCF training has no effect on SCM fatigue or cervical flexion strength. Neither exercise approach changes SCM activation during a functional task, indicating that training of cervical muscles should include functional postures and tasks.

Selected Exercises for Patients With Neck Pain With Movement Coordination Impairments

The exercise prescription is guided by identified cervicothoracic and regional impairments and integrated with other strategies of a multimodal approach, including manual techniques, AROM, and self-care. Based upon rapid changes in muscle properties and muscle activity in response to acute and chronic neck pain, Jull et al[658] offered basic principles for a specific exercise approach:

- Exercise begins early in the process and should not provoke pain.
- Exercises should address specific changes in muscle and sensorimotor function with emphasis on precision in the motor learning process.
- Training should be functional and task-specific.
- Repetition is necessary for appropriate movement and control.
- Patient education and adherence are vital components.[658]

The next section discusses exercises for both low-load and high-load training programs. The low load exercises are pain-free and can be introduced early in the plan of care, incorporating principles of motor learning and progression to functional exercises. Many exercises are performed initially in the same manner as tested during the examination. A detailed description to address neuromuscular impairments through a progressive motor learning and training program is described in Jull et al.[658] Exercises are prescribed to address a patient's individual impairments related to activity limitation. Not all exercises are appropriate for all patients.

Deep Neck Flexors

Training of the DNF begins in supine with craniocervical flexion (CCF) or head nodding (the ability to nod "Yes"; see Figure 6-53). The first step is correct performance of CCF or rotation of the cranium through activation of the longus capitis and longus colli without excessive activation of the superficial flexors. A diaphragmatic breathing pattern is preferred since upper costal breathing results in higher SCM activity.[509] CCF is performed pain-free and slowly with precision and control while palpating the SCM and AS for excessive activation. Common patterns of poor performance include the following:

- Cervical retraction
- Excessive SCM or AS activation
- Jaw clenching or jaw depression
- Breath holding or upper chest breathing
- Poor control by overshooting on return to neutral[658]

Cues such as "slide the back of your head up the table," "lengthen the back of your neck," or "look down as you begin to nod" may assist with correct performance. CCF performance during slow expiration reduces SCM activity in patients with upper chest breathing patterns[509] or diaphragmatic breathing exercises may be necessary. The patient may need instruction in the rest position of the mandible with the lips together, teeth slightly apart, and the anterior one third of the tongue resting on the roof of the mouth behind the upper incisors. Initial practice occurs 2 to 3 times per day for 10 repetitions, 10 seconds each.[658]

The next step is low-level endurance training of the DNF. Pressure biofeedback is used, starting at the pressure level at which the patient is able to perform CCF correctly, which is usually 20 to 22 or 24 mm Hg. The goal is to hold the pressure steady for 10 seconds with 10 repetitions toward a goal of 30 mm Hg.[183] Poor performance is indicated by fluctuation of the needle or inability to sustain the pressure. Practice is encouraged twice daily with training performed short of fatigue.[658] After practice with eyes open, patients close the eyes and attempt to relocate the position in preparation for practice at home. Supervised practice is necessary in addition to a home program.[658] When able to attain neutral upright posture, patients may progress to CCF in sitting or standing and train to ensure active CCF occurs rather than eccentric lowering by the cervical extensors.[585] Preliminary findings suggest that DNF training in sitting with an upright, neutral spinal posture and a neck lengthening maneuver improve the pattern of SCM activity during the CCF test, inferring

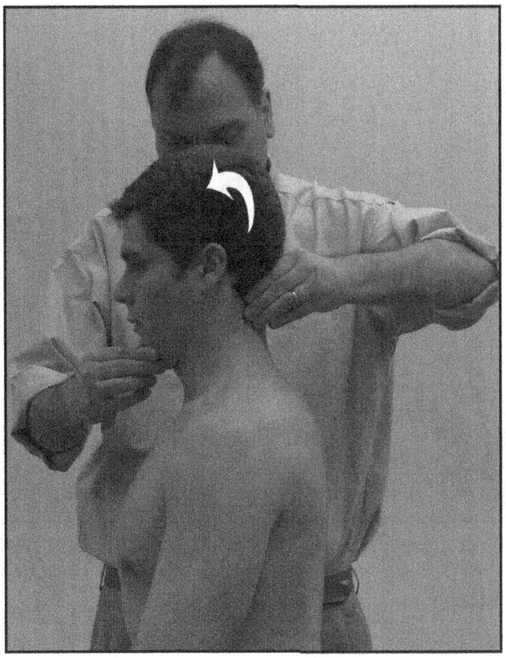

Figure 6-88. Deep neck flexor training in sitting—neck lengthening maneuver.

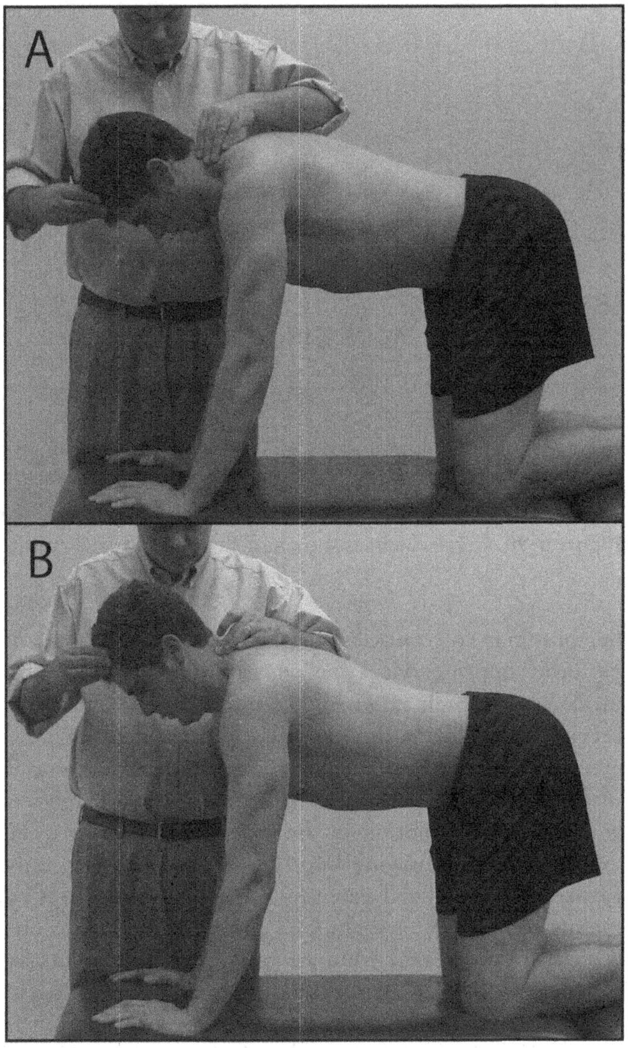

Figure 6-89. Deep neck extensor training in quadruped: (A) craniocervical neutral and (B) craniocervical extension.

an increase in DNF activation after training.[659] Exercise instruction includes cues to lengthen the cervical spine by gently lifting the base of the head from the top of the neck (Figure 6-88). Exercises are held for 10 seconds and performed every 15 to 20 minutes during the waking day. Exercises are supervised 2 times per week. DNF activation sitting is beneficial as an effective means of increasing practice and repetitions throughout the day as part of a motor learning approach.[659]

Deep Neck Extensors

Cervical extensors have a superficial group (splenius capitis [SpC] and semispinalis capitis [SCa] and a deep group, semispinalis cervicis [SCe] and multifidus [Mf]). The superficial group spans the entire cervical spine before attaching to the head and the deeper group spans only C2 to C7 vertebrae.[660] Impairments in the cervical extensors have been identified in patients with neck pain,[62,661-664] but little is known about extensor muscle activation during exercise or the best way to train cervical extensors. Using functional MRI, Elliott et al[665] examined isometric neck extensor muscle activity in healthy subjects during 2 different extension exercises. The extension exercises were performed in prone with the head in craniocervical neutral (CCN; Figure 6-89A) and craniocervical extension (CCE; Figure 6-89B) at 20% maximum voluntary contraction (MVC). Preliminary findings suggest that both deep and superficial extensor muscles are activated at 20% of MVC loads, but greater levels of superficial activity are observed when the exercise incorporates CCE, supporting a theory that the SCa is a primary extensor of the head and neck.[665]

O'Leary et al[660] compared the same exercise conditions as Elliott et al[665] in subjects with MNP and healthy controls. Compared with the healthy controls, less deep muscle (Mf/SCe) activity was observed in the Mf/SCe and SpC muscles lower in the cervical spine during the CCN exercise condition, suggesting the CCN exercise may be more useful for identifying extensor muscle deficits in patients with neck pain. The authors suggest the differences in patients with neck pain may represent a change in motor control strategy that warrants further study.[660]

Considering the results of the previous 2 studies,[660,665] Jull et al[658] described a protocol for initial training of the SO and neck extensor muscles in quadruped or prone-on-elbows or prone over a ball. For lower loads, patients can lean forward against a wall or counter top. Patients must first be able to attain a neutral spine posture in 4-point kneeling and an optimal scapular position. In this position, all cervical extensor muscles work to support the head and neck against gravity. To bias the craniocervical extensors

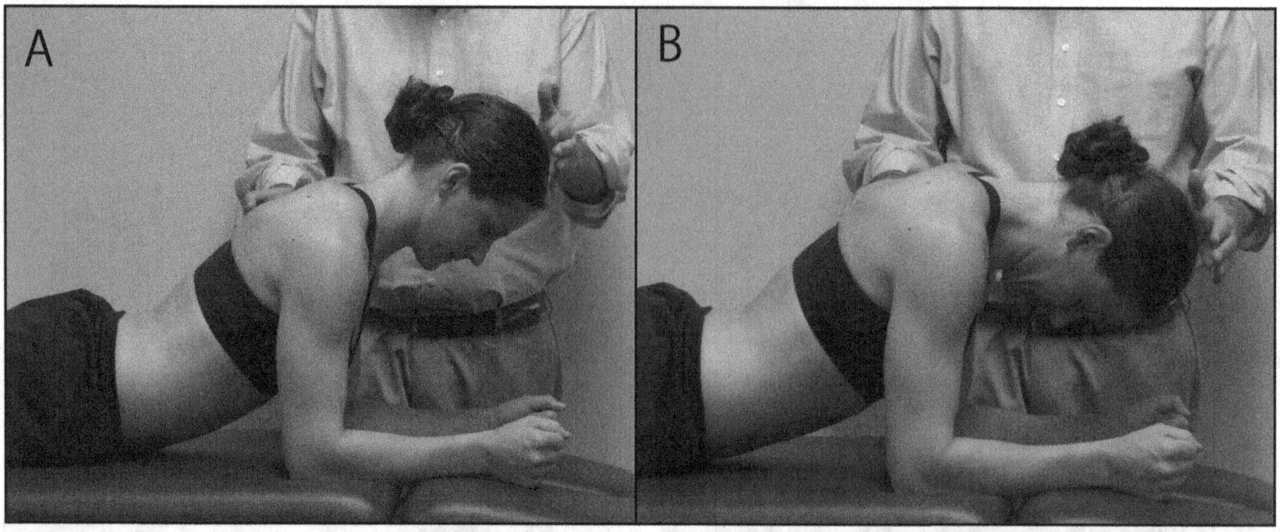

Figure 6-90. Cervical extensor training in prone: (A) start position and (B) eccentric lowering into flexion and return to neutral.

(ie, posterior SO muscles; see Figure 6-89), the patient performs upper cervical flexion, extension, and rotation 40 degrees to each side while keeping the mid and lower cervical spine in neutral. To bias the superficial cervical extensors (Figure 6-90), a neutral, upper cervical spine is maintained while the patient performs cervical extension with the axis of motion in the lower cervical spine. The exercise starts by moving into flexion and returning only to neutral. Superficial extensor activity is minimized by maintaining CCN or slight CCF and avoiding CCE. The exercise is progressed from neutral toward extension by instructing the patient to curl the head and neck backwards without lifting the chin. The range of extension is progressively increased. A small pain-free exercise dose of 5 repetitions in each direction as tolerated is initiated as long as quality of movement is maintained and progressed to 3 sets of 10 repetitions. The exercise may be progressed to include isometric contraction to train low-load endurance.[658]

If the patient is unable to perform in prone, cervical extensor training begins in supine with gentle 20% MVC isometric exercise. The position is the same for DNF training with the cervical spine in neutral. The patient gently presses the head into the table without CCE (ie, lifting the chin) and CCF while visualizing a curling back motion of the head and neck. The motion is not cervical retraction. The exercise is progressed to low-load sustained contraction for endurance training and then into the prone position.[658]

Active Postural Education[658]

The benefits of education and active practice of assuming a neutral, upright posture are discussed in the Lumbar Spine chapter and is inherently necessary for proper cervical spine posture. Patients are not instructed to sit up straight. Postural correction begins in sitting by first positioning the pelvis anteriorly to create a normal lumbar lordosis. Thoracic and cervical postures are then corrected as needed by a gentle lift of the sternum to reduce an increased thoracic kyphosis, or by a gentle depression of the sternum to relax an extended thoracic spine. Scapular position is addressed through manual cues and active correction. Cervical postural correction may be guided by asking the patient to lengthen the back of the neck by imagining a gentle occipital lift or lifting the occiput 1 mm off of the atlas.[658] A gentle occipital lift facilitates activation of the longus colli.[666] The specific components of postural correction may need to be practiced as individual skills. Patients are asked to repeat active postural correction as an exercise every 15 minutes throughout the day, holding for 10 seconds while continuing activities in sitting or standing.[658] To facilitate cocontraction of the DNF and deep neck extensors, self-resisted isometric exercises may be performed in sitting. The patient first assumes neutral spine posture and adds gentle resistance on the side of the head, using eye movement to facilitate the direction of rotation to both sides in a controlled slow activation of 10% of maximum.[658] Additional directions of extension, flexion, and lateral flexion may be added as needed.

Cervical Spine Extension Control[658]

In sitting or standing, cervical extension is initiated by cervical extensors and requires early eccentric control of the cervical flexors; movement on return to neutral trains concentric flexor control and is initiated by craniocervical flexors to facilitate activation of the DNF. Patients should be able to perform craniocervical flexion endurance exercises at 28 to 30 mm Hg as a prerequisite to cervical extension training. The patient is asked to look to the ceiling and follow it backward to slowly extend past the plane of the shoulder, staying in a pain-free range with good control and return to neutral, beginning with craniocervical flexion (Figure 6-91A). A return to neutral initiated with

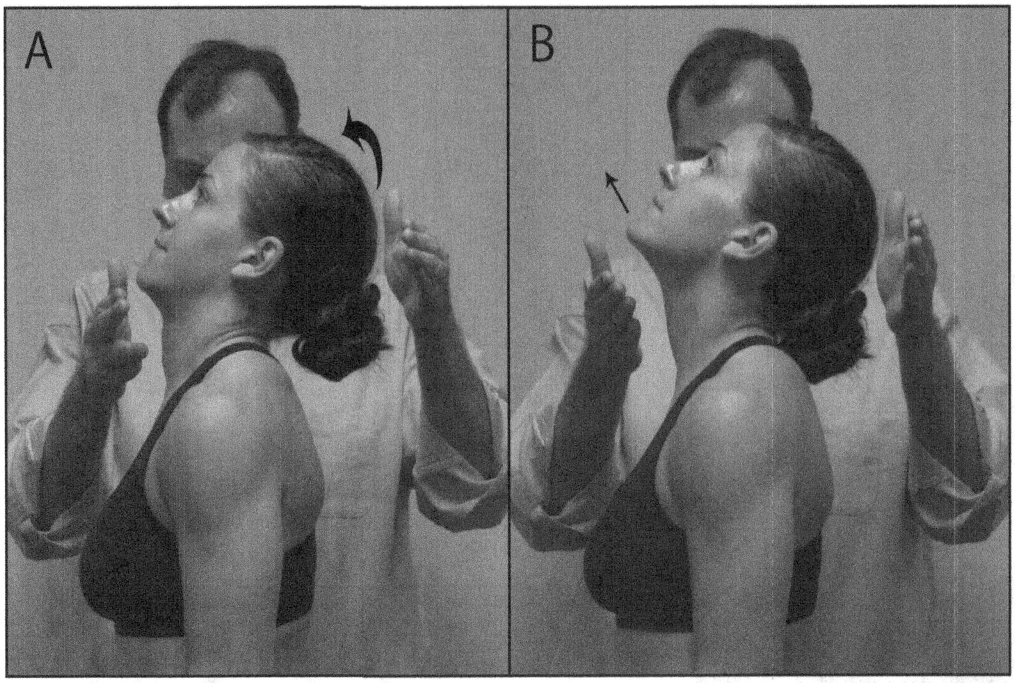

Figure 6-91. Cervical spine extension control in sitting: (A) return to neutral with craniocervical flexion and (B) return to neutral with upper cervical extension suggests deep neck flexor weakness.

upper cervical extension suggests DNF weakness (Figure 6-91B). The range of extension is gradually increased as control improves.[658] To begin strength and endurance training, isometric holds are added in different portions of the range. The clinician supports the head in extension and the patient relaxes. The patient then initiates a head lift by looking down with CCF and by just lifting the weight of the head off of the clinician's hand, holding for 5 seconds before returning to neutral. Repetitions are increased as well as increasing the range of extension requirements.[658]

Cervical Spine Control With Arm Movement[658]

As the patient regains control and endurance of the deep cervical muscles in supine and upright postures, progression begins, using upper extremity movement and loads required for functional activities or described as aggravating by the patient. Task-specific exercises, such as working at a computer (Figure 6-92) or daily home activities, are started using a small range of arm elevation. The patient maintains neutral upright posture and optimal scapular positioning during the task. Progression adds speed of movement or resistance to the arm movement and increases range of elevation based on the demands of the task.[658] Functional activities require the ability to maintain cervical spine neutral as well as to have segmental control during head and neck movements.[591]

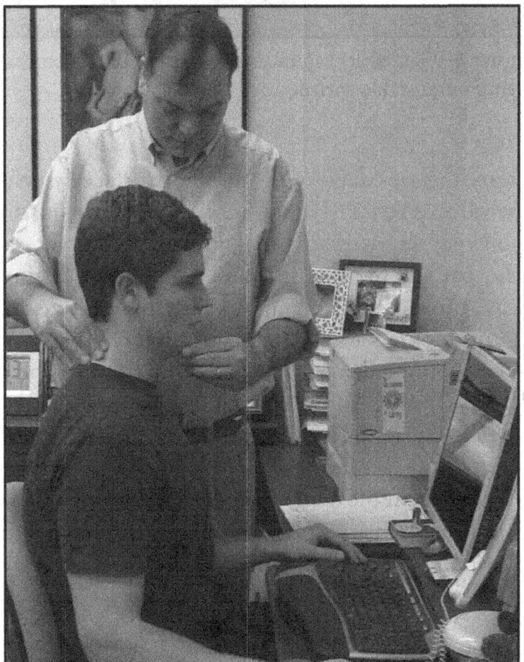

Figure 6-92. Cervical spine control with arm movement at computer.

Maintaining Cervical Spine Neutral With Arm Movement

Each patient begins in a position appropriate to their clinical presentation. Patients are instructed to begin in CCF to actively stabilize prior to extremity movement and repeat this exercise to work on timing. For endurance, a cervical neutral posture is maintained throughout the movements. Patients with poor control or an irritable presentation begin in supine on a mat and are progressed to half or full foam roll. Progression continues to sitting

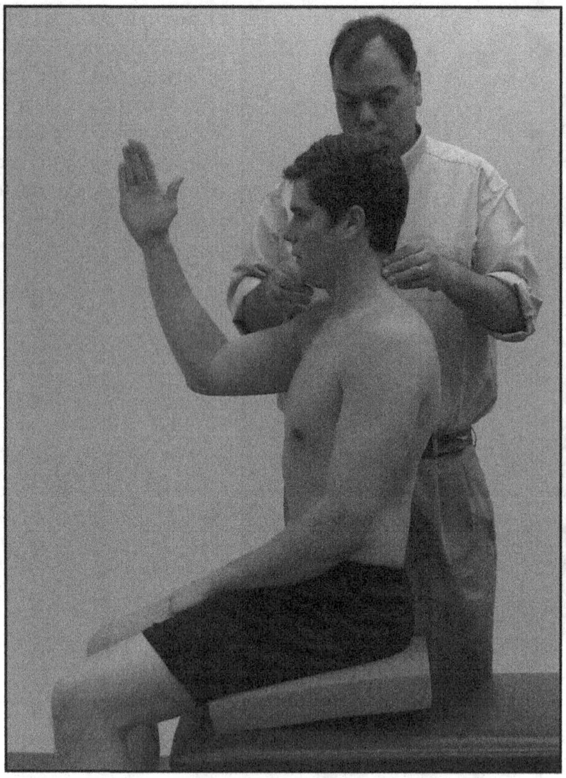

Figure 6-93. Cervical spine control with arm movement—sitting on unstable surface.

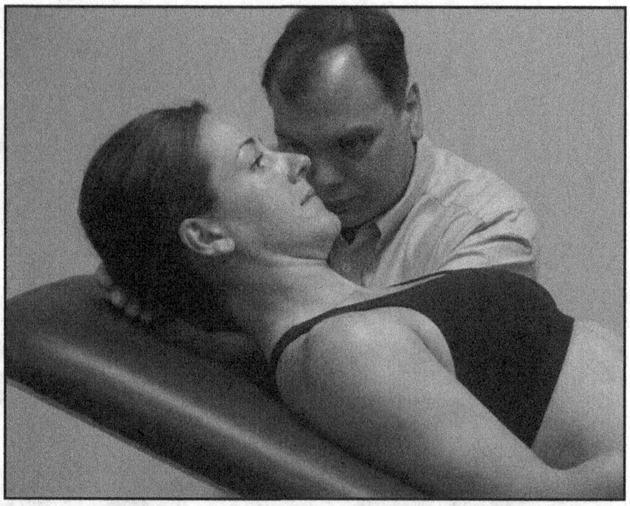

Figure 6-94. Deep neck flexor training on inclined surface.

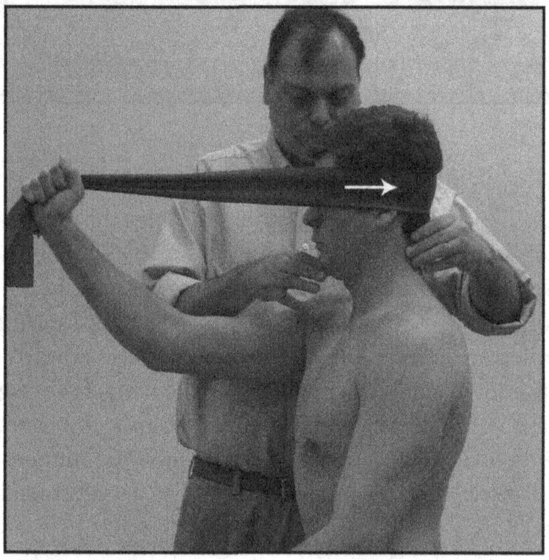

Figure 6-95. Extension strength training with elastic resistance.

and standing on stable and unstable surfaces, such as a ball or wobble board (Figure 6-93). Use of the quadruped position may be used to simulate work positions, requiring the patient to lean forward.[585] Patients begin with the least provocative arm movements (ie, below shoulder level) and progress to challenging spinal control. Bilateral arm elevation challenges anterior translation in the neck. Unilateral flexion or abduction challenge lateral neck translation. Speed of movement provides additional stress to maintaining cervical spine neutral. Setting the DNF prior to each arm movement emphasizes timing and motor control. Progression with resistance, using free weights or elastic bands, targets scapular stabilizers with emphasis on quality.[585]

Segmental Control with Active Range of Motion Exercise

Low-load exercises are initiated early in rehabilitation in nonweightbearing or supine, with pillow support if needed. Rotation is performed in supine, beginning with setting the DNF prior to controlling motion into rotation. Rotation and lateral flexion can be performed in standing with the head in contact with the wall as feedback to maintain the plane of motion and cervical spine neutral.[585] Segmental flexion and extension control were discussed previously in sitting and prone.

Strength and Endurance Training

Higher load progression strategies facilitate more superficial muscle activation and are not initially indicated for patients with high pain and disability levels or with long-standing bracing strategies.[585] Patient symptoms should be mild and stable prior to adding higher loads with age, gender, and functional requirements considered prior to initiation and slow progression to higher muscles forces to the cervical spine.[658] Jull et al[658] recommended training cervical flexor strength, beginning in supine with pillows. The patient sets the DNF prior to just lifting the head from the surface and holds for 1 to 2 seconds for 5 repetitions. Repetitions, sets, and hold time are used to progress. Pillows are removed so that the patient has to lift from a flat surface. An inclined surface is also used and gradually moved toward horizontal (Figure 6-94). Extension strength training in craniocervical neutral, using resistance bands, is performed in sitting, standing or quadruped (Figure 6-95). Patients who participate in general exercise and fitness programs should be observed for cervical spine control during these activities and adjustments made as needed.[658] As discussed above, the strengthening program designed by Ylinen et al[651,652] is an example of high-load strategy general exercise program.

Somatosensory Deficits

Exercises for patients with deficits in cervical proprioception, eye movement control, and balance include cervical relocation practice, eye following, gaze stability, eye-head coordination and balance.[658] Prescription is based on the level of impairment assessed during the examination, with exercises performed 2 to 3 times per day without provocation or worsening of symptoms. A temporary increase in dizziness to onset only may be allowed, but monitored closely.[658]

Cervical joint position sense is trained by cervical relocation practice, which involves relocating the head back to a neutral posture and to predetermined positions in all directions with eyes open and closed. A laser pointer attached to the head provides feedback (see Figure 6-87) with the patient positioned 1 m from a wall. The laser beam is lined up with a point on the wall, indicating the neutral head posture. The point is relocated after movement and progresses to following a moving target at a set speed, distance and repetition with eyes closed.[658] Tracing a figure or pattern on the wall combines eye and head control with position sense.[585]

Some patients with severe symptoms, such as pain or dizziness, may need to start in supine and progress to sitting and standing for eye movement control. Eye follow exercises keep the head still and move only the eyes to a target, such as a pen moving slowly side to side or up and down. Dosage begins at 10 seconds and progresses to 30 seconds of sustained practice (5 times per day).[658] Progression includes rotating the trunk 45 degrees, increasing the speed, moving to standing, or combining with balance exercises.[658] Gaze stability involves head movement while the eyes are fixed on a stationary object. The head is moved in all directions. Progression includes moving to standing, use of swimming goggles to restrict peripheral vision, increasing head movement speed, or focus on an object in a busy background. To simulate daily gaze stability needed for driving or shopping in a grocery store, gaze fixation is practiced in sitting or standing on an unstable surface, while walking and turning the head,[114] or tandem walking and turning directions.[585]

Examples of eye-head coordination exercise in sitting include (a) rotating the head and eyes together in the same direction (left and right and up or down), (b) moving the eyes first to focus on an object followed by the head, (c) moving the eyes first to focus between 2 objects followed by the head, and (d) moving the eyes and head in opposite directions.[658] Progression includes standing, increased speed, increased range of movements, and performance with balance exercise.[658] In standing, the start position may be comfortable stance, narrow base, tandem, or single leg stance, progressing from eyes open to eyes closed and stable to unstable surfaces. Walking is progressed in different directions while moving the head and increasing speed. Safety in balance training is important for home practice and for the elderly, whiplash disorders, and severe deficits.[658]

Summary of Neck Pain With Movement Coordination Impairments Classification

Therapeutic exercise to address neuromuscular deficits in patients with neck pain is necessary to provide optimal recovery since muscular impairments are generic to neck pain patients regardless of etiology. Current research supports a low-load, motor control approach and a high-load, general strengthening and endurance approach to reduce pain and activity limitations. A multimodal approach combining MT, exercise, and advice is supported for most patients, but the focus of the exercise program is guided by diagnostic classification, examination findings, and patient expectations and goals. A summary of neck pain with movement coordination impairments is provided in Table 6-3.

Neck Pain With Headache Classification

The neck pain with headache classification is associated with the ICD conditions: headache and cervicocranial syndrome.[15] ICF categories are as follows: (a) body functions—pain in the head and neck, (b) body structure—joints of the head and neck region, muscles of head and neck region, and (c) activities and participation—maintaining a body position, specified as maintaining the head in a flexed or an extended position.[15]

Clinical findings obtained during the history for neck pain with headache include noncontinuous unilateral neck pain and associated (ie, referred) headache, and headache precipitated or aggravated by neck movements or sustained positions. Examination findings include unilateral headache associated with neck and SO area symptoms aggravated by neck movements or positions, headache produced or aggravated with provocation of the ipsilateral or involved posterior cervical soft tissue and motion segments, restricted cervical ROM, restricted upper cervical segmental mobility, and poor performance on the CCF test.[12,15,25,183] ICF terminology impairment of body function includes headache reproduced with provocation of involved upper cervical segments, limited cervical ROM, restricted upper cervical mobility, and strength and endurance deficits of the DNF muscles.[15] Matched interventions include cervical mobilization and manipulation, muscle lengthening procedures, and coordination, strengthening, and endurance exercise.[15,667]

Differential Diagnosis

Fourteen different types and further subtypes of headache documented by the International Headache Society[668] make differential diagnosis a challenge. Tension-type headache has a global prevalence of 38%,[668] 10% with migraine,[668] and 2.5% to 4.2% with CGH.[669,670] Other headaches that may be amenable to PT are associated with occipital neuralgia and TMD disorders.[671]

The first step in diagnosis of a CGH is to exclude headaches due to a nonmusculoskeletal cause. Some serious or life threatening headaches (ie, tumor, meningitis, temporal arteritis, and carotid artery dissection) outside the scope of PT practice can mimic headaches that are appropriate for PT intervention. Therefore, a thorough history and physical examination are vital to reveal red flags that may identify serious pathology. A detailed description of differential diagnosis of headaches is available for review.[672] Red flags that may require referral to a medical specialist for additional testing include the following:

- Sudden-onset headache (ie, thunderclap)
- Worsening pattern of headache
- Change in pattern of previous headaches
- Fixed laterality
- Triggered by cough, exertion, or postural change
- Nocturnal or early morning onset
- New onset after age 50
- Systemic symptoms and signs (ie, fever, rash, and stiff neck)
- Seizures
- Papilledema or optic disc swelling
- Focal neurologic symptoms or signs other than typical visual or sensory migraine aura
- New pain level, especially when described as the worst ever
- Personality change or cognitive impairment
- No response to seemingly appropriate treatment[673]

CGH is thought to arise from a musculoskeletal dysfunction of the upper 3 cervical segments. Pain originating in the neck can be referred to the head or perceived as pain in the head by convergence of sensory afferents from the upper 3 cervical segments in the trigeminocervical nucleus, which descends in the spinal cord to the C3 to C4 level. Characteristics of headaches may assist with differential diagnosis, but some features are common among headache types.

The diagnostic utility of history taking in patients with headache is very limited. Detsky et al[674] developed a preliminary CPR relevant to the diagnosis of migraine headache. Five factors make up the CPR:

1. Is it a pulsating headache?
2. Does it last between 4 and 72 hours without medication?
3. Is it unilateral?
4. Is there nausea?
5. Is the headache disabling or disruptive of daily activities?[674]

If "yes" is the answer to 4 or more of the questions, the +LR is 24 (95% CI: 1.5 to 388); 3 out of 5 yes answers, +LR is 3.5 (95% CI: 1.3 to 9.2); 1 or 2 out of 5, +LR is 0.42 (95% CI: 0.32 to 0.52). The best predictors to assist with clinical decision making are the following descriptors: pulsating, duration of 4 to 72 hours, unilateral, nausea, and disabling.[674] Table 6-14 is a summary of clinical criteria[668,675] for CGH, tension-type headache (TTH), and migraine-type headaches.

After the history, the clinician plans the examination with consideration of SINSS and test procedures necessary to rule in or rule out competing hypotheses. Physical examination findings are not well defined in the clinical criteria section of Table 6-14. Neck pain is commonly associated with headache, and persons with chronic cervical musculoskeletal symptoms have a high prevalence of headache.[676] Two clinical criteria—reduced range of neck movement and pain elicited by external pressure over the occipital or SO region on the same side as the headache, are not specific to patients with CGH, meaning these findings could be present in persons with or without CGH. Considering that any structure innervated by the upper 3 cervical nerves is a potential source of headache, the physical examination must include the spinal motion segments, muscular system, and neural structures.[476]

Musculoskeletal impairments are present in patients with headache, but vary according to the headache type. The relationship between posture and CGH is unclear. Forward head posture was associated with CGH in one study,[57] but other studies found no differences among migraine, CGH, and persons without headache.[12,402] Static forward head posture is not predictive of response to PT.[103] Impairments of muscle length[80,402,511,677] and trigger points[677] have been associated with CGH. Sensorimotor disturbances, such as joint position sense are not different among persons with migraine, TTH, or CGH.[62]

In persons reporting a single type of headache, certain musculoskeletal impairments are characteristic of persons with CGH, but not TTH or migraine. Restricted ROM—with palpable upper cervical joint dysfunction from the occiput to C4 during PAIVM—and impairment in the CCF test demonstrated 100% sensitivity and 94% specificity to identify CGH and in distinguishing CGH

Table 6-14. Summary of Clinical Criteria of Cervicogenic, Tension-Type Headache, and Migraine[a]

CERVICOGENIC HEADACHE[683]	*TENSION-TYPE HEADACHE*[683]	*MIGRAINE WITHOUT AURA*[683]
A. Pain referred from the neck and perceived in 1 or more head regions and/or face, fulfilling C and D B. Clinical, lab, and/or imaging evidence of a cervical spine disorder known or accepted as a valid cause of headache C. Evidence that pain is due to a neck disorder based on at least 1 of the following: o Clinical signs that implicate a source of neck pain o Abolition of headache after diagnostic blockade D. Pain resolves within 3 months of successful treatment of the causative disorder	Episodic: • At least 10 episodes occurring <1 day/month on average (<12 days/year) and fulfilling criteria 2 to 4 Frequent episodic: • At least 10 episodes occurring on ≥1 but <15 days/month for at least 3 months • Headache lasts from 30 minutes to 7 days • Headache has at least 2 of the following: o Bilateral location o Pressing/tightening (nonpulsating) quality o Mild or moderate intensity o Not aggravated by routine activity (walking or stairs) • Both of the following: o No nausea or vomiting o No more than 1 of photophobia or phonophobia • Not attributed to another disorder	• Headache attacks lasting 4 to 72 hours (untreated or unsuccessfully treated) • Headache has at least 2 of the following: o Unilateral location o Pulsating quality o Moderate or severe intensity o Aggravations by or causing avoidance of routine activity (walking or stairs) • During headache at least 1 of the following: o Nausea and/or vomiting o Photophobia and phonophobia • Not attributed to another disorder • Having had at least 5 attacks of headache fulfilling these criteria
CERVICOGENIC HEADACHE[685]	*TENSION-TYPE HEADACHE*[683]	*MIGRAINE WITH AURA*[683]
A. Symptoms/signs of neck involvement: o Precipitation of the head pain similar to the usual occurring one: o By neck movement and/or sustained awkward head posture o By external pressure over the upper cervical or occipital region on the symptomatic side o Restriction of neck ROM o Ipsilateral neck, shoulder, or arm pain of vague nonradicular or occasionally radicular nature	Chronic • Headache occurring on > 15 days/month on average for > 3 months per year and fulfilling criteria 2 to 4 • Headache lasts for hours or may be continuous • Same as for episodic • Both of the following: o No more than 1 of photophobia, phonophobia, or mild nausea o Neither moderate or severe nausea or vomiting • Not attributed to another disorder	• At least 2 attacks of criteria B to D • Aura with at least 1 of the following but no motor weakness: o Fully reversible visual symptoms (flickering lights or loss of vision) o Fully reversible sensory symptoms (pins/needles, or numbness) o Fully reversible speech disturbance • At least 2 of the following: o Homonymous visual and/or unilateral sensory symptoms o At least 1 aura symptom develops over ≥5 minutes and/or different aura symptoms in succession over ≥5 minutes o Each symptom lasts ≥5 or ≤60 minutes

(continued)

TABLE 6-14 (CONTINUED). SUMMARY OF CLINICAL CRITERIA OF CERVICOGENIC, TENSION-TYPE HEADACHE, AND MIGRAINE

CERVICOGENIC HEADACHE[685]	*TENSION-TYPE HEADACHE[683]*	*MIGRAINE WITH AURA[683]*
B. Confirmatory evidence by diagnostic anesthetic blockades C. Unilaterality of the head pain without side shift For a CGH diagnosis, one or more aspects of point I must be present with Ia sufficient to serve as a sole criterion for positivity or Ib and Ic combined		• Headache fulfilling B to D for migraine without aura begins during aura or follows aura within 60 minutes • Not due to another disorder

ROM indicates range of motion; CGH, cervicogenic headache.

from migraine and TTH.[62] ROM was limited in extension and right and left rotation and SCM activation was significantly greater in the final 3 stages of the CCF test. In persons who report 2 or more intermittent headaches, Amiri et al[661] suggested that CGH can be differentiated with more confidence if a pattern of cervical musculoskeletal impairment involves symptomatic dysfunction in the upper cervical joints, restricted cervical motion, and DNF deficits identified by the CCF test. No differences in measures of cervical musculoskeletal impairment are present between control subjects and subjects with non-CGH.[661]

The presence of cervical musculoskeletal impairments was examined by Zito et al[12] in 27 subjects with CGH, 25 with migraine with aura, and 25 control subjects. The CGH group had significantly less range of cervical flexion and extension, significantly higher painful upper cervical joint dysfunction assessed manually, and muscle tightness of the UT, scalenes, SO extensors, and levator scapulae. Performance on the CCF test was not significantly different. No differences among groups were observed in static posture, pressure pain threshold over different cervical sites, neural tissue mechanosensitivity, and cervical joint position sense. Two measures—manual examination at C1 to C2 segment and pectoralis muscle length—discriminated the CGH group from the migraine and control subjects with 80% sensitivity.[12] Hall et al[479] studied the reliability of manual examination and frequency of symptomatic upper cervical motion segment dysfunction above C4. Manual examination using PAIVM and PPIVM shows good reliability with the C1 to C2 segment being the most symptomatic segment followed by C2 to C3 and occiput to C1.[479]

The cervical flexion rotation test (CFRT; Figure 6-96) is commonly used to identify C1 to C2 dysfunction. The CFRT is performed in supine with the cervical spine fully flexed. In this position, the range of rotation is about 40 to 44 degrees to each side.[678] Subjects with C1 to C2 dysfunction have significantly less rotation.[478,678] In differentiating subjects with CGH from asymptomatic controls or subjects with migraine with aura,[480] the CFRT has Sn (0.91) and Sp (0.90). The test is considered positive if the range is limited to 32 degrees or less.[478] In a more heterogeneous population, the CFRT demonstrated Sn (0.90), Sp (>0.88), and κ = 0.85.[476] Measurements of the CFRT are stable over time (2, 4, and 14 days), with a MDC of at least 7 degrees.[479] Comparison of CFRT mean ROM deficits to the involved side in subjects with CGH (25 degrees), migraine (42 degrees), and multiple headache forms (35 degrees) revealed clinically significant

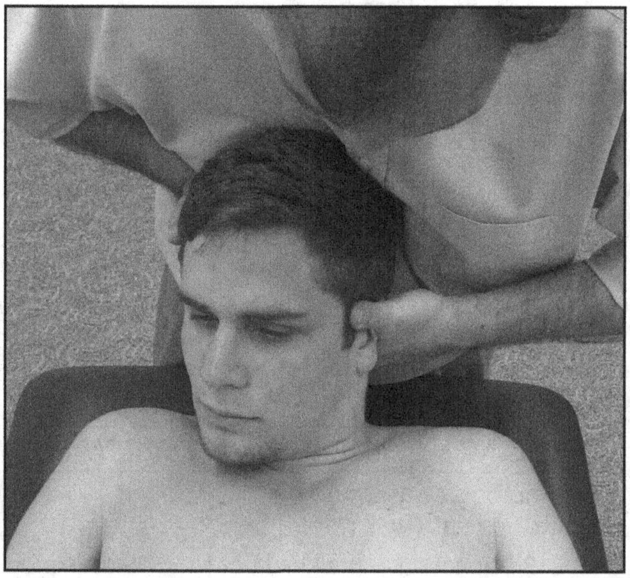

Figure 6-96. Cervical flexion rotation test.

differences, but a negative CFRT does not rule out the potential for CGH.[679] Migraine with or without aura appears to have minimal effect on ROM. ROM to the symptomatic side during the CFRT is significantly reduced in subjects with CGH when compared to subjects with migraine or multiple headache forms. The CFRT cutoff value for a positive test is ROM less than 30 degrees for differentiation among headache groups.[679]

The presence of neural tissue mechanosensitivity or peripheral nerve sensitization in persons with CGH is reported as a 7% to 10% incidence.[12] An antalgic posture of upper cervical extension with reduced upper cervical flexion that is worse in the long sitting position is a typical presenting pattern. In supine, passive upper cervical flexion is also reduced. Palpation of the lesser or greater occipital nerves or third occipital nerve is provocative. Neural tissue is implicated by repeating upper cervical flexion in supine with the arms positioned in abduction or the lower limbs in a straight leg raise position.[476] Hall et al[476] suggested that identification of a neural sensitization pattern is important since these patients may not respond adequately to joint mobilization and motor control exercise alone.

A pattern of restricted range of movement with palpable upper cervical joint dysfunction and impairment in the DNF provides a high degree of certainty to distinguish a CGH from migraine and TTH. Similarly, absence of these impairments suggests that a cervical musculoskeletal disorder is highly unlikely as the cause of a patient's headache. Current research has identified musculoskeletal impairments in persons with chronic TTH, such as muscle trigger points,[680] impairment of the DNF,[689] atrophy of the deep cervical extensors,[682] and sensitization of neural tissues.[683] Information from the history and physical examination provides support for a diagnostic classification of CGH, TTH, migraine and mixed presentations to guide initial intervention. The differentiation of headache types and the presentation of mixed headache forms require careful examination of the cervicothoracic motion segments, muscular system, and neural tissues and continued evaluation of the response to treatment. High quality randomized trials related to the effectiveness of MT and exercise for managing CGH or TTH are limited.

Evidence for Neck Pain With Headache and Matched Intervention

Systematic Reviews—Intervention

Systematic review[684] of the effectiveness of MT for CGH concludes that physiotherapy (consisting of spinal manipulative therapy and specific exercise and spinal manipulative therapy provided by chiropractors) might be an effective treatment. Despite mixed results, a review by Posadzki and Ernst[685] suggested that spinal manipulation is more effective in reducing headache frequency, intensity, and duration than PT (ie, electrotherapy, ultrasound, TENS), gentle massage, drug therapy, or no intervention. Based on a review of 3 randomized controlled trials of low quality, current research does not support the use of spinal manipulation for the treatment of migraine headaches.[686] For TTH, insufficient evidence exists to support or refute the efficacy of PT, exercise, or spinal manipulation.[687]

To help prevent chronic recurrent headaches, a Cochrane Review[688] concluded that, for migraine, spinal manipulation may be effective in the short term—similar to use of the drug amitriptyline. The Review also found weak evidence for the use of pulsating electromagnetic fields and TENS. For chronic TTH, amitriptyline is more effective than spinal manipulation. However, spinal manipulation is superior in the short term after cessation of both treatments. Therapeutic touch, cranial electrotherapy, TENS, and a combination of self-massage, TENS, and stretching may be effective for TTH. For episodic TTH, adding spinal manipulation to massage is not effective. For CGH, both spinal manipulation and low intensity endurance exercise may be effective. All treatments appear to be associated with little risk of serious adverse effects.[688]

Randomized Controlled Trials—Intervention

A preliminary CPR provides the potential to identify those patients with chronic TTH who are likely to experience short-term, 1-month follow-up success following muscle trigger point (TrP) therapy and low-load exercise training.[689] The probability of a successful intervention at one month follow-up increased from 54% to 87.4% (+LR = 5.9) for patients with all of the following variables:

- Less headache duration (ie, less than 8.5 hours per day
- Less headache frequency (ie, less than 5.5 days per week)
- Lower body pain assessed by the SF-36 questionnaire (ie, less than 47/100 points)
- Higher vitality SF-36 (ie, more than 47.5/100 points)[689]

Success was based on a 50% reduction on at least one headache variable of intensity, frequency or duration, and self-report perceived recovery. Patients received 6 sessions of TrP therapy that consisted of different approaches, such as pressure release, muscle energy, or soft tissue techniques, which were applied in order to inactivate active muscle trigger points. Additionally, patients performed a low-load exercise program for DNF and extensor muscles in a slow and controlled manner, using craniocervical flexion and extension (10 repetitions in each direction) daily. Additional studies with a larger sample size are needed for validation.[689]

Craniocervical flexion exercise, as part of a multimodal approach, including cervical mobilization, also appears effective for patients with TTH. The study was a multicenter randomized controlled trial with 81 patients classified as TTH (see Table 6-14) who were assigned to an exercise group (EG) and a control group (CG) for a 6-week intervention.[690] The EG received massage, postural correction, low-velocity cervical mobilization at the physical therapist's discretion, and a low-load endurance craniocervical flexion training (CCF) program. The CCF program consisted of craniocervical flexion exercises using a 150-cm elastic band for resistance. The elastic band was positioned at the craniocervical region of the patient's neck, with the other side fixed somewhat above the horizontal. While in sitting with a neutral spine posture, craniocervical flexion was performed, slightly elongating the cervical spine in a slow, controlled manner through various ranges of motion, resistance, and speeds incorporating isometric contractions. The exercises were performed twice daily for 10 minutes per session. The control group received massage, postural correction, and cervical mobilization, but not the CCF program. At 6 weeks, both groups showed significantly reduced headache frequency, duration, and intensity, but at 6 months only the EG showed significantly reduced headache frequency, intensity, duration, and reduced medication intake. In contrast at 6 months, the CG showed significant increase in headache parameters and no reduction in medication use.[690]

Research currently supports a role for spinal manipulation and exercise in the management of chronic CGH. A multicenter, prospective, and randomized controlled trial[183] examined the role of cervical manipulation and low-load exercise alone and in combination in the management of chronic CGH of moderate intensity versus a control group receiving no treatment. Two hundred subjects were randomized into 4 groups: manipulative therapy, exercise therapy, combined therapy, and a control group. Manipulative therapy consisted of both low velocity and high velocity techniques. Exercise consisted of low-load endurance exercises to train cervicoscapular muscles. Treatment consisted of 8 to 12 30-minute sessions over 6 weeks. Data were collected at baseline, 7 weeks and at 3, 6, and 12 months. Subjects and therapists were not blinded, but outcome assessors were blinded for collection of non-self-reported data. Outcome measures were change in headache frequency, headache duration and intensity, assessment of DNF muscle function, and medication usage. Compared to controls, all groups improved with regard to frequency and intensity. Manipulation plus exercise was superior to exercise alone in regard to headache duration. Only the groups receiving exercise demonstrated improved cervical muscle function.[183]

In addition to cervical mobilization and manipulation plus exercise, a sustained natural apophyseal glide procedure provides additional support for home exercise in the management of CGH. Hall et al[586] examined the effect of a C1 to C2 sustained natural apophyseal glide (SNAG; see Figure 6-74) on CGH in 32 subjects with CGH and a limitation in the cervical flexion rotation test (CFRT). Subjects were randomized to receive a C1 to C2 SNAG or placebo treatment. After 2 clinic sessions for instruction and practice, the C1 to C2 SNAG was performed for 2 repetitions, 2 times per day, as a home program. Outcomes were measured at 1 month and 12 months. Headache index scores improved significantly more in the self-SNAG group at 4 weeks and were maintained at 1 year. Self-report or treatment benefit favored the self-SNAG group over placebo treatment.[479] In persons with CGH and a positive CFRT, the C1 to C2 self-SNAG may be an effective home exercise component for self-management.[586]

Exercise programs that emphasize both strength and endurance and mobilization are effective in a mixed population of chronic headache types. Ylinen et al[691] compared the effectiveness of 3 12-month training programs on headache and upper extremity pain in patients with chronic neck pain. In this study, headaches were not classified, but persons who suffered from migraines more often than 2 times per month were excluded. One hundred and eighty female office workers were divided into 3 groups: (1) strength group (SG), (2) endurance group (EG), and (3) control group (CG)—with each group further divided by headache intensity. Each group began with a 2-day institutional rehabilitation program for instruction in a home exercise program of 5 45-minute sessions per week, with every other session performed at only half intensity to avoid overload. The EG exercised the neck flexor muscles by using a head lift in supine for 3 sets of 20 repetitions. The SG group pushed against an elastic band in the sitting position (forwards, backwards, and obliquely to the right and left) for 1 set of 15 repetitions. Both groups performed dynamic exercises consisting of dumbbell shrugs, presses, curls, bent-over rows, flys, and pullovers. The EG used a pair of dumbbells (2 kg each) and performed 3 sets of 20 repetitions for each exercise throughout the training period. The SG group used an individually adjusted single dumbbell for 1 set of 15 repetitions for each exercise at the highest possible load. Both training groups performed the same exercises in the same way for the trunk and leg muscles against their body-weight for a single series of squats, sit-ups, and back extension exercises. Each training session was completed by stretching for the neck, shoulder, and upper limb muscles. Both training groups also received 4 sessions of PT, consisting of massage and mobilization to reduce neck pain and to enable those with severe neck pain to perform the physical exercises effectively. The CG did aerobic exercise 3 times a week for 30 minutes and after instruction performed the same stretching exercise for 20 minutes at home with no additional treatments. All 3 groups exercised 3 times per week at home. Control visits to check SG and EG, and motivate participants to continue exercise training, were conducted after 2 and 6 months from the baseline assessment. At the 12-month follow-up, headache decreased by 69% in SG, 58% in the EG, and 37% in the CG compared to baseline. Neck pain diminished most in the SG with the most severe headache

(P < .001). Upper extremity pain decreased by 58% in the SG, 70% in the EG, and 21% in the CG. All 3 groups had decreased headache, but the CG with stretching alone was less effective than when combined with muscle endurance and strength training.[691]

Summary of Neck Pain With Headache Classification (see Table 6-2)

Criteria to assist with differential diagnosis of CGH, migraine, and TTH (according to the International Headache Society) are provided in Table 6-14. Additional clinical findings related to examination of the posture, cervicothoracic segmental motion, axioscapular muscle performance, and altered neurodynamics aid in the diagnosis of headache types appropriate for PT intervention and to guide overall management. While additional research is needed, current evidence supports the effectiveness of MT and therapeutic exercise for CGH headache and TTH.[183,586,684,685,687,689-691]

Whiplash-Associated Disorders Classification

Due to the potential for acceleration-deceleration mechanisms of injury, whiplash-associated disorders (WAD) usually occur during motor vehicle collisions (MVC), but are also known to occur during sporting events, such as skiing. The head and cervicothoracic regions may undergo large single or multiplanar motions, resulting in injury to associated spinal structures, such as bony elements, intervertebral discs, zygapophyseal joints, ligaments, muscles, and neural tissues. WAD is characterized as a complex and heterogeneous condition with a variety of clinical presentations related to motor, sensorimotor, and sensory deficits and psychological distress. Immediate onset of symptoms is common, but often symptoms are delayed up to 12 to 15 hours.[692] A primary complaint is neck pain that may refer to the head or extremities, interscapular, thoracic, or low back regions. Additional symptoms may include headache, visual disturbances, paresthesia, anesthesia, weakness, and poor balance, concentration, and memory.[103,693] Current research related to examination and treatment of acute, subacute, and chronic WAD is directed towards understanding the underlying mechanisms related to the physical and psychological impairments.[47,89,257,694-696] The initial classification for WAD into 4 groups is presented in Table 6-5, as described by the Quebec Task Force (QTF),[29] with WAD II being the most common classification, but outcomes of this group vary from full recovery at 6 months to persistent moderate or severe symptoms. Based on emerging evidence and a need to consider all aspects of WAD, a proposed adaptation to WAD II, including physical and psychological factors, is presented in Table 6-6.[295] Improved classification assists with focusing treatment strategies toward the underlying mechanisms to improve outcomes and prevent transition to a chronic state.[696]

Motor and Sensorimotor Impairments and Whiplash-Associated Disorders

Loss of cervical ROM is common to all patients with WAD within 1 month of injury.[40] Subjects who recover or report lesser pain and disability, as measured by the neck pain and disability index, regain cervical ROM within 2 to 3 months of injury.[89] However, subjects with persistent moderate or severe levels of pain and disability continue to show ROM deficits at 2 to 3 years.[275] Altered patterns of muscle activation in the cervical spine and shoulder girdle occur early, with greater deficits in those with higher levels of pain and disability[257] and persist in those with chronic symptoms as well as those who recover.[257,275] Structural changes of fatty infiltrates in both the deep and superficial cervical muscles are higher in subjects with WAD compared to asymptomatic controls.[697,698] The cause and relevance of these changes are unknown, but may represent deficits in motor function.[696] Impairments in joint positioning error are greater in patients with moderate or severe pain and disability and in patients with chronic WAD[89,102] with balance and eye movement control deficits present in patients with persistent WAD.[116,361] Patients with sensorimotor disturbances are also more likely to have complaints of dizziness.[116,369] Rehabilitation should be directed to identified impairments.[696]

Sensory Impairments and Whiplash-Associated Disorders

Sensory disturbances in both acute and chronic WAD are most likely central nervous system features of hyperexcitability or enhanced pain processing.[114,696] Pain thresholds to pressure, thermal, electrical, and light touch stimuli are decreased[35,699] and found locally over the area of injury and in remote uninjured areas, such as the upper or lower extremities.[35] While motor impairments are present, regardless of severity of pain and disability, sensory impairments are associated with high levels of self-reported pain and disability[696] and present very soon after injury.[35] Lower pain thresholds to pressure and thermal stimuli are present in areas remote to the cervical pain in chronic WAD, but not in idiopathic neck pain.[36,253,700] Likewise, widespread hyperaesthesia (ie, elevated detection levels) to vibration, thermal and electrical stimuli are present in WAD, but not idiopathic neck pain. The early onset of sensory hypersensitivity is associated with poor functional recovery,[260,275] poor responsiveness to PT,[47] impaired sympathetic vasoconstriction,[701] and stress-related factors.[701]

Psychological Factors and Whiplash-Associated Disorders

Psychological distress is present in acute and chronic WAD and includes affective disturbance, anxiety, depression, and behavioral problems, such as fear of movement[255] with ongoing distress associated with persistence of pain and disability.[696] Posttraumatic stress, however, is one factor that might be unique to patients with neck pain associated with WAD[696] with prognostic capability for poor functional recovery at 6 months and 2 years postinjury, as measured by the IES (see Figure 6-6).[40,258,275]

Consideration for Assessment in Whiplash-Associated Disorders

A detailed history is performed to rule out any red flag conditions and should include the NDI (see Figure 6-5) since higher levels of pain (ie, VAS greater than 7/10) and disability (NDI greater than 20/50) are features of prolonged recovery.[696] The IES should be included as a measure of posttraumatic stress. A score of greater than 26 at 6 weeks postinjury may indicate the need for a psychological referral.[702] Physical examination is performed as guided by the history. Other factors predictive of poor outcome, such as complaints of reduced cervical ROM and cold hyperalgesia, should be assessed.[114,696] A thorough description the patient's symptoms and nature of the pain are important. To identify neuropathic pain, use of the S-LANSS (see Figure 4-127) has shown that 20% of patients presenting with acute WAD have a predominantly neuropathic pain condition related to items of higher pain and disability,[703] such as burning pain in the neck, hyperalgesia to manual pressure, and electrical shock-like pain. Pressure algometry for mechanical pain threshold, cold hyperalgesia (such as time to pain threshold for ice application),[704] and the response to light touch to determine the presence of allodynia[696] can be included as sensory assessments, but validity of these sensory function tests is not agreed upon.[695] Assessment of cervical ROM, motor, and sensorimotor dysfunction of the cervical and shoulder girdle, and neurological examination were discussed earlier. Diagnostic classification may include a WAD grade according to the Quebec Task Force, with inclusion of the motor, sensorimotor, and sensory impairments as well as psychological factors. Poor prognostic indicators should be identified, such as high initial disability (NDI greater than 20/50), high initial pain scores (VAS greater than 7/10), education level, low self-efficacy, and cold sensitivity.[705]

Considerations for Management and Whiplash-Associated Disorders

For acute WAD, clinical guidelines advocate a supportive approach of patient education, reassurance, advice to remain active as usual, simple exercises as appropriate (ie, ROM, muscle reeducation),[702] and simple analgesics.[702,705] Motor Accidents Authority 2007 guidelines[702] do not recommend prescribed rest for more than 4 days, immobilization collars, spray and stretch, steroid injections, magnetic necklaces, and other interventions, such as Pilates, Feldenkrais, Alexander Technique, massage, and homeopathy. Additional research is needed to determine the best approach for acute WAD. Considering the complexity of patients with chronic WAD, a multidisciplinary approach may be required. Research is scarce relative to strategies for optimal PT management.[702]

A best practice review for the management of WAD during the acute (less than 2 weeks), subacute (2 to 12 weeks), and chronic (longer than 12 weeks) stages is summarized as follows.[705-707] Recommendations for interventions during the acute stage of WAD included the following[706]:

- Education alone does not provide a significant benefit, but oral and video information may be more effective than pamphlets
- Immobilization with a soft collar is less effective than active exercise and no more effective than advice to act as usual
- Active exercise results in reduced pain intensity and may improve ROM
- The use of pulsed electromagnetic field therapy and acupuncture are not supported
- Some evidence supports methylprednisolone infusion, but no firm conclusions are possible[706]

Current evidence does not provide support for early intervention over natural recovery in the acute phase since no early management approach has been shown to lessen the incidence of transition to persistent symptoms. However, in some patients, a delay between onset of injury and the start of therapy presents an increased risk to develop chronic symptoms.[707]

Recommendations for interventions for the subacute stage of WAD included the following:

- Supervised exercise may be more effective than unsupervised exercise in the short term.
- Earlier therapy appears more effective than later therapy.
- Fitness and aggressive work-hardening programs may be counterproductive or detrimental to recovery.
- An interdisciplinary approach of psychological counseling and exercise may be more effective in reducing pain and sick leave than passive therapy modalities.

- Interdisciplinary treatment may result in an earlier return to work.
- Some evidence supports thoracic and cervical joint manipulation in the short-term for pain relief and improved motion, but definitive conclusions cannot be made.
- Botulinum toxin injections do not appear to be more effective than placebo.[708]

Active exercise is recommended to decrease pain and increase motion in the subacute stage. In 25 subjects with subacute WAD, and 6 weeks after onset of the injury, Ask et al[519] compared the effectiveness of 2 exercise programs: (a) motor control training (MCT), and (b) general endurance and strength training (GEST) over a 6-week period for 6 to 10 sessions. The MCT group followed a motor relearning program.[86] The GEST group followed a modified program, according Ylinen et al.[651] Both exercise programs were described in detail earlier in this chapter. No statistically significant differences in any outcomes were noted between groups. About 50% of subjects in both groups showed a clinically important change in perceived disability at 6 weeks and at 1 year. For pain related variables, within group differences were noted at 6 weeks, but not at 1 year. The protocol lacked a comparison control group, but both programs resulted in similar improvements in the short and long terms, though a large proportion of subjects in both groups still had pain and disability at 1 year,[519] suggesting the possibility of additional impairments that were not addressed by exercise or subgroups 6 weeks after WAD.

Because sensory impairments are associated with high levels of self-reported pain and disability,[696] and present very soon after injury,[35] pain provocation from manual or exercise interventions may serve to maintain and prolong the central hypersensitivity, and delay or prevent recovery in the long term.[709] Patients with sensory hypersensitivity should be managed with care, avoiding pain provocation through graded activity levels slowly increased as tolerated by the individual.[658] The effects of spinal MT on cold hyperalgesia are unknown.[658] Pharmacological management has been suggested for pain hypersensitivity, but optimal pharmacological agents are not known.[98]

For patients classified as chronic WAD II with mean symptoms present for at least a year, Jull et al[47] conducted a prospective randomized controlled trial to compare the effectiveness of self-management to a multimodal PT intervention. Both groups emphasized nonprovocative management over 10 weeks. The PT group received between 10 to 15 PT sessions of low velocity mobilization techniques, low load exercises aimed at reeducation of the cervical flexors and extensors, and scapular muscles, incorporated into postural and function activities, retraining of kinesthetic sense, education, and ergonomic advice. The exercises were continued at home. The self-management group received a booklet about education of whiplash, assurance on recovery, the need to stay active, ergonomic advice, and a description of the exercise program to be performed twice daily. The multimodal PT group reported significantly greater reduction in neck pain and disability (effect size 0.48), perceived benefits of treatment, and perceived relief of symptoms on the VAS. No differences were noted in range of movement between groups. Both groups improved similarly by about 10 degrees in all planes. Significant improvement was also noted in the PT group for performance on the CCFT, but not in the self-management group, suggesting the need for skilled supervision of this exercise program. Preliminary subgroup analysis reveals that subjects with both widespread mechanical and cold hyperalgesia have the least improvement and discontinued the trial with persistent moderate neck pain and disability, which may indicate a poor response to PT management alone or the need for an alternative intervention. Despite the fact that a subgroup of patients showed the least improvement, an effect size of 0.48 warrants the use of PT in the management of patients with chronic WAD.[47]

Best practice recommendations for noninvasive interventions during the chronic WAD stage include the following[710]:

- Exercise programs are effective in reducing pain but not in the long term.
- Specific exercise protocols (as discussed above) appear to be effective, but more research is needed.
- The majority of studies support interdisciplinary intervention of PT and psychological counseling intervention.
- Evidence to support joint manipulation is insufficient.
- Limited evidence supports myofeedback training.
- Gestalt therapy, Rosen method bodywork, and craniosacral therapy are not supported.[710]
- Considering a review of surgical and injection-based interventions for chronic WAD, the strongest research supports radiofrequency neurotomy for whiplash-related pain, although the relief is not permanent.[711]

Different forms of exercise seem to be modestly effective in some patients with acute, subacute, or chronic WAD, suggesting that exercise prescription can be improved through specific dosage to address individual impairments.[712] Mobility exercises improve range of movement and control deficits, but do not improve activation patterns or endurance capacity.[660] Changes in cervical motor control and posture improve with low-load motor relearning rather than strength training.[87,655] Strength and endurance factors require higher load training.[88] Sensorimotor deficits, such as joint position error, require head relocation exercises[112] as opposed to muscle training programs. A trial currently in progress may provide answers for optimal dosage and specificity of exercise in chronic WAD.[713]

Neurophysiology of pain education appears to be a promising strategy to affect motor performance, disability levels, pain behavior, and pain thresholds—at least in the short term. An A-B-C single-case design, with 6 patients with chronic WAD I and II, studied the effects of only 2 sessions of neurophysiology of pain education.[714] At 6 weeks, a significant decrease occurred in kinesiophobia, the passive coping strategy of resting, self-rated disability, and photophobia. Significantly increased pain pressure thresholds and improved pain-free movement performance were observed for the Neck Extension Test and ULNDT.[714] All 6 patients improved significantly for the pain pressure threshold at the trapezius, whereas only 5 out of 6 improved in the lower extremity.

Acute and chronic WAD are both associated with augmented central pain processing, stress system responses, and motor and psychological factors. Exercise, education, reassurance, and advice to act as usual are the recommended interventions in the acute stage. MT, exercise, and interdisciplinary programs are emerging approaches that demonstrate benefits of decreased pain and disability in patients with chronic WAD without sensory hypersensitivity. The presence of mechanical and cold hypersensitivity and posttraumatic stress may require additional interventions.[696] Psychological factors, such as posttraumatic stress, may be involved in central hypersensitivity.[715] Cold pain hyperalgesia of thresholds less than 13°C predict a pathway to more severe pain and disability, meaning patients with higher pain and disability are more likely to show higher posttraumatic stress symptoms.[326] Fatty infiltrates in the cervical extensor muscles are higher in moderate to severe pain and disability compared to persons who recover or have mild disability at 3 and 6 months, demonstrating a link between structural muscle changes and transition to a chronic stage. The effect of pain intensity on muscle fatty infiltrate may be mediated by posttraumatic stress symptoms.[716] Physical, psychological, and nociceptive processes seem to be interrelated, leaving many questions related to intervention.[715] Further research is needed to determine the best interventions to address the complex and heterogeneous nature of WAD.

Surgical Management of Cervical Radiculopathy and Myelopathy

Degenerative changes in the cervical spine are often asymptomatic, but, in 10% to 15% of cases, may present as compression of the spinal cord or nerve roots as CM or radiculopathy.[23,717] Conservative care usually results in successful outcomes with surgical management reserved for patients with progressive neurological deficit and intractable pain. The goals of the surgery are decompression of the neural tissues, alleviation of pain, and prevention of deformity by maintaining or supplementing spinal stability. Many surgical techniques are available through anterior, posterior or circumferential approaches with or without fusion of the vertebrae[718,719] Descriptions of these procedures are available by Schenk and Wise.[719] Cervical spine surgical procedures are costly and associated with complications.

Nikolaidis et al[720] reported death rates range from 0% to 1.8%, with other complications, such as difficulty swallowing breathing, esophageal perforation, carotid or vertebral artery trauma or neutral tissue injury in 1% to 8% of patients and progression to a chronic pain status.

A Cochrane Review[720] compared only 2 trials related to the outcomes for cervical surgery and conservative management. The first trial compared surgical and conservative management for CR.[721] At 3 months postsurgery, the surgical group had superior outcomes in terms of pain reduction of 29% in VAS compared to physiotherapy, which had 19% reduction in VAS, or hard collar immobilization 4% reduction in VAS. No significant differences were observed among groups at 1 year for pain—with a 30% reduction in the surgical group, 17% in the physiotherapy group and 16% in the hard collar group. Surgically treated patients had better outcomes related to sensory loss at 4 months, but at 16 months there were no significant differences. These results confirm a short-term benefit from surgery compared with physiotherapy or immobilization in terms of pain relief with an apparent lack of treatment benefit at one year. The results of this study[721] are similar to a community-based epidemiological survey of 561 patients where a spontaneous symptomatic improvement within 5 years from the onset of symptoms was reported in 75% of patients with CR.[238]

The second trial of 68 patients with mild functional deficit, associated with CM, allocated patients by coin to surgery or conservative treatment.[722] No significant differences between surgery and conservative treatment were found at 3 years following intervention.[720] Reported success rates for anterior cervical discectomy and fusion are generally high (92%, 80%, and 65% for 1-level, 2-level, and 3-level procedures, respectively).[723] However, biomechanical studies show increased stress at the unfused adjacent segment resulting in degenerative changes above or below the level of the fusion.[723] The occurrence of symptomatic disease at adjacent segments has been analyzed by survey over a 10-year period, with incidence rates after fusion reported at a rate of 2.9% per year, or 25% total.[723] Galbraith et al[718] noted that the results of operative treatment for CM are generally better in patients who undergo early decompression. In 146 patients, Suri et al[724] observed significantly greater motor recovery after surgery in patients with symptoms less than 1 year compared to patients with longer duration symptoms.

The following is a comprehensive summary of the best evidence related to invasive management of neck pain. A review by Carragee et al[725] condensed evidence for injections and surgical treatment of neck pain in the absence of serious destructive, inflammatory, or neoplastic processes:

- "Intraarticular steroid injections or radiofrequency neurotomy for neck pain are not supported.
- Anterior cervical fusion or cervical disc arthroplasty for neck pain without radiculopathy or serious underlying pathology is not supported.
- Epidural or selective nerve root injections with corticosteroids is supported for short-term symptomatic improvement of cervical radicular symptoms, but the need or rate of open surgery for these patients may not decrease.
- Relatively rapid and substantial pain and impairments are reliably reduced 6 to 12 weeks after surgical treatment for radiculopathy, but it is not clear if the long-term outcomes are superior compared to nonoperative measures.
- In patients with neck without primary radicular pain, early results of cervical disc arthroplasty show similar early outcomes compared with anterior discectomy and fusion surgery with long term viability of the prosthesis not yet demonstrated.
- Testing has been inadequate to support surgery for upper cervical ligamentous injury after whiplash."[725(pS191)]*

The goals of cervical fusion are to decompress the neural tissues, alleviate pain, and prevent deformity by maintaining or enhancing spinal stability with an end result of loss of functional cervical ROM. A newer procedure of cervical disc arthroplasty (CDA) has similar goals, but in contrast, has a goal of preserving segmental motion. In the short term, outcomes for CDA are similar to anterior single level cervical discectomy with fusion.[726,727] Quan et al[728] reported on long-term outcomes for 21 patients who experienced 1 or 2 level CDA for radiculopathy. At 8 years' follow-up, the Bryan (Medtronic Sofamor Danek) cervical disc arthroplasty has favorable results for preserving of motion and satisfactory clinical outcome in the majority of cases. However, complications of heterotopic ossification in 48% of operated segments result in restricted range of movement of the prosthesis.[728] Within a 2-year follow-up of cervical disc arthroplasty and cervical fusion, the effectiveness and safety of both procedures appear to be similar.[729]

When degenerative changes in the cervical spine become symptomatic in the form of CR or myelopathy, conservative care usually results in successful outcomes with invasive procedures reserved for patients with progressive neurological deficits and intractable pain. Many surgical procedures are available (with not one approach known to be superior to another). These results of most research confirm a short-term benefit from surgery compared with conservative management of pain relief with similar outcomes observed at 1 year. In the presence of neurological deficits, motor recovery may be greater in patients who undergo early decompression surgery.

Postsurgical Rehabilitation

Evidence-based guidelines are lacking with respect to postsurgical rehabilitation. Communication with the surgeon related to the surgical procedure, precautions or guidelines for progression, follow-up surgical appointments, and expected outcomes from the surgeon's and patient's perspective are all necessary to plan an appropriate evaluation for the patient. The outpatient evaluation process is the same as discussed earlier in this chapter, keeping in mind the stage of tissue healing, severity, irritability, nature, stage and stability of the patient's presentation, and the patient's response to examination. An appropriate rationale for the plan of care, clinical reasoning process, and PT evaluation is individualized to each patient's needs.

Postoperative referrals for rehabilitation vary considerably from no rehabilitation to immediate postop rehabilitation, delay until fusion occurs, or on an as-needed basis. A standardized approach does not exist for postoperative surgery rehabilitation related to the cervical spine, and wide variation exists in outpatient rehabilitation evaluation and management strategies with no guidelines known to be superior to another. In the absence of research describing optimal criteria for postsurgical rehabilitation related to the cervical spine, the clinician relies on the clinical reasoning process, tissue healing, the surgical procedure, surgeon prescription, applied sciences, and the patient to guide clinical decision making.

Summary

Current evidence favors use of a diagnostic classification system that identifies subgroups of patients who are most likely to respond to specific interventions with the potential to maximize outcomes. Neck pain clinical practice guidelines (described by Childs et al[15] and linked to the ICF by incorporating ICF impairments of body function terminology) recommend the following subgroup classifications: (a) neck pain with mobility deficits, (b) neck pain with radiating pain, (c) neck pain with movement coordination impairment, and (d) neck pain with headaches. Whiplash associated disorders are described as a separate classification.

*Reprinted from *J Manipulative Physiol Ther*, 32(2), Carragee EJ, Hurwitz EL, Cheng I, et al, Treatment of neck pain. Injections and surgical interventions: results of bone and joint decade 2000-2010 task force on neck pain and its associated disorders, S176-S193, Copyright 2009, with permission from Elsevier.

Diagnostic classification that guides PT intervention is not a protocol. Subgroups are continually evolving based on emerging research. Not all patients will fit neatly into one classification or may not fit at all into the classification system. In this situation, clinicians utilize clinical reasoning to prioritize criteria and relevant impairments in deciding on the best initial individualized treatment. Continued assessment and reassessment of the patient's response to treatment provide additional criteria for reclassification and progression of treatment. Considering the complex nature of neck pain, patients will present with criteria from more than one subgroup and most likely require multimodal treatment.

Multimodal intervention could mean an interdisciplinary approach or one therapist. Self-report outcome measures should be assessed throughout the plan of care to determine treatment effectiveness and progression. Patient education, advice, and reassurance vary, but, where appropriate, a simple explanation should include: neck pain as a musculoskeletal problem without signs of a serious disorder, a good prognosis for recovery in general, and the importance of active participation and self-care. Preventative strategies for altering work or recreational activities may be helpful.[114] Education about pain physiology may be needed and relevant psychosocial issues should be addressed. Patients presenting with high severity and irritability are unlikely to tolerate a complete examination. In this population, PT management is initially directed toward pain relief, rather than provocative MT and exercise procedures. Pharmaceutical pain management in the acute pain state for patients with moderate or severe pain and neurogenic pain or central sensitization should be addressed with a medical professional. Neurological signs and symptoms must be carefully monitored. As the severity and irritability of a neck disorder lessen, additional testing provides an initial diagnostic classification. Using an evidence-based framework, individual patient management is guided by the initial classification, clinician expertise, and patient expectations, as well as the nature and extent of the impairments in the sensory, motor, and psychological systems.[11]

Recommendations of the neck pain clinical practice guidelines[15] include (1) combined cervical mobilization and manipulation with exercise are more effective in decreasing neck pain, headache, and disability than mobilization or manipulation alone, and (2) thoracic spine manipulation can be used for patients with primary complaints of neck pain and for decreasing pain and disability in patients with neck pain and associated arm pain.[15] Systematic review[610] on MT and exercise for neck pain suggested that, compared to no treatment, MT and exercise result in clinically important long-term improvements in pain, function, and global perceived effect, MT and exercise provide greater short-term pain relief than exercise alone, but not in the long-term for all outcomes in subacute and chronic neck pain with or without CGH, and MT and exercise are superior to MT alone for reducing pain and improving quality of life for chronic neck pain. Evidence related to MT and exercise for radiculopathy is limited. Acute and chronic WAD are associated with augmented central pain processing, stress system responses, motor, sensorimotor, and psychological factors. Exercise, education, reassurance, and advice to act as usual are the mainstays of acute intervention. MT, exercise, and interdisciplinary programs are emerging approaches that demonstrate benefits of decreased pain and disability in patients with chronic WAD without sensory hypersensitivity. The presence of mechanical and cold hypersensitivity and posttraumatic stress require additional research-based management strategies.[712]

Subgroup classification of patients with spinal pain continues to evolve based on current research. Not all patients fit neatly into one classification and some do not fit at all into a classification system. However, the process of diagnostic classification is necessary to ensure early appropriate care and to improve and sustain outcomes. The clinician continues to use an evidence-based framework and clinical reasoning process to prioritize criteria, classification, and relevant impairments in deciding on the best initial treatment for the individual patient. Continual assessment and reassessment of the patient's response to treatment guides treatment progression, targeting the patient's functional recovery.

The Appendix section provides case studies for each region (Appendices H and I—cervical pain) to illustrate the clinical reasoning framework. Each case study allows for practice taking a history and planning a physical examination. The data from the history and physical examination are then synthesized using current best evidence to determine appropriate diagnostic classification, prognosis, and initial management strategies. The case study process provides an opportunity to practice using clinical reasoning and an evidence-based framework.

References

1. Haldeman S, Carroll L, Cassidy JD, Schubert J, Nygren A. The Bone and Joint Decade 2000-2010 Task Force on Neck Pain and Its Associated Disorders: executive summary. *Spine.* 2008;33(4 suppl):S5-S7.
2. Bovim G, Schrader H, Sand T. Neck pain in the general population. *Spine.* 1994;19:1307-1309.
3. Côté P, Cassidy JD, Carroll L. The factors associated with neck pain and its related disability in the Saskatchewan population. *Spine.* 2000;25:1109-1117.
4. Côté P, Cassidy JD, Carroll L. The Saskatchewan Health and Back Pain Survey. The prevalence of neck pain and related disability in Saskatchewan adults. *Spine.* 1998;23:1689-1698.
5. Linton SJ, Ryberg M. Do epidemiological results replicate? The prevalence and health-economic consequences of neck and back pain in the general population. *Eur J Pain.* 2000;4:347-354.

6. Palmer KT, Walker-Bone K, Griffin MJ, et al. Prevalence and occupational associations of neck pain in the British population. *Scand J Work Environ Health.* 2001;27:49-56.
7. Côté P, Cassidy JD, Carroll lH, Kristman V. The annual incidence and course of neck pain in the general population: a population-based cohort study. *Pain.* 2004;112:267-273.
8. Holmstrom EB, Lindell J, Moritz U. Low back and neck/shoulder pain in construction workers: occupational workload and psychosocial risk factors. Part 2: relationship to neck and shoulder pain. *Spine.* 1992;17:672-677.
9. van der Donk J, Schouten JS, Passchier J, van Romunde LK, Venkenburg HA. The associations of neck pain with radiological abnormalities of the cervical spine and personality traits in a general population. *J Rheumatol.* 1991;18:1884-1889.
10. Jette AM, Smith K, Haley SM, Davis KD. Physical therapy episodes of care for patients with low back pain. *Phys Ther.* 1994;74:101-110; discussion 110-105.
11. Uthaikhup S, Sterling M, Jull G. Cervical musculoskeletal impairment is common in elders with headaches. *Man Ther.* 2009;14(6):636-641.
12. Zito G, Jull G, Sotry I. Clinical tests of musculoskeletal dysfunction in the diagnosis of cervicogenic headache. *Man Ther.* 2006:11:118-129.
13. Hogg-Johnson S, van der Velde G, Carroll LJ, et al. The burden and determinants of neck pain in the general population. Results of the Bone and Joint Decade 2000-2010 Task Force on Neck Pain and Its Associated Disorders. *Spine.* 2008;33(4S):S39-S51.
14. Carroll LJ, Hogg-Johnson S, van der Velde G, et al. Course and prognostic factors for neck pain in the general population. Results of the Bone and Joint Decade 2000-2010 Task Force on Neck Pain and Its Associated Disorders. *Spine.* 2008;33(Suppl):S75-S82.
15. Childs JD, Cleland JA, Elliott JM, et al. Neck pain: clinical practice guidelines linked to the international classification of functioning, disability and health. *J Orthop Sports Phys Ther.* 2008;38(9):A1-A34.
16. Di Fabio RP, Boissonnault W. Physical therapy and health-related outcomes for patients with common orthopaedic diagnoses. *J Orthop Sports Phys Ther.* 1998;27:219-230.
17. Borghouts JA, Koes BW, Bouter LM. The clinical course and prognostic factors of non-specific neck pain: a systematic review. *Pain.* 1998;77:1-13.
18. Hoving JL et al. Manual Therapy, Physical therapy or continued care by a general practitioner for patients with neck pain: a randomized controlled trial. *Ann Inter Med.* 2002;136:713-722.
19. Pransky G, Benjamin K, Hill-Fotouhi C, et al. Outcomes in work-related upper extremity and low back injuries: results of a retrospective study. *Am J Ind Med.* 2000;37:400-409.
20. Barnsley L, Lord S, Bogduk N. Clinical review: whiplash injury. *Pain.* 1994;58:283-307.
21. Bunketorp L, Nordholm L, Carlsson J. A descriptive analysis of disorders in patients 17 years following motor vehicle accidents. *Eur Spine J.* 2002;11:227-234.
22. Wright A, Mayer TG, Gatchel RJ. Outcomes of disabling cervical spine disorders in compensation injuries. A prospective comparison to tertiary rehabilitation response for chronic lumbar spinal disorders. *Spine.* 1999;24:178-183.
23. Teresi LM, Lufkin RB, Reicher MA, et al. Asymptomatic degenerative disk disease and spondylosis of the cervical spine: MR imaging. *Radiology.* 1987;164(1):83-88.
24. Ernst CW, Stadnik TW, Peeters E, Breucq C, Osteaux MJC. Prevalence of annular tears and disc herniations on MR images of cervical spine in symptom free volunteers. *EJR.* 2005;55:409-414.
25. Fritz JM, Brennan GP. Preliminary examination of a proposed treatment-based classification system for patients receiving physical therapy interventions for neck pain. *Phys Ther.* 2007;87:513-524.]
26. Guzman J, Haldeman S, Carroll L, et al. Clinical practice implications of the Bone and Joint Decade 2000-2010 Task Force on Neck Pain and Its Associated Disorders: from concepts and findings to recommendations. *Spine.* 2008;33(4S):S199-S233.
27. Bogduk N. Neck pain. *Aust Fam Phys.* 1984;13:26-30.
28. Bogduk N, McGuirk B. *Management of Acute and Chronic Neck Pain: An Evidence Based Approach. Pain Research and Clinical Management.* 1st ed. Philadelphia, PA: Elsevier; 2006:3-20. In: Misailidou V, Paraskevi M, Beneka A, Karagiannidis A, GOgolias G. Assessment of patients with neck pain: a review of definitions, selection criteria, and measurement tools. *J Chiropractic Med.* 2010;9:49-59.
29. Spitzer WO, Skovron ML, Salmi LR et al. Scientific monograph of the Quebec Task Force on Whiplash-Associated Disorders: redefining "whiplash" and its management. *Spine.* 1995;20:1S-73S.
30. International Association for the Study of Pain (IASP®). *IASP® Task Force for Taxonomy. Pain Terminology.* Seattle, WA: Author; 2004.
31. Wang WTJ, Olson SL, Campbell AH, Hanten SP, Gleeson PB. Effectiveness of physical therapy for patients with neck pain: an individualized approach using a clinical decision-making algorithm. *Am J Phys Med Rehabil.* 2003;82(3):203-218; quiz 219-211.
32. Sheather-Reid, Cohen M. Psychophysical evidence for a neuropathic component of chronic neck pain. *Pain.* 1998;75:341-347.
33. Kasch H, Stengaard-Pederson K, Arendt-Nielsen L et al Pain thresholds and tenderness in neck and head following acute whiplash injury: a prospective study. *Cephalalgia.* 2001;21:189-197.
34. Sterling M, Jull G, Vicenzino B et al. Characterisation of acute whiplash-associated disorders. *Spine.* 2004;29:182-188.
35. Sterling M, Jull G, Vicenzino et al. Sensory hypersensitivity occurs soon after whiplash injury and is associated with poor recovery. *Pain.* 2003;104;509-517.
36. cott D, Jull G, Sterling M. Sensory hypersensitivity is a feature of chronic whiplash-associated disorders but no chronic idiopathic neck pain. *Clin J Pain.* 2005;21:175-181.
37. Bovim G. Cervicogenic headache, migraine, and tension-type headache. Pressure pain threshold measurements. *Pain.* 1992;51:169-173.
38. Chien A, Eliav E, Sterling M. Hypoaesthesia occurs with sensory hypersensitivity in chronic whiplash: indication of a minor peripheral neuropathy? *Man Ther.* 2008;14(2):138-146.
39. Sterling M, Jull G, Vicenzino B et al. Physical and psychological factors predict outcome following whiplash injury. *Pain.* 2005;114:141-148.
40. Sterling M, Jull G, Kenardy J. Physical and psychological predictors of outcomes following whiplash injury maintain predictive capacity at long term follow-up. *Pain.* 2006;122:102-108.
41. Sterling M Jull G Wright A. The effect of musculoskeletal pain on motor activity and control. *J Pain.* 2001;2:135-145.
42. Vicenzino B, Collins D, Benson H, et al. An investigation of the interrelationship between manipulative therapy induced hypoalgesia and sympathoexcitation. *J Manipul Physiol Ther.* 1998;21:448-453.
43. Hoving J, Koes B, de Vet H et al Manual therapy, physical therapy or continued care by a general practitioner for patients with neck pain. *Ann Intern Med.* 2004;136:713-722.

44. Ylinen J, Takala E, Kautianen H et al. Effecct of long-term neck muscle training on pressure pain threshold; a randomized controlled trial. *Eur J Pain*. 2005;9:673-681.
45. Gracely R, Lynch S, Bennett G. Painful neuropathy: altered central processing maintained dynamically by peripheral input. *Pain*. 1992;51:175-194.
46. Devor M. Central versus peripheral substrates of persistent pain: which contributes more? *Behav Brain Sci*. 1997;20:446-447.
47. Jull G, Sterling M, Kenardy J, et al. Does the presence of sensory hypersensitivity influence outcomes of physical rehabilitation for chronic whiplash? A preliminary RCT. *Pain*. 2007;129:28-34.
48. Dall'Alba P, Sterling M, Treleavan J, et al. Cervical range of motion discriminates between asymptomatic persons and those with whiplash subjects. *Spine*. 2001;26:2090-2094.
49. Zwart JA. Neck mobility in different headache disorders. *Headache*. 1997;37:6-11.
50. Dvorak J, Froehlich D, Penning L, et al. Functional radiographic diagnosis of the cervical spine: flexion/extension. *Spine*. 1988;13:748-755.
51. Panjabi MM. The stabilizing system of the spine. Part II. Neutral zone and instability hypothesis. *J Spinal Disord*. 1992;5:390-396.
52. Panjabi MM, Lydon c, Vasavada A, et al. On the understanding of clinical instability. *Spine*. 1994;19:2642-2650.
53. Placzek JD, Pagett BT, Roubal PJ, et al. The influence of the cervical spine on chronic headache in women: a pilot study. *J Manual Manipul Ther*. 1999;7:33-39.
54. Vernon HT, Aker P, Aramenko M, et al. Evaluation of neck muscle strength with a modified sphygmomanometer dynamometer: reliability and validity. *J Manipul Physio Ther*. 1992;15:343-349.
55. Barton PM, Hayes KC. Neck flexor muscle strength, efficiency, and relaxation times in normal subjects and subjects with unilateral neck pain and headache. *Arch Phys Med Rehabil*. 1996;77:680-687.
56. Silverman JL, Rodriquez AA, Agre JC. Quantitative cervical floor strength in healthy subjects and in subjects with mechanical neck pain. *Arch Phys Med Rehabil*. 1991;72:679-681.
57. Watson DH, Trott PH. Cervical headache: an investigation of natural head posture and upper cervical flexor muscle performance. *Cephalalgia*. 1993;13:272-284.
58. O'Leary S, Jull G Kim M et al. Craniocervical flexor muscle impairment at maximal, moderate, and low loads is a feature of neck pain. *Man Ther*. 2007;12:34-39.
59. Jull G, Kristjansson E, Dall'Alba P. Impairment in the cervical flexors: a comparison of whiplash and insidious onset neck pain patients. *Man Ther*. 2004;9:89-94.
60. Airi M, Jull G, Bullock-Saxton J, et al. Cervical musculoskeletal impairment in frequent intermittent headache. Part 2: subjects with multiple headaches. *Cephalalgia*. 2007;27:891-898.
61. Chiu TT, Law E, Chiu TH. Performance of the craniocervical flexion test in subjects with and without chronic neck pain. *J Orthop Sports Phys Ther*. 2005;35:567-571.
62. Jull G, Amiri M, Bullock-Saxton J et al. Cervical musculoskeletal impairment in frequent intermittent headache. Part 1: subjects with single headaches. *Cephalalgia*. 2007;24:793-802.
63. Jull GA. Deep cervical flexor muscle dysfunction in whiplash. *J Musculoskel Pain*. 2000;8:143-154.
64. Falla D, Jull G, Hodges PW. Patients with neck pain demonstrate reduced electromyographic activity of the deep cervical flexor muscles during performance of the craniocervical flexion test. *Spine*. 2004;29:2108-2114.
65. Fernandez-de-las Penas C, Falla D, Arendt-Nielsen L, et al. Cervical muscle co-contraction in isometric contraction is enhanced in chronic tension type headache patients. *Cephalalgia*. 2008;28(7):744-751.
66. Johnston V, Jull G, Souvlis T, et al. Alterations in cervical muscle activity in functional and stressful tasks in female office workers with neck pain. *Eur J Appl Physiol*. 2008;103(3):253-264.
67. Lukasiewicz A, McClure P, Michener L, et al. Comparison of 3-dimensional scapular position and orientation between subjects with and without shoulder impingement. *J Orthop Sports Phys Ther*. 1999;29:574-586.
68. Nederhand MJ MJ, Hermens H, Izerman MJ, et al. Cervical muscle dysfunction in the chronic whiplash associated disorder grade 2: the relevance of the trauma. *Spine*. 2002;27:1056-1061.
69. Falla D. Jull G, Hodges PW. Feedforward activity of the cervical flexor muscles during voluntary arm movements is delayed in chronic neck pain. *Exp Brain Res*. 2004;157:43-48.
70. Falla D, Rainoldi A, Merletti R, et al. Spatiotemporal evaluation of neck muscle activation during postural perturbations in healthy subjects. *J Electromyogr Kinesiol*. 2004;14:463-474.
71. Falla D, Farina D, Graven-Nielsen T. Experimental muscle pain results in reorganization of coordination among trapezius muscle subdivisions during repetitive shoulder flexion. *Exp Brain Res*. 2007;178:385-393.
72. Ge HY, Arendt-Nielsen L Farina D, et al. Gender-specific differences in electromyographic changes and perceived pain induced by experimental muscle pain during sustained contraction of the upper trapezius muscle. *Muscle Nerve*. 2005;32:726-733.
73. Madeleine P, Leclerc F, Arendt-Nielsen L, et al. Experimental muscle pain changes the spatial distribution of upper trapezius muscle activity during sustained contraction. *Clin Neurophysiol*. 2006;117:2436-2445.
74. Falla D, Farina D, Kanstrup Dahl M, et al Muscle pain induces task-dependent changes in cervical agonist/antagonist activity. *J App Physiol*. 2007;102:601-609.
75. Svensson P, Wang K, Sessle BJ, et al. Associations between pain and neuromuscular activity in human jaw and neck muscles. *Pain*. 2004;109:225-232.
76. Uhlig Y, Weber BR, Grob D et al. Fiber composition and fiber transformations in neck muscles of patients with dysfunction of the cervical spine. *J Orthop Res*. 1995;13:240-249.
77. Gore DR, Sepic SB, Gardner GM, et al. Neck pain: a long-term follow-up of 205 patients. *Spine*. 1987;12:1-5.
78. Falla D, Farina D. Neural and muscular factors associated with motor impairment in neck pain. *Curr Rheumatol Rep*. 2007;9(6):497-502.
79. Elliott J, Jull G, Noteboom JT, et al. Fatty infiltration in the cervical extensor muscles in persistent whiplash-associated disorders: a magnetic resonance imaging analysis. *Spine*. 2006;31:847-855.
80. Treleaven J, Jull G, Atkinson L. Cervical musculoskeletal dysfunction in post-concussional headache. *Cephalalgia*. 1994;14:273-279.
81. Kristjansson E. Reliability of ultrasonography for the cervical multifidus muscles in asymptomatic and symptomatic subjects. *Man Ther*. 2004;9:83-88
82. Andary MT, Hallgren RC, Greenman PE, et al. Neurogenic atrophy of suboccipital muscles after a cervical injury: a case study. *Am J Phys Med Rehabil*. 1998;77:545-549.
83. Hallgren RC, Greenman PE, Rechtien JJ. Atrophy of suboccipital muscles in patients with chronic pain: a pilot study. *J Am Osteopath Assoc*. 1994;94:1032-1038.

84. McPartland JM, Brodeur RR, Hallgren RC. Chronic neck pain, standing balance, and suboccipital muscle atrophy: a pilot study. *J Manipul Physiol Ther.* 1997;20:24-29.
85. Falla D, Rainoldi A, Merletti R, et al. Myoelectric manifestations of sternocleidomastoid and anterior scalene muscle fatigue in chronic neck pain patients. *Clin Neurophysiol.* 2003;114:488-495.
86. Jull G, Falla D, Treleaven J, et al. A therapeutic exercise approach for cervical disorders. In: Boyling JD, Jull G, eds. *Grieve's Modern Manual Therapy: The Vertebral Column.* 3rd ed. Edinburgh, London: Elsevier; 2004:451-470.
87. Falla D, Jull G, Russell T, et al. Effect of neck exercise on sitting posture in patients with chronic neck pain. *Phys Ther.* 2007;87:408-417.
88. Falla D, Jull G, Hodges P, et al An endurance-strength training regime is effective in reducing myoelectric manifestations of cervical flexor muscle fatigue in females with chronic neck pain. *Clin Neurophysiol.* 2006;117:828-837.
89. Sterling M, Jull G, Vincenzino B et al. Development of motor dysfunction following whiplash injury. *Pain.* 2003;103:65-73.
90. Peterson BW. Current approaches and future directions to understanding control of head movement. Brain mechanisms for the integration of posture and movement. *Prog Brain Res.* 2004;143:369-381.
91. Heikkila H, Astrom PG. Cervicocephalic kinesthetic sensibility in patients with whiplash injury. *Scand J Rehabil Med.* 1996;28:133-138.
92. Karlberg M, Johansson R, Magnusson M, et al. Dizziness of suspected cervical origin distinguished by posturographic assessment of human postural dynamics. *J Vestibul Res Equil.* 1996;6:37-47.
93. Peterson B, Goldberg J, Bilotto G, et al. Cervicocollic reflex: its dynamic properties and interaction with vestibular reflexes. *J Neurophysiol.* 1985;54:90-108.
94. Revel M, Andre-Deshays C, Minguet M. Cervicocephalic kinesthetic sensibility in patients with cervical pain. *Arch Phys Med Rehabil.* 1991;72:288-291.
95. Thunberg J, Hellstrom F, Solander P, et al. Influences on the fusimotor-muscle spindle system from chemosensitive nerve endings in the cervical facet joints in the cat; possible implications for whiplash induced disorders. *Pain.* 2001;91:15-22.
96. Wenngren B, Pederson J, Sjolander P, et al. Bradykinin and muscle stretch alter contralateral cat neck muscle spindle output. *Neurosci Res.* 1998;32:119-229.
97. Le Pera D, Graven-Nielsen T, Valeriani M, et al. Inhibition of motor syste excitability at cortical and spinal level by tonic muscle pain. *Clin Neurophysiol.* 2001;112:1633-1641.
98. Curatolo M, Petersen-Felix S, Arendt-Nielsen L, et al. Central hypersensitivity in chronic pain after whiplash injury. *Clin J Pain.* 2001;17:306-315.
99. Seaman D. Dysafferentation: a novel term to describe the neuropathological effects of joint complex dysfunction: a look at likely mechanisms of symptoms generation: in reply. *J Manipul Physiol Ther.* 1999;22:493-494.
100. Passatore M, Roatta S. Influence of sympathetic nervous system on sensorimotor function: whiplash associated disorders (WAD) as a model. *Eur J Appl Physiol.* 2006;98:423-449.
101. Humphreys BK, Bolton J, Peterson C, et al. A cross-sectional study of the association between pain and disability in neck pain patients with dizziness of suspected cervical origin. *J Whiplash Relat Disord.* 2003;1:63-73.
102. Treleaven J, Jull G, Sterling M. Dizziness and unsteadiness following whiplash injury: characteristic features and relationship with cervical joint position error. *J Rehabil Med.* 2003;35:36-43.
103. Jull G Stanton W. Predictors of responsiveness to physiotherapy treatment of cervicogenic headache. *Cephalalgia.* 2005;25:101-108.
104. Rubin AM, Woolley SM, Dailey VM, et al. Postural stability following mild head or whiplash injuries. *Am J Otol.* 1995;16:216-221.
105. Hildingsson C, Wenngren BI, Toolanen G. Eye motility dysfunction after soft-tissue injury of the cervical spine: a controlled, prospective study of 38 patients. *Acta Orthop Scand.* 1993;64:129-132.
106. Gimse R, Bjorgen IA, Tjell C, et al. Reduced cognitive functions in a group of whiplash patients with demonstrated disturbances in the posture control system. *J Clin Exp Neurophsychol.* 1997;19:838-849.
107. Tjell C, Rosenhall U. Smooth pursuit neck torsion test: a specific test for cervical dizziness. *Am J Otol.* 1998;19:76-81.
108. Treleaven J, Jull G, Low Choy N. The relationship of cervical joint position error to balance and eye movement disturbances in persistent whiplash. *Man Ther.* 2006;11:99-106.
109. Michaelson P, Michaelson M, Jaric S, et al. Vertical posture and head stability in patients with chronic neck pain. *J Rehabil Med.* 2003;35:229-235.
110. Field S. Treleaven J, Jull G. Standing balance: a comparison between idiopathic and whiplash-induced neck pain. *Man Ther.* 2008;13(3):183-191.
111. Poole E, Treleaven J, Jull G. The influence of neck pain on balance and gait parameters in community dwelling elders. *Man Ther.* 2008;13(4):317-324.
112. Revel M, Minguet M, Gregoy P, Vaillant J, Manuel JL. Changes in cervicocephalic kinesthesia after a proprioceptive rehabilitation program in patients with neck pain: a randomized controlled study. *Arch Phys Med Rehabil.* 1994;75:895-899.
113. Mergner T,Schweigart G, Botti F, et al. Eye movements evoked by proprioceptive stimulation along the body axis in humans. *Exp Brain Res.* 1998;120;450-460.
114. Jull G, Sterling M, Falla D, Treleaven J, O'Leary S. *Whiplash, Headache, and Neck Pain. Research-Based Directions for Physical Therapies.* New York, NY: Churchill Livingstone; 2008.
115. Hildingsson C, Toolanen G. Outcomes after soft-tissue injury of the cervical spine: a prospective study of 93 car-accident victims. *Acta Orthop Scand.* 1990;61:357-359.
116. Treleaven J, Jull G, Low Choy N. Smooth pursuit neck torsion test in whiplash associated disorders- relationship to self-reports of neck pain and disability, dizziness and anxiety. *J Rehabil Med.* 2005;37:219-223.
117. Treleaven J, Low Choy N, Jull G, et al. Comparison of postural control disturbance between subjects with persistent whiplash associated disorder and subjects with vestibular pathology associated with acoustic neuroma. *Arch Phys Med Rehabil.* 2008;89(3):522-530.
118. Sackett DL, Rennie D. The science of the art of the clinical examination. *JAMA.* 1992;267(19):2650-2652.
119. Bogduk N. The anatomy and pathophysiology of neck pain. *Phys Med Clin N Amer.* 2011:22(3):367-382.
120. Nordin M, Carragee EJ, Hogg-Johnson S, et al. Assessment of neck pain and its associated disorders. Results of the bone and joint decade 2000-2010 task force on neck pain and its associated disorders. *Spine.* 2008;33(4S):S101-S122.
121. Abdu WA, Provencher M. Primary bone and metastatic tumors of the cervical spine. *Spine.* 1998;23(24):2767- 2777.
122. Bohlman HH, Sachs BL, Carter JR, Riley L, Robinson RA. Primary neoplasms of the cervical spine. Diagnosis and treatment of twenty-three patients. *J Bone Joint Surg [Am].* 1986;68:483-493.

123. Harrington KD. Metastatic disease of the spine: current concepts review. *J Bone Joint Surg [Am]*. 1986;68:1110-15.
124. Rao S, Davis RF. Cervical spine metastases. In: Editorial Committee, eds. *The Cervical Spine*. 3rd ed. Philadelphia, PA: Lippincott-Raven Publishers, 1998;603-18. In: Abdu WA, Provencher M. Primary bone and metastatic tumors of the cervical spine. *Spine*. 1998;23(24):2767-2777.
125. Aebi M. Spinal metastasis in the elderly. *Eur Spine J*. 2003;12(suppl 2):S202-S213.
126. Jenis LG, Dunn EJ, An HS. Metastatic disease of the cervical spine. A review. *Clin Orthop*. 1999;359:89-103.
127. Kovach SG, Huslig EL. Shoulder pain and Pancoast tumor: A diagnostic dilemma. *J Manipulative Physiol Ther*. 1984;7(1):25-31.
128. Goodman CC, Snyder TEK. *Differential Diagnosis for Physical Therapists. Screening for Referral*. St. Louis, MO: Saunders; 2007.
129. Henschke N, Maher CG, Refshauge KM. Screening for malignancy in low back pain: a systematic review. *Eur Spine J*. 2007;16(10):1673-1679.
130. Deyo RA, Diehl AK, Cancer as a cause of back pain: frequency, clinical presentation, and diagnostic strategies. *J Gen Intern Med*. 1988:3(3):230-238.
131. Acosta FL Jr, Chin CT, Quinones-Hinojosa A, Ames CP, Weinstein PR, Chou D. Diagnosis and management of adult pyogenic osteomyelitis in the cervical spine. *Neurosurg Focus*. 2004;17(6):E2.
132. Schimmer RC, Jeanneret C, Nunley PD, Jeanneret B. Osteomyelitis of the cervical spine: a potentially dramatic disease. *J Spinal Disord Tech*. 2002;15(2):110-117.
133. Barnes B, Alexander JT, Branch CL Jr. Cervical osteomyelitis: a brief review. *Neurosurg Focus*. 2004;17(6):E11.
134. Gouliouris T, Aliyu SH, Brown NM. Spondylodiscitis: update on diagnosis and management. *J Antimicrob Chemother*. 2010;65(Suppl3):iii11-24.
135. Modic MT, Feiglin DH, Piraino DW, et al. Vertebral osteomyelitis: assessment using MR. *Radiology*. 1985;157:157-166.
136. Heller CA, Stanley P, Lewis-Jones B, et al. Value of x ray examinations of the cervical spine. *BMJ*. 1983;287:1276-1278.
137. Johnson MJ, Lucas GL. Value of cervical spine radiographs as a screening tool. *Clin Orthop*. 1997;340:102-108.
138. Davenport M. Cervical spine fracture in emergency medicine. *Medscape Reference*. http://emedicine.medscape.com/article/824380-clinical. Accessed January 16, 2012.
139. Leucht P, Fischer K, Muhr G, Mueller EJ. Epidemiology of traumatic spine fractures. *Injury*. 2009;40(2):166-172.
140. Stiell IG, Wells GA, Vandemheen KL. The Canadian C-spine Rule for radiography in alert and stable trauma patients. *JAMA*. 2001;286:1841-1848.
141. Stiell IG, Clement CM, McKnight RD, et al. The Canadian C-spine Rule versus the NEXUS low-risk criteria in patients with trauma. *New Engl J Med*. 2003;349:2510-2518.
142. Kerry R, Taylor AJ. Cervical arterial dysfunction: knowledge and reasoning for manual physical therapist. *J Orthop Sports Phys Ther*. 2009;39(5):378-387.
143. Lee VH, Brown RD JR. Mandrekar JN, Mokri B. Incidence and outcomes of cervical artery dissection: a population-based study. *Neurology*. 2006;67(10):1809-1812.
144. Touze E, Randoux B, Meary E, Arquizan C, Meder JF, Mas JL. Aneurysmal forms of cervical artery dissection: associated factors and outcome. *Stroke*. 2001;32(2):418-423.
145. Hart RG, Easton JD. Dissections of cervical and cerebral arteries. *Neurol Clin*. 1983;1(1):155-182.
146. Rivett DA. The vertebral artery and vertebrobasilar insufficiency. In: Boyling JD, Jull GA, eds. *Grieve's Modern Manual Therapy: The Vertebral Column*. Edinburgh, UK: Churchill Livingstone; 2005:257-273.
147. Rubenstein SM, Peerdeman SM, van Tulder MW. Riphagen I, Haldeman S. A systematic review of the risk factors for cervical artery dissection. *Stroke*. 2005;36(7):1575-1580.
148. Caso V, Paciaroni M, Bogousslavsky J. Environmental factors and cervical artery dissection. *Front Neurol Neurosci*. 2005;20:44-53.
149. Zetterling M, Carlstrom C, Konrad P. Internal carotid artery dissection. *Acta Neurological Scandinavia*. 2000;101:1-7.
150. Kerry R, Taylor AJ. Cervical arterial dysfunction assessment and manual therapy. *Man Ther*. 2006;11:243-253.
151. Arnold M, Bousser MG. Clinical manifestations of vertebral artery dissection. *Front Neurol Neurosci*. 2005;20:77-86.
152. Baumgartner RW, Bogousslasky. Clinical manifestations of carotid artery dissection. *Front Neurol Neurosci*. 2005;20:70-76.
153. Arnold M, Bousser MG. Carotid and vertebral artery dissection. *Practical Neurology*. 2005;5:100-109.
154. Asavasopon S, Jankoski J, Godges JJ. Clinical diagnosis of vertebrobasilar insufficiency: resident's case problem. *J Orthop Sports Phys Ther*. 2005;35(10):645-650.
155. Thanvi B, Munshi SK, Dawson SL, Robinson TG. Carotid and vertebral artery dissection syndromes. *Postgraduate Medical Journal*. 2005;81:383-388.
156. Silbert PL, Mokri B, Schievink WI. Headache and neck pain in spontaneous internal carotid and vertebral artery dissections. *Neurology*. 1995;45(8):1517-1522.
157. Saeed AB, Shuaib A, Al-Sulaiti G, Emery D. Vertebral dissection: warning symptoms, clinical features and prognosis in 26 patients. *Can J Neurol Sci*. 2000;27(4):292-296.
158. Biousse V, D'Anglejan-Chatillon J, Massiou H, et al. Head pain in nontraumatic carotid artery dissection: a series of 65 patients. *Cephalalgia*. 1994;14:33-36.
159. Coman WB. Dizziness related to ENT conditions. In: Grieve GP, ed. *Grieve's Modern Manual Therapy of the Vertebral Column*. Edinburgh, UK: Churchill-Livingstone; 1986:303-314.
160. Cassidy D, Boyle E, Côté P, He Y, Hogg-Johnson S, Silver F, et al. Risk of vertebrobasilar stroke and chiropractic care. Results of a population-based case control and case-crossover study. *Spine*. 2008;33(4S):S176e83.
161. Rivett D, Shirley D, Magarey M, Refshauge K; Australian Physiotherapy Association (APA). *Clinical Guidelines for Assessing Vertebrobasilar Insufficiency in the Management of Cervical Spine Disorders*. Victoria, Australia: Australian Physiotherapy Association; 2006:2. http://www.whitmore-physiotherapy.com/downloads/Level_3_Upper/APA_VBI_Guidelines.pdf. Accessed September 22, 2013.
162. Childs JD, Flynn TW, Fritz JM, P, et al. Screening for vertebrobasilar insufficiency in patient with neck pain: manual therapy decision-making in the presence of uncertainty. *J Orthop Sports Phys Ther*. 2005;35:300-306.
163. Kerry R, Taylor AJ, Mitchell J, McCarthy C, Brew J. Manual therapy and cervical arterial dysfunction, directions for the future: a clinical perspective. *J Man Manip Ther*. 2008;16(1):39-48.
164. Thiel H Rix G. Is it time to stop functional pre-manipulative testing of the cervical spine? *Man Ther*. 2005;10(2):154-158.
165. Bronfort G, Evans R, Anderson AV, Svendsen KH, Bracha Y, Grimm RH. Spinal manipulation, medication, or home exercise with advice for acute and subacute neck pain. A randomized trial. *Ann Intern Med*. 2012;156:1-10.

166. Huijbregts P, Vidal P. Dizziness in orthopaedic physical therapy practice: classification and pathophysiology. *J Man Manip Ther.* 2004;12(4):199-214.
167. Wrisley DM, Sparto PJ, Whitney SL, Furman JM. Cervicogenic dizziness: a review of diagnosis and treatment. *J Orthop Sports Phys Ther.* 2000;30(12):755-766.
168. Vidal P, Huijbregts P. Dizziness in orthopaedic physical therapy practice: history and physical examination. *J Man Manip Ther.* 2005;13(4):222-251.
169. Drachman DA, Hart CW. An approach to the dizzy patient. *Neurology.* 1972;22:323-334.
170. Eaton DA, Roland PS. Dizziness in the older adult. Part 2. *Geriatrics.* 2003;58:46-52.
171. Sloan PD, Coeytaux RR, Beck RS, Dallara J. Dizziness: state of the science. *Ann Intern Med.* 2001;134:823-832.
172. Witting MD, Gallagher K. Unique cutpoints for sitting-to-standing orthostatic vital signs. *Am J Emerg Med.* 2003;21:45-47.
173. The Consensus Committee of the American Autonomic Society and the American Academy of Neurology. Consensus statement on the definition of orthostatic hypotension, pure autonomic failure, and multiple system atrophy. *Neurology.* 1996;46:1470.
174. Reid SA, Rivett DA. Manual therapy treatment for cervicogenic dizziness: a systemic review. *Man Ther.* 2005;10:4-13.
175. Taylor AJ, Kerry R. A system based approach to risk assessment of the cervical spine prior to manual therapy. *Int J Osteopath Med.* 2010;13:85-93.
176. Savitz SI, Caplan LR. Current concepts: vertebrobasilar disease. *N Engl J Med.* 2005;325:2618e26.
177. Biesinger E. Vertigo caused by disorders of the cervical vertebral column. *Adv Otorhinolaryngol.* 1988;39:44-51.
178. Schenk R, Coons BL, Bennett SE, Huijbregts PA. Cervicogenic dizziness: a case report illustrating orthopaedic manual and vestibular physical therapy comanagement. *J Man Manip Ther.* 2006;14(3):E56-E68.
179. Swinkels RA, Oostendorp RA. Upper cervical instability: fact or fiction? *J Manipulative Physiol Ther.* 1996;19:185-194.
180. Pope MH, Frymoyer JW, Krag MH. Diagnosing instability. *Clin Orthop.* 1992;279:60-67.
181. Vo P, MacMillan M. The aging spine: clinical instability. *South Med J.* 1994;87:S26-S35.
182. Dobbs A. Manual therapy assessment of cervical instability. *Orthop Phys Ther Clin North Am.* 2001;10:431-454.
183. Jull G, Trott P, Potter H, et al. A randomized controlled trial of exercise and manipulative therapy for cervicogenic headache. *Spine.* 2002;27:1835-1843.
184. Petersen SM. Articular and muscular impairments in cervicogenic headache: a case report. *J Orthop Sports Phys Ther.* 2003;33:21-30.
185. Maigne JY, Lapeyre E, Morvan G, Chatellier G. Pain immediately upon sitting down and relieved by standing up is often associated with radiologic lumbar instability or marked anterior loss of disc space. *Spine.* 2003;28:1327-1334.
186. Aspinall W. Clinical testing for the craniovertebral hypermobility syndrome. *J Orthop Sports Phys Ther.* 1990;12:47-54.
187. Dai L. Disc degeneration and cervical instability: correlation of magnetic resonance imaging with radiography. *Spine.* 1998;23:1734-1738.
188. Panjabi MM, Lydon C, Vasavada A, et al. On the understanding of clinical instability. *Spine.* 1994;19:2642-2650.
189. Oxland TR, Panjabi MM. The onset and progression of spinal injury: a demonstration of neutral zone sensitivity. *J Biomech.* 1992;25:1165-1172.
190. Cook C, Brismée JM, Fleming R, Sizer PS Jr. Identifiers suggestive of clinical cervical spine instability: a Delphi study of physical therapists. *Phys Ther.* 2005;85(9):895-906.
191. Pettman E. Stress tests of the craniovertebral joints. In: Boyling J, Palastanga N, eds. *Grieve's Modern Manual Therapy: The Vertebral Column.* Edinburgh, UK: Churchill Livingstone; 1994:529-538.
192. Niere KR, Torney SK. Clinicians' perceptions of minor cervical instability. *Man Ther.* 2004;9(3):144-150.
193. Reiter MF, Boden SD. Inflammatory disorders of the cervical spine. *Spine.* 1998;23:2755-2766.
194. Bouchard-Chabot A, Liote F. Cervical spine involvement in rheumatoid arthritis. A review. *Joint Bone Spine.* 2002;69(2):141-154.
195. Neva MH, Hakkinen A, Makinen H, Hannonen P, Kauppi M, Sokka T. High prevalence of symptomatic cervical spine subluxation in patients with rheumatoid arthritis waiting for orthopaedic surgery. *Ann Rheum Dis.* 2006;65(7):884-888.
196. Neva MH, Kaarela K, Kauppi M. Prevalence of radiological changes in the cervical spine: a cross sectional study after 20 years from presentation of rheumatoid arthritis. *J Rheumatol.* 2000;27(1):90-93.
197. Younes M, Belghali S, Kriaa S, et al. Compared imaging of the rheumatoid cervical spine: prevalence study and associated factors. *Joint Bone Spine.* 2009;76(4):361-368.
198. Narvaez JA, Narvaez J, Serrallonga M, et al. Cervical spine involvement in rheumatoid arthritis: correlation between neurological manifestations and magnetic resonance imaging findings. *Rheumatology.* 2008;47(12):1814-1819.
199. Nguyen HV, Ludwig SC, Silber J, et al. Rheumatoid arthritis of the cervical spine. *Spine J.* 2004;4(3):329-334.
200. Dreyer SK. Boden SD. Natural history of rheumatoid arthritis of the cervical spine. *Clin Orthop Rel Res.* 1999;366:98-106.
201. Delamarter RB, Bolman HH. Postmortem osseous and neuropathologic analysis of the rheumatoid cervical spine. *Spine.* 1994;19:2267-2274.
202. Boden SD, Dodge LD, Bohlman HH, Rechtine GR. Rheumatoid arthritis of the cervical spine. A long term analysis with predictors of paralysis and recovery. *J Bone Joint Surg Am.* 1993;75(9):1282-1297.
203. Pellicci PM, Ranawat CS, Tsairis P, Bryan WJ. A prospective study of the progression of rheumatoid arthritis of the cervical spine. *J Bone Joint Surg Am.* 1981;63:342-350.
204. Collins DN, Barnes L, Fitzrandolph R. Cervical spine instability in rheumatoid patients having total hip or knee arthroplasty. *Clin Orthop Rel Res.* 1991;272:127-135.
205. Fujiwara K, Fujimoto M, Owaki H, et al. Cervical lesions related to the systemic progressions in rheumatoid arthritis. *Spine.* 1998;23(19):2051-2056.
206. El Maghraoui A, Bensabbah R, Bahiri R, Bezza A, Guedira N, Hajjaj-Hassouni N. Cervical spine involvement in ankylosing spondylitis. *Clin Rheumatol.* 2003;37(9):813-819.
207. Lee JY, Kim JI, Park JY, et al. Cervical spine involvement in longstanding ankylosing spondylitis. *Clin Exp Rheumatol.* 2005;23(3):331-338.
208. Holden W. Taylor S, Stevens H, Wordsworth P, Bowness P. Neck pain is a major clinical problem in ankylosing spondylitis, and impacts on driving and safety. *Scand J Rheumatol.* 2005;34(2):159-160.
209. Koivikko MP, Koskinen SK. MRI of cervical sine injuries complicating ankylosing spondylitis. *Skeletal Radiol.* 2008;37(9):813-819.
210. Westerveld LA, Verlaan JJ, Oner FC. Spinal fractures in patients with ankylosing spinal disorders: a systematic review of the literature on treatment, neurological status and complications. *Eur Spine J.* 2009;18(2)145-156.

211. Canto JG, Shlipak MG, Rogers WJ, et al. Prevalence, clinical characteristics, and mortality among patients with myocardial infarctions presenting without chest pain. *JAMA.* 2000;283(24):3223-3229.
212. Coven DL, Yang EH. Acute coronary syndrome. *Medscape Reference.* http://emedicine.medscape.com/article/1910735-overview. Accessed: January 20, 2012.
213. De Von HA, Zerwic JJ. Differences in the symptoms associated with unstable angina and myocardial infarction. *Prog Dardiovasc Nurs.* 2004;19(1):6-11.
214. Goldberg R, Goff D, Cooper L, et al. Age and sex difference I presentation of symptoms among patients with acute coronary disease: the react trial. Rapid early action for coronary treatment. *Coron Artery Dis.* 2000;11(5):399-407.
215. Goodman CC, Boissonnault WG, Fuller K. *Pathology: Implications for the Physical Therapist.* 2nd ed. Philadelphia, PA: WB Saunders; 2003:408.
216. Pope JH, Afderheide TP, Ruthazer R, et al. Missed diagnoses of acute cardiac ischemia in the emergency department. *N Engl J Med.* 2000;342(16):1163-1170.
217. Matz PG, Anderson PA, Holly LT, et al. The natural history of cervical spondylotic myelopathy. *J Neurosurg Spine.* 2009;11(2):104-111.
218. Chiles BW, Leonard MA, Choudhri HF, Cooper PR. Cervical spondylotic myelopathy: patterns of neurological deficit and recovery after anterior cervical decompression. *Neurosurg.* 1999;44:762-769; discussion 769-770.
219. Dvorak J. Epidemiology, physical examination, and neurodiagnostics. *Spine.* 1998;23:2663-2673.
220. Montgomery DM, Brower RS. Cervical spondylotic myelopathy. Clinical syndrome and natural history. *Orthop Clin North Am.* 1992;23:487-493.
221. Shamji MF, Cook C, Pietrobon R, Tackett S, Brown C, Isaacs RE. Impact of surgical approach on complication and resource utilization of cervical spine fusion: a nationwide perspective. *Spine J.* 2009;9:31-38.
222. Bartels RH, Verbeek AL, Grotenhuis JA. 2007 Design of Lamifuse: a randomized, multi-centre controlled trial comparing laminectomy without or with dorsal fusion for cervical myeloradiculopathy. *BMC Musculoskel Dis.* 2007;8:111.
223. Harrop JS, Hanna A, Silva MT, Sharan A. Neurological manifestations of cervical spondylosis: an overview of signs, symptoms, and pathophysiology. *Neurosurgery.* 2007;60(1 Suppl 1):S14-S20.
224. Cook C, Roman M, Stewart KM, Leithe LG, Isaacs R. Reliability and diagnostic accuracy of clinical special tests for myelopathy in patients seen for cervical dysfunction. *J Orthop Sports Phys Ther.* 2009;39:172-178.
225. Polston DW. Cervical radiculopathy. *Neurol Clin.* 2007;25(2):373-385.
226. Thongtrangan I, Le H, Park J, Kim DH. Cauda equine syndromes in patients with low lumbar fractures. *Neurosurg Focus.* 2004;16:e6.
227. Cook CE, Cook AE. Cervical spine myelopathy, radiculopathy, and myeloradiculopathy. In: Fernandas de las Penas C, Cleland J, Huijbregts P, eds. *Neck and Arm Pain Syndromes: Evidence-Informed Screening, Diagnosis, and Management in Manual Therapy.* Burlington, MA: Elsevier; 2011:123-139.
228. Denno JJ, MeadowsGR. Early diagnosis of cervical spondylotic myelopathy: a useful clinical sign. *Spine.* 1991;16:1353-1355.
229. Cook CE, Hegedus E, Pietrobon R, Goode A. A pragmatic neurological screen for patients with suspected cord compressive myelopathy. *Phys Ther.* 2007;87:1233-1242.
230. Young WF. Cervical spondylotic myelopathy: a common cause of spinal cord dysfunction in older persons. *Am Fam Physician.* 2000;62:1064-1070, 1073.
231. Estanol BV, Marin OS. Mechanism of the inverted supinator reflex. A clinical and neurophysiological study. *J Neurol Neurosurg Psychiatry.* 1976;39:905-908.
232. de Freitas GR, Andre C. Absence of the Babinski sign in brain death—a prospective study of 144 cases. *J Neurol.* 2005;252:106-107.
233. Cook C, Wilhelm M, Cook AE, Petrosino C, Isaacs R. Clinical tests for screening and diagnosis of cervical spine myelopathy: a systematic review. *J Manipulative Physiol Ther.* 2011;34:539-546.
234. Cook C, Brown C, Isaacs R, Roman M, Davis S, Richardson W. Clustered clinical findings for a diagnosis of cervical spine myelopathy. *J Man Manip Ther.* 2010:18(4):175-180.
235. Fukushima T, Ikata T, Taoka Y, Takata S. Magnetic resonance imaging study on spinal cord plasticity in patients with cervical compression myelopathy. *Spine.* 1991;16:S534-S538.
236. Wainner RS, Gill H. Diagnosis and nonoperative management of cervical radiculopathy. *J Orthop Sports Phys Ther.* 2000;30:728-744.
237. Rao R. Neck pain, cervical radiculopathy, and cervical myelopathy: pathophysiology, natural history, and clinical evaluation. *J Bone Joint Surg Am.* 2002;84:1872-1881.
238. Radhakrishnan K, Litchy WJ, O'Fallon M, Kurlan LT. Epidemiology of cervical radiculopathy. A population based study from Rochester, Minnesota, 1976 through 1990. *Brain.* 1994;117:325-335.
239. Wolff MW, Levine LA. Cervial radiculopathies: conservative approaches to management. *Phys Med Rehabil Clin N Am.* 2002;13(3):589-608.
240. Rhee JM, Yoon T, Riew DK. Cervial radiculopathy. *J Am Acad Orthop Surg.* 2007;15(8):486-494.
241. Henderson CM, Hennessy RG, Shuey HM Jr, Shackelford EG. Posterior-lateral foraminotomy as an exclusive operative technique for cervical radiculopathy: a review of 846 consecutively operated cases. *Neurosurgery.* 1983;13:504-512.
242. Tanaka Y, Kokuubn S, Sato T, Ozawa K. Diagnostic indices of involved nerve root in cervical radiculopathy. *J Bone Joint Surg (Br).* 2002;84-B(Supp_III):245-246.
243. Tanaka Y, Kokubun S, Sata T, Ozawa H. Cervical roots as origin of pain in the neck or scapular regions. *Spine.* 2006;31(17):E568-E573.
244. Cook C, Hegedus E. *Orthopaedic Physical Examination Tests: An Evidence-Based Approach.* Upper Saddle River, NJ: Prentice Hall; 2008:26-56.
245. Wainner RS, Fritz JM, Irrgang JJ, Boninger ML, Delitto A, Allison S. Reliability and diagnostic accuracy of the clinical examination and patient self-report measures for cervical radiculopathy. *Spine.* 2003;28(1):52-62.
246. Rubinstein SM, Pool JJM, van Tulder MW, Riphagen II, de Vet HCW. A systematic review of the diagnostic accuracy of provocative tests of the neck for diagnosing cervical radiculopathy. *Eur Spine J.* 2007;16:307-319.
247. Nederland M, IJzerman MJ, Hermens HJ, Turk DC, Zilvold G. Predictive value of fear avoidance in developing chronic neck pain disability: consequences for clinical decision making. *Arch Phys Med Rehabil.* 2004;85:496-501.
248. Bot SDM, van der Waal JM, Terwee CB, et al. Predictors of outcome in neck and shoulder symptoms. *Spine.* 2005;30(16):E459-E470.
249. Coté P, Cassidy JD, Carroll L, Frank JW, Bombardier C. A systematic review of the prognosis of acute whiplash and a new conceptual framework to synthesize the literature. *Spine.* 2001;19:E445-E458.

250. Kasch H, Flemming W, Jensen T. Handicap after acute whiplash injury. *Neurology.* 2001;56:1637-1643.
251. Kamper SJ, Rebbeck TJ, Maher CG, McAuley JH, Sterling M. Course and prognostic factors of whiplash: a systematic review and metaanalysis. *Pain.* 2008;138:617-629.
252. Raak R, Wallin M. Thermal thresholds and catastrophizing in individuals with chronic pain after whiplash injury. *Biol Res Nurs.* 2006;8:138-146.
253. Elliott J, Sterling M, Noteboom JT, Darnell R, Galloway G, Jull G. Fatty infiltrate in the cervical extensor muscles is not a feature of chronic, insidious-onset neck pain. *Clin Radiol.* 2008;63:681-687.
254. Johnston V, Jimmieson NL, Jull G, Souvlis T. Contribution of individual, workplace, psychosocial and physiological factors to neck pain in female office workers. *Eur J Pain.* 2009;13(9):985-991.
255. Williamson E, Williams M, Gates S, Lamb SE. A systematic literature review of psychological factors and the development of late whiplash syndrome. *Pain.* 2008;135:20-30.
256. George SZ, Fritz JM, Erhard RE. A comparison of fear-avoidance beliefs in patients wit lumbar spine and cervical spine pain. *Spine (Phila Pa 1976).* 2001;26(19):2139-2145.
257. Sterling M, Kenardy J, Jull G, Vicenzino B. The development of psychological changes following whiplash injury. *Pain.* 2003;106:481-489.
258. Buitenhuis J, DeJong J, Jaspers J, Groothoff J. Relationship between posttraumatic stress disorder symptoms and the course of whiplash complaints. *J Psychosom Res.* 2006;61:681-689.
259. Kamper SJ, Maher CG, Costa L, McAuley JH, Hush JM, Sterling M. Does fear of movement mediate the relationship between pain intensity and disability in patients following whiplash injury? A prospective longitudinal study. *Pain.* 2012;153:113-119.
260. Buitenhuis J, Spanjer, Fidler V. Recovery from acute whiplash: the role of coping styles. *Spine.* 2003;28:896-901.
261. Carroll L, Cassidy D, Coté P. The role of pain coping strategies in prognosis after whiplash injury: passive coping predicts slowed recovery. *Pain.* 2006;124:18-26.
262. Mercado A, Carroll L, Cassidy D, Coté P. Passive coping is a risk factor for disabling neck or low back pain. *Pain.* 2005;117:51-57.
263. Hurwitz E, Goldstein M, Morgenstern H, Chiang L. The impact of psychosocial factors on neck pain and disability outcomes among primary care patients: results from the UCLA neck pain study. *Dis Rehabil.* 2006;28:1319-1329.
264. Peebles J, McWIlliam L, MacLennan R. A comparison of symptoms checklist 90-revised profiles from patients with chronic pain from whiplash and patients with other musculoskeletal injuries. *Spine.* 2001;26:766-770.
265. Wenzel H, Haug T, Mykletun A, Dahl A. A population study of anxiety and depression among persons who report whiplash traumas. *J Psychosom Res.* 2002;53:831-835.
266. Vernon H, Mior S. The Neck Disability Index: a study of reliability and validity. *J Manipulative Physiol Ther.* 1991;14:409-415.
267. Westaway M, Stratford P, Binkley J. The patient-specific functional scale: validation of its use in persons with neck dysfunction. *J Orthop Sports Phys Ther.* 1998;27:331-338.
268. Jaeschke R, Singer J, Guyatt G. Measurement of health status. Ascertaining the minimal clinically important difference. *Control Clin Trials.* 1989;10:407-415.
269. Waddell G, Newton M, Henderson I, et al. A Fear-Avoidance Beliefs Questionnaire (FABQ) and the role of fear-avoidance beliefs in chronic low back pain and disability. *Pain.* 1993;52:157-168.
270. Horowitz M, Wilner N, Alvarez W. Impact of event scale: a measure of subjective stress. *Psychosom Med.* 1979;41:209-218.
271. Tesio L, Alpini D, Cesarani A, et al. Short form of the Dizziness Handicap Inventory. *Am J Phys Medical Rehabil.* 1999;78:233-241.
272. Kori S, Miller R, Todd D. Kinesiophobia: a new view of chronic pain behavior. *Pain Manag.* 1990;Jan/Feb:35-43.
273. Bennett M, Smith B, Torrance N, et al. The S-LANSS score for identifying pain of predominantly neuropathic origin: validation for use in clinical and postal research. *J Pain.* 2005;6:149-158.
274. Vernon H. The Neck Disability Index: state-of-the- art, 1991-2008. *J Manipulative Physiol Ther.* 2008;31:491-502.
275. Sterling M, Jull G, Kenardy J. Physical and psychological factors maintain long-term predictive capacity post-whiplash injury. *Pain.* 2006;122:102-108.
276. MacDermid JC, Walton EM, Avery S, et al. Measurement properties of the neck disability index: a systematic review. *J Orthop Sports Phys Ther.* 2009;39(5):400-417.
277. Young BA, Walker MJ, Strunce JB, Boyles RE, Whitman JM, Childs JD. Responsiveness of the neck disability index in patients with mechanical neck disorders. *Spine J.* 2009;9:802-808.
278. Young IA, Cleland JA, Michener LA, Brown C. Reliability, construct validity, and responsiveness of the neck disability index, patient-specific functional scale, and numeric pain rating scale. *Am J Phys Med Rehabil.* 2010;89(10):831-839.
279. Ferriera ML, Borges BM, Rezende IL, et al. Are neck pain scales and questionnaires compatible with the international classification of functioning, disability and health? A systematic review. *Disabil Rehabil.* 2010;32(19):1539-1546.
280. Cleland JA, Fritz JM, Whitman JM, Palmer JA. The reliability and construct validity of the Neck Disability Index and patient specific functional scale in patients with cervical radiculopathy. *Spine.* 2006;31(5):598-602.
281. Costa LOP, Maher CG, Latimer J, et al. Clinimetric testing of three self-report outcome measures for low back pain patients in Brazil: which one is the best? *Spine.* 2008;33:2459-2463.
282. Cleland JA, Childs JD, Fritz JM, Whitman JM, Eberhart SL. Development of a clinical prediction rule for guiding treatment of a subgroup of patients with neck pain: use of thoracic spine manipulation, exercise, and patient education. *Phys Ther.* 2007;87(1):9-23.
283. Cleland JA, Childs JD, Mcae M, Palmer JA, Stowell T. Immediate effects of a thoracic manipulation in patients with neck pain: a randomized clinical trial. *Man Ther.* 2005;10:127-135.
284. Puentedura EJ, Landers MR, Cleland JA, Mintken P, Huijbregts P, Fernandez-de-las-Peñas C. Thoracic spine thrust manipulation versus cervical spine thrust manipulation in patients with acute neck pain: a randomized clinical trial. *J Orthop Sports Phys Ther.* 2011;41(4):208-220.
285. Kamper SJ, Maher CG, Mackay G. Global rating of change scales: a review of strengths and weaknesses and considerations for design. *J Man Manip Ther.* 2009;17(3):163-170.
286. Cleland JA, Fritz JM, Childs JD: Psychometric properties of the fear-avoidance beliefs questionnaire and Tampa scale of kinesiophobia in patients with neck pain. *Am J Phys Med Rehabil.* 2008;87:109-117.
287. Landers MR, Creger RV, Baker CV, Stutelberg KS. The use of fear-avoidance beliefs and nonorganic signs in predicting prolonged disability in patients with neck pain. *Man Ther.* 2008;13:239-248.

288. Karlehagen S, Malt U, Hoff H, Tibell E, Herrstromer U, Hildingson K. The effect of major railway accidents on the psychological health of train drivers. *J Psychosom Res.* 1993;37:807-817.
289. Joseph S. Psychometric evaluation of Horowitz's impact of event scale: a review. *J Trauma Stress.* 2000;13(1):101-113.
290. Sterling M, Kenardy J, Jull G, Vicenzino B. The development of psychological changes following whiplash injury. *Pain.* 2003;106:481-489.
291. Corcoran K, Fischer J. *Measures for Clinical Practice: A Sourcebook.* 3rd ed. Vol 2 Adults. New York, NY: The Free Press; 1994.
292. Sundin EC, Horowitz MJ. Impact of Event Scale: psychometric properties. *Br J Psych.* 2002;180:205-209.
293. Weiss DS, Marmar CR. The Impact of Event Scale: revised. In: Wilson JP, Keane TM, eds. *Assessing Psychological Trauma and PTSD.* New York, NY: Guilford; 2007:399-411.
294. Forbes D, Creamer M, Phelps A, et al. Australian guideline for the treatment of adults with acute stress disorders and post-traumatic stress disorder. *Aust N Z J Psychiatry.* 2007;41(8):637-648.
295. Sterling M. A proposed new classification system for whiplash associated disorders: implications for assessment and management. *Man Ther.* 2004;9:60-70.
296. Rekola KE, Keinanen-Kiukaanniemi S, Takala J. Use of primary health services in sparsely populated country districts by patients with musculoskeletal symptoms: consultations with a physician. *J Epidemiol Community Health.* 1993;47:153-157.
297. Holm LW, Carroll LR, Cassidy JD, et al. The burden and determinants of neck pain in whiplash-associated disorders after traffic collisions. *Spine.* 2008;33(4S):S52-S59.
298. Carroll LF, Holm LW Hogg-Johnson S, et al. Course and prognostic factors for neck pain in whiplash-associated disorders (WAD). *Spine.* 2008;33(4s):S83-S92.
299. Côté P, van der Velde G, Cassidy JD, et al. The burden and determinants of neck pain in workers. Results of the bone and joint decade 2000-2010 task force on neck pain and its associated disorders. *Spine.* 2008;33(4S):S60-S74.
300. Korhonen T, Ketola R, Toivonen R, et al. Work related and individual predictors for incident neck pain among office employees working with video display units. *Occup Environ Med.* 2003;60:475-782.
301. Luime JJ, Koes BW, Miedem HS, et al. High incidence and recurrence of shoulder and neck pain in nursing home employees was demonstrated during a 2-year follow-up. *J Clin Epidemol.* 2005;58:407-413.
302. Carroll LJ, Hogg-Johnson S, Côté P, et al. Course and prognostic factors for neck pain in workers. Results of the bone and joint decade 2000-2010 task force on neck pain and its associated disorders. *Spine.* 2008:33(4S):S93-S100.
303. Boissonnault WG, Bass C. Pathological origins of trunk and neck pain: part I. Pelvic and abdominal visceral disorders. *J Orthop Sports Phys Ther.* 1990;12:192-207.
304. Merskey H, Bogduk N, eds. *Classification of Chronic Pain. Descriptions of Chronic Pain Syndromes and Definition of Pain Terms.* 2nd ed. Seattle, WA: IASP Press; 1994:103-111.
305. Bogduk N. On the definitions and physiology of back pain, referred pain, and radicular pain. *Pain.* 2009;147:17-19.
306. Arendt-Nielsen L, Graven-Nielsen T, Drewes AM. Referred poain and hyperalgesia related to muscle and visceral pain. *Technical Corner from IASP Newsletter.* 1998;Jan/Feb.
307. Arendt-Nielsen L, Svensson P. Referred muscle pan: basic and clinical findings. *Clin J Pain.* 2001;17(1):11-19.
308. Dwyer A, Aprill C, Bogduk N. Cervical zygapophysial joint pain patterns. I: a study in normal volunteers. *Spine.* 1990:15:453-457.
309. Aprill C, Dwyer A, BOgduk N. Cervical zygapophyseal joint pain patterns. II: a clinical evaluation. *Spine.* 1990;15:458-461.
310. Fukui S, Ohseto K, Shiotani M, et al. Referred pain distribution of the cervical zygapophyseal joints and cervical dorsal rami. *Pain.* 1996;68:79-83.
311. Cloward RB. Cervical discography. A contribution to the aetiology and mechanism of neck, shoulder and arm pain. *Ann Surg.* 1959;130:1052-1064.
312. Schellhas KP, Smith MD, Gundry CR, et al. Cervical discogenic pain: prospective correlation of magnetic resonance imaging and discography in asymptomatic subjects and pain sufferers. *Spine.* 1996;21:300-312.
313. Grubb SA, Kelly CK. Cervical discography: clinical implications from 12 years of experience. *Spine.* 2000;25:1382-1389.
314. Bogduk N, Aprill C. On the nature of neck pain, discography and cervical zygapophysial joint pain. *Pain.* 1993;54:213-217.
315. Dreyfuss P, Michaelsen M, Fletcher D. Atlantooccipital and lateral atlanto-axial joint pain patterns. *Spine.* 1994;19:1125-1131.
316. Cooper G, Bailey B, Bogduk N. Cervical zygapophysial joint pain maps. *Pain Medicine.* 2007;8(4):344-353.
317. Slipman CW, Plastaras C, Patel R, et al. Provocative cervical discography symptom mapping. *Spine J.* 2005;5:381-388.
318. Slipman CW, Plastaras CT, Palmitier RA, et al. Symptom provocation of fluoroscopically guided cervical nerve root stimulation: are dynatomal maps identical to dermatomal maps? *Spine.* 1998;23:2235-2242.
319. IASP® Taxonomy. Updated in 2011 by the IASP® Taxonomy Working Group based on Merskey H, Bogduk N, eds. *Classification of Chronic Pain.* 2nd ed. Part III. Seattle, WA: IASP Press; 1994. http://www.iasp-pain.org/AM/Template.cfm?Section=General_Resource_Links&Template=/CM/HTMLDisplay.cfm&ContentID=2035. Accessed January 31, 2012.
320. Baron R, Binder A, Wasner G. Neuropathic pian: diagnosis, pathophysiological mechanisms, and treatment. *Lancet Neurol.* 2010;9(8):807-819.
321. Melzack R, Coderre TJ, Katz J, Vaccarino AL. Central neuroplasticity and pathological pain. *Ann N Y Acad Sci.* 2001;933:157-174.
322. Meeus M, Nijs J. Central sensitization: a biopsychosocial explanation for chronic widespread pain in patients with fibromyalgia and chronic fatigue syndrome. *Clin Rheumatol.* 2007;26(4):465-473.
323. Nijs J, Van Houdenhove B, Oostendorp RAB. Recognition of central sensitization in patients with musculoskeletal pain: application of pain neurophysiology in manual therapy practice. *Man Ther.* 2010;15:135-141.
324. Cleland JA, Childs JD, Whitman JM. Psychometric properties of the Neck Disability Index and Numeric Pain Rating Scale in patients with mechanical neck pain. *Arch Phys Med Rehabil.* 2008;89:69-74.
325. Bot SD, van der Waal JM, Terwee CB, et al. Predictors of outcome in neck and shoulder symptoms a cohort study in general practice. *Spine.* 2005;30:E459-E470.
326. Sterling M, Hendrikz J, Kenardy J. Developmental trajectories of pain and disability and PTSD symptoms following whiplash injury. *Pain.* 2010;159(1):22-28.
327. Drottning M, Staff PH, Sjaastad O. Cervicogenic headache (CEH) after whiplash injury. *Cephalagia.* 2002;22:165-171.
328. Carroll LJ, Cassidy JD, Côté P. The role of pain coping strategies in prognosis after whiplash injury: passive coping predicts slowed recovery. *Pain.* 2006;124:18-26.

329. Boissonnault WG. Patient health history including identification of health risk factors. In: Boissonnault WG. *Primary Care for the Physical Therapist: Examination and Triage.* Philadelphia, PA: Saunders; 2005:70.
330. Mäntyselkä P, Kautiainen H, Vanhala M. Prevalence of neck pain in subjects with metabolic syndrome: a cross-sectional population-based study. *BMC Musculoskelet Disord.* 2010;11:171.
331. Rubin DI. Epidemiology and risk factors for spine pain. *Neurol Clin.* 2007;25:353-371.
332. Billek-Sawhney B, Sawhney R. Cardiovascular considerations in outpatient orthopedic physical therapy [abstract]. *J Orthop Sports Phys Ther.* 1998:27:57.
333. Scherer SA, Noteboom JT, Flynn TW. Cardiovascular assessment in the orthopaedic practice setting. *J Orthop Sports Phys Ther.* 2005;35:730-737.
334. Douglass AB, Bope ET. Evaluation and treatment of posterior neck pain in family practice. *J Am Board Fam Pract.* 2004;17:S13-S22.
335. Hurwitz EL, Carragee EJ, van der Belde G, et al. Treatment of neck pain: noninvasive interventions. Results of the bone and joint decade 2000-2010 task force on neck pain and its associated disorders. *Spine.* 2008;33(4S):S123-S152.
336. Barnsley L, Lord SM, Wallis BJ, et al. Lack of effect of intraarticular corticosteroids for chronic pain in the cervical zygapophyseal joints. *N Engl J Med.* 1994;330:1047-1050.
337. Pettersson K, Toolanen G. High-dose methylprednisolone prevents extensive sick leave after whiplash injury. A prospective, randomized, double blind study. *Spine.* 1998;23:984-989.
338. Kearney PM, Baigent C, Godwin J, et al. Do selective cyclo-oxygenase-2 inhibitors and traditional non-steroidal anti-inflammatory drugs increase the risk of atherothrombosis? Meta-analysis of randomized trials. *BMJ.* 2006;332:1302-1308.
339. Hernandez-Diaz S, Rodriguez LA. Association between non-steroidal anti-inflammatory drugs and upper gastrointestinal tract bleeding/perforation: an overview of epidemiologic studies published in the 1990s. *Arch Intern Med.* 2000;160:2093-2099.
340. Guzman J, Haldeman S, Carroll LJ, et al. Clinical practice implications for the bone and joint decade 2000-2010 task force on neck pain and its associate disorders. From concepts and findings to recommendations. *Spine.* 2008;33(4S):S199-S213.
341. Eyre A. Overview and comparison of the NEXUS and Canadian C-spine rules. *Am J Clin Med.* 2006;3:12-15.
342. Matsumoto M, Fujimura Y, Suzuki N, et al. MRI of cervical intervertebral discs in asymptomatic subjects. *J Bone Joint Surg Br.* 1998;80:19-24.
343. Boden SD, McCowin PR, Davis DO, et al. Abnormal magnetic-resonance scans of the cervical spine in asymptomatic subjects. A prospective investigation. *J Bone Joint Surg Am.* 1990;72:1178-1184.
344. Lehto IJ, Tertti MO, Komu ME, et al. Age-related MRI changes at 0.1 T in cervical discs in asymptomatic subjects. *Neuroradiology.* 1994;36:49-53.
345. Oxford Dictionaries Online. Oxford University Press. http://oxforddictionaries.com/definition/expectation?region=us. Accessed February 2, 2012.
346. Bialosky JE, Bishop MD, Cleland JA. Individual expectation: an overlooked, but pertinent factor in the treatment of individuals experiencing musculoskeletal pain. *Phys Ther.* 2010;90(9):1345-1355.
347. Barron CJ, Moffett JA, Potter M. Patient expectations of physiotherapy: definitions, concepts, and theories. *Physiother Theor Pract.* 2007;23(1):37-46.
348. American Academy of Orthopaedic Manual Physical Therapists. *Orthopaedic Manual Physical Therapy: Description of Advanced Clinical Practice.* Tallahassee, FL: Author; 2009:11-61.
349. Cook C, Hegedus E. Diagnostic utility of clinical tests for spinal dysfunction. *Man Ther.* 2011;16:21-25.
350. Wise CH, Schenk RJ. Clinical decision making in the application of cervical spine manipulation. In: *Cervical and Thoracic Pain: Evidence for Effectiveness of Physical Therapy. Independent Study Course 21.1.5.* La Crosse, WI: Orthopaedic Section, APTA, Inc; 2011:15-23.
351. Leal M, Dennison B. Best evidence for examination and treatment of the cervical spine. In: *Cervical and Thoracic Pain: Evidence for Effectiveness of Physical Therapy. Independent Study Course 21.1.5.* La Crosse, WI: Orthopaedic Section, APTA, Inc; 2011:14.
352. LaBan MM, Green ML. "Young" cervical spinal stenotic: a review of 118 patients younger than 51 years of age. *Am J Phys Med Rehabil.* 2004;83:162-165.
353. Poole E, Treleaven J, Jull G. The influence of neck pain on balance and gait parameters in community-dwelling elders. *Man Ther.* 2008;13:317-324.
354. Falla D, Jull G, Rainoldi A, Merletti R. Neck flexor muscle fatigue is side specific in patients with unilateral neck pain. *Eur J Pain.* 2004;8(1):71-77.
355. Enwemeka CS, Bonet IM, Ingle JA, Prudhithumrong S, Ogbahon FE, Gbenedio NA. Postural correction in persons with neck pain. (II. Integrated electromyography of the upper trapezius in three simulated neck positions.) *J Orthop Sports Phys Ther.* 1986;8:240-242.
356. Bonney RA, Corlett EN. Head posture and loading of the cervical spine. *Appl Ergon.* 2002;33:415-417.
357. O'Leary S, Falla D, Elliott JM, Jull G. Muscle dysfunction in cervical spine pain: implications for assessment and management. *J Orthop Sports Phys Ther.* 2009;39(5):324e33.
358. Madeleine P. On functional motor adaptations: from the quantification of motor strategies to the prevention of musculoskeletal disorders in the neck-shoulder region. *Acta Physiologica (Oxford).* 2010;199(s699):1-46.
359. Griegel-Morris P, Larson K, Mueller-Klaus K, Oatis CA. Incidence of common postural abnormalities in the cervical, shoulder and thoracic regions and their association with pain in two age groups of healthy subjects. *Phys Ther.* 1992;72:425-431.
360. Braun BL. Postural differences between asymptomatic men and women and craniofacial pain patients. *Arch Phys Med Rehabil.* 1991;72:653-656.
361. Haughie LJ, Fiebert IM, Roach KE. Relationship of forward head posture and the cervical backward bending to neck pain. *J Man Manip Ther.* 1995;3:91-97.
362. Hanten WP, Olson SL, Russel JL, Lucio RM, Campbell AH. Total head excursion and resting head posture: normal and patients comparisons. *Arch Phys Med Rehabil.* 2000;81:62-66.
363. Harrison AL, Barry-Greb T, Wojtowicz G. Clinical measurement of head and shoulder posture variables. *J Orthop Sports Phys Ther.* 1996;23:353-361.
364. Cleland JA, Childs JD, Fritz JM, Whitman JM. Interrater reliability of the history and physical examination in patients with mechanical neck pain. *Arch Phys Med Rehabil.* 2006;87:1388-1395.
365. Silva AG, Punt TD, Johnson MI. Reliability and validity of head posture assessment by observation and a four-category scale. *Man Ther.* 2010;15:490-495.
366. Silva AG, Punt TD, Sharples P, Vilas-Boas JP, Johnson MI. Head posture and neck pain of chronic nontraumatic origin: a comparison between patients and pain-free persons. *Arch Phys Med Rehabil.* 2009;90:669-674.

367. Lau KT, Cheung KY, Chan KB, Chan MH, Lo KY, Chiu TTW. Relationships between sagittal postures of thoracic and cervical spine, presence of neck pain, neck severity and disability. *Man Ther.* 2010;10:457-462.
368. Yip CHT, Chiu TTW, Poon ATK. The relationship between head posture and severity and disability of patients with neck pain. *Man Ther.* 2008;13:148-154.
369. Treleaven J. Jull G, Low CHoy N. Standing balance in persistent whiplash: a comparison between subjects with and without dizziness. *J Rehabil Med.* 2005;37:224-229.
370. Stokell R, Yu A, Williams K, Treleaven J. Dynamic and functional balance tasks in subjects with persistent whiplash: a pilot trial. *Man Ther.* 2011;16:394-398.
371. Szeto GPY, Straker L, Raine S. A field comparison of neck and shoulder postures in symptomatic and asymptomatic office workers. *Applied Ergonomics.* 2002;33:75-84.
372. Szeto GPY, Strker LM, O'Sullivan PB. A comparison of symptomatic and asymptomatic office workers performing monotonous keyboard work: 2: Neck and shoulder kinematics. *Man Ther.* 2005;10(4):281-291.
373. Sobush DC, Simoneau GG, Dietz KE, et al. The Lennie test for measuring scapular position in healthy young adult females: a reliability and validity study. *J Orthop Sports Phys Ther.* 1996;23:39-50.
374. Ludewig PM, Phadke V, Braman J, Hassett DR, Cieminski CJ, LaPrade RF. Motion of the shoulder complex during multiplanar humeral elevation. *J Bone Joint Surg Am.* 2009;91:378-389.
375. McClure PW, Michener LA, Sennett BJ, et al. Direct 3-dimensional measurement of scapular kinematics during dynamic movements in vivo. *J Shoulder Elbow Surg.* 2001;10:269-277.
376. Ludewig PM, Cook TM. Alterations in shoulder kinematics and associated muscle activity in people with symptoms of shoulder impingement. *Phys Ther.* 2000;80(3):276-291.
377. Ludewig PM, Behrens SA, Meyer SM, et al. Three-dimensional clavicular motion during arm elevation: reliability and descriptive data. *J Orthop Sports Phys Ther.* 2004;34:140-149.
378. Kibler WB, Sciascia A. Current concepts: scapular dyskinesis. *Br J Sports Med.* 2010;44:300-305.
379. Ha S, Kwon O, Yi C, Jeon H, Lee W. Effects of passive correction of scapular position on pain, proprioception, and range of motion in neck-pain patients with bilateral scapular downward-rotation syndrome. *Man Ther.* 2011;16:585-589.
380. Van Dillen LR, McDonell MK, Susco TM, Sahrmann SA. The immediate effect of passive scapular elevation on symptoms with active neck rotation in patients with neck pain. *Clin J Pain.* 2007;23(8):641-647.
381. Eriksson PO,Häggman-Henrikson B, Nordh E, Zafar H. Coordinated mandibular and head-neck movements during rhythmic jaw activities in man. *J Dent Res.* 2000;79:1378-1384.
382. Walker N, Bohannon RW, Cameron D. Discriminant validity of temporomandibular joint range of motion obtained with a ruler. *J Orthop Sports Phys Ther.* 2000;30:484-492.
383. Okeson JP. *Management of Temporomandibular Disorders and Occlusion.* 6th ed. St. Louis, MO: Mosby Elsevier; 2007.
384. Ho S. *The Temporomandibular Joint: Physical Therapy Patient Management Utilizing Current Evidence. Concepts of Orthopaedic Physical Therapy.* 3rd ed. La Crosse, WI: Orthopaedic Section Inc; 2011: Orthopaedic Section Independent Study Course series 12.2.
385. Kibler WB, Sciascia A, Dome D. Evaluation of apparent and absolute supraspinatus strength in patients with shoulder injury using the scapular retraction test. *Am J Sports Med.* 2006;34:1643-1647.
386. Tate AR, Kareha S, Irwin D, McClure PW. Effect of the scapula reposition test on shoulder impingement symptoms and elevation strength in overhead athletes. *J Orthop Sports Phys Ther.* 2008;38(1):4-11
387. Caneiro JP, O'Sullivan P, Burnett A, et al. The influence of different sitting postures on head/neck posture and muscle activity. *Man Ther.* 2010; 15(1):54-60.
388. Falla D, O'Leary S, Fagan A, Jull G. Recruitment of the deep cervical flexor muscles during a postural-correction exercise performed in sitting. *Man Ther.* 2007;12(2):139-143.
389. Edmondston SJ, Sharp M, Symes A, Alhabib N, Allison GR. Changes in mechanical load and extensor muscle activity in the cervicothoracic spine induced by sitting posture modification. *Ergonomics.* 2011;54(2):179-186.
390. Hodges PW, Ferreira PH, Ferreira ML. Lumbar spine: treatment of instability and disorders of movement control. In: Magee DJ, Zachazewski JE, Quillen WS. *Pathology and Intervention in Musculoskeletal Rehabilitation.* St. Louis, MO: Saunders Elsevier; 2009:389-425.
391. Bogduk N, Mercer S. Biomechanics of the cervical spine. I: normal kinematics. *Clin Biomech.* 2000;15:633-648.
392. Mercer SR, Bogduk N. Joints of the cervical vertebral column. *J Orthop Sports Phys Ther.* 2001;31:174-182.
393. Magee DJ. *Orthopedic Physical Assessment.* 4th ed. Philadelphia, PA: Saunders, Elsevier; 2002:133-135.
394. Vasavada AN, Peterson BW, Delp SL. Three-dimensional spatial tuning of neck muscle activation in humans. *Exp Brain Res.* 2002;147:437-448.
395. Peck D, Buxton DF, Nitz A. A comparison of spindle concentrations in large and small muscles acting in parallel combinations. *J Morphol.* 1984;180:243-252.
396. Boyd-Clark LC, Briggs CA, Galea MP. Comparative histochemical composition of muscle fibers in a pre- and a postvertebral muscle of the cervical spine. *J Anat.* 2001;199:709-716.
397. Boyd-Clark LC, Briggs CA, Galea MP. Muscle spindle distribution, morphology, and density in longus colli and multifidus muscle of the cervical spine. *Spine.* 2002;27:694-701.
398. Conley MS, Meyer RA, Bloomberg JJ, et al. Noninvasive analysis of human neck muscle function. *Spine.* 1995;20:2505-2512.
399. Roy RR, Ishihara A. Overview: functional implications of the design of skeletal muscles. *Acta Anat.* 1997;159:75-77.
400. Van Mameren H, Drukker J, Sanches H, Beursgens J. Cervical spine motion in the sagittal plane. (I). Range of motion of actually performed movements, an X-ray cinematographic study. *Eur J Morph.* 1990;28:47-68.
401. Maynoux Behnamou MA, Revel M, Vallee C. Selective electromyography of dorsal neck muscles in humans. *Exp Brain Res.* 1997;113:353-360.
402. Dumas JP, Arsenault AB, Boudreau G, et al. Physical impairments in cervicogenic headache: traumatic versus nontraumatic onset. *Cephalalgia.* 2001;21:884-893.
403. Zwart JA. Neck mobility in different headache disorders. *Headache.* 1997;37:6-11.
404. Chiu TT, Lam T-H, Hedley AJ. Correlation among physical impairments, pain, disability, and patient satisfaction in patients with chronic neck pain. *Arch Phys Med Rehabil.* 2005;86:534-540.
405. Riddle DL, Stratford PW. Use of generic versus region-specific functional status measures on patients with cervical spine disorders. *Phys Ther.* 1998;78:951-963.
406. Rudolfsson T, Björklund M, Djupsjöbacka M. Range of motion in the upper and lower cervical spine in people with chronic neck pain. *Man Ther.* 2012;17:53-59.

407. Norre ME. Neurophysiology of vertigo with special reference to cervical vertigo: a review. *Acta Belg Med Phys.* 1986;9:183-194.
408. Phillipszoon A. Neck torsion nystagmus. *Pract Oto-Rhino-Laryngologist.* 1963;25:339-344.
409. Oosterveld WJ, Kortschot HW, Kingma GG, DeJong JMBV, Saatci MR. Electronystagmographic findings following cervical whiplash injuries. *Acta Otolaryngol (Stockh).* 1991:111:201-205.
410. Norre ME. Cervical vertigo: diagnostic and semiological problem with special emphasis upon "cervical nystagmus." *Acta Otorhinolaryngol Belg.* 1987;41:436-452.
411. Clendaniel RA, Landel R. Non-vestibular diagnosis and imbalance: cervicogenic dizziness. In: Herdman SJ. *Vestibular Rehabilitation.* 3rd ed. Philadelphia, PA: F.A. Davis Company; 2007;467-484.
412. Herdman SJ. *Vestibular Rehabilitation.* 3rd ed. Philadelphia, PA: F.A. Davis Company; 2007.
413. Bhattacharyya N, Baugh RF, Orvidas L, et al. Clinical practice guideline: benign paroxysmal positional vertigo. *Otolaryngol Head Neck Surg.* 2008;139:S47-S81.
414. Halker R, Barrs D, Wellik K, Wingerchuk, Demaerschalk BM. Establishing a diagnosis of benign paroxysmal positional vertigo through the Dix-Hallpike and side-lying maneuvers: a critically appraised topic. *The Neurologist.* 2008;14(3):201-204.
415. Whitney SL, Morris LO. Multisensory impairment in older adults: evaluation and intervention. In: Calhoun KH, Eibling DE, eds. *Geriatric Otolaryngology.* New York, NY: Taylor and Francis; 2006:115.
416. Whitney SL, Marchetti GF, Morris LO. Usefulness of the dizziness handicap inventory in the screening for benign paroxysmal positional vertigo. *Otol Neurotol.* 2005;26:1027-1033.
417. Lind B, Sihlbom H, Nordwall A, Malchau H. Normal range of motion of the cervical spine. *Arch Phys Med Rehabil.* 1989;20:692-695.
418. Youdas M, Garrett TR, Suman VJ, et al. Normal range of motion of the cervical spine: an initial goniometric study. *Phys Ther.* 1992;72:770-780.
419. de Koning CHP, van den Heuvel SP, Staal JB, Smits-Engelsman BCM, Henddriks EJM. Clinimetric evaluation of active range of motion measures in patients with non-specific neck pain: a systematic review. *Eur Spine J.* 2008;17:905-921.
420. Piva SR, Erhard R, Childs JF, Browder D. Inter-tester reliability of passive inter-vertebral and active movements of the cervical spine. *Man Ther.* 2006;11:321-330.
421. Tuttle N. Do changes within a manual therapy treatment session predict between-session changes for patients with cervical spine pain? *Aust J Physiother.* 2005;51(1):43-48.
422. McKenzie R, May S. *The Cervical and Thoracic Spine Mechanical Diagnosis and Therapy.* Vol 1. Raumati Beach, New Zealand: Spinal Publications New Zealand Ltd; 2006:171-282.
423. Norlander S, Aste-Norlander U, Nordgren B, Sahlstedt B. Mobility in the cervicothoracic motion segment: an indicative factor of musculo-skeletal neck-shoulder pain. *Scan J Rehab Med.* 1996;28(4):183-192.
424. Norland S, Gustavssono BA, Lindell J, Nordgren B. Reduced mobility in the cervicothoracic motion segment: a risk factor for musculoskeletal neck-shoulder pain: a two-year prospective follow-up study. *Scan J Rehab Med.* 1997;29(3):167-174.
425. Norlander S, Nordgren B. Clinical symptoms related to musculoskeletal neck-shoulder pain and mobility in the cervicothoracic spine. *Scan J Rehab Med.* 1998;30:243-251.
426. Browder DA, Erhard RE, Piva SR. Intermittent cervical traction and thoracic manipulation for management of mild cervical compressive myelopathy attributed to cervical herniated disc: a case series. *J Orthop Sports Phys Ther.* 2004;34:701-712.
427. Fernández-de-las-Peñas C, Palomeque-del-Cerro L, Rodriguez-Blanco C, Gomez-Conesa A, Miangolarra-Page JC. Changes in neck pain and active range of motion after a single thoracic spine manipulation in subjects presenting with mechanical neck pain: a case series. *J Manipulative Physiol Ther.* 2007;30:312-320.
428. Costello M. Treatment of a patient with cervical radiculopathy using thoracic spine thrust manipulation, soft tissue mobilization, and exercise. *J Man Manip Ther.* 2008;16:129-135.
429. Gonzalez-Iglesias J, Fernández-de-las-Peñas C, Cleland JA, Alburquerque-Sendin F, Palomeque-del-Cerro L, Mendez-Sanchez R. Inclusion of thoracic spine thrust manipulation into an electro-therapy/thermal program for the management of patients with acute mechanical neck pain: a randomized clinical trial. *Man Ther.* 2009;14:306-313.
430. Gonzalez-Iglesias J, Fernández-de-las-Peñas C, Cleland JA, Gutierrez-Vega Mdel R. Thoracic spine manipulation for the management of patients with neck pain: a randomized clinical trial. *J Orthop Sports Phys Ther.* 2009;39(1):20-27.
431. Cleland JA, Mintken PE, Carpenter K, et al. Examination of a clinical prediction rule to identify patients with neck pain likely to benefit from thoracic spine thrust manipulation and a general cervical range of motion exercise: multi-center randomized clinical trial. *Phys Ther.* 2010;90:1239-1250.
432. Cross KM, Kuenze C, Grindstaff T, Hertel J. Thoracic spine thrust manipulation improves pain, range of motion,and self-reported function in patients with mechanical neck pain: a systematic review. *J Orthop Sports Phys Ther.* 2011;41(9):633-642.
433. McKenzie R, May S. *The Cervical and Thoracic Spine Mechanical Diagnosis and Therapy.* Vol 2. Raumati Beach, New Zealand: Spinal Publications New Zealand Ltd; 2006:171-282.
434. Childs JD, Fritz JM, Piva SR, Whitman JM. Proposal of a classification system for patients with neck pain. *J Orthop Sports Phys Ther.* 2004;34:686-696.
435. Clare A, Adams R., Maher C. Reliability of McKenzie classification of patients with cervical or lumbar pain. *J Manipulative Physiol Ther.* 2005;28:122-127.
436. Schenk R, Bhaidani T, Boswell M, Kelley J, Kruchowky T. Inclusion of mechanical diagnosis and therapy (MDT) in the management of cervical radiculopathy: a case report. *J Man Manip Ther.* 2008;16(1):E2-E8.
437. Edward BC. Combined movements in the cervical spine (C2-C7) their value in examination and technique choice. *Aust J Physiother.* 1980;26(5):165-171.
438. McCarthy C. *Combined Movement Theory: Rational Mobilization and Manipulation of the Vertebral Column.* New York, NY: Churchill Livingstone, Elsevier Limited; 2010:111-164.
439. Bertilson BC, Grunnesjö M, Strender LE. Reliability of clinical tests in the assessment of patients with neck/shoulder problems: impact of history. *Spine.* 2003;28(19):2222-2231.
440. Rubinstein SM, Pool JJM, van Tulder MW, Riphagen II, de Vet HCW. A systematic review of diagnostic accuracy of provocative tests of the neck for diagnosing cervical radiculopathy. *Eur Spine J.* 2007;16:307-319.
441. Sanders RJ, Hammond SL, Rao NM. Thoracic outlet syndrome: a review. *Neurologist.* 2008;14(6):365-373.

442. Stalka S. Thoracic outlet syndrome. In: Fernández de las Peñas C, Cleland J, Huijbregts P. *Neck and Arm Pain Syndromes. Evidence-Informed Screening, Diagnosis and Management.* New York, NY: Churchill Livingstone Elsevier Inc; 2011:141-152.
443. Watson LA, Pizzari T, Balster S. Thoracic outlet syndrome part 1: clinical manifestations, differentiation and treatment pathways. *Man Ther.* 2009;14(6):586-595.
444. Watson LA, Pizzari T, Balster S. Thoracic outlet syndrome part 2: conservative management of thoracic outlet. *Man Ther.* 2010;15(4):305-314.
445. Mackinnon SE, Novak CB. Thoracic outlet syndrome. *Curr Probl Surg.* 2002;39(11):1070-1145. In: Watson LA, Pizzari T, Balster S. Thoracic outlet syndrome part 2: conservative management of thoracic outlet. *Man Ther.* 2010;15(4):305-314.
446. Gillard J, Pérez-Cousin M, Hachulla E, et al. Diagnosing thoracic outlet syndrome: contribution of provocative tests, ultrasonography, electrophysiology, and helical computed tomography in 48 patients. *Joint Bone Spine.* 2001;68(5):416-424.
447. Hooper TL, Denton J, McGalliard MK, Brismée JM, Sizer PS. Thoracic outlet syndrome: a controversial clinical condition. Part 1: anatomy, and clinical examination/diagnosis. *J Man Manip Ther.* 2010;18(2):74-83.
448. Hooper TL, Denton J, McGalliard MK, Brismée JM, Sizer PS. Thoracic outlet syndrome: a controversial clinical condition. Part 2: non-surgical and surgical management. *J Man Manip Ther.* 2010;18(3):132-138.
449. Plewa MC, Delinger M. The false-positive rate of thoracic outlet syndrome shoulder maneuvers in healthy subjects. *Acad Emerg Med.* 1998;5:337-342.
450. Howard M, Lee C, Dellon AL. Documentation of brachial plexus compression (in the thoracic inlet) utilizing provocative neurosensory and muscular testing. *J Reconstr Microsurg.* 2003;19:303-312.
451. Nord KM, Kapoor P, Fisher J, et al. False positive rate of thoracic outlet syndrome diagnostic maneuvers. *Electromyogr Clin Neurophysiol.* 2008;48:67-74.
452. Rayan GM, Jensen C. Thoracic outlet syndrome: provocative examination maneuvers in a typical population. *J Shoulder Elbow Surg.* 1995;4:113-117.
453. Quintner JL. A study of upper limb pain and paresthesia following neck injury in motor vehicle accidents: assessment of the brachial plexus tension test of Elvey. *Br J Rheumatol.* 1989;28:528-533.
454. Greening J, Dilley A, Lynn B. In vivo study of nerve movement and mechanosensitivity of the median nerve in whiplash and non-specific arm pain patients. *Pain.* 2005;115:248-253.
455. Bohannon, RW. Comfortable and maximum walking speed of adults aged 20-79 years: reference values and determinants. *Age Ageing.* 1997;26(1):15-19.
456. Marchetti GF, Whitney SL, Blatt PJ, Morris LO, Vance JM. Temporal and spatial characteristics of gait during performance of the Dynamic Gait Index in people with and people without balance or vestibular disorders. *Phys Ther.* 2008;88(5):640-651.
457. Kristjansson E, Treleaven J. Sensorimotor function and dizziness in neck pain: implications for assessment and management. *Man Ther.* 2009;39(5):364-377.
458. Tjell C, Tenenbaum A, Sandstrom S. Smooth pursuit neck torsion test: a specific test for whiplash associated disorders? *J Whiplash Rel Disorders.* 2002;1:9-24.
459. Grip H, Jull G, Treleaven J. Head eye co-ordination using simultaneous measurement of eye in head and head in space movements: potential for use in subjects with a whiplash injury. *J Clin Mon Computing.* 2009;23:31-40.
460. Mintken PE, Metrick L, Flynn T. Upper cervical ligament testing in a patient with os odontoideum presenting with headaches. *J Orthop Sports Phys Ther.* 2008;38(8):465-475.
461. Aspinall W. Clinical testing for the craniovertebral hypermobility syndrome. *J Orthop Sports Phys Ther.* 1990;12:47-54.
462. Uitvlugt G, Indenbaum S. Clinical assessment of atlantoaxial instability using the Sharp-Purser test. *Arthritis Rheum.* 1988;31(7):918-922.
463. Cleland JA, Koppenhaver S. *Netter's Orthopaedic Clinical Examination: An Evidence-Based Approach.* Philadelphia, PA: Saunders, Elsevier Inc; 2011:115.
464. Osmotherly PG, Rivett DA, Rowe LJ. The anterior shear and distraction tests for craniocervical instability. An evaluation using magnetic resonance imaging. *Man Ther.* 2012;17(5):416-421. Epub 2012 May 3.
465. Pettman E. Stress tests of the craniovertebral joints. In: Boyling JD, Palastanga N, eds. *Grieve's Modern Manual Therapy: The Vertebral Column.* 2nd ed. Edinburgh, Scotland: Churchill Livingstone; 1994:529-537.
466. Beeton K. Instability in the upper cervical region: clinical presentation, radiological and clinical testing. *Man Ther.* 1995;27:19-32.
467. Osmotherly PG, Rivett DA, Rose LJ. Imaging integrity: an evaluation using magnetic resonance. *Phys Ther.* 2012;92:718-725.
468. Fjellner A, Bexander C, Faleij R, Strender LE. Interexaminer reliability in physical examination of the neck. *J Manipulative Physiol Ther.* 1999;22:511-516.
469. Pool JJ, Hoving JL, de Vet HC, van Mameren H, Bouter LM. The interexaminer reproducibility of physical examination of the cervical spine. *J Manipulative Physiol Ther.* 2004;27:84-90.
470. Jull G, Zito G, Trott P, Potter H, Shirley D. Inter-examiner reliability to detect painful upper cervical joint dysfunction. *Aust J Physiother.* 1997;43:125-129.
471. Jull G, Bogduk N, Marsland A. The accuracy of manual diagnosis for cervical zygapophyseal joint pain syndromes. *Med Journal of Australia.* 1988;148:233-236.
472. Maitland G, Hengeveld E, Banks K, English K. *Maitland's Vertebral Manipulation.* 6th ed. Boston, MA: Butterworth-Heinemann; 2002:249-258.
473. Greenman PE. *Principles of Manual Medicine.* 3rd ed. Philadelphia, PA: Lippincott Williams and Wilkins; 2003:202-228, 539-544.
474. Bogduk N. Cervicogenic headache: anatomic basis and pathophysiologic mechanisms. *Curr Pain Headache Rep.* 2001;5:382-386.
475. Aprill C, Axinn MJ, Bogduk N. Occipital headaches stemming from the lateral atlanto-axial (C1-C2) joint. *Cephalalgia.* 2002;22:15-22.
476. Hall T, Briffa K, Hopper D. Clinical evaluation of cervicogenic headache: a clinical perspective. *J Man Manip Ther.* 2008;16:73-80.
477. Hall TM, Robinson KW, Fujinawa O, Akasaka K, Pyne EA. Intertester reliability and diagnostic validity of the cervical flexion-rotation test. *J Manipulative Physiol Ther.* 2008;31:293-300.
478. Ogince M, Hall T, Robinson K, Blackmore AM. The diagnostic validity of the cervical flexion-rotation test in C1-C2-related cervicogenic headache. *Man Ther.* 2007;12:256-262.
479. Hall T, Briffa K. Hopper D, Robinson K. Long-term stability and minimal detectable change of the cervical flexion-rotation test. *J Orthop Sports Phys Ther.* 2010;40(4):225-229.
480. Panjabi MM, Cholewicki J, Nibu K, Grauer J, Babat LB, Dvorak J. Critical load of the human cervical spine: an in vitro experimental study. *Clin Biomech (Bristol, Avon).* 1998;13:11-17.

481. Conley MS, Meyer RA, Bloomberg JJ, et al. Noninvasive analysis of human neck muscle function. *Spine.* 1995;20:2505-2512.
482. Boyd-Clark L, Briggs C, Galea M. Comparative histochemical composition of muscle fibres in a pre- and a costovertebral muscle of the cervical spine. *J Anat.* 2001;199:709-716.
483. Boyd-Clark L, Briggs C, Galea M. Muscle spindle distribution, morphology, and density in longus colli and multifidus muscle of the cervical spine. *Spine.* 2002;27:694-701.
484. Peck D, Buxton DF, Nitz A. A comparison of spindle concentrations in large and small muscles acting in parallel combinations. *J Morphol.* 1984;180:243-252.
485. Falla D, Bilenkij G Jull G. Patients with chronic neck pain demonstrate altered patterns of muscle activation during performance of a functional upper limb task. *Spine.* 2004;29:1436-1440.
486. Hallgren RC, Greenman PE, Rechtien JJ. Atrophy of suboccipital muscles in patients with chronic pain: a pilot study. *J Am Osteopath Assoc.* 1994;94:1032-1038.
487. McPartland JM, Brodeur RR, Hallgren RC: Chronic neck pain, standing balance, and suboccipital muscle atrophy—a pilot study. *J Manipulative Physiol Ther.* 1997;20:24-29.
488. DeLoose V, van den Oord M, Keser I, et al. MRI study of the morphometry of the cervical musculature in F-16 pilots. *Aviat Space Environ Med.* 2009;80:727-731.
489. Larsson SE, Bengtsson A, Bodegard L, et al. Muscle changes in work-related chronic myalgia. *Acta Orthop Scand.* 1998;59:552-556.
490. Larsson B, Bjork J, Kadi F, et al. Blood supply and oxidative metabolism in muscle biopsies of female cleaners with and without myalgia. *Clin J Pain.* 2004;20:440-446.
491. Larsson R, Cai H, Zhang Q, et al. Visualization of chronic neck-shoulder pain: impaired microcirculation in the upper trapezius muscle in chronic cervico-brachial pain. *Occup Med (London).* 1998;48:189-194.
492. Uhlig Y, Weber BR, Grob D, Muntener M. Fiber composition and fiber transformations in neck muscles of patients with dysfunction of the cervical spine. *J Orthop Res.* 1995;13:240-249.
493. Jull GA, O'Leary SP, Falla DL. Clinical assessment of the deep cervical flexor muscles: the craniocervical flexion test. *J Man Manip Physio Ther.* 2008;31(7):525-533.
494. Fernández-de-las-Peñas C, Falla D, Arendt-Nielsen L, Farina D. Cervical muscle coactivation in isometric contractions is enhanced in chronic tension-type headache patients. *Cephalalgia.* 2008;28:744-751.
495. Lindstrøm R, Schomacher J, Farina D, et al. Association between neck muscle coactivation, pain, and strength in women with neck pain. *Man Ther.* 2011;16:80-86.
496. Johnston V, Jull G, Darnell R, et al. Alterations in cervical muscle activity in functional and stressful tasks in female office workers with neck pain. *Eur J Appl Physiol.* 2008;103:253-264.
497. Falla D, Farina D. Muscle fiber conduction velocity of the upper trapezius muscle during dynamic contraction of the upper limb in patients with chronic neck pain. *Pain.* 2005;116:138-145.
498. Fredin Y, Elert J, Britschgi N, Nyberg V, Vaher A, Gerdle B. A decreased ability to relax between repetitive muscle contractions in patients with chronic symptoms after whiplash trauma of the neck. *J Musculoskel Pain.* 1997;5:55-70.
499. Falla D, Jull G, Edwards S, Koh K, Rainoldi A. Neuromuscular efficiency of the sternocleidomastoid and anterior scalene muscles in patients with chronic neck pain. *Disabil Rehabil.* 2004;26:712-717.
500. Wenngren BI, Pettersson K, Lowenhielm G, Hildingsson C. Eye motility and auditory brainstem response dysfunction after whiplash injury. *Acta Otolaryngol.* 2002;122:276-283.
501. Madeleine P, Nielsen M, Arendt-Nielsen L. Characterization of postural control deficit in whiplash patients by means of linear and nonlinear analyses: a pilot study. *J Electromyogr Kinesiol.* 2011;21:291-297.
502. Strimpakos N. The assessment of the cervical spine. Part 2: strength and endurance/fatigue. *J Bodyw Mov Ther.* 2011;15:217-430.
503. Grimmer K. Measuring the endurance capacity of the cervical short flexor muscle group. *Aust J Physiother.* 1994;40:251-254.
504. Domenech MA, Sizer PS, Dedrick GS, McGalliard MK, Brismee JM. The deep neck flexor endurance test: normative data scores in health adults. *PMR.* 2011;3:105-110.
505. Harris KD, Heer DM, Roy TC, et al. Reliability of a measurement of neck flexor muscle endurance. *Phys Ther.* 2005;85:1349-1355.
506. O'Leary S, Falla D, Jull G, Vicenzino B. Muscle specificity in tests of cervical flexor muscle performance. *J Electromyogr Kinesiol.* 2007;17:35-40.
507. Sterling M, Jull G, Vicenzino B, Kenardy J, Darnell R. Development of motor system dysfunction following whiplash injury. *Pain.* 2003;103:65-73.
508. Falla D, Jull G, Hodges P. Training the cervical muscle with prescribed motor tasks does not change muscle activation during a functional activity. *Man Ther.* 2008;13:507-512.
509. Cagnie B, Danneels L, Cools A, Dickx N, Cambier D. The influence of breathing type, expiration and cervical posture on the performance of the craniocervical flexion test in healthy subjects. *Man Ther.* 2008;13:232-238.
510. Jull G, Barrett C, Magee R, et al. Further characterization of muscle dysfunction in cervical headache. *Cephalalgia.* 1999;19:179-185.
511. Lindstroem R, Graaven-Nielsen T, Falla D. Current pain and fear of pain contribute to reduced maximum voluntary contraction of neck muscles in patients with chronic neck pain. *Arch Phys Med Rehabil.* 2012;93(11):2042-2048.
512. Chiu TT, Sing KL. Evaluation of cervical range of motion and isometric neck muscle strength: reliability and validity. *Clin Rehabil.* 2002;16:851-858.
513. Ylinen J, Salo P, Nykanen M, Kautianinen H. Kakkinen A. Decreased isometric neck strength in women with chronic neck pain and the repeatability of neck strength measurements. *Arch Phys Med Rehabil.* 2004;85:1303-1308.
514. Ylinen J, Takala EP, Kautiainen H, et al. Association of neck pain, disability and neck pain during maximal effort with neck muscle strength and range of movement in women with chronic non-specific neck pain. *Eur J Pain.* 2004;8:473-478.
515. Prushansky T, Gepstein R, Gordon C, Dvir Z. Cervical muscles weakness in chronic whiplash patients. *Clin Biomech (Bristol, Avon).* 2005;20:794-798.
516. Cagnie B, Dickx N, Peeters I, et al. The use of functional MRI to evaluate cervical flexor activity during different cervical flexion exercises. *J Appl Physiol.* 2008;104:230-235.
517. De Loose V, Van den OM, Burnotte F, et al. Functional assessment of the cervical spine in F-16 pilots with and without neck pain. *Aviat Space Environ Med.* 2009;80:477-481.
518. O'Leary S, Falla D, Hodges PW, Jull G, Vicenzino B. Specific therapeutic exercise of the neck induces immediate local hypoalgesia. *J Pain.* 2007;8:832-839.
519. Ask T, Strand LI, Skouen JS. The effect of two exercise regimes; motor control versus endurance/strength training for patients with whiplash-associated disorders: a randomized controlled pilot study. *Clin Rehabil.* 2009;23:812-823.

520. Dvir Z, Prushansky T. Cervical muscles strength testing: methods and clinical implications. *J Manipulative Physiol Ther.* 2008;31:518-524.
521. Kendall FP, McCreary EK, Provance PG. *Muscles Testing and Function.* 4th ed. Baltimore, MD: Williams and Wilkins; 1993:314-319.
522. Bohannon RW. Literature reporting normative data for muscle strength measured by hand-held dynamometry: a systematic review. *Isokinet Exerc Sci.* 2011;19:143-147.
523. van der Ploeg RJO, Fidler V, Oosterhuis HGGH. Handheld myometry: reference values. *J Neurol Neurosurg Psychiatry.* 1991;54:244-247.
524. Phillips BA, Lo SK, Mastaglia FL. Muscle force measured using "break" testing with a hand-held myometer in normal subjects aged 20-69 years. *Arch Phys Med Rehabil.* 2000;81:653-661.
525. Beenakker EAC, van der Hoeven JH, Fock JM, Maurits NM. Reference values of maximum isometric muscle force obtained in 270 children aged 4-16 years by hand-held dynamometry, *Neuromusc Disord.* 2011;11:441-446.
526. Mayer TG, Barnes D, Kishino ND, et al. Progressive isoinertial lifting evaluation: I. A standardized protocol and normative database. *Spine.* 1988;13:993-997. Erratum in *Spine.* 1990;15(1):5.
527. Horneij E, Homstrom E, Hemborg B, Isberg PE, Ekdahl CH. Interrater reliability and between-days repeatability of eight physical performance tests. *Adv Physiother.* 2002;4:146-160.
528. Ljungquist T, Jensen IB, Nygren Å, Harms-Ringdahl K. Physical performance tests for people with long-term spinal pain: aspects of construct validity. *J Rehabil Med.* 2003;35:69-75.
529. Page P, Frank CC, Lardner R. *Assessment and Treatment of Muscle Imbalance. The Janda Approach.* Champaign, IL: Benchmark Physical Therapy Inc; 2010:105-108.
530. Bershin JF, Maguire K. Levator scapulae action during shoulder movement. A possible mechanism of shoulder pain of cervical origin. *Aus J Physiother.* 1986;32:101-106.
531. Lewis JS and Valentine RE. The pectoralis minor length test: a study of the intrarater reliability and diagnostic accuracy in subjects with and without shoulder symptoms. *BMC Musculoskeletal Disorders.* 2007;8:64.
532. Borstad JD. Measurement of pectoralis minor muscle length: validation and clinical application. *J Orthop Sports Phys Ther.* 2008;38(4):169-174.
533. Shacklock M. Neurodynamics. *Physiotherapy.* 1995;81:9-16.
534. Shacklock M. Improving application of neurodynamic (neural tension) testing and treatments: a message to researchers and clinicians. *Man Ther.* 2005;10:175-179.
535. Butler DS. *The Sensitive Nervous System.* Adelaide, Australia: NOI Publications; 2000;48-173, 311-341.
536. Breig A, Marions O. Biomechanics of the lumbosacral nerve roots. *Acta Radiol Diagn (Stockh).* 1963;1:1141-1160.
537. Breig A, El-Nadi AF. Biomechanics of the cervical spinal cord. Relief of contact pressure on and overstretching of the spinal cord. *Acta Radiol Diagn (Stockh).* 1966;4(6):602-624.
538. Mellesi H. The nerve gap: theory and clinical practice. *Hand Clin.* 1986;2:651-663.
539. Ogata K Naito M. Blood flow of peripheral nerve: effects of dissection, stretching and compression. *J Hand Surg (Br).* 1986;11(1):10-14.
540. Driscoll PJ, Glasby MA, Lawson GM. An in vivo study of peripheral nerves in continuity: biomechanical and physiological responses to elongation. *J Orthop Res.* 2002;20(2):370-375.
541. Wall EJ, Massie JB, Kwan MK, et al. Experimental stretch neuropathy. *J Bone Joint Surg Br.* 1992;74(1):126-129.
542. Rydevik B, Lundborg G, Bagge U. Effects of graded compression on intraneural blood flow: an in-vivo study on rabbit and tibial nerve. *J Hand Surg.* 1981;6:3-12.
543. Nee RJ, Butler D. Management of peripheral neuropathic pain: integrating neurobiology, neurodynamics and clinical evidence. *Phys Ther Sport.* 2006;7:36-49.
544. Nee RJ, Jull GA, Vicenzino B, Coppieters MW. The validity of upper-limb neurodynamic tests for detecting peripheral neuropathic pain. *J Orthop Sports Phys Ther.* 2012;42(5):413-424. Epub 2012 Mar 8.
545. Kenneally M, Rubenach H, Elvey R. The upper limb tension test: the SLR test of the arm. In: Grant R, ed. *Physical Therapy of the Cervical and Thoracic Spine.* New York, NY: Churchill Livingstone; 1988:167-194.
546. Lohkamp M, Small K. Normal response to upper limb neurodynamic test 1 and 2A. *Man Ther.* 2011;16:125-130.
547. Raney NH, Petersen EJ, Smith TA, et al. Development of a clinical prediction rule to identify patients with neck pain likely to benefit from cervical traction and exercise. *Eur Spine J.* 2009;18(3):382-391.
548. Coveney B, Trott P, Kneebone C, Shacklock MC. The response to the upper limb tension test in carpal tunnel sufferers. In: Proceedings of the Tenth Biennial Conference of the Manipulative Physiotherapists' Association of Australia, Melbourne; 1997:31-33.
549. Vanti C, Bonfiglioli R, Calabrese M, Marinelli F, Violante FS, Pillastrini P. Relationship between interpretation and accuracy of the upper limb neurodynamic test I in carpal tunnel syndrome. *J Manipulative Physiol Ther.* 2012;35:54-63.
550. Yaxley GA, Jull GA. A modified upper limb tension test: an investigation of responses in normal subjects. *Aust J Physiother.* 1991;37:143-152.
551. Yaxley GA, Jull GA. Adverse tension in the neural system: a preliminary study of tennis elbow. *Aust J Physiother.* 1993;39:15-22.
552. Flanagan M. Normative responses to the ulnar nerve bias tension test. University of South Australia, Adelaide; 1993. In: Butler DS. *The Sensitive Nervous System.* Adelaide, Australia: NOI Publications; 2000;48-173;311-341.
553. Garmer DA, Jones MA, McHorse KJ, Keely G. *The Ulnar Nerve Bias Upper Limb Neurodynamic Tension Test: An Investigation of Responses in Asymptomatic Subjects.* Alexandria, VA: American Physical Therapy Association; 2002. http://apps.apta.org/Custom/abstracts/pt2002/abstractsPt2002.cfm?pubNo=PL-RR-176-F. Accessed September 22, 2013.
554. Covill LG, Petersen SM. Upper extremity neurodynamic tests: range of motion asymmetry may not indicate impairment. *Physiother Theor Pract.* 2012;28(7):535-541.
555. Hollerwöger D. Methodological quality and outcomes of studies addressing manual cervical spine examinations: a review. *Man Ther.* 2006;11:93-98.
556. Stochkendahl H, Christensen J, Hartvigsen W, Vach M, Haas L. Manual examination of the spine: a systematic review of reproducibility. *J Manipul Physiol Ther.* 2006;29:475-485.
557. Lee RYW, McGregor AH, Bull AMJ, Wragg P. Dynamic response of the cervical spine to posteroanterior mobilization. *Clin Biomech.* 2005;20:228-231.
558. Hall T, Briffa K, Hopper D, Robinson K. Reliability of manual examination and frequency of symptomatic cervical motion segment dysfunction in cervicogenic headache. *Man Ther.* 2010;15(6):542-546.
559. Mottram SL, Woledge RC, Morrissey D. Motion analysis study of a scapular orientation exercise and subjects' ability to learn the exercise. *Man Ther.* 2009:14:13-18.
560. Mottram SL. Dynamic stability of the scapula. *Man Ther.* 1997;2:123-131.

561. Wegner S, Jull G, O'Leary S, Johnston V. The effect of a scapular postural correction strategy on trapezius activity in patients with neck pain. *Man Ther.* 2010;15:562-566.
562. Page P, Frank CC, Lardner. Evaluation of movement patterns. In: Page P, Frank CC, Lardner R. *Assessment and Treatment of Muscle Imbalance. The Janda Approach.* Champaign, IL: Human Kinetics; 2010:90-91.
563. American College of Radiology Appropriateness Criteria 2011. http://www.acr.org/SecondaryMainMenuCategories/quality_safety/app_criteria.aspx. Accessed March 9, 2012.
564. Spitzer WO, Skovron ML, Salmi LR, et al. Scientific monograph of the Quebec Task Force on Whiplash-Associated Disorders: redefining "whiplash" and its management. *Spine.* 1995;20(8Suppl):1S-73S.
565. Boutin RD, Steinbach LS, Finnesey K. MR imaging of degenerative diseases in the cervical spine. *Magn Reson Imaging Clin N Am.* 2000;8(3):471-490.
566. Chen CJ, Hsu HL, Niu CC, et al. Cervical degenerative disease at flexion-extension MR imaging: prediction criteria. *Radiology.* 2003;227(1):136-142.
567. Kaale BR, Krakenes J, Albrektsen G, Wester K. Whiplash associated disorders impairment rating: neck disability index score according to severity of MRI findings of ligaments and membranes in the upper cervical spine. *J Neurotrauma.* 2005;22(4):466-475.
568. Johansson BH. Whiplash injuries can be visible by functional magnetic resonance imaging. *Pain Res Manag.* 2006;11(3):197-199.
569. Krakenes J, Kaale BR. Magnetic resonance imaging assessment of craniovertebral ligaments and membranes after whiplash trauma. *Spine (Phila Pa 1976).* 2006;31(24):2820-2826.
570. Ichihara D, Okada E, Chiba K, et al. Longitudinal magnetic resonance imaging study on whiplash injury patients: minimum 10-year follow-up. *J Orthop Sci.* 2009;14(5):602-610.
571. Myran R, Kvistad KA, Nygaard OP, Andresen H, Folvik M, Zwart JA. Magnetic resonance imaging assessment of the alar ligaments in whiplash injuries: a case-control study. *Spine (Phila Pa 1976).* 2008;33(18):2012-2016.
572. Vetti N, Krakenes J, Eide GE, Rorvik J, Gilhus NE, Espeland A. MRI of the alar and transverse ligaments in whiplash-associated disorders (WAD) grades 1-2: high-signal changes by age, gender, event and time since trauma. *Neuroradiology.* 2009;51(4):227-235.
573. Myran R, Kvistad KA, Nygaard OP, Andresen H, Folvik M, ZwartJA. Magnetic resonance imaging assessment of the alar ligaments in whiplash injuries: a case-control study. *Spine (Phila Pa 1976).* 2008;33(18):2012-2016.
574. Aprill C, Bogduk N. The prevalence of cervical zygapophyseal joint pain. A first approximation. *Spine.* 1992;17(7):744-747.
575. Werneke M, Hart DL, Cook D. A descriptive study of the centralization phenomenon. A prospective analysis. *Spine.* 1999;24:676-683.
576. Hoving IL, De Vet HC, Koes BW, et al. Manual therapy, physical therapy, or continued care by the general practitioner for patients with neck pain; long term results from a pragmatic randomized clinical trial. *Clin J Pain.* 2006;22:370-377.
577. Tseng YL, Wang WT, Chen WY, Hou TJ, Chen TC. Lieu FK. Predictors for the immediate responders to cervical manipulation in patients with neck pain. *Man Ther.* 2006;11:306-315.
578. Bowler N, Shamley D, Davies R. The effect of a simulated manipulation position on internal carotid and vertebral artery blood flow in healthy individuals. *Man Ther.* 2011;16:87-93.
579. Puentedura EJ, Cleland JA, Landers MR, Mintken PE, Louw A, Fernández-de-las Peñas C. Development of a clinical prediction rule to identify patients with neck pain likely to benefit from thrust joint manipulation to the cervical spine. *J Orthop Sports Phys Ther.* 2012;42(7):577-592.
580. Olson KA. *Manual Physical Therapy of the Spine.* St. Louis, MO: Saunders; 2009:288-291.
581. Gibbons P, Tehan P. *Manipulation of the Spine, Thorax, and Pelvis. An Osteopathic Perspective.* 3rd ed. Philadelphia, PA: Churchill Livingstone, Elsevier; 2010:103-139.
582. Mintken PE, Cleland JA, Carpenter KJ, Bieniek ML, Keirns M, Whitman JM. Some factors predict successful short-term outcomes in individuals with shoulder pain receiving cervicothoracic manipulation: a single-arm trial. *Phys Ther.* 2010;91(1):26-42. Epub 2009 Dec 3.
583. Cleland JA, Markowski AM, Childs JD. The cervical spine: physical therapy patient management utilizing current evidence. In: *Independent Study Course 16.2.2. Current Concepts of Orthopaedic Physical Therapy.* 2nd ed. La Crosse, WI: Orthpedic Section, APTA, Inc; 2006:25-41.
584. Fryer G. Muscle energy approaches. In: Fernández de las Peñas C, Cleland J, Huijbregts P. *Neck and Army Pain Syndromes. Evidence-Informed Screening, Diagnosis, and Management.* New York, NY: Churchill Livingstone, Elsevier Ltd; 2011:439-454.
585. Kennedy C. Therapeutic exercise for mechanical neck pain. In: Fernández de las Peñas C, Cleland J, Huijbregts P. *Neck and Army Pain Syndromes. Evidence-Informed Screening, Diagnosis, and Management.* New York, NY: Churchill Livingstone, Elsevier Ltd; 2011:185-200.
586. Hall T, Chan HT, Christensen L, Odenthal B, Wells C, Robinson K. Efficacy of a C1-C2 self-sustained natural apophyseal glide (SNAG) in the management of cervicogenic headache. *J Orthop Sports Phys Ther.* 2007;37:100-107.
587. Bookhout MR. Greenman PE. *Principles of Exercise Prescription.* Woburn, MA: Butterworth-Heinemann Medical; 2002; In: Childs JD, Whitman JM, Fritz JM, Piva SR, Young B. *Lower Cervical Spine. Home Study Course 13.3.1. Physical Therapy for the Cervical Spine and Temporomandibular Joint.* La Crosse, WI: Orthopedic Section, APTA, Inc; 2003:31-34.
588. Coronado RA, Gay CW, Bialosky JE, Carnaby GD, Bishop MD, George SZ. Changes in pain sensitivity following spinal manipulation: a systematic review and meta-analysis. *J Electromyogr Kinesiol.* 2012;22(5):752-767.
589. Coronado RA, Bialosky JE, Cook CE. The temporal effects of a single session of high-velocity, low-amplitude thrust manipulation on subjects with spinal pain. *Phys Ther Rev.* 2010;15:1-7.
590. Childs JD, Fritz JM, Flynn TW, et al. A clinical prediction rule to identify patients with low back pain most likely to benefit from spinal manipulation: a validation study. *Ann Intern Med.* 2004;141(12):920-928.
591. Cleland JA, Glynn P, Whitman JM, Eberhart SL, MacDonald C, Childs JD. Short-term effects of thrust versus nonthrust mobilization/manipulation directed at the thoracic spine in patients with neck pain: a randomized clinical trial. *Phys Ther.* 2007;87(4):431-440.
592. Flynn T, Fritz J, Whitman J, et al. A clinical prediction rule for classifying patients with low back pain who demonstrate short-term improvement with spinal manipulation. *Spine (Phila Pa 1976).* 2002;27(24):2835-2843.
593. Fritz JM, Childs JD, Flynn TW. Pragmatic application of a clinical prediction rule in primary care to identify patients with low back pain with a good prognosis following a brief spinal manipulation intervention. *BMC Family Practice.* 2005;6(1):29.
594. Moulson A, Watson T. A preliminary investigation into the relationship between cervical SNAGS and sympathetic nervous system activity in the upper limbs of an asymptomatic population. *Man Ther.* 2006;11:214-224.

595. Perry J, Green A. An investigation into the effects of a unilaterally applied lumbar mobilisation technique on peripheral sympathetic nervous system activity in the lower limbs. *Man Ther.* 2008;13:492-499.
596. Vicenzino B, Collins D, Benson H, Wright A. An investigation of the interrelationship between manipulative therapy-induced hypoalgesia and sympathoexcitation. *J Manip Physiol Ther.* 1998;21:448-453.
597. Sterling M, Jull G, Wright A. Cervical mobilisation: concurrent effects on pain, sympathetic nervous system activity and motor activity. *Man Ther.* 2001;6:72-81.
598. Coppieters MW, Stappaerts KH, Wouters LL, Janssens K. The immediate effects of a cervical lateral glide treatment technique in patients with neurogenic cervicobrachial pain. *J Orthop Sports Phys Ther.* 2003;33:369-378.
599. Petersen N, Vicenzino B, Wright A. The effects of a cervical mobilization technique on sympathetic outflow to the upper limb in normal subjects. *Physiother Theory Pract.* 1993;9:149-156.
600. Chiu TW, Wright A. To compare the effects of different rates of application of a cervical mobilisation technique on sympathetic outflow to the upper limb in normal subjects. *Man Ther.* 1996;1:198-203.
601. Coppieters MW, Stappaerts KH, Wouters LL, Janssens K. Aberrant protective force generation during neural provocation testing and the effect of treatment in patients with neurogenic cervicobrachial pain. *J Manip Physiol Ther.* 2003;26:99-106.
602. Saranga J, Green A, Lewis J, Worsfold C. Effect of a cervical lateral glide on the upper limb neurodynamic test 1: a blinded placebo-controlled investigation. *Physiotherapy.* 2003;89:678-684.
603. Schmid A, Brunner F, Wright A, Bachmann LM. Paradigm shift in manual therapy? Evidence for a central nervous system component in the response to passive cervical joint mobilization. *Man Ther.* 2008;13:387-396.
604. Hegedus EJ, Goode A, Butler RJ, Slaven E. The neurophysiological effects of a single session of spinal joint mobilization: does the effect last? *J Man Manip Ther.* 2011;19(3):143-151.
605. Vicenzino B, Collins D, Wright A. The initial effects of a cervical spine manipulative physiotherapy treatment on the pain and dysfunction of lateral epicondylalgia. *Pain.* 1996;68:69-74.
606. Kanlayanaphotporn R, Chiradejnant A, Vachalathiti R. Immediate effects of the central posteroanterior mobilization technique on pain and range of motion in patients with mechanical neck pain. *Disabil Rehabil.* 2010;32:622-628.
607. Kanlayanaphotporn R, Chiradejnant A, Vachalathiti R. The immediate effects of mobilization technique on pain and range of motion in patients presenting with unilateral neck pain: a randomized controlled trial. *Arch Phys Med Rehabil.* 2009;90:187-192.
608. Lee RY, McGregor AH, Bull AMJ, Wragg P. Dynamic response of the cervical spine to posteroanterior mobilization. *Clin Biomech.* 2005;20:228-231.
609. Gross A, Miller J, D'Sylva J, et al. Manipulation or mobilization for neck pain: a Cochrane Review. *Man Ther.* 2010;15:315-333.
610. Miller J, Gross A, D'Sylva J, et al. Manual therapy and exercise for neck pain: a systematic review. *Man Ther.* 2010;15:334-354.
611. Leaver AM, Maher CG, Herbert RD, et al. A randomized controlled trial comparing manipulation with mobilization for recent onset neck pain. *Arch Phys Med Rehabil.* 2010;91:1313-1318.
612. Walker JM, Boyles RE, Young BA, et al. The effectiveness of manual physical therapy and exercise for mechanical neck pain. A randomized clinical trial. *Spine.* 2008;33(22):2371-2378.
613. Boyles RE, Walker MJ, Young BA, Strunce JB, Wainner RS. The addition of cervical thrust manipulations to a manual physical therapy approach in patients treated for mechanical neck pain: a secondary analysis. *J Orthop Sports Phys Ther.* 2010;40(3):133-140.
614. Puentedura EJ, Landers MR, Cleland JA, Mintken P, Huijbregts P, Fernández-de-las-Peñas C. Thoracic spine thrust manipulation versus cervical spine thrust manipulation in patients with acute neck pain: a randomized clinical trial. *J Orthop Sports Phys Ther.* 2011;41(4):208-220.
615. Dunning JR, Cleland JA, Waldrop MA, et al. Upper cervical and upper thoracic thrust manipulation versus nonthrust mobilization in patients with mechanical neck pain: a multicenter randomized clinical trial. *J Orthop Sports Phys Ther.* 2012;42(1):5-18.
616. Bronført G, Evans R, Anderson AV, Svendsen KH, Bracha Y, Grimm RH. Spinal manipulation, medication, or home exercise with advice for acute and subacute neck pain. *Ann Intern Med.* 2012;156:1-10.
617. Guzman J, Hurwitz EL, Carroll LJ, et al; Bone and Joint Decade 2000-2010 Task Force on Neck Pain and Its Associated Disorders. A new conceptual model of neck pain: linking onset, course, and care: the Bone and Joint Decade 2000-2010 Task Force on Neck Pain and Its Associated Disorders. *Spine (Phila Pa 1976).* 2008;33:S14-S23.
618. Hoving JL, Koes BW, de Vet HCW, et al. Manual therapy, physical therapy, or continued care by a general practitioner for patients with neck pain. A randomized, controlled trial. *Ann Intern Med.* 2002;136:713-722.
619. Korthals-de Bos IBC, Hoving JL, van Tulder MW, et al. Effectiveness of physiotherapy, manual therapy, and general practitioner care for neck pain: economic evaluation alongside a randomised controlled trial. *BMJ.* 2003;325:911-914.
620. Bronfort G, Evans R, Nelson B, Goldsmith CH. A randomized clinical trial of exercise and spinal manipulation for patients with chronic neck pain. *Spine.* 2001;26:788-799.
621. Evans R, Bronfort G, Nelson B, Aker PD, Goldsmith CH, Vernon H. Two-year follow-up of a randomized clinical trial of spinal manipulation and two types of exercise for patients with chronic neck pain. *Spine.* 2002;27:2383-2389.
622. Evans R, Bronfort G, Schulz C, et al. Supervised exercise with and without spinal manipulation perform similarly and better than home exercise for chronic neck pain: a randomized controlled trial. *Spine (Phila Pa 1976).* 2012;37(11):903-914.
623. Walser RF, Meserve BB, Boucher TR. et al. The effectiveness of thoracic spine manipulation for management of musculoskeletal conditions: a systematic review and meta-analysis of randomized clinical trials. *J Man Manip Ther.* 2009;17(4):237-246.
624. Cleland JA, Whitman JM, Fritz JM, Palmer JA. Manual physical therapy, cervical traction, and strengthening exercises in patients with cervical radiculopathy: a case series. *J Orthop Sports Phys Ther.* 2005;35:802-811.
625. Carpenter KJ, Mintken P, Cleland JA. Evaluation of outcomes in patients with neck pain treated with thoracic spine manipulation and exercise: a case series. *N Z J Physiother.* 2009;37:71-80.
626. Fernández-de-las-Peñas C, Fernández- Carnero J, Fernández AP, Lomas-Varga R, Miangolarra-Page JC. Dorsal manipulation in whiplash injury treatment: A randomized controlled trial. *J Whiplash Rel Disord.* 2004;3(2):55-72.

627. Fernández-de-Las-Peñas C, Palomeque-del-Cerro L, Rodríguez-Blanco C, Gómez-Conesa A, Miangolarra-Page JC. Changes in neck pain and active range of motion after a single thoracic spine manipulation in subjects with mechanical neck pain: a case series. *J Manipulative Physiol Ther.* 2007;30(4):312-320.
628. Browder DA, Erhard RE, Piva SR, et al. Intermittent cervical traction and thoracic manipulation for management of mild cervical compressive myelopathy attributed to cervical herniated disc: a case series. *J Orthop Sports Phys Ther.* 2004;34:701-712.
629. Pho C, Godges JJ. Management of whiplash-associated disorder addressing thoracic and cervical spine impairments: a case report. *J Orthop Sports Phys Ther.* 2004;34(9):511-523.
630. Costello M. Treatment of a patient with cervical radiculopathy using thoracic spine thrust manipulation, soft tissue mobilization, and exercise. *J Man Manp Ther.* 2008;16(3):129-135.
631. González-Iglesias J, Fernández-de-las-Peñas C, Cleland JA, Gutiérrez-Vega MR. Thoracic spine manipulation for the management of patients with neck pain: a randomized clinical trial. *J Orthop Sports Phys Ther.* 2009;39:20-27.
632. González-Iglesias J, Fernández-de-las-Peñas C, Cleland JA, Alburquerque-Sendín F, Palomeque-del-Cerro L, Mendes-Sanchez R. Inclusion of thoracic spine thrust manipulation into an electro-therapy/thermal program for the management of patients with acute mechanical neck pain: a randomized clinical trial. *Man Ther.* 2009;14:306-313.
633. Lau HMC, Chiu TTW, Lam TH. The effectiveness of thoracic manipulation on patients with chronic mechanical neck pain: a randomized controlled trial. *Man Ther.* 2011;16:141-147.
634. Kroeling P, Gross A, Goldsmith CH, et al. Electrotherapy for neck pain. *Cochrane Database Syst Rev.* 2009;(4):CD004251.
635. Gross A, Forget M, St. George K, et al. Patient education for neck pain. *Cochrane Database Syst Rev.* 2012;3:CD005106.
636. Salt E, Wright C, Kelly S, Dean A. A systematic literature review on the effectiveness of non-invasive therapy for cervicobrachial pain. *Man Ther.* 2011;16:53-65.
637. Boyles R, Toy P, Mellon J, Hayes M, Hammer B. Effectiveness of manual physical therapy in the treatment of cervical radiculopathy: a systematic review. *J Man Manip Ther.* 2011;19(3):135-142.
638. Ragonese J. A randomised trial comparing manual physical therapy therapeutic exercises, to a combination of therapies for the treatment of cervical radiculopathy. *Orthopaedic Practice.* 2009;21(3):71-75.
639. Young I, Michener L, Cleland J, Arnold J, Aguilera A, Snyder A. Manual therapy, exercise, and traction for patients with cervical radiculopathy: a randomized clinical trial. *Phys Ther.* 2009;89(7):632-642.
640. Forbush SW, Cox T, Wilson E. Treatment of patients with degenerative cervical radiculopathy using a multimodal conservative approach in a geriatric population: a case series. *J Orthop Sports Phys Ther.* 2011;41(10):723-733
641. Cleland JA, Fritz JM, Whitman JM, Heath R. Predictors of short-term outcome in people with a clinical diagnosis of cervical radiculopathy. *Phys Ther.* 2007;87:1619-1632.
642. Langevin P, Roy JS, Desmeules F. Cervical radiculopathy: study protocol of a randomized clinical trial evaluating the effect of mobilizations and exercises targeting the opening of intervertebral foramen. *BMC Musculoskelet Disord.* 2012;13:10.
643. Werneke M, Hart DL. Centralization phenomenon as a prognostic factor for chronic low back pain and disability. *Spine.* 2001;26:758-765.
644. Kjellman G, Öberg B. A randomized clinical trial comparing general exercise, McKenzie treatment and a control group in patients with neck pain. *J Rehabil Med.* 2002;34:183-190.
645. Klaber-Moffett JK, Jackson DA, Gardiner ED, et al. Randomized trial of two physiotherapy interventions for primary care neck and back pain patients: "McKenzie" vs brief physiotherapy pain management. *Rheumatology.* 2006;45:1514-1421.
646. Attal N, Bouhissera D. Can pain be more or less neuropathic? *Pain.* 2004;110:510-511.
647. Allison GT, Nagy BM, Hall T. A randomized clinical trial of manual therapy for cervicobrachial pain syndrome: a pilot study. *Man Ther.* 2002;7(2):95-102.
648. Nee RJ, Vicenzino, Jull GA, Cleland JA, Coppieters MW. Neural tissue management provides immediate clinically relevant benefits without harmful effects for patients with nerve-related neck and arm pain: a randomized trial. *J Physiotherapy.* 2012;58:23-31.
649. Nee R, Vicenzino B, Jull G, Cleland J, Coppieters M. A novel protocol to develop a prediction model that identifies patients with nerve-related neck and arm pain who benefit from the early introduction of neural tissue management. *Contemporary Clinical Trials.* 2011;32:760-770.
650. Berg HE, Berggren G, Tesch PA. Dynamic neck strength training effect on pain and function. *Arch Phys Med Rehab.* 1994;75:661-665.
651. Ylinen J, Takala EP, Nykanen M, et al. Active neck muscle training in the treatment of chronic neck pain in women: a randomized controlled trial. *JAMA.* 2003;289:2509-2516.
652. Ylinen J, Häkkinen A, Nykänen M, Kautiainen H, Takala EP. Neck muscle training in the treatment of chronic neck pain: a three-year follow-up study. *Eura Medicophys.* 2007;43:161-169.
653. Chiu TTW, Lam TH, Hedley AJ. A randomized controlled trial on the efficacy of exercise for patients with chronic neck pain. *Spine.* 2005;30(1):E1-E7.
654. Jull G, Falla D, Hodges P, Vicenzino B. Cervical flexor muscle retraining: physiological mechanisms of efficacy. In: Proceedings of the 2nd International Conference on Movement Dysfunction. Edinburgh, Scotland; 2005.
655. Jull GA, Fall D, Vicenzino B, Hodges PW. The effect of therapeutic exercise on activation of the deep cervical flexor muscles in people with chronic neck pain. *Man Ther.* 2009;14:696-701.
656. Jull G, Falla D, Treleaven J, Hodges P, Vicenzino B. Retraining cervical joint position sense: the effect of two exercise regimes. *J Orthop Res.* 2007;25:404-412.
657. Uthaikhup S, Jull G , Sungkarat S, Treleaven J. The influence of neck pain on sensorimotor function in the elderly. *Arch Gerontol Geriatr.* 2012;55(3):667-672.
658. Jull G, Sterling M, Falla D, Treleaven J, O'Leary S. Therapeutic exercise for cervical disorders: practice pointers. In: *Whiplash, Headache and Neck Pain. Research-Based Directions for Physical Therapists.* New York, NY: Churchill Livinstone, Elsevier Limited; 2008:207-229.
659. Beer A, Treleaven J, Jull G. Can a functional postural exercise improve performance in the craniocervical flexion test? A preliminary study. *Man Ther.* 2012;17(3):219-224.
660. O'Leary S, Cagnie B, Reeve A, Jull G, Elliott JM. Is there altered activity of the extensor muscles in chronic mechanical neck pain? A functional magnetic resonance imaging study. *Arch Phys Med Rehabil.* 2011;92:929-934.
661. Amiri M, Jull G, Bullock-Saxton J, Darnell R, Lander C. Cervical musculoskeletal impairment in frequent intermittent headache. Part 2: subjects with concurrent headache types. *Cephalalgia.* 2007;27:891-898.

662. Fernández-de-las-Peñas C, Albert-Sanchís JC, Buil M, Benitez JC, Alburquerque-Sendín F. Cross-sectional area of cervical multifidus muscle in females with chronic bilateral neck pain compared to controls. *J Orthop Sports Phys Ther.* 2008;38:175-180.
663. Fernández-de-Las-Peñas C, Bueno A, Ferrando J, Elliott JM, Cuadrado ML, Pareja JA. Magnetic resonance imaging study of the morphometry of cervical extensor muscles in chronic tension-type headache. *Cephalalgia.* 2007;27:355-362.
664. Elliott J, Jull G, Noteboom JT, Galloway G. MRI study of the cross-sectional area for the cervical extensor musculature in patients with persistent whiplash associated disorders (WAD). *Man Ther.* 2008;13:258-265.
665. Elliott JM, O'Leary SP, Cagnie B, Durbridge G, Danneels L, Jull G. Craniocervical orientation affects muscle activation when exercising the cervical extensors in healthy subjects. *Arch Phys Med Rehabil.* 2010;91:1418-1422.
666. Fountain FP, Minear WL, Allison PD. Function of longus colli and longissimus cervicis muscles in man. *Arch Phys Med Rehabil.* 1966;47:665-669. In: *Whiplash, Headache and Neck Pain. Research-Based Directions for Physical Therapists.* New York, NY: Churchill Livinstone, Elsevier Limited; 2008:218.
667. Mintken PE, Cleland J. In a 32-year-old woman with chronic neck pain and headaches. Will an exercise regimen be beneficial for reducing her reports of neck pain and headaches? *Phys Ther.* 2012;92(5):1-7.
668. International Headache Society. The International Classification of Headache Disorders. 2nd ed. *Cephalalgia.* 2004;24(Suppl1):9-160.
669. Haldeman S, Dagenais S. Cervicogenic headaches: a critical review. *Spine J.* 2001;1:31-46.
670. Sjaastad O, Bakketeig LS. Prevalence of cervicogenic headache: Vaga study of headache epidemiology. *Acta Neurol Scand.* 2008;117:170-183.
671. Huijbregts PA. Clinical reasoning in the diagnosis: history taking in patient with headache. In: Fernández-de-las-Peñas C, Nielsen LA, Gerwin RD. *Tension-Type and Cervicogenic Headache: Pathophysiology, Diagnosis, and Management.* Boston, MA: Jones and Bartlett Publishers: 2010:133-151.
672. Fernández-de-las-Peñas C, Nielsen LA, Gerwin RD. *Tension-Type and Cervicogenic Headache: Pathophysiology, Diagnosis, and Management.* Boston, MA: Jones and Bartlett Publishers: 2010.
673. Cuadrado ML, Pareja JA. Medical approach to headaches. In: Fernández-de-las-Peñas C, Nielsen LA, Gerwin RD. *Tension-Type and Cervicogenic Headache: Pathophysiology, Diagnosis, and Management.* Boston, MA: Jones and Bartlett Publishers: 2010:15-20.
674. Detsky ME, McDonald DR, Baerlocher MO, Tomlinson GA, McCrory DC, Booth CM. Does this patient with headache have a migraine or need neuroimaging? *JAMA.* 2006;296(10):1274-1283.
675. Sjaastad O, Fredriksen TA, Pfaffenrath V. Cervicogenic headache: diagnostic criteria. The Cervicogenic Headache International Study Group. *Headache.* 1998;38:442-445.
676. Hagen K, Einarsen C, Zwart J, Svebak S, Bovim G. The co-occurrence of headache and musculoskeletal symptoms amongst 51,050 adults in Norway. *Eur J Neurol.* 2002;9:527-533.
677. McDonnell M, Sahrmann S, Van Dillen L. A specific exercise program and modification of postural alignment for the treatment of cervicogenic headache: a case report. *J Orthop Sports Phys Ther.* 2005;35:3-15.
678. Hall T, Robinson K. The flexion-rotation test and active cervical mobility: a comparative measurement study in cervicogenic headache. *Man Ther.* 2004;9:197-202.
679. Hall TM, Briffa K, Hopper D, Robinson K. Comparative analysis and diagnostic accuracy of the cervical flexion-rotation test. *J Headache Pain.* 2010;11(5):391-397.
680. Fernández-de-las-Penas C, Cuadrado ML, Arendt-Nielsen L, Simons DG, Pareja JA. Myofascial trigger points and sensitisation: an updated pain model for tension type headache. *Cephalalgia.* 2007;27:383-393.
681. Fernández-de-las-Penas C, Perez-de-Heredia M, Molero-Sanchez A, Miangolarra-Page JC. Performance of the craniocervical flexion test, forward head posture, and headache clinical parameters in patients with chronic tension type headache: a pilot study. *J Orthop Sports Phys Ther.* 2007;37:33-39.
682. Fernández-de-las-Penas C, Bueno A, Ferrando J, Elliott JM, Cuadrado ML, Pareja JA. Magnetic resonance imaging of the morphometry of cervical extensor muscles in chronic tension type headache. *Cephalalgia.* 2007;27:355-362.
683. Fernández-de-las-Penas C, Coppieters MW, Cuadrado ML, Pareja JA. Patients with chronic tension type headache demonstrate increased mechanosensitivity of the supraorbital nerve. *Headache.* 2008;48:570-577.
684. Chaibi A, Russell MB. Manual therapies for cervicogenic headache: a systematic review. *J Headache Pain.* 2012;13(5):351-359.
685. Posadzki P, Ernst E. Spinal manipulations for cervicogenic headaches: a systematic review of randomized clinical trials. *Headache: The Journal of Head and Face Pain.* 2011;51(7):1132-1139.
686. Posadzki P, Ernst E. Spinal manipulations fro the treatment of migraine: a systematic review of randomized clinical trials. *Cephalalgia.* 2011;31(8):964-970.
687. Fernández-de-las-Peñas C, Alonso-Blanco C, Cuadrado ML, Miangolarra JC, Barriga FJ, Pareja JA. Are manual therapies effective in reducing pain from tension-type headache? A systematic review. *Clin J Pain.* 2006;22:278-285.
688. Brønfort G, Nilsson N, Haas M, et al. Noninvasive physical treatments for chronic/recurrent headache. *Cochrane Database Syst Rev.* 2004;(3):CD001878.
689. Fernández-de-las-Peñas C, Cleland JA, Cuadrado ML, Pareja JA. Predictor variables for identifying patients with chronic tension type headache who are likely to achieve short-term success with muscle trigger point therapy. *Cephalalgia.* 2008;28(3):264-275.
690. Van Ettekoven H, Lucas C. Efficacy of physiotherapy incliding a craniocervical training programme for tension-type headache: a randomized clinical trial. *Celphalalgia.* 2006;26(8):983-991.
691. Ylinen J Nikander R, NykänenM, Kautiainen H, Häkkinen A. Effect of neck exercises on cervicogenic headache: a randomized controlled trial. *J Rehabil Med.* 2010;42(4):344-349.
692. Provinciali L, Baroni M. Clinical approaches to whiplash injuries: a review. *Crit Rev Phys Rehabil Med.* 1999;11:339-368.
693. Barnsley L, Lord S, Bogduk N. The pathophysiology of whiplash. *Spine.* 1998;12:209-242.
694. Woolf CJ, Decosterd I. Implications of recent advances in the understanding of pain pathophysiology for the assessment of pain in patients. *Pain.* 1999;(Suppl 6):S141-147.
695. Jensen TS, Baron R. Translation of symptoms and signs into mechanisms in neuropathic pain. *Pain.* 2003;102:1-8.
696. Sterling M. Whiplash associated disorders. In: Fernández-de-las-Peñas C, Cleland J, Huijbregts P. *Neck and Arm Pain Syndromes: Evidence-Informed Screening, Diagnosis and Management.* Philadelphia, PA: Elsevier Ltd; 2011:112-122.
697. Elliott J, Jull G, Noteboom T, Darnell R, Galloway G, Givvon W. Fatty infiltration in the cervical extensor muscles in persistent whiplash associated disorders: an MRI analysis. *Spine.* 2006;31:E847-851.

698. Elliott J, O'Leary S, Sterling M, Hendrikz J, Pedler A, Jull G. MRI findings of fatty infiltrate in the cervical flexors in chronic whiplash. *Spine.* 2010;35:948-954.
699. Raak R, Wallin M. Thermal thresholds and catastrophizing in individuals with chronic pain after whiplash injury. *Biology Research Nursing.* 2006;8:138-146.
700. Chien A, Eliav E, Sterling M. Sensory hypoaesthesia is a feature of chronic whiplash but no chronic idiopathic neck pain. *Man Ther.* 2010;15:48-53.
701. Sterling M, Kenardy J. The relationship between sensory and sympathetic nervous system changes and acute posttraumatic stress following whiplash injury: a prospective study. *J Psychosom Res.* 2006;60:387-393.
702. Motor Accidents Authority. *Summary Guidelines for the Management of Acute Whiplash-Associated Disorder for Health Professionals.* 2nd ed. Sydney, Australia: Author; 2007. https://www.maa.nsw.gov.au/getfile.aspx?Type=document&ID=35276&ObjectType=3&ObjectID=3202. Accessed September 22, 2013.
703. Sterling M, Pedler A. A neuropathic pain component is common in acute whiplash and associated with a more complex clinical presentation. *Man Ther.* 2009;14:173-179.
704. Cathcart S, Pritchard D. Reliability of pain threshold measurement in young adults. *J Headache Pain.* 2006;7:21-26.
705. *Clinical Guidelines for Best Practice Management of Acute and Chronic Whiplash Associated Disorders: Clinical Resource Guide.* TRACsa: Trauma and Injury Recovery, South Australia: Adelaide; 2008. http://www.mac.sa.gov.au/xstd_files/Whiplash-Clinical-Guidelines.pdf. Accessed May 25, 2012.
706. Teasell RW, McClure JA, Walton D, et al. A research synthesis of therapeutic interventions for whiplash-associated disorder (WAD): part 2—interventions for acute WAD. *Pain Res Manag.* 2010;15(5):295-304.
707. Dufton JA, Kopec JA, Wong H, et al. Prognostic factors associated with minimal improvement following acute whiplash-associated disorders. *Spine.* 2006;31:E757-E765.
708. Teasell RW, McClure JA, Walton D, et al. A research synthesis of therapeutic interventions for whiplash-associated disorder (WAD): part 3—interventions for subacute WAD. *Pain Res Manag.* 2010;15(5):305-312.
709. Sterling M, Kenardy J. Physical and psychological aspects of whiplash: important considerations for primary care assessment. *Man Ther.* 2008;14:173-179.
710. Teasell R W, McClure JA, Walton D, et al. A research synthesis of therapeutic interventions for whiplash-associated disorder (WAD): part 4—noninvasive interventions for chronic WAD. *Pain Res Manag.* 2010;15(5):313-322.
711. Teasell R W, McClure JA, Walton D, et al. A research synthesis of therapeutic interventions for whiplash-associated disorder (WAD): part 5—surgical and injection-based interventions for chronic WAD. *Pain Res Manag.* 2010;15(5):323-334.
712. Jull G. Considerations in the physical rehabilitation of patients with whiplash-associated disorders. *Spine.* 2011;36:S286-S291.
713. Michaleff Z, Maher C, Jull G, et al. A randomised clinical trial of a comprehensive exercise program for chronic whiplash: trial protocol. *BMC Musculoskel Dis.* 2009;10:49.
714. Van Oosterwijck J, Nijs J, Meeus M, et al. Pain neurophysiology education improves cognitions, pain thresholds, and movement performance in people with chronic whiplash: a pilot study. *J Rehabil Res Dev.* 2011;48(1):43-58.
715. Sterling M, Whiplash-associated disorder: musculoskeletal pain and related clinical findings. *J Man Manip Ther.* 2011;19(4):194-200.
716. Elliott J, Pedler A, Kenardy J, Galloway G, Jull G, Sterling M. The temporal development of fatty infiltrates in the neck muscles following whiplash injury: an association with pain and posttraumatic stress. *PLoS One.* 2011;6:e21194.
717. Bednarik J, Kadanka Z, Dusek L, et al. Presymptomatic spondylotic cervical cord compression. *Spine.* 2004;29(20):2260-2269.
718. Galbraith JG, Butler JS, Dolan AM, O'Byrne JM. Operative outcomes for cervical myelopathy and radiculopathy. *Adv Orthop.* 2012;2012:919153.
719. Schenk RJ, Wise CJ. *Cervical and Thoracic Spine: Postoperative Management. Cervical and Thoracic Pain: Evidence for Effectiveness of Physical therapy. Home Study Monograph 21.1.6.* La Crosse WI: Orthopaedic Section of American Physical Therapy Association; 2010.
720. Nikolaidis I, Fouyas IP, Sandercock PAG, Statham PF. Surgery for cervical radiculopathy or myelopathy. *Cochrane Database Syst Rev.* 2010;(1):CD001466.
721. Persson LCG, Carlsson C-A, Carlsson JY. Long-lasting cervical radicular pain managed with surgery, physiotherapy, or a cervical collar. A prospective, randomized study. *Spine.* 1997;22(7):751-758.
722. KadaAŁka Z, Mareš M, BednaÅ™ík J, et al. Approaches to spondylotic cervical myelopathy. Conservative versus surgical results in a 3-year follow up study. *Spine.* 2002;27(20):2205-2211.
723. Hilibrand A, Carlson G, Palumbo M, Jones P, Bohlman H. Radiculopathy and myelopathy at segments adjacent to the site of a previous anterior cervical arthrodesis. *J Bone Joint Surg.* 1999;81(4):519-528.
724. Suri A, Chabbra RPS, Mehta VS, Gaikwad S, Pandey RM. Effect of intramedullary signal changes on the surgical outcome of patients with cervical spondylotic myelopathy. *Spine J.* 2003;3(1):33-45.
725. Carragee EJ, Hurwitz EL, Cheng I, et al. Treatment of neck pain. Injections and surgical interventions: results of bone and joint decade 2000-2010 task force on neck pain and its associated disorders. *J Manipulative Physiol Ther.* 2009;32:S176-S193.
726. Murrey D, Janssen M, Delamarter R, et al. Results of the prospective, randomized, controlled multicenter Food and Drug Administration investigational device exemption study of the ProDisc-C total disc replacement versus anterior discectomy and fusion for the treatment of 1-level symptomatic cervical disc disease. *Spine J.* 2009;9(4):275-286.
727. Nabhan A, Ahlhelm F, Shariat D, et al. The ProDisc-C prothesis: clinical and radiological experience 1 year after surgery. *Spine.* 2007;32(18):1935-1941.
728. Quan GMY, Vital JM, Hansen SM, Pointillart V. 8 year clinical and radiological follow-up of the Bryan cervical disc arthroplasty. *Spine.* 2010;36(8):639-646.
729. Cepoiu-Martin M, Faris P, Lorenzetti D, Prefontaine E, Noseworhty T, Sutherland L. Artificial cervical disc arthroplasty: a systematic review. *Spine (Phila Pa 1976).* 2011 Dec 1;36(25):E1623-E1633.

Please visit www.routledge.com/9781556429323 to access additional material.

Appendix A

Case Study for Limited Examination

Patient Profile: 28 y/o male, Caucasian; 3rd grade school teacher; sits, stands, and bends through the day; unable to work yesterday and today; jogs 5 miles, 4 days per week, gardening and yard work on the weekends. Direct Access. ODI: 40%. FABQPA: 18; FABQW: 29

Chief Complaint: Constant low back pain with radiation into right leg

Description of Symptoms

- P1 = constant, variable deep ache
- NPRS = best 1/10, worst 4/10 over past 24 hours
- P2 = constant, variable deep burning
- NPS = best 1/10, worst 3/10
- P1 and P2 occur together
- No numbness or tingling

History of Current Problem (Present Episode)

Onset 2 days ago getting out of the car after a 4-hour drive; first noted LBP getting out of the car, had difficulty standing up straight after the drive. LBP continued that evening and through the night; woke up in the morning with LBP and burning in the leg. No current treatment except over-the-counter Aleve and resting in bed with a pillow under knees; reports his leg pain is worse this morning

Past History (Previous Episode of Similar Problem)

Denies previous history of low back or leg pain

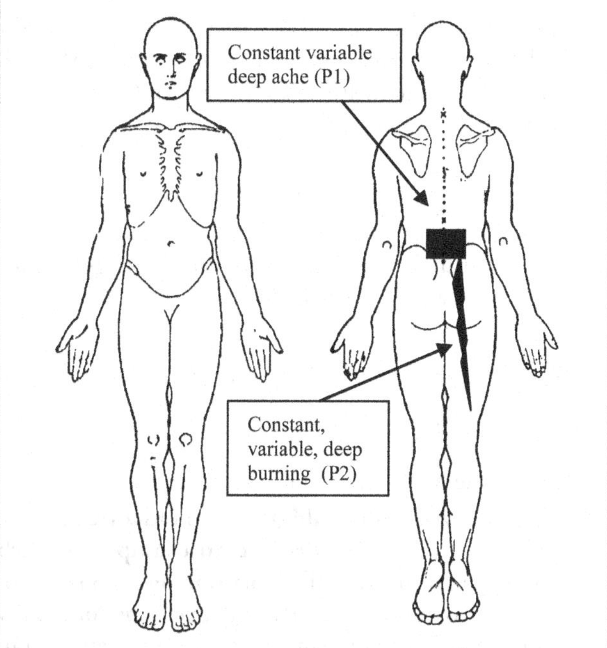

Stetts DM, Carpenter JG. *Physical Therapy Management of Patients With Spinal Pain: An Evidence-Based Approach (pp 589-590).*

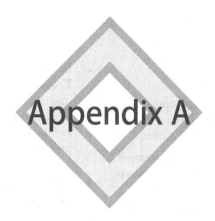

Aggravating Factors

- Getting out of bed, difficulty straightening up—increased LBP and leg burning, seemed to ease to 1/10 with walking around the house for 1 to 2 minutes
- Tried sitting to eat breakfast this morning, increased LBP and leg burning after 5 minutes, had to stand up and walk for 1 to 2 minutes
- Needed help getting dressed this morning with slacks and shoes due to pain in back and right leg
- Walking to PT clinic (100 feet) increased pain in low back and leg, settled to 1/10 after 5 minutes standing

Easing Factors

- Supine with pillow under knees or side-lying on the left side
- Hasn't tried lying on stomach; normally sleeps on left side or stomach

24-Hour Behavior

- Woke up 1 time last night, quickly returned to sleep with change of position; has been resting in bed most of the time since onset; woke this morning with LBP 1/10 and leg pain, both 2/10

Medical Screening Questionnaire

- Excellent general health; denies current or past medical problems. Fractured right ankle playing basketball at age 16, treated with short leg cast for 6 weeks; fully recovered; no imaging or medications

Patient Expectations

- Expects full recovery; wants to return to jogging program and weekend gardening

Case A: Clinical Reasoning Guide to Plan the Physical Examination

Analyze the data from the history.

1. **Are the symptoms mild (0 to 3), moderate (4 to 6), or severe (7 to 10)? Provide an example for each symptom and the self-report outcome score.** Both symptoms are severe at 4/10, unable to perform daily activities such as dressing, and unable to work. ODI: 40%. FABQPA: 18; FABQW: 29
2. **Is the presentation irritable or nonirritable? Provide an example for each symptom.** Uncertain due to decreased activity level but will err on the side of an irritable disorder (symptoms are easy to provoke and constant). Has constant 1/10 LBP and leg burning; increased LBP and leg burning after 5 minutes, had to stand up and walk to ease
3. **What is the nature of the disorder (musculoskeletal, nonmusculoskeletal, or both)? Provide rationale.**
   a. Musculoskeletal disorder, no red, first episode
4. **What is your working diagnostic hypothesis or classification?**
   a. **Primary hypothesis(es):** Acute LBP with mobility deficits and referred/radicular pain into lower extremity
   b. **Secondary hypothesis(es):** Screen (session 1, 2, or 3) hip, lower thoracic spine, sacroiliac regions
   c. **Precautions or contraindications:** No contraindications. Caution indicated due to constant pain, acute nature, severity, and irritability; leg symptoms were worse this morning
5. **What is the stage of the disorder?** Acute
6. **What is the stability of the disorder?** LBP unchanged, leg pain worse this morning
7. **What tests and measures (region/structures) should be completed on session 1?**
   a. Functional activities: gait, posture (standing, sitting)
   b. Specific movements: AROM to point of increase in symptoms; repeated movements; PAIVM PRN
   c. Neurological examination: attempt reflexes, sensation; MMT may be restricted to L4-S1 if nonprovocative
   d. Special tests: defer to next visit
   e. Limited examination: looking to find pain-easing positions or movements or classification for acute LBP
8. **What is the diagnosis/classification/prognosis at the end of the physical examination?**
9. **What is your intervention/reassessment for session 1?**
10. **What evidence (research, expertise, patient preferences) supports your decision?**
11. **Are there potential risk factors/concerns contributing to the condition?** Advice to remain active, education related to sitting and gardening ergonomics. Risk factors: off work × 2 days; potential radicular pain; yellow flags present: FABQPA and FABQW

Appendix B

Case Study for Full Examination

Patient Profile: 28 y/o male, Caucasian; 3rd grade school teacher; sits, stands, and bends through the day, still working full time. Jogs 5 miles, 4 days per week, gardening and yard work on the weekends; only able to jog about 1 mile before he has to stop due to LBP, walks for ½ mile, and then continues again. Direct Access. ODI: 25/50; FABQPA: 9; FABQW: 18

Chief Complaint: Intermittent low back pain with radiation into right leg

Description of Symptoms

- P1 = intermittent, deep ache
- NPRS = best 0/10, worst 4/10 over past 24 hours
- P2 = intermittent, deep burning
- NPS = best 0/10, worst 3/10
- P1 and P2 occur together; P1 comes on first then P2
- No numbness or tingling

History of Current Problem (Present Episode)

Onset 2 weeks ago getting out of the car after a 4-hour drive; first noted LBP getting out of the car, had difficulty standing up straight after the drive; LBP continued that evening and through the night; woke up in the morning with LBP and burning in the leg. No current treatment except over-the-counter Aleve for 1 week; tried to stay active and continued working. Overall, low back and leg pain are improving, no longer constant over past week

Past History (Previous Episode of Similar Problem)

Denies previous history of low back or leg pain

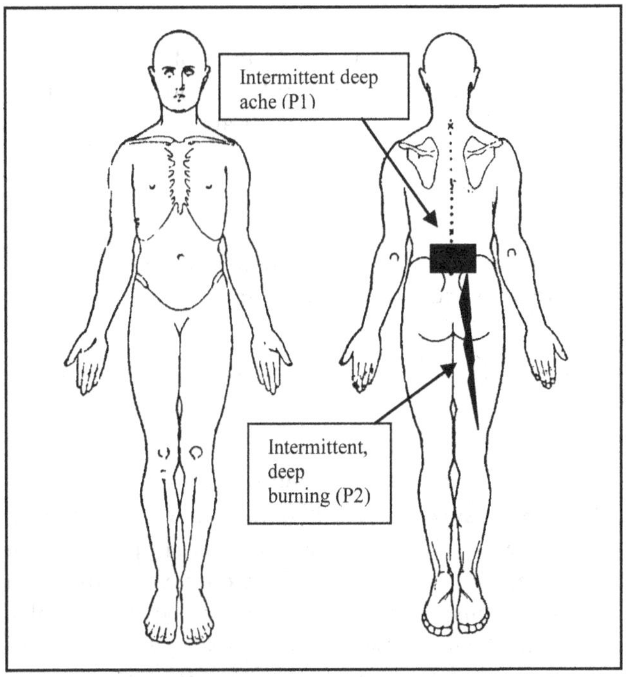

Stetts DM, Carpenter JG. *Physical Therapy Management of Patients With Spinal Pain: An Evidence-Based Approach (pp 591-592).*

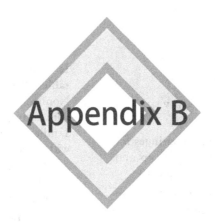

Aggravating Factors

- Getting out of bed, no pain, stiff, difficulty straightening up, eases with 30 sec of walking
- Sitting × 20 minutes, bring on LBP; if continues for 5 minutes, leg burning starts, had to stand up and walk for 15 sec for all symptoms to settle to 0/10
- Bending to put socks on and tie shoes brings back and leg pain in the morning; settles immediately when upright
- Jogging 1 mile, stops due to onset LBP, walks ½ mile to ease pain, then jogs again until LBP starts, repeats until 5 miles

Easing Factors

- Supine with pillow under knees or side-lying on the left side
- Normally sleeps on left side or stomach, hasn't tried recently

24-Hour Behavior

- Sleeps through the night; occasionally wakes if rolls onto stomach but returns quickly to sleep. Wakes only with low back stiffness; no worse by the end of the day

Medical Screening Questionnaire

- Excellent general health; denies current or past medical problems. Fractured right ankle playing basketball at age 16, treated with short leg cast for 6 weeks; fully recovered; no imaging or medications

Patient Expectations

- Expects full recovery and return to regular jogging program and weekend gardening.

Case B: Clinical Reasoning Guide to Plan the Physical Examination

Analyze the data from the history.

1. **Are the symptoms mild (0 to 3), moderate (4 to 6), or severe (7 to 10)? Provide an example for each symptom and the self-report outcome score.** Both symptoms are mild to moderate at 0/10 to 4/10, able to perform daily activities and able to work, but limited in jogging for exercise; ODI: 20%
2. **Is the presentation irritable or nonirritable? Provide an example for each symptom.** Nonirritable. Symptoms are intermittent, provoked with sitting for 20 minutes, bending, and jogging for 1 mile. Both symptoms, if provoked, settle quickly within seconds, except after jogging, which takes longer. Jogging is a repetitive, vigorous activity. Physical examination is unlikely to produce forces equivalent to jogging for 1 mile
3. **What is the nature of the disorder (musculoskeletal, nonmusculoskeletal, or both)? Provide rationale.**
    a. Musculoskeletal disorder, no red or yellow flags, first episode
4. **What is your working diagnostic hypothesis(es)/classification?**
    a. **Primary hypothesis(es):** Subacute LBP with mobility deficits with referred/radicular pain into lower extremity
    b. **Secondary hypothesis(es):** Screen (session 1, 2, or 3) hip, lower thoracic spine, sacroiliac regions
    c. **Precautions or contraindications:** No contraindications. Caution with burning pain referred to leg but settles quickly. Nonsevere, nonirritable
5. **What is the stage of the disorder?** Subacute
6. **What is the stability of the disorder?** LBP and leg burning improving over the past week
7. **What tests and measures (region/structures) should be completed on session 1?**
    a. Functional activities: gait, posture (standing, sitting)
    b. Specific movements: AROM/PROM, overpressure, repeated movements, PAIVM, screen hip/SI/T-spine
    c. Neurological examination: yes
    d. Special tests: SLR
    e. Full examination as needed to reach diagnosis and treatment threshold
8. **What is the diagnosis/classification/prognosis at the end of the physical examination?**
9. **What is your intervention/reassessment for session 1?**
10. **What evidence (research, expertise, patient preferences) supports your decision?**
11. **Are there potential risk factors/concerns contributing to the condition?** Advice to remain active, education related to sitting and gardening ergonomics. Risk factors: age, expectations, working, first episode, no yellow flags

Appendix C

Case Study for Low Back Pain

Patient Profile: 30 y/o male; engineer, unemployed for 4 wks due to layoff; currently looking for employment; married with no children; plays chess 2 to 3× per week and enjoys reading; no regular exercise. Referred from orthopedic surgeon. ODI: 38%; FABQPA: 12; FABQW: 20

Chief Complaint: Right LBP (L4-5 pain) spreads into R buttock and posterior thigh to knee

Description of Symptoms

- R L4-5 deep ache, constant, variable 1/10 to 4/10
- R buttock to post thigh, diffuse burning, intermittent 2/10
- No other lower quarter symptoms; no N/T
- No abdominal complaints, no B/B complaints

History of Current Problem (Present Episode)

Onset 12 days ago; started after rising from sitting position; back, buttock, and thigh symptoms came on at the same time, limiting activities but no treatment; symptoms are not getting worse. Hasn't been to chiropractor yet, orthopedic surgeon said to try PT first

Past History (Previous Episode of Similar Problem)

Three similar episodes over past 5 years, treated with bed rest, brace, chiropractic manipulation over 4 weeks; 100% recovered between episodes

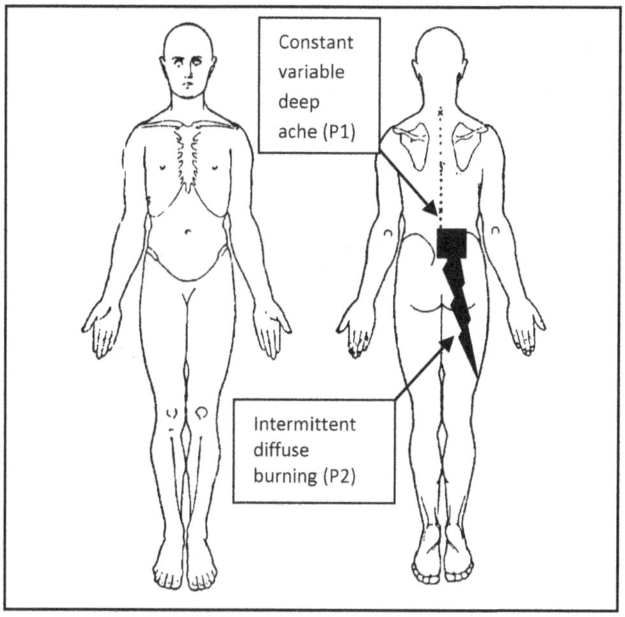

Aggravating Factors:

- Bending increases LBP and brings on butt and post thigh pain; settles with return to upright
- Sitting increases LBP and brings on butt and post thigh pain after 30 minutes; settles with walking for 5 minutes
- Prolonged standing increases LBP only after 15 minutes; settles with walking for 5 minutes
- Difficulty standing upright initially after sitting due to pain and stiffness; has to walk about 10 steps to get upright

Easing Factors

- Walking, lying face down

24-Hour Behavior

- Wakes at night when he turns over due to back pain; goes back to sleep quickly
- AM: mild stiffness, 1/10 LBP only after waking

Systems Review, PMH, PSH, Imaging, Medications, and Special Questions Revealed the Following

- General health: excellent
- Systems review: negative
- Medications/steroids: none
- PMH/PSH: negative
- X-ray of lumbar spine: negative

Patient Expectations and Goals

- Decrease LBP and leg pain since he does a lot of sitting at work and needs to find employment
- Expects full recovery similar to previous episodes

Case C: Analyze the Data From the History to Plan the Physical Examination

1. **Are the symptoms mild (0 to 3), moderate (4 to 6), or severe (7 to 10)? Provide an example for each symptom.** Intensity of symptoms and impact on function. Self-report outcome scores. ODI: moderate (39%); NPRS: 1/10 to 4/10
2. **Is the presentation irritable or nonirritable? Provide an example for each symptom.** Mild to moderate since sitting 30 minutes provokes symptoms that ease in 5 minutes; symptoms produced by bending ease when upright
3. **What is the nature of the condition (musculoskeletal, nonmusculoskeletal, or both)?**
4. **Data from the history that support a working diagnosis(es)/classification(s):**

LBP With Mobility Deficits	LBP With Movement Coordination Deficits	LBP With Related/ Referred LE Pain	Traction	Other
• Onset < 16 days; FABQW not < 19; no pain below knee • Successful prior treated with chiropractic manipulation	• Age <40 • Recurrent episodes	• Direction-specific preference extension subgroup • Worse with flexion activities and postures • Better with extension activities such as walking	• Post thigh pain could be somatic (nociceptive) or radicular (neurogenic)	• Low FABQ • No red flags

5. **What is your initial working diagnostic hypothesis or classification?**
   a. **Primary hypothesis (region to examine in detail):** LBP with related/referred LE pain; extension subgroup; rule out radicular component
   b. **Secondary hypothesis may include region(s) to screen for sessions 1, 2, 3:**
      - LBP with mobility deficits: screen hip and pelvic girdle
      - LBP with movement coordination deficits: recurrent episodes
   c. **Precautions or contraindications to your examination:** None
   d. **What is the stage of the disorder?** Acute to subacute on chronic
6. **What is the stability of the disorder?** Staying the same
7. **Are there potential risk factors (psychosocial, ergonomic, expectations, etc, contributing) to the condition?** Postures at work, playing chess, and reading; address importance of regular exercise
8. **What tests and measures (region/structures) should be completed on session 1?** Observation, gait, posture, AROM, repeated movements, neurological

screen LE, palpation, PAIVM, screen hip and pelvis, SLR; others depending on response

a. **Physical examination findings Case C** (*Note*: Some tests may be optional at therapist discretion)
   - o Observation/gait/posture: Gait: decreased trunk rotation; decreased lumbar lordosis; pelvis level; no lateral shift
   - o Rest symptoms: 2/10 R LBP, 0/10 buttock pain, 1/10 R post thigh pain
   - o Neuro: Bilateral: normal sensory to light touch; DTRs: 2+ AJ/KJ bilateral; MMT: 5/5
   - o AROM lumbar spine, OP end feel, PRN:
     - Flex: 45° increase R LBP/post thigh pain, produces buttock pain
     - Ext: 5° increase R LBP, decrease buttock/thigh pain
     - LF L: full range, no effect; OP soft tissue stretch
     - LF R: 15° increase R LBP/thigh pain, produces buttock pain
   - o Repeated movements:
     - REIS: Increase R LBP, abolished R buttock/thigh pain after 15 reps, ROM increased
     - REIL: Centralized pain at L5, but does not abolish; no buttock or thigh pain
   - o Optional:
     - FIL: Increase R LBP/thigh pain, produces butt pain
     - RFIL: Increase R LBP/thigh pain, produces and increases buttock pain after 2 reps
   - o Special tests:
     - R SLR: Increase R LBP, buttock, post thigh pain at 60°, DF increase R butt pain
     - L SLR: 75°, DF: no effect
   - o Slump: not tested
   - o Optional (could be deferred to day #2):
     - Muscle length: Hip: Short rectus femoris on right (prone knee flexion 70° with hip in neutral)
     - Muscle strength: Not tested; need to assess core stability within next 2 visits
   - o Palpation/passive segmental mobility testing:
     - PPIVM: Not examined
     - PAIVM: Central PA R at L5-S1 > L4-5 hypomobile, local central LBP; unilateral PA at L5-S1 > L4-5 hypomobile, local pain on R
   - o Joint clearing hip, pelvis, other LE:
     - SIJ provocation tests: Negative
     - Hip: ER/IR prone (60/45° bilaterally); other not tested

9. **Data from physical examination that supports a working diagnosis(es)/classification(s)**

LBP With Mobility Deficits	LBP With Movement Coordination Deficits	LBP With Related/ Referred LE Pain	Traction	Other
• AROM limited ext, flex, R LF • PAIVM: central and unilateral on R hypo • Lumbar PA hypomobility • 1 Hip > 35 IR • 4/5 on CPR	• Trunk muscle performance not assessed • Complete within next 2 to 3 visits	• Repeated extension centralizes • Repeated flexion peripheralizes	• Normal neuro	• +SLR: sensitized neural tissue—altered mobility • SIJ provocation negative—could be deferred • Muscle length—short hip flexors

10. **What is the PT diagnosis/classification/prognosis at the end of the physical examination?**
    a. LBP with related/referred LE pain: Direction-specific exercise: extension subgroup
    b. LBP with mobility deficits: L4-5, L5-S1
    c. Altered neural tissue mobility

11. **What is your intervention/reassessment? What evidence informs your decision?** Options: Meets 4/5 criteria for supine lumbopelvic regional or side-lying rotational manipulation; defer manipulation in favor of repeated movements due to centralization and continue to assess at next session
    a. **Intervention Options**
       - o Continue repeated movement
       - o Strategy to abolish LBP
       - o Progress based on patient response
       - o REIL with sag

- o REIL with clinical overpressure
- o PAIVM: Central L4-5, L5-S1

b. **Reassessment**

- o REIS in standing after REIL

12. **What is your plan of care for session 1?**

a. Adherence to end-range REIL 10 reps every 2 to 3 hours; avoid flexion

b. Advice on maintenance of lumbar lordosis in sitting, standing postures

c. Minimize sitting throughout the day

d. Education on transitional movement sit-to-stand, stand-to-sit, standing

e. Discussion of prognosis and self-management

Appendix D

Case Study for Low Back Pain

Patient Profile: 45 y/o male; works as a systems programmer and is still able to work; pain only limits his workout routine of spinning class 2× per week and general weight training 3× per week; he is unable to exercise since start of pain. Patient referral is direct access. ODI: 20%; FABQPA: 12; FABQW: 10

Chief Complaint: L LBP and left groin pain

Description of Symptoms

- Intermittent deep, sharp pain low back and groin, both symptoms come on at the same time
- Best 0/10, worst 5/10; now 0/10
- No N/T or other LE symptoms; no B/B problems

History of Current Problem (Present Episode)

Onset 2 weeks ago suddenly after getting up off the floor, both LB and groin pain came on at the same time when getting up; had been lying on his stomach on the floor reading a magazine for about 30 minutes. No current treatment, not getting worse

Past History (Previous Episode of Similar Problem)

Three to five episodes of LBP over past 2 years; last 2 episodes have been within past 8 months, seems to be getting more frequent. Treated in the past with medication, exercise, and manipulation. Manipulation seems to be the only treatment that has helped in the past; full recovery between episodes

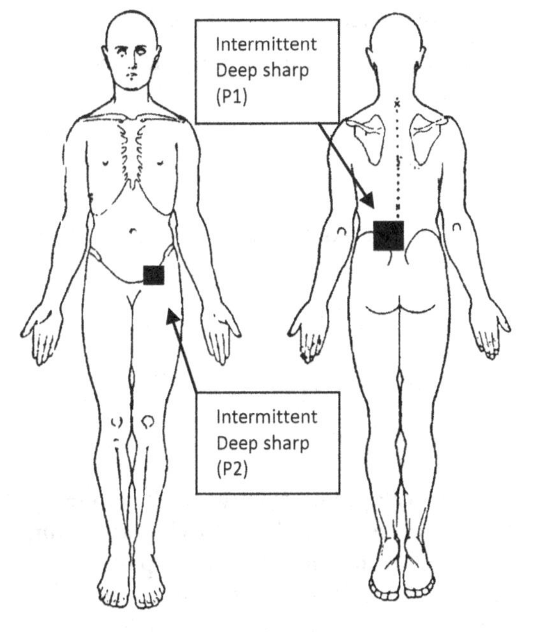

Stetts DM, Carpenter JG. *Physical Therapy Management of Patients With Spinal Pain: An Evidence-Based Approach (pp 597-600).*

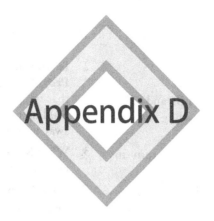

Aggravating Factors

- Getting into and out of car reproduces LBP and groin pain, which eases after transition to standing or walking a few steps
- Bending produces LBP, which eases on return to upright
- Bending to the right also produces LBP, which eases on return to upright
- Sitting has no effect on symptoms; he has an ergonomic chair and moves frequently throughout the day

Easing Factors

- Standing and walking; tried ice, but it doesn't help

24-Hour Behavior

- AM: no pain or stiffness except when bending
- Day: no worse except when necessary to bend forward or to right
- End of day about the same without night pain when sleeping

Systems Review and Special Questions Reveal the Following

- General health: excellent
- Medications/steroids: Tylenol PRN
- Previous imaging: 3 months ago, normal radiographs of lumbar spine

Patient Expectations and Goals

- Return to workout routine and decrease repeated onsets of LBP

Case D: Analyze the Data From the History to Plan the Physical Examination

1. **Are the symptoms mild (0 to 3), moderate (4 to 6), or severe (7 to 10)? Provide an example for each symptom.** Intensity of symptoms and impact on function. Self-report outcome scores. ODI: mild/moderate 20/50; NPRS: 0/10 to 5/10
2. **Is the presentation irritable or nonirritable? Provide an example for each symptom.** Mild such that symptoms are easily produced and ease quickly; bending reproduces symptoms, but the symptoms go away immediately when upright
3. **What is the nature of the condition (musculoskeletal, nonmusculoskeletal, or both)?**
4. **Data from the history that support a working diagnosis(es)/classification(s):**

LBP With Mobility Deficits	LBP With Movement Coordination Deficits	LBP With Related/ Referred LE Pain	Traction	Other
• No pain below knee • FABQW <19 • Recent onset • Previous treatment with manipulation plus exercise successful	• Recurrent and more frequent episodes	• Sitting has no effect on symptoms, but bending produces LBP • Ease: standing and walking	• No neurological symptoms	• Hip pain: possibly related to LBP • SIJ refers to groin • Low FABQ • No red flag

5. **What is your initial working diagnostic hypothesis or classification?**
   a. **Primary hypothesis (region to examine in detail):** LBP with mobility deficits; mobilization/manipulation plus exercise.
   b. **Secondary hypothesis may include region(s) to screen for sessions 1, 2, 3:** Hip screen; LBP with movement coordination deficits: recurrent episodes
   c. **Precautions or contraindications to your examination:** None
   d. **What is the stage of the disorder?** Subacute (onset 2 weeks ago) on chronic
6. **What is the stability of the disorder?** Staying the same; recurrences are more frequent
7. **Are there potential risk factors (psychosocial, ergonomic, expectations, etc, contributing) to the condition?** Posture during exercise, lumbopelvic stability while weight training, transitions in and out of care; low FABQ

8. **What tests and measures (region/structures) should be completed on session 1?** Observation, gait, posture, AROM, repeated movements, hip screen, SLR, palpation, PAIVM, assess trunk muscle performance of ADIM; neuro today or defer to day 2; SIJ provocation if time or defer to day 2
   a. **Physical examination findings Case D** (*Note*: Some tests may be optional at therapist discretion)
      - Observation/gait/posture: no postural deviations; pelvis level, gait normal
      - Rest symptoms: 0/10 L low back and groin
      - AROM lumbar spine, OP end feel, PRN:
        - Flex: full range with L LBP at end range and painful arc on return to upright (aberrant movement)
        - Ext: full range, OP normal
        - LF L: 25° OP normal
        - LF R: 15° L LBP & groin pain
      - Repeated movements:
        - REIS: No effect
        - RFIS: Limited and end range LBP and groin pain increased with continued painful arc, but no worse
      - Neuro screen LE: Bilateral: normal sensory to light touch
        - DTRs: 2+ AJ/KJ bilateral
        - MMT: 5/5
      - Palpation/passive segmental mobility testing:
        - PPIVM: F/R SB: L4-L5 hypomobile
        - PAIVM: Central PA L3, L4 hypomobile/local pain; unilateral PA: L L3-L4/L4-L5: hypomobile local pain
      - Special tests:
        - SLR: 70° bilateral, HS stretch; DF added, no change
      - Slump: Not tested
      - Prone instability: Negative
      - Muscle length: Not tested
      - Muscle performance LE: Not tested; Core: ADIM: excessive IO/EO contraction bilaterally by palpation
      - Screen: pelvis: Pain provocation tests negative
      - Screen: hip: Normal ROM, symmetrical: F, IR, ER, F/Add with OP; IR prone bilaterally 25°
      - Other LE: Not tested

9. **Data from physical examination that supports a working diagnosis(es)/classification(s)**

LBP With Mobility Deficits	LBP With Movement Coordination Deficits	LBP With Related/ Referred LE Pain	Traction	Other
• AROM: Flex/R LF limited painful • Central/ unilateral PA PAIVM hypomobile • PPIVM limited painful: F, R SB hypomobile • Hip IR 25 bilaterally, normal ROM with OP • 4/5 on CPR	• Painful arc on return from flexion • Prone instability test negative • Poor ADIM performance excessive superficial contraction	• No centralization or peripheralization • Repeated movement RFIS limited with end range pain only, increased but no worse	• Neuro normal	• SIJ provocation negative • Hip AROM and OP normal

10. **What is the PT diagnosis/classification/prognosis at the end of the physical examination?**
    a. Left LBP with mobility deficits and referred pain to left hip: mobilization/manipulation plus exercise classification
    b. Left LBP with movement coordination deficits: poor TrA with ADIM, painful arc, recurrent episodes, increasing frequency

11. **What is your intervention/reassessment? What evidence informs your decision?** Options: Meets 4/5 criteria for supine lumbopelvic regional or side-lying rotational manipulation; secondarily, LBP with movement coordination deficits (ADIM, prone instability test)
    a. **Intervention Options**
       - Lumbopelvic regional manipulation or side-lying rotational manipulation
    b. **Reassessment**
       - AROM: Flex, R LF
       - PAIVM, PPIVM F, R SB
       - Performance during ADIM
       - If successful, instruct in-home exercise program to improvement in mobility (flexion and/or R SB)

- o Instruction on neutral spine posture and ADIM if improved after manipulation or may need additional assessment and instruction at second session

12. **What is your plan of care for session 1?**
    a. Education on prognosis, adherence to exercise program, ergonomics for moving in/out of car, return to exercise routine, and self-care
    b. Continue to assess trunk/hip/and lower extremity muscle length and performance with 2 to 3 sessions

Appendix E

Case Study for Pelvic Girdle Pain

Patient Profile: 32 y/o female; pediatric nurse; married, 3 children (8, 4, and 2); currently unable to work; daily activities include domestic activities and caring for her children; no regular exercise. ODI: 38%; FABQPA: 24

Chief Complaint: Right LBP

Description of Symptoms

- Intermittent R LBP pain with some referral to posterior hip
- 6/10 today; average 5/10; best 0/10; 5/10 average for 3 months

History of Current Problem (Present Episode)

Gradual onset during 3rd pregnancy with worse pain following child birth, which has not gone away; all treatment has not helped and made symptoms worse. Previous treatment of manipulation made it worse; stabilization exercises had no effect on her pain, but a physical therapist diagnosed a hypertonic pelvic floor, which was treated with relaxation, breathing, and aerobic exercise that also made it worse, with a new problem of stress incontinence. Overall, nothing has changed over the past 3 months

Past History (Previous Episode of Similar Problem)

Similar pain with first 2 pregnancies, but pain went away after child birth without treatment

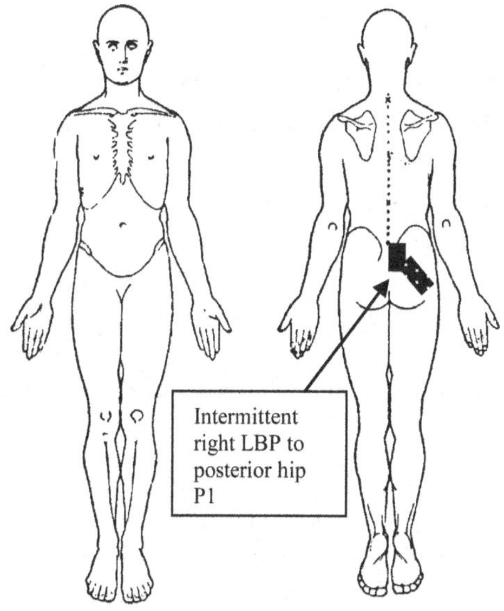

Stetts DM, Carpenter JG. *Physical Therapy Management of Patients With Spinal Pain: An Evidence-Based Approach (pp 601-604).*

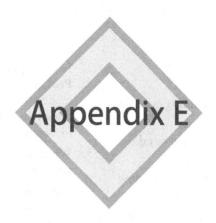

Aggravating Factors:

- Sitting for 30 minutes, eased by standing without weight on right leg in 1 to 2 minutes
- Standing on right leg after 10 minutes eased by taking weight off the right leg 1 to 2 minutes
- Walking greater than 10 minutes eased by standing on the left leg or sitting for 1 to 2 minutes
- Previous stabilizing exercises and physioball workouts
- Lifting and carrying child for 5 minutes eases in 1 to 2 minutes by sitting

Easing Factors

- Avoids provoking activities due to belief that producing pain causes damage to her low back
- Rest; unloading of right leg and nonweightbearing

24-Hour Behavior

- Sleeps through the night
- No pain on waking until she has been up walking or standing for 10 minutes
- Worse throughout day, varies with loading activities

Systems Review and Special Questions Reveal the Following

- Medical history: negative
- Medications/steroids: NSAIDs and Tylenol regularly
- Feels depressed due to conflicting advice on how to manage problem
- Imaging: x-rays and CT show no abnormalities; blood tests negative

Patient Expectations and Goals

- Find out what the problem is and return to work

Case E: Analyze the Data From the History to Plan the Physical Examination

1. **Are the symptoms mild (0 to 3), moderate (4 to 6), or severe (7 to 10)? Provide an example for each symptom.** Intensity of symptoms and impact on function. Self-report outcome scores. ODI: moderate (39%); NPRS: 0/10 to 6/10
2. **Is the presentation irritable or nonirritable? Provide an example for each symptom.** Mild to moderate since sitting 30 minutes provokes symptoms that ease in <5 minutes; symptoms produced by bending ease when upright
3. **What is the nature of the condition (musculoskeletal, nonmusculoskeletal, or both)?**
4. **Data from the history that support a working diagnosis(es)/classification(s):**

LBP With Mobility Deficits	LBP With Movement Coordination Deficits	LBP With Related/ Referred LE Pain	Pelvic Girdle Pain	Other
• No support; made worse with chiropractic manipulation	• Age <40 • Chronic pain • Postpartum onset • No worse with stabilization exercises • Worse without stabilization (relaxation)	• Does not appear to be a directional preference • Standing, sitting, and walking • Avoids loading on the right side	• Onset associated with pregnancy • 3 pregnancies • No worse with stabilization • Worse without stabilization	• FABQPA • Depression • No red flags

5. **What is your initial working diagnostic hypothesis or classification?**
   a. **Primary hypothesis (region to examine in detail):** Right pelvic girdle pain; peripherally mediated with reduced force closure; cognitive psychosocial factors resulting in central sensitization
   b. **Secondary hypothesis may include region(s) to screen for sessions 1, 2, 3:** LBP with movement coordination deficits: recurrent episodes
   c. **Precautions or contraindications to your examination:** None
   d. **What is the stage of the disorder?** Chronic
6. **What is the stability of the disorder?** Staying the same
7. **Are there potential risk factors (psychosocial, ergonomic, expectations, etc, contributing) to the condition?** Postures at home and caring for children, depression, fear-avoidance beliefs and behavior
8. **What tests and measures (region/structures) should be completed on session 1?** Observation, gait, posture, AROM, repeated movements, neurological screen LE, palpation, PAIVM, screen hip and

pelvis, lumbopelvic muscle performance, SLR; others depending on response

a. **Physical examination findings Case E**
   - o Observation/gait/posture:
     - Posture: Pelvis anterior to thorax; avoids WB on right leg
     - Decreased tone: Abdominal wall, right gluteal muscles
     - Gait: Positive Trendelenburg on R
     - Pelvis: Appears level; able to put weight on both sides without pain for 2 minutes
   - o Sitting posture: Slumped with weight shift to left buttock
   - o Rest symptoms: 0/10
   - o AROM lumbar spine, OP end feel, PRN:
     - Flex: Full ROM, no pain; on return poor control of posterior pelvic rotation (walks up thighs)
     - Ext: Full, no pain
     - LF L: Full, no pain
     - LF R: Full, no pain
   - o Repeated movements:
     - REIS: 10 reps no symptoms
     - RFIS: Not tested due to poor control
     - Neuro: Normal
   - o Special tests:
     - Standing flexion/seated flexion: Symmetrical
     - Standing hip flexion test/Stork/Gillet
     - Hip flexion phase: R = normal; L = unable to test due to + Trendelenburg on R
     - Stance/support phase: L = normal; R = anterior tilt of pelvis, + Trendelenburg with pain; the test was repeated with postural realignment and SIJ compression to ilium, which reduced pain
     - SLR bilateral: 70 HS pulling sensation; adding DF = no change in pulling sensation
     - + ASLR on R: Moderate heaviness on R 3/5; with manual compression: 0/5
     - Prone instability test: Negative
   - o Muscle performance:
     - TrA: Bilaterally performs ADIM with breath holding and bracing; pelvic floor: not tested
     - Multifidi at L5-S1: Unable to palpate with ADIM; poor lumbopelvic control with prone arm lift
   - o Muscle strength: Hip ext and abd on R: 3/5; hip ext and abd on L: 5/5
   - o Passive segmental mobility testing:
     - PAIVM: Central PA/Unilateral PA L5 to L1 normal except pain with central PA at L5-S1
     - Palpation: Painful inferior to R PSIS and over R gluteus maximus and piriformis
   - o Joint clearing hip, pelvis, other LE:
     - SIJ provocation: (–) Gap/compression, + thigh thrust, + Gaenslen's test, + sacral thrust on R
     - Hip: Clear to AROM, PROM, OP: full range, no effect

9. **Data from physical examination that supports a working diagnosis(es)/classification(s)**

LBP With Mobility Deficits	LBP With Movement Coordination Deficits	LBP With Related/ Referred LE Pain	Pelvic Girdle Pain	Other
	• Aberrant AROM		• Posture • +Trendelenburg • +3/5 SIJ provocation • No centralization or peripheralization • +Standing hip flexion test stance phase • +ASLR (reduced force closure); failed load transfer through LE • Poor motor control deep system (ADIM) • Weak hip extension and abduction	

10. **What is the PT diagnosis/classification/prognosis at the end of the physical examination?**
    a. Postpartum, pelvic girdle pain: peripherally mediated with reduced force closure
    b. Cognitive psychosocial factors resulting in central sensitization
11. **What is your intervention/reassessment? What evidence informs your decision?** Lumbopelvic motor learning approach to enhance force closure of

loading through the right lower extremity and pelvic girdle; initially, a motor control approach is preferred because of the response of breath holding and bracing (excessive superficial muscle activation) neurophysiology of pain education; graded exercise and activity approach

a. **Intervention Options**
   - o Begin neurophysiology of pain education
   - o Explain motor control approach and rationale based on the patient's exam findings
   - o Previous stabilization program most likely resulted in over utilization of the superficial system rather than developing a balance between systems
   - o Begin to establish goals
   - o Begin postural instruction to facilitate the deep muscle activation in upright position

b. **Reassessment**
   - o Reassess ADIM
   - o Instruct in proper performance of ADIM

12. **What is your plan of care for session 1?**
   a. Advice on maintenance of neutral spine posture through the day
   b. ADIM prescription
   c. Discussion of prognosis and self-management

Appendix F

Case Study for Thoracic Spinal Pain

Patient Profile: 60 y/o female; retired teacher; walks 45 minutes a day 6× per week, likes to garden occasionally, but has not done much activity over the last 2 days since the pain started. Self-referral. PSFS: dressing 4/10, reaching 3/10, sleeping 6/10 = total 13/30; FABQPA: 12; FABQW: 10

Chief Complaint: Mid back pain between shoulder blades

Description of Symptoms

- Central, intermittent ache in mid upper back
- Best 0/10, worst 8/10; now 2/10
- Denies numbness/tingling, balance, dizziness; neck, shoulder, or head pain

History of Current Problem (Present Episode)

Onset 2 days ago. Immediately after painting a door frame overhead for about 20 minutes, pain came on in upper mid back. Went to ER and given Tylenol #3 and told to see family doctor if pain persists; x-rays were normal. Has been resting in bed trying to get in comfortable position since onset and pain has decreased quite a bit

Past History (Previous Episode of Similar Problem)

No pain like this previously. Has had previous low back pain but resolved with Tylenol

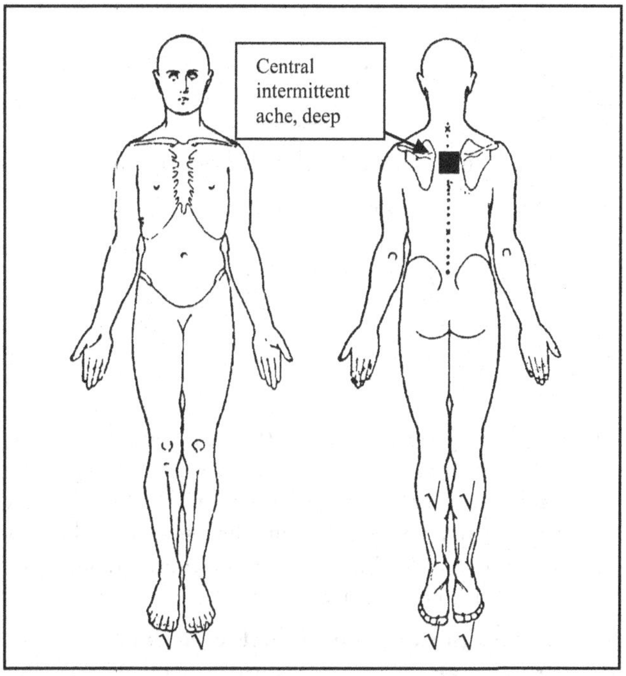

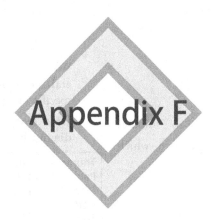

Aggravating Factors:

- Looking up in shower eases with return
- Putting on an overhead sweater eases in 1 to 2 minutes
- Reaching overhead in closet with right arm, which eases with lowering her arm

Easing Factors

- Bending forward to put on shoes or bending neck down to read

24-Hour Behavior

- AM: wakes with pain; difficulty finding a comfortable position to sleep; unable to lay flat
- Wakes 1× a night, sleeps L side-lying for comfort

Systems Review and Special Questions Reveal the Following

- General health: excellent; denies difficulty with balance, gait, or sensation
- Takes calcium supplement to prevent osteoporosis
- Hysterectomy 8 years ago
- Recent DEXA scan reveals no osteoporosis, only mild osteopenia

Patient Expectations and Goals

- Return to walking and gardening
- Help with finding a comfortable position to sleep
- No communication barriers

Case F: Analyze the Data From the History to Plan the Physical Examination

1. **Are the symptoms mild (0 to 3), moderate (4 to 6), or severe (7 to 10)? Provide an example for each symptom.** Intensity of symptoms and impact on function. Self-report outcome scores. Mild, but activities self-limited. Pain is intermittent. Has low PSFS with home tasks; NPRS: 2/10
2. **Is the presentation irritable or nonirritable? Provide an example for each symptom.** Mild; symptoms are easy to produce with looking up or reaching and go away quickly
3. **What is the nature of the condition (musculoskeletal, nonmusculoskeletal, or both)?** No red flags; specific onset
4. **Data from the history that support a working diagnosis(es)/classification(s):**

Thoracic Pain With Mobility Deficits—Thoracic Spine and Rib Cage	Thoracic Hypomobility With Shoulder Impairments and With Upper Extremity Referred Pain	Direction-Specific Exercise for Thoracic Spinal Pain	Thoracic Hypomobility With Neck Pain or LBP	Thoracic Clinical Instability; Other
• Recent onset • Thoracic extension activity limitations • Looking up • Reaching • Unable to lay on her back		• Symptoms produced with extension • Ease with flexion	• No complaints of neck or LBP	• No red flags • Low FABQ • X-rays normal • Recent bone scan

5. **What is your initial working diagnostic hypothesis or classification?**
   a. **Primary hypothesis (region to examine in detail):** Thoracic spinal pain with mobility deficits
   b. **Secondary hypothesis may include region(s) to screen for sessions 1, 2, 3:**
      - Thoracic pain referred from the cervical spine
      - Screen shoulder girdle region
   c. **Precautions or contraindications to your examination:** Full examination as needed to reach diagnosis and treatment threshold; monitor patient response closely. Caution with the use of manipulation due to osteopenia
   d. **What is the stage of the disorder?** Acute
6. **What is the stability of the disorder?** Getting better
7. **Are there potential risk factors (psychosocial, ergonomic, expectations, etc, contributing) to the condition?** Gradual return to exercise, posture/positions during household tasks. Risk factors: age, osteopenia, previous LBP history

8. **What tests and measures (region/structures) should be completed on session 1?** Observation, gait, posture, cervical AROM, thoracic AROM, repeated movements, PAIVM (cervical and thoracic), screen shoulder; neuro exam today or defer to next session; no indications for neurological exam
   a. **Physical examination findings Case F** (*Note*: Some tests may be optional at therapist discretion)
      - o Observation/gait/posture: Forward head, thoracic kyphosis, increased lumbar lordosis. Unable to correct posture to neutral due to limited mobility, but symptoms do not change. Gait normal. Respiration pattern normal
      - o Rest symptoms: 2/10 mid-back pain
      - o Functional activities: Reaching overhead with arm increases pain to 3/10; no increased pain with deep breathing
      - o Shoulder girdle:
        - AROM R flexion: 150° increased central, thoracic pain
        - AROM L flex: 160°, OP no pain capsular end feel
      - o AROM cervical spine:
        - F: Full range, no change in resting pain
        - E: Full range, increased thoracic pain at end range
        - L LF: Full range, no change in resting pain
        - R LF: Full range, no change in resting pain
        - L Rot: Full range, no change in resting pain
        - R Rot: Full range, increased thoracic pain at end range
      - o AROM thoracic spine, OP end feel, PRN:
        - Flexion: Full range, pain decreases to 1/10
        - Extension: 10°, increases pain @ end range pain
        - L lateral flexion: Full range , no change in resting pain
        - R lateral flexion: Full range, no change in resting pain
        - L Rot: Full range, no change in resting pain
        - R Rot: Moderately limited with increased pain at end range
      - o Repeated movements:
        - Flex: 1/10 pain after 10 rep, no better
        - Ext: Pain at end range, but no worse (remains at 2/10) after 10 reps
        - L Rot: 1/10 pain after 10 reps, no better
        - R Rot: Pain at end range, but no worse (remains at 2/10) after 10 reps
      - o Palpation/passive segmental mobility testing:
        - Palpation: Tenderness at T5-T6 on R
        - PPIVM: T5-T6 extension and right rotation hypomobile
        - PAIVM: Central T4-T5/T5-T6 with central local pain; unilateral PA T4-T5/T5-T6 hypomobile with local pain on R; PA right rib 5 hypomobile with local pain
        - PAIVM cervical: central PA C4-C7, hypomobile with no change in thoracic resting pain

9. **Data from physical examination that supports a working diagnosis(es)/classification(s)**

Thoracic Pain With Mobility Deficits—Thoracic Spine and Rib Cage	Thoracic Hypo-mobility With Shoulder Impairments and With Upper Extremity Referred Pain	Direction-Specific Exercise for Thoracic Spinal Pain	Thoracic Hypo-mobility With Neck Pain or LBP	Thoracic Clinical Instability; Other
• AROM limited painful: ext & R rot • PPIVM and PAIVM hypomobile • No centralization or peripheralization	• Right shoulder hypomobility produced thoracic pain • Requires additional testing for clarification		• Limited cervical exam did not produce neck pain • Asymptomatic cervical hypomobility	

10. **What is the PT diagnosis/classification/prognosis at the end of the physical examination?**
    a. Acute thoracic pain with hypomobility deficits
    b. Right shoulder flexion limitation

11. **What is your intervention/reassessment? What evidence informs your decision?** Options: Thoracic mobilization or muscle energy techniques to improve mobility and decrease pain; favor mobilization due to osteopenia, monitor resting symptoms closely; reassess, if improved, AROM to maintain and improve mobility

    a. **Intervention Options**
       - o PAIVM: Central PA at hypomobile segments
       - o PAIVM: unilateral at hypomobile segments
       - o MET to improve thoracic extension/right rotation
       - o Central thoracic SNAG

    b. **Reassessment**
       - o Reassess thoracic extension, right rotation, and shoulder flexion

12. **What is your plan of care for session 1?**

    a. If decreased pain and increase mobility, AROM to improve extension and right rotation

    b. Begin to facilitate neutral upright posture in sitting and standing

    c. Problem-solve position for sleeping at night

    d. Discuss prognosis, advice to remain active, and return to walking progression

Appendix G

Case Study for Thoracic Spinal Pain

Patient Profile: 26 y/o male; works as a welder in an automobile factory; plays recreational basketball and softball; runs 5 days per week, 5 to 6 miles. Still able to work but has decreased running to about 2 miles and is not playing softball; PSFS: bending forward 6/10, twist to grab seat belt 4/10, lifting tool chest from floor at work 5/10 = total 15/30; FABQPA: 9; FABQW: 18

Chief Complaint: Mid back pain between shoulder blades extends to L ribs

Description of Symptoms

- Constant sharp and pinching in mid back
- Denies any UE/LE symptoms; no abdominal or chest pain
- Now 4/10, worst 6/10, best 2/10
- Denies numbness/tingling, bowel or bladder problems, dizziness; neck, shoulder, or head pain

History of Current Problem (Present Episode)

Onset 2 weeks ago. After bending forward to assemble a piece of equipment at work, had difficulty returning to upright after injury; had been working in a bent position for several hours before the injury. Went to company nurse who sent patient to physician. X-rays ordered were normal. Appointment set up for patient to have steroid injections. Given pain medication; the pain seems to be getting better slowly

Past History (Previous Episode of Similar Problem)

No previous back pain

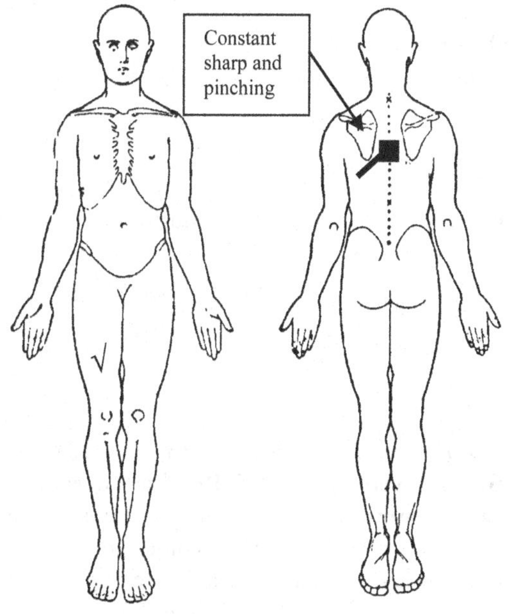

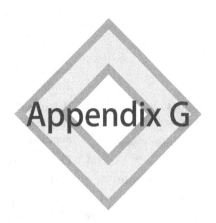

Aggravating Factors:

- Bending forward with difficulty returning to upright coming up to correct posture increases, ease 10 sec
- Grabbing seat belt with right hand in driver's seat (twisting to left) increases pain for 1 minute
- Picking up toolbox from floor at work increases pain for 2 minutes
- Looking up or turning the neck right or left does not change symptoms

Easing Factors

- Leaning back to look up including working overhead
- Lifting boxes above head
- Temporary relief with pain medication

24-Hour Behavior

- Night: feels better sleeping on stomach and worse on either side
- Takes medication to aid falling asleep
- Better in the morning with stiffness
- Worse at end of day and does a lot of bending

Systems Review and Special Questions Reveal the Following

- General health: undergoing test for potential hypothyroidism
- Systems review/PSH: all negative

Patient Expectations and Goals

- Work and run without pain and return to softball

Case G: Analyze the Data From the History to Plan the Physical Examination

1. **Are the symptoms mild (0 to 3), moderate (4 to 6), or severe (7 to 10)? Provide an example for each symptom.** Intensity of symptoms and impact on function. Self-report outcome scores. Moderate, constant pain; impacts work and recreational activity
2. **Is the presentation irritable or nonirritable? Provide an example for each symptom.** Mild to moderate; symptoms are easy to produce with bending or twisting and goes away within 1 to 2 minutes
3. **What is the nature of the condition (musculoskeletal, nonmusculoskeletal, or both)?** No red flags; pending tests for hypothyroidism
4. **Data from the history that support a working diagnosis(es)/classification(s):**

Thoracic Pain With Mobility Deficits—Thoracic Spine and Rib Cage	Thoracic Hypo-mobility With Shoulder Impairments and With Upper Extremity Referred Pain	Direction-Specific Exercise for Thoracic Spinal Pain	Thoracic Hypo-mobility With Neck Pain or LBP	Thoracic Clinical Instability; Other
• Recent onset • Activity limitations • Bending, twisting		• Worse with flexion • Better with extension	• No complaints of neck or LBP	• No red flags • Low FABQ • X-rays normal

5. **What is your initial working diagnostic hypothesis or classification?**
   a. **Primary hypothesis (region to examine in detail):**
      - Thoracic spinal pain with mobility deficits
      - Direction-specific exercise classification for thoracic spinal pain with subgroup extension

   b. **Secondary hypothesis may include region(s) to screen for sessions 1, 2, 3:**
      - Thoracic pain referred from the cervical spine
      - Screen shoulder girdle region

   c. **Precautions or contraindications to your examination:** None except caution with constant pain. Examine as needed to diagnosis and treatment threshold; monitor patient response closely

   d. **What is the stage of the disorder?** Acute
6. **What is the stability of the disorder?** Getting better
7. **Are there potential risk factors (psychosocial, ergonomic, expectations, etc, contributing) to the condition?** Gradual return to exercise, posture, positions at work; no yellow flags
8. **What tests and measures (region/structures) should be completed on session 1?** Observation, gait, posture, cervical AROM, thoracic AROM, repeated movements, PAIVM thoracic, screen shoulder; neuro exam today or defer to next session since no indications for neurological exam

a. **Physical examination findings Case G**
  - Observation/gait/posture: Forward head posture, thoracic kyphosis lumbar kyphosis; able to assume neutral upright posture slowly but has increased pain initially that then eases to 2/10; respiratory pattern normal; resting scapular position symmetrical
  - Rest symptoms: 4/10 thoracic pain with referral to left ribs
  - Functional activities: No change with deep breathing
  - Shoulder girdle: AROM, no pain, OP normal with symmetrical scapula movement
  - Cervical AROM: Full range all directions with OP, no increase in resting symptom
  - Repeated cervical retraction: 10 repetitions, no change in resting symptoms
  - Repeated cervical flexion: 10 repetitions, no change in resting symptoms
  - AROM thoracic spine, OP end feel, PRN:
    - Flex: 45° increased to 5/10
    - Ext: 10° increased to 5/10
    - L LF: 10° increased to 5/10
    - R LF: Full range, no increase in pain from resting
    - L Rot: Moderate limitation, pain increased to 5/10
    - R Rot: Full range, no increase in pain from resting
  - Repeated movements:
    - Flex: 6 repetitions, increased all pain to 6/10
    - Ext: Pain decreased to 1/10 after 15 repetitions, abolished rib pain and centralized thoracic pain, range of motion increased
    - REIL: 10 repetitions, pain remained at 1/10 centralized in thoracic spine
  - Palpation/passive segmental mobility testing:
    - Palpation: Tender, increased muscle tone bilateral T4-T8
    - PAIVM: Central PA T4-T8 hypomobile with sharp pain that spread to the left ribs. Unilateral PA T4-T8 hypomobile on left produced local pain

9. **Data from physical examination that supports a working diagnosis(es)/classification(s)**

Thoracic Pain With Mobility Deficits—Thoracic Spine and Rib Cage	Thoracic Hypomobility With Shoulder Impairments and With Upper Extremity Referred Pain	Direction-Specific Exercise for Thoracic Spinal Pain	Thoracic Hypomobility With Neck Pain or LBP	Thoracic Clinical Instability; Other
• AROM limited painful: flex, L LF, L rot • PAIVM hypomobile • Shoulder and neck screen clear		• Centralization with repeated extension • Shoulder and neck screen clear		

10. **What is the PT diagnosis/classification/prognosis at the end of the physical examination?** Acute thoracic pain, direction-specific extension subgroup; centralization with repeated extension
11. **What is your intervention/reassessment? What evidence informs your decision?** Options: Repeated thoracic extension in sitting or REIL; monitor resting symptoms closely; home exercise program repeated thoracic extension
    a. **Intervention Options**
      - Repeated thoracic extension in sitting
      - Repeated extension in lying
      - PAIVM: Central PA at hypomobile segments
      - PAIVM: Unilateral at hypomobile segments

    b. **Reassessment**
      - Reassess thoracic extension
12. **What is your plan of care for session 1?**
    a. Repeated thoracic extension, 10 reps every 2 to 3 hours
    b. Postural education; avoid flexion
    c. Activity modification
    d. Discuss prognosis and return to exercise progression

Appendix H

Case Study for Cervical Pain

Patient Profile: 40 y/o male; graphic designer; hobbies include running, bicycling, and working on old sports cars. Runs or cycles 3× per week for 30 minutes. Has stopped cycling for about 1 week. NDI: 20/50; FABQPA: 12; FABQW: 9

Chief Complaint: Intermittent deep ache in R neck lower neck that occasionally becomes sharp; burning in R upper trap area and R shoulder region

Description of Symptoms

- R lower neck pain, intermittent sharp (0/10 to 5/10)
- Burning R upper trap and right shoulder region (0/10 to 3/10)
- No thoracic/chest; left neck, facial, or head pain
- No numbness or tingling; no headache or dizziness

History of Current Problem (Present Episode)

One week ago, woke with stiff neck, unable to extend or turn to right; no trauma but reports increase in desk and computer work in past month preparing for a special project. Severe pain felt in the R neck and shoulder area that persisted for 2 days. He is now 30% improved in that the intensity is decreased and he has some increased mobility

Past History (Previous Episode of Similar Problem)

3 previous episodes in the past 5 years. In all cases, it went away without treatment in 2 to 3 days. He experiences occasional R neck pain/stiffness and mild dull R ache occasionally between episodes. MVA 15 years ago resulted in "whiplash"; recovered in 2 months with PT heat, massage, and traction

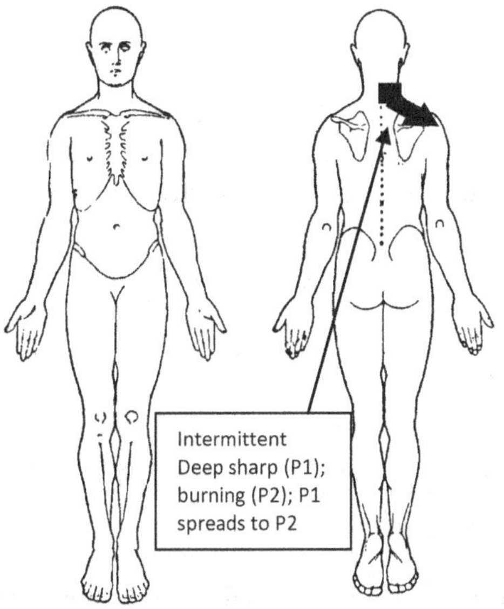

Stetts DM, Carpenter JG. *Physical Therapy Management of Patients With Spinal Pain: An Evidence-Based Approach (pp 613-616).*

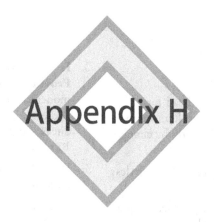

Aggravating Factors:

- Working under the car with arms overhead for more than 15 minutes produces pain in R neck and upper trap area burning pain; settles in 5 minutes by changing position
- Backing out car R rotation, R neck pain; settles immediately by changing position
- Computer work more than 2 hours, produces upper trap and shoulder burning pain; settles in 10 min if stops working
- No pain with running
- Cycling brings on all symptoms after 25 minutes; settles in 5 minutes after hot shower

Easing Factors

- Hot shower and rest

24-Hour Behavior

- PM: no complaints in evening; sleeps through the night
- AM: neck stiff in morning; eases with hot shower. Occasionally wakes with severe stiffness (unable to rotate)
- Day: depends on computer work during day

Systems Review and Special Questions Reveal the Following

- General health: excellent
- Systems review: all negative, except x-rays show narrowed C5-6 disc space
- Medications/steroids: Advil PRN with some relief

Patient Expectations and Goals

- Return to cycling without pain

Case H: Analyze the Data From the History to Plan the Physical Examination

1. **Are the symptoms mild (0 to 3), moderate (4 to 6), or severe (7 to 10)? Provide an example for each symptom.** Intensity of symptoms and impact on function. Self-report outcome scores. NDI: mild/mod 20/50; NPRS: 0/10 to 5/10
2. **Is the presentation irritable or nonirritable? Provide an example for each symptom.** Mild to moderate such that symptoms are easily produced and ease quickly; overhead work, turning neck reproduces symptoms, but the symptoms go away in 5 to 10 seconds or immediately when upright
3. **What is the nature of the condition (musculoskeletal, nonmusculoskeletal, or both)?**
4. **Data from the history that support a working diagnosis(es)/classification(s):**

Neck Pain With Mobility Deficits	Neck Pain With Movement Coordination Impairments	Neck Pain With Radiating Pain	Neck Pain With Headache	Other: WAD, Altered Neurodynamics
• Recent onset, no pain below shoulder • Unilateral symptoms	• Recurrent episodes • History of WAD	• Neck pain with referred pain to shoulder girdle region • Could be somatic or radicular • Extension activities are provocative • No neurological symptoms	• No complaints of neck or LBP	• No red flags • Low FABQ • Chronic

5. **What is your initial working diagnostic hypothesis or classification?**
   a. **Primary hypothesis (region to examine in detail):** Neck pain with mobility deficits: extension movements painful and limited with referral to UE
   b. **Secondary hypothesis may include region(s) to screen for sessions 1, 2, 3:**
      - Neck pain with radiating pain: pain referred to shoulder girdle could be somatic or radicular
      - Neck pain with movement coordination deficits: recurrent episodes and history of WAD
   c. **Precautions or contraindications to your examination:** None
   d. **What is the stage of the disorder?** Acute on chronic
6. **What is the stability of the disorder?** Getting better
7. **Are there potential risk factors (psychosocial, ergonomic, expectations, etc, contributing) to the condition?** Posture during work and exercise; low FABQ

8. **What tests and measures (region/structures) should be completed on session 1?** Observation, gait, posture, AROM, repeated movements, shoulder screen, neuro, PAIVM (cervical and thoracic), assess deep neck flexors, palpation
   a. **Physical examination findings Case H** (*Note*: Some tests may be optional at therapist discretion)
      - o Observation/gait/posture: Forward head posture, shoulder girdle protracted, slightly elevated; postural correction does not alter symptoms; gait normal
      - o Rest symptoms: None
      - o Neuro: WNL
      - o AROM cervical spine:
         - F: 40° pulls in R upper trap area
         - E: 20° R neck pain spreads to R UT area
         - LF L: 20° "pulling" sensation right lateral neck
         - LF R: 10° sharp right neck pain
         - ROT L: full range, "pull" right lateral neck and upper trap area with overpressure
         - ROT R: 45° sharp neck pain R, OP quickly spreads to UT area
      - o Repeated movements:
         - Retraction in sitting × 15 reps; increase R neck at end range, no worse
         - Repeated flexion: × 15; no effect other than pulling in R upper trap area
      - o Right and left shoulder AROM:
         - Flexion/abduction/horizontal adduction: full range, OP slight ache over right acromioclavicular area, no neck pain IR/ER: normal range, OP no effect
      - o Muscle length: (optional day 1)
         - Upper trapezius and levator scapulae: mild stiffness on R compared to L, no pain
      - o Special tests: Compression/distraction/ Spurling (optional):
         - Spurling test deferred since extension, R LF, and R rot produce neck pain and referred pain to shoulder area
         - Cervical rotation lateral flexion: full range bilaterally
      - o PAIVMs/passive segmental mobility testing:
         - Soft tissue thickness, R upper trapezius, levator scapulae
         - Central PA C5, local central pain; hypomobile, spreads to R UT area
         - Central PA C6 Stiff, local central pain
         - Unilateral PA C5-C6 hypomobile, "familiar pain" spreads to UT area
         - T1-T4 central, stiff, no pain; T3-5 unilateral R > L stiffness
         - PPIVM: mod loss of R LF, R ROT, EXT at C5/6
         - In extension at C5/6, translation to the left, restricted
         - 1st rib inferior glide: normal bilaterally

9. **Data from physical examination that supports a working diagnosis(es)/classification(s)**

Neck Pain With Mobility Deficits	Neck Pain With Movement Coordination Impairments	Neck Pain With Radiating Pain	Neck Pain With Headache	Other: WAD, Altered Neuro-dynamics
• AROM limited: ext, R LF, R Rot and painful • Repeated movements • No worse—end range only; repeated flexion did not peripheralize • PAIVM/ PPIVM hypomobile cervical and thoracic • No radicular symptoms • Muscle length asymmetrical	• Recurrent episodes • History of WAD • DNF not assessed this session	• Cervical ext, R LF, R rot produce local and radiating pain • No neurological signs		• No red flags • Low FABQ • Chronic • Neuro-dynamics not examined

10. **What is the PT diagnosis/classification/prognosis at the end of the physical examination?**
    a. Neck pain with mobility deficits: ext, R LF, R rot, and limited with referral to UE
    b. Neck pain with movement coordination deficits: recurrent episodes and history of WAD requires further examination cervicothoracic motor control
    c. Neck pain with radiating pain: continue to monitor neurological status requires neurodynamics examination to rule out neurogenic component

11. **What is your intervention/reassessment? What evidence informs your decision?** Options: Manual therapy and exercise to thoracic and cervical spine

    a. **Intervention Options**

    - Thoracic spine mobilization/manipulation
    - Cervical spine (downslope/closing) mobilization manipulation/MET
    - MET for upper trapezius/levator scapulae

    b. **Reassessment**

    - AROM: Ext, R LF, R rot; shoulder elevation
    - PAIVM/PPIVM
    - If successful, instruct in-home exercise program of mobility exercises as indicated by response to intervention
    - Instruction on neutral spine posture to facility DNF and multifdus activation in upright postures

12. **What is your plan of care for session 1?**

    a. Education on prognosis, adherence to exercise program, ergonomics at work and during exercise

    b. Continue to assess cervicothoracic/shoulder girdle regions for mobility deficits and movement coordination impairments within 2 to 3 sessions

    c. Discuss prognosis and recurrences and progression for return to cycling

Appendix I

Case Study for Cervical Pain

Patient Profile: 24 y/o female; graduate student, personal trainer on weekends, waitress 2 nights per week; still able to work; elliptical aerobics and weight training 3× per week; has stopped weight training but able to do elliptical training. NDI: 18/50, referred from family practice MD; FABQPA: 12; FABQW: 18

Chief Complaint: Central/right lower cervical pain, refers to posterior right shoulder and arm above elbow

Description of Symptoms

- Intermittent deep ache, central/R neck and arm; starts at neck and then travels into R arm
- No numbness/tingling, headache, dizziness
- No other upper quarter symptoms
- Arm: best 0/10, worst 3/10, now 2/10; neck, best 0/10, worst 6/10, now 4/10

History of Current Problem (Present Episode)

Four months ago, woke with a sore, stiff neck, gradual spread into right arm over next month; no treatment because of classes—overall, the problem is staying the same

Past History (Previous Episode of Similar Problem)

No previous history of neck or arm symptoms

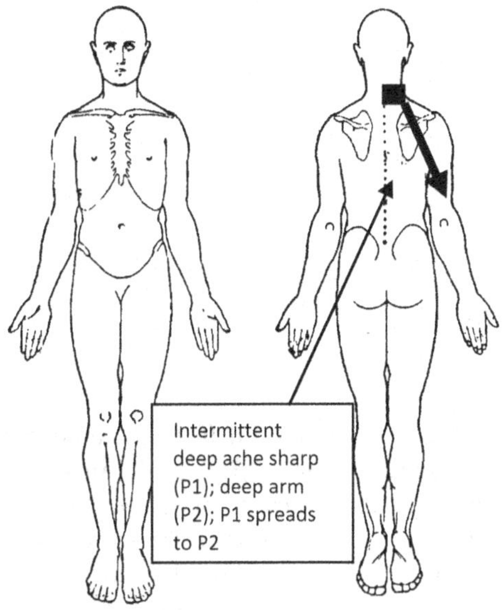

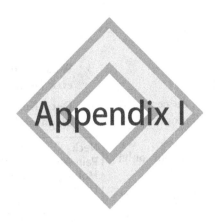

Aggravating Factors

- Sitting 45 minutes at computer brings on central/R neck pain and arm pain; eases in 2 minutes if stands and walks around
- Turning L to R brings on central/R neck pain only; eases when she stops movement
- Looking up to put makeup in the morning increases central/R neck pain only
- Use of both UE overhead does not affect symptoms

Easing Factors

- Lying down

24-Hour Behavior

- Worse through the day if does a lot of computer work
- Is able to sleep through the night without pain
- AM: decreased arm and neck pain; usually wakes without pain

Systems Review and Special Questions Reveal the Following

- General health: excellent
- No surgical history or past medical history
- Medications/steroids: Tylenol PRN

Patient Expectations and Goals

- Eliminate the pain; return to workouts
- Learn how to prevent pain from coming back

Case I: Analyze the Data From the History to Plan the Physical Examination

1. **Are the symptoms mild (0 to 3), moderate (4 to 6), or severe (7 to 10)? Provide an example for each symptom.** Intensity of symptoms and impact on function. Self-report outcome scores. NDI: mild/mod 18/50; NPRS: 0/10 to 6/10 arm; 0 to 3 neck
2. **Is the presentation irritable or nonirritable? Provide an example for each symptom.** Mild to moderate such that symptoms are easily produced and go away quickly; turning neck and looking up reproduce symptoms, but the symptoms go away in up to 1 to 2 minutes
3. **What is the nature of the condition (musculoskeletal, nonmusculoskeletal, or both)?**
4. **Data from the history that support a working diagnosis(es)/classification(s):**

Neck Pain With Mobility Deficits	Neck Pain With Movement Coordination Impairments	Neck Pain With Radiating Pain	Neck Pain With Headache	Other: WAD, Altered Neurodynamics
• Unilateral symptoms • With referral to UE • Activity limitations due to pain and mobility	• Chronic stage • 4 months since onset	• Neck pain with referred pain to UE • Could be somatic or radicular • Extension activities are provocative • No neurological symptoms but pain into arm above elbow		• No red flags • Low FABQ • Remains active

5. **What is your initial working diagnostic hypothesis or classification?**
   a. **Primary hypothesis (region to examine in detail):** Neck pain with mobility deficits: extension movements painful and limited with referral to UE
   b. **Secondary hypothesis may include region(s) to screen for sessions 1, 2, 3:**
      - Neck pain with radiating pain; pain referred to shoulder girdle could be somatic or radicular
      - Neck pain with movement coordination deficits: first episode, but chronic stage
   c. **Precautions or contraindications to your examination:** None
   d. **What is the stage of the disorder?** Chronic, but first episodes
6. **What is the stability of the disorder?** Staying the same
7. **Are there potential risk factors (psychosocial, ergonomic, expectations, etc, contributing) to the condition?** Posture during classes, computer, work activities, and exercise; low FABQ
8. **What tests and measures (region/structures) should be completed on session 1?** Observation, gait, posture, AROM, repeated movements, shoulder

screen, neuro, PAIVM (cervical and thoracic), assess deep neck flexors, palpation.

a. **Physical examination findings Case I** (*Note*: Some tests may be optional at therapist discretion)
   - o Observation/gait/posture: Gait normal; poor sitting posture: easily corrected to neutral, no effect on symptoms
   - o Standing posture: Good; no deformity noted
   - o Rest symptoms: Central and lower right cervical pain at C6-7 (4/10); arm pain 2/10
   - o Neuro: normal C4-T1 (MMT, sensation to LT, DTRs)
   - o TMJ/shoulder/AC screen other:
     - TMJ AROM: normal, no symptoms
     - Shoulder AROM: F, ABD, HBB, HBH, OP; symmetrical bilaterally; no symptoms
     - Resisted static tests: Abd, ER, IR, elbow flexion: 5/5 no pain
   - o AROM cervical spine:
     - F: 60°, OP normal
     - E: 50°, increase central/lower R neck pain with pain during movement and poor eccentric control
     - LF L: 45°, OP normal
     - LF R: 35°, increase central/lower R neck pain at end range
     - ROT L: 80°, increase R neck pain
     - ROT R: 70°, increase all symptoms with pain during movement, but no worse
   - o Repeated movements:
     - Seated
     - Protrusion: increased R arm pain, no worse
     - Repeated protrusion: increased R neck and arm pain, worse × 3 reps
     - Retraction: increase neck/R arm pain, now worse
     - Repeated retraction: abolished R arm pain, R neck pain is 5/10 (15 reps)
     - Repeated retraction, OP: abolished R arm pain, R neck pain is 4/10 (10 reps)
     - Retraction/extension: decrease R neck pain, but no better (still 4/10) R neck pain
     - Repeated retraction in supine: abolished R arm pain and centralized neck pain (3/10)
   - o Reassessment:
     - Repeated retraction with OP in sitting: centralized neck (2/10)
     - Extension AROM: 60°, central/lower R neck pain; remains better
     - R ROT: 80, central/lower R neck pain only; remains better
   - o Special tests:
     - Passive segmental mobility testing
     - PPIVM: Not examined
     - PAIVM: Not examined this session due to centralization with repeated movements
     - Palpation: Local PVM tenderness and increased tissue tension at C4-C7 on R

9. **Data from physical examination that supports a working diagnosis(es)/classification(s)**

Neck Pain With Mobility Deficits	Neck Pain With Movement Coordination Impairments	Neck Pain With Radiating Pain	Neck Pain With Headache	Other: WAD, Altered Neuro-dynamics
• AROM limited: ext, R LF, R rot and painful • No radicular symp-toms • PAIVM, PPIVM not assessed	• DNF and motor control not assessed this session	• Central-ization with repeated exten-sion • No neu-rological signs		• No red flags • Low FABQ • Chronic • Neuro-dynam-ics not examined

10. **What is the PT diagnosis/classification/prognosis at the end of the physical examination?**
    a. Neck pain with radiating pain: extension subgroup for repeated movements classification; continue to monitor neurological status; requires neurodynamics examination to rule out neurogenic component
    b. Reassess for cervicothoracic mobility deficits based on patient response to current intervention and chronic stage
    c. Reassess for movement coordination impairments

11. **What is your intervention/reassessment? What evidence informs your decision?** Options: Repeated movement for extension subgroup based on response of centralization

a. **Intervention Options**
   - o Repeated retraction in supine
   - o Repeated retraction in sitting with OP
   - o Patient education on adherence to exercise prescription; avoid flexion
   - o Instruction on neutral spine posture to facility DNF and multifidus activation in upright postures

12. **What is your plan of care for session 1?**
    a. Education on prognosis, adherence to exercise program, ergonomics at computer, work and during exercise
    b. Continue to assess cervicothoracic/shoulder girdle regions for mobility deficits and movement coordination impairments within 2 to 3 sessions
    c. Discuss prognosis and recurrences and progression for return weight training

Index

Printed in the United States
by Baker & Taylor Publisher Services